HANDBOOK OF INDIVIDUAL DIFFERENCES IN SOCIAL BEHAVIOR

Handbook of
INDIVIDUAL DIFFERENCES IN SOCIAL BEHAVIOR

■ ● ▲ ◆ ■ ● ▲ ◆

edited by
Mark R. Leary
Rick H. Hoyle

THE GUILFORD PRESS
New York   London

© 2009 The Guilford Press
A Division of Guilford Publications, Inc.
72 Spring Street, New York, NY 10012
www.guilford.com

Printed in the United States of America

This book is printed on acid-free paper.

Last digit is print number: 9   8   7   6   5   4   3   2   1

Library of Congress Cataloging-in-Publication Data

Handbook of individual differences in social behavior / edited by Mark R. Leary, Rick H. Hoyle.
   p. cm.
  Includes bibliographical references and index.
  ISBN 978-1-59385-647-2 (hardcover)
  1. Social psychology. 2. Human behavior. I. Leary, Mark R. II. Hoyle, Rick H.
  HM1033.H355 2009
  302.5′4—dc22

                                        2008053706

About the Editors

Mark R. Leary, PhD, is Professor of Psychology and Neuroscience at Duke University. His research interests include self-awareness, interpersonal motivation and emotion, and the interfaces of social and clinical psychology. He is a Fellow of the American Psychological Association, the Association for Psychological Science, and the Society for Personality and Social Psychology, and was the founding editor of the journal *Self and Identity.*

Rick H. Hoyle, PhD, is Professor of Psychology and Neuroscience at Duke University. The primary focus of his research is the investigation of basic cognitive, affective, and social processes relevant to self-regulation. He is a Fellow of the American Psychological Association, the Association for Psychological Science, the Society for the Psychological Study of Social Issues, and the Division of Evaluation, Measurement, and Statistics of the American Psychological Association.

Contributors

Vanessa T. Anderson, PhD, Department of Psychology, Columbia University, New York, New York

John C. Barefoot, PhD, Behavioral Medicine Research Center, Department of Psychiatry, Duke University, Durham, North Carolina

Robert F. Bornstein, PhD, Derner Institute, Adelphi University, Garden City, New York

Jennifer K. Bosson, PhD, Department of Psychology, University of South Florida, Tampa, Florida

Stephen H. Boyle, PhD, Behavioral Medicine Research Center, Department of Psychiatry, Duke University, Durham, North Carolina

Pablo Briñol, PhD, Department of Social Psychology, Universidad Autónoma de Madrid, Madrid, Spain

John T. Cacioppo, PhD, Center for Cognitive and Social Neuroscience and Department of Psychology, University of Chicago, Chicago, Illinois

Charles S. Carver, PhD, Department of Psychology, University of Miami, Coral Gables, Florida

David E. Conroy, PhD, Departments of Kinesiology and Human Development and Family Studies, Pennsylvania State University, University Park, Pennsylvania

Susan E. Cross, PhD, Department of Psychology, Iowa State University, Ames, Iowa

Claudia Dalbert, PhD, Department of Educational Psychology, Martin Luther University of Halle-Wittenberg, Halle, Germany

Ed Diener, PhD, Department of Psychology, University of Illinois at Urbana–Champaign, Champaign, Illinois

Geraldine Downey, PhD, Department of Psychology, Columbia University, New York, New York

John Duckitt, PhD, Department of Psychology, University of Auckland, Auckland, New Zealand

Alice H. Eagly, PhD, Department of Psychology, Northwestern University, Evanston, Illinois

Grant Edmonds, BA, Department of Psychology, University of Illinois at Urbana–Champaign, Champaign, Illinois

Andrew J. Elliot, PhD, Department of Clinical and Social Sciences in Psychology, University of Rochester, Rochester, New York

Jennifer V. Fayard, BA, Department of Psychology, University of Illinois at Urbana–Champaign, Champaign, Illinois

Allan Fenigstein, PhD, Department of Psychology, Kenyon College, Gambier, Ohio

Patrick H. Finan, MA, Department of Psychology, Arizona State University, Tempe, Arizona

Shira Fishman, MA, Department of Psychology, University of Maryland, College Park, Maryland

Eugene M. Fodor, PhD, Department of Psychology, Clarkson University, Potsdam, New York

Paul T. Fuglestad, BA, Department of Psychology, University of Minnesota, Minneapolis, Minnesota

Adrian Furnham, DSc, DPhil, DLitt, Department of Psychology, University College London, London, United Kingdom

William G. Graziano, PhD, Department of Psychological Science, Purdue University, West Lafayette, Indiana

Erin E. Hardin, PhD, Department of Psychology, Texas Tech University, Lubbock, Texas

Louise C. Hawkley, PhD, Center for Cognitive and Social Neuroscience and Department of Psychology, University of Chicago, Chicago, Illinois

Craig A. Hill, PhD, Department of Psychology, Indiana University–Purdue University Fort Wayne, Fort Wayne, Indiana

Ronald R. Holden, PhD, Department of Psychology, Queens University, Kingston, Ontario, Canada

Rick H. Hoyle, PhD, Department of Psychology and Neuroscience, Duke University, Durham, North Carolina

Joshua J. Jackson, BS, Department of Psychology, University of Illinois at Urbana–Champaign, Champaign, Illinois

Daniel N. Jones, MA, Department of Psychology, University of British Columbia, Vancouver, British Columbia, Canada

Kristine M. Kelly, PhD, Department of Psychology, Western Illinois University, Macomb, Illinois

Pelin Kesebir, MA, Department of Psychology, University of Illinois at Urbana–Champaign, Champaign, Illinois

Arie W. Kruglanski, PhD, Department of Psychology, University of Maryland, College Park, Maryland

Randy J. Larsen, PhD, Department of Psychology, Washington University in St. Louis, St. Louis, Missouri

Mark R. Leary, PhD, Department of Psychology and Neuroscience, Duke University, Durham, North Carolina

Chris Loersch, MA, Department of Psychology, Ohio State University, Columbus, Ohio

Michael J. McCaslin, MA, Department of Psychology, Ohio State University, Columbus, Ohio

Robert R. McCrae, PhD, National Institute on Aging, National Institutes of Health, Baltimore, Maryland

Jenna Meints, BS, Department of Psychology, University of Illinois at Urbana–Champaign, Champaign, Illinois

Mario Mikulincer, PhD, School of Psychology, Interdisciplinary Center, Herzliya, Israel

Rowland S. Miller, PhD, Department of Psychology and Philosophy, Sam Houston State University, Huntsville, Texas

Kristin Neff, PhD, Department of Educational Psychology, University of Texas at Austin, Austin, Texas

Julie K. Norem, PhD, Department of Psychology, Wellesley College, Wellesley, Massachusetts

Jennifer Passey, MA, Department of Psychology, Queens University, Kingston, Ontario, Canada

Delroy L. Paulhus, PhD, Department of Psychology, University of British Columbia, Vancouver, British Columbia, Canada

Benjamin Peterson, PhD, Department of Psychology, University of Utah, Salt Lake City, Utah

Richard E. Petty, PhD, Department of Psychology, Ohio State University, Columbus, Ohio

Kavita S. Reddy, MA, Department of Psychology, Columbia University, New York, New York

William Revelle, PhD, Department of Psychology, Northwestern University, Evanston, Illinois

Frederick Rhodewalt, PhD, Department of Psychology, University of Utah, Salt Lake City, Utah

Brent W. Roberts, PhD, Department of Psychology, University of Illinois at Urbana–Champaign, Champaign, Illinois

Rainer Romero-Canyas, PhD, Department of Psychology, Columbia University, New York, New York

Michael F. Scheier, PhD, Department of Psychology, Carnegie Mellon University, Pittsburgh, Pennsylvania

Phillip R. Shaver, PhD, Department of Psychology, University of California Davis, Davis, California

Mark Snyder, PhD, Department of Psychology, University of Minnesota, Minneapolis, Minnesota

Jeffrey Stuewig, PhD, Department of Psychology, George Mason University, Fairfax, Virginia

Peter Suedfeld, PhD, Department of Psychology, University of British Columbia, Vancouver, British Columbia, Canada

Angelina R. Sutin, PhD, Laboratory of Personality and Cognition, National Institute on Aging, National Institutes of Health, Baltimore, Maryland

William B. Swann, Jr., PhD, Department of Psychology, University of Texas at Austin, Austin, Texas

Berna Gercek Swing, MS, Department of Psychology, Iowa State University, Ames, Iowa

June Price Tangney, PhD, Department of Psychology, George Mason University, Fairfax, Virginia

Howard Tennen, PhD, Department of Community Medicine, University of Connecticut Health Center, Farmington, Connecticut

Todd M. Thrash, PhD, Department of Psychology, College of William and Mary, Williamsburg, Virginia

Renée M. Tobin, PhD, Department of Psychology, Illinois State University, Normal, Illinois

William Tov, PhD, School of Social Sciences, Singapore Management University, Singapore

Thomas A. Widiger, PhD, Department of Psychology, University of Kentucky, Lexington, Kentucky

Joshua Wilt, MA, Department of Psychology, Northwestern University, Evanston, Illinois

Wendy Wood, PhD, Department of Psychology and Neuroscience, Duke University, Durham, North Carolina

Kerstin Youman, MA, Department of Psychology, George Mason University, Fairfax, Virginia

Alex J. Zautra, PhD, Department of Psychology, Arizona State University, Tempe, Arizona

Marvin Zuckerman, PhD, Department of Psychology, University of Delaware, Newark, Delaware

Preface

Historically, psychologists and other scientists who study human behavior have tended to fall into one of two camps that are characterized by the kind of psychological variability in which they are most interested. Some researchers are predominantly interested in how people's thoughts, emotions, and behaviors vary across situations. These researchers tend to use experimental methods in which features of a controlled setting are varied to study the effects of these situational variations on participants' responses. If we are interested in knowing whether changes in temperature affect aggression or how differences in group size influence conformity, experiments will tell us whether variations in temperature or group size—features of the situation—cause behavior to vary.

Other behavioral researchers are more interested in understanding how thoughts, emotions, and behaviors vary across people. Looking beyond situational influences, we can easily see that people differ in their characteristic ways of thinking, feeling, and behaving. On virtually any psychological dimension one can imagine, people differ from one another—in their typical degree of confidence, enjoyment of social activities, fear of public speaking, trust in other people, desire for approval, comfort with uncertainty, dominance, self-control, cheerfulness, achievement motivation, self-esteem, pursuit of novel experiences, tendency to experience various emotions (such as shame, anger, loneliness, or embarrassment), and so on. Researchers interested in these individual differences have tended to use correlational methods to examine how differences among people relate to their thoughts, emotions, behaviors, or physiological responses.

Although these two camps have sometimes skirmished over the merits of focusing on situational versus dispositional variables, a full understanding of psychological processes requires devoting attention to both. Although trained as experimental social psychologists, both of us have found over the years that our own work has benefited from attention to both situational influences and individual differences in people's personalities, and we have difficulty imagining any topic that does not require a dual focus on situational and dispositional variables. We do not mean to suggest that every investigator must necessarily focus on situational and dispositional variables but, rather, that a complete understanding of virtually any phenomenon requires attention to both. As Lewin (1936) observed, behavior is indeed a function of both the person and the environment.

As we have considered the role of personality in our own theorizing and research, we have often felt the need for articles or chapters that provided an overview of what is known about a particular personality variable. Our goal in editing the *Handbook of Individual Differences in Social Behavior* was to provide a relatively comprehensive examination of nearly 40 personality variables that have been studied by behavioral researchers. Dozens, if not hundreds, of personality attributes have been studied, and, by necessity, we had to be selective. But we hope that the *Handbook* includes the personality variables that researchers currently find to be the most interesting, important, and useful. Some of these variables—such as extraversion, neuroticism, and achievement motivation—have been studied extensively for decades. Other variables—such as desire for control, self-compassion, and embarrassability—have been examined in fewer studies. The literature on each is summarized by an acknowledged expert—the researcher who either first popularized the construct, developed a commonly used measure of it, or conducted influential research.

Although the study of individual differences is sometimes regarded as the purview of personality psychology, researchers cutting a wide swath across the social and behavioral sciences have in fact shown an interest in dispositional factors. Individual differences have been studied not only by social and personality psychologists, but also by researchers in developmental, clinical, educational, counseling, health, organizational, political, cognitive, and sport psychology, as well as by researchers in marketing, management, law, education, political science, sociology, psychiatry, nursing, and social work. We hope that this book serves as an invaluable resource for scholars and students across all areas of social and behavioral science.

MARK R. LEARY, PhD
RICK H. HOYLE, PhD

Reference

Lewin, K. (1936). *Principles of topological psychology.* New York: McGraw-Hill.

Contents

Contents   **xv**

PART VI. SELF-RELATED DISPOSITIONS

PART I

INTRODUCTION

CHAPTER 1

■ ● ▲ ◆ ■ ● ▲ ◆

Situations, Dispositions, and the Study of Social Behavior

MARK R. LEARY
RICK H. HOYLE

In a discipline with few propositions about which nearly everyone agrees, Lewin's (1936) dictum that behavior is a function of both the person and the situation enjoys widespread support. Even the most extreme psychodynamic or personological psychologist could not argue that situations exert no influence whatsoever on people's behaviors, nor could diehard behaviorists seriously deny that attributes within the person contribute to how he or she responds to situational influences. We find it hard to imagine that any contemporary behavioral scientist could seriously question Lewin's notion that thought, emotion, and behavior depend both on "the state of the person and at the same time on the environment, although their relative importance is different in different cases" (p. 12).

Even so, debates have arisen regarding the relative influence of situational and dispositional variables on psychological processes, and researchers interested in the effects of situations and those interested in trait-like characteristics of the person have at times had an uneasy relationship with each other. Historically, this tension has been seen clearly in the relationship between social psychologists, who have traditionally stressed the impact of situational forces, and personality psychologists, who have focused on traits and processes operating within the individual's psyche.

This rift was not apparent in the earliest years of scientific psychology. Wundt, Titchener, Terman, and other founders of the field considered the role of both situational and dispositional variables in their research. But the dominance of behaviorism during the middle part of the 20th century led mainstream research psychologists to focus on situational factors and, in extreme cases, to deny that intrapersonal factors play any role in behavior. At about the same time, the influence of psychodynamic approaches and the emergence of personality psychology as a separate field of investigation led other researchers to highlight intrapersonal variables. Indeed, although Gordon Allport (1937), the founder of scientific personality psychology, acknowledged the importance of both situations and personality, he also argued that personality and social psychology should be independent fields. As a result of these forces, social and personality psychologists worked largely in ignorance of each other's work and often at cross-purposes for over 50 years.

Methodological Barriers

Part of the schism was fueled by mere differences in intellectual interests, with social psychologists being interested in situations and personality psychologists in dispositions and intrapsychic processes. But part of the rift also stemmed from differences in the prevailing research paradigms that dominated social and personality psychology during most of the 20th century. Social psychologists relied primarily on experimental methods in which participants were randomly assigned to experimental conditions that consisted of variations in the social situation. In fact, the classic experiments in social psychology—many of them conducted by founders of the field such as Asch, Sherif, Schachter, Festinger, and Milgram—exemplified the experimental approach and provided the dominant research paradigm for future generations of social psychologists that exists to this day.

The social psychologists' reliance on experimental studies, typically conducted under controlled laboratory conditions, emerged not only from their inherent interest in situational influences on behavior but also from a philosophy of science that viewed experimental work as inherently more "scientific" than other research approaches. Because research that relied solely on descriptive or correlational methods, in which there is no random assignment of participants to conditions controlled by the researcher, was unable to draw firm conclusions about the causal relationships between purported antecedents and consequences, it was viewed as less rigorous, definitive, and thus "scientific" than research that employed true experiments. The experimentalists' perspective on the proper way to conduct psychological research led social psychologists to look askance at much of the research in personality psychology, which relied primarily on descriptive and correlational methods.

The correlational tradition had a long and respected history from the earliest days of psychometrics and differential psychology in the early part of the 20th century. Galton, Pearson, Spearman, and others made contributions to the development of statistical methods that could be used to understand relationships among existing variables (e.g., correlation and factor analysis) and then used these methods to study individual differences in intellectual, psychological, and physical characteristics. But as social psychologists looked at results from correlational research, they saw mostly confounded variables and indefinite causal conclusions.

Conversely, when personality psycholo-gists considered the research of their social-psychological colleagues, they suspected that the effects of any particular experimental treatment were rarely, if ever, obtained on every participant in the experiment. The findings in social psychology were based on comparisons of the means of participants' responses in various experimental conditions, and such comparisons obscured the fact that participants in a particular condition differed among themselves in how they responded to the independent variable. Because social psychologists were interested primarily in between-group situational effects, these individual differences were relegated to the error term of their statistical tests—with no effort to determine why some people reacted differently to the independent variable than others.

When Lee Cronbach gave his presidential address to the American Psychological Association in 1957, he addressed this entrenched schism between researchers who rely on experimental versus correlational approaches. Cronbach observed that the field of psychology had fractured into two distinct disciplines—one defined by the experimental method and the other defined by correlational approaches. Furthermore, he noted that psychology was severely "limited by the dedication of its investigators to one or the other method of inquiry rather than to scientific psychology as a whole" (1957, p. 671), even though the primary difference between those who subscribe to each of these "two disciplines of scientific psychology" merely concerned whether the variability that they sought to explain preexists in the world or is created through experimental manipulations.

The Person–Situation Debate

Differences in scientific approach were accompanied by lively debates regarding the relative importance of situational versus dispositional factors in understanding behavior. Although a foreshadowing of this controversy can be seen earlier (Ichheisser, 1943), the opening volley was fired in Mischel's (1968) critique of the trait concept (and of personality psychology more generally). After critically reviewing 50 years of research that showed only small correlations in people's behaviors across situations and time, Mischel concluded that "highly generalized behavioral consistencies have not been demonstrated and the concept of personality traits as broad response dispositions is thus untenable" (p. 145). His recommendation that psychologists abandon their efforts to explain behavior with traits and focus instead on situations was embraced by many social psychologists. For example, after posing a scenario asking the reader to predict whether a hypothetical person, John, will help someone he sees slumped in a doorway, Ross and Nisbett (1991) concluded:

> A half century of research has taught us that in this situation, and in most other novel situations, one cannot predict *with any accuracy* how particular people will behave. At least one cannot do so using information about an individual's personal dispositions or even about that individual's past behavior. ... While knowledge about John is of surprisingly little value in predicting whether he will help the person slumped in the doorway, details concerning the specifics of the situation would be invaluable. (pp. 2–3, emphasis added)

The effects of Mischel's (1968) book were powerful and immediate. For example, the percentage of articles published in the *Journal of Personality and Social Psychology* (*JPSP*) that included any reference to individual differences, whether alone or in combination with experimental manipulations, dropped from 50% to about 30% from 1966 to 1977 (Swann & Seyle, 2005). During the same time period, the percentage of articles in *JPSP* that reported purely experimental studies rose from about 50% to nearly 70%.

At the same time, a great deal of time, energy, and ink were devoted to analyzing Mischel's (1968) claims more deeply. This discussion led to four important conclusions about the respective influences of situational and dispositional factors and the relationships among them (for overviews, see Bem & Funder, 1978; Cervone, Caldwell, & Orom, in press; Epstein & O'Brien, 1985; Kenrick & Dantchik, 1983; Magnusson & Endler, 1977; Snyder & Ickes, 1985).

First, Mischel's (1968) most damning argument was that correlations between measures of personality and of behavior (and between measures of behavior collected on different occasions) typically hover around .30, seeming to reflect a very weak relationship. However, evidence emerged that the strength of situational effects on behavior were comparably low. In an early documentation of this point, Funder and Ozer (1983) calculated the correlation effect sizes for some well-known situational effects in social psychology (including classic studies of forced compliance, bystander intervention, and obedience) and found that all fell under .40. Other researchers have documented the same conclusion, suggesting that the strength of the relationships between measured dispositions and behavior are comparable to those between situational manipulations and behavior.

Second, Epstein (1979, 1983) noted that a single measure of behavior is not a reliable indicator of a person's general behavioral tendencies. As a result, the magnitude of correlations between measures of personality and specific behaviors are attenuated by measurement error, which lowers the strength of statistical effects. When behaviors are aggregated across situations (just as self-report responses are aggregated across the items on a personality questionnaire), behavioral measures are more reliable, correlations are notably larger, and personality does a better job of predicting behavior.

Third, research began to show that personality relates more strongly to behavior in some situations than in others. In "strong" situations that constrain people's behavior and provide clear cues regarding how people should behave, most people tend to act similarly. In contrast, when "weak," unstructured, or novel situations offer few cues or norms to guide behavior, large individual differences emerge (Caspi & Moffitt, 1993; Ickes, 1982). Importantly, the laboratory situations that researchers create to study individual differences typically constrain behavior (and thus the manifestation of traits) because they are rigidly controlled, often with independent variables that are intentionally designed to exert a strong influence on people's behavior. Even when situations are strong, however, we often still see individual differences. Even in experiments with powerful manipulations, such as Milgram's (1963) studies of obedience to authority, large individual differences in the degree to which participants disobeyed the experimenter were observed (Packer, 2008).

Fourth, theorists noted a fallacy in the reasoning of those, including Mischel (1968), who used small personality–behavior correlations to argue that situational factors play a more powerful role in behavior than personality. They noted that the fact that personality and behavior tend to correlate .30 does not indicate that any of the remaining variance is produced by the situation. Perhaps more important, they pointed out that the strength of situational and dispositional effects are not inversely related to one another, as one might assume. Contrary to first appearances, behavior can simultaneously be strongly affected by situational factors and also demonstrate strong evidence of individual differences.

An example may help to make this point. Imagine that we administer a measure of dispositional fearfulness—the degree to which people tend to feel anxious and afraid—to a sample of 100 participants. We then randomly assign them to either an experimental condition in which they are threatened with painful electric shocks or to a control condition in which no threat is present and ask them to rate how anxious they feel. An analysis of the between-group differences in anxiety would undoubtedly show a very strong effect of experimental condition indicating that participants who were threatened with shocks reported more anxiety on average than those who were not. At the same time, however, correlating participants' pretest fearfulness scores with their anxiety ratings (whether correlated within each condition or for the entire sample) would undoubtedly reveal a large correlation between dispositional fearfulness and how much anxiety participants reported while they waited to be shocked. In such a case, a strong situational effect is revealed via between-group differences in state anxiety, and a strong personality effect is revealed via correlations between a measure of personality and state anxiety.

Funder (2006) demonstrated this effect empirically. Using data from Funder and Colvin (1991), he showed that, across 62 behaviors that were measured across two situations, 20 behaviors differed significantly between the two situations at the same time that 37 behaviors showed significant within-person stability. Furthermore, the correlation between the magnitude of between-situation differences and cross-situational stability in behavior was –.01, showing that the relationship between situational influences and behavior was independent of the relationship between personality influences and behavior. Fleeson (2001, 2004) similarly showed that strong cross-situational consistencies in people's modal or typical level of a trait are, at the same time, accompanied by large variability in their reactions across different situations.

Considerations such as these not only helped to lead personality psychologists out of their crisis of confidence but also induced many social psychologists to consider personality more seriously in their own work. By the mid-1980s, the percentage of articles in *JPSP* that involved personality had regained their precrisis levels. In 2002, the last year for which data are available, just over half of the articles in *JPSP* included some measure of personality (Swann & Selye, 2005).

Uses of Personality Variables in Behavioral Research

Most social psychologists now acknowledge that dispositional factors predict variation in people's thoughts, feelings, and behaviors that cannot be explained by situational factors and that a consideration of personality can thus contribute to our understanding of social-psychological phenomena. Researchers differ in the degree to which they incorporate personality variables into their own work, but, overall, social psychology is more amenable to the study of personality than ever before (Swann & Selye, 2005). Specifically, individual-difference variables can be used to address five basic types of questions about social thought, emotion, and behavior.

Main Effects

The simplest and most straightforward questions about the relationship between personality and social behavior involve "main effect" relationships between a particular disposition and some socially relevant thought, emotion, or behavior. In its simplest form, these kinds of studies simply correlate trait measures of personality with measures of particular behaviors, cognitions, emotions, or physiological reactions. For example, in a study designed to understand aspects of political behavior, Bizer and colleagues (2004) found that individual differences in the need to evaluate—the tendency to chronically evaluate aspects of one's life and environment—predicted the degree to which people relied on party identification to form attitudes toward political candidates, the likelihood of voting in national and state elections, and the degree to which participants had emotional reactions to political candidates. Main-effect findings such as these show how features of people's personalities relate to social-psychological phenomena.

Another strain of main-effect research involves correlations between two or more personality characteristics that are relevant to social behavior. For example, in a study that focused on the question of whether individual differences in religiosity are distinct from individual differences in spirituality, Saucier and Skrzypińska (2006) found that individual differences in subjective spirituality were positively correlated with private self-consciousness and absorption, but traditional religiousness was not. In contrast, traditional religiousness correlated with right-wing authoritarianism, but subjective spirituality did not. In studies such as these, relationships among various individual-difference measures that are relevant to social-psychological phenomena are examined.

Much of the research that has been conducted on gender differences also falls in this category. Although not a "personality" attribute per se, gender is certainly a potent individual-difference variable that relates to a wide array of socially relevant thoughts, emotions, and behaviors (see Wood & Eagly, Chapter 8, this volume). The wealth of data regarding how women and men differ is reflected in the growing number of meta-analyses that have examined gender differences in aggression, leadership, communication, jealousy, conversational interruptions, and other interpersonal behaviors (e.g., Eagly & Johnson, 1990; Harris, 2003; Hyde, 1984).

Of course, these main-effect analyses of the relationship between personality and socially relevant outcomes can become much more complex as researchers investigate multiple predictors of various outcomes, examine possible interactions among individual-difference variables in predicting behavior, and test mediational and path-analytic models.

Testing Theories about Situations

The fact that a particular experimental manipulation influences some behavior of interest often does not provide a great deal of insight into the causes of the obtained effect. Even when the experiment was designed to test a particular theory, obtaining results consistent with hypotheses does not unequivocally support the theory's explanation, because one cannot prove the antecedent of a logical argument (the theory-based predictions) by affirming the consequent (obtaining results that support the hypothesis). Results may appear to support a hypothesis for reasons other than those that the theory specifies, and science is filled with examples of empirical findings that appeared to support a theory that was eventually shown to be false (Wallach & Wallach, 1998).

One strategy for exploring the possible mechanisms underlying a particular experimental effect involves determining whether a particular personality variable moderates the effects of an experimental manipulation in the manner predicted by theory. In such instances, the researcher is not primarily interested in the personality variable per se but uses it as a methodological tool to test a hypothesis regarding a situational effect. Imagine, for example, that we are testing the hypothesis that a particular situational effect on behavior is caused by the fact that the situation increases people's concerns about being rejected by other people. If, prior to manipulating the independent variable(s) of interest, we obtain participants' scores on a dispositional measure of rejection sensitivity (Downey & Feldman, 1996), we can examine whether people who score low versus high in rejection sensitivity respond differently to the experimental manipulation, as they would be expected to do if the effect somehow involves concerns with rejection.

Testing Theories about Dispositions

A parallel strategy may be used to test hypotheses about the nature of a particular personality disposition. Historically, personality researchers have been interested primarily in main-effect hypotheses about dispositions, which they have tested by correlating scores on a personality scale with other scales or by comparing how people

who score low versus high on the scale behave in some situation.

However, our understanding of the cognitive, emotional, or behavioral features of
a personality variable can be enhanced by
studying how people who score differently
on the personality variable respond across
various experimentally created situations.
For example, to examine how optimists versus pessimists process negative emotional
stimuli differently, Isaacowitz (2005) had
participants complete a self-report measure
of optimism. Participants then viewed three
types of visual stimuli while their eye movements were tracked. Optimists showed selective inattention to the most negative stimuli,
and this relationship remained significant
after controlling for the effects of neuroticism, anxiety, and other variables. In studies
such as this, experimentally manipulating
features of the participants' environment (in
this case the nature of visual stimuli) provides insight into the nature of the personality variable of interest.

The strategy of combining manipulated
independent variables and measured personality variables in a single study may result in
precisely the same research design whether
one is primarily interested in understanding
the situational or the dispositional effects. In
both cases, one is interested in the interaction of the experimental manipulation and
the measured trait, and whether we say that
the personality variable moderated the effects of the independent variable or the independent variable moderated the effects of the
personality variable depends on our focus.

State and Trait Convergence

Certain situational variables create differences in people's psychological states that
are conceptually analogous to the individual
differences that we see among people who
possess different levels of a personality trait.
For example, just as mildly versus severely
threatening situations elicit different levels
of state anxiety, trait-like differences exist
in the degree to which people are generally
anxious. Likewise, certain situations increase people's motivation to obtain social
approval, and certain people are dispositionally more motivated to obtain approval than
are others.

When conceptually analogous states and
traits exist, much can be learned by examining similarities and differences in how low
versus high levels of the state and low versus
high levels of the trait manifest in thoughts,
emotions, behaviors, or physiological reactions. For example, we can learn a great deal
about anxiety both by assessing people's reactions to experimentally manipulated low
and high threat and by comparing the reactions of people who score low versus high on
a measure of trait anxiety. Similarly, we can
study the relationship between the motive to
obtain social approval and some behavior,
either by experimentally varying factors that
influence the desire for approval or by measuring individual differences in the need for
approval.

When the results of experimental studies
of states converge with those of correlational
studies of traits, we have greater confidence
that we understand the processes involved.
And, when they do not converge (and they
often do not), interesting questions arise regarding why the state and trait operational
definitions of seemingly analogous constructs are not equivalent.

State-by-Trait Interactions

Most social psychologists realize that, because people differ in their reactions to social stimuli, almost every general statement
about the effects of a particular situational
factor is at best incomplete and at worst
misleading or wrong. Likewise, personality psychologists seem to understand that,
although general predictions can be made
on the basis of a person's position on a particular trait dimension, how people actually
behave at any moment is typically influenced
to some degree by the situation in which
they are found. Thus explaining virtually
any thought, emotion, or behavior at a given
moment in time requires attention to both
situational and dispositional factors.

Furthermore, situational and dispositional factors not only exert separate, additive
influences on people's responses but also can
potentially interact in a statistical sense in
that the effects of a particular situation may
vary across levels of a trait or the effects of
a trait may vary across situations. In fact,
a particular trait may relate to behavior in
only some situations, and a particular situation may influence the reactions of only people with a certain personality characteristic
(Bem & Funder, 1978). Thus many studies

in social and personality psychology test for person–situation (or trait-by-state) interactions.

Behavioral researchers tend to love statistical interactions, which, for some reason, tend to connote the presence of a more sophisticated and elegant psychological process than the mere presence of simultaneous main effects. Yet, although interactions between situations and dispositions are often interesting and informative, they are also notoriously difficult to obtain, and, when they occur, they tend to be quite small relative to main effects (Chaplin, 1997; Keppel, 1982). Several factors contribute to the weakness of person–situation interactions. First, the reliability of an interaction term is almost always lower than the reliability of its constituents (Bohrnstedt & Marwell, 1977). Because the strength of a statistical effect is attenuated by measurement error, the lower reliability of interaction terms decreases the likelihood that interactions will be detected even if they are present (McClelland & Judd, 1993). Furthermore, statistical models that include interaction terms have lower degrees of freedom for the error term than models that contain main effects only, so that statistical significance is less likely.

We would add to these documented considerations the possibility that we live in a predominantly main-effect world. Although people undoubtedly respond differently from each other in any particular situation, those differences are often scaled similarly across situations. Thus, rather than finding interactions in which the effects of a situation are different for some people than for others, we often find two main effects that reveal a situational influence that increases or decreases everyone's reactions while the variability among people remains constant. In any case, for these and other reasons, statistical interactions between situations and personality are relatively rare relative to main effects, and those that do occur generally account for relatively little variance.

Personality and situational influences can combine, influence, and interact with one another in much more complicated ways than through simple statistical interactions between experimental manipulations and measured personality variables. Proponents of "interactionism" point to the fact that situational and personality influences are mutually interdependent (Endler, 1983; Endler &

Magnusson, 1976; Endler & Parker, 1992). The two sets of influences not only combine to influence or predict behavioral outcomes as just described, but they also influence one another in a dynamic, reciprocal fashion. In dynamic interactionism (Endler, 1983), the distinction between antecedents and consequences (and independent and dependent variables) may not be appropriate because situations and traits mutually influence one another in a variety of ways. For example, a person's traits can change the nature of a situation, such as when a highly agreeable person creates a friendly and cooperative social environment or an aggressive child instigates widespread hostility on a previously peaceful playground. Furthermore, people with different personality predispositions sometimes choose different kinds of social settings (Snyder & Ickes, 1985). Unlike in experimental settings in which people are thrust into situations that they did not pick, in everyday life people have a certain degree of flexibility and freedom to gravitate toward situations that are consistent with their personalities. Once people are in those self-selected situations, one finds it meaningless to ask whether their behavior is a function of the situations or of their personalities, because personality has determined the situation. Likewise, personality traits can change when people are in certain situations. For instance, the classic Bennington study showed that students became less conservative during their college experience and remained less conservative for years afterward (Newcomb, Koenig, Flacks, & Warwick, 1967).

Fortunately, the development of structural equation modeling and related statistical modeling strategies provides for the first time a way to approach modeling these complex, reciprocal influences. As described by Hoyle and Leary (Chapter 2, this volume), if data are gathered strategically (i.e., repeatedly, with appropriate spacing, across time and situations), it is possible to model the strong, dynamic version of interactionism that its proponents advocate (Endler & Parker, 1992).

Nonlinearity

A relatively uncharted direction for research on the interplay of personality and social behavior is the modeling of nonlinear relations. Following up on our suggestion that, for the most part, people inhabit a main-effect world, we suspect that the relationships between variables in that world are, by and large, linear. However, just as interaction effects add nuance (and sometimes significant variance accounted for) to models of personality and social behavior, the addition of nonlinear terms to statistical models may add richness and subtlety to our understanding of the relationship between dispositions and behavior.

Nonlinear relations can range from relatively straightforward curvilinear effects evaluated using power polynomials in multiple regression and trend analysis in analysis of variance to complex dynamical systems that attempt to model the "chaos" and "catastrophe" evident in human social behavior (e.g., Tesser & Achee, 1994; Vallacher, Nowak, & Kaufman, 1994). An example of work in which potential curvilinear relations are explored is Jorm and Christensen's (2004) study of the relations between religiosity and Eysenck's three-factor model of personality. In addition to a modest linear relation with one factor, they found quadratic relations with all three factors, indicating similarity in the personalities of individuals at the highest and lowest levels of religiosity. Tesser and Achee (1994) identified a number of instances of catastrophe in the prediction of social behaviors. In such cases, a seemingly linear relation between two variables quickly changes direction at a particular point before returning to a linear form like that before the "catastrophe." Such dynamical systems analyses also offer a compelling means of connecting seemingly disparate levels of analysis, such as neurobiology and personality (Mandell & Selz, 1995). Such findings contribute to conceptual models that offer more precise and nuanced accounts of individual differences in social behavior.

Conclusions

We find it difficult to imagine scientists in any other discipline falling into a controversy that would be equivalent to the traditional schism between social and personality psychologists. Would one branch of physics declare that the most important topics in the field involved the nature of matter but that forces such as gravitation were unimport-

ant, while another branch declared that only the forces that acted on matter were worth studying (and that those forces could be studied without reference to the characteristics of matter itself)? Can we imagine one group of chemists being interested only in chemical structure and another group being interested only in interactions among chemicals without considering the structure of the constituents? Could meteorologists function if some studied only the properties of relatively static weather systems and others studied only the forces that act on them? Fortunately, most behavioral scientists now agree that the rift between social psychologists and personality psychologists has been misguided and detrimental to a full understanding of socially relevant thought, emotion, and behavior.

This rapprochement does not mean that we should all start studying precisely the same things, of course. We need specialists in personality structure and process, as well as those who specialize in studying the effects of the "actual, imagined, or implied presence of others" (Allport, 1968, p. 3). But, in trying to understand the phenomena that constitute the science of human psychology, devoting attention to both situational and dispositional factors is the optimal strategy.

References

Allport, G. W. (1937). *Personality: A psychological interpretation*. New York: Holt, Rinehart & Winston.

Allport, G. W. (1968). The historical background of modern social psychology. In G. Lindzey & E. Aronson (Eds.), *Handbook of social psychology* (Vol. 1, 2nd ed., pp. 1–80). Reading, MA: Addison-Wesley.

Bem, D., & Funder, D. (1978). Predicting more of the people more of the time: Assessing the personality of situations. *Psychological Review, 85,* 485–501.

Bizer, G. Y., Krosnick, J. A., Holbrook, A. L., Wheeler, S. C., Rucker, D. D., & Petty, R. E. (2004). The impact of personality on cognitive, behavioral, and affective political processes: The effects of need to evaluate. *Journal of Personality, 72,* 995–1027.

Bohrnstedt, G. W., & Marwell, G. (1977). The reliability of products of two random variables. In K. F. Schussler (Ed.), *Sociological methodology: 1978* (pp. 254–273). San Francisco: Jossey-Bass.

Caspi, A., & Moffitt, T. E. (1993). When do individual differences matter?: A paradoxical theory of personality coherence. *Psychological Inquiry, 4,* 247–271.

Cervone, D., Caldwell, T. L., & Orom, H. (in press). Beyond person and situation effects: Intraindividual personality architecture and its implications for the study of personality and social behavior. In F.

Rhodewalt (Ed.), *Frontiers of social psychology: Personality and social behavior.* New York: Psychology Press.

Chaplin, W. F. (1997). Personality, interactive relations, and applied psychology. In R. Hogan, J. Johnson, & Briggs, S. (Eds.), *Handbook of personality psychology* (pp. 873–890). San Diego, CA: Academic Press.

Cronbach, L. J. (1957). The two disciplines of scientific psychology. *American Psychologist, 12,* 671–684.

Downey, G., & Feldman, S. I. (1996). Implications of rejection sensitivity for intimate relationships. *Journal of Personality and Social Psychology, 70,* 1327–1343.

Eagly, A. H., & Johnson, B. T. (1990). Gender and leadership style: A meta-analysis. *Psychological Bulletin, 108,* 233–256.

Endler, N. S. (1983). Interactionism: A personality model, but not yet a theory. In M. M. Page (Ed.), *Nebraska Symposium on Motivation 1982: Personality—Current theory and research* (pp. 155–200). Lincoln: University of Nebraska Press.

Endler, N. S., & Magnusson, D. (1976). Toward an interactional psychology of personality. *Psychological Bulletin, 83,* 956–974.

Endler, N. S., & Parker, J. D. A. (1992). Interactionism revisited: Reflections on the continuing crisis in the personality area. *European Journal of Personality, 6,* 177–198.

Epstein, S. (1979). The stability of behavior: I. On predicting most of the people much of the time. *Journal of Personality and Social Psychology, 37,* 1097–1126.

Epstein, S. (1983). Aggregation and beyond: Some basic issues on the prediction of behavior. *Journal of Personality, 51,* 360–392.

Epstein, S., & O'Brien, E. J. (1985). The person–situation debate in historical and current perspective. *Psychological Bulletin, 98,* 513–537.

Fleeson, W. (2001). Towards a structure- and process-integrated view of personality: Traits as density distributions of states. *Journal of Personality and Social Psychology, 80,* 1011–1027.

Fleeson, W. (2004). Moving personality beyond the person–situation debate: The challenge and opportunity of within-person variability. *Current Directions in Psychological Science, 13,* 83–87.

Funder, D. C. (2006). Towards a resolution of the personality triad: Persons, situations, and behaviors. *Journal of Research in Personality, 40,* 21–34.

Funder, D. C., & Colvin, C. R. (1991). Explorations in behavioral consistency: Properties of persons, situations and behaviors. *Journal of Personality and Social Psychology, 52,* 773–794.

Funder, D. C., & Ozer, D. J. (1983). Behavior as a function of the situation. *Journal of Personality and Social Psychology, 44,* 107–112.

Harris, C. R. (2003). A review of sex differences in sexual jealousy, including self-report data, psychophysiological responses, interpersonal violence, and morbid jealousy. *Personality and Social Psychology Review, 7,* 102–128.

Hyde, J. S. (1984). How large are gender differences in aggression?: A developmental meta-analysis. *Developmental Psychology, 20,* 722–736.

Ichheisser, G. (1943). Misinterpretations of personality in everyday life and the psychologist's frame of reference. *Character and Personality, 12,* 145–160.

Ickes, W. (1982). A basic paradigm for the study of personality, roles, and social behavior. In W. Ickes & E. Knowles (Eds.), *Personality, roles, and social behavior* (pp. 305–331). New York: Springer-Verlag.

Isaacowitz, D. M. (2005). The gaze of the optimist. *Personality and Social Psychology Bulletin, 31,* 407–415.

Jorm, A. F., & Christensen, H. (2004). Religiosity and personality: Evidence for nonlinear associations. *Personality and Individual Differences, 36,* 1433–1441.

Kenrick, D. T., & Dantchik, A. (1983). Interactionism, idiographics, and the social psychological invasion of personality. *Journal of Personality, 51,* 286–307.

Keppel, G. (1982). *Design and analysis: A researcher's handbook* (2nd ed.). Englewood Cliffs, NJ: Prentice-Hall.

Lewin, K. (1936). *Principles of topological psychology.* New York: McGraw-Hill.

Magnusson, D., & Endler, N. S. (1977). Interactional psychology: Present status and future propsects. In D. Magnusson & N. S. Endler (Eds.), *Personality at the crossroads: Current issues in trait psychology* (pp. 3–35). Hillsdale, NJ: Erlbaum.

Mandell, A. J., & Selz, K. A. (1995). Nonlinear dynamical patterns as personality theory for neurobiology and psychiatry. *Psychiatry, 58,* 371–390.

McClelland, G. H., & Judd, C. M. (1993). Statistical difficulties of detecting interactions and moderator effects. *Psychological Bulletin, 114,* 376–389.

Milgram, S. (1963). Behavioral study of obedience. *Journal of Abnormal and Social Psychology, 67,* 371–378.

Mischel, W. (1968). *Personality and assessment.* New York: Wiley.

Newcomb, T. M., Koenig, K. E., Flacks, R., & Warwick, D. P. (1967). *Persistence and change.* New York: Wiley.

Packer, D. J. (2008). Identifying systematic disobedience in Milgram's obedience experiments. *Perspectives on Psychological Science, 3,* 301–308.

Ross, L., & Nisbett, R. E. (1991). *The person and the situation.* New York: McGraw-Hill.

Saucier, G., & Skrzypińska, K. (2006). Spiritual but not religious?: Evidence for two independent dispositions. *Journal of Personality, 74,* 1257–1292.

Snyder, M., & Ickes, W. (1985). Personality and social behavior. In G. Lindzey & E. Aronson (Eds.), *Handbook of social psychology* (3rd ed., pp. 883–947). New York: Random House.

Swann, W. B., Jr., & Seyle, C. (2005). Personality psychology's comeback and its emerging symbiosis with social psychology. *Personality and Social Psychology Bulletin, 31,* 155–165.

Tesser, A., & Achee, J. (1994). Aggression, love, conformity, and other social psychological catastrophes. In R. R. Vallacher & A. Nowak (Eds.), *Dynamical systems in social psychology* (pp. 96–109). San Diego, CA: Academic Press.

Vallacher, R., Nowak, A., & Kaufman, J. (1994). Intrinsic dynamics of social judgment. *Journal of Personality and Social Psychology, 67,* 20–34.

Wallach, M. A., & Wallach, L. (1998). When experiments serve little purpose: Misguided research in mainstream psychology. *Theory and Psychology, 8,* 183–194.

CHAPTER 2

■ ● ▲ ◆ ■ ● ▲ ◆

Methods for the Study
of Individual Differences in Social Behavior

RICK H. HOYLE
MARK R. LEARY

Research on the relationships between individual-difference variables and social behavior poses many methodological challenges, the most fundamental of which involves how to measure personality dispositions in ways that are both accurate and sensitive. However, given that each chapter in this volume provides information about the most reliable and valid measures of each construct and that virtually all of these measures have been shown to be valid across a variety of research contexts and participant populations, this chapter focuses primarily on methods for studying individual differences in social behavior, assuming that acceptable measures are available.

Although we do not discuss how suitable measures of individual differences are developed and validated, we begin the chapter with a section on how such measures are used. As we see it, regardless of the methodological strategy researchers adopt, they must answer four questions in order to decide how best to use valid measures of personality in studies of socially relevant thought, behavior, and emotion:

- Does the research question call for trait or state measurement?
- Should measurement be at a general or a specific level?

- Which mode of measurement best suits the sample and research question?
- Is one measure of the variable of interest enough?

In the remainder of this section, we highlight the primary issues to be considered when answering each of these questions for a given study.

Trait versus State Measurement

Individual differences (or traits) are characteristics of people that are relatively stable across time and situations. Although traits show some degree of stability, situations increase or decrease the likelihood that a particular individual-difference variable will predict thoughts, emotions, or behaviors at a given point in time in the same way that specific situations "afford" certain thoughts, feelings, and behaviors (Gibson, 1977). Particular traits will predict a specific outcome in certain situations but not in others. Furthermore, although an individual's characteristic level of a trait may predict his or her general tendency to respond in a certain fashion, his or her actual reactions may vary markedly as a function of situational influences (Fleeson, 2001). For some research questions, this momentary or situated reaction, not the characteristic or dispositional form, is of interest. In such cases, a state measure is the appropriate choice. Alternatively, if the research question concerns participants' characteristic standing on a psychological characteristic, then a trait measure is appropriate.

For some responses, separate trait and state measures have been developed. For example, the State–Trait Anxiety Inventory allows the assessment of both the "transitory emotional state" of anxiety and "relatively stable individual differences" in the degree to which people tend to experience anxiety (Spielberger, 1983). Another widely used instrument with which state and trait measurement is possible is the Positive and Negative Affect Schedule, on which respondents can be asked to rate on a single set of adjectives their feelings either "during the past week" (i.e., trait) or "right now, at this moment" (i.e., state; Watson, Clark, & Tellegen, 1988). A similar tack has been taken with the Self-Esteem Scale (Rosenberg, 1965). Although this scale is typically regarded as a measure of trait self-esteem, researchers have used it to assess state self-esteem by asking respondents to indicate the extent to which the statements about their self-worth apply "at the moment" that they complete the scale (e.g., Kernis, Grannemann, & Barclay, 1989). Often, researchers find it beneficial to assess a construct at both a trait and a state level so that the relationship between general tendencies and specific behaviors can be examined.

General versus Specific Measurement

Individual differences can be measured at varying levels of specificity, from very general (e.g., trait anxiety) to highly specific (e.g., trait anxiety regarding interactions with people of the other sex). Typically, the specificity of the measure used should fall at a point along this continuum that corresponds to the level of specificity at which other variables in the study are measured. The practice of matching the specificity of measurement of variables follows from the principle of compatibility originally proposed in studying relations between attitudes and behavior (Fishbein & Ajzen, 1975). Indeed,

across a range of studies, relationships between attitudes and behaviors are strongest when the context and specificity of the measures are compatible (Kim & Hunter, 1993). For instance, predictions of the use of birth control pills improve markedly when the specificity of the predictor and outcome are comparable. Predictions of the use of birth control pills from people's self-reported attitudes ranges from $r = .08$ for attitude toward birth control in general to $r = .32$ for attitude toward birth control pills to $r = .52$ for attitudes toward use of birth control pills to $r = .57$ for attitude toward using birth control pills in the next 2 years (Davidson & Jaccard, 1979). Similarly, one solution to the problem of low observed correlations between personality and behavior (Mischel, 1968) is to aggregate behaviors to produce a variable at a level of generality that is similar to standard measures of personality traits (Epstein, 1980). For example, extraversion is more appropriately used as a predictor of trends in behavior in social settings across time and situations than of any single instance of extraverted behavior. In studies of individual differences in social behavior, the principle of compatibility dictates that, to the extent possible, the individual-difference variable should be measured at a level of specificity that corresponds to the specificity of the measure of the variables to be predicted.

Unlike the development of state-level counterparts to trait measures, the development of specific measures from general measures (and vice versa) is not straightforward. A fundamental concern involves determining the appropriate dimensions that should be used to parse the general construct to produce more specific variants. A rich example is global versus domain-specific self-esteem. Several researchers have attempted to parse global self-esteem into more specific "types" by identifying a relatively small number of dimensions on which people characteristically evaluate themselves, such as physical appearance, social skills, and academic competence (e.g., Fleming & Courtney, 1984; Harter, 1988). However, these dimensions can be further decomposed into even more specific areas of self-evaluation, such as particular features of one's appearance (e.g., Franzoi & Shields, 1984) or specific academic subjects (Marsh & O'Neill, 1984). Following from the principle of compatibility, these more specific variants are most fruitfully used when other variables in the study are equally specific.

Moving in the other direction—from specific to general—is more straightforward. Measures of particular behaviors or of domain-specific self-reports can be aggregated (i.e., typically summed or averaged) to produce measures of general tendencies that are comparable in level of specificity with general measures of personality. For instance, the seven specific domains in which contingency of self-worth is measured by the Contingencies of Self-Worth Scale (Crocker, Luhtanen, Cooper, & Bouvrette, 2003) can be aggregated into two more general domains—internal versus external contingencies—and these two domains can be further aggregated into a measure of overall contingency of self-worth. This general measure would be compatible with more general measures of other constructs, such as global self-esteem and overall adjustment.

Measurement Modality

When planning studies to examine links between individual differences and social behavior, researchers should consider the optimal way to administer the measures. The number of options for assessing traits continues to increase as technology expands and access to this technology improves. The traditional paper-and-pencil approach is giving way to computer administration on either stand-alone or locally networked computers or via server over the World Wide Web. Significant advantages of computer-based administration are low cost (e.g., no photocopying, postage, or data entry), the ability to shuffle the order of items or scales easily, and, if needed, the ability to score measures on the fly so that subsequent aspects of the study can be tailored to each participant's score on a particular measure. Computer administration also allows seamless integration of questionnaires with audio and video stimuli. However, these benefits are offset by the need for participants to have access to a computer and the Internet, the potential for lost data due to computer malfunction, the inability of researchers to control the conditions under which people complete the measures over the Web, and, in some instances,

concerns about the confidentiality of sensitive information that is transmitted over a network.

Both paper-and-pencil and computer-administered measures assume that respondents can read and understand what they are asked to do. When these assumptions are not reasonable or when self-administration is not viable for other reasons, administration of measures by a researcher is preferred. Although the relative cost of this modality is high, it generally yields a high response rate and high-quality data. Drawbacks to this modality include the potential for interviewer bias, concerns about anonymity, the time required to interview respondents individually, and cost.

Because all measurement modalities have shortcomings, it is worrisome that the overwhelming majority of published research on individual differences in social behavior is based on self-administered paper-and-pencil questionnaires. To help address concerns with the ubiquity of paper-and-pencil measurement, measures should be validated across modalities of administration. When measures perform comparably no matter how they are completed by respondents, researchers have added faith in the validity of the measures and are equipped to disentangle modality-specific biases from genuine relations between variables by using multiple modes of collecting data across studies in a research program (Campbell, 1969). They also are in a position to choose the measurement modality that best fits the study population (e.g., college students, the poor, the mentally ill), the setting (e.g., research lab, participants' homes, school), and research question (e.g., simple associations, change over time, variability across situations) without concern for validity.

Multiple Measures

No single measure fully captures the construct that it operationally defines—a frequent but misguided assumption known as definitional operationism (Campbell, 1969). For example, no measure of extraversion truly, accurately, and completely assesses extraversion. Moreover, all measures are influenced to some degree by extraneous factors such as social desirability or biases in how particular respondents use the response scales. For this reason, it is unwise for research findings to be based on only one measure of key constructs. Ideally, multiple measures should be used across (or within) studies in a research literature or program, measures that differ not only in content but also in modality of administration, reporters (e.g., self, peer, parent, teacher), and means of responding. Findings that obtain across measures (particularly if the measures differ in response format or mode of administration) are presumably more robust and replicable than those based on a single measure. Moreover, when effect sizes are combined across such studies, the average should converge on the true effect size, that is, the effect size uncontaminated by particular method effects.

The use of multiple measures can take various forms that address different concerns about the reliance on a single measure. In one form, which addresses concerns about the degree to which a single measure covers the full content of a construct, two or more measures of the same construct are used. For instance, three different self-report measures of self-esteem ensure greater coverage of the construct and provide a means of removing sources of bias that differ across measures. Despite these important payoffs, this strategy does not deal with any biases that are related to self-reports of self-esteem in general. Alternatively, a single measure might be used but completed by two or more reporters (i.e., collateral reports). For instance, severity of depressive symptoms might be assessed by asking a parent and a teacher to complete the instrument for each participant, as well as the participant him- or herself. This strategy does not address concerns about the content coverage of the measure, but it addresses concerns about the validity of self-reports. A third strategy is to use two or more measures that differ in content coverage, modality, and/or reporter. For example, anxiety might be measured through paper-and-pencil or computer-administered self-reports, assessment of relevant physiological markers, and trained judges' coding of participants' videotaped behavior in the presence of an anxiety-inducing stimulus. If anxiety as measured in these various ways correlates similarly to measures of social behavior, then the researcher can conclude

that the effect is not due to a measurement or method artifact.

Although using different measures and measurement strategies across studies addresses concerns across a program of research or a research literature, it is advantageous to include multiple measures and strategies in individual studies when possible. Referring back to the anxiety example, if these three measures—a self-report, physiological marker, and judges' rating—were gathered in a single study, their commonality could be modeled as a latent variable (e.g., using structural equation modeling), which then is correlated with other variables. In this application, one assumes that, although each measure is subject to various extraneous influences that undermine its reliability, the three measures share in common the influence of anxiety. By separating this commonality from unique and random error, one is left with a relatively pure representation of the construct. Assuming significantly different content and measurement strategies, any effects obtained using this approach cannot be attributed to the idiosyncrasies of individual measures or measurement strategies (cf. DeShon, 1998).

Methodological Strategies

The goal of sound measurement is an operational definition of the individual-difference variable that allows an accurate estimate of the magnitude and form of the relationship between the variable and relevant social thoughts, emotions, or behaviors. Yet even the most careful and complete measurement strategy does not ensure that this goal is met. Measurement is undertaken in the context of a methodological strategy and, as with measurement, no methodological strategy is perfect. Consequently, the strongest evidence is obtained when different methodological approaches are used to estimate or model the relationships between individual differences and social-psychological outcomes. In this section, we outline a set of principles for choosing and evaluating findings from research methods that are commonly used to study individual differences in social behavior. We then describe four categories of methodological strategies for such research.

Principles

In the ideal research program on the relationships between personality and social behavior, findings that are generated using various measures, measurement modalities, and methodological strategies converge on the true effect size and form; that is, the relations generally do not need to be qualified with reference to how the constructs are measured or the study conducted. In terms of maximizing the contribution of methods to this effort, we offer these overarching principles:

• Although no method is perfect, virtually all methods are useful at some point in the process of building a body of evidence relevant to understanding the relationships between individual differences and social behaviors. For this reason, we do not recommend avoiding any credible method altogether but, rather, suggest matching methodological strategy with the goals of the research program at a given point in its development.

• The reports of findings from individual studies should acknowledge shortcomings in the methodology, understanding that no methodology is without fault and that subsequent studies should replicate the findings using alternative methods with complementary strengths.

• Because individual differences co-occur, a major goal in using any methodological strategy is to isolate variance due to the individual difference of interest from other personality variables and from transient influences. Inferences should take into account the degree to which isolation has been accomplished and, when it clearly has not, researchers should acknowledge plausible alternative explanations of their findings.

• When the goal of a particular study is causal inference, a number of conditions must be met before casualty can be inferred. Because these conditions are sometimes difficult to meet in a single study, the evidence necessary for a firm causal conclusion often must accrue across a number of studies, each designed to satisfy one or more of the necessary conditions. As such, strong causal inferences typically are advisable only after numerous studies have been conducted that address the various conditions necessary for causal inference.

With these principles as context, we now describe three categories of methodological strategies for research on individual differences in social behavior.

Cross-Sectional Strategies

Easily the most straightforward approach to studying individual differences in social behavior is one in which the individual-difference variable, any extraneous variables to be ruled out or moderators to be considered, and the outcomes of interest are measured at one point in time. In the typical implementation of this cross-sectional strategy, data are collected using a single mode of measurement (e.g., paper and pencil, Web administration, interview). This strategy has many advantages. It is relatively low in cost in terms of materials, space, and personnel. Data can be collected from a large number of respondents in a relatively short period of time. And data on many variables can be obtained in a single study. Furthermore, if the measures are computer administered, the data are, in effect, input by the participants, making it possible to move from data collection to report writing in a few weeks. For these reasons, cross-sectional studies have become a staple in research in personality and social psychology.

These compelling advantages must be weighed against the significant limitations, however. Foremost among these is the inability to nonarbitrarily sequence variables in statistical models of the data. Because data on all variables are gathered at one point in time, usually in one sitting, it is impossible to use the data to convincingly evaluate relationships using statistical methods that assume sequence or causal ordering (such as structural equation modeling). In addition, it is likely that some portion of the covariance between variables is attributable to the fact that they were assessed under precisely the same circumstances, with the respondent in precisely the same physical and psychological state. Because all variables are assessed simultaneously, typically using a single mode of measurement, statistical relations are almost certainly overestimated, and what appears as covariance between variables is, in part (potentially even entirely), due to shared method and situation variance. Concerns about the inability to sequence variables in statistical models and about inflated estimates of covariance are significant, and they limit the potential contribution of cross-sectional studies to a general understanding of the role of individual differences in social behavior.

Nonetheless, there is a place for cross-sectional studies. The first question to be settled when undertaking any new line of research is simply whether and how the variables of interest are associated, and more complex studies typically await a cross-sectional assessment of this question. The large sample sizes typical of cross-sectional research, coupled with the fact that most variables are measured on quasi-continuous scales, allow efficient evaluations of the relations among variables, including those attributable to moderation by other variables. Cross-sectional studies often include a large number of variables, allowing the use of statistical approaches (e.g., multiple regression analysis) that isolate the personality variable of interest from other variables with which it is correlated. Thus, early in a research program, when the strength and form of relations involving an individual difference are not clear, cross-sectional studies are useful—even ideal.

Under certain circumstances and for certain research questions, more sophisticated cross-sectional strategies are available that allow firmer inferences. For example, when one's hypothesis concerns the behavior of a population rather than the behavior of individuals within the population, one can model changes in behavior associated with situational "interruptions" (either due to naturally occurring events or planned interventions) by repeatedly randomly sampling (without replacement) from the population over time. For example, Palmgreen, Donohew, Lorch, Hoyle, and Stephenson (2001) found that when the population of young viewers in a television market is divided into subgroups of individuals low and high in sensation seeking, the high-sensation-seeking group is both more likely to use illicit substances and to be influenced by antidrug media campaigns than the low-sensation-seeking group.

A variation on this strategy is to draw (ideally, random) samples of different ages from a population at a single point in time, thereby incorporating time as reflected in age in the design. For instance, Schultz and Moore (1988) compared loneliness scores and correlates for high school students, college undergraduates, and retirees with the goal of shedding light on age-related changes in loneliness. These variations on the one-shot cross-sectional study offer some of the benefits of strategies that explicitly incorporate time, but the findings they yield must be interpreted with caution. For instance, comparisons of different age groups are subject to cohort effects, in which putative age effects are actually due to history and context effects. Similarly, in cross-sectional time-series studies, events may transpire during the course of a study that alter the state of the population (e.g., September 11, 2001), obfuscating effects of the event of interest. Thus, although both cross-sectional time-series and age-based cross-sectional strategies offer benefits beyond those of one-shot cross-sectional studies, isolating the influence of specific variables remains a concern.

Experimental Strategies

Although also subject to limitations, experimental strategies overcome many of the shortcomings of cross-sectional strategies. A major benefit of well-designed experiments is the isolation of the putative cause from alternative causal factors, accomplished by randomly assigning participants to levels of the independent variables and manipulating one or more independent variables. Experimental methods also address concerns about sequence in directional relations between variables. Because standing on the independent variables is attributable to a random process that occurs at a known moment in time (i.e., the introduction of the independent variable), it cannot be attributed to other systematic sources. As such, if the independent variable is statistically associated with scores on other variables, the only logical inference is that the independent variable is antecedent to those variables in a causal sequence. This does not rule out the possibility that, if the roles of the variables were reversed in another study so that the independent variable was measured and one of the other variables manipulated, we might also observe a relation. Such a pattern would indicate a bidirectional relation between the variables.

Research using experimental methods often is undertaken in "laboratory" conditions, a typically artificial setting in which the experimenter controls the situational variables that might influence the participant during the experiment. Experiments need not occur in such settings, however, and the field experiment is a compelling strategy that brings to bear on a research question the strengths of the experimental method in a setting in which the behaviors of interest might typically be enacted.

A true experiment involving only individual differences is not possible, because research participants self-select to levels of the individual difference, bringing with them unknown other characteristics that cannot be ruled out as alternative explanations. Thus the usefulness of experimental methods as a means of isolating causal variables is lost. However, researchers often combine manipulated independent variables and measured personality variables in the same study in what has been called an *expericorr* design (Leary, 2008). (They are called *expericorr* because they possess features of both a true experiment and a cross-sectional correlation design.) In such designs, participants are pretested on the personality variable of interest and then randomly assigned to experimental conditions. Such designs allow researchers to explore the possibility that the personality variable moderates reactions to the independent variable such that participants who score differently on the personality measure respond differently to the independent variable.

Traditionally, such moderation effects were tested by splitting participants into low versus high groups using a median split, then entering this dichotomous personality variable, along with the manipulated independent variable(s), into an analysis of variance and testing the personality-by-independent-variable interaction. This analytical approach is now strongly discouraged because of evidence that converting a rich continuous personality variable into a dichotomy throws away a great deal of informative variability and greatly reduces the power of statistical tests (MacCallum, Zhang, Preacher, & Rucker, 2002; more on this later). Tests of personality moderation should be conducted using moderated multiple regression in which the continuity of the

personality scores is preserved (see Aiken & West, 1991).

The strength of experimental designs that include personality characteristics can be increased by measuring and covarying one or more other personality variables that are potentially confounded with the personality variable of interest. Imagine, for example, that one is interested in how people who vary in need for power (the personality variable of interest) respond to a manipulated threat to their authority (the independent variable). Because need for power is likely correlated with need for control, one might wish to eliminate the confounding effects of control motivation from the findings. To do so, one could pretest participants on both need for power and control motivation and then covary (i.e., partial) control motivation from analyses that test effects involving need for power. Doing so would ensure that any obtained effects were not due to control motivation and thus were more likely to reflect individual differences in need for power. This inference is tentative, however, because other unidentified traits that correlate with need for power might be responsible for any obtained effects.

An increasingly common use of experimental strategies for research on individual differences involves tests of statistical mediation. In the measurement-of-mediation strategy (Spencer, Zanna, & Fong, 2005), the putative cause is manipulated as an independent variable, and, prior to or concurrent with the dependent variables, putative mediators (i.e., intervening variables) of the relationship between the independent and dependent variables are measured. Mediational hypotheses assume a strict sequence of causal influences from independent variable to mediator to dependent variable. When the measurement-of-mediation approach is implemented using experimental methods, the temporal order from the independent variable to mediator is fixed; however, the sequence from mediator to the outcome variable is not. The reason is that the mediator is measured rather than manipulated. Because the mediator serves as both an outcome variable (to the independent variable) and an antecedent variable (to the dependent variable), this problem cannot be solved in a single experiment. Instead, a pair of experiments is required. In the first, the effect of the independent variable on the mediator is evaluated. In the second, the effect of the mediator on the dependent variable is evaluated. Because the mediator is measured in the first instance and manipulated in the second, this strategy requires a measure and a manipulation that have been shown to be equivalent operational definitions of the mediator (e.g., private self-awareness; Fejfar & Hoyle, 2000).

Because, under the right conditions, experiments can isolate causal variables and establish sequence in the relations between variables, one might be tempted to conclude that experimental strategies are always preferred over other strategies for studying individual differences in social behavior. However, as with all methodological strategies, experimental methods have significant limitations. For example, in contrast with cross-sectional studies, experimental studies are relatively costly in terms of space, personnel, and the amount of time required to complete data collection. Furthermore, many topics cannot be studied experimentally because of ethical or logistical constraints. For example, one could not conduct an experimental study of the relationship between parental punitiveness and children's authoritarianism because doing so would require randomly assigning parents to punish their children with varying degrees of severity. In such cases, the best we can do is to measure hypothesized causes and outcomes and model their relationships.

Strategies That Incorporate Time

If sequencing the temporal order of variables is a goal and experimental manipulation is not feasible, then nonexperimental strategies that incorporate time are an attractive alternative. In the prototypical use of this strategy, a hypothesized cause measured at one point in time is related to an outcome measured at a later point in time. (If mediation is also of interest, then an intermediate assessment of the hypothesized mediator is required.) It is important to recognize that the simple form of this strategy—in which each variable is measured only at the time it is hypothesized to operate in the psychological process—is inadequate for establishing temporal sequence. The reason is that a portion of the variance in the measures is typically stable, and, by definition, stable

variance is not a function of other variables in the model. Thus, for example, in a study in which individual differences in rejection sensitivity are measured at Time 1 and aspects of social interaction are assessed 2 weeks later at Time 2, the statistical relation between rejection sensitivity and social behaviors might reflect nothing more than covariance between stable components of the two variables rather than the fact that rejection sensitivity was antecedent to behaviors observed in social interactions. Precisely the same findings might have been obtained had rejection sensitivity and social behavior been measured concurrently.

This concern is addressed rather simply by measuring social interaction concurrent with rejection sensitivity at both Time 1 and Time 2. In so doing, the stable component of social interaction can be statistically estimated and separated from the component that is subject to change. By including the measure of rejection sensitivity at the second assessment, it is possible both to estimate the degree of stability in sensitivity to rejection and to entertain the possibility that, to some degree, social interaction causes people to be more attuned to rejection. Panel studies (often called cross-lagged panel designs), in which all measures are administered at all points in time, allow for persuasive tests of sequence (Farrell, 1994). Using data from such studies, cross-lagged panel analyses can be used to test directly for sequence (Hoyle & Robinson, 2003). For example, Farrell (1994) measured anger and alcohol use on three occasions and used cross-lagged panel analysis to show that the relation between anger and alcohol use can be attributed solely to the effect of anger on alcohol use; when stability of these constructs is controlled, there is no lagged effect of alcohol use on anger.

At least two additional concerns must be addressed if longitudinal strategies are to be used effectively in studies of individual differences in social behavior. One concern stems from the fact that research participants are not randomized to levels of the variables, and therefore those variables are not isolated from other variables to which observed relations might be attributed. Thus, as with cross-sectional studies, statistical methods of isolation must be used. An additional complication is that the variables of interest are measured more than once, raising the question of whether the variables to be controlled must be measured repeatedly as well. If the influence of these confounding variables is expected to vary by time—either because scores on the variable change or because the variable's influence on other variables of interest varies from one time to the next—then they must be measured repeatedly and included in the statistical analysis at the appropriate place in the model. If the variables to be controlled are fixed characteristics of research participants (e.g., genotype), then they need be measured only once, preferably at the initial assessment, but possibly at any of the assessments.

A second concern is the spacing of assessments. The goal of repeated assessment is to observe and model change. On the one hand, if the amount of time between assessments is too short, it is possible that change attributable to or moderated by personality characteristics might not be observed. On the other hand, if the lag is too long, multiple, undetected changes might take place between assessments. Looking across the large number of longitudinal studies in the literature, it would seem that time between assessments is more a function of convenience or convention than a reasoned decision based on hypotheses about the timing of a well-articulated causal process. The strongest longitudinal studies are those in which the spacing between assessments is thoughtfully and strategically determined.

For individual differences that are studied during a time at which they are still emerging or developing, studies that use time to model trajectories of change are useful. If the individual-difference variable is measured on three or more occasions, latent growth modeling can be used to distinguish research participants in terms of their patterns of change over time (Bollen & Curran, 2005). For instance, data on dispositional optimism could be obtained from a sample of children at the beginning and end of their last year of middle school and first year of high school. Trajectories of change across these four assessments could be estimated and the characteristic form (e.g., linear, curvilinear) determined. In the simplest case, the characteristic form is linear and defined by two parameters—an intercept and a slope. It is typical to estimate these parameters for the sample as a whole, but in latent growth models they can be estimated for each research participant. Variance in these parameters reflects the fact that participants vary in their intercepts (often, though not always, defined as the first time point) and vary in the slopes of their trajectories. These slopes can be treated like traditional variables in statistical models and used as predictors, outcomes, or simple correlates. Also, through the use of growth mixture modeling, participants can be grouped in terms of similarity in growth parameters and these groups used to define and study subpopulations (Muthén & Muthén, 2000).

Strategies for Studying Processes as They Naturally Occur

To this point we have described strategies by which summary reports on dispositions and behavior are provided in hindsight (cross-sectional and panel studies) or by which behaviors are observed in settings controlled by the researcher (experimental studies). In the former case, it is possible that research participants do not, or cannot, accurately recall prior thoughts, feelings, or behaviors. In the latter case, it is possible that the controlled environment, although powerful, does not readily generalize to the social environments about which inferences are to be made. Both of these shortcomings are addressed using strategies that allow the collection of data on many occasions as the events and processes of interest occur in the course of everyday life.

Research using these methods is particularly well suited to the study of individual differences when conceptualized as the typical response of the individual to behavioral contingencies in the immediate, experienced environment (Mischel, Shoda, & Mendoza-Denton, 2002). Although traditional measures of individual differences provide a summary of these responses, they are not suitable for capturing the typical expression of the individual difference and the processes that account for its influence on behavior. For this endeavor, research strategies are required that allow the detection of within-person variance in situated behavioral contingencies, expression of individual differences, and behavior.

One such strategy is experience sampling (Conner, Barrett, Tugade, & Tennen, 2007). In the prototypic application of experience sampling, the experiences (i.e., thoughts, feelings, behaviors) of a relatively small number of individuals are sampled across time and naturally occurring situations. The sampling can be random, scheduled, or contingent. Random sampling is accomplished by equipping research participants with an electronic device that signals them a set number of times each day at random to provide data. In the earliest uses of this strategy, participants carried pagers that signaled them in response to randomly timed calls by research personnel (e.g., Csikszentmihalyi, Larson, & Prescott, 1977). Borrowing the colloquial terms for pagers, these studies came to be known as *beeper studies*. By randomly sampling the experience of selected individuals, these studies allow the researcher to draw inferences about the more general experience of the individual.

In other applications, akin to the panel studies described earlier, research participants are assessed at predetermined times (e.g., morning, evening) each day for several days. Signaling is required, but it may be done by simply programming alarms on wristwatches or mobile telephones. Because specific aspects of experience often are of interest to researchers (and these may or may not be captured by random or scheduled sampling), it may be more efficient to peg data collection to the occurrence of specific events. For instance, if the research question concerns social interaction, the researcher is interested in the experience of research participants only when they are engaged in social interactions. Event-contingent sampling cannot be signaled by devices or the research team. Instead, it requires that research participant be trained to recognize relevant situations and accept the responsibility of providing data when those situations arise. Data from three decades of research using this strategy indicate that research participants are generally reliable and responsible in this role.

It is not uncommon for experience sampling studies to engage research participants for 2 weeks, sampling six to eight times each day. The researcher then possesses 80 to 100 (or more) observations of each research participant. How are these data to be used in research on individual differences? In some research applications, descriptive information at the level of the individual is of primary interest. For example, a researcher might be interested in the mean level of positive affect, as well as in cross-situational variability around that value, for each research participant (e.g., Fleeson, 2004). Alternatively, these descriptive statistics can be studied in relation to other situated variables (e.g., location at the time of reporting) or, in multilevel applications, in relation to dispositions and other individual differences.

These strategies for studying naturally occurring experience as it happens offer an intriguing alternative to strategies such as cross-sectional or longitudinal studies, but they are not without complications and limitations. Experience-sampling studies can be costly. They require signaling equipment, frequent interaction (planned and unplanned) with research participants during data collection, and expertise with statistical methods for analyzing nested data. Although methods have become more refined and equipment more reliable, it still is not uncommon to lose data from participants due to equipment malfunction or unexpected events in the lives of individual participants that alter their typical experience or make it difficult for them to faithfully provide data. Because research participants provide data on numerous occasions, they cannot be asked too much each time lest the experience of participating in the study intrude on and alter their typical experience. The concern about isolation of key variables that we have highlighted throughout the chapter applies in these studies as well. People cannot be randomized to situations; therefore, we cannot distinguish between characteristics of situations influencing their behavior and their choice of those situations as opportunities to behave in desired ways. Because all variables are measured on all occasions, the concern about sequencing of variables can be addressed using methods described earlier for panel studies.

A Nod to Data Analysis

Although our focus is methods, not analysis, the choice of method often dictates or constrains the choice of analysis. For instance, data from cross-sectional studies typically are continuous, making them ill suited for mean-comparison analytical strategies that assume factors with two or three levels. Data generated from panel studies with three or more assessments are not conducive to analysis using typical strategies such as multiple regression analyses. And the nonindependence in data from experience-sampling studies requires the use of analytical strategies appropriate for such data. In light of this inherent link between how variables are measured and how they are analyzed, we recommend factoring data analysis concerns into decisions about how data will be collected.

In addition, we recommend accounting fully for the manner in which data were collected when analyzing them. Said differently, researchers should avoid forcing data to fit an analytical strategy that was chosen without consideration for the methodological strategy by which the data were collected and the characteristics of those data. As noted, a frequent and counterproductive form of this error is dichotomization of variables measured on a continuum to allow means comparisons (e.g., using ANOVA), a strategy that persists despite the well-documented loss in statistical power and potential increase in Type I errors (Fitzsimons, 2008). If the nature of the research question and the state of the literature point to comparisons of means, then data should be collected in a form that anticipates this analysis, or, better, strategies should be used for generating estimated means from analyses appropriate for continuously measured variables (Aiken & West, 1991).

Other ill-advised data-analytic choices are better categorized as missed opportunities than as outright errors. For example, if, as we have advised, multiple measures (preferably measured using different modes) of key constructs are included, then the data analysis should capitalize on this strength by modeling a latent variable that captures commonality in the measures while removing uniqueness and random error. At a more basic level, if multiple items are available for specific constructs, then a similar separation of commonality and error can be done in data analysis, ensuring that effect size estimates are not attenuated by some forms of error. In short, the benefits of conscientious measurement are not realized until the data have been analyzed using methods that take full advantage of the measurement strategy.

As a final word of caution related to the association between methodological strategy and data analysis, we note the importance of drawing inferences from statistical results that fully account for the strengths of the methodological strategy used to generate the data. Sophisticated statistical methods cannot overcome the limitations of research methods, as sometimes is assumed. For instance, the most elegant and nuanced structural equation model estimated on cross-sectional data cannot overcome the fact that research participants self-selected to levels on all variables and were assessed at one point in time. Conversely, the strengths of research methods sometimes necessitate only rudimentary statistical analyses, as in carefully designed experiments and research questions that focus on a specific pattern of means. This interplay between method and analysis requires that researchers keep one in mind when considering the other.

Conclusions

The strength and informativeness of evidence bearing on the relationships between individual differences and socially relevant responses is a direct result of the methodological strategies by which that evidence was produced. In this chapter, we have attempted to convey that all methods have strengths and limitations that make them more or less useful, depending on the research question and constraints that are imposed by the topic, research context, and sample. The strongest bodies of evidence are those in which the individual difference of interest has been measured in multiple ways using multiple modes of measurement and studied using a range of methodological strategies. This systematic and thorough approach to studying individual differences in social behavior ensures that variance and covariance attributable to the way in which they are measured and studied is not confused as variance and covariance attributable to the individual difference itself. Moreover, thoughtful designs and analyses make possible research syntheses that generate unbiased estimates of the magnitude and form of relationships between individual differences and other variables. These estimates then allow more precise statements about individual differences in theoretical models of their development and influence.

References

Aiken, L. S., & West, S. G. (1991). *Multiple regression: Testing and interpreting interactions.* Thousand Oaks, CA: Sage.

Bollen, K. A., & Curran, P. J. (2005). *Latent curve models: A structural equation perspective.* New York: Wiley.

Campbell, D. T. (1969). Definitional versus multiple operationalism. *Et Al., 2,* 14–17.

Conner, T. S., Barrett, L. F., Tugade, M. M., & Tennen, H. (2007). Idiographic personality: The theory and practice of experience sampling. In R. W. Robins, R. C. Fraley, & R. F. Krueger (Eds.), *Handbook of research methods in personality psychology* (pp. 79–96). New York: Guilford Press.

Crocker, J., Luhtanen, R. K., Cooper, M. L., & Bouvrette, S. (2003). Contingencies of self-worth in college students: Theory and measurement. *Journal of Personality and Social Psychology, 85,* 894–908.

Csikszentmihalyi, M., Larson, R., & Prescott, S. (1977). The ecology of adolescent experience. *Journal of Youth and Adolescence, 6,* 218–294.

Davidson, A. R., & Jaccard, J. (1979). Variables that moderate the attitude–behavior relation: Results of a longitudinal study. *Journal of Personality and Social Psychology, 37,* 1364–1379.

DeShon, R. P. (1998). A cautionary note on measurement error corrections in structural equation models. *Psychological Methods, 4,* 412–423.

Epstein, S. (1980). The stability of behavior: II. Implications for psychological research. *American Psychologist, 35,* 790–806.

Farrell, A. D. (1994). Structural equation modeling with longitudinal data: Strategies for examining group differences and reciprocal relationships. *Journal of Consulting and Clinical Psychology, 62,* 477–487.

Fejfar, M. C., & Hoyle, R. H. (2000). Effect of private self-awareness on negative affect and self-referent attribution: A quantitative review. *Personality and Social Psychology Review, 4,* 132–142.

Fishbein, M., & Ajzen, I. (1975). *Beliefs, attitude, intention, and behavior: An introduction to theory and research.* Reading, MA: Addison-Wesley.

Fitzsimons, G. (2008). Death to dichotomizing [Editorial]. *Journal of Consumer Research, 35*(1), 5–8.

Fleeson, W. (2001). Towards a structure- and process-integrated view of personality: Traits as density distributions of states. *Journal of Personality and Social Psychology, 80,* 1011–1027.

Fleeson, W. (2004). Moving personality beyond the person–situation debate: The challenge and the opportunity of within-person variability. *Current Directions in Psychological Science, 13,* 83–87.

Fleming, J. S., & Courtney, B. E. (1984). The dimensionality of self-esteem: II. Hierarchical facet model for revised measurement scales. *Journal of Personality and Social Psychology, 46,* 404–421.

Franzoi, S. L., & Shields, S. A. (1984). The Body-Esteem Scale: Multidimensional structure and sex differences in a college population. *Journal of Personality Assessment, 48,* 173–178.

Gibson, J. J. (1977). The theory of affordances. In R. Shaw & J. Bransford (Eds.), *Perceiving, acting, and knowing: Toward an ecological psychology* (pp. 67–82). Hillsdale, NJ: Erlbaum.

Harter, S. (1988). *Manual for the Adolescent Self-Perception Profile.* Denver, CO: Author.

Hoyle, R. H., & Robinson, J. I. (2003). Mediated and moderated effects in social psychological research: Measurement, design, and analysis issues. In C. Sansone, C. Morf, & A. T. Panter (Eds.), *Handbook of methods in social psychology* (pp. 213–233). Thousand Oaks, CA: Sage.

Kernis, M. H., Grannemann, B. D., & Barclay, L. C. (1989). Stability of self-esteem: Assessment, correlates, and excuse-making. *Journal of Personality, 60,* 621–644.

Kim, M.-S., & Hunter, J. E. (1993). Relationships among attitudes, behavioral intentions, and behavior: A meta-analysis of past research: Part 2. *Communication Research, 20,* 331–364.

Leary, M. R. (2003). *Introduction to behavioral research methods* (5th ed.). Boston: Allyn & Bacon.

MacCallum, R. C., Zhang, S., Preacher, K. J., & Rucker, D. D. (2002). On the practice of dichotomization of quantitative variables. *Psychological Methods, 7,* 19–40.

Marsh, H. W., & O'Neill, R. (1984). Self Description Questionnaire III: The construct validity of multidimensional self-concept ratings by late adolescents. *Journal of Educational Measurement, 21,* 153–174.

Mischel, W. (1968). *Personality and assessment.* New York: Wiley.

Mischel, W., Shoda, Y., & Mendoza-Denton, R. (2002). Situation-behavior profiles as a locus of consistency in personality. *Current Directions in Psychological Science, 11,* 50–54.

Muthén, B., & Muthén, L. (2000). Integrating person-centered and variable-centered analysis: Growth mixture modeling with latent trajectory classes. *Alcoholism: Clinical and Experimental Research, 24,* 882–891.

Palmgreen, P., Donohew, L., Lorch, E. P., Hoyle, R. H., & Stephenson, M. T. (2001). Television campaigns and adolescent marijuana use: Tests of sensation seeking targeting. *American Journal of Public Health, 91,* 292–295.

Rosenberg, M. (1965). *Society and the adolescent self-image.* Princeton, NJ: Princeton University Press.

Schultz, N. R., Jr., & Moore, D. (1988). Loneliness: Differences across three age levels. *Journal of Social and Personal Relationships, 5,* 275–284.

Spencer, S. J., Zanna, M. P., & Fong, G. T. (2005). Establishing a causal chain: Why experiments are often more effective than mediational analyses in examining psychological processes. *Journal of Personality and Social Psychology, 89,* 845–851.

Spielberger, C. D. (1983). *Manual for the State–Trait Anxiety Inventory (STAI).* Palo Alto, CA: Consulting Psychologists Press.

Watson, D., Clark, L. A., & Tellegen, A. (1988). Development and validation of brief measures of positive and negative affect: The PANAS Scales. *Journal of Personality and Social Psychology, 47,* 1063–1070.

PART II

■ ● ▲ ◆

INTERPERSONAL DISPOSITIONS

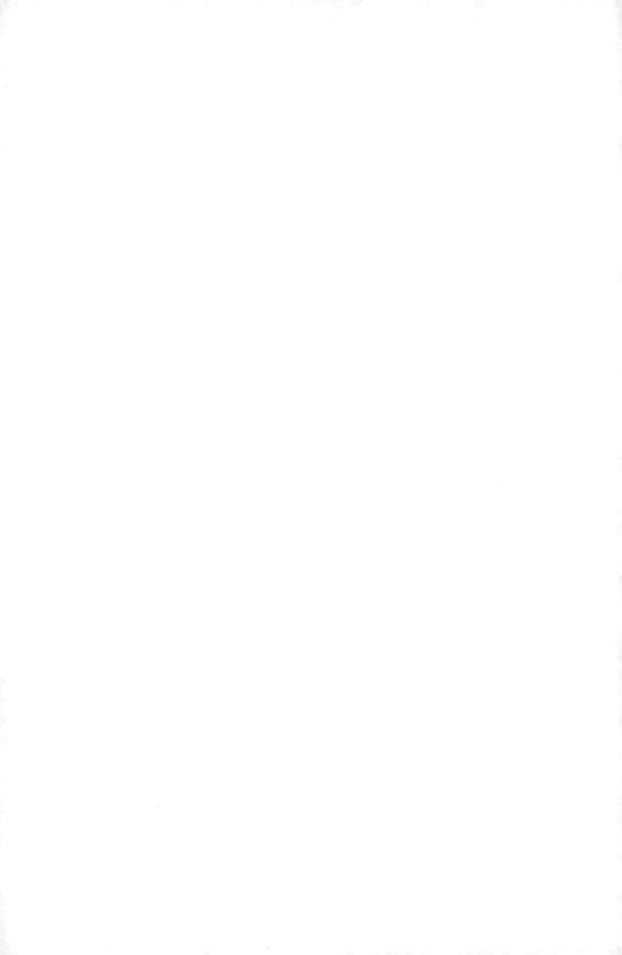

CHAPTER 3

■ ● ▲ ◆ ■ ● ▲ ◆

Extraversion

JOSHUA WILT
WILLIAM REVELLE

For at least 2,500 years, some people have been described as more bold, assertive, and talkative than others. For almost equally long, this set of behaviors has been thought to have a biological basis and to be socially important. Although our taxometric techniques have changed and our theories of biology are more advanced, the question of the causal basis, as well as the behavioral consequences, of the trait dimension that has come to be called *extraversion–introversion*[1] remains vitally important.

In general, there are at least three basic characteristics of extraversion that make it important to study. First, extraversion has emerged as one of the fundamental dimensions of personality (Costa & McCrae, 1992a; Digman, 1990; Eysenck & Himmelweit, 1947; Goldberg, 1990; Norman, 1963). As such, it has the potential to explain the covariation of a wide variety of behaviors, which is one of the central concerns for the field of personality (Funder, 2001). Second, extraversion predicts effective functioning and well-being across a wide variety of domains (Ozer & Benet-Martínez, 2006), from cognitive performance (Matthews, 1992) and social endeavors (Eaton & Funder, 2003) to socioeconomic status (Roberts, Kuncel, Shiner, Caspi, & Goldberg, 2007). Third, extraversion predicts risk and also resilience for different forms

of psychopathology (Trull & Sher, 1994; Widiger, 2005).

The ABCDs of Personality

We previously have proposed that personality can be conceptualized as the coherent patterning over time and space of Affect, Behavior, Cognition, and Desire (Ortony, Norman, & Revelle, 2005; Revelle, 2008). We believe that this model can be applied to specific trait complexes such as extraversion, and thus we structure this chapter around these four domains of effective functioning.

The remainder of the chapter is organized as follows. First, we present a brief history of the interest in extraversion. Second, we summarize taxometric approaches to the measurement of extraversion. Third, the main focus of the chapter is devoted to recent and current trends in research on extraversion, structured around the "ABCDs" of extraversion. Fourth, we offer directions for future research.

Extraversion from Theophrastus to Eysenck

Tyrtamus of Lesbos, known as Theophrastus for his speaking ability (Morley, 1891),

27

asked a fundamental question of personality theory that is still of central concern to us today:

> Often before now have I applied my thoughts to the puzzling question—one, probably, which will puzzle me for ever—why it is that, while all Greece lies under the same sky and all the Greeks are educated alike, it has befallen us to have characters so variously constituted. (Theophrastus, 1909, p. 77)

The "characters" of Theophrastus are often used to summarize the lack of coherence of early personality trait description, although it is possible to organize his characters into a table (Table 3.1) that looks remarkably similar to equivalent tables of the late 20th century (John, 1990; John & Srivastava, 1999). The taxonomy developed by Theophrastus used antiquated terms; however, it is easy to see that some of them bear close resemblance to the adjectives used in contemporary approaches in describing extraversion.

Another noteworthy personality taxonomy that captured an extraversion dimension was the model of the four temperaments described by Hippocrates and Galen, which was later reorganized into two dimensions (changeability and excitability) by Wundt (Wundt & Judd, 1897). The choleric and sanguine temperaments can be characterized as being more changeable, whereas the melancholic and phlegmatic temperaments are less changeable. The changeability dimension was later conceptualized as extraversion by Eysenck (1981; Eysenck & Himmelweit, 1947); see Stelmack and Stalikas (1991) for a review. Presaging current efforts to explain personality dimensions, a physiological basis for the four temperaments was proposed (blood for sanguine, yellow bile for choleric, black bile for melancholic, and phlegm for phlegmatic). In contrast to the similarity of old and new taxometric approaches to extraversion, the contemporary physiological differences (Canli, 2004) thought to underlie extraversion differ quite dramatically from the bodily humors.

Although people were recognized as falling at a certain level on behavioral dimensions resembling extraversion as far back as 2,500 years ago, it was not until C. G. Jung (1921/1971) that the words *extraversion* and *introversion* were brought into the popular terminology of psychology. However, Jung did not emphasize a continuous extraversion dimension but rather conceptualized extraverts and introverts as different types of people. For Jung, extraverts were more focused on the outer world and introverts on their own inner mentality. He also associated ex-

TABLE 3.1. The Characters of Theophrastus and the Adjectives of the Big Five Show Remarkable Similarity

Big Five				
Extraversion	Agreeableness	Conscientiousness	Neuroticism	Openness
talkative	sympathetic	organized	tense	wide interests
assertive	kind	thorough	anxious	imaginative
active	appreciative	planful	nervous	intelligent
energetic	affectionate	efficient	moody	original
-quiet	-cold	-careless	-stable	-commonplace
-reserved	-unfriendly	-disorderly	-calm	-simple
-shy	-quarrelsome	-frivolous	-contented	-shallow
-silent	-hard-headed	-irresponsible	-unemotional	-unintelligent
		Characters of Theophrastus		
talker	anxious to please	-hostile	coward	-stupid
chatty	flatterer	-shameless	grumbler	-superstitious
boastful	-unpleasant	-distrustful	mean	-boor
arrogant	-outcast	-avaricious	unseasonable	-gross
garrulous	-offensive	-reckless	feckless	ironical

Note. Big Five adjectives from John (1990). The characters of Theophrastus are from Jebb's (1909) translation. Words with the symbol "-" are reverse scored.

traversion with hysterical disorders and introversion with what today would be called mood disorders. Although the credit is usually given to Jung for originating the modern term *extraversion*, the less known but very important work of Gerard Heymanns (Eysenck, 1992) had already identified extraversion more accurately as a dimension (rather than a type) along a continuum of "strong" and "weak" functioning. It is also Heymanns whom we should credit with the integration of psychometric methods with experimental approaches to personality and with situating psychological research in the hypothetico-deductive method. Standing on the shoulders of Heymanns and those who came before him, Hans Eysenck demonstrated the importance of extraversion as a fundamental dimension of personality in a series of experimental and taxometric studies in the late 1940s and early 1950s (Eysenck, 1952; Eysenck & Himmelweit, 1947).

The Measurement of Extraversion

The descriptive tradition in personality, as mentioned before, has its roots in Theophrastus and Galen. In the 20th century, psychologists began serious efforts to measure the major dimensions of personality, and all such efforts have identified extraversion as a major dimension.

Mid-20th-Century Taxonomies

Eysenck was one of the first to try to describe the core features of extraversion with scales developed to assess personality, the Maudsley Personality Questionnaire (MPQ; Eysenck, 1959), the Eysenck Personality Inventory (EPI; Eysenck & Eysenck, 1968), the Eysenck Personality Questionnaire (EPQ; Eysenck & Eysenck, 1975), and the Eysenck Personality Profiler (EPP; Eysenck & Wilson, 1991). Some of the items for the MPQ and EPI were adapted from Guilford (Guilford & Zimmerman, 1949), which led to an interesting debate as to the proper structure of extraversion. The instrument Guilford developed to measure personality, the Guilford–Zimmerman Temperament Survey (GZTS; Guilford & Zimmerman, 1949), identifies a higher order factor called Introversion–Extraversion, which reflects a

dimension similar to Jung's in that Introversion is described by reflective behavior. However, the Extraversion pole of this scale is similar to EPI Extraversion, as extraverts are described as lacking restraint and exhibiting impulsive behavior. Another higher order factor identified by the GZTS is called Social Activity, which contains aspects similar to the sociability part of Eysenck's extraversion. Subsequent analyses of the structure of the EPI and the EPQ showed that the biggest difference is that extraversion in the EPI contains a roughly equivalent amount of sociability and impulsivity items, whereas the EPQ contains many more sociability than impulsivity items (Rocklin & Revelle, 1981).

Raymond Cattell laid the foundation for modern lexical analysis when he factor-analyzed paragraph descriptors based on Allport and Odbert's (1936) list of traits (extracted from an unabridged dictionary) to derive 16 primary personality factors (Cattell, 1946), five of which cluster together to form a higher order factor of Extraversion (Cattell, 1957). The content of Cattell's Extraversion contains aspects of Eysenck's, Gray's, and Guilford's conceptualizations of extraversion, as Cattell's extravert is described as highly impulsive, social, and ascendant.

Current Taxonomies

The Big Five

Warren Norman (1963) derived what has come to be called the Big Five (Goldberg, 1990) factors of personality from a factor analysis of English adjectives taken from the dictionary. Norman's work was based on the prior work of Fiske (1949) and Tupes and Christal (1961) on peer ratings and his own work on peer ratings, based on the paragraph descriptors of Cattell. (These five factors, called Surgency—similar to extraversion—Agreeableness, Conscientiousness, Neuroticism, and Openness, have since been observed in the languages of many different cultures; Goldberg, 1990.) Many of the adjectives have high loadings on two (not one or three) factors (Hofstee, De Raad, & Goldberg, 1992), so that pairs of the Big Five dimensions have a circumplex structure. This structure is measured by the Abridged Big Five Circumplex (AB5C), which contains items that have a primary loading on one factor and secondary loading on a second one. In the AB5C, Surgency is described mainly by the disposition to engage in *approach behavior*.

The Five-Factor Model

Costa and McCrae's (1992b; McCrae & Costa, 1997) five-factor model (FFM) of personality consists of personality dimensions similar to the Big Five and also identifies extraversion as a primary factor. The FFM assumes a hierarchical structure, with each higher order factor seen as the aggregate of six lower order facets. In the case of extraversion, the facets are warmth, gregariousness, assertiveness, activity, excitement seeking, and positive emotion. The FFM is primarily associated with the Neuroticism–Extraversion–Openness Personality Inventory—Revised (NEO PI-R) and the NEO Five-Factor Inventory (NEO FFI) (Costa & McCrae, 1992b). The core feature of extraversion in the FFM is thought to be the disposition to engage in *social behavior*.

The Smaller Seven

Tellegen (1985) also took terms from the dictionary and subjected them to factor analysis; the resulting taxonomy of personality consisted of seven factors, five of which resemble the Big Five and FFM and two that reflect positive evaluation and negative evaluation. Tellegen divided extraversion into lower order facets—well-being, social potency, social closeness, and achievement—that are measured by the Multidimensional Personality Questionnaire (MPQ; Tellegen, 1982). In this taxonomy, *positive emotionality* constitutes the core of extraversion.

Socioanalytic Theory

Another personality theory with seven factors in which extraversion appears is Hogan's (1982) socioanalytic theory. This theory differs from the other descriptive taxonomies in that, instead of viewing traits as entities within a person, they are instead seen as aspects of a person's reputation. In this scheme, sociability and ambition serve

as markers of social adaptation and form a higher order factor resembling extraversion. The causal mechanism thought to give rise to *sociability* and *ambition* are the evolutionary pressures "to get along" and "get ahead" (Hogan, 1982).

HEXACO

Sharing socioanalytic theory's emphasis on evolutionary adaptation is the HEXACO (X = extraversion) model of personality (Ashton & Lee, 2001), which adds Honesty to the Big Five factors. The core feature of extraversion is thought to be *active engagement in social endeavor*, which is assumed to be one of the common tasks for humans in evolutionary history (Ashton, Lee, & Paunonen, 2002). The HEXACO model divides extraversion into four facets labeled *expressiveness, liveliness, sociability,* and *social boldness*.

Biological Distinctions

Although there is a divide between the biological and descriptive traditions, efforts to reconcile these views are emerging. DeYoung, Quilty, and Peterson (2007) developed the Big Five Aspects Scales (BFAS), which measure the lexically derived factors of personality using biologically informed theory. In the BFAS, extraversion is divided into two aspects that supposedly have different genetic underpinnings, *enthusiasm* and *assertiveness*. One advantage of the BFAS is that items are highly correlated within aspects but only moderately correlated between aspects.

Summary: Measurement

The appearance of extraversion in lexically, behaviorally, and biologically derived taxonomies is suggestive evidence that it is one of the most noticeable and important descriptors of personality. Although there are not as many inventories measuring extraversion as there are investigators, it sometimes seems that way (Table 3.2). Many of the early studies used scales made up of items of complete sentences created by the Eysencks (the MPQ, EPI, EPQ, EPP), but more recent studies have tended to use either the sentence format of the NEO-PI-R and NEO-FFI or the adjectives of the Big Five Markers (BFM;

TABLE 3.2. Commonly Used Inventories Measuring Extraversion

Inventory	Abbreviation	Authors	Year
Abridged Big Five Circumplex	AB5C	Hofstee, De Raad, & Goldberg	1992
Big Five Markers	BFM	Goldberg	1992
Big Five Inventory	BFI	John, Donahue, & Kentle	1991
Big 5 Aspect Scales	BFAS	DeYoung, Quilty, & Peterson	2007
Eysenck Personality Inventory	EPI	H. J. Eysenck & S. B. Eysenck	1968
Eysenck Personality Questionnaire	EPQ	S. B. Eysenck & H. J. Eysenck	1975
Eysenck Personality Profiler	EPP	Eysenck & Wilson	1991
Five-Factor Nonverbal Personality Questionnaire	FF-NPQ	Paunonen & Ashton	2002
Guilford–Zimmerman Temperament Study	GZTS	Guilford & Zimmerman	1949
HEXACO Personality Inventory	HEXACO-PI	Lee & Ashton	2004
International Personality Item Pool	IPIP	Goldberg	1999
Maudsley Personality Questionnaire	MPQ	Eysenck	1959
Multidimensional Personality Questionnaire	MPQ	Tellegen	1982
NEO Personality Inventory—Revised	NEO PI-R	Costa & McCrae	1992b
NEO Five-Factor Inventory	NEO FFI	Costa & McCrae	1992b
Riverside Behavioral Q-Sort	RBQ	Funder, Furr, & Colvin	2000

Goldberg, 1992) (see Table 3.3). With the release of the open-source collaboratory, the International Personality Item Pool (IPIP; Goldberg, 1999; Goldberg et al., 2006), which emphasizes phrases rather than sentences or adjectives, it is now possible to create scales targeted at all the other commonly used inventories or to create new scales such as the BFAS (DeYoung et al., 2007). A "consumer's guide" comparing the IPIP to most of the larger inventories has also been published (Grucza & Goldberg, 2007).

Theoretical Approaches

It is obvious that conceptualizations of extraversion differ from investigator to investigator; however, because it seems nearly certain that one of the fundamental dimensions of human personality contains extraversion content, it is important to determine where this dimension has its basis. No two researchers did more to advance this cause than Hans Eysenck and Jeffrey Gray. We now review their seminal work and famous debate and then transition to contemporary evolutionary, neurological, and temperamental approaches to explaining extraversion.

Hans Eysenck

Hans Eysenck modernized the study of extraversion through both experimental and psychometric approaches. Eysenck long argued that the major dimensions of human personality have a biological basis. His first attempt to explain extraversion was based on the notions of excitation and inhibition (Eysenck, 1957), which were thought to influence the acquisition and extinction of behavior (Hull, 1943; Pavlov, 1927). Specifically, Eysenck proposed that introverts had higher cortical excitability than extraverts and thus would condition more efficiently. The conditioning model underwent significant revision and was reformulated as the now-famous arousal hypothesis of extraversion (Eysenck, 1967). The central tenet of arousal theory is that introverts have lower thresholds for arousal in the ascending reticular activating system (ARAS) than extraverts. The ARAS is a feedback loop connecting the cortex to the reticular activating system. The beauty of the arousal theory of extraversion is that it led to two direct and testable hypotheses about performance differences between extraverts and introverts. First, from the Yerkes–Dodson "law" (Ye-

TABLE 3.3. Representative Items from Extraversion Scales Emphasize Affective and Behavioral Aspects

Inventory	ABCD	Item
AB5C	A	Radiate joy
BFI	A	I see myself as someone who is full of energy.
GZTS	A	You are a happy-go-lucky individual.
HEXACO-PI	A	Am usually active and full of energy
MPQ (Multidimensional)	A	Have a lot of fun
NEO-FFI	A	I really enjoy talking to people.
BFAS	B	Am the first to act
BFM	B	Talkative
EPI	B	Do you like going out a lot?
EPQ	B	Do you like telling jokes and funny stories to your friends?
EPP	B	Would you prefer to fight for your beliefs than let an important issue go unchallenged?
FF-NPQ	B	Picture of person riding a bucking horse
IPIP	B	Am the life of the party
MPQ (Maudsley)	B	Do you like to mix socially with people?
NEO-PI-R	B	I am dominant, forceful, and assertive.

rkes & Dodson, 1908), extraverts should outperform introverts in highly arousing situations (because extraverts should be less prone to overarousability), and introverts should outperform extraverts in low-arousal situations (because introverts should be less prone to underarousability). For an elegant test of this hypothesis within subjects, see Anderson (1990). Second, based on Wundt's notion that people try to maintain moderate arousal (Wundt & Judd, 1897), extraverts should, on average, respond more and faster (in order to increase their arousal) than introverts during performance tasks. Indeed, the explanation of extraverted behavior as arousal seeking provided a compelling explanation for extraverts' use of stimulant drugs (cigarettes), sexual activities, and social interaction.

Jeffrey Gray and Reinforcement Sensitivity Theory

Over the past 50 years, Eysenck's hypotheses have generated thousands of studies yielding varying degrees of support (Matthews & Gilliland, 1999). More interesting and more conducive to scientific progress than tests of a single theory is the emergence of competing theories. This happened when

Jeffrey Gray proposed an alternative causal theory of extraversion, reinforcement sensitivity theory (RST; Gray, 1970, 1981, 1982). Based on animal research, the original formulation of RST postulated the existence of three separate neural systems underlying behavior: (1) the behavioral approach system (BAS), (2) the behavioral inhibition system (BIS), and (3) the fight–flight system (FFS). The primary emphasis was on the effects of the BIS and BAS. Sensitivity of the BAS was thought to underlie trait impulsivity, and sensitivity of the BIS was thought to underlie trait anxiety. These traits were conceptualized as primary traits that together could explain Eysenck's higher order factor of Extraversion. Eysenck's Extraversion was thought by Gray to be Impulsivity minus Anxiety. Similar to Eysenck's theory, RST makes predictions about performance, but these predictions are more complicated and harder to generalize to human research because RST was founded on animal data. However, RST does make straightforward predictions regarding learning and affect: Because extraverts should be more sensitive to reward than introverts, extraverts should condition faster to rewarding stimuli and experience more positive affect than introverts.

The Eysenck–Gray Debate

Eysenck's and Gray's theories were at the forefront of research on extraversion for nearly 30 years, generating a wide range of studies employing various methodologies. An excellent review of the vast body of literature motivated by these theories is provided by Matthews and Gilliland (1999). Most of that review lies outside the scope of this chapter, but we do present a simplified summary of findings that have relevance to our previous discussion. Eysenck's early theory of conditioning has not received support, as both extraverts and introverts show conditioning advantages in different situations. Eysenck's arousal theory, however, has received a moderate amount of support, as introverts have been shown to be more aroused than extraverts in general, although Revelle, Humphreys, Simon, and Gilliland (1980) suggest that this might be true only in the morning. In support of Gray's theory, extraverts experience more positive affect than introverts; this finding has been one of the most robust in all of personality psychology (Lucas, Diener, Grob, Suh, & Shao, 2000). Also in support of Gray's theory, most research suggests that extraverts condition faster to rewarding stimuli (although Zinbarg & Revelle, 1989, show complex interactions with anxiety). Since the time of the Matthews and Gilliland review, Gray's theory has undergone drastic revisions that are beyond the scope of this chapter (Corr, 2008; Gray & McNaughton, 2000; Smillie, 2008; Smillie, Pickering, & Jackson, 2006). Eysenck and Gray were pioneers in the investigation of extraversion, and it is doubtless that their legacies will live on, with new advances in biological theory about extraversion in the years to come.

Contemporary Evolutionary, Neurological, and Temperamental Approaches

Research has sought to elucidate causes for the extraversion dimension at different levels of analysis. From the most distal to the most proximal explanations proposed for extraversion, we address its evolutionary, neurological, and temperamental underpinnings, as we believe that understanding broad higher order traits such as extraversion require analysis at all of these levels.

Evolution and Genetics

It has been claimed that evolutionary theory must anchor personality theory, as Buss (1995) proposed that personality dimensions evolved to deal with domain-specific tasks in the social environment. Two of the most important evolutionary tasks, in Buss's view, can be succinctly summarized as "getting along" and "getting ahead" (note the similarity to socioanalytic theory). Based on the universality of these tasks, it is assumed that all humans developed behavioral approach and avoidance systems (the former is associated with the extraversion continuum).

In criticism of evolutionary theory of personality, Tooby and Cosmides (1990) argue that such between-person variations would not exist in characteristics under selective pressure. In response, different explanations for between-person variations have been put forward. Individual variation in approach behavior (and thus extraversion) could have arisen out of the variety of social niches that people can occupy (Buss, 1995). There are a variety of ways for people to navigate the social environment, and different levels of personality traits reflect different ways to deal with the social environment (MacDonald, 1995). Nettle (2006) points out two general flaws with the Tooby and Cosmides argument. First, if a characteristic is determined from multiple genes (as is assumed for personality traits), it will take an incredibly long time to minimize variations in such constructs. Second, many adaptations along the same dimension can be equally beneficial. Tradeoffs can occur at different levels on the extraversion continuum (Nettle, 2005, 2006). At high levels of extraversion, people might be more likely to mate and succeed socially, but they might also be more likely to die from risky behavior. At low levels of extraversion, these probabilities are reversed. Nettle (2005) cleverly addressed the common criticism that psychological theories based on evolution cannot be tested by actually testing and finding support for the tradeoff hypothesis for IPIP extraversion. Extraverts do have more mates but also die earlier than introverts (Nettle, 2005). As would be expected for traits with evolutionary bases, and as is true for most personality traits, extraversion is moderately heritable, h^2 = .45–.50, with little if any shared environmental influence (Bouchard & Loehlin, 2001). Support for extraversion as having a substantial genetic basis is also garnered from the finding that extraversion can be identified in many animal species; additionally, each FFM facet of extraversion displays moderately high heritability, and the relationships between extraversion facets are largely accounted for by genetic factors (Jang, Livesley, Angleitner, Riemann, & Vernon, 2002). There is some evidence that heritability for extraversion declines with age (Bouchard & Loehlin, 2001), which logically means that the environment becomes a more important source of extraversion variation as people grow older. Finding that extraversion is heritable is the first step in uncovering specific genetic pathways that influence extraversion's development. For example, recent research has identified genes that account for between-person variation in extraversion, one likely candidate being *ADH4* (Luo, Kranzler, Zuo, Wang, & Gelernter, 2007).

Extraversion and Brain Function/Structure

Genes do not act directly on behavior; genetic effects are mediated by brain function and structure (Revelle, 1995). Eysenck and Gray were the first to detail complex theories about how this might be the case for extraversion, and recent empirical investigations continue to advance our understanding of the neurobiological basis of extraversion.

The Dopaminergic Hypothesis of Agentic Extraversion

Recently, Depue (1995) developed a novel theory for a subcomponent of extraversion labeled *agentic extraversion* because it encompasses the achievement and ascendance aspects of extraversion (Depue & Collins, 1999).[2] Depue's theory closely resembles Gray's original RST in that a behavioral facilitation system (BFS)—the function of which is to increase the salience of positive stimuli—is thought to be a causal basis for agentic extraversion (Depue, 1995; Depue & Collins, 1999). Depue's model of behavioral

facilitation is a threshold model in that dopamine must reach a certain level for approach behavior to be elicited. Thus approach behavior is thought to depend on one's tonic level of dopamine, as well as one's phasic level (Depue, 1995). At present, evidence for this model is inconsistent. The first support for the theory was the finding that extraversion, as measured by the MPQ (Tellegen, 1982), correlated with prolactin indicators of dopamine functioning in 11 women (Depue, Luciana, Arbisi, Collins, & Leon, 1994); this finding was subsequently replicated with a larger sample (Depue, 1995). Other studies do not support Depue's theory. For example, Fischer, Wik, and Fredrikson (1997) measured extraversion with a German adaptation (Ruch & Hehl, 1989) of the EPQ-R (S. B. Eysenck, Eysenck, & Barrett, 1985) and found that extraversion was negatively correlated with subcortical brain activity in the caudate nucleus and the putamen, areas that have high concentrations of dopamine terminals. As it stands, the dopaminergic hypothesis provides an exciting avenue along which to pursue the biological basis of agentic extraversion. Newly developed ways to measure dopaminergic functioning noninvasively, such as with electroencephalography (EEG), may serve to increase the rate at which research determines the relationships between agentic extraversion and dopamine (Wacker, Chavanon, & Stemmler, 2006).

Neurophysiological and Neuroanatomical Underpinnings of Extraversion

It is clear from the section on measurement in this chapter that extraversion has a positive affect component, but the biological mechanisms underlying this association are not well known. In an excellent review, Canli (2004) describes neuroimaging studies conducted with the aim of elucidating the extraversion–positive affect association. Across a wide range of tasks, functional magnetic resonance imaging (fMRI) analysis revealed that extraversion as measured with the NEO-PI-R was associated with greater activation in numerous areas of the brain (amygdala, caudate, mediofrontal gyrus, right fusiform gyrus) when positive stimuli, but not negative stimuli, were presented. One important implication of these studies, noted by Canli, is that personality factors such as extraversion are likely to be widely distributed in the brain.

Recent studies have added to our knowledge about the activation patterns that correlate with extraversion and have sought to explain such patterns. EPQ extraversion has been associated with activation in the lateral prefrontal cortex, lateral parietal cortex, and right anterior cingulate cortex; each of these brain areas is associated with task-focused self-control and discrepancy detection (Eisenberger, Lieberman, & Satpute, 2005). Haas, Omura, Amin, Constable, and Canli (2006) determined that the NEO-PI-R facets of excitement seeking and warmth accounted for the association noted between extraversion and anterior cingulate cortex activity (Canli, 2004; Eisenberger et al., 2005). Two other novel findings from this work were that extraversion predicted functional connectivity to the anterior cingulate and that this association was mediated by the facets of warmth, gregariousness, and positive emotions. The studies discussed up to this point have focused on predicting brain activity during task engagement. Deckersbach and colleagues (2006) recently extended these findings by showing that, at rest, extraversion measured by the NEO-FFI is associated with greater activity in the orbitofrontal cortex, which might play a part in shifting attention to positive incentives.

Differences in brain structures are also associated with extraversion, and such differences may have diverse implications for psychopathology, learning, and behavior. Magnetic resonance imaging (MRI) studies have shown that NEO-PI-R extraversion is positively correlated with gray matter in the left amygdala (Omura, Constable, & Canli, 2005); as reductions in amygdalar gray matter predict depression, this finding may suggest that extraversion is a protective factor against depression (Omura et al., 2005). NEO-FFI extraversion and thickness of orbitofrontal cortex are associated, and extinction of fear retention mediates the path from orbitofrontal thickness to extraversion (Rauch et al., 2005), suggesting that brain structure influences extraversion by influencing learning processes. One way that brain structure relates to specific components of extraverted behavior is illustrated by the finding that NEO-FFI extraversion is inversely related to thickness of the right anterior prefrontal cortex and the right fusiform gyrus; low thickness in these areas has been suggested as underlying impulsive and disinhibited behavior (Wright et al., 2006).

Temperament

It is clear that extraversion is associated with structure and function across many areas of the brain. The fact that extraversion has a strong biological component suggests that precursors of trait extraversion should appear early in development. The study of temperament shows this to be the case. Temperament refers to individual differences in reactivity and self-control that arise from a constitutional basis (Durbin, Klein, Hayden, Buckley, & Moerk, 2005; Rothbart, 1981). A temperament dimension of extraversion—positive affect (PA)—has been identified in infants as young as 3 months, in middle childhood, and even into adulthood (Rothbart, Ahadi, & Evans, 2000). As its name implies, this dimension shares characteristics with the extraversion personality trait. For example, one study that factor-analyzed lower order components of temperament found that a higher order extraversion/PA factor included sociability and positive affect components, as well as regulatory components such as inhibitory control (Evans & Rothbart, 2007). The inclusion of regulatory aspects makes temperamental extraversion/PA especially interesting to study in the context of dynamic cognitive and behavioral processes (Evans & Rothbart, 2007). In one of the few studies to use a dynamic design, Derryberry and Reed (1994) found that adult extraversion/PA temperament (measured with a short version of the EPQ) predicted difficulty in shifting attention away from positive stimuli but not from negative stimuli. It is interesting to note that the previous findings hark back to notions from Eysenck's and Gray's conceptualizations of extraversion. Inhibitory control overlaps considerably with Eysenck's emphasis on the impulsivity component of extraversion (Eysenck, 1967), and RST (Gray & McNaughton, 2000) explicitly predicts that extraversion should relate to attentional biases toward positive stimuli and approach behavior.

Extraversion and the ABCDs

The previous sections can be thought of as the ontogeny of a trait, starting off as genes, developing into biological structures and systems, and then being expressed early in life as temperament. We view the fully developed, higher order traits such as the Big Five as characteristic patterns of affect, behavior, cognition, and desire.

How Do Extraverts Feel?

It is well established that extraverts feel higher levels of positive affect than introverts (Costa & McCrae, 1980; Lucas & Baird, 2004; Watson & Clark, 1992). The relationship between trait extraversion and trait positive affect has emerged in many cultures with many different methods (Lucas & Baird, 2004), with the average correlation found to be around $r = .40$ (Lucas & Fujita, 2000). Not only do measures of trait extraversion predict trait positive affect, but trait extraversion also predicts aggregated momentary positive affect (Costa & McCrae, 1992a; Spain, Eaton, & Funder, 2000), as well as single ratings of current positive affect (Lucas & Baird, 2004; Uziel, 2006). This means that extraverts are happier than introverts in general, over short time frames, and even in the moment.

It has even been proposed that extraversion is at its core the tendency to experience positive affect (Watson & Clark, 1997), and there is some evidence to support this claim. The covariation of extraversion components is accounted for by positive affect; once positive affect is removed, the other components of extraversion do not correlate with each other. A similar finding reported recently that extraversion facets that reflect reward sensitivity load on a higher order Extraversion factor that accounts for the correlations between the other facets of extraversion (Lucas & Baird, 2004). Not only does trait extraversion predict trait positive affect, but both traits also predict similar outcomes such as social activity, leadership, and number of friends (Watson & Clark, 1997).

The evidence linking extraversion and positive affect is very strong; however, at least three findings suggest that it would be rash to conceptualize extraversion and positive affect as redundant constructs. First, they share only about 30% of the total variance between constructs (Watson, 2000). Second, behavioral content is better represented than positive affect in measures of extraversion (Pytlik Zillig, Hemenover, & Dienstbier, 2002). Third, a study by Ashton and colleagues (2002) used the same method as in Lucas and colleagues (2000) and showed that the tendency to behave in ways that attract social attention accounts for the common variance among NEO-PI-R Extraversion facets.

Extraversion and positive affect might not be the same construct, but the robust relationship between the two calls for explanation. The explanations that have been offered can be grouped into those postulating either a primarily structural or an instrumental basis for the relationship. A structural explanation means that extraverts possess some quality or characteristic that leads them to experience more happiness than introverts. The general structural explanation is described by the affect-threshold model (Rosenberg, 1998), which can be divided into the affect-level model (Gross, Sutton, & Ketelaar, 1998) and the affect-reactivity model (Larsen & Ketelaar, 1991; Strelau, 1987). The affect-threshold model states that extraverts have a lower threshold for experiencing positive affect than introverts; that is, it should require less positive stimulation to elicit positive affect from extraverts than from introverts. This model is general in that it does not distinguish between two ways that equal positive stimulation could lead to more positive affect for extraverts. The first way is described by the affect-level model (Gross et al., 1998), which states that because extraverts are closer to experiencing positive affect than introverts at baseline, they require relatively less positive stimulation to feel good. The second way is described by the affect-reactivity model, which states that extraverts and introverts could feel the same amount of positive affect at baseline but that extraverts react more strongly to positive stimuli than introverts do. It is clear that the affect-reactivity model has its roots in RST (Corr, 2008; Gray, 1970, 1981, 1982).

Testing the two models requires identifying circumstances under which they make conflicting predictions. In the affect-level model, it is assumed that extraverts have a higher tonic level of positive affect; thus it predicts that extraverts should be happier than introverts in negative-, neutral-, and positive-valence situations. The affect-reactivity model assumes that extraverts and introverts have similar tonic levels of positive affect but that extraverts react more strongly to positive stimuli; thus it predicts that extraverts should be happier than introverts in positive-valence situations only. Gross and colleagues (1998) found support for both models in their seminal investigation, manipulating situation valence with positive, neutral, and negative film clips. Recently, a meta-analysis of six studies revealed that the accuracy of each model depends on situational properties (Lucas & Baird, 2004). In support of the affect-level model, extraverts were happier in neutral situations. In support of the affect-reactivity model, extraverts' activated positive affect (e.g., being awake, alert) but not pleasant positive affect was more reactive to positive stimulation. An even more complex picture emerges when the interaction of extraversion with neuroticism on affective reactivity is taken into account, as emotionally stable extraverts react to positive stimuli more strongly than neurotic extraverts (Rogers & Revelle, 1998).

Another class of explanations for the extraversion–positive affect relationship posits instrumental origins. Instrumental explanations assume that the relationship between extraversion and positive affect is based on differences in what extraverts and introverts do in their daily lives.

Sociability theory (Watson, 1988; Watson, Clark, McIntyre, & Hamaker, 1992) posits both instrumental and structural explanations for the extraversion–positive affect relationship. Sociability theory's intuitive instrumental hypothesis is that extraverts are happier than introverts because they engage in more social activities; the complementary structural explanation is that extraverts enjoy social activities more than introverts. Some evidence has been found in support of sociability theory, as Argyle and Lu (1990) found that extraverts participate in more social activities than introverts and that the amount of social activity partially mediated the extraversion–happiness relationship. Some evidence, however, contradicts sociability theory. Pavot, Diener, and Fujita (1990) found that extraverts and introverts

spend the same amount of time in social situations and that introverts experience just as much happiness as extraverts in social situations. It has been found that extraverts are happier than introverts across a variety of both social and nonsocial situations (Diener, Sandvik, Pavot, & Fujita, 1992). The between-person extraversion–positive affect relationship has recently been extended to existing within persons as well. A within-person relationship means that an individual's momentary positive affect depends on momentary levels of extraversion, or *state* extraversion (Fleeson, Malanos, & Achille, 2002). Fleeson and colleagues (2002) found that all participants, regardless of trait-level extraversion, were happier the more extraverted they acted. Recent studies continue to support the strong link between state extraversion and state positive affect. Participants felt more positive affect in experiments in which participants were instructed to act extraverted, suggesting that state extraversion causes state positive affect (McNiel & Fleeson, 2006). Additionally, state extraversion was found to mediate the relationship between approach goals and state positive affect (Heller, Komar, & Lee, 2007).

How Do Extraverts Behave?

In the field of personality psychology, primary importance has been placed on explaining behavior (Funder, 2001). According to Funder, despite the importance, little research has actually been conducted toward this aim; Funder (2001) even explicitly offered extraversion as an example of a trait that has not been investigated in relationship to actual behavior. However, this seems be a very narrow definition of behavior, restricted to laboratory situations, for it ignores the earlier work of Eysenck, who examined the factor structures of behavioral observations (Eysenck & Himmelweit, 1947), and the even earlier work of Heymans (Eysenck, 1992); but it *would* include the German Observational Study of Adult Twins project (GOSAT; Borkenau, Riemann, Angleitner, & Spinath, 2001) and Antill's (1974) observational study of talking behavior as a function of extraversion and group size. Recently, research has begun to address the important goal of elucidating the content of extraverted behavior.

As it is expected that personality traits manifest themselves in behavior (Funder, 2001), the most straightforward hypothesis (relating to extraversion) resulting from this expectation is that trait extraversion should at least predict aggregate state extraversion. What little research exists suggests that individuals with higher levels of trait extraversion are indeed predisposed to enact more extraversion states (Heller et al., 2007; Schutte, Malouff, Segrera, Wolf, & Rodgers, 2003). Research on how extraversion relates to more discrete categories of behavior is also lacking, a fact that motivated the development of the Riverside Behavioral Q-Sort (RBQ) as a remedy (Funder, Furr, & Colvin, 2000). The RBQ contains a list of behavioral items that can be rated for how much they describe a participant's behavior in social interactions. In a study using the RBQ, extraversion measured with the NEO-PI (Costa & McCrae, 1985) predicted behaviors that can be characterized as energetic, bold, socially adept, and secure (Funder et al., 2000). Also driven by the paucity of behavioral research, Paunonen and colleagues (Paunonen, 2003) predicted various behavioral categories on the Behavioral Report Form (Paunonen & Ashton, 2001) from extraversion as measured by the NEO-PI-R, the NEO-FFI, and the Five-Factor Nonverbal Personality Questionnaire (FF-NPQ; Paunonen & Ashton, 2002). Across scales, extraversion reliably predicted alcohol consumption, popularity, parties attended, dating variety, and exercise (Paunonen, 2003).

One limitation of the research on specific behavior described thus far is that the behaviors were not collected in natural environments. An exciting new methodology called Big EAR (electronically activated recorder; Mehl & Pennebaker, 2003) circumvents this problem. Big EAR is simply a small recording device that is programmed to turn on and off throughout the day, recording for a few minutes at a time, producing objective data in natural environments. In a study using Big EAR to investigate behavioral correlates of extraverts, as well as judges' folk theories of extraverted behavior, it was found that extraversion as measured by the Big Five Inventory (BFI; John & Srivastava, 1999) related to talking to and spending time with people; additionally, judges rated people who were more talkative and social as more extraverted (Mehl, Gosling, & Pennebaker, 2006).

Although some research has been done on how personality predicts actual behavior, there has been almost no research on how personality affects dynamic patterns of behavior in different situations. However, Eaton and Funder (2003) were able to conduct a study that revealed how extraversion influences dynamic social interactions. As in other studies, it was found that extraverts behaved more socially than introverts; it was also found that extraverts influence the behavior, affect, and interpersonal judgments of those with whom they interacted, generally creating a more positive social environment. The question of why extraverts are so socially adept is unresolved at this time, but one intriguing possibility is that extraverts have certain abilities that are lacking in introverts. Support for this notion comes from a study that measured extraversion with the EPI and found that extraverts are better at nonverbal decoding than introverts when it is a secondary task (Lieberman & Rosenthal, 2001), as may be the case in social situations.

How Do Extraverts Think?

Individual differences in behavior can be assessed in various categories, as described previously; in contrast, individual differences in cognition are reflected in the different ways that people categorize the world. Extraversion has been found to predict differences in categorization across various tasks. Broadly speaking, extraversion relates to a relatively positive view of the world, as extraverts judge neutral events more positively than introverts do (Uziel, 2006). Extraversion predicts categorization of words by their positive affective quality rather than their semantic quality (Weiler, 1992). For example, extraverts are more likely to judge the words *hug* and *smile* as more similar than the words *smile* and *face*. Extraversion also predicts judging positive valence words, for example, *truth* and *honesty*, as more similar than negative valence words, for example, *grief* and *death*, although extraverts are not faster to categorize positive words than negative words by valence (Rogers & Revelle, 1998). This finding suggests a categorization advantage for positive valence only when processes are competing. Extraversion also does not relate to classifying rewards faster than threats; however, among people scoring low on IPIP extraversion, quickness to classify threatening stimuli was related to experiencing negative affect in daily life (Robinson, Meier, & Vargas, 2005). In this study, quickness to classify threatening stimuli did not relate to negative affect among individuals scoring high in extraversion, suggesting that extraversion might be a protective factor against sensitivity to threat.

One concern that might be raised is that concurrent mood might be responsible for the cognitive differences described here. An example of how mood affects cognition is given by a study finding that state positive affect predicts classification of objects by their broad, global features over their local features (Gasper & Clore, 2002). Studies examining the combined effects of extraversion and positive affect are in their beginning stages, and, as such, results are quite complicated as this point. Although EPQ Extraversion had a positive main effect on choosing positive-valence homophones over neutral homophones, on completing open-ended stories with more positive tone, and on recalling more positive than neutral or negative words in a free-recall task, this effect was positively moderated by current positive affect when positive affect was experimentally induced, but not when mood was allowed to vary freely (Rusting, 1999). A different study found that an extraversion composite consisting of the EPQ, BAS/BIS scales, and the Generalized Reward and Punishment Expectancy Scales (GRAPES; Ball & Zuckerman, 1990) was related to beliefs that positive events were more likely in the future (Zelenski & Larsen, 2002). Extraversion in this study did not interact with naturally occurring or experimentally manipulated positive mood, but a unique main effect of positive affect emerged when mood was experimentally manipulated. Future research will need to employ clever methods in order to clarify the complex relationships of extraversion and positive affect to cognition.

What Do Extraverts Want?

Comparatively little work has examined motives and goals that are associated with extraversion. Initial investigation into this area revealed that extraversion is generally associated with high motivation for social contact, power, and status (Olson & Weber, 2004), personal strivings (Emmons, 1986) for intimacy and interdependence (King, 1995), and wishing for higher levels of positive affect and interpersonal contact (King & Broyles, 1997).

It was recently suggested that the correct level of abstraction for investigating the relationship between desire and a broad, higher order trait such as extraversion is probably not at the relatively narrow level of concepts such as personal strivings and wishes but rather at the broad level of major life goals (Roberts & Robins, 2000). At this level, NEO-FFI extraversion relates to having more economic (e.g., status and accomplishment), political (e.g., influencing and leading), and hedonistic (e.g., fun and excitement) goals (Roberts & Robins, 2000). These findings were subsequently replicated in another study finding that NEO-FFI extraversion was related to social goals (Roberts & Robins, 2004). This study also determined that positive increases in extraversion in early adulthood were related to assigning increased importance to economic, aesthetic, social, economic, political, and hedonistic goals. These initial findings suggest that motivation, especially at the level of broad life goals, is an area ripe for important discoveries that is largely untapped at this point.

Extraversion and Psychopathology

In general, the importance of studying the relationships between normal personality and psychopathology rests on the possibility that personality factors could indicate early and persistent risk for the development of psychopathology (Krueger, Caspi, Moffitt, Silva, & McGee, 1996; Markon, Krueger, & Watson, 2005). Recently renewed interest in the relationships between normal and abnormal personality have led to investigations of how extraversion relates to various forms of psychopathology (Widiger, 2005).

As a general dimension of personality, extraversion most obviously has implications for personality disorders; a personality disorder is defined by the DSM-IV-TR as "an enduring pattern of inner experience and behavior" that is "stable and of long duration, and its onset can be traced back at least to adolescence or early adulthood" (American Psychiatric Association, 2000, p. 689). In general, low extraversion is negatively correlated with the presence of personality disorders, but this finding is not universal, as there are some studies implicating high extraversion in certain personality disorders (Widiger, 2005); see Costa and Widiger (2002) for a diverse set of reviews. That both high and low extraversion relate to personality disorders is reminiscent of Nettle's suggestion that both poles of normal personality dimensions involve costs and benefits (Nettle, 2006).

Although Hans Eysenck had examined the importance of extraversion in psychiatric diagnoses (Eysenck & Himmelweit, 1947) and continued to emphasize the application of normal personality traits to psychopathology (Eysenck, 1957), recent investigations of the relationships between normal personality and psychopathology outside of the personality disorders began in earnest with the groundbreaking study of Trull and Sher (1994). They measured normal personality with the NEO-FFI and showed that low extraversion, unique among the FFM dimensions, predicted depression and anxiety. Krueger and colleagues (1996) examined how MPQ (Tellegen, 1982) dimensions were related to psychological disorders; in regard to extraversion, the Social Closeness scale was negatively related to conduct disorder, affective disorders, and substance use disorders, whereas the Social Potency scale was positively related to conduct disorder and substance abuse disorders. More recent research has looked specifically at extraversion's role in anxiety and depressive disorders, with one study finding EPI Extraversion to be negatively related to anxiety and major depressive disorder but that the relationship to anxiety did not remain when statistically controlling for gender, age, and education (Jylha & Isometsa, 2006).

Extraversion and the Future

It is an exciting time to be investigating extraversion, as significant advances are accruing at a fast rate in various content areas, spurred on by the use of a wide range of the cutting-edge research methods. We are optimistic that the coming research on extraversion will prove even more innovative and important, and we offer three areas that promise to be particularly fruitful. First, research should investigate how extraversion is implicated in ongoing functioning. We echo Funder's call for more behavioral studies employing both self- and other reports (Funder, 2001), as well as the continued development of unobtrusive methods such as Big EAR (Mehl & Pennebaker, 2003). Of particular interest will be studies that investigate social processes in terms of the dynamic state manifestations of behavior, feelings, thoughts, and desires. A second area of investigation that we believe shows great promise is testing the new RST (Gray & McNaughton, 2000). We believe that RST could become the unifying theory for extraversion research, as it has implications for studies at every level of personality research, from genetics and brain structure to patterns of thoughts and behavior. We encourage future investigations to integrate research between different levels in the attempt to elucidate mediating pathways; for example, it may be possible to find genetic markers of brain structures that are implicated in the BIS, BAS, and FFS (Corr, 2008; Smillie, 2008). The third area we highlight is the growing availability of public-domain personality assessments, specifically the IPIP item pool (Goldberg et al., 2006). The ability to obtain a large quantity of data in a relatively short period of time (Goldberg et al., 2006) makes public-domain assessment the method of choice for investigating the following questions: What extraversion scales and items have the best predictive validity for various domains such as health, occupational success, and interpersonal functioning? What are the lower order facets or aspects that extraversion encompasses? How does extraversion content fit into higher order factors of personality? The first data using public domain assessment to address these questions have recently been reported (DeYoung et al., 2007; Grucza & Goldberg, 2007; Revelle, Wilt, & Rosenthal, in press).

Conclusion

Greek philosophers intuited that one fundamental way in which people differed was their propensity to act bold, talkative, and assertive. Twenty-five hundred years later, psychologists armed with advanced psychometric techniques are building a scientific paradigm around the construct in which the Greeks were interested. Rooted in one's genes, brain structure and function, and early temperament is the personality trait of extraversion. Similar to any other personality trait, extraversion is expressed in individual differences in a person's characteristic patterns of feelings, actions, thoughts, and goals. We are encouraged by the recent progress and growing interest in extraversion, and we are confident that, as personality theory and research methods continue to become more accurate and precise, an even greater array of extraversion's implications across a wide variety of social, occupational, and clinical contexts will be revealed.

Acknowledgment

We would like to thank Allen Rosenthal for help with earlier drafts.

Notes

1. Although occasionally one will see extroversion–introversion, the preferred spelling in psychological research is extraversion–introversion. For purposes of brevity, we refer to the bipolar dimension of introversion–extraversion by referring to just one end of it, extraversion.
2. The neurobiology of Depue's "affiliative extraversion," encompassing warmth and social closeness, has only recently received research attention but is generally thought to be based on opiate functioning (Depue & Morrone-Strupinsky, 2005)

References

Allport, G. W., & Odbert, H. S. (1936). Trait names: A psycholexical study. *Psychological Monographs, 47*(211).

American Psychiatric Association. (2000). *Diagnostic and statistical manual of mental disorders* (4th ed., text rev.). Washington, DC: Author.

Anderson, K. J. (1990). Arousal and the inverted-*u* hypothesis: A critique of Neiss's reconceptualizing arousal. *Psychological Bulletin, 107*(1), 96–100.

Antill, J. K. (1974). The validity and predictive power of introversion–extraversion for quantitative aspects of conversational patterns. *Dissertation Abstracts International, 35*(1-B), 532

Argyle, M., & Lu, L. (1990). The happiness of extraverts. *Personality and Individual Differences, 11*(10), 1011–1017.

Ashton, M. C., & Lee, K. (2001). A theoretical basis for the major dimensions of personality. *European Journal of Personality, 15*(5), 327–353.

Ashton, M. C., Lee, K., & Paunonen, S. V. (2002). What is the central feature of extraversion?: Social attention versus reward sensitivity. *Journal of Personality and Social Psychology, 83*(1), 245–251.

Ball, S. A., & Zuckerman, M. (1990). Sensation seeking, Eysenck's personality dimensions and reinforcement sensitivity in concept formation. *Personality and Individual Differences, 11*(4), 343–353.

Borkenau, P., Riemann, R., Angleitner, A., & Spinath, F. M. (2001). Genetic and environmental influences on observed personality: Evidence from the German observational study of adult twins. *Journal of Personality and Social Psychology, 80*(4), 655–668.

Bouchard, T. J., & Loehlin, J. C. (2001). Genes, evolution, and personality. *Behavior Genetics, 31*(3), 243–273.

Buss, D. M. (1995). Evolutionary psychology: A new paradigm for psychological science. *Psychological Inquiry, 6*(1), 1–30.

Canli, T. (2004). Functional brain mapping of extraversion and neuroticism: Learning from individual differences in emotion processing. *Journal of Personality, 72*(6), 1105–1132.

Cattell, R. B. (1946). *Description and measurement of personality.* Oxford, UK: World Book.

Cattell, R. B. (1957). *Personality and motivation structure and measurement.* Oxford, UK: World Book.

Corr, P. J., & McNaughton, N. (2008). The reinforcement sensitivity theory. In P. J. Corr (Ed.), *The reinforcement sensitivity theory of personality* (pp. 155–187). Cambridge, UK: Cambridge University Press.

Costa, P. T., & McCrae, R. R. (1980). Influence of extraversion and neuroticism on subjective well-being: Happy and unhappy people. *Journal of Personality and Social Psychology, 38*(4), 668–678.

Costa, P. T., & McCrae, R. R. (1985). *NEO PI professional manual.* Odessa, FL: Psychological Assessment Resources.

Costa, P. T., & McCrae, R. R. (1992a). Four ways five factors are basic. *Personality and Individual Differences, 13*(6), 653–665.

Costa, P. T., & McCrae, R. R. (1992b). *NEO PI-R professional manual.* Odessa, FL: Psychological Assessment Resources.

Costa, P. T., & Widiger, T. A. (2002). *Personality disorders and the five-factor model of personality* (2nd ed.). Washington, DC: American Psychological Association.

Deckersbach, T., Miller, K. K., Klibanski, A., Fischman, A., Dougherty, D. D., Blais, M. A., et al. (2006). Regional cerebral brain metabolism correlates of neuroticism and extraversion. *Depression and Anxiety, 23*(3), 133–138.

Depue, R. A. (1995). Neurobiological factors in personality and depression. *European Journal of Personality, 9*(5), 413–439.

Depue, R. A., & Collins, P. F. (1999). Neurobiology of the structure of personality: Dopamine, facilitation of incentive motivation, and extraversion. *Behavioral and Brain Sciences, 22*(3), 491–569.

Depue, R. A., Luciana, M., Arbisi, P., Collins, P., & Leon, A. (1994). Dopamine and the structure of personality: Relation of agonist-induced dopamine activity to positive emotionality. *Journal of Personality and Social Psychology, 67*(3), 485–498.

Depue, R. A., & Morrone-Strupinsky, J. V. (2005). A neurobehavioral model of affiliative bonding: Implications for conceptualizing a human trait of affiliation. *Behavioral and Brain Sciences, 28*(3), 313–395.

Derryberry, D., & Reed, M. A. (1994). Temperament and attention: Orienting toward and away from positive and negative signals. *Journal of Personality and Social Psychology, 66*(6), 1128–1139.

DeYoung, C. G., Quilty, L. C., & Peterson, J. B. (2007). Between facets and domains: 10 aspects of the Big Five. *Journal of Personality and Social Psychology, 93*(5), 880–896.

Diener, E., Sandvik, E., Pavot, W., & Fujita, F. (1992). Extraversion and subjective well-being in a U.S. national probability sample. *Journal of Research in Personality, 26*(3), 205–215.

Digman, J. M. (1990). Personality structure: Emergence of the five-factor model. *Annual Review of Psychology, 41*, 417–440.

Durbin, C., Klein, D. N., Hayden, E. P., Buckley, M. E., & Moerk, K. C. (2005). Temperamental emotionality in preschoolers and parental mood disorders. *Journal of Abnormal Psychology, 114*(1), 28–37.

Eaton, L. G., & Funder, D. C. (2003). The creation and consequences of the social world: An interactional analysis of extraversion. *European Journal of Personality, 17*(5), 375–395.

Eisenberger, N. I., Lieberman, M. D., & Satpute, A. B. (2005). Personality from a controlled processing perspective: An fMRI study of neuroticism, extraversion, and self-consciousness. *Cognitive, Affective and Behavioral Neuroscience, 5*(2), 169–181.

Emmons, R. A. (1986). Personal strivings: An approach to personality and subjective well-being. *Journal of Personality and Social Psychology, 51*(5), 1058–1068.

Evans, D. E., & Rothbart, M. K. (2007). Developing a model for adult temperament. *Journal of Research in Personality, 41*(4), 868–888.

Eysenck, H. J. (1952). *The scientific study of personality*. London: Routledge & Kegan Paul.

Eysenck, H. J. (1957). *The dynamics of anxiety and hysteria: An experimental application of modern learning theory to psychiatry*. Oxford, UK: Praeger.

Eysenck, H. J. (1959). The "Maudsley Personality Inventory" as determinant of neurotic tendency and extraversion. *Zeitschrift fur Experimentelle und Angewandte Psychologie, 6*, 167–190.

Eysenck, H. J. (1967). *The biological basis of personality*. Springfield, IL: Thomas.

Eysenck, H. J. (1981). General features of the model. In H. J. Eysenck (Ed.), *A model for personality* (pp. 1–37). Berlin, Germany: Springer-Verlag.

Eysenck, H. J. (1992). *A hundred years of personality research, from Heymans to modern times*. Houten, The Netherlands: Bohn.

Eysenck, H. J., & Eysenck, S. B. G. (1968). *Manual for the Eysenck Personality Inventory*. San Diego, CA: Educational and Industrial Testing Service.

Eysenck, H. J., & Himmelweit, H. T. (1947). *Dimensions of personality: A record of research carried out in collaboration with H. T. Himmelweit [and others]*. London: K. Paul, Trench.

Eysenck, H. J., & Wilson, G. D. (2000). *The Eysenck Personality Profiler* (Version 6). Worthing, UK: Psi-Press.

Eysenck, S. B., & Eysenck, H. J. (1975). *Manual of the Eysenck Personality Questionnaire*. London: Hodder & Stoughton.

Eysenck, S. B., Eysenck, H. J., & Barrett, P. (1985). A revised version of the Psychoticism scale. *Personality and Individual Differences, 6*(1), 21–29.

Fischer, H., Wik, G., & Fredrikson, M. (1997). Extraversion, neuroticism and brain function: A PET study of personality. *Personality and Individual Differences, 23*(2), 345–352.

Fiske, D. W. (1949). Consistency of the factorial structures of personality ratings from different sources. *Journal of Abnormal and Social Psychology, 44*, 329–344.

Fleeson, W., Malanos, A. B., & Achille, N. M. (2002). An intraindividual process approach to the relationship between extraversion and positive affect: Is acting extraverted as "good" as being extraverted? *Journal of Personality and Social Psychology, 83*(6), 1409–1422.

Funder, D. C. (2001). Personality. *Annual Review of Psychology, 52*, 197–221.

Funder, D. C., Furr, R., & Colvin, C. (2000). The Riverside Behavioral Q-Sort: A tool for the description of social behavior. *Journal of Personality, 68*(3), 451–489.

Gasper, K., & Clore, G. L. (2002). Attending to the big picture: Mood and global versus local processing of visual information. *Psychological Science, 13*(1), 34–40.

Goldberg, L. R. (1990). An alternative "description of personality": The Big-Five factor structure. *Journal of Personality and Social Psychology, 59*(6), 1216–1229.

Goldberg, L. R. (1992). The development of markers for the Big-Five factor structure. *Psychological Assessment, 4*(1), 26–42.

Goldberg, L. R. (1999). A broad-bandwidth, public domain, personality inventory measuring the lower-level facets of several five-factor models. In I. Mervielde, I. Deary, F. De Fruyt, & F. Ostendorf (Eds.), *Personality psychology in Europe* (Vol. 7, pp. 7–28). Tilburg, The Netherlands: Tilburg University Press.

Goldberg, L. R., Johnson, J. A., Eber, H. W., Hogan, R., Ashton, M. C., Cloninger, C. R., et al. (2006). The International Personality Item Pool and the future of public-domain personality measures. *Journal of Research in Personality, 40*(1), 84–96.

Gray, J. A. (1970). The psychophysiological basis of introversion–extraversion. *Behaviour Research and Therapy, 8*(3), 249–266.

Gray, J. A. (1981). A critique of Eysenck's theory of personality. In H. J. Eysenck (Ed.), *A model for personality* (pp. 246–277). Berlin, Germany: Springer-Verlag.

Gray, J. A. (1982). *Neuropsychological theory of anxiety: An investigation of the septal-hippocampal system*. Cambridge, UK: Cambridge University Press.

Gray, J. A., & McNaughton, N. (2000). *The neuropsychology of anxiety: An enquiry into the functions of the septo-hippocampal system (2nd ed.). Oxford, UK: Oxford University Press.

Gross, J. J., Sutton, S. K., & Ketelaar, T. (1998). Relations between affect and personality: Support for the affect-level and affective reactivity views. *Personality and Social Psychology Bulletin, 24*(3), 279–288.

Grucza, R. A., & Goldberg, L. R. (2007). The comparative validity of 11 modern personality inventories: Predictions of behavioral acts, informant reports, and clinical indicators. *Journal of Personality Assessment, 89*(2), 167–187.

Guilford, J. P., & Zimmerman, W. S. (1949). *The Guilford–Zimmerman temperament survey.* Oxford, UK: Sheridan Supply.

Haas, B. W., Omura, K., Amin, Z., Constable, R., & Canli, T. (2006). Functional connectivity with the anterior cingulate is associated with extraversion during the emotional Stroop task. *Social Neuroscience, 1*(1), 16–24.

Heller, D., Komar, J., & Lee, W. B. (2007). The dynamics of personality states, goals, and well-being. *Personality and Social Psychology Bulletin, 33*(6), 898–910.

Hofstee, W. K., De Raad, B., & Goldberg, L. R. (1992). Integration of the big five and circumplex approaches to trait structure. *Journal of Personality and Social Psychology, 63*(1), 146–163.

Hogan, R. (1982). A socioanalytic theory of personality. In R. A. Dienstbier & M. M. Page (Eds.), *Personality: Current theory and research. Nebraska Symposium on Motivation* (Vol. 30, pp. 55–89). Lincoln: University of Nebraska Press.

Hull, C. L. (1943). *Principles of behavior: An introduction to behavior theory.* Oxford, UK: Appleton-Century.

Jang, K. L., Livesley, W., Angleitner, A., Riemann, R., & Vernon, P. A. (2002). Genetic and environmental influences on the covariance of facets defining the domains of the five-factor model of personality. *Personality and Individual Differences, 33*(1), 83–101.

John, O. P. (1990). The "Big Five" factor taxonomy: Dimensions of personality in the natural language and in questionnaires. In L. A. Pervin & O. P. John (Eds.), *Handbook of personality: Theory and research* (pp. 66–100). New York: Guilford Press.

John, O. P., Donahue, E. M., & Kentle, R. L. (1991). *The Big Five Inventory—Versions 4a and 54.* Berkeley: Institute of Personality and Social Research, University of California, Berkeley.

John, O. P., & Srivastava, S. (1999). The Big Five trait taxonomy: History, measurement, and theoretical perspectives. In L. A. Pervin & O. P. John (Eds.), *Handbook of personality: Theory and research* (2nd ed., pp. 102–138). New York: Guilford Press.

Jung, C. G. (1971). *Psychological types: Collected works* (Vol. 6). Princeton, NJ: Princeton University Press. (Original work published 1921)

Jylha, P., & Isometsa, E. (2006). The relationship of neuroticism and extraversion to symptoms of anxiety and depression in the general population. *Depression and Anxiety, 23*(5), 281–289.

King, L. A. (1995). Wishes, motives, goals, and personal memories: Relations of measures of human motivation. *Journal of Personality, 63*(4), 985–1007.

King, L. A., & Broyles, S. J. (1997). Wishes, gender, personality, and well-being. *Journal of Personality, 65*(1), 49–76.

Krueger, R. F., Caspi, A., Moffitt, T. E., Silva, P. A., & McGee, R. (1996). Personality traits are differentially linked to mental disorders: A multitrait–multidiagnosis study of an adolescent birth cohort. *Journal of Abnormal Psychology, 105*(3), 299–312.

Larsen, R. J., & Ketelaar, T. (1991). Personality and susceptibility to positive and negative emotional states. *Journal of Personality and Social Psychology, 61*(1), 132–140.

Lee, K., & Ashton, M. C. (2004). Psychometric properties of the HEXACO personality inventory. *Multivariate Behavioral Research, 39*(2), 329–358.

Lieberman, M. D., & Rosenthal, R. (2001). Why introverts can't always tell who likes them: Multitasking and nonverbal decoding. *Journal of Personality and Social Psychology, 80*(2), 294–310.

Lucas, R. E., & Baird, B. M. (2004). Extraversion and emotional reactivity. *Journal of Personality and Social Psychology, 86*(3), 473–485.

Lucas, R. E., Diener, E., Grob, A., Suh, E. M., & Shao, L. (2000). Cross-cultural evidence for the fundamental features of extraversion. *Journal of Personality and Social Psychology, 79*(3), 452–468.

Lucas, R. E., & Fujita, F. (2000). Factors influencing the relation between extraversion and pleasant affect. *Journal of Personality and Social Psychology, 79*(6), 1039–1056.

Luo, X., Kranzler, H. R., Zuo, L., Wang, S., & Gelernter, J. (2007). Personality traits of agreeableness and extraversion are associated with *ADH4* variation. *Biological Psychiatry, 61*(5), 599–608.

MacDonald, K. (1995). Evolution, the five-factor model, and levels of personality. *Journal of Personality, 63*(3), 525–567.

Markon, K. E., Krueger, R. F., & Watson, D. (2005). Delineating the structure of normal and abnormal personality: An integrative hierarchical approach. *Journal of Personality and Social Psychology, 88*(1), 139–157.

Matthews, G. (1992). Extroversion. In A. P. Smith & D. M. Jones (Eds.), *Handbook of human performance: Vol. 3. State and trait* (pp. 95–126). San Diego, CA: Academic Press.

Matthews, G., & Gilliland, K. (1999). The personality theories of H. J. Eysenck and J. A. Gray: A comparative review. *Personality and Individual Differences, 26*(4), 583–626.

McCrae, R. R., & Costa, P. T. (1997). Personality trait structure as a human universal. *American Psychologist, 52*(5), 509–516.

McNiel, J., & Fleeson, W. (2006). The causal effects of extraversion on positive affect and neuroticism on negative affect: Manipulating state extraversion and state neuroticism in an experimental approach. *Journal of Research in Personality, 40*(5), 529–550.

Mehl, M. R., Gosling, S. D., & Pennebaker, J. W. (2006). Personality in its natural habitat: Manifestations and implicit folk theories of personality in daily life. *Journal of Personality and Social Psychology, 90*(5), 862–877.

Mehl, M. R., & Pennebaker, J. W. (2003). The sounds of social life: A psychometric analysis of students' daily social environments and natural conversations. *Journal of Personality and Social Psychology, 84*(4), 857–870.

Morley, H. (1891). *Character writings of the seventeenth century.* London: Kessinger.

Nettle, D. (2005). An evolutionary approach to the extraversion continuum. *Evolution and Human Behavior, 26*(4), 363–373.

Nettle, D. (2006). The evolution of personality variation in humans and other animals. *American Psychologist, 61*(6), 622–631.

Norman, W. T. (1963). Toward an adequate taxonomy of personality attributes: Replicated factors structure in peer nomination personality ratings. *Journal of Abnormal and Social Psychology, 66*(6), 574–583.

Olson, K. R., & Weber, D. A. (2004). Relations between big five traits and fundamental motives. *Psychological Reports, 95*(3), 795–802.

Omura, K., Constable, R., & Canli, T. (2005). Amygdala gray matter concentration is associated with extraversion and neuroticism. *NeuroReport, 16*, 1905–1908.

Ortony, A., Norman, D. A., & Revelle, W. (2005). Effective functioning: A three-level model of affect, motivation, cognition, and behavior. In J. Fellous & M. Arbib (Eds.), *Who needs emotions?: The brain meets the machine* (pp. 173–202). New York: Oxford University Press.

Ozer, D. J., & Benet-Martínez, V. (2006). Personality and the prediction of consequential outcomes. *Annual Review of Psychology, 57*, 401–421.

Paunonen, S. V. (2003). Big five factors of personality and replicated predictions of behavior. *Journal of Personality and Social Psychology, 84*(2), 411–422.

Paunonen, S. V., & Ashton, M. C. (2001). Big five factors and facets and the prediction of behavior. *Journal of Personality and Social Psychology, 81*(3), 524–539.

Paunonen, S. V., & Ashton, M. C. (2002). *The nonverbal assessment of personality: The NPQ and the FF-NPQ.* Ashland, OH: Hogrefe & Huber.

Pavlov, I. P. (1927). *Conditioned reflexes: An investigation of the physiological activity of the cerebral cortex.* Oxford, UK: Oxford University Press.

Pavot, W., Diener, E., & Fujita, F. (1990). Extraversion and happiness. *Personality and Individual Differences, 11*(12), 1299–1306.

Pytlik Zillig, L. M., Hemenover, S. H., & Dienstbier, R. A. (2002). What do we assess when we assess a Big 5 trait?: A content analysis of the affective, behavioral and cognitive processes represented in the Big 5 personality inventories. *Personality and Social Psychology Bulletin, 28*(6), 847–858.

Rauch, S. L., Milad, M. R., Orr, S. P., Quinn, B. T., Fischl, B., & Pitman, R. K. (2005). Orbitofrontal thickness, retention of fear extinction, and extraversion. *NeuroReport, 16*, 1909–1912.

Revelle, W. (1995). Personality processes. *Annual Review of Psychology, 46*, 295–328.

Revelle, W. (2008). The contribution of reinforcement sensitivity theory to personality theory. In P. J. Corr (Ed.), *The reinforcement sensitivity theory of personality* (pp. 508–527). Cambridge, UK: Cambridge University Press.

Revelle, W., Humphreys, M. S., Simon, L., & Gilliland, K. (1980). The interactive effect of personality, time of day and caffeine: A test of the arousal model. *Journal of Experimental Psychology: General, 109*, 1–31.

Revelle, W., Wilt, J., & Rosenthal, A. (in press). Personality and cognition: The personality–cognition link. In A. Gruszka, G. Matthews, & B. Szymura (Eds.), *Handbook of individual differences in cognition: Attention, memory and executive control.* New York: Springer.

Roberts, B. W., Kuncel, N. R., Shiner, R., Caspi, A., & Goldberg, L. R. (2007). The power of personality: The comparative validity of personality traits, socioeconomic status, and cognitive ability for predicting important life outcomes. *Perspectives on Psychological Science, 2*(4), 313–345.

Roberts, B. W., & Robins, R. W. (2000). Broad dispositions, broad aspirations: The intersection of personality traits and major life goals. *Personality and Social Psychology Bulletin, 26*(10), 1284–1296.

Roberts, B. W., & Robins, R. W. (2004). Person–environment fit and its implications for personality development: A longitudinal study. *Journal of Personality, 72*(1), 89–110.

Robinson, M. D., Meier, B. P., & Vargas, P. T. (2005). Extraversion, threat categorizations, and negative affect: A reaction time approach to avoidance motivation. *Journal of Personality, 73*(5), 1397–1436.

Rocklin, T., & Revelle, W. (1981). The measurement of extraversion: A comparison of the Eysenck Personality Inventory and the Eysenck Personality Questionnaire. *British Journal of Social Psychology, 20*(4), 279–284.

Rogers, G. M., & Revelle, W. (1998). Personality, mood, and the evaluation of affective and neutral word pairs. *Journal of Personality and Social Psychology, 74*(6), 1592–1605.

Rosenberg, E. L. (1998). Levels of analysis and the organization of affect. *Review of General Psychology, 2*(3), 247–270.

Rothbart, M. K. (1981). Measurement of temperament in infancy. *Child Development, 52*(2), 569–578.

Rothbart, M. K., Ahadi, S. A., & Evans, D. E. (2000). Temperament and personality: Origins and outcomes. *Journal of Personality and Social Psychology, 78*(1), 122–135.

Ruch, W., & Hehl, F. J. (1989, June). *Psychometric properties of the German version of the EPQ-R.* Paper presented at the 4th annual meeting of the International Society for the Study of Individual Differences. Heidelberg, Germany.

Rusting, C. L. (1999). Interactive effects of personality and mood on emotion-congruent memory and judgment. *Journal of Personality and Social Psychology, 77*(5), 1073–1086.

Schutte, N. S., Malouff, J. M., Segrera, E., Wolf, A., & Rodgers, L. (2003). States reflecting the big five dimensions. *Personality and Individual Differences, 34*(4), 591–603.

Smillie, L. D. (2008). What is reinforcement sensitivity?: Neuroscience paradigms for approach–avoidance processes in personality. *European Journal of Personality, 22*(5), 359–384.

Smillie, L. D., Pickering, A. D., & Jackson, C. J. (2006). The new reinforcement sensitivity theory: Implications for personality measurement. *Personality and Social Psychology Review, 10*(4), 320–335.

Spain, J. S., Eaton, L. G., & Funder, D. C. (2000). Perspectives on personality: The relative accuracy of self versus others for the prediction of emotion and behavior. *Journal of Personality, 68*(5), 837–867.

Stelmack, R. M., & Stalikas, A. (1991). Galen and the humour theory of temperament. *Personality and Individual Differences, 12*(3), 255–263.

Strelau, J. (1987). Emotion as a key concept in temperament research. *Journal of Research in Personality, 21*(4), 510–528.

Tellegen, A. (1982). *Brief manual for the Differential Personality Questionnaire.* Minneapolis: University of Minnesota.

Tellegen, A. (1985). Structures of mood and personality and their relevance to assessing anxiety, with an emphasis on self-report. In A. H. Turna & J. D. Maser (Eds.), *Anxiety and the anxiety disorders* (pp. 681–706). Hillsdale, NJ: Erlbaum.

Theophrastus. (1909). *The characters of Theophrastus* (R. C. Jebb, Trans. & J. E. Sandys, Ed.). London: Macmillan.

Tooby, J., & Cosmides, L. (1990). On the universality of human nature and the uniqueness of the individual: The role of genetics and adaptation. *Journal of Personality, 58*(1), 17–67.

Trull, T. J., & Sher, K. J. (1994). Relationship between the five-factor model of personality and Axis I disorders in a nonclinical sample. *Journal of Abnormal Psychology, 103*(2), 350–360.

Tupes, E. C., & Christal, R. E. (1961). *Recurrent personality factors based on trait ratings* (USAF ASD Tech. Rep. No. 61-97). Lackland Air Force Base, TX: U.S. Air Force.

Uziel, L. (2006). The extraverted and the neurotic glasses are of different colors. *Personality and Individual Differences, 41*(4), 745–754.

Wacker, J., Chavanon, M.-L., & Stemmler, G. (2006). Investigating the dopaminergic basis of extraversion in humans: A multilevel approach. *Journal of Personality and Social Psychology, 91*(1), 171–187.

Watson, D. (1988). Intraindividual and interindividual analyses of positive and negative affect: Their relation to health complaints, perceived stress, and daily activities. *Journal of Personality and Social Psychology, 54*(6), 1020–1030.

Watson, D. (2000). *Mood and temperament.* New York: Guilford Press.

Watson, D., & Clark, L. A. (1992). On traits and temperament: General and specific factors of emotional experience and their relation to the five-factor model. *Journal of Personality, 60*(2), 441–476.

Watson, D., & Clark, L. A. (1997). Extraversion and its positive emotional core. In R. Hogan, J. Johnson, & S. Briggs (Eds.), *Handbook of personality psychology* (pp. 767–793). San Diego, CA: Academic Press.

Watson, D., Clark, L. A., McIntyre, C. W., & Hamaker, S. (1992). Affect, personality, and social activity. *Journal of Personality and Social Psychology, 63*(6), 1011–1025.

Weiler, M. A. (1992). *Sensitivity to affectively valenced stimuli.* Unpublished doctoral dissertation, Northwestern University.

Widiger, T. A. (2005). Five factor model of personality disorder: Integrating science and practice. *Journal of Research in Personality, 39*(1), 67–83.

Wright, C. I., Williams, D., Feczko, E., Barrett, L. F., Dickerson, B. C., Schwartz, C. E., et al. (2006). Neuroanatomical correlates of extraversion and neuroticism. *Cerebral Cortex, 16*(12), 1809–1819.

Wundt, W., & Judd, C. H. (1897). *Outlines of psychology.* Oxford, UK: Engelmann.

Yerkes, R., & Dodson, J. (1908). The relation of strength of stimuli to rapidity of habit-formation. *Journal of Comparative Neurology and Psychology, 18*, 459–482.

Zelenski, J. M., & Larsen, R. J. (2002). Predicting the future: How affect-related personality traits influence likelihood judgments of future events. *Personality and Social Psychology Bulletin, 28*(7), 1000–1010.

Zinbarg, R., & Revelle, W. (1989). Personality and conditioning: A test of four models. *Journal of Personality and Social Psychology, 57*(2), 301–314.

CHAPTER 4

■ ● ▲ ◆ ■ ● ▲ ◆

Agreeableness

WILLIAM G. GRAZIANO
RENÉE M. TOBIN

Agreeableness is an abstract, higher level summary term for a set of relations among connected lower level characteristics. It describes individual differences in being likeable, pleasant, and harmonious in relations with others. Research shows that persons who are described by others as "kind" are also described as "considerate" and "warm," implicating a superordinate dimension that is relatively stable over time and related to a wide range of thoughts, feelings, and social behaviors. Agreeableness is one of the five major dimensions of personality in the Big Five, the one most concerned with how individuals differ in their orientations toward interpersonal relationships. Agreeableness appears in free descriptions and in ratings in every cultural group studied so far. For example, when Kohnstamm, Halverson, Mervielde, and Havill (1998) asked parents from 11 different cultural groups to describe their own children, approximately 50% of the free descriptions involved agreeableness and extraversion. Cultures differed, of course, in the importance assigned to agreeableness, but all groups described it.

Agreeableness as a Moderator

One way to conceptualize agreeableness is as a *moderator* of various kinds of interpersonal behaviors. If persons differ in their motivation to maintain positive relationships with others (Graziano & Eisenberg, 1997), then we can expect persons who show higher levels of such motivation to perform more positive, constructive behaviors in various behavioral domains than their peers. This approach was a reasonable starting place to begin a program of scientific work, and it helped uncover several important findings on conflict, cooperation, helping, and prejudice. We review some of these findings subsequently. The moderator approach has some limitations, however, as a means of linking individual differences to interpersonal behaviors. First, interpersonal behaviors are determined to a large extent by expectations about the likely reactions of interaction partners (Kelley et al., 2003). However highly motivated Person A might be to cooperate, when A develops expectations that cooperative behaviors will be met by exploitation by Person B, expectations can redirect the underlying cooperative motivation (e.g., Graziano, Hair, & Finch, 1997). Second, personality can operate indirectly through its potent influence on the self-selection of situations. Self-selection processes should be especially striking for interpersonal behaviors, even to the point of masking potential moderation by personality variables. For example, one of the most fundamental principles of interpersonal attraction is reciprocity. People tend to like persons who like them. At a process level, this principle is almost certainly true, but it is also true that some people are liked by virtually everyone. Liking is both a personal and an interpersonal process. Presumably people would avoid environments containing persons they do not like. However, if we looked closely at the mutuality of liking in group of people in vivo, we would discover a lower match than expected. Some people would have friends and interaction partners with whom they seemed not to match.

These considerations apply directly to agreeableness. Persons high in agreeableness are well liked and popular with their peers, in part because they project positivity onto others and make excuses for others' shortcomings (Graziano & Tobin, 2002). Persons high in agreeableness expect others to be pleasant and likeable and appear to elicit such behavior from their partners. This pattern is consistent with the reciprocity of attraction principle, but it suggests the need to look past the personality moderator approach. In particular, it points to the need for attention to social interdependence and to other social-cognitive processes underlying interpersonal interaction. The Person × Situation approach is a step in that direction (Graziano, Habashi, Sheese, & Tobin, 2007). That is, rather than treating agreeableness as a variable that merely raises or lowers the level of situational effects, agreeableness enters the stage as an equal partner. In some cases, the presence of persons at different levels of agreeableness can fundamentally alter the situations themselves. We discuss this in the section on cooperation and competition.

Historical Origins of Agreeableness

From ancient times, writers have commented on the value of agreeableness in social relationships (e.g., Aristotle's *Akrasia*). In modern scientific research, agreeableness has a curious history relative to many other recognized dimensions of personality. Unlike the supertraits of extraversion and neuroticism, agreeableness did not initially receive systematic empirical research because of deductive top-down theorizing about its link to biology or to especially conspicuous social behaviors (Feigl, 1970). Instead, systematic research

on agreeableness began as a result of reliable empirical regularities arising in descriptions of others and later in self-descriptions (Digman & Takemoto-Chock, 1981). Because of its bottom-up empirical origins, there were debates about its correlates and even a suitable label for this hypothetical construct. Other labels used to describe the dimension are *tender-mindedness, friendly compliance versus hostile noncompliance, likeability, communion*, and even *love versus hate*.

Labeling constructs has consequences. For example, the term *compliance* has a process-based meaning in social psychology that often places it on a continuum of social influence with internalization and identification (e.g., Petty & Wegener, 1999). That variety of compliance is considerably different from the one used more casually in personality to imply tendencies to follow rules and norms. Friendly compliance might imply a general conforming personality, but there is no experimental or even correlational evidence that persons high in agreeableness are more responsive to social influence per se.

Recently, Habashi and Wegener (2008) manipulated the quality of arguments (strong vs. weak) in a study of persuasive communication. They found that persons low in agreeableness were less influenced by persuasive communications than their peers high in agreeableness, regardless of the quality of argument. For persons high in agreeableness, however, strong arguments led to greater attitude change than weak arguments. Taken together, these data suggest that agreeableness is related to being *responsive* to others, including their communications. Responsiveness may be a prerequisite for social influence, but it is certainly not the same construct as compliance.

Another issue related to the labeling of compliance is socially desirable responding. Virtually every positive self-report marker or statement for agreeableness is more socially desirable than its supposed bipolar opposite. *Warm* and *kind* are more desirable than *cold* and *unkind*. It is possible that agreeableness primarily indexes self-favoring bias and social desirability rather than basic individual differences in social dispositions, but the data do not support this interpretation. First, agreeableness differences initially entered the scientific literature through regularities in observer ratings (e.g., Digman &

Takemoto-Chock, 1981). Observer ratings are not entirely invulnerable to social desirability problems, but their bias problems will be different from those affecting self-report. When observer ratings and self-report converge despite differences in bias, as is the case with agreeableness ratings, it suggests some validity for both assessment methods.

Second, the empirical literature does not support a self-favoring-bias artifact explanation. In three studies using observational, correlational, and experimental methods (N = 979), Graziano and Tobin (2002) found that other dimensions of the Big Five (Conscientiousness, Neuroticism) had more significant correlations with various indexes of self-favoring bias (impression management, self-deception, all three self-monitoring factors) than Agreeableness. Some measures of self-favoring bias (self-deception) were unrelated to agreeableness. A social relations analysis (Kenny, 1996) also found that, by a ratio of almost 4:1, the larger part of agreeableness variance was in the perceiver effect, relative to the target effect. That is, the larger source of variance in rated agreeableness was due to perceivers' attributing the qualities of agreeableness to targets. In another study participants were randomly assigned to conditions in which they were told that it was bad to be agreeable or good to be agreeable or were given no instructions. Participants actually *increased* their self-ratings of agreeableness when they were told it was a bad quality. If agreeableness is somehow related to self-favoring bias, being seen in a socially positive light is not a major part of it. Overall, these and other outcomes suggest that agreeableness effects are probably not artifacts of self-favoring bias.

Other measurement issues have implications for construct validity. One is the assumed dimensionality of the construct itself. High internal consistency and even coherent loadings in factor analyses do not guarantee that one and only one dimension underlies phenotypic expressions of agreeableness. At least conceptually, the pattern of behavior exhibited by persons low in agreeableness may require a set of variables completely different from those used to describe the behaviors exhibited by persons high in agreeableness. Operationally, is a person low in agreeableness merely a person who is a deficient version of a person high in agreeableness? Perhaps persons high in agreeableness are enhanced versions of persons low in agreeableness. Exactly what process do persons low in agreeableness lack that persons high in agreeableness possess? (For a parallel discussion of the dimensionality of self-monitoring, see Graziano & Waschull, 1995, pp. 238–242). This issue is discussed for the case of agreeableness in the sections on helping, on prejudice, and on the overall motivational model of agreeableness.

As we inch upward from the soil of observation toward theory, another issue involves configurations of personality dimensions. In talking about agreeableness, it may not be safe to ignore other aspects of personality, whether they are correlated with agreeableness or not (e.g., Goldberg, 1999). Is it reasonable to expect the same pattern of, say, aggressive behavior from persons high in agreeableness who are also high in extraversion as from persons high in agreeableness who are high in neuroticism (but not extraversion)? Research showed that retaliatory aggression was related (inversely) to agreeableness (Gleason, Jensen-Campbell, & Richardson, 2004), but is there a configural aspect to this story? Their rationale was derived from a different interactive theoretical perspective, but Ode, Robinson, and Wilkowski (2008) presented data showing that at higher levels of agreeableness, the anger–neuroticism link was considerably reduced. In a set of studies, Ode and Robinson (2008) found a similar moderating effect for agreeableness on the relation between neuroticism and depressive symptoms. Similarly, in a resistance-to-temptation study, Jensen-Campbell and Graziano (2005) showed that higher levels of conscientiousness could partially compensate for lower levels of agreeableness (and vice versa) in predicting cheating in adolescents. Interestingly, in all of these cases the substantive, focal concern was affect regulation. The configuration of personality patterns (vs. one personality dimension at a time) is at the leading edge of personality theory and measurement, generally under the rubric of the Abridged Big Five Circumplex (AB5C), but it clearly suggests avenues for refinement of our understanding of links among personality dimensions and their collective relation with behavior (De Raad, 2000; De Raad, Hendriks, & Hofstee, 1994). For the purpose of this chapter, however, we do not discuss AB5C issues unless immediately relevant to the topic. The configuration issue is important in the discussion of our new motivational approach to agreeableness.

Measuring Agreeableness

Agreeableness differences can be measured through observation by knowledgeable informants such as spouses (Costa & McCrae, 1988), employment supervisors (Hogan, Hogan, & Roberts, 1996), and teachers (e.g., Digman & Takemoto-Chock, 1981). Agreeableness may even be manipulated experimentally as an independent variable (Jensen-Campbell, Graziano, & West, 1995). However, the method most commonly used is self-report, and this can be accomplished through several different instruments. Goldberg (1992) offered a set of adjective markers that can be used even with children (Graziano, Jensen-Campbell, Steele, & Hair, 1998). Goldberg and his colleagues have translated their instruments into many different languages (see *http:// ipip.ori.org/newItemTranslations.htm*). Another option is to use questionnaire-format measures such as the Big Five Inventory (BFI; John & Srivastava, 1999), the International Personality Item Pool (IPIP; Goldberg et al., 2006), or one of the versions of the NEO (Costa & McCrae, 1988). Overall, the measures show some differences, but more remarkable is their convergence. An individual scoring high on agreeableness on the Goldberg markers is likely to score high on the BFI as well (John & Srivastava, 1999).

Confidence that most Big Five instruments can measure agreeableness is enhanced by evidence that such measures converge positively with corresponding individual differences in prosocial motives and negatively with antisocial tendencies, suggesting that personality differences and motives are related systematically (e.g., Finch, Panter, & Caskie, 1999). Evidence for divergent validity also supports the claim that agreeableness warrants research as a separate construct. The simple correlation between agreeableness and sex varies from sample to sample and across age groups. In self-report data from college-age students, in our samples of 300 or more, the correlation rarely exceeds .15 (vs. sex and extraversion at .20). Among children, teachers rate girls as more agreeable than boys, but in self-reports from the same children, we find little evidence that boys and girls consistently differ. Agreeableness is correlated more highly with psychological femininity (but not psychological masculinity) than with biological sex per se. This is consistent with the Spence and Helmreich (1979) view that psychological femininity is tied closely to interpersonal and expressive motives and interests in relationships (Lenney, 1991). We find no evidence that minority children differ systematically from majority children in agreeableness (Graziano et al., 1998; Hair & Graziano, 2003). Usually, agreeableness is correlated negatively with neuroticism, in the range of −.20 to −.30.

The process of searching for measurement artifacts and correlates of agreeableness could be endless apart from the focus provided by relevant theory (Feigl, 1970). Some guidance comes from work on personality development. Agreeableness may be tied distinctively to systems of self-regulation, especially as they apply to frustration regulation in social relations (Jensen-Campbell & Graziano, 2005; Jensen-Campbell & Malcolm, 2007).

Ahadi and Rothbart (1994) offer a developmental hypothesis linking an early-appearing temperamental process, effortful control, to subsequent personality structure in children, adolescents, and adults. They propose that effortful control is part of a common developmental system underlying two of the major dimensions in the Big Five structural model of personality, namely Agreeableness and Conscientiousness (Graziano, 1994; Graziano & Eisenberg, 1997). Specifically, Rothbart and her colleagues (e.g., Rothbart & Bates, 2006; Rothbart & Posner, 1985) proposed that effortful control modulates other temperament systems as the frontal cortex matures. Effortful control is related to early-appearing differences in the ability to sustain and shift attention and the ability to initiate and inhibit action voluntarily (e.g., Kochanska, Murray, & Coy, 1997). Effortful control seems to be related to the ability to suppress a dominant behavior to perform a subdominant response or even an opposing dominant response, as is commonly the case for agreeableness. Jensen-Campbell and colleagues (2002) found that both agreeableness and conscientiousness were associated with traditional assessments of self-regulation (e.g., on Stroop and Wisconsin Card Sorting tasks).

Agreeableness and Interpersonal Behaviors

Like most psychological constructs, agreeableness can be understood in terms of thoughts, feelings, and behaviors that are related to it (Shadish, Cook, & Campbell, 2002). Overall, agreeableness seems to be positively related to adaptive social behaviors (e.g., conflict resolution, emotional responsiveness, helping behavior) and negatively related to maladaptive social behaviors (i.e., prejudice, stigmatization). In this section we discuss the links between agreeableness and four classes of interpersonal behaviors: interpersonal conflict, interpersonal cooperation, helping and prosocial behavior, and prejudice. First, we focus on these four classes of interpersonal behavior because each involves important elements of social motivation and social cognition. If humans did not live communally and had no prospect of continuing interaction with each other, then each day would become a totally new blank slate, as in *Groundhog Day*, the movie starring Bill Murray. There would be little utility to social cognition and efforts to understand the motivation of others. With the prospect of future interaction and social exchange, any given act of bias, helping, or conflict has implications for future interaction. These implications inspire researchers to search for underlying motives.

Second, each of these types of behaviors has been linked to processes of control and regulation. It makes sense to look for the fingerprints of agreeableness in behaviors containing elements of control and regulation. Third, in keeping with Kurt Lewin's general theoretical perspectives, we assume that interpersonal behaviors share basic underlying processes, so classification into discrete classes serves only a temporary pragmatic function (see Graziano & Waschull, 1995). Nevertheless, each of these kinds of interpersonal behavior has a distinct behavioral topography. Our starting position was that if agreeableness is related to differences in motivation for maintaining positive relations

with others (Graziano & Eisenberg, 1997) and if such motivation reflects underlying processes of control and regulation (Jensen-Campbell et al., 2002; Jensen-Campbell, Knack, Waldrip, & Campbell, 2007; Tobin, Graziano, Vanman, & Tassinary, 2000), then in each of these domains agreeableness would be an important moderator of behavioral output. In each case, outcomes pointed toward the need for more complicated ways of conceptualizing each of the classes of interpersonal behaviors. Fourth, stronger experimental studies linking agreeableness to interpersonal processes have entered the literature, enhancing the credibility of the suggestive (but inherently weaker) correlational studies. These experimental studies receive special attention.

Agreeableness and Conflict

Theoretically, agreeableness maps onto the major motivational system of communion, or the desire for unity, intimacy, and solidarity with others (Wiggins, 1991). Consistent with this theoretical link, Graziano, Jensen-Campbell, and Hair (1996) found that most people tend to endorse negotiation and disengagement tactics in resolving conflict but that the difference between persons low in agreeableness and persons high in agreeableness was maximal when destructive tactics (e.g., power assertion tactics such as physical force) were at issue. In particular, persons low in agreeableness reported that destructive tactics were generally more acceptable than did persons high in agreeableness. Furthermore, individuals high in agreeableness tended to perceive less conflict in their social interactions, report more liking of interaction partners, and elicit less conflict from their partners. They are perceived by others as displaying less tension in their interactions relative to their peers.

Building on these findings, Jensen-Campbell and Graziano (2001) conducted multimethod research, including a diary study, examining agreeableness as a moderator of middle-school children's conflict patterns. Consistent with their previous work, individuals high in agreeableness reported engaging in more constructive conflict resolution tactics in their day-to-day interactions relative to their peers. Thus, across age ranges and methodologies, agreeableness is linked to positive resolution of conflict, presumably because of its underlying motivation to get along with others.

Agreeableness and Cooperation

Agreeableness is related to behavior in competitive and cooperative situations. Graziano and colleagues (1997) examined patterns of cooperative and competitive behaviors in triads of college students. Overall, agreeableness was related negatively to competitiveness in groups and related positively to expectations of harmonious group interactions. Graziano and colleagues also found that competitiveness mediates the relation between agreeableness and cooperation, indicating that individuals low in agreeableness tend to view themselves as less interdependent with other group members and to respond with more competitive behaviors relative to their high-agreeable peers. Similar relations were also found earlier in development with 115 triads of school-age children (Tobin, Schneider, Graziano, & Pizzitola, 2002). In both age groups, persons high in agreeableness seem to transform competitive situations into cooperative ones. This transformation is easier to accomplish if other group members are also high in agreeableness.

Agreeableness and Helping

Agreeableness also plays an important role in the experience of positive emotions within the context of interpersonal relationships. Among the five dimensions of personality, agreeableness is the only one that is significantly correlated with both of the major aspects of prosocial emotions, namely empathic concern and personal distress. Zero-order correlations between agreeableness and measures of self-reported empathy are consistently strong and positive (e.g., Graziano, Habashi, et al., 2007). Beyond self-reports, agreeableness has also been connected to prosocial behaviors, such as volunteering to help others in need. In the first of a set of studies, Graziano, Habashi, and colleagues (2007) found that individuals high in agreeableness are more likely to report willingness to help a wider range of others than those low in agreeableness when presented with scenarios in which they may offer to help a sibling, a friend, or a stranger.

Studies 2 and 3 translated the findings from this vignette study into laboratory-based experiments in which participants were given opportunities to volunteer help to a person in need. Using Batson's Katie Banks paradigm (Coke, Batson, & McDavis, 1978), Graziano, Habashi, and colleagues found that individuals high in agreeableness offered to help outgroup members (i.e., a student from a different university) more often than did individuals low in agreeableness. They also offered help more often than their low-agreeable counterparts even when their attention was directed experimentally to the technical aspects (rather than the emotional aspects) of the situation, demonstrating that an other-focused, empathic response is more automatic in persons high in agreeableness relative to their peers. Results of Study 3 shed additional light on the relation between agreeableness and helping by demonstrating that empathic concern, but not personal distress, mediates this relation in the technical-focus condition.

Graziano, Habashi, and colleagues (2007, Study 4) extended this line of research by experimentally manipulating not only the focus of participants' attention (emotional vs. technical aspects) but also the cost of helping. They found that when the cost of helping is high, asking participants low in agreeableness to focus on the emotional aspects of the situation reduces their willingness to help. When cost of helping is low, however, the opposite pattern was obtained for individuals low in agreeableness: Persons low on this personality dimension increased their helping when the cost of helping was low and they were instructed to focus on emotion. Thus, when costs are low, a reminder to pay attention to others' emotions facilitates helping behavior in people low in agreeableness, whereas this same reminder decreases helping behavior when greater costs of helping are placed on people low in agreeableness. These findings indicate that helping may be increased in persons who ordinarily do not offer to do so when the costs to them are low. In contrast, the request to focus on emotions as opposed to the technical aspects of the situation did not yield a similar reduction in helping for individuals high in agreeableness when the cost of helping was either high or low. Taken together, the Graziano, Habashi, and colleagues studies demonstrated important links among agreeableness, empathy, and helping behavior. Thus research indicates that the motives underlying agreeableness are related to greater experience of empathy and that this emotional experience is, in turn, related to increased willingness to help.

Agreeableness and Prejudice

Agreeableness-related responsiveness motives have also been linked to biases in reactions to others. Graziano, Bruce, Sheese, and Tobin (2007) investigated whether the motives underlying agreeableness lead individuals to respond differentially to persons from a stigmatized group (e.g., persons who are overweight). In a five-study program, these researchers first examined how agreeableness was related to perceived social norms and personal endorsements of prejudice toward over 100 potential targets of prejudice. They found that individuals high in agreeableness did not differ from their peers in terms of their understanding of the social norms related to the acceptability of holding prejudiced feelings toward these groups; however, they did differ in their personal endorsement of such prejudice. That is, individuals high in agreeableness reported less negative reactions to most groups, including traditional targets of prejudice (e.g., homosexuals, Jews, Hispanics) relative to their peers. Thus the findings support the hypothesis that agreeableness is related to prejudiced reactions, at least in terms of verbal self-reports.

Moving beyond these self-reports, Graziano, Bruce, and colleagues (2007) used an established experimental paradigm (Snyder & Haugen, 1994) to investigate prejudicial reactions to specific interaction partners. In this study, participants were partnered with an unknown female participant for a "getting acquainted conversation." Before the conversation, participants were provided with a photograph of the supposed partner. This photograph was digitally altered so that the partner appeared either overweight or of typical weight. Participants reported their prejudicial reactions to their partners using a social-distance measure following the conversations. Male participants low in agreeableness responded with the most prejudicial reactions, but only when partnered

with an overweight woman. In Study 3, the authors replicated and extended these findings by demonstrating that these prejudicial responses translated into discriminatory behaviors. Participants were presented with a photograph of either a typical or overweight partner who was ostensibly similar to the participant in personality and were given the opportunity to change partners without penalty. Graziano, Bruce, and colleagues found that only men low in agreeableness indicated a desire to switch partners, and they only did so when paired with an overweight female partner.

The remaining two studies by Graziano, Bruce, and colleagues (2007) focused on identifying conditions under which persons high in agreeableness may be more likely to exhibit the prejudicial responses shown by individuals low in agreeableness. In Study 4, providing a justification for expressing prejudice (i.e., the partner expressed counternormative negative sentiments about their university) yielded increased prejudicial responding from individuals high in agreeableness, but only when they were paired with overweight female partners. Although persons high in agreeableness increased their prejudicial responding in this condition, overall, participants low in agreeableness expressed stronger prejudicial reactions than their high-agreeable counterparts. A similar pattern of results was obtained in a fifth study, when participants were provided with an even greater justification for the expression of prejudice, namely that the ostensible interaction partner created additional work for the participant. Individuals high in agreeableness expressed prejudice toward overweight partners relative to typical weight partners, but only when the partner was at fault for a mistake that led to additional workload for the participants. In contrast, individuals low in agreeableness expressed more negative reactions to their partners regardless of the cause of additional work.

Emotional Processes Underlying Agreeableness and Interpersonal Behavior

Agreeableness may not be highly related to other major structural dimensions of personality, but it is probably related to other dispositions, perhaps due to overlapping regulatory processes. Intuitively, one might expect empathy to be one component of agreeableness. Studies show that agreeableness is related to dispositional empathy. Persons high in agreeableness report greater ease in seeing the world through others' eyes (perspective taking) and feeling the suffering of others (empathic concern), but not necessarily in experiencing self-focused negative emotions (personal distress) when observing victims in sorrow. Past research showed that these cognitive and emotional processes are related to overt helping, so we might expect persons high in agreeableness to offer more help and aid to others, even to strangers, than do their peers. Recent empirical research supports the claim that agreeableness is related to both empathic concern and helping (e.g., Graziano, Habashi, et al., 2007).

Moving further away from intuition toward theory, agreeableness seems to be related to frustration control. Due to their motivation to maintain good relations with others, persons high in agreeableness are probably more willing or better able to regulate the inevitable frustrations that come from interacting with others. As discussed previously, theorists proposed that agreeableness (along with its conceptual cousin, conscientiousness) may have its developmental origins in an early-appearing temperamental process called effortful control (Jensen-Campbell et al., 2002, 2007; Tobin et al., 2000). Indeed, Haas, Omura, Constable, and Canli (2007) found that agreeableness is related to activation of the right lateral prefrontal cortex following exposure to negative emotional stimuli. These results suggest that individuals high in agreeableness automatically engage in emotion regulation processes when exposed to negative stimuli.

When examining the experience, expression, and regulation of emotion, psychologists historically have focused on links to extraversion and neuroticism. Recent empirical work, however, indicates that agreeableness is also connected to emotional processes, particularly in interpersonal situations. In a three-study set, Tobin and colleagues (2000) examined the relations among agreeableness, emotion experience, and emotion regulation using self-report, psychophysiological, and observational methods. They found that individuals high in agreeableness

experienced stronger emotional reactions to evocative stimuli and exerted greater efforts to regulate these emotions than their peers. These results were obtained in the context of communicating about their reactions to viewing negative images selected from the International Affective Picture System (e.g., burn victims, a baby with a facial tumor) (Lang, Bradley, & Cuthbert, 1995). Building on this work, Tobin, Kieras, and Graziano (2003) found a similar relation between agreeableness and emotion regulation in school-age children using the disappointing gift paradigm (Cole, 1986; Saarni, 1984). They found that children high in agreeableness displayed less negative affect when receiving an undesirable gift than did children low in agreeableness. Thus agreeableness has been linked to greater responsiveness and regulation of negative emotions in both children and adults.

Agreeableness as a Set of Motivational Processes

In the first comprehensive review of agreeableness as a distinct psychological construct, Graziano and Eisenberg (1997) proposed that agreeableness could be defined in motivational terms. Specifically, they proposed that agreeableness indexed individual differences in the motivation to maintain positive relations with others. Subsequent research supported this approach but also suggested the need for refinements and elaborations. First, we observe striking parallels in the way agreeableness relates to the two seemingly opposite social behaviors of prejudice and helping. Despite their different emphases and focuses, and despite behavior-genetic evidence that prosocial and antisocial systems may be different (e.g., Krueger, Hicks, & McGue, 2001), the specific behaviors of prejudice and helping both include approach and avoidance processes. A common motivational system including agreeableness may underlie both forms of behavior. Second, some anomalies and curiosities within each of these two research literatures may be explained by applying a *dual-process model* to fit both literatures. One component of the dual process is agreeableness. Dual-process and multiprocess models are prominent in the literatures on prejudice (Pryor, Reeder,

Yeadon, & Hesson-McInnis, 2004) and on helping (Batson, 1991; Dijker & Koomen, 2007), but the processes may be more general than previously recognized. Third, further clarification of the apparent anomalies in the two literatures can be obtained using a dual-process, sequential-opponent motivational system that incorporates agreeableness. We describe such a model here.

Let us first consider some of these anomalies, curiosities, and striking parallels. Research on the social psychology of prejudice lives in almost total isolation from research on helping and altruism. At first glance, this makes sense. After all, prejudice is a negative, even antisocial behavior, whereas helping is a positive, constructive, prosocial activity. With closer inspection, however, the separate-but-equal status is harder to justify. First, the small number of researchers who are active in both areas (e.g., Dovidio, 1984) have found a few processes that seem to affect both prejudice and helping. Perhaps the most conspicuous example is the ingroup–outgroup status of the victim (e.g., Graziano, Habashi, et al., 2007; Piliavin, Dovidio, Gaertner, & Clark, 1982). Members of outgroups are often targets of prejudice, and they are also less likely to receive help. Digging a bit deeper, we find half-hidden assumptions about processes that apply to both areas. Prejudice and helping are relationship phenomena, usually operating at the initiation phase of interpersonal attraction, at least as investigated by social psychologists (Graziano & Bruce, 2008). Even within more focused debates about interpersonal processes (e.g., Byrne, 1997; Rosenbaum, 1986), the typical assumption was that target persons were placed along a single continuum of positive to negative affect (Graziano & Bruce, 2008).

Agreeableness research may help us understand the links between prejudice and prosocial behavior. In particular, findings involving agreeableness allow us to see connections between these two sets of behaviors that are not obvious. We elaborate on this point later. For now, we note that even without agreeableness, we can see connections between the two. In addition to a few common influential variables and processes, both literatures acknowledge the possibility that phenomena in the prejudice and helping literatures contain elements of both approach and avoidance. In the helping area, studies show that "messy victims" (such as those who are bleeding) seem to activate avoidance that blocks helping (e.g., Piliavin, Callero, & Evanset, 1982). In Batson's (1991) empathy–altruism model, self-focused personal distress seems to block helping, especially when escape from the helping situation is relatively easy (Batson et al., 1981). In the stigma literature, Pryor and colleagues (2004) showed that people often have an initially negative reflexive reaction to outgroup members. Within 300–500 milliseconds, however, corrective reflective processes can come online and suppress the avoidance. The nature of the Pryor paradigm makes it clear that both reflexive avoidance and reflective approach are operative.

From a theoretical perspective, apparent anomalies within each of these two areas are more informative than are similarities. In Batson's empathy–altruism approach, noted previously, the self-focused emotion of personal distress undermines helping, whereas the victim-focused emotion of empathic concern promotes helping. This relation has been demonstrated in experimental studies that manipulate perspective taking. Technically, empathy refers to a set of related components that include personal distress, empathic concern, and perspective taking (Davis, 1996). The last of these three provides a distinctively cognitive process that is relatively easy to manipulate experimentally. In the typical experiment using the Batson paradigm, operationally the affective processes of empathic concern are elicited from research participants by manipulating their focus of attention (e.g., Coke et al., 1978; Toi & Batson, 1982).

The apparent anomaly here is that virtually all studies that have measured both personal distress and empathic concern find that they are correlated *positively*, not negatively (e.g., Batson, O'Quin, Fultz, Vanderplas, & Isen, 1983; Graziano, Habashi, et al., 2007). For present purposes, we note that Batson and colleagues (1983) attempted to address this problem by categorizing "preponderant motives." Because personal distress and empathic concern are both present in participants (and are correlated positively), Batson and colleagues assigned participants to conditions based on their single most dominant motive (see pp. 711–712).

Thus Batson and his colleagues recognize the operation of two potentially opposing motives linked to avoidance and approach. Here we expand on this conceptualization by connecting these avoidance and approach motives to individual differences in agreeableness.

Another set of curiosities involves overcompensation. The prejudice literature shows that often (but not always), research participants may provide exceptionally larger offers of help, assistance, or other benefits to outgroup members than to ingroup members (Dijker & Koomen, 2007). As noted previously, Pryor and colleagues (2004) found evidence of deliberative compensation. If Pryor and colleagues are describing general processes extending beyond prejudice and stigmatization, then overcompensation may be the result of two interdependent motivation processes that occur in sequence. In the specific cases studied so far, the reflective processes generally lead away from prejudice toward prosocial behavior. At least in theory, there is no prior reason to assume that reflective processes per se lead to prosocial action, but agreeableness provides us with a motivational structure to support these observations. Because the literature as a whole shows less liking for outgroup members, overcompensation results suggest that at least two motivational processes are involved in the outcome. Two likely candidates are approach and avoidance, and these processes theoretically connect to agreeableness.

Another apparent anomaly comes from the Batson empathy–altruism model. It may appear to be a tangent at this point, but its relevance is explained in the subsequent integration section. The research literature shows that many (maybe even most) forms of helping are motivated by self-interest (Batson, 1991; Cialdini et al., 1987). What is still controversial is the frequency of helping motivated solely for the benefit of the victim. Batson (1991) argued that the motives underlying most acts of helping are difficult to discern because helping can relieve the provider's distress, as well as the victim's. One situation, however, allows a clearer delineation of helper's motives. If a potential helper can readily escape but still chooses to help, then altruistic, other-oriented motives are now more plausible. This logic im-

plicitly sets high standards for altruism and does not allow for the operation of multiple motives. Given these limitations, the basic proposition receives only mixed empirical support (Schroeder, Dovidio, Sibicky, Matthews, & Allen, 1988). In some cases, the ease of escape seems to matter little (e.g., Eisenberg et al., 1989; Habashi, 2008). At the least, the inconsistency in the effectiveness of the easy–difficult escape manipulations is an anomaly. As we see later, differences in agreeableness help us confront this apparent anomaly.

Another set of curiosities is associated with individual differences in motivation. The quests for the "prejudiced personality" (Allport, 1954; Graziano, Bruce, et al., 2007) and the "altruistic personality" (Batson, Bolen, Cross, & Neuringer-Benefiel, 1986; Carlo, Eisenberg, Troyer, Switzer, & Speer, 1991; Graziano & Eisenberg, 1997; Penner, Fritzsche, Craiger, & Friefeld, 1995) have long histories. That many individual differences moderate helping or prejudice is no longer controversial (Dovidio, Piliavin, Schroeder, & Penner, 2006; Penner, Dovidio, Piliavin, & Schroeder, 2005). More controversial is the generality of the influence of any given individual difference. For example, Pryor and colleagues (2004) found that prejudiced reactions to an HIV victim were moderated by individual differences on the Heterosexual Attitudes toward Homosexuals scale (Larson, Reed, & Hoffman, 1980), but there was no evidence that this individual difference moderated prejudice against ex-convicts. Part of the problem is theoretical. It is not clear precisely what mechanisms are responsible for mediation. Ideally, a single motive or set of motives would be identified that cut across substantive topic areas and provide a unifying thread. As noted previously, Graziano and colleagues (Graziano, Bruce, et al., 2007; Graziano, Habashi, et al., 2007) found evidence that a shared mechanism links personality, namely agreeableness, with both helping and prejudice.

A final curiosity involved empathy as an emotion. Some studies treat empathy as a category of emotion (e.g., Batson, 1991), whereas other studies treat it as part of a dimension based on negative-to-positive emotion (e.g., Piliavin et al., 1982). As noted previously, empirical work suggests that empathy as a construct has a complex structure consisting of both affective and cognitive processing (Davis, 1996). Within this structural approach, affect is further differentiated into a self-focused element and an other-focused element (Eisenberg et al., 1989). In some research, the cognitive component is used to activate the affective components. In Batson's theory, perspective taking enhances empathic concern but inhibits personal distress. This makes intuitive sense, but it seems to assume that empathic concern and personal distress are separate categories of emotion or are negatively correlated. Furthermore, even from a dimensional approach to emotion, what is the affective valence of emotion once it is aroused? Is it primarily negative or positive (e.g., Davis, 1996)? Perhaps its initial activation is experienced as negative, but if help can be provided, it becomes positive. We discuss this subsequently.

One step toward integrating these divergent issues and building a model of agreeableness may be found in work by Dijker and Koomen (2007). They proposed an innovative, integrative approach to stigmatization that included two evolved, preverbal systems of motivation. Each of these two reflects human evolutionary history. The older component is a fight-or-flight system that we carry as part of our paleoreptilian heritage. Encounters with "unusual cases" ("deviance" in Dijker & Koomen, 2007) activate this system without conscious deliberation, priming a system that impels individuals to flee from danger or to fight if forced to do so. The second system is newer in evolutionary time and is part of the parental care system associated with kin selection (Hamilton, 1964; Trivers, 1972). Furthermore, the two motivational systems have the capacity to elicit characteristic emotions when exposed to certain specific environmental triggers. Because humans evolved in small groups of genetically related individuals, aggressive reactions to unusual cases had to be inhibited. Some of the unusual cases probably involved kin, for whom repair of deviance would be more beneficial than aggression or exclusion. The care system has the capacity to suppress the fight–flight system.

The theoretical system presented by Dijker and Koomen (2007) may be expanded further toward agreeableness. Let us assume that agreeableness is the psychological manifestation of the care system. If this is correct, then agreeableness may not only relate to sympathetic caregiving to the weak and disadvantaged but may also operate to suppress the responses associated with the more primitive fight–flight system. Put differently, some agreeableness phenomena may be fairly direct expressions of care and others may be a product of care-based suppression of fight–flight. Concretely, persons high in agreeableness may feel empathic concern directly for victims of misfortune (Graziano, Habashi, et al., 2007), but they may also suppress (perhaps effortfully) negative reactions to traditional targets of prejudice generated by their fight–flight systems (Graziano, Bruce, et al., 2007).

Taking the system a bit further past description, let us assume some connections between the fight–flight and care systems of potential relevance to agreeableness. If we assume that both fight–flight and care systems are present in almost all people (but at varying strengths) and that fight–flight occurs faster than care on exposure to an environmental oddity, the two may operate as opponents to each other's preponderant responsive activation tendencies. If so, we can generate explanations for apparent paradoxes and anomalies. In the helping context, personal distress may inhibit prosocial acts because it is part of fight–flight, not care. Empathic concern promotes helping because it is part of care. Despite having opposite effects on helping, both personal distress and empathic concern are present in most people, explaining the positive correlation. Personal distress is the first response to a victim because it is connected to the faster fight–flight system. If there is an opportunity for easy escape from the victim when personal distress is high, then the victim will not receive help. If escape cannot occur quickly, or if the observer must remain in proximity to the victim, then enough time may pass for the slower empathic-concern system to become active. This would suppress the fight–flight system and increase chances the victim would receive help. This account would explain why outcomes of research on ease–difficulty of escape are unstable. The key variable—the time interval between exposure to the victim and the window of opportunity for escape—is unmeasured.

Going one step further, the system we describe may be a case of the opponent-process model of motivation presented by Solomon and his colleagues (Solomon, 1980; Solomon & Corbit, 1974). In a search of the published literature, we could locate only two applications of the Solomon opponent-process model to either helping or prejudice (Baumeister & Campbell, 1999; Piliavin et al., 1982). In both cases, the focus of attention was primarily on Solomon's opponent explanation for cycles of addictive behavior. Our version of the opponent approach is presented in Figure 4.1. In keeping with Solomon, the first process activated is labeled Process A. Its activation is virtually automatic, a kind of unconditioned response to the onset of an environmental stimulus. It remains active while the evocative stimulus is present and ends when the stimulus is removed. The second process activated is an opponent, labeled Process B. It is slower to come on line but persists well after Process A ends. Because A and B are opponents but A occurs first and more quickly in response to an environmental event for some brief part of the sequence, Process A operates in almost pure form (without an opponent). Concretely, if Process A is personal distress and Process B is empathic concern, then the first response to a victim should be unopposed personal distress. If escape is possible in this interval, the victim will not receive help. By the same logic, initial reactions to unusual cases (e.g., victims of misfortune), as well as to members of outgroups, would be personal distress and avoidance. With time, however, Process B can be activated, opposing the processes of Process A. These opponent processes may be what Pryor and colleagues (2004) index in their behavior correction research. Initial negative reactions are replaced by more positive ones.

The Solomon opponent-process approach offers several additional insights relevant to agreeableness. Repeated exposure to the evocative (unconditioned) stimuli produces systematic changes in the relative strengths of Process A and Process B. Process A becomes weaker, and Process B becomes stronger. The prototype is drug addiction, in which repeated exposure to substances such as cocaine create smaller and shorter states of euphoria and longer states of withdrawal. In the present application, repeated exposure to victims of misfortune should lead to smaller and shorter periods of personal distress and, at least in theory, to longer states

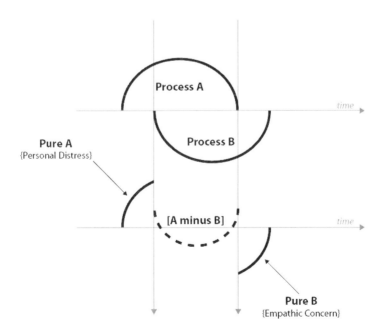

FIGURE 4.1. Opponent-process model of motivation. From Solomon and Corbit (1974). Copyright 1974 by the American Psychological Association. Adapted by permission.

of empathic concern. This connection might explain why there are individual differences and why they appear in the forms that they do. In most of these cases, the kinds of individual differences in motivation for helping reported by Oliner and Oliner (1988) and by others reflect the fact that the helpers had repeated exposure to various kinds of "unusual cases" of people earlier in their lives.

The Solomon approach also raises important questions about the conceptual status of large individual differences such as agreeableness, the decomposition of molar social behavior into constituent components, and the role of time in the expression of complex social behavior. Regarding the first of these questions, at some level each individual is born prepared for a life trajectory by a set of inherited tendencies and motivation systems. Evolution may have left us with two powerful motive systems in fight–flight and care (Dijker & Koomen, 2007), but there are probably individual differences in the relative strength of fight–flight and care motivations. Observers might detect and label these socially important behavioral differences as neuroticism and agreeableness, respectively. At this point, we might be satisfied to build structural models or to collect data showing intercorrelations among variables such as care, agreeableness, and some other disposition, such as self-esteem. Such an approach would grossly underestimate the dynamic quality of the major dispositions and probably the range of influence of the individual difference under consideration. That being said, repeated exposure to certain kinds of environmental events alters the basic parameters of the inherited dispositions and motives.

Regarding the second question, the expression of such complex social behavior as helping is almost certainly the outcome of several different but related systems. When these systems operate at the same time, one system may reduce the influence of another. In the opponent-process model, the influence of Process A is much reduced once Process B is activated. From observing a single episode of helping or prejudice, a researcher might conclude that a single process is operative, but it is likely that the process is better studied only by observing the operation of the components over time.

The opponent-process model linking agreeableness to interpersonal behaviors and to more general self-regulatory processes (Tobin & Graziano, 2006) is novel, so many unanswered questions remain. Is agreeableness tied to the care system only or to fight–flight as well? Is it tied to both personal distress and empathic concern, to both prejudice and the suppression of prejudice, or to just one of these elements in each pair? We believe that the opponent-process approach to agreeableness allows us to anticipate phenomena that cannot be found elsewhere. Here we offer a few tentative ideas.

To the best of our knowledge, no empirical research has addressed the issue of delayed helping (but see Penner et al., 1995). In general, a common assumption is that the influence of a manipulation of victim need, mood state, or empathic concern will dissipate for most or all people over time. That is, rates of helping are affected by the interval between provision of information and the request for help and the opportunity to provide it. Note the analogue to the correction of prejudice outcomes reported by Pryor and colleagues (2004). If the opponent-process system operates roughly as described here, then some forms of helping may be greater after a short delay than they are following an immediate request. The initial fight–flight reaction may come under the control of the opponent care system, in effect disinhibiting helping with time. Undoubtedly, we would also see characteristic emotions, such as relief at finally having an opportunity to provide assistance. Based on the previous rationale, we would also expect persons high in agreeableness to offer more help, sooner and with less influence of delay, than persons low in agreeableness. At this point, such conjectures are speculative. Whatever outcomes do appear, it is clear that agreeableness and its associated motives for maintaining positive relationships with others will play a role in our deeper understanding of interpersonal processes.

Acknowledgments

This research was supported in part by grants from the National Science Foundation and the National Institutes of Health. We thank Meara

M. Habashi, Lauri A. Jensen-Campbell, John B. Pryor, Michael D. Robinson, and Brad E. Sheese for helpful suggestions and comments. We dedicate this chapter to the memory of John Digman, who encouraged us to conduct focal research on agreeableness.

References

Ahadi, S. A., & Rothbart, M. K. (1994). Temperament, development, and the Big Five. In C. F. Halverson, Jr., G. A. Kohnstamm, & R. P. Martin (Eds.), *The developing structure of temperament and personality from infancy to adulthood* (pp. 189–207). Hillsdale, NJ: Erlbaum.

Allport, G. W. (1954). *The nature of prejudice*. New York: Doubleday.

Batson, C. D. (1991). *The altruism question: Toward a social-psychological answer*. Hillsdale, NJ: Erlbaum.

Batson, C. D., Bolen, M. H., Cross, J. A., & Neuringer-Benefiel, H. E. (1986). Where is the altruism in the altruistic personality? *Journal or Personality and Social Psychology, 50*, 212–220.

Batson, C. D., Duncan, B. D., Ackerman, P., Buckley, T., & Birch, K. (1981). Is empathic emotion a source of altruistic motivation? *Journal of Personality and Social Psychology, 40*, 290–302.

Batson, C. D., O'Quin, K., Fultz, J., Vanderplas, M., & Isen, A. M. (1983). Influence of self-reported distress and empathy on egoistic versus altruistic motivation to help. *Journal of Personality and Social Psychology, 45*, 706–718.

Baumeister, R. F., & Campbell, W. K. (1999). The intrinsic appeal of evil: Sadism, sensational thrills, and threatened egotism. *Personality and Social Psychology Review, 3*, 210–221.

Byrne, D. (1997). An overview (and underview) of research and theory within the attraction paradigm. *Journal of Social and Personal Relationships, 14*, 417–431.

Carlo, G., Eisenberg, N., Troyer, D., Switzer, G., & Speer, A. L. (1991). The altruistic personality: In what contexts is it apparent? *Journal of Personality and Social Psychology, 61*, 450–458.

Cialdini, R. B., Schaller, M., Houlihan, D., Arias, K., Fultz, J., & Beaman, A. L. (1987). Empathy-based helping: Is it selflessly or selfishly motivated? *Journal of Personality and Social Psychology, 52*, 749–758.

Coke, J. S., Batson, C. D., & McDavis, K. (1978). Empathic mediation of helping: A two-stage model. *Journal of Personality and Social Psychology, 36*, 752–766.

Cole, P. M. (1986). Children's spontaneous control of facial expression. *Child Development, 57*, 1309–1321.

Costa, P. T., & McCrae, R. R. (1988). Personality in adulthood: A six-year longitudinal study of self-reports and spouse ratings on the NEO Personality Inventory. *Journal of Personality and Social Psychology, 54*(5), 853–863.

Davis, M. H. (1996). *Empathy: A social psychological approach*. Boulder, CO: Westview Press.

De Raad, B. (2000). *The Big Five personality factors: The psycholexical approach to personality*. Seattle, WA: Hogrefe & Huber.

De Raad, B., Hendriks, A. A. J., & Hofstee, W. K. B. (1994). The Big Five: A tip of the iceberg of individual differences. In C. F. Halverson, Jr., G. A. Kohnstamm, & R. P. Martin (Eds.), *The developing structure of temperament and personality from infancy to adulthood* (pp. 91–109). Hillsdale, NJ: Erlbaum.

Digman, J. M., & Takemoto-Chock, N. K. (1981). Factors in the natural language of personality: Re-analysis, comparison, and interpretation of six major studies. *Multivariate Behavioral Research, 16*(2), 149–170.

Dijker, A. J. M., & Koomen, W. (2007). *Stigmatization, tolerance, and repair: An integrative psychological analysis of responses to deviance*. New York: Cambridge University Press.

Dovidio, J. (1984). Helping behavior and altruism: An empirical and conceptual overview. In L. Berkowitz (Ed.), *Advances in experimental social psychology* (Vol. 17, pp. 362–427). New York: Academic Press.

Dovidio, J., Piliavin, J. A., Schroeder, D. A., & Penner, L. (2006). *The social psychology of prosocial behavior*. Mahwah, NJ: Erlbaum.

Eisenberg, N., Fabes, R. A., Miller, P. A., Fultz, J., Shell, R., Mathy, R. M., et al. (1989). Relation of sympathy and personal distress to prosocial behavior: A multimethod study. *Journal of Personality and Social Psychology, 57*, 55–66.

Feigl, H. (1970). The "orthodox" view of theories: Remarks in defense as well as critique. In M. Radner & S. Winokur (Eds.), *Minnesota studies in the philosophy of science: Analyses of theories and methods of physics and psychology* (pp. 3–16). Minneapolis: University of Minnesota Press.

Finch, J. F., Panter, A. T., & Caskie, G. I. L. (1999). Two approaches for identifying shared personality dimensions across methods. *Journal of Personality, 67*, 407–438.

Gleason, K. A., Jensen-Campbell, L. A., & Richardson, D. S. (2004). Agreeableness as a predictor of aggression in adolescence. *Aggressive Behavior, 30*(1), 43–61.

Goldberg, L. R. (1992). The development of markers of the Big Five factor structure. *Psychological Assessment, 4*, 26–42.

Goldberg, L. R. (1999). A broad-bandwidth, public domain, personality inventory measuring the lower-level facets of several five-factor models. In I. Mervielde, I. Deary, F. De Fruyt, & F. Ostendorf (Eds.), *Personality psychology in Europe* (Vol. 7, pp. 7–28). Tilburg, The Netherlands: Tilburg University Press.

Goldberg, L. R., Johnson, J. A., Eber, H. W., Hogan, R., Ashton, M. C., Cloninger, C. R., et al. (2006). The International Personality Item Pool and the future of public-domain personality measures. *Journal of Research in Personality, 40*(1), 84–96.

Graziano, W. G. (1994). The development of Agreeableness as a dimension of personality. In C. F. Halverson, Jr., G. A. Kohnstamm, & R. P. Martin (Eds.), *The developing structure of temperament and personality from infancy to adulthood* (pp. 339–354) Hillsdale, NJ: Erlbaum.

Graziano, W. G., & Bruce, J. W. (2008). Attraction

and the initiation of relationships: A review of the empirical literature. In S. Sprecher, A. Wenzel, & J. Harvey (Eds.), *Handbook of relationship initiation* (pp. 269–295). New York: Psychology Press.

Graziano, W. G., Bruce, J. W., Sheese, B. E., & Tobin, R. M. (2007). Attraction, personality, and prejudice: Liking none of the people most of the time. *Journal of Personality and Social Psychology, 93,* 565–582.

Graziano, W. G., & Eisenberg, N. (1997). Agreeableness: A dimension of personality. In R. Hogan, J. Johnson, & S. Briggs (Eds.), *Handbook of personality psychology* (pp. 795–824). San Diego, CA: Academic Press.

Graziano, W. G., Habashi, M. M., Sheese, B. E., & Tobin, R. M. (2007). Agreeableness, empathy, and helping: A person × situation perspective. *Journal of Personality and Social Psychology, 93,* 583–599.

Graziano, W. G., Hair, E. C., & Finch, J. F. (1997). Competitiveness mediates the link between personality and group performance. *Journal of Personality and Social Psychology, 73,* 1394–1408.

Graziano, W. G., Jensen-Campbell, L. A., & Hair, E. C. (1996). Perceiving interpersonal conflict and reacting to it: The case for Agreeableness. *Journal of Personality and Social Psychology, 70,* 820–835.

Graziano, W. G., Jensen-Campbell, L. A., Steele, R. G., & Hair, E. C. (1998). Unknown words in self-reported personality: Lethargic and provincial in Texas. *Personality and Social Psychology Bulletin, 24,* 893–905.

Graziano, W. G., & Tobin, R. M. (2002). Agreeableness: Dimension of personality or social desirability artifact? *Journal of Personality, 70,* 695–727.

Graziano, W. G., & Waschull, S. B. (1995). Social development and self-monitoring. In N. Eisenberg (Ed.), *Social development* (pp. 233–260). Thousand Oaks, CA: Sage.

Haas, B. W., Omura, K., Constable, R. T., & Canli, T. (2007). Is automatic emotion regulation associated with agreeableness? A perspective using a social neuroscience approach. *Psychological Science, 18,* 130–132.

Habashi, M. M. (2008). *Separating altruistic and egoistic motives for helping: An individual difference approach.* Unpublished doctoral dissertation, Purdue University.

Habashi, M. M., & Wegener, D. (2008). *Preliminary evidence that agreeableness is more closely related to responsiveness than conformity.* Unpublished manuscript, Purdue University.

Hair, E. C., & Graziano, W. G. (2003). Self-esteem, personality, and achievement in high school: A prospective longitudinal study in Texas. *Journal of Personality, 71,* 971–994.

Hamilton, W. D. (1964). The genetical evolution of social behaviour: I, II. *Journal of Theoretical Biology, 7,* 1–32.

Hogan, R., Hogan, J., & Roberts, B. W. (1996). Personality measurement and employment decisions: Questions and answers. *American Psychologist, 51*(5), 469–477.

Jensen-Campbell, L. A., & Graziano, W. G. (2001). Agreeableness as a moderator of interpersonal conflict. *Journal of Personality, 69,* 323–361.

Jensen-Campbell, L. A., & Graziano, W. G. (2005).

Two faces of temptation: Differing motives for self-control. *Merrill–Palmer Quarterly, 51,* 287–324.

Jensen-Campbell, L. A., Graziano, W. G., & West, S. G. (1995). Dominance, prosocial orientation, and female preferences: Do nice guys really finish last? *Journal of Personality and Social Psychology, 68,* 427–440.

Jensen-Campbell, L. A., Knack, J. M., Waldrip, A. M., & Campbell, S. D. (2007). Do Big Five personality traits associated with self-control influence the regulation of anger and aggression? *Journal of Research in Personality, 41*(2), 403–424.

Jensen-Campbell, L. A., & Malcolm, K. T. (2007). The importance of conscientiousness in adolescent interpersonal relationships. *Personality and Social Psychology Bulletin, 33*(3), 368–383.

Jensen-Campbell, L. A., Rosselli, M., Workman, K. A., Santisi, M., Rios, J. D., & Bojan, D. (2002). Agreeableness, conscientiousness and effortful control processes. *Journal of Research in Personality, 36,* 476–489.

John, O. P., & Srivastava, S. (1999). The Big Five trait taxonomy: History, measurement, and theoretical perspectives. In L. A. Pervin & O. P. John (Eds.), *Handbook of personality: Theory and research* (2nd ed., pp. 102–138). New York: Guilford Press.

Kelley, H. H., Holmes, J. G., Kerr, N. L., Reis, H. T., Rusbult, C. E., & Van Lange, P. A. M. (2003). *An atlas of interpersonal situations.* New York: Cambridge University Press.

Kenny, D. A. (1996). The design and analysis of social-interaction research. *Annual Review of Psychology, 47,* 59–86.

Kochanska, G., Murray, K., & Coy, K. C. (1997). Inhibitory control as a contributor to conscience in childhood: From toddler to early school age. *Child Development, 68,* 263–277.

Kohnstamm, G. A., Halverson, C. F., Jr., Mervielde, I., & Havill, V. L. (1998). Analyzing parental free description of child personality. In G. A. Kohnstamm, C. F. Halverson, Jr., I. Mervielde, & V. L. Havill (Eds.), *Parental description of child personality: Developmental antecedents of the Big Five?* (pp. 1–19). Mahwah, NJ: Erlbaum.

Krueger, R. F., Hicks, B. N., & McGue, M. (2001). Altruism and antisocial behavior: Independent tendencies, unique personality correlates, distinct etiologies. *Psychological Science, 12,* 397–402.

Lang, P. J., Bradley, M. M., & Cuthbert, B. N. (1995). *International Affective Picture System (IAPS): Technical manual and affective ratings.* Gainesville: University of Florida, Center for Research in Psychophysiology.

Larson, K. S., Reed, M., & Hoffman, S. (1980). Attitudes of heterosexuals toward homosexuals: A Likert-type scale and construct validity. *Journal of Sex Research, 16,* 245–257.

Lenney, E. (1991). Sex roles: The measurement of masculinity, femininity and androgyny. In J. P. Robinson, P. R. Shaver, & L. S. Wrightsman (Eds.), *Measures of personality and social psychological attitudes: Vol. 1. Measures of social psychological attitudes* (pp. 573–660). San Diego, CA: Academic Press.

Ode, S., & Robinson, M. D. (2008). *Can agreeableness turn gray skies blue?: A role for agreeable-*

ness in moderating neuroticism-linked depression. Manuscript submitted for publication.

Ode, S., Robinson, M. D., & Wilkowski, B. M. (2008). Can one's temper be cooled?: A role for agreeableness in moderating Neuroticism's influence on anger and aggression. *Journal of Research in Personality, 42*, 295–311.

Oliner, S. P., & Oliner, P. M. (1988). *The altruistic personality: Rescuers of Jews in Nazi Germany.* New York: Free Press.

Penner, L. A., Dovidio, J., Piliavin, J. A., & Schroeder, D. A. (2005). Prosocial behavior: Multilevel perspectives. *Annual Review of Psychology, 56*, 356–392.

Penner, L. A., Fritzsche, B. A., Craiger, J. P., & Freifeld, T. S. (1995). Measuring the prosocial personality. In J. N. Butcher & C. D. Spielberger (Eds.), *Advances in personality assessment* (Vol. 10, pp. 147–163). Hillsdale, NJ: Erlbaum.

Petty, R. E., & Wegener, D. T. (1999). The elaboration likelihood model: Current status and controversies. In S. Chaiken & Y. Trope (Eds.), *Dual-process theories in social psychology* (pp. 41–72). New York: Guilford Press.

Piliavin, J. A., Callero, P. L., & Evanset, D. E. (1982). Addiction to altruism?: Opponent-process theory and habitual blood donation. *Journal of Personality and Social Psychology, 43*, 1200–1213.

Piliavin, J. A., Dovidio, J., Gaertner, S., & Clark, R. D. (1982). *Emergency intervention.* New York: Academic Press.

Pryor, J. B., Reeder, G. D., Yeadon, C., & Hesson-McInnis, M. (2004). A dual-process model of reactions to perceived stigma. *Journal of Personality and Social Psychology, 87*(4), 436–452.

Rosenbaum, M. (1986). The repulsion hypothesis: On the nondevelopment of relationships. *Journal of Personality and Social Psychology, 51*, 1156–1166.

Rothbart, M. K., & Bates, J. E. (2006). Temperament. In N. Eisenberg, W. Damon, & R. M. Lerner (Eds.), *Handbook of child psychology: Vol. 3. Social, emotional, and personality development* (6th ed., pp. 99–166). Hoboken, NJ: Wiley.

Rothbart, M. K., & Posner, M. I. (1985). Temperament and the development of self-regulation. In L. C. Hartlage & C. F. Telzrow (Eds.), *The neuropsychology of individual differences: A developmental perspective* (pp. 93–123). New York: Plenum Press.

Saarni, C. (1984). An observational study of children's attempts to monitor their expressive behavior. *Child Development, 55*, 1504–1513.

Schroeder, D. A., Dovidio, J. F., Sibicky, M. E., Matthews, L. L., & Allen, J. L. (1988). Empathic concern and helping behavior: Egoism or altruism?

Journal of Experimental Social Psychology, 24, 333–353.

Shadish, W., Cook, T. D., & Campbell, D. T. (2002). *Experimental and quasi-experimental designs for generalized causal inference.* Boston: Houghton Mifflin.

Snyder, M., & Haugen, J. A. (1994). Why does behavioral confirmation occur? A functional perspective on the role of the perceiver. *Journal of Experimental Social Psychology, 30*, 218–246.

Solomon, R. (1980). The opponent-process theory of acquired motivation: The costs of pleasure and the benefits of pain. *American Psychologist, 35*, 691–712.

Solomon, R. L., & Corbit, J. D. (1974). An opponent-process theory of motivation: I. Temporal dynamics of affect. *Psychological Review, 57*, 119–145.

Spence, J. T., & Helmreich, R. L. (1979). The many faces of androgyny: A reply to Locksley and Colton. *Journal of Personality and Social Psychology, 37*, 1037–1042.

Tobin, R. M., & Graziano, W. G. (2006). Development of regulatory processes through adolescence: A review of recent empirical studies. In D. Mroczek & T. Little (Eds.), *Handbook of personality development* (pp. 263–283). Mahwah, NJ: Erlbaum.

Tobin, R. M., Graziano, W. G., Vanman, E. J., & Tassinary, L. G. (2000). Personality, emotional experience, and efforts to control emotions. *Journal of Personality and Social Psychology, 79*, 656–669.

Tobin, R. M., Kieras, J. E., & Graziano, W. G. (2003, April). *Parental influence and individual differences in children's emotional responses.* Poster presented at the meeting of the Society for Research in Child Development, Tampa, FL.

Tobin, R. M., Schneider, W. J., Graziano, W. G., & Pizzitola, K. M. (2002, February). *Nice kids in competitive situations.* Poster presented at the meeting of the Society for Personality and Social Psychology, Savannah, GA.

Toi, M., & Batson, C. D. (1982). More evidence that empathy is a source of altruistic motivation. *Journal of Personality and Social Psychology, 43*, 281–292.

Trivers, R. (1972). Parental investment and sexual selection. In B. Campbell (Ed.), *Sexual selections and the descent of man: 1871–1971* (pp. 136–179). Chicago: Aldine.

Wiggins, J. S. (1991). Agency and communion as conceptual coordinates for the understanding and measurement of interpersonal behavior. In W. Grove & D. Cicchetti (Eds.), *Thinking clearly about psychology: Essays in honor of Paul E. Meehl* (pp. 89–113). Minneapolis: University of Minnesota Press.

CHAPTER 5

■ ● ▲ ◆ ■ ● ▲ ◆

Attachment Styles

PHILLIP R. SHAVER
MARIO MIKULINCER

Attachment theory (Ainsworth, Blehar, Waters, & Wall, 1978; Bowlby, 1969/1982) was initially proposed as a way of understanding why close relationships in the family and the loss of such relationships are among the most important determinants of later social adjustment and mental health. The originator of the theory, John Bowlby, was a British psychoanalyst with an unusual interest in ethology and cognitive and developmental psychology. He was fortunate to form a working relationship with an American developmental psychologist, Mary Ainsworth, who added psychometric and research skills to Bowlby's astute clinical observations and exceptional ability to integrate diverse scientific literatures in the service of what, by today's standards, is a "grand theory."

The key components of the theory are few, and they are relatively easy to describe:

1. Humans and other primates evolved behavioral and motivational systems that allow them to survive and reproduce, despite vulnerabilities associated with being born prematurely, taking a long time to develop to maturity, and needing the protection, assistance, and cooperation of other species members across the lifespan.

2. One of these behavioral systems, the attachment system, is responsible for establishing primary social connections and calling on them in times of stress or difficulty.

3. The history of a person's close relationships shapes the parameters of his or her attachment system, leaving an important residue in the form of "internal working models" of self, partners, and relationships. This developmental process results in each person having a measurable "attachment style" (Hazan & Shaver, 1987) that influences the nature and outcomes of subsequent relationships, including those with romantic/sexual partners, close friends, offspring, and even coworkers and subordinates in social organizations (e.g., Davidovitz, Mikulincer, Shaver, Ijzak, & Popper, 2007).

In this chapter we describe the theory in more detail, explain how its key constructs are measured in studies of adolescents and adults, and provide a brief summary of research findings. A much more detailed account of the theory and the research it has generated can be found in our book, *Attachment in Adulthood* (Mikulincer & Shaver, 2007a).

Attachment Theory: Basic Concepts

The Attachment Behavioral System

In *Attachment and Loss*—one of the most cited series of books in contemporary psychology—Bowlby (1973, 1980, 1969/1982) attempted to map and understand the profound impact that the quality of early relationships with primary caregivers has on personality development and individual differences in social behavior across the lifespan. As a psychoanalyst, Bowlby was well aware that Freud and his followers had already explored this issue, but he was also aware that his fellow psychoanalysts had not effectively integrated their work and their interpretive approach to human problems with the rest of scientific psychology and psychiatry. By considering a vast array of empirical and theoretical writings ranging from clinical observations of infants deprived of maternal care to primate ethology and Piaget's theory of cognitive development, Bowlby came to the conclusion that a person's fundamental sense of safety, self-worth, coping efficacy, and well-being rests on the quality of his or her social interactions with close relationship partners, beginning with primary caregivers in infancy. He also concluded that when a person does not have reliable, trustworthy, supportive relationships with close others, personality development is distorted in ways that have serious negative consequences.

In explaining the motivational processes involved in personality development, which Freud attempted to do using concepts such as sexual and aggressive "drives" or "instincts," Bowlby (1969/1982) borrowed from primate ethology the concept of *behavioral systems*—species-universal, biologically evolved neural programs that organize behavior in ways that increase the likelihood of survival and reproduction. He portrayed these systems as similar to cybernetic control systems, which do not follow drive principles. According to Bowlby, one of the key behavioral systems is the *attachment system*, which has the biological function of protecting a person (especially during infancy and early childhood) from danger by ensuring that he or she maintains proximity to caring and supportive others (whom Bowlby, 1969/1982, called *attachment figures*). In Bowlby's view, the need to seek out and maintain proximity to attachment figures evolved in relation to

the prolonged dependence of human infants on "stronger and wiser" others (often, but not always, parents), who could defend them from predators and other dangers. Because human (and other primate) infants seem naturally to look for and gravitate toward *particular* others (those who are familiar and, at least sometimes, helpful) and to prefer them over alternative caregivers, Bowlby used the terms *affectional bond* and *attachment*, which is the reason for calling his formulation *attachment theory*. Although the attachment system is most important and most visible in behavior during the early years of life, Bowlby (1988) claimed that it is active across the lifespan and is frequently manifested in seeking support and love from close relationship partners. This inspired various researchers (e.g., Main, Kaplan, & Cassidy, 1985; Shaver, Hazan, & Bradshaw, 1988) to extend the theory into the domain of adult relationships.

The purported goal of the attachment system is to maintain a sense of safety or security (called "felt security" by Sroufe & Waters, 1977). In Bowlby's (1969/1982) view, the attachment behavioral system is particularly activated by events that threaten the sense of security, such as encounters with actual or symbolic threats or noticing that an attachment figure is not sufficiently near, interested, or responsive. In such cases, a person is automatically motivated to seek and reestablish actual or symbolic proximity to an attachment figure (a process Bowlby, 1969/1982, called the attachment system's "primary strategy"). These bids for proximity persist until protection and security are attained. The attachment system is then deactivated, and the person can calmly and coherently return to other activities, which Bowlby considered to be under the control of other behavioral systems (e.g., exploration, affiliation, caregiving). In infancy, attachment-system activation includes nonverbal expressions of distress, need, and desire for proximity (e.g., crying, calling) and locomotor behaviors aimed at reestablishing and maintaining proximity (Ainsworth et al., 1978). In adulthood, the primary attachment strategy does not necessarily require actual proximity-seeking behavior, although often such behavior is initiated; it can also involve the internal activation of comforting mental representations of relationship partners who regularly provide care and protection (Mikulincer & Shaver, 2004). These cognitive representations can create a sense of safety and security and help a person deal successfully with threats.

Individual Differences in Attachment-System Strategies

Although nearly all children are born with normal attachment systems, which motivate them to pursue proximity and security from an attachment figure in times of need, the quality of attachment-system functioning also depends on the availability of such a figure in times of need; his or her sensitivity and responsiveness to bids for closeness, comfort, and support; and his or her ability and willingness to alleviate distress and provide a secure base from which the child can return calmly to other activities (Bowlby, 1973, 1988). As Cassidy (1999) noted, "Whereas nearly all children become attached (even to mothers who abuse them; Bowlby, 1956), not all are securely attached" (p. 7). According to attachment theory, the quality of interactions with attachment figures in times of need is the major cause of individual differences in attachment-system functioning. (There may also be genetic causes, as shown recently by Crawford et al., 2007, and Donnellan, Burt, Levendosky, & Klump, 2008, a possibility that was mentioned early on by Bowlby, 1969/1982.)

When an attachment figure is available, sensitive, and responsive to an individual's proximity bids, the individual is likely to feel an inner sense of security—a sense that the world is a safe place, that others are helpful when called on, and that it is possible to explore the environment curiously and confidently and engage rewardingly with other people. This sense is an inner signal that the attachment system is functioning well and that proximity seeking is an effective emotion-regulatory strategy. Moreover, people acquire important procedural knowledge about distress management, which becomes organized around a relational script (Waters, Rodrigues, & Ridgeway, 1998; Waters & Waters, 2006). The secure form of this script includes the following if–then propositions: "If I encounter an obstacle and/or become distressed, then I can approach a significant other for help; he or she is likely

to be available and supportive; I will experience relief and comfort as a result of proximity to this person; I can then return to other activities."

When an attachment figure is not physically or emotionally available in times of need, not responsive to one's bids for proximity, or poor at alleviating distress or providing a secure base, attachment-system functioning is disrupted, and the individual does not experience comfort, relief, or felt security. Rather, the distress that initially activated the system is compounded by serious doubts about the feasibility of attaining a sense of security: "Is the world a safe place or not? Can I trust others in times of need? Do I have the resources necessary to manage my own negative emotions?" These worries about self and others can maintain the attachment system in a continually activated state, keep a person's mind preoccupied with threats and the need for protection, and interfere drastically with other activities.

Frustrating interactions with inadequately available or unresponsive attachment figures indicate that the attachment system's operating parameters need to be adjusted. This implies that certain *secondary attachment strategies* need to be adopted rather than continuing to rely only on the primary strategy, confident proximity seeking. Attachment theorists (e.g., Cassidy & Kobak, 1988; Main, 1990) have emphasized two such secondary strategies: *hyperactivation* and *deactivation* of the attachment system. Hyperactivating strategies emerge from interactions with attachment figures who are sometimes responsive but only unreliably so, placing the attached person on a partial reinforcement schedule that seems to reward energetic, strident, noisy proximity bids because they sometimes seem to succeed. In such cases, people do not easily give up on proximity seeking, and in fact they intensify it as a way to demand the attachment figure's love and support. The main goal of these strategies is to get an attachment figure, viewed as unreliable or insufficiently available and responsive, to pay attention and provide protection or support. The chosen way to pursue this goal is to maintain the attachment system in a chronically activated state. This involves exaggerating appraisals of danger and signs of attachment-figure unavailability and intensifying demands for attention, affection, and assistance. When repeatedly practiced, this secondary strategy becomes what we call an anxious attachment style.

Deactivating strategies are another reaction to an attachment figure's unavailability, and they seem to arise in conjunction with attachment figures who disapprove of and punish closeness and expressions of need or vulnerability. In such relationships, an individual learns to expect better outcomes if signs of need and vulnerability are hidden or suppressed, proximity bids are weakened or blocked, the attachment system is deactivated despite a sense of security not being achieved, and attempts are made to handle threats by oneself (a strategy Bowlby, 1969/1982, called "compulsive self-reliance"). The primary goal of deactivating strategies is to keep the attachment system down-regulated to avoid the distress caused by an attachment figure's unavailability or rejection. This deactivation requires denying attachment needs, steering clear of closeness and interdependence in relationships, and distancing oneself from threats that might cause unwanted activation of the attachment system.

Attachment Working Models

Beyond characterizing individual differences in attachment-system functioning during interactions with attachment figures, Bowlby (1973) also proposed that such interactions can be incorporated into mental structures that eventually become relatively stable personality patterns. At the core of these mental structures are what Bowlby called *internal working models*. The term *working* has two meanings in attachment theory. One is that the models are not static representations but rather are the basis of social expectations, inferences about the likely outcomes of alternative social behaviors, and behavioral programs that can be enacted in relationships. The other meaning of *working* is that the models are based on past experiences and can be revised based on new experiences. This characteristic is what makes personality change and successful relationship-oriented psychotherapy possible (Bowlby, 1988).

Bowlby thought that interactions with attachment figures were stored in at least two kinds of working models: representations of attachment figures' responses (*working models of others*) and representations of the self's lovability and competence (*working models of self*). He argued that "if an individual is to draw up a plan to achieve a set-goal not only does he have to have some sort of working model of his environment, but he must have also some working knowledge of his own behavioral skills and potentialities" (1969/1982, p. 112). Thus the attachment system, once it has been activated repeatedly during interactions with a specific attachment figure, includes representations of the availability, responsiveness, and sensitivity of such a figure, as well as representations of the self's own capabilities for mobilizing the attachment figure's support and one's feelings of being loved and valued by this figure.

Because working models, at least initially, are based on the internalization of specific interactions with a particular attachment figure, a person can hold multiple working models that differ in the outcome of the interaction (success or failure to attain security) and the strategy used to deal with the distress caused by attachment-figure unavailability (hyperactivating or deactivating, anxious or avoidant). Like other cognitive representations, these working models form excitatory and inhibitory associations with each other (e.g., experiencing or thinking about a security attainment activates memories of congruent episodes of successful proximity bids and renders memories of attachment-figure unavailability less accessible), and these associations favor the formation of more abstract and generalized representations of a relationship with a specific partner. Thus models with a specific attachment figure (relationship-specific models) are created, and through excitatory and inhibitory links with models representing interactions with other attachment figures, even more generic working models are formed to summarize different kinds of relationships. The result of this process can be conceptualized as a hierarchical associative memory network that includes episodic memories, relationship-specific models, and generic models of security attainment, hyperactivation, and deactivation. As a result, with respect to a particular relationship and across different relationships, most people can sometimes think about interpersonal relations in secure terms and at other times think about them in less secure terms. In a 2003 paper, Overall, Fletcher, and Friesen provided empirical support for this hierarchical structure of attachment working models.

Each working model within the hierarchical network differs in cognitive accessibility—that is, in the ease with which it can be activated and used to guide the functioning of the attachment system in a given social interaction. As with other cognitive representations, the strength or accessibility of each model is determined by the amount of experience on which it is based, the number of times it has been applied in the past, and the density of its connections with other working models (e.g., Baldwin, 1992; Shaver et al., 1996). At a relationship-specific level, the model representing the typical interaction with an attachment figure has the highest accessibility in subsequent interactions with that person. At a generic level, the model that represents interactions with major attachment figures (e.g., parents and romantic partners) becomes the most chronically accessible working model and has the strongest effect on attachment-system functioning across relationships and over time.

Consolidation of a chronically accessible working model is the most important psychological process accounting for the enduring, long-term effects on personality functioning of attachment-relevant interactions during infancy, childhood, and adolescence (Bowlby, 1973; Fraley, 2002; Waters, Merrick, Treboux, Crowell, & Albersheim, 2000). Given a fairly consistent pattern of interactions with primary caregivers during childhood, the most representative or prototypical working models of these interactions become part of a person's implicit procedural knowledge, tend to operate automatically and unconsciously, and are resistant to change. Thus what began as representations of specific interactions with a primary caregiver during childhood become core personality characteristics; they tend to be applied in new situations and relationships, and they shape the functioning of the attachment system in adulthood.

The Concept of Attachment Style

According to attachment theory (Bowlby, 1988; Mikulincer & Shaver, 2007a), a particular history of attachment experiences and the resulting consolidation of chronically accessible working models lead to the formation of relatively stable individual differences in the operating parameters of the attachment system. These stable and generalized individual differences can be empirically examined by measuring a construct called *attachment style*—a person's characteristic pattern of expectations, needs, emotions, and behavior in social interactions and close relationships (Hazan & Shaver, 1987). Depending on how it is measured, attachment style characterizes the way people behave in a particular relationship (relationship-specific style) or across relationships (global attachment style).

The concept of attachment style, although not given that name, was first proposed by Ainsworth (1967) to describe infants' patterns of responses to separations from and reunions with their mothers in a laboratory "Strange Situation" assessment procedure. Based on this procedure, infants were classified into one of three style categories: secure, anxious, or avoidant. Main and Solomon (1990) later added a fourth category, "disorganized/disoriented," which included odd, awkward behavior and unusual fluctuations between anxiety and avoidance. Ainsworth and colleagues (1978) noticed that the different infant attachment patterns can be arrayed in a two-dimensional space based on the anxiety and avoidance dimensions. This possibility has also been pursued in subsequent studies of romantic and global attachment styles.

Infants classified as secure seem to possess chronically accessible working models of secure attachment, and their pattern of responses to separation and reunion reflects a stable sense of attachment security. Specifically, they react to separation from their mothers with overt expressions of distress but then recover quickly and continue to explore the environment with interest. When reunited with their mothers, they greet them with joy and affection, respond positively to being held, and initiate contact with them (Ainsworth et al., 1978). Avoidant infants seem to hold chronically accessible working models of unsuccessful proximity bids organized around attachment-system deactivation. During separation and reunion episodes, they show little distress when separated from their mothers and seem to actively avoid them on reunion (Ainsworth et al., 1978). Anxious infants also seem to hold chronically accessible working models of frustrated proximity bids, but these models seem to be organized around attachment-system hyperactivation. These infants show overt expressions of distress and despair during separation episodes and conflictual, angry responses toward their mothers on reunion (Ainsworth et al., 1978). The two different insecure patterns can be viewed as defensive styles, one based on attempting to shut down or deactivate the attachment system in order to avoid punishment or frustration and the other based on attempting to escalate the expression of negative emotion until a more security-enhancing response from an attachment figure is attained.

In the 1980s, researchers from different psychological fields (developmental, clinical, personality, and social psychology) constructed new measures of attachment style in order to extend attachment research into adolescence and adulthood. Based on a developmental and clinical approach, Main and her colleagues (George, Kaplan, & Main, 1985; Main et al., 1985; see Hesse, 2008, for a review) devised the Adult Attachment Interview (AAI) to study adolescents' and adults' mental representations of attachment to their parents during childhood. In the AAI, interviewees answer open-ended questions about their childhood relationships with parents and are classified into three categories paralleling Ainsworth's infant typology: "secure" (or free and autonomous with respect to attachment), "dismissing" (of attachment), or "preoccupied" (with attachment). A person is classified as secure if he or she describes parents as available and responsive and if his or her memories of relationships with parents are presented in a clear, convincing, and coherent manner. Dismissing individuals play down the importance of attachment relationships and tend to recall few concrete episodes of emotional interactions with their parents. Preoccupied people are entangled in worries and angry feelings about parents and, although they can easily retrieve negative memories, they have trouble discussing them coherently without becoming overwhelmed and disorganized by anger or anxiety. In recent years, new categories have been added to the AAI coding system, because some adults seem either to be unresolved with respect to traumas or losses or to be unclassifiable into any of the major attachment categories. These patterns, which would take us beyond our space limitations to discuss, are associated with having a child with the new, fourth attachment pattern, "disorganized/disoriented" (Main & Solomon, 1990), which in turn is most strongly related to later psychopathology. These issues are among the most actively studied by clinically oriented attachment researchers because of their applied significance.

Despite the great value of the AAI as a method of studying adults' attachment patterns, the interview is difficult to administer and score, and it focuses almost exclusively on an adult's early relationships with parents. Taking a different path into the domain of adult attachment, Hazan and Shaver (1987; Shaver et al., 1988) applied Bowlby's ideas to the study of romantic relationships. Because they developed their ideas within the framework of personality–social psychology, they began with a simple self-report measure of adult attachment style. This measure consisted of three brief descriptions of feelings and behaviors in romantic relationships that were intended to be adult analogues of the three infant attachment styles identified by Ainsworth et al. (1978). Participants were asked to read the three descriptions and then place themselves into one of the three attachment categories according to their predominant feelings and behavior in romantic relationships. The three descriptions were:

Secure: I find it relatively easy to get close to others and am comfortable depending on them and having them depend on me. I don't worry about being abandoned or about someone getting too close to me.

Avoidant: I am somewhat uncomfortable being close to others; I find it difficult to trust them completely, difficult to allow myself to depend on them. I am nervous when anyone gets too close, and often others want me to be more intimate than I feel comfortable being.

Anxious: I find that others are reluctant to get as close as I would like. I often worry that my partner doesn't really love me or won't want to stay with me. I want to get very close to my partner, and this sometimes scares people away.

Hazan and Shaver's (1987, 1990) initial studies were followed by hundreds of others that used the simple forced-choice self-report measure to examine the interpersonal and intrapersonal correlates of adult attachment style (see Mikulincer & Shaver, 2007a, for a review). Over time, attachment researchers made methodological and conceptual improvements to the original self-report measure, improvements that included using Likert (agree–disagree) scales to rate the extent to which each of the three prototypes described one's experiences in romantic relationships (e.g., Levy & Davis, 1988); decomposition of the descriptions into separate items that formed multi-item scales (e.g., Collins & Read, 1990; Feeney & Noller, 1990); splitting the avoidant category into "dismissing" and "fearful" subtypes, thus moving from a three- to a four-category classification scheme (Bartholomew & Horowitz, 1991); and rewording the instructions and items to examine global attachment style in close relationships generally (not just romantic relationships), as well as relationship-specific styles (e.g., Baldwin, Keelan, Fehr, Enns, & Koh Rangarajoo, 1996; La Guardia, Ryan, Couchman, & Deci, 2000). (The history of this kind of measurement is spelled out in detail in Chapter 4, Mikulincer & Shaver, 2007a.)

Today, adult attachment researchers working from a personality–social perspective largely agree that attachment styles are best conceptualized as regions in a two-dimensional (anxiety-by-avoidance) space. The two dimensions are consistently obtained in factor analyses of attachment measures (e.g., Brennan, Clark, & Shaver, 1998). Moreover, Fraley and Waller (1998) demonstrated that dimensional representations of attachment style are more accurate than categorical representations. The first dimension, attachment-related *anxiety*, is concerned with a strong desire for closeness and protection, intense worries about partner availability and one's own value to the partner, and the use of hyperactivating strategies for dealing with insecurity and distress. The second dimension, attachment-related *avoidance*, is concerned with discomfort with closeness and dependence on relationship partners, preference for emotional distance and self-reliance, and the use of deactivating strategies to deal with insecurity and distress.

People who score low on both dimensions are said to be secure or to have a secure attachment style. They enjoy a chronic sense of attachment security, trust in partners and expectations of partner availability and responsiveness, comfort with closeness and interdependence, and constructive ways of coping with threats and stressors. People who score high on both dimensions (labeled "fearful avoidants" by Bartholomew & Horowitz, 1991) are especially low in trust and seem more likely than other people to have been hurt or abused in important relationships (Shaver & Clark, 1994).

The two attachment-style dimensions can be measured with the 36-item Experiences in Close Relationships inventory (ECR; Brennan et al., 1998), which is reliable in both the internal-consistency and test–retest senses and has high construct, predictive, and discriminant validity (Crowell, Fraley, & Shaver, 1999). Eighteen items tap the avoidance dimension (e.g., "I try to avoid getting too close to my partner"; "I prefer not to show a partner how I feel deep down"), and 18 tap the anxiety dimension (e.g., "I need a lot of reassurance that I am loved by my partner"; "I resent it when my partner spends time away from me"). (Slightly revised but similar versions of the scales, labeled the ECR-R, were created by Fraley, Waller, & Brennan, 2000.) The two scales were conceptualized as independent and have been found to be empirically uncorrelated in most studies. Hundreds of studies using self-report measures of adult attachment style, some based on three categories, some on four categories, and some on two dimensions, have found theoretically coherent attachment-style variations in relationship quality, interpersonal behavior, self-esteem, social cognitions, emotion regulation, ways of coping with stress, and mental health. In the remaining sections of this chapter, we provide brief examples of these studies (for a comprehensive review, see Mikulincer & Shaver, 2007a).

Individual Differences Related to Attachment Style

Relationship Quality

In the original studies of adult attachment style, Hazan and Shaver (1987) provided initial evidence for an association between a person's attachment style (measured with the three-category measure reproduced earlier in this chapter) and the way he or she construes experiences of romantic love. Specifically, they found that people who classified themselves as securely attached reported that their love relationships were friendly, warm, trusting, and supportive; they emphasized intimacy as the core feature of these relationships; and they said they believed in the existence of romantic love and the possibility of maintaining intense love over a long time period. People with an avoidant style described their romantic relationships as low in warmth, lacking friendly interactions, and low in emotional involvement; and they said that romantic love fades with time. In contrast, people who reported an anxious attachment style described their romantic relationships in terms of obsession and passion, strong physical attraction, desire for union with the partner, and proneness to fall in love quickly and perhaps indiscriminately. At the same time, they characterized their lovers as untrustworthy and inadequately supportive; they confessed to intense bouts of jealousy and anger toward romantic partners, as well as worries about rejection and abandonment. Subsequent studies have replicated and extended these initial findings, indicating that anxiously attached individuals are less confident than their more secure counterparts about being able to establish successful relationships (e.g., Carnelley & Janoff-Bulman, 1992; Pietromonaco & Carnelley, 1994) and more likely to emphasize potential losses when thinking about relationships (Boon & Griffin, 1996).

There is good evidence that secure individuals tend to maintain more stable romantic relationships than insecure people (either anxious or avoidant) and report higher levels of relationship satisfaction and adjustment (see Mikulincer & Shaver, 2007a). This pattern has been consistently obtained in studies of both dating and married couples and cannot be explained by other personality factors, such as the "Big Five" personality traits or self-esteem (Mikulincer, Florian, Cowan, & Cowan, 2002; Noftle & Shaver, 2006). For example, Davila, Karney, and Bradbury (1999) collected data every 6 months for 3 years from newlywed couples and found that changes in husbands' and wives' reports of secure attachment predicted concurrent changes in both partners' reports of marital satisfaction. Studies have also linked attachment security with greater intimacy (e.g., Collins & Read, 1990; Feeney & Noller,

1990), stronger relational commitment (e.g., Shaver & Brennan, 1992; Simpson, 1990), and stronger relational cohesion (Mikulincer & Florian, 1999).

Attachment style seems to be involved in several interpersonal processes that facilitate or hinder the maintenance of a satisfactory couple relationship. For example, several studies have found that higher scores along the attachment anxiety or avoidance dimension are associated with less constructive, less mutually sensitive patterns of dyadic communication (e.g., Feeney, 1994; Fitzpatrick, Fey, Segrin, & Schiff, 1993). Moreover, secure partners have been found to maintain more positive patterns of nonverbal communication (expressiveness, pleasantness, attentiveness) than less secure partners (e.g., Guerrero, 1996; Tucker & Anders, 1998) and to be more accurate in expressing their feelings and noticing their partners' nonverbal signals (e.g., Feeney, 1994). A person's attachment style has also been related to the methods couples adopt to manage interpersonal tensions and conflicts (e.g., Gaines et al., 1997; Scharfe & Bartholomew, 1995). Specifically, secure people rely more heavily on effective conflict resolution strategies—compromising and integrating their own and their partners' positions. They also display greater accommodation when responding to partners' anger or criticism. In contrast, insecure people tend to rely on less effective conflict resolution strategies that leave conflicts unresolved and may even lead to conflict escalation. Whereas anxious hyperactivating strategies lead people to intensify conflict, avoidant deactivating strategies lead people to distance themselves from conflictual interactions and to avoid engaging with their partners.

Attachment style is also associated with sexual motivation and sexual behavior, as would be expected based on Bowlby's (1969/1982) contention that the attachment behavioral system and the sexual behavioral system are intertwined in romantic/sexual relationships (e.g., Brennan & Shaver, 1995; Mikulincer & Shaver, 2007b; Tracy, Shaver, Albino, & Cooper, 2003). Attachment security is associated with sexual satisfaction and is conducive to genuine intimacy in sexual situations, including sensitivity and responsiveness to a partner's wishes and openness to mutual sexual exploration. In contrast, avoidant individuals tend to remain emotionally detached during sexual activities, and anxiously attached individuals tend to hyperactivate sex-related worries and engage in sex primarily to placate a partner, feel accepted, and avoid abandonment (Brassard, Shaver, & Lussier, 2007; Davis, Shaver, & Vernon, 2004; Schachner & Shaver, 2004).

Insecurely attached people's approach to sexual activities can also hinder marital satisfaction by fostering relational tensions related to fidelity, betrayal, and jealousy. For example, Schachner and Shaver (2002) found that avoidant attachment is associated with "mate poaching"—attempts to attract someone who is already in a relationship and being open to being "poached" by others—and with low scores on a relationship exclusivity scale. In contrast, the tendency of anxious individuals to hyperactivate vigilance and concern regarding the possibility of losing their sexual partners can lead to intense bouts of jealousy, which in turn endanger relationship stability and quality. There is extensive evidence that anxiously attached individuals are prone to jealousy and tend to be overwhelmed by jealous feelings (e.g., Guerrero, 1998; Sharpsteen & Kirkpatrick, 1997). Furthermore, they tend to report high levels of suspicion and to cope with them by engaging in intensive partner surveillance (Guerrero, 1998).

Interpersonal Interactions

People differing in attachment style seem to differ in the way they construe and experience interpersonal exchanges. In six studies, the Rochester Interaction Record (RIR; Reis & Wheeler, 1991) was used to examine attachment-style differences in daily interpersonal interactions over the course of 1 to 2 weeks (Kafetsios & Nezlek, 2002; Kerns & Stevens, 1996; Pierce & Lydon, 2001; Pietromonaco & Barrett, 1997; Sibley, Fischer, & Liu, 2005; Tidwell, Reis, & Shaver, 1996). As compared with secure people, avoidant ones reported lower levels of satisfaction, intimacy, self-disclosure, supportive behaviors, and positive emotions during daily interactions, as well as higher levels of negative emotions (e.g., boredom, tension). In addition, Tidwell and colleagues (1996) found that more avoidant people interacted less often and for shorter times with oppo-

site-sex partners. As compared with secure people, anxious ones reported higher levels of negative emotions and feelings of rejection, especially when interacting with opposite-sex partners. Tidwell and colleagues also found that attachment anxiety was associated with more variability or lability in emotional responses and closeness-promoting behavior. Thus, whereas avoidant people seemed to steer clear of intimate exchanges and feel uninvolved, tense, and bored during daily interactions, more anxious people experienced and displayed greater levels of distress and more ups and downs across interactions. This finding fits well with other evidence concerning anxious people's ambivalence and the strong influence of perceived availability or unavailability of attachment figures on their emotional reactions (e.g., Bartz & Lydon, 2006; Pierce & Lydon, 2001).

Interestingly, Gallo and Matthews (2006) showed that insecurely attached people's negative experiences of daily interpersonal interactions tend to be manifested in cardiovascular responses. Attachment anxiety was associated with less pleasant and more conflictual interpersonal exchanges and, more important, with heightened ambulatory diastolic and systolic blood pressure during interactions with friends. Avoidant attachment was associated with heightened ambulatory diastolic blood pressure during conflictual interpersonal interactions. These findings suggest that attachment insecurities amplify stress-related physiological reactions to daily interpersonal interactions.

A person's attachment style also shapes his or her reactions to specific kinds of interpersonal exchanges. For example, extensive evidence documents attachment-style differences in the ways people react to others' offenses and hurtful behaviors. These studies have consistently linked attachment security with functional, constructive expressions of anger (nonhostile protests) and attachment insecurity with less functional forms of anger, such as animosity, hostility, vengeful criticism, or vicious retaliation (e.g., Mikulincer, 1998b; Rholes, Simpson, & Orina, 1999; Shaver, Mikulincer, Lavy, & Cassidy, in press; Simpson, Rholes, & Phillips, 1996). In addition, more avoidant people tend to be less inclined to forgive a hurtful partner and more likely to withdraw or seek revenge

(Mikulincer, Shaver, & Slav, 2006). They also reported more intense feelings of vulnerability or humiliation, a stronger sense of relationship deterioration, and less empathy and understanding associated with forgiving the offending partner.

Mikulincer, Shaver, and Slav (2006) provided initial evidence that people differing in attachment style also differ in the way they react to episodes in which another person behaves positively toward them. Compared with less avoidant people, those scoring high on avoidance were less disposed to feel gratitude. Moreover, when avoidant people were asked to recall a time when they felt grateful to a relationship partner, they tended to remember more negative experiences, involving more narcissistic threats (e.g., "I felt I was risking my personal freedom"; "I thought I was giving up my dignity") and distrust, and less happiness and love. These negative responses reflect avoidant people's unwillingness to depend on or be supported by others or to express emotions, such as gratitude, that can be interpreted as indicating relational closeness or interdependence.

Attachment style is also associated with a person's attitudes and behaviors during episodes in which another person expresses signs of distress and neediness. Several studies have shown that attachment security is associated with higher scores on self-report scales tapping responsiveness to a relationship partner's needs (e.g., Feeney, 1996; Kunce & Shaver, 1994) and more supportive actual behaviors toward a distressed partner (e.g., Fraley & Shaver, 1998; Simpson, Rholes, & Nelligan, 1992). In addition, Westmaas and Silver (2001) found that avoidant attachment was associated with negative attitudes toward a person who had been diagnosed with cancer and that attachment anxiety was associated with high levels of distress during an interaction with the ill person. Mikulincer and colleagues (2001) and Mikulincer, Shaver, Gillath, and Nitzberg (2005) found that both dispositional and situationally augmented attachment security were associated with heightened empathy and compassion for a suffering individual.

There is also evidence that attachment security is associated with prosocial values. Mikulincer and colleagues (2003) reported that chronic and contextually augmented attachment security was associated with stronger endorsement of personal values reflecting concern for other people's welfare. In addition, Gillath and colleagues (2005) found that avoidant attachment was negatively associated with engagement in various altruistic activities, such as caring for older adults and donating blood. Although attachment anxiety was not related to overall involvement in such volunteer activities, it was associated with more self-enhancing or self-soothing motives for volunteering (e.g., to feel better about oneself, to enjoy a sense of belonging). Overall, these studies indicate that attachment insecurities interfere with prosocial feelings and behaviors.

Attachment Sources of Self-Esteem

As mentioned earlier, Bowlby (1973) argued that children construct a model of themselves while interacting with attachment figures in times of need. During episodes of attachment-figure availability, children can easily perceive themselves as valuable, lovable, and special when they are valued, loved, and regarded as special by a caring attachment figure. Moreover, they learn to view themselves as active, strong, and competent, because they can effectively mobilize a parent's support and restore emotional equanimity. In this way, interactions with responsive others and the resulting sense of attachment security become primary sources of feelings of self-worth and mastery.

Adult attachment research consistently shows that attachment security is strongly associated with positive self-representations. As compared with anxiously attached people, secure ones report higher self-esteem (e.g., Bartholomew & Horowitz, 1991; Mickelson, Kessler, & Shaver, 1997), view themselves as more competent and efficacious (e.g., Cooper, Shaver, & Collins, 1998), and possess more optimistic expectations about their ability to cope with stressful events (e.g., Berant, Mikulincer, & Florian, 2001; Cozzarelli, Sumer, & Major; 1998). Attachment security is also associated with having a coherent, balanced, and well-organized model of self. In a series of studies, Mikulincer (1995) found that, although participants with secure attachment styles tended to recall more positive than negative self-relevant traits, they had ready cognitive access to both positive and negative self-attributes in a Stroop task. In addition, they revealed a highly differentiated and integrated self-organization in trait-sorting tasks and had relatively small discrepancies between actual-self representations and self-standards (ideal-self and ought-self representations). That is, attachment security not only encourages positive self-appraisals but also seems to allow people to tolerate weak points in the self and integrate them within a coherent and overall positive self-structure.

According to attachment theory, both of the secondary attachment strategies (anxious hyperactivation and avoidant deactivation) distort a person's sense of self-worth, but in different ways. Whereas hyperactivating strategies negatively bias anxious people's sense of self-esteem, deactivating strategies favor defensive processes of self-enhancement and self-inflation. On the one hand, anxious hyperactivating strategies cause attention to be directed to self-relevant sources of distress (e.g., thoughts about personal weaknesses) and exacerbate self-defeating self-presentational tendencies, which involve emphasizing helplessness and vulnerability as a way of eliciting other people's compassion and support. On the other hand, avoidant deactivating strategies divert attention away from self-relevant sources of distress and encourage the adoption of a self-reliant attitude, which requires exaggeration of strengths and self-worth.

In studies of these defensive biases, Mikulincer (1998a) examined the way people differing in attachment style also differ in their self-appraisals following threatening and neutral situations. Participants with an avoidant attachment style made more positive self-appraisals following threatening as compared with neutral situations. In contrast, anxiously attached participants reacted to threat with self-devaluation, making more negative self-appraisals following threatening as compared with neutral conditions. Mikulincer noted that introducing contextual factors that inhibited defensive tendencies (e.g., a "bogus pipeline" device that measures "true feelings about things") inhibited avoidant participants' self-inflation response, as well as anxious participants' self-devaluation response. That is, insecure people's self-appraisals seemed to be strategic defensive maneuvers aimed at convincing

other people of the strength of the avoidant self or the neediness of the anxious self.

Attachment Sources of Person Perception

Extensive evidence links attachment security to positive perceptions of relationship partners. As compared with insecure individuals, securely attached people have more positive views of their romantic partners (e.g., Collins & Read, 1990), perceive their partners as more supportive (e.g., Collins & Read, 1990), and feel more trusting and affectionate toward their partners (e.g., Collins & Read, 1990; Simpson, 1990). Attachment security is also associated with positive expectations concerning partner behaviors (e.g., Baldwin, Fehr, Keedian, Seidel, & Thompson, 1993; Baldwin et al., 1996). For example, Baldwin and colleagues (1993) examined the cognitive accessibility of expectations concerning partner's behaviors in a lexical-decision task and found that secure people had poorer access to negative partner behaviors (e.g., partner being hurtful) than anxious and avoidant people. Attachment security is also associated with more positive explanations of a relationship partner's behavior (e.g., Collins, 1996; Mikulincer, 1998a). Collins (1996) asked participants to explain hypothetical negative behaviors of a romantic partner and found that more secure individuals were more likely to attribute partner's negative behaviors to unintentional, unstable, and highly specific causes and less likely to provide explanations that had negative implications for relationship stability.

In contrast, insecure people tend to describe specific friends and romantic partners in negative terms and also hold negative views of humanity in general. For example, Collins and Read (1990) reported that anxiously attached people were more likely to believe that others are difficult to understand and that they have little control over their lives. These authors also found that avoidant individuals were less likely than other people to believe that human beings are altruistic, willing to stand up for their beliefs, or able to control their lives. Subsequent studies have found that these negative views are also manifested in insecure people's lack of esteem for and acceptance of others (e.g., Luke, Maio, & Carnelley, 2004; Shaver et al., 1996), doubts about other people's trustworthiness (e.g., Cozzarelli, Hoekstra, & Bylsma, 2000), and lack of respect for relationship partners (Frei & Shaver, 2002).

Secondary attachment strategies are also likely to bias person perception. Avoidant individuals, who want to maintain distance from others and view themselves as strong and perfect, are also likely to view themselves as distinctive, unique, and better than other people. In contrast, anxiously attached people, who want to be loved and accepted, are likely to perceive themselves as more like others, especially in sharing similar problems, so they can more easily feel connected to others. For example, Mikulincer, Orbach, and Iavnieli (1998) found that whereas anxious individuals were more likely than their secure counterparts to perceive others as similar to themselves and to exhibit a false-consensus bias in both trait and opinion descriptions, avoidant individuals were more likely than secure individuals to perceive others as dissimilar to them and to exhibit a false-distinctiveness bias. Mikulincer and colleagues also found that anxious individuals reacted to threats by generating self-descriptions that were more similar to their partners' self-descriptions. Avoidant individuals, in contrast, reacted to the same threats by generating self-descriptions that were less similar to their partners' and by forgetting more of the traits they and their partners shared.

Emotion Regulation, Coping with Stress, and Mental Health

According to attachment theory, interactions with available attachment figures and the resulting sense of attachment security provide actual and symbolic contexts in which to learn constructive emotion regulation strategies. Beyond strengthening a person's confidence in the effectiveness of proximity bids and support seeking, episodes of attachment-figure availability facilitate the adoption of other constructive regulatory strategies mentioned earlier in this chapter: acknowledgment and display of distress, positively reappraising the distress-eliciting situation, and engaging in instrumental problem solving.

Interactions with emotionally accessible and responsive others provide the context in which a child learns that acknowledgment and display of emotions are functional steps toward restoring emotional equanimity and that one can feel comfortable exploring, acknowledging, and expressing one's own emotions (Cassidy, 1994). In adult attachment research, there is extensive evidence that secure people, as compared with less secure ones, tend to score higher on self-report and behavioral measures of emotional expressiveness (e.g., Feeney, 1995; Searle & Meara, 1999) and self-disclosure (e.g., Keelan, Dion, & Dion, 1998; Mikulincer & Nachshon, 1991). For example, Mikulincer and Nachshon (1991) content-analyzed participants' face-to-face verbal disclosures of personal information to another person and found that secure participants disclosed more intimate and emotion-laden information than avoidant participants. Moreover, using a biographical memory task in which participants were asked to recall specific, early memories of positive and negative emotions, Mikulincer and Orbach (1995) found that secure participants had more ready mental access to painful memories of anger, sadness, and anxiety than avoidant people. When compared with anxious people, secure people still had better access to positive memories of happiness and experienced less automatic spread of memories of other negative emotional experiences.

According to attachment theory, interactions with available and supportive attachment figures promote and reaffirm optimistic and hopeful appraisals of person–environment transactions. During positive interactions with good attachment figures, children gradually become convinced that distress is manageable, that external obstacles can be overcome, and that restoration of emotional equanimity is only a matter of time. As a result, secure people can make self-soothing reappraisals of aversive events that help them resolve distressing episodes with less strain than is experienced by less secure people. Indeed, as compared with anxious and avoidant people, secure people have been consistently found to hold more optimistic appraisals of stressful events (e.g., Berant et al., 2001; Birnbaum, Orr, Mikulincer, & Florian, 1997; Mikulincer & Florian, 1998). For example, Berant and colleagues (2001) found that securely attached mothers of infants who were diagnosed with congenital heart defects reported more positive appraisals of motherhood-related tasks, both immediately after the diagnosis and 1 year later, than anxious or avoidant mothers. Six years later, the effects of insecure mothers on their children with congenital heart defects were evident in both objective and projective measures administered to the then 7-year-old children (Berant, Mikulincer, & Shaver, 2008).

Experiences of attachment-figure availability also offer opportunities to learn that one's own instrumental actions are often able to reduce distress. For example, a child learns that his or her bids for proximity alter a partner's behavior and result in the restoration of emotional equanimity. As a result, security-providing interactions strengthen a person's reliance on active, instrumental approaches to problem solving. In support of this view, secure people have been found to rely on problem-focused strategies while coping with stressful events (e.g., Lussier, Sabourin, & Turgeon, 1997; Mikulincer & Florian, 1998). This constructive approach to emotion regulation was illustrated by Mikulincer (1998b), who found that secure participants' recollections of personal experiences of anger were characterized by adaptive problem-solving actions aimed at repairing the relationship with the instigator of anger.

Attachment security promotes what Lazarus (1991) called a "short circuit of threat," sidestepping the interfering and dysfunctional aspects of emotions while retaining their functional, adaptive qualities. Efficient management of distress results in more and longer periods of positive mood, thereby rendering mood disorders, maladjustment, and psychopathology less likely. Indeed, several studies have documented positive associations between secure attachment and measures of well-being (e.g., Berant et al., 2001; Birnbaum et al., 1997) and negative associations between security and symptoms of depression, anxiety, and hostility (e.g., Cooper et al., 1998; Mickelson et al., 1997). Mikulincer, Shaver, and Horesh (2006) also found that both dispositional measures of attachment security and contextual manipulations of the sense of attachment security are associated with lower levels of posttraumatic symptoms (e.g., intrusion of traumatic thoughts) among people who were exposed to the traumas of war or terrorism.

Unlike relatively secure people, those who are avoidant cannot readily engage in optimal problem solving because this often requires opening knowledge structures to new information, admitting frustration and possible defeat, dealing with uncertainty and confusion, and running freely through one's memories without attempting to block attachment-system activation (Mikulincer, 1997). Avoidant people often prefer to dissociate their emotions from their thoughts and actions, using what Lazarus and Folkman (1984) called "distancing coping." This requires suppression of emotion-eliciting thoughts, repression of painful memories, diversion of attention from emotion-related material, and inhibition of verbal and nonverbal expressions of emotion. For anxiously attached people, in contrast, negative emotions can be congruent with their goal of attachment-system hyperactivation. In the process of emotion regulation, anxious people tend to engage in effortful attempts to generate and intensify emotional states. These states include every emotion that plays a role in activating the attachment system— threats, dangers, and negative interactions with attachment figures. They also include emotions that emphasize a person's wounds and incompetence, such as sadness, anxiety, shame, and guilt, because these make it natural to insist on attachment figures' attention and care (Cassidy, 1994).

These emotion regulation patterns have now been well documented in empirical studies of attachment style and ways of coping with stressful events (see Mikulincer & Florian, 1998; Mikulincer & Shaver, 2007a). In these studies, higher avoidance scores are associated with higher scores on measures of coping by distancing, and attachment anxiety is associated with higher scores on measures of emotion-focused coping. For example, Mikulincer and Orbach (1995) reported that attachment avoidance was associated with a repressive coping style, Feeney (1995) reported that avoidance was related to behavioral blunting (seeking distractions when dealing with stress), and Mikulincer and Florian (1998) found that people who classified themselves as anxiously attached tended to report more frequent task-related, ruminative worries after failing cognitive tasks than were reported by their secure and avoidant counterparts.

These emotion regulation strategies are also manifested in the ways people cope with attachment-related threats. For example, Fraley and Shaver (1997) found attachment-style differences in the suppression of separation-related thoughts. Participants wrote continuously about whatever thoughts and feelings they were experiencing while being asked to suppress thoughts about their romantic partners' leaving them for someone else. Attachment anxiety was associated with poorer ability to suppress separation-related thoughts—more frequent thoughts of breakup following the suppression task and higher skin conductance during the task. In contrast, more avoidant people were better able than less avoidant individuals not only to stop thinking about separation but also to reduce the intensity of their autonomic responses to these thoughts.

In a series of studies examining the experience and management of death anxiety (e.g., Mikulincer & Florian, 2000; Mikulincer, Florian, & Tolmacz, 1990), anxious individuals were found to intensify death concerns and to keep death-related thoughts active in memory. In contrast, avoidant individuals tended to suppress death concerns and to dissociate their conscious claims from their unconscious anxiety. Although avoidance was related to low levels of self-reported fear of death, it was also related to heightened death anxiety on projective Thematic Apperception Test (TAT) stories.

Avoidant people's dissociative tendencies were also documented by Mikulincer (1998b), who found that avoidant individuals, as compared with secure ones, reacted to anger-eliciting episodes with lower levels of self-reported anger and higher levels of physiological arousal (heart rate). Two other studies examined access to emotions during the AAI, finding that avoidant people expressed fewer negative feelings during the interview but displayed higher levels of physiological arousal (heightened electrodermal activity; Dozier & Kobak, 1992).

Attachment theorists view insecure people's modes of emotion regulation as risk factors that reduce resilience in times of stress and contribute to emotional problems and poor adjustment. Indeed, a large number of studies have shown that attachment anxiety is associated with global distress, depression, anxiety, eating disorders, substance abuse, conduct disorders, and severe personality disorders (see Mikulincer & Shaver, 2007a). However, for avoidance, the findings are more complex. On the one hand, a host of studies yielded no significant associations between avoidant attachment and self-report measures of well-being and global distress (see Mikulincer & Shaver, 2007a). On the other hand, several studies indicate that avoidant attachment is associated with a pattern of depression characterized by perfectionism, self-punishment, and self-criticism (e.g., Zuroff & Fitzpatrick, 1995), heightened reports of somatic complaints (e.g., Mikulincer, Florian, & Weller, 1993), a hostile view of other people (e.g., Mikulincer, 1998b), substance abuse and conduct disorders (e.g., Brennan & Shaver, 1995; Cooper et al., 1998; Mickelson et al., 1997), and schizoid and avoidant personality disorders (e.g., Brennan & Shaver, 1998).

In addition, whereas no consistent association has been found in community samples between avoidant attachment and emotional problems, studies that focus on highly demanding and distressing events reveal that avoidance is related to greater reported distress. For example, in studies assessing mothers' long-term reactions to the births of infants with congenital heart defects, avoidance, as assessed at the times of the initial diagnoses of the infants' disorders, was the most potent predictor of maternal distress 1 and 7 years later (Berant et al., 2001, 2008). It seems that avoidant attachment may contribute to mental health under fairly normal circumstances characterized by only mild encounters with stressors. Under highly demanding conditions, however, deactivating strategies seem to collapse, and in such cases avoidant individuals may exhibit high levels of distress and emotional problems. This conclusion is supported by two laboratory studies (Mikulincer, Dolev, & Shaver, 2004) that showed that the addition of a demanding cognitive task, which had previously been shown to interfere with mental suppression (e.g., Wegner, Erber, & Zanakos, 1993), impaired avoidant individuals' ability to block the activation of attachment-related worries. Specifically, under high-load conditions, avoidant participants resembled their anxiously attached counterparts, exhibiting high accessibility of separation-related thoughts and negative self-representations.

Concluding Remarks

As we hope to have shown in this relatively brief but jam-packed trip through the large and still exploding adult attachment literature, Bowlby and Ainsworth's theory has been an extremely rich and seminal source of ideas for empirical research in personality and social psychology. Despite the many lines of research we have summarized, the attachment field is much broader than we have indicated, including impressive longitudinal studies running from infancy to adulthood (Grossmann, Grossmann, & Waters, 2005). The entire field is analyzed in the two editions of the *Handbook of Attachment* (Cassidy & Shaver, 1999, 2008). Anyone wishing to gain a reasonably complete picture of the field has a great deal of reading to do.

Although there are many well-replicated research findings in the various streams of attachment research, there are still numerous controversies and conundrums in the field. First and foremost is the problem of nonconvergent measures of adult attachment styles. For example, a recent review of studies (Roisman, Holland, et al., 2007) based on both the AAI and self-report measures of adult attachment, such as the ECR, found little convergence between the two kinds of measures, even though some of the studies revealed substantial associations (e.g., Shaver, Belsky, & Brennan, 2000). Given that both kinds of measures are based on the same theory, it is not yet clear why both yield coherent support for the theory without being strongly related to each other.

Second, it is still unclear whether categorical or dimensional measures of adult attachment make the most sense, theoretically and psychometrically. The AAI uses a categorical classification system, but the ECR and similar self-report measures are based on continuous dimensions. Roisman, Fraley, and Belsky (2007) recently showed that the AAI, especially the distinction between secure and avoidant attachment, should be scored dimensionally, an argument Fraley and Spieker (2003) made earlier with respect to Ainsworth's Strange Situation.

Third, there has always been controversy about the possible role of genes, in addition to social experience, in determining adult attachment patterns. There is now preliminary evidence that classifications and scores on both the AAI (Torgerson, Grova, & Sommerstad, 2007) and the ECR (Crawford et al., 2007) are influenced by genetic factors, as are classifications based on the Strange Situation (Bakermans-Kranenburg & van IJzendoorn, 2007). The degree of genetic influence remains to be clarified.

Fourth, measures such as the ECR are related to scores on the "Big Five" personality factors (e.g., Donnellan et al., 2008; Noftle & Shaver, 2006), and those relations are due in part to shared genetic influences (Crawford et al., 2007; Donnellan et al., 2008). Attachment anxiety, not surprisingly, is substantially correlated with Neuroticism, and avoidance is often significantly negatively correlated with Agreeableness and Extraversion. Yet many studies of associations between attachment styles, or attachment-style dimensions, and other variables find predicted attachment effects even when scores on Big Five trait measures are statistically controlled (e.g., Erez, Mikulincer, van IJzendoorn, & Kroonenberg, 2008; Noftle & Shaver, 2006), so attachment insecurities and major personality factors are not simply redundant.

Given these controversies and many as yet unaddressed questions about personality and relationships, the future of adult attachment research seems bright. Bowlby and Ainsworth's theory is an example of the utility of grand theories even in a field that is increasingly guided by discrete, focused research questions. By putting together several key theoretical innovations and research advances of his era, Bowlby was able to retain some of the insights of Freudian psychoanalytic theory while building bridges to other theories and to empirical research findings. The same kinds of innovations and advances have been repeatedly demonstrated in post-Darwinian biology, which is perhaps the best professional model for empirical psychology. It seems likely that the broad swath of phenomena addressed by attachment theory—that is, the formation of personality in the crucible of interpersonal relationships and the shaping of such relationships by personality factors—will be repeatedly reconceptualized in future versions of what is currently called attachment theory.

References

Ainsworth, M. D. S. (1967). *Infancy in Uganda: Infant care and the growth of love.* Baltimore: Johns Hopkins University Press.

Ainsworth, M. D. S., Blehar, M. C., Waters, E., & Wall, S. (1978). *Patterns of attachment: Assessed in the Strange Situation and at home.* Hillsdale, NJ: Erlbaum.

Bakermans-Kranenburg, M. J., & van IJzendoorn, M. H. (2007). Genetic vulnerability or differential susceptibility in child development: The case of attachment. *Journal of Child Psychology and Psychiatry, 48,* 1160–1173.

Baldwin, M. W. (1992). Relational schemas and the processing of social information. *Psychological Bulletin, 112,* 461–484.

Baldwin, M. W., Fehr, B., Keedian, E., Seidel, M., & Thompson, D. W. (1993). An exploration of the relational schemata underlying attachment styles: Self-report and lexical decision approaches. *Personality and Social Psychology Bulletin, 19,* 746–754.

Baldwin, M. W., Keelan, J. P. R., Fehr, B., Enns, V., & Koh Rangarajoo, E. (1996). Social-cognitive conceptualization of attachment working models: Availability and accessibility effects. *Journal of Personality and Social Psychology, 71,* 94–109.

Bartholomew, K., & Horowitz, L. M. (1991). Attachment styles among young adults: A test of a four-category model. *Journal of Personality and Social Psychology, 61,* 226–244.

Bartz, J. A., & Lydon, J. E. (2006). Navigating the interdependence dilemma: Attachment goals and the use of communal norms with potential close others. *Journal of Personality and Social Psychology, 91,* 77–96.

Berant, E., Mikulincer, M., & Florian, V. (2001). The association of mothers' attachment style and their psychological reactions to the diagnosis of infant's congenital heart disease. *Journal of Social and Clinical Psychology, 20,* 208–232.

Berant, E., Mikulincer, M., & Shaver, P. R. (2008). Mothers' attachment style, their mental health, and their children's emotional vulnerabilities: A seven-year study of mothers of children with congenital heart disease. *Journal of Personality, 76,* 31–66.

Birnbaum, G. E., Orr, I., Mikulincer, M., & Florian, V. (1997). When marriage breaks up: Does attachment style contribute to coping and mental health? *Journal of Social and Personal Relationships, 14,* 643–654.

Boon, S. D., & Griffin, D. W. (1996). The construction of risk in relationships: The role of framing in decisions about intimate relationships. *Personal Relationships, 3,* 293–306.

Bowlby, J. (1956). The growth of independence in the young child. *Royal Society of Health Journal, 76,* 587–591.

Bowlby, J. (1973). *Attachment and loss: Vol. 2. Separation: Anxiety and anger.* New York: Basic Books.

Bowlby, J. (1980). *Attachment and loss: Vol. 3. Sadness and depression.* New York: Basic Books.

Bowlby, J. (1982). *Attachment and loss: Vol. 1. Attachment.* New York: Basic Books. (Original work published 1969)

Bowlby, J. (1988). *A secure base: Clinical applications of attachment theory.* London: Routledge.

Brassard, A., Shaver, P. R., & Lussier, Y. (2007). Attachment, sexual experience, and sexual pressure in romantic relationships: A dyadic approach. *Personal Relationships, 14,* 475–494.

Brennan, K. A., Clark, C. L., & Shaver, P. R. (1998). Self-report measurement of adult attachment: An integrative overview. In J. A. Simpson & W. S. Rholes (Eds.), *Attachment theory and close relationships* (pp. 46–76). New York: Guilford Press.

Brennan, K. A., & Shaver, P. R. (1995). Dimensions of adult attachment, affect regulation, and romantic relationship functioning. *Personality and Social Psychology Bulletin, 21,* 267–283.

Brennan, K. A., & Shaver, P. R. (1998). Attachment styles and personality disorders: Their connections to each other and to parental divorce, parental death, and perceptions of parental caregiving. *Journal of Personality, 66,* 835–878.

Carnelley, K. B., & Janoff-Bulman, R. (1992). Optimism about love relationships: General vs. specific lessons from one's personal experiences. *Journal of Social and Personal Relationships, 9,* 5–20.

Cassidy, J. (1994). Emotion regulation: Influences of attachment relationships. *Monographs of the Society for Research in Child Development, 59,* 228–283.

Cassidy, J. (1999). The nature of the child's ties. In J. Cassidy & P. R. Shaver (Eds.), *Handbook of attachment: Theory, research, and clinical applications* (pp. 3–20). New York: Guilford Press.

Cassidy, J., & Kobak, R. R. (1988). Avoidance and its relationship with other defensive processes. In J. Belsky & T. Nezworski (Eds.), *Clinical implications of attachment* (pp. 300–323). Hillsdale, NJ: Erlbaum.

Cassidy, J., & Shaver, P. R. (Eds.). (1999). *Handbook of attachment: Theory, research, and clinical applications.* New York: Guilford Press.

Cassidy, J., & Shaver, P. R. (Eds.) (2008). *Handbook of attachment: Theory, research, and clinical applications* (2nd ed.). New York.

Collins, N. L. (1996). Working models of attachment: Implications for explanation, emotion, and behavior. *Journal of Personality and Social Psychology, 71,* 810–832.

Collins, N. L., & Read, S. J. (1990). Adult attachment, working models, and relationship quality in dating couples. *Journal of Personality and Social Psychology, 58,* 644–663.

Cooper, M. L., Shaver, P. R., & Collins, N. L. (1998). Attachment styles, emotion regulation, and adjustment in adolescence. *Journal of Personality and Social Psychology, 74,* 1380–1397.

Cozzarelli, C., Hoekstra, S. J., & Bylsma, W. H. (2000). General versus specific mental models of attachment: Are they associated with different outcomes? *Personality and Social Psychology Bulletin, 26,* 605–618.

Cozzarelli, C., Sumer, N., & Major, B. (1998). Mental models of attachment and coping with abortion. *Journal of Personality and Social Psychology, 74,* 453–467.

Crawford, T. N., Livesley, W. J., Jang, K. L., Shaver, P. R., Cohen, P., & Ganiban, J. (2007). Insecure attachment and personality disorder: A twin study of adults. *European Journal of Personality, 21,* 191–208.

Crowell, J. A., Fraley, R. C., & Shaver, P. R. (1999). Measurement of adult attachment. In J. Cassidy & P. R. Shaver (Eds.), *Handbook of attachment: Theory, research, and clinical applications* (pp. 434–465). New York: Guilford Press.

Davidovitz, R., Mikulincer, M., Shaver, P. R., Ijzak, R., & Popper, M. (2007). Leaders as attachment figures: Their attachment orientations predict leadership-related mental representations and followers' performance and mental health. *Journal of Personality and Social Psychology, 93,* 632–650.

Davila, J., Karney, B. R., & Bradbury, T. N. (1999). Attachment change processes in the early years of marriage. *Journal of Personality and Social Psychology, 76,* 783–802.

Davis, D., Shaver, P. R., & Vernon, M. L. (2004). Attachment style and subjective motivations for sex. *Personality and Social Psychology Bulletin, 30,* 1076–1090.

Donnellan, M. B., Burt, S. A., Levendosky, A. A., & Klump, K. L. (2008). Genes, personality, and attachment in adults: A multivariate behavioral genetic analysis. *Personality and Social Psychology Bulletin, 34,* 3–16.

Dozier, M., & Kobak, R. (1992). Psychophysiology in attachment interviews: Converging evidence for deactivating strategies. *Child Development, 63,* 1473–1480.

Erez, A., Mikulincer, M., van IJzendoorn, M. H., & Kroonenberg, P. M. (2008). Attachment, personality, and volunteering: Placing volunteerism in an attachment-theoretical framework. *Personality and Individual Differences, 44,* 64–74.

Feeney, J. A. (1994). Attachment style, communication patterns, and satisfaction across the life cycle of marriage. *Personal Relationships, 1,* 333–348.

Feeney, J. A. (1995). Adult attachment and emotional control. *Personal Relationships, 2,* 143–159.

Feeney, J. A. (1996). Attachment, caregiving, and marital satisfaction. *Personal Relationships, 3,* 401–416.

Feeney, J. A., & Noller, P. (1990). Attachment style as a predictor of adult romantic relationships. *Journal of Personality and Social Psychology, 58,* 281–291.

Fitzpatrick, M. A., Fey, J., Segrin, C., & Schiff, J. L. (1993). Internal working models of relationships and marital communication. *Journal of Language and Social Psychology, 12,* 103–131.

Fraley, R. C. (2002). Attachment stability from infancy to adulthood: Meta-analysis and dynamic modeling of developmental mechanisms. *Personality and Social Psychology Review, 6,* 123–151.

Fraley, R. C., & Shaver, P. R. (1997). Adult attachment and the suppression of unwanted thoughts. *Journal of Personality and Social Psychology, 73,* 1080–1091.

Fraley, R. C., & Shaver, P. R. (1998). Airport separations: A naturalistic study of adult attachment dynamics in separating couples. *Journal of Personality and Social Psychology, 75,* 1198–1212.

Fraley, R. C., & Spieker, S. J. (2003). Are infant attachment patterns continuously or categorically distributed? A taxometric analysis of Strange Situation behavior. *Developmental Psychology, 39,* 387–404.

Fraley, R. C., & Waller, N. G. (1998). Adult attachment patterns: A test of the typological model. In J. A. Simpson & W. S. Rholes (Eds.), *Attachment theory and close relationships* (pp. 77–114). New York: Guilford Press.

Fraley, R. C., Waller, N. G., & Brennan, K. A. (2000). An item-response theory analysis of self-report measures of adult attachment. *Journal of Personality and Social Psychology, 78,* 350–365.

Frei, J. R., & Shaver, P. R. (2002). Respect in close relationships: Prototype definition, self-report assessment, and initial correlates. *Personal Relationships, 9,* 121–139.

Gaines, S. O., Jr., Reis, H. T., Summers, S., Rusbult, C. E., Cox, C. L., Wexler, M. O., et al. (1997). Impact of attachment style on reactions to accommodative dilemmas in close relationships. *Personal Relationships, 4,* 93–113.

Gallo, L. C., & Matthews, K. A. (2006). Adolescents' attachment orientation influences ambulatory blood pressure responses to everyday social interactions. *Psychosomatic Medicine, 68,* 253–261.

George, C., Kaplan, N., & Main, M. (1985). *The Adult Attachment Interview.* Unpublished manuscript, University of California, Berkeley.

Gillath, O., Shaver, P. R., Mikulincer, M., Nitzberg, R. A., Erez, A., & van IJzendoorn, M. H. (2005). Attachment, caregiving, and volunteering: Placing volunteerism in an attachment-theoretical framework. *Personal Relationships, 12,* 425–446.

Grossmann, K. E., Grossmann, K., & Waters, E. (Eds.). (2005). *Attachment from infancy to adulthood: The major longitudinal studies.* New York: Guilford Press.

Guerrero, L. K. (1996). Attachment-style differences in intimacy and involvement: A test of the four-category model. *Communication Monographs, 63,* 269–292.

Guerrero, L. K. (1998). Attachment-style differences in the experience and expression of romantic jealousy. *Personal Relationships, 5,* 273–291.

Hazan, C., & Shaver, P. R. (1987). Romantic love conceptualized as an attachment process. *Journal of Personality and Social Psychology, 52,* 511–524.

Hazan, C., & Shaver, P. R. (1990). Love and work: An attachment-theoretical perspective. *Journal of Personality and Social Psychology, 59,* 270–280.

Hesse, E. (2008). The Adult Attachment Interview: Protocol, method of analysis, and empirical studies. In J. Cassidy & P. R. Shaver (Eds.), *Handbook of attachment: Theory, research, and clinical applications* (2nd ed., pp. 552–598). New York: Guilford Press.

Kafetsios, K., & Nezlek, J. B. (2002). Attachment styles in everyday social interaction. *European Journal of Social Psychology, 32,* 719–735.

Keelan, J. R., Dion, K. K., & Dion, K. L. (1998). Attachment style and relationship satisfaction: Test of a self-disclosure explanation. *Canadian Journal of Behavioral Science, 30,* 24–35.

Kerns, K. A., & Stevens, A. C. (1996). Parent–child attachment in late adolescence: Links to social relations and personality. *Journal of Youth and Adolescence, 25*, 323–342.

Kunce, L. J., & Shaver, P. R. (1994). An attachment-theoretical approach to caregiving in romantic relationships. In K. Bartholomew & D. Perlman (Eds.), *Advances in personal relationships: Attachment processes in adulthood* (Vol. 5, pp. 205–237). London: Kingsley.

La Guardia, J. G., Ryan, R. M., Couchman, C. E., & Deci, E. L. (2000). Within-person variation in security of attachment: A self-determination theory perspective on attachment, need fulfillment, and well-being. *Journal of Personality and Social Psychology, 79*, 367–384.

Lazarus, R. S. (1991). *Emotion and adaptation.* New York: Oxford University Press.

Lazarus, R. S., & Folkman, S. (1984). *Stress, appraisal, and coping.* New York: Springer.

Levy, M. B., & Davis, K. E. (1988). Love styles and attachment styles compared: Their relations to each other and to various relationship characteristics. *Journal of Social and Personal Relationships, 5*, 439–471.

Luke, M. A., Maio, G. R., & Carnelley, K. B. (2004). Attachment models of the self and others: Relations with self-esteem, humanity esteem, and parental treatment. *Personal Relationships, 11*, 281–303.

Lussier, Y., Sabourin, S., & Turgeon, C. (1997). Coping strategies as moderators of the relationship between attachment and marital adjustment. *Journal of Social and Personal Relationships, 14*, 777–791.

Main, M. (1990). Cross-cultural studies of attachment organization: Recent studies, changing methodologies, and the concept of conditional strategies. *Human Development, 33*, 48–61.

Main, M., Kaplan, N., & Cassidy, J. (1985). Security in infancy, childhood, and adulthood: A move to the level of representation. *Monographs of the Society for Research in Child Development, 50*, 66–104.

Main, M., & Solomon, J. (1990). Procedures for identifying infants as disorganized/disoriented during the Ainsworth Strange Situation. In M. T. Greenberg, D. Cicchetti, & M. Cummings (Eds.), *Attachment in the preschool years: Theory, research, and intervention* (pp. 121–160). Chicago: University of Chicago Press.

Mickelson, K. D., Kessler, R. C., & Shaver, P. R. (1997). Adult attachment in a nationally representative sample. *Journal of Personality and Social Psychology, 73*, 1092–1106.

Mikulincer, M. (1995). Attachment style and the mental representation of the self. *Journal of Personality and Social Psychology, 69*, 1203–1215.

Mikulincer, M. (1997). Adult attachment style and information processing: Individual differences in curiosity and cognitive closure. *Journal of Personality and Social Psychology, 72*, 1217–1230.

Mikulincer, M. (1998a). Adult attachment style and affect regulation: Strategic variations in self-appraisals. *Journal of Personality and Social Psychology, 75*, 420–435.

Mikulincer, M. (1998b). Adult attachment style and individual differences in functional versus dysfunc-tional experiences of anger. *Journal of Personality and Social Psychology, 74*, 513–524.

Mikulincer, M., Dolev, T., & Shaver, P. R. (2004). Attachment-related strategies during thought suppression: Ironic rebounds and vulnerable self-representations. *Journal of Personality and Social Psychology, 87*, 940–956.

Mikulincer, M., & Florian, V. (1998). The relationship between adult attachment styles and emotional and cognitive reactions to stressful events. In J. A. Simpson & W. S. Rholes (Eds.), *Attachment theory and close relationships* (pp. 143–165). New York: Guilford Press.

Mikulincer, M., & Florian, V. (1999). The association between spouses' self-reports of attachment styles and representations of family dynamics. *Family Process, 38*, 69–83.

Mikulincer, M., & Florian, V. (2000). Exploring individual differences in reactions to mortality salience: Does attachment style regulate terror management mechanisms? *Journal of Personality and Social Psychology, 79*, 260–273.

Mikulincer, M., Florian, V., Cowan, P. A., & Cowan, C. P. (2002). Attachment security in couple relationships: A systemic model and its implications for family dynamics. *Family Process, 41*, 405–434.

Mikulincer, M., Florian, V., & Tolmacz, R. (1990). Attachment styles and fear of personal death: A case study of affect regulation. *Journal of Personality and Social Psychology, 58*, 273–280.

Mikulincer, M., Florian, V., & Weller, A. (1993). Attachment styles, coping strategies, and posttraumatic psychological distress: The impact of the Gulf War in Israel. *Journal of Personality and Social Psychology, 64*, 817–826.

Mikulincer, M., Gillath, O., Halevy, V., Avihou, N., Avidan, S., & Eshkoli, N. (2001). Attachment theory and reactions to others' needs: Evidence that activation of the sense of attachment security promotes empathic responses. *Journal of Personality and Social Psychology, 81*, 1205–1224.

Mikulincer, M., Gillath, O., Sapir-Lavid, Y., Yaakobi, E., Arias, K., Tal-Aloni, L., et al. (2003). Attachment theory and concern for others' welfare: Evidence that activation of the sense of secure base promotes endorsement of self-transcendence values. *Basic and Applied Social Psychology, 25*, 299–312.

Mikulincer, M., & Nachshon, O. (1991). Attachment styles and patterns of self-disclosure. *Journal of Personality and Social Psychology, 61*, 321–331.

Mikulincer, M., & Orbach, I. (1995). Attachment styles and repressive defensiveness: The accessibility and architecture of affective memories. *Journal of Personality and Social Psychology, 68*, 917–925.

Mikulincer, M., Orbach, I., & Iavnieli, D. (1998). Adult attachment style and affect regulation: Strategic variations in subjective self–other similarity. *Journal of Personality and Social Psychology, 75*, 436–448.

Mikulincer, M., & Shaver, P. R. (2004). Security-based self-representations in adulthood: Contents and processes. In W. S. Rholes & J. A. Simpson (Eds.), *Adult attachment: Theory, research, and clinical implications* (pp. 159–195). New York: Guilford Press.

Mikulincer, M., & Shaver, P. R. (2007a). *Attachment*

in adulthood: Structure, dynamics, and change. New York: Guilford Press.

Mikulincer, M., & Shaver, P. R. (2007b). A behavioral systems perspective on the psychodynamics of attachment and sexuality. In D. Diamond, S. J. Blatt, & J. D. Lichtenberg (Eds.), *Attachment and sexuality* (pp. 51–78). New York: Analytic Press.

Mikulincer, M., Shaver, P. R., Gillath, O., & Nitzberg, R. A. (2005). Attachment, caregiving, and altruism: Boosting attachment security increases compassion and helping. *Journal of Personality and Social Psychology, 89,* 817–839.

Mikulincer, M., Shaver, P. R., & Horesh, N. (2006). Attachment bases of emotion regulation and posttraumatic adjustment. In D. K. Snyder, J. A. Simpson, & J. N. Hughes (Eds.), *Emotion regulation in families: Pathways to dysfunction and health* (pp. 77–99). Washington, DC: American Psychological Association.

Mikulincer, M., Shaver, P. R., & Slav, K. (2006). Attachment, mental representations of others, and gratitude and forgiveness in romantic relationships. In M. Mikulincer & G. S. Goodman (Eds.), *Dynamics of romantic love: Attachment, caregiving, and sex* (pp. 190–215). New York: Guilford Press.

Noftle, E. E., & Shaver, P. R. (2006). Attachment dimensions and the Big Five personality traits: Associations and comparative ability to predict relationship quality. *Journal of Research in Personality, 40,* 179–208.

Overall, N. C., Fletcher, G. J. O., & Friesen, M. D. (2003). Mapping the intimate relationship mind: Comparisons between three models of attachment representations. *Personality and Social Psychology Bulletin, 29*(12), 1479–1493.

Pierce, T., & Lydon, J. (2001). Global and specific relational models in the experience of social interactions. *Journal of Personality and Social Psychology, 80,* 613–631.

Pietromonaco, P. R., & Barrett, L. F. (1997). Working models of attachment and daily social interactions. *Journal of Personality and Social Psychology, 73,* 1409–1423.

Pietromonaco, P. R., & Carnelley, K. B. (1994). Gender and working models of attachment: Consequences for perceptions of self and romantic relationships. *Personal Relationships, 1,* 63–82.

Reis, H. T., & Wheeler, L. (1991). Studying social interaction with the Rochester Interaction Record. In M. P. Zanna (Ed.), *Advances in experimental social psychology* (Vol. 24, pp. 270–318). San Diego, CA: Academic Press.

Rholes, W. S., Simpson, J. A., & Orina, M. (1999). Attachment and anger in an anxiety-provoking situation. *Journal of Personality and Social Psychology, 76,* 940–957.

Roisman, G. I., Fraley, R. C., & Belsky, J. (2007). A taxometric study of the Adult Attachment Interview. *Developmental Psychology, 43,* 675–686.

Roisman, G. I., Holland, A., Fortuna, K., Fraley, R. C., Clausell, E., & Clarke, A. (2007). The Adult Attachment Interview and self-reports of attachment style: An empirical rapprochement. *Journal of Personality and Social Psychology, 92,* 678–697.

Schachner, D. A., & Shaver, P. R. (2002). Attachment style and human mate poaching. *New Review of Social Psychology, 1,* 122–129.

Schachner, D. A., & Shaver, P. R. (2004). Attachment dimensions and motives for sex. *Personal Relationships, 11,* 179–195.

Scharfe, E., & Bartholomew, K. (1995). Accommodation and attachment representations in young couples. *Journal of Social and Personal Relationships, 12,* 389–401.

Searle, B., & Meara, N. M. (1999). Affective dimensions of attachment styles: Exploring self-reported attachment style, gender, and emotional experience among college students. *Journal of Counseling Psychology, 46,* 147–158.

Sharpsteen, D. J., & Kirkpatrick, L. A. (1997). Romantic jealousy and adult romantic attachment. *Journal of Personality and Social Psychology, 72,* 627–640.

Shaver, P. R., Belsky, J., & Brennan, K. A. (2000). The Adult Attachment Interview and self-reports of romantic attachment: Associations across domains and methods. *Personal Relationships, 7,* 25–43.

Shaver, P. R., & Brennan, K. A. (1992). Attachment styles and the "Big Five" personality traits: Their connections with each other and with romantic relationship outcomes. *Personality and Social Psychology Bulletin, 18,* 536–545.

Shaver, P. R., & Clark, C. L. (1994). The psychodynamics of adult romantic attachment. In J. M. Masling & R. F. Bornstein (Eds.), *Empirical perspectives on object relations theories* (pp. 105–156). Washington, DC: American Psychological Association.

Shaver, P. R., Hazan, C., & Bradshaw, D. (1988). Love as attachment: The integration of three behavioral systems. In R. J. Sternberg & M. Barnes (Eds.), *The psychology of love* (pp. 68–99). New Haven, CT: Yale University Press.

Shaver, P. R., Mikulincer, M., Lavy, S., & Cassidy, J. (in press). Understanding and altering hurt feelings: An attachment-theoretical perspective on the generation and regulation of emotions. In A. L. Vangelisti (Ed.), *Feeling hurt in close relationships*. New York: Cambridge University Press.

Shaver, P. R., Papalia, D., Clark, C. L., Koski, L. R., Tidwell, M., & Nalbone, D. (1996). Androgyny and attachment security: Two related models of optimal personality. *Personality and Social Psychology Bulletin, 22,* 582–597.

Sibley, C. G., Fischer, R., & Liu, J. H. (2005). Reliability and validity of the revised Experiences in Close Relationships (ECR-R) self-report measure of adult romantic attachment. *Personality and Social Psychology Bulletin, 31,* 1524–1536.

Simpson, J. A. (1990). Influence of attachment styles on romantic relationships. *Journal of Personality and Social Psychology, 59,* 971–980.

Simpson, J. A., Rholes, W. S., & Nelligan, J. S. (1992). Support seeking and support giving within couples in an anxiety-provoking situation: The role of attachment styles. *Journal of Personality and Social Psychology, 62,* 434–446.

Simpson, J. A., Rholes, W. S., & Phillips, D. (1996). Conflict in close relationships: An attachment perspective. *Journal of Personality and Social Psychology, 71,* 899–914.

Sroufe, L. A., & Waters, E. (1977). Attachment as an organizational construct. *Child Development, 48,* 1184–1199.

Tidwell, M. C. O., Reis, H. T., & Shaver, P. R. (1996).

Attachment, attractiveness, and social interaction: A diary study. *Journal of Personality and Social Psychology, 71,* 729–745.

Torgerson, A. M., Grova, B. K., & Sommerstad, R. (2007). A pilot study of attachment patterns in adult twins. *Attachment and Human Development, 9,* 127–138.

Tracy, J. L., Shaver, P. R., Albino, A. W., & Cooper, M. L. (2003). Attachment styles and adolescent sexuality. In P. Florsheim (Ed.), *Adolescent romance and sexual behavior: Theory, research, and practical implications* (pp. 137–159). Mahwah, NJ: Erlbaum.

Tucker, J. S., & Anders, S. L. (1998). Adult attachment style and nonverbal closeness in dating couples. *Journal of Nonverbal Behavior, 22,* 109–124.

Waters, E., Merrick, S., Treboux, D., Crowell, J., & Albersheim, L. (2000). Attachment security in infancy and early adulthood: A twenty-year longitudinal study. *Child Development, 71,* 684–689.

Waters, H. S., Rodrigues, L. M., & Ridgeway, D. (1998). Cognitive underpinnings of narrative attachment assessment. *Journal of Experimental Child Psychology, 71,* 211–234.

Waters, H. S., & Waters, E. (2006). The attachment working models concept: Among other things, we build script-like representations of secure base experiences. *Attachment and Human Development, 8,* 185–197.

Wegner, D. M., Erber, R., & Zanakos, S. (1993). Ironic processes in the mental control of mood and mood-related thoughts. *Journal of Personality and Social Psychology, 65,* 1093–1104.

Westmaas, J., & Silver, R. C. (2001). The role of attachment in responses to victims of life crises. *Journal of Personality and Social Psychology, 80,* 425–438.

Zuroff, D. C., & Fitzpatrick, D. K. (1995). Depressive personality styles: Implications for adult attachment. *Personality and Individual Differences, 18,* 253–265.

CHAPTER 6

■ ● ▲ ◆ ■ ● ▲ ◆

Interpersonal Dependency

ROBERT F. BORNSTEIN

Interpersonal dependency—the tendency to rely on other people for protection and support even in situations in which autonomous functioning is warranted—is one of the more widely studied traits in social, personality, and clinical psychology, with more than 1,000 published studies during the past 50 years (Bornstein, 2005). Individual differences in dependency not only predict important features of social behavior (e.g., help seeking, conformity, suggestibility) but also have implications for illness risk (Bornstein, 1998c), health service use (Tyrer, Mitchard, Methuen, & Ranger, 2003), compliance with medical and psychotherapeutic regimens (Poldrugo & Forti, 1988), and success in adjusting to the physical and emotional challenges of aging (Baltes, 1996).

This chapter reviews research on the interpersonal dynamics of interpersonal dependency. Following a brief overview of classic and contemporary theoretical models and the most widely used dependency assessment tools, research on dependency as a social construct is discussed. As the ensuing review shows, the construct of dependency is more complex than psychologists initially thought, with investigations in this area shaped by two distinct trends. First, although dependent people often exhibit acquiescent, compliant behavior, studies suggest that in certain situations they may actually behave quite actively—even aggressively. Second, although high levels of interpersonal dependency are associated with social and psychological impairment in a variety of contexts, in certain settings high levels of dependency may actually enhance adjustment and functioning.

Conceptualizing Dependency

The first influential theoretical model of interpersonal dependency came from psychoanalytic theory, wherein a dependent personality orientation was conceptualized as the product of "oral fixation"—continued preoccupation during adulthood with the events and developmental challenges of the infantile oral stage. As Freud (1908/1959, p. 167) noted, "one very often meets with a type of character in which certain traits are very strongly marked while at the same time one's attention is arrested by the behavior of these persons in regard to certain bodily functions." Thus classical psychoanalytic theory postulated that the orally fixated (or oral dependent) person would: (1) continue to rely on others for nurturance, guidance, protection, and support and (2) exhibit behaviors in adulthood that mirror those of the oral stage (e.g., preoccupation with activities of the mouth, reliance on food and eating as a strategy for coping with anxiety).

Empirical support for the classical psychoanalytic model of dependency was mixed (see Bornstein, 1996), and gradually this perspective was supplanted by an object relations model wherein dependency was conceptualized as resulting from the internalization of a mental representation of the self as weak and ineffectual (Blatt, 1974). Retrospective and prospective studies of parent–child interactions confirmed that those parenting styles that cause children to perceive themselves as powerless and vulnerable are in fact associated with high levels of interpersonal dependency later in life (Baker, Capron, & Azorloza, 1996; Blatt & Homann, 1992). Specifically, overprotective and authoritarian parenting, alone or in combination, are associated with the development of a dependent personality, in part because of the impact these two parenting styles have on the child's sense of self. Overprotective parenting teaches children that they are fragile and weak and must look outward to others for protection from a harsh and threatening environment. Authoritarian parenting, by contrast, teaches the child that the way to get by in life is to accede passively to others' demands and expectations (see Bornstein, 1993, 2005, for detailed reviews of studies in this area).

Behavioral and social learning models called psychologists' attention to the role that learning—including observational learning—may play in the etiology and dynamics of dependency-related responding. As Ainsworth (1969) pointed out, intermittent reinforcement of dependency-related behavior will propagate this behavior over time and across situation; as Bandura (1977) noted, modeling—including symbolic modeling—can facilitate this learning/reinforcement process. Building on these initial social learning models, later researchers showed that traditional gender role socialization practices may help account for the higher levels of overt dependent behavior exhibited by women relative to men insofar as dependent responding is discouraged more strongly in boys than in girls in most Western societies (Cross, Bacon, & Morris, 2000). Analyses of cultural variations in dependency further indicated that traditionally sociocentric

cultures (e.g., India, Japan) have tended to be more tolerant of dependency in adults than are more individualistic cultures (e.g., America, Great Britain), wherein dependency is associated with immaturity, frailty, and dysfunction (Johnson, 1993; Yamaguchi, 2004).

Combining key elements of extant theoretical frameworks, Bornstein (1992, 1993, 1996, 2005) delineated an interactionist model wherein interpersonal dependency is conceptualized in terms of four primary components: (1) *cognitive* (i.e., a perception of oneself as powerless and ineffectual coupled with the belief that others are comparatively powerful and potent); (2) *motivational* (i.e., a strong desire to obtain and maintain relationships with potential protectors and caregivers); (3) *affective* (i.e., fear of abandonment, fear of negative evaluation by figures of authority); and (4) *behavioral* (i.e., use of relationship-facilitating self-presentation strategies to strengthen ties to others and preclude abandonment and rejection). The links among these four components of dependency are illustrated in Figure 6.1.

As Figure 6.1 shows, three variables (parenting style, gender role socialization, and cultural norms regarding achievement and relatedness) are central to the etiology of a dependent personality style, leading to the construction of a "helpless self-concept." This helpless self-concept is the linchpin of a dependent personality orientation—the psychological mechanism from which all other manifestations of dependency originate. First, a perception of oneself as powerless and ineffectual helps create the motivational component of dependency: If one views oneself as weak and ineffectual, then one's desire to curry favor with potential caregivers and protectors will increase. These dependency-related motivations in turn give rise to dependency-related behaviors (e.g., ingratiation, supplication) and to affective responses that reflect the dependent person's core beliefs about the self. Finally, as the feedback loop in the right half of Figure 6.1 indicates, dependency-related affective responses actually reinforce the dependent person's perception of the self as powerless and ineffectual. Thus, when a dependency-related affective response (e.g., fear of abandonment by a valued other) occurs, the helpless self-concept is primed (i.e., brought into working memory),

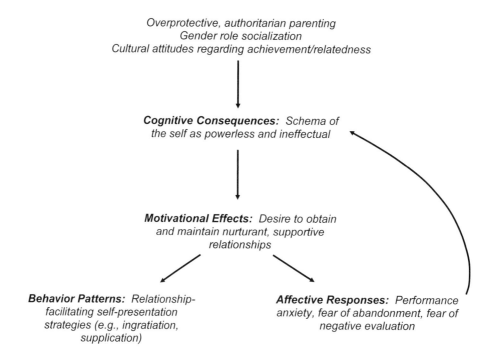

FIGURE 6.1. An interactionist model of interpersonal dependency. As this figure shows, dependent personality traits reflect the interplay of cognitive, motivational, emotional, and behavioral features, all of which stem from early learning and socialization experiences within and outside the family.

and dependency-related responding is more likely to occur (see Bornstein, Ng, Gallagher, Kloss, & Regier, 2005).

Although several researchers have examined links between dependency and attachment to ascertain whether interpersonal dependency may be best conceptualized in terms of a characteristic pattern of attachment-related behavior, for the most part results in this area have been inconclusive. Some investigations have found high levels of interpersonal dependency to be associated with an insecure attachment style (Collins & Read, 1990; Pincus & Wilson, 2001), but others have found that dependent children and adults tend to show preoccupied or secure attachment (see Meyer & Pilkonis, 2005; Sperling & Berman, 1991). Differences in the findings obtained in these studies may be due in part to the different populations assessed and different attachment-style measures used (Bornstein, 2005), but given researchers' interest in attachment-based models of personality and interpersonal functioning, continued exploration of

dependency–attachment links is clearly warranted.

Assessing Dependency

Because interpersonal dependency is of interest to social, personality, and clinical psychologists, numerous measures of dependency have been developed during the past several decades; at least 30 different measures are currently in use (Bornstein, 1999, 2005). The vast majority of these are either self-report or free-response tests.

Self-Report Scales

Self-report dependency scales typically consist of a series of dependency-related self-statements, each of which is evaluated by the respondent using a true–false or Likert rating scale. Most self-report dependency tests are fairly transparent, so respondents (especially psychologically minded respondents) are at least partially aware that test items are tapping dependency-related traits, attitudes, and behaviors. For this reason self-report measures are best conceptualized as assessing *self-attributed dependency needs*—dependency needs that the respondent sees in him- or herself and is willing to acknowledge when asked. Among the more widely used self-report dependency tests are Hirschfeld and colleagues' (1977) Interpersonal Dependency Inventory (IDI, which yields a single score reflecting overall level of dependency); Pincus and Gurtman's (1995) 3-Vector Dependency Inventory (3VDI, which yields separate scores for three dependency subtypes—Exploitable, Submissive, and Love Dependency); and Bornstein and colleagues' (2003) Relationship Profile Test (RPT, which includes three subscales measuring Destructive Overdependence, Dysfunctional Detachment, and Healthy Dependency).

Free-Response Measures

In contrast to the situation involving self-report scales, a single free-response measure—Masling, Rabie, and Blondheim's (1967) Rorschach Oral Dependency (ROD) scale—has dominated dependency research for the past several decades, being used in more than 80% of studies involving free-response dependency scores. As with all free-response tests, the ROD scale requires respondents to provide open-ended descriptions of ambiguous stimuli (in this case, Rorschach inkblots); these descriptions are then scored for the proportion of responses containing oral and/or dependent imagery. Although free-response tests in general (and the Rorschach in particular) have been the subject of considerable controversy in recent years, construct validity data for the ROD scale are quite strong, and Rorschach proponents and critics alike acknowledge the utility of the scale as a measure of interpersonal dependency (see, e.g., Hunsley & Bailey, 1999). Because the purpose of the ROD scale is not obvious, ROD scores are unaffected by respondents' degree of insight regarding their underlying dependency needs or by self-presentation and self-report biases. ROD scores are best conceptualized as assessing *implicit dependency needs*—dependency needs that the person might not be aware of but that nonetheless help shape dependency-related responding.

Test Score Convergences and Discontinuities

For many years researchers viewed self-report and free-response tests as alternative methods for assessing the strength of a psychological need or motive. However, as McClelland, Koestner, and Weinberger (1989) pointed out, the traditional view of self-report and free-response test scores as equivalent and interchangeable is inaccurate. McClelland and colleagues (1989, pp. 698–699) noted instead that "measures of implicit motives provide a more direct readout of motivational and emotional experiences than do self-reports that are filtered through analytic thought and various concepts of self and others, [because] implicit motives are more often built on early, prelinguistic affective experiences whereas self-attributed motives are more often built on explicit teaching by parents as to what values or goals it is important for a child to pursue."

A key corollary of McClelland and colleagues' (1989) framework is that even when self-report and free-response dependency tests show evidence of good concurrent and predictive validity, scores on these tests should be only modestly intercorrelated because they tap different psychological processes and assess different manifestations of dependency. Support for this corollary came from two meta-analyses. First, Bornstein (1999) assessed the behaviorally referenced validity coefficients of widely used dependency scales, finding that the mean validity coefficient (r) for self-report tests (number of studies = 54) was .26, whereas the mean validity coefficient for free-response tests (number of studies = 32) was .37. These validity coefficients are comparable to those typically obtained when trait-based measures are pooled across different contexts, settings, and dimensions of trait-related behavior (see Baldwin & Sinclair, 1996; Mischel, Shoda, & Mendoza-Denton, 2002). Second, Bornstein (2002) found that in published studies wherein both types of dependency measures were used (number of studies = 12), the mean self-report/free-response test score correlation was .24.

The modest intercorrelations of self-report and free-response dependency tests provide an opportunity to examine naturally occurring discontinuities between implicit and self-attributed dependency needs. Although many people score consistently high or consistently low on these two measures and may therefore be described as being generally *dependent* or *nondependent*, others obtain inconsistent scores on self-report and free-response tests. Some people obtain high free-response scores but low self-report scores; these people have *unacknowledged dependency strivings*. In contrast, some people obtain low free-response scores but high self-report scores; these people may be described as having a *dependent self-presentation*.

Self-attributed dependency needs seem to best predict mindful, goal-directed dependent behavior, whereas implicit dependency needs predict more spontaneous, reflexive expressions of dependency. Using an in vivo experience sampling methodology over 4 weeks, Bornstein (1998a) found that college students who were *dependent* or showed a *dependent self-presentation* made a large number of direct requests for help from professors, friends, and family members; in contrast, college students with *unacknowledged dependency strivings* made few direct requests but many indirect requests for help (e.g., hinting to roommates that they needed assistance on a homework assignment, implying that a ride to the mall was needed without explicitly asking for a ride). A second experiment demonstrated that when participants completed self-report and free-response dependency tests (the IDI and the ROD scale) and then took part in a laboratory problem-solving task in which they were permitted to ask an experimenter for assistance, the way in which the task was labeled altered the predictive power of the two dependency scales. When the laboratory task was identified to participants as a measure of help seeking, number of requests for assistance was more strongly related to IDI than to ROD scores, but when the task was identified as a measure of problem solving, number of requests for assistance was more strongly related to ROD than to IDI scores (Bornstein, 1998a). Apparently, the way participants perceive and interpret a given situation will determine whether dependency-related behavior is best predicted by self-report or free-response dependency scores (see also Bornstein, 2005, for a discussion of this issue).

Although self-report and free-response dependency scales differ in myriad ways, they do have one important feature in common: On both types of measures a low score merely reflects an absence of dependent behavior; it does not necessarily indicate high levels of autonomous, independent, or counterdependent behavior. Increasingly, theoreticians and researchers conceptualize dependency, autonomy, and independence as distinct constructs, with *autonomy* characterized by self-confidence, self-directedness, and healthy connectedness and *independence* characterized by some degree of isolation and detachment, along with an unwillingness to rely on or be influenced by others (see Bornstein, 2005, and Bornstein et al., 2003, for detailed discussions of these three personality styles).

Dependency as a Social Construct

Although there have been about a half dozen investigations exploring discontinuities between implicit and self-attributed dependency needs (Bornstein, 1998a, 1998b, 2007; Bornstein, Bowers, & Bonner, 1996a, 1996b), the vast majority of studies to date have used a single self-report or free-response measure to assess level of dependency and examine links between dependency and various indices of social behavior. Following a brief summary of seminal theoretical writings on the interpersonal correlates and consequences of dependency, empirical studies of dependency and social behavior are reviewed.

The Traditional View: Dependency as Passivity

Kraepelin (1913) and Schneider (1923) were among the first theoreticians to discuss the dependency–passivity link, but the notion that high levels of dependency are associated with a compliant, acquiescent stance in interpersonal interactions was popularized primarily by psychoanalytic theorists who wrote extensively on this topic during the first decades of the 20th century. Abraham (1927, p. 400) summarized nicely the prevailing view of dependency at that time when he argued that dependent persons "are dominated by the belief that there will always be some kind person—a representative of the mother, of course—to care for them and give them everything they need. This optimistic belief condemns them to inactivity … they make no kind of effort, and in some cases they even disdain to undertake a breadwinning occupation." Twenty years later Fromm (1947, p. 62) extended this characterization of the dependent person, noting that these individuals "are dependent not only on authorities for knowledge and help, but on people in general for any kind of support. They feel lost when alone because they feel that they cannot do anything without help. It is characteristic of these people that their first thought is to find somebody else to give them needed information rather than make even the slightest effort on their own."

Given these views, it is not surprising that throughout much of the 20th century social research emphasized the passive aspects of dependency, documenting links between dependency and suggestibility (Jakubczak & Walters, 1959; Tribich & Messer, 1974), help seeking (Diener, 1967; Shilkret & Masling, 1981), interpersonal yielding in an Asch-type paradigm (Kagan & Mussen, 1956; Masling, Weiss, & Rothschild, 1968), and compliance with the perceived expectations of experimenters (Weiss, 1969) and professors (Masling, O'Neill, & Jayne, 1981). Even today researchers tend to focus primarily on the passive, acquiescent features of interpersonal dependency (e.g., Leising, Sporberg, & Rehbein, 2006; Vittengl, Clark, & Jarrett, 2003).

From Pervasive Passivity to Goal-Driven Activity

When Bornstein, Masling, and Poynton (1987) conducted a modified replication of Masling and colleagues' (1968) yielding experiment, an unexpected pattern emerged. In Bornstein and colleagues' study, dependent and nondependent undergraduates were selected using the ROD scale. Same-sex pairs consisting of one dependent and one nondependent student were constructed, and participants were informed that they were taking part in a study of the decision-making process. They were asked to determine individually the gender of 10 poets after reading brief poem excerpts; the experimenter then compared the two participants' judgments and selected three poems on which they had disagreed. The experimenter asked the two participants to discuss these three poems for 10 minutes and come to a consensus decision regarding the gender of the poets.

In line with previous results in this area, Bornstein and colleagues (1987) expected that the dependent participants would change their opinions in the majority of dyads, but in fact the opposite occurred: In 35 of 50 dyads (70%) the nondependent participant yielded to the initial opinion of the dependent participant on at least two of the three poems. Postexperiment interviews provided some insight regarding the psychological processes that led to this unexpected pattern: A majority of dependent participants indicated that they chose not to alter their initial opinions because they wanted to impress the experimenter (who—in contrast to the typical Asch paradigm—was aware of the participant's initial opinion before the discussions took place). In other words, when confronted with choosing between impressing a figure of authority by holding their ground or accommodating a peer by yielding, the dependent participants opted to stand by their initial opinions and impress the authority figure.

Context-Driven Variability in Responding

Following Bornstein and colleagues' (1987) study, researchers became increasingly interested in identifying contextual cues that help shape dependency-related behavior. A study by Bornstein, Riggs, Hill, and Calabrese (1996) was among the first to document some of these cues. In Bornstein and colleagues' investigation, same-sex pairs of college students were brought to the laboratory and told they were taking part in a study of the personality–creativity link. Each pair consisted of one dependent and one nondependent student, classified using Hirschfeld and colleagues' (1977) IDI. The two students were told that because they had obtained similar personality profiles in an earlier testing (actually the dependency prescreening), they were expected to obtain comparable creativity scores.

Half the participants were told that their creativity test data would be seen only by the other student (the *no-authority* condition); the remaining participants were told their tests would be reviewed by two psychology professors who would contact them later in the semester to discuss their results (the *authority* condition). Participants were then given several opportunities to engage in behaviors they believed would enhance or undermine their test performance (e.g., choosing to do many or few practice items before taking the test, choosing to listen to relaxing or distracting music while being tested).

The results of the experiment were clear: Dependent students "self-handicapped" (i.e., did few practice items, chose distracting background music) in the *no-authority* condition, because their primary goal in this situation was to be liked by the peer. However, dependent students "self-enhanced" (i.e., did many practice items, chose relaxing background music) in the *authority* condition, because their primary goal had changed: Now, impressing the professors became more important than getting along with a peer. Nondependent students' behavior was unaffected by authority condition.

These findings illustrate the predictable variability in dependency-related behavior and confirm that this variability is largely a function of the dependent person's perceptions of interpersonal risks and opportunities. With no authority figure present, being liked by a peer was paramount, but once a figure of authority entered into the equation, impressing this person became more important than getting along with a peer. Thus dependent students exhibited a very rational social influence strategy: They chose to curry favor with the person best able to offer protection and support over the long term.

Using a very different paradigm, Thompson and Zuroff (1998, 1999) assessed context-driven variability in mothers' responses to their adolescent sons and daughters. In their first investigation Thompson and Zuroff (1998) divided a sample of mothers into dependent and nondependent groups, then provided each mother false feedback regarding her daughter's problem-solving skill (competence) and desire to partner with her mother on a problem-solving task (autonomy). Dependent mothers responded to their daughters' autonomy and competence with authoritarian behavior and negative performance feedback but provided positive feedback under conditions of low daughter competence. When Thompson and Zuroff (1999) replicated this study with mother–son pairs, a similar pattern emerged, with dependent mothers providing the most positive feedback to sons who displayed average competence and low autonomy. Apparently dependent mothers are threatened by competent and autonomous behaviors in their sons and daughters and respond to these behaviors by subtly undermining their offspring's confidence through negative feedback.

An Interactionist Perspective on Dependency

These findings, taken together, confirm that dependency-related responding is proactive, goal-driven, and guided by beliefs and expectations regarding the self, other people, and self–other interactions. Thus the behavior of dependent persons varies considerably from situation to situation, but the dependent person's underlying cognitions and motives remain constant. With this in mind, it is not surprising that dependent college students who believe they performed well on a major-specific aptitude test choose to wait significantly longer than high-performing nondependent college students to go over their test results with one of their major professors (approximately 15 minutes for the dependent students versus 8 minutes for nondependent students). These waiting-time differences increase when the dependent student's helpless self-concept is activated via a series of subliminal lexical primes (Bornstein, 2006b, Experiment 1). However, when participants are informed that the professor who is to go over their test results with them will be leaving the college at the end of the semester (and therefore cannot offer future help and support), dependent–nondependent waiting-time differences disappear (Bornstein, 2006b, Experiment 2).

Other examples of goal-driven "active dependency" emerge in the medical and academic arenas. For example, studies indicate that dependent women show shorter latencies than nondependent women in seeking medical help following detection of a serious medical symptom (e.g., a possible lump in the breast), in part because the dependent women are more comfortable seeking help from potential caregivers (Greenberg & Fisher, 1977). Dependent patients also adhere more conscientiously than nondependent patients to medical and psychotherapeutic treatment regimens (Fisher, Winne, & Ley, 1993; Poldrugo & Forti, 1988). Other investigations indicate that dependent college students are more willing than nondependent students to seek advice from professors and advisors when they are having difficulty with class material. As a result, dependent college students have significantly higher grade point averages than nondependent college students with similar demographic backgrounds and comparable Scholastic Aptitude Test (SAT) scores (Bornstein & Kennedy, 1994).

These findings should not be taken to suggest that all active manifestations of dependency lead to positive outcomes. On the contrary, dependent elementary school students who make frequent contact with the teacher are perceived by classmates as being clingy and demanding, and these students tend to score low on peer ratings of sociometric status and high on self-report measures of loneliness (Mahon, 1982; Overholser, 1992; Wiggins & Winder, 1961). Other studies suggest that dependency-related insecurity can lead to difficulties in friendships and romantic relationships and increased conflict with college roommates (Mongrain, Lubbers, & Struthers, 2004; Mongrain, Vettese, Shuster, & Kendal, 1998). Dependent psychiatric patients tend to have a higher number of "pseudo-emergencies" than nondependent patients (Emery & Lesher, 1982) and to overuse medical and consultative services when hospitalized (O'Neill & Bornstein, 2001), a pattern also displayed by dependent nursing home residents (Baltes, 1996).

In addition, studies consistently show that highly dependent men are at significantly increased risk for perpetrating partner abuse, in part because these men are fearful of being abandoned by their partner (Bornstein, 2006a; Holtzworth-Monroe, Stuart, & Hutchinson, 1997; Kane, Staiger, & Ricciardelli, 2000). As a result they tend to overperceive abandonment risk, becoming jealous of even casual contacts between their partner and other men (Babcock, Costa, Green, & Eckhardt, 2004). Murphy, Meyer, and O'Leary (1994, p. 734) described this dependency–abuse dynamic well when they

noted that high levels of interpersonal dependency "contribute to an escalating cycle of coercive control regulated by changes in emotional distance. Although coercive tactics may engender short-term behavioral compliance or intense emotional reunion, a frequently coerced partner is likely to withdraw emotionally … in the long run. As the batterer's emotional vulnerabilities are further activated, he may engage in more intense, frequent, and diverse coercive behavior."

Conclusion

In some ways the evolution of research on interpersonal dependency has paralleled the broader changes taking place in social psychology during the past 50 years. What was once conceptualized as a personality pattern that manifested itself consistently across different contexts and settings has come to be seen in a more nuanced way, as a set of traits that may be expressed very differently depending on the opportunities and constraints characterizing different situations. What was once conceptualized primarily in terms of expressed behavior has come to be understood in terms of the synergistic interplay of underlying cognitive, motivational, and affective processes. And like many variables in social psychology that were initially conceptualized as reflecting flaws or deficits in functioning (e.g., high self-monitoring, external locus of control), interpersonal dependency has come to be seen as a personality style that can impair adjustment in certain ways but enhance it in others.

Two trends characterize research on interpersonal dependency today. First, researchers have begun to explore the possibility that there are trait-like individual differences in the degree to which people express underlying dependency needs in adaptive (versus maladaptive) ways. The concept of *healthy dependency* overlaps with several other constructs in psychology, sociology, and medicine, including compensatory dependency (Baltes, 1996), connectedness (Clark & Ladd, 2000), and mature dependency (Baumeister & Leary, 1995). Research on healthy dependency is still in its infancy, but studies suggest that in contrast to unhealthy dependency (which is characterized by intense, unmodulated dependency strivings exhibited indiscriminately across a broad range of situations), healthy dependency is characterized by dependency strivings that— even when strong—are exhibited selectively (i.e., in some contexts but not others) and flexibly (i.e., in situation-appropriate ways). In general, people with a healthy dependent personality orientation show greater insight into their dependency needs than do unhealthy dependent persons, better social skills, more effective impulse control, greater cognitive complexity, and a more mature defense and coping style (see Bornstein, 2005, and Pincus & Wilson, 2001, for reviews of research in this area).

Second, researchers have devoted increasing attention to exploring the mental representations and information processing dynamics associated with a dependent personality orientation. In the former realm, researchers have documented features of the dependent person's self-concept (Mongrain, 1998), representations of significant others (Pincus & Wilson, 2001), and internal working models of self–other interactions (Meyer & Pilkonis, 2005). In the latter realm, researchers have assessed the impact of subliminal lexical priming on dependency-related interpersonal Stroop latencies (Bornstein et al., 2005), the impact of self-relevant personality trait feedback (both accurate and false) on perceptions of dependency-related Rorschach imagery (Bornstein, 2007), and cognitive distortions associated with positively and negatively toned experiences in close relationships (Mongrain et al., 1998). Given the impact of dependency-related cognitions on the motivational, affective, and behavioral sequelae of interpersonal dependency, continued exploration of these cognitive features is needed.

References

Abraham, K. (1927). The influence of oral erotism on character formation. In C. A. D. Bryan & A. Strachey (Eds.), Selected papers on psycho-analysis (pp. 393–406). London: Hogarth Press.

Ainsworth, M. D. S. (1969). Object relations, dependency, and attachment: A theoretical review of the infant–mother relationship. Child Development, 40, 969–1025.

Babcock, J. C., Costa, D. M., Green, C. E., & Eckhardt, C. I. (2004). What situations induce intimate partner violence?: A reliability and validity study of the Proximal Antecedents to Violent Episodes scale. Journal of Family Psychology, 18, 433–442.

Baker, J. D., Capron, E. W., & Azorloza, J. (1996). Family environment characteristics of persons with histrionic and dependent personality disorders. Journal of Personality Disorders, 10, 82–87.

Baldwin, M. W., & Sinclair, L. (1996). Self-esteem and "if … then" contingencies of interpersonal acceptance. Journal of Personality and Social Psychology, 71, 1130–1141.

Baltes, M. M. (1996). The many faces of dependency in old age. Cambridge, UK: Cambridge University Press.

Bandura, A. (1977). Self-efficacy: Toward a unifying theory of behavior change. Psychological Review, 84, 191–215.

Baumeister, R. F., & Leary, M. R. (1995). The need to belong: Desire for interpersonal attachment as a fundamental human motivation. Psychological Bulletin, 117, 497–529.

Blatt, S. J. (1974). Levels of object representation in anaclitic and introjective depression. Psychoanalytic Study of the Child, 29, 107–157.

Blatt, S. J., & Homann, E. (1992). Parent–child interaction in the etiology of dependent and self-critical depression. Clinical Psychology Review, 12, 47–91.

Bornstein, R. F. (1992). The dependent personality: Developmental, social, and clinical perspectives. Psychological Bulletin, 112, 3–23.

Bornstein, R. F. (1993). The dependent personality. New York: Guilford Press.

Bornstein, R. F. (1996). Beyond orality: Toward an object relations/interactionist reconceptualization of the etiology and dynamics of dependency. Psychoanalytic Psychology, 13, 177–203.

Bornstein, R. F. (1998a). Implicit and self-attributed dependency needs: Differential relationships to laboratory and field measures of help-seeking. Journal of Personality and Social Psychology, 75, 778–787.

Bornstein, R. F. (1998b). Implicit and self-attributed dependency needs in dependent and histrionic personality disorders. Journal of Personality Assessment, 71, 1–14.

Bornstein, R. F. (1998c). Interpersonal dependency and physical illness: A meta-analytic review of retrospective and prospective studies. Journal of Research in Personality, 32, 480–497.

Bornstein, R. F. (1999). Criterion validity of objective and projective dependency tests: A meta-analytic assessment of behavioral prediction. Psychological Assessment, 11, 48–57.

Bornstein, R. F. (2002). A process dissociation approach to objective–projective test score interrelationships. Journal of Personality Assessment, 78, 47–68.

Bornstein, R. F. (2005). The dependent patient: A practitioner's guide. Washington, DC: American Psychological Association.

Bornstein, R. F. (2006a). The complex relationship between dependency and domestic violence: Converging psychological factors and social forces. American Psychologist, 61, 595–606.

Bornstein, R. F. (2006b). Self-schema priming and desire for test performance feedback: Further evaluation of a cognitive/interactionist model of interpersonal dependency. Self and Identity, 5, 110–126.

Bornstein, R. F. (2007). Might the Rorschach be a projective test after all?: Social projection of an undesired trait alters Rorschach Oral Dependency scores. *Journal of Personality Assessment, 88,* 354–367.

Bornstein, R. F., Bowers, K. S., & Bonner, S. (1996a). Effects of induced mood states on objective and projective dependency scores. *Journal of Personality Assessment, 67,* 324–340.

Bornstein, R. F., Bowers, K. S., & Bonner, S. (1996b). Relationships of objective and projective dependency scores to sex role orientation in college student participants. *Journal of Personality Assessment, 66,* 555–568.

Bornstein, R. F., & Kennedy, T. D. (1994). Interpersonal dependency and academic performance. *Journal of Personality Disorders, 8,* 240–248.

Bornstein, R. F., Languirand, M. A., Geiselman, K. J., Creighton, J. A., West, M. A., Gallagher, H. A., et al. (2003). Construct validity of the Relationship Profile Test: A self-report measure of dependency–detachment. *Journal of Personality Assessment, 80,* 64–74.

Bornstein, R. F., Masling, J. M., & Poynton, F. G. (1987). Orality as a factor in interpersonal yielding. *Psychoanalytic Psychology, 4,* 161–170.

Bornstein, R. F., Ng, H. M., Gallagher, H. A., Kloss, D. M., & Regier, N. G. (2005). Contrasting effects of self-schema priming on lexical decisions and interpersonal Stroop task performance: Evidence for a cognitive/interactionist model of interpersonal dependency. *Journal of Personality, 73,* 732–761.

Bornstein, R. F., Riggs, J. M., Hill, E. L., & Calabrese, C. (1996). Activity, passivity, self-denigration, and self-promotion: Toward an interactionist model of interpersonal dependency. *Journal of Personality, 64,* 637–673.

Clark, K. E., & Ladd, G. W. (2000). Connectedness and autonomy support in parent–child relationships: Links to children's socioemotional orientation and peer relationships. *Developmental Psychology, 36,* 485–498.

Collins, N. L., & Read, S. J. (1990). Adult attachment, working models, and relationship quality in dating couples. *Journal of Personality and Social Psychology, 58,* 644–663.

Cross, S. E., Bacon, P. L., & Morris, M. L. (2000). The relational-interdependent self-construal and relationships. *Journal of Personality and Social Psychology, 78,* 791–808.

Diener, R. G. (1967). Prediction of dependent behavior in specified situations from psychological tests. *Psychological Reports, 20,* 103–108.

Emery, G., & Lesher, E. (1982). Treatment of depression in older adults: Personality considerations. *Psychotherapy, 19,* 500–505.

Fisher, P., Winne, P. H., & Ley, R. G. (1993). Group therapy for adult women survivors of child sexual abuse: Differentiation of completers versus dropouts. *Psychotherapy, 30,* 616–624.

Freud, S. (1959). Character and anal erotism. In J. Strachey (Ed. & Trans.), *The standard edition of the complete psychological works of Sigmund Freud* (Vol. 9, pp. 167–176). London: Hogarth Press. (Original work published 1908)

Fromm, E. (1947). *Man for himself.* New York: Rinehart.

Greenberg, R. P., & Fisher, S. (1977). The relationship between willingness to adopt the sick role and attitudes toward women. *Journal of Chronic Disease, 30,* 29–37.

Hirschfeld, R. M. A., Klerman, G. L., Gough, H. G., Barrett, J., Korchin, S. J., & Chodoff, P. (1977). A measure of interpersonal dependency. *Journal of Personality Assessment, 41,* 610–618.

Holtzworth-Monroe, A., Stuart, G. L., & Hutchinson, G. (1997). Violent versus nonviolent husbands: Differences in attachment patterns, dependency, and jealousy. *Journal of Family Psychology, 11,* 314–331.

Hunsley, J., & Bailey, J. M. (1999). The clinical utility of the Rorschach: Unfulfilled promises and an uncertain future. *Psychological Assessment, 11,* 266–277.

Jakubczak, L. F., & Walters, R. H. (1959). Suggestibility as dependency behavior. *Journal of Abnormal and Social Psychology, 59,* 102–107.

Johnson, F. A. (1993). *Dependency and Japanese socialization.* New York: New York University Press.

Kagan, J., & Mussen, P. (1956). Dependency themes on the TAT and group conformity. *Journal of Consulting Psychology, 20,* 29–32.

Kane, T. A., Staiger, P. K., & Ricciardelli, L. A. (2000). Male domestic violence: Attitudes, aggression, and interpersonal dependency. *Journal of Interpersonal Violence, 15,* 16–29.

Kraepelin, E. (1913). *Psychiatrie: Ein lehrbuch.* Leipzig, Germany: Barth.

Leising, D., Sporberg, D., & Rehbein, D. (2006). Characteristic interpersonal behavior in dependent and avoidant personality disorder can be observed within very short interaction sequences. *Journal of Personality Disorders, 20,* 319–330.

Mahon, N. E. (1982). The relationship of self-disclosure, interpersonal dependency, and life changes to loneliness in young adults. *Nursing Research, 31,* 343–347.

Masling, J. M., O'Neill, R. M., & Jayne, C. (1981). Orality and latency of volunteering to serve as experimental subjects. *Journal of Personality Assessment, 45,* 20–22.

Masling, J. M., Rabie, L., & Blondheim, S. H. (1967). Obesity, level of aspiration, and Rorschach and TAT measures of oral dependence. *Journal of Consulting Psychology, 31,* 233–239.

Masling, J. M., Weiss, L. R., & Rothschild, B. (1968). Relationships of oral imagery to yielding behavior and birth order. *Journal of Consulting and Clinical Psychology, 32,* 89–91.

McClelland, D. C., Koestner, R., & Weinberger, J. (1989). How do self-attributed and implicit motives differ? *Psychological Review, 96,* 690–702.

Meyer, B., & Pilkonis, P. A. (2005). An attachment model of personality disorders. In M. F. Lenzenweger & J. F. Clarkin (Eds.), *Major theories of personality disorder* (2nd ed., pp. 231–281). New York: Guilford Press.

Mischel, W., Shoda, Y., & Mendoza-Denton, R. (2002). Situation–behavior profiles as a locus of consistency in personality. *Current Directions in Psychological Science, 11,* 50–54.

Mongrain, M. (1998). Parental representations and support-seeking behaviors related to dependency and self-criticism. *Journal of Personality, 66,* 151–173.

Mongrain, M., Lubbers, R., & Struthers, W. (2004). The power of love: Mediation of rejection in roommate relationships of dependents and self-critics. *Personality and Social Psychology Bulletin, 30,* 94–105.

Mongrain, M., Vettese, L. C., Shuster, B., & Kendal, N. (1998). Perceptual biases, affect, and behavior in the relationships of dependents and self-critics. *Journal of Personality and Social Psychology, 75,* 230–241.

Murphy, C. M., Meyer, S. L., & O'Leary, K. D. (1994). Dependency characteristics of partner assaultive men. *Journal of Abnormal Psychology, 103,* 729–735.

O'Neill, R. M., & Bornstein, R. F. (2001). The dependent patient in a psychiatric inpatient setting: Relationship of interpersonal dependency to consultation and medication frequencies. *Journal of Clinical Psychology, 57,* 289–298.

Overholser, J. C. (1992). Interpersonal dependency and social loss. *Personality and Individual Differences, 13,* 17–23.

Pincus, A. L., & Gurtman, M. B. (1995). The three faces of interpersonal dependency: Structural analysis of self-report dependency measures. *Journal of Personality and Social Psychology, 69,* 744–758.

Pincus, A. L., & Wilson, K. R. (2001). Interpersonal variability in dependent personality. *Journal of Personality, 69,* 223–251.

Poldrugo, F., & Forti, B. (1988). Personality disorders and alcoholism treatment outcome. *Drug and Alcohol Dependence, 21,* 171–176.

Schneider, K. (1923). *Die psychopathischen personlichkeiten.* Vienna, Austria: Deuticke.

Shilkret, C. J., & Masling, J. M. (1981). Oral dependence and dependent behavior. *Journal of Personality Assessment, 45,* 125–129.

Sperling, M. B., & Berman, W. H. (1991). An attachment classification of desperate love. *Journal of Personality Assessment, 56,* 45–55.

Thompson, R., & Zuroff, D. C. (1998). Dependent and self-critical mothers' responses to adolescent autonomy and competence. *Personality and Individual Differences, 24,* 311–324.

Thompson, R., & Zuroff, D. C. (1999). Dependent and self-critical mothers' responses to adolescent sons' autonomy and competence. *Journal of Youth and Adolescence, 28,* 365–384.

Tribich, D., & Messer, S. (1974). Psychoanalytic character type and status of authority as determiners of suggestibility. *Journal of Consulting and Clinical Psychology, 42,* 842–848.

Tyrer, P., Mitchard, S., Methuen, C., & Ranger, M. (2003). Treatment-rejecting and treatment-seeking personality disorders: Type R and Type S. *Journal of Personality Disorders, 17,* 263–268.

Vittengl, J. R., Clark, L. A., & Jarrett, R. B. (2003). Interpersonal problems, personality pathology, and social adjustment after cognitive therapy for depression. *Psychological Assessment, 15,* 29–40.

Weiss, L. R. (1969). Effects of subject, experimenter, and task variables on compliance with the experimenter's expectation. *Journal of Projective Techniques and Personality Assessment, 33,* 247–256.

Wiggins, J. S., & Winder, C. L. (1961). The Peer Nomination Inventory. *Psychological Reports, 9,* 643–677.

Yamaguchi, S. (2004). Further clarifications of the concept of *amae* in relation to dependence and attachment. *Human Development, 47,* 28–33.

CHAPTER 7

■ ● ▲ ◆ ■ ● ▲ ◆

Machiavellianism

DANIEL N. JONES
DELROY L. PAULHUS

Early in the 16th century, Niccolo Machiavelli acted as chief political advisor to the ruling Medici family in Florence, Italy. The details of his counsel are well known because Machiavelli laid them out for posterity in his 1513 book, *The Prince*. The gist of his advice for maintaining political control is captured in the phrase "the end justifies the means." According to Machiavelli, a ruler with a clear agenda should be open to any and all effective tactics, including manipulative interpersonal strategies such as flattery and lying.

Four centuries later, these ideas struck a chord with the personality psychologist Richard Christie, who noticed that Machiavelli's political strategies had parallels in people's everyday social behavior. Christie and his colleagues at Columbia University identified a corresponding personality syndrome, which they dubbed *Machiavellianism*. The label was chosen to capture a duplicitous interpersonal style assumed to emerge from a broader network of cynical beliefs and pragmatic morality. Christie applied his psychometric expertise to develop a series of questionnaires designed to tap individual differences in Machiavellianism. Those questionnaires, along with the research supporting their construct validity, were presented in Christie and Geis's (1970) book, *Studies in Machiavellianism*. Of these measures, by far the most popular

has been the Mach IV.[1] Used in more than 2,000 cited studies, the scale has proved valuable in studying manipulative tendencies among student, community, and worker samples. The follow-up version, Mach V, was designed as an improvement but, in the end, raised more problems than it solved (Wrightsman, 1991).

The only comprehensive review of the research literature on Machiavellianism was published 20 years later by Fehr, Samsom, and Paulhus (1992). Rather than recapitulate that review, our strategy here is to summarize its conclusions and springboard into the subsequent research. Our emphasis is on the Christie tradition primarily focused on research using his scales. We conclude by discussing new directions in theory and research on Machiavellianism.

The Character of Machiavellians

Their Motivation

The 1992 review by Fehr and colleagues described Machiavellian motivation as one of cold selfishness or pure instrumentality. Rather than having a unique set of goals, individuals high in Machiavellianism (referred to casually as "Machs") were assumed to have typical intrinsic motives (e.g., sex, achievement, and sociality). Whatever the motives, Machs pursue them in duplicitous ways.

This view has required some adjustment based on recent work wherein Machs were asked about their motivations. Compared to low Machs, high Machs gave high priority to money, power, and competition (Stewart & Stewart, 2006) and relatively low priority to community building, self-love, and family concerns (McHoskey, 1999). Machs admitted to a focus on unmitigated achievement and winning at any cost (Ryckman, Thornton, & Butler, 1994). Note that this distinctive motivational profile does not necessarily conflict with the original view of Machs as purely instrumental: After all, money seeking and power seeking tend to maximize instrumental benefits in the long run.

Their Abilities

Because of their success at interpersonal manipulation, it is often assumed that Machiavellians have superior intelligence, especially with regard to understanding people in social situations (Davies & Stone, 2003). However, the lack of relation between Machiavellianism and IQ has been clearly established (e.g., Paulhus & Williams, 2002; Wilson, Near, & Miller, 1996). As a result, researchers have turned to possible links with more specific cognitive abilities, in particular, mind reading and emotional intelligence.

The assumption that Machiavellians have a more advanced "theory of mind" has stirred a new commotion of developmental research. An advanced theory of mind is said to facilitate "mind reading" in the sense of anticipating what others are thinking in interpersonal interactions (Davies & Stone, 2003; McIlwain, 2003; Repacholi, Slaughter, Pritchard, & Gibbs, 2003). To date, however, research has failed to support the putative link with Machiavellianism (Loftus & Glenwick, 2001; Paal & Bereczkei, 2007).

Even more disappointing, associations of Machiavellianism with emotional intelligence (EQ) have actually turned out to be *negative*. This pattern applies to overall scores on both performance and questionnaire measures of EQ (Austin, Farrelly, Black, & Moore, 2007). Most relevant are two key facets of EQ—the ability to empathize with other people and the ability to recognize others' emotions. Both empathy (Carnahan & McFarland, 2007; Loftus &

Glenwick, 2001; Paal & Bereczkei, 2007; Wastell & Booth, 2003) and emotion recognition (Simon, Francis, & Lombardo, 1990) have shown consistent negative correlations with Machiavellianism.

In sum, the assumption that Machs have superior mental abilities—whether it be IQ, EQ, or mind reading—is not supported by the data. Indeed, one should be cautious about concluding from Machs' willingness to manipulate others that they are naturally skilled at the task. Instead, we argue here that any manipulative abilities that Machiavellians possess derive from superior impulse regulation rather than any special cognitive ability.

How Machs Are Perceived by Others

The 1992 review reported mixed results with respect to how Machs are perceived by others, and more recent research has attempted to clarify that ambiguity. On the one hand, the developmental literature suggests that young Machiavellians may be well adjusted and even well liked (Hawley, 2003; Newcomb, Bukowski, & Pattee, 1993). Even as adults, they are sometimes preferred as leaders (Coie, Dodge, & Kupersmidt, 1990) and debate partners (Wilson, Near, & Miller, 1998). Notwithstanding those exceptions, Machiavellian behaviors among adults generally draw strong disapproval (Falbo, 1977).

One moderating variable may be the social role for which the Machiavellian is being rated. Wilson and colleagues (1998) showed that high Machs were seen as less desirable for most forms of social interaction (e.g., confidant, good friend, business partner) but may be more desirable as debate partners. Consistent with that finding are two studies of presidential personalities. Ratings of archival data indicated that presidents seen as more Machiavellian were also seen as having higher levels of drive and poise (Simonton, 1986). A follow-up to that research indicated that presidents who were viewed as more Machiavellian were also seen as more desirable leaders, with high ratings on charisma and effectiveness (Deluga, 2001).

A recent review by Wilson and colleagues (1996) offered a second possible moderating variable—time delay. They argued that Machiavellians pursue short-term manipulative social strategies and thus fool some people some of the time; but repeat offenses lead to resentment and social exclusion over time. To date, no empirical evidence supports these claims. Furthermore, as explained subsequently, we dispute the idea that Machiavellians prefer short-term over long-term strategies.

Their Personalities and Psychological Adjustment

Self-Monitoring

A personality construct sharing many features of Machiavellianism is self-monitoring (Snyder, 1974). Although both constructs involve social manipulation, Machiavellianism also harbors the darker features of cynical worldviews and amorality. In the original publication of the self-monitoring scale, Snyder (1974) emphasized their distinctiveness, and subsequent research confirmed that the two traits correlate only in the .20–.33 range (Bolino & Turnley, 2003; Fehr et al., 1992; Leone & Corte, 1994).

Locus of Control

The 1992 review indicated (counterintuitively) that Machiavellians have an external locus of control; that is, they feel that external forces control people's behavior and outcomes. More recent studies have reported the same pattern (Gable & Dangello, 1994; O'Connor & Morrison, 2001; Yong, 1994). Along with Paulhus (1983), we consider that conclusion to be misleading. None of these studies partitioned perceived control into its three spheres of engagement—personal, interpersonal, and sociopolitical. Paulhus showed that these three aspects of perceived control have quite different relations with Machiavellianism. Machs' apparent external locus of control derives entirely from the sociopolitical factor: Machs are simply endorsing their cynical view of others' competence (see also McHoskey et al., 1999). That is, they perceive other people as weak and as having little control over their situations.

In contrast, Machiavellians score quite high on measures of interpersonal control. In this sphere, Machs believe that they can manipulate others to get what they want. We encourage other researchers to include

the three subscales instead of a global measure of locus of control. Further clarification would be provided by a measure that distinguished perceptions of control by oneself ("I can control … ") from perceptions of control among others ("People can control … ").

Worldviews

One might expect a positive association between Machiavellianism and authoritarianism because a condescending attitude toward outgroups is central to both constructs. The 1992 review, however, concluded that overall associations are weak. The exception was a positive correlation between authoritarianism and the Mach IV Moral Views subscale, which taps tough-mindedness. That link is understandable because intolerance of personal weakness is an element of the authoritarian personality (Christie, 1991).

Since then, the only direct study failed to find an overall association between Machiavellianism and authoritarianism, although both measures predicted the willingness to volunteer for a study on "prison life," as well as endorsement of pragmatic sociopolitical views (Carnahan & McFarland, 2007). Indirect research also indicates links with specific aspects of conservatism and authoritarianism (Christie, 1991). For example, Machiavellianism has been linked to traditional attitudes toward women in the workplace (Valentine & Fleischman, 2003). As noted later, Machs also score relatively low on communal values (Trapnell & Paulhus, in press; Watson & Morris, 1994). In sum, the worldview of Machs is one of pragmatic tough-mindedness.

Mental Health

An analysis of the links between psychopathology and Machiavellianism must first acknowledge the distinction between Axis I and Axis II disorders. We defer our discussion of Axis II (personality disorders) to a subsequent section and deal here with Axis I disorders, primarily mood and anxiety disorders.

The 1992 review indicated a consistent positive association between Machiavellianism and anxiety. Even Christie and Geis (1970) were suspicious that this counterintuitive association was artifactual, resulting from the willingness of Machs to disclose negative feelings. Wrightsman (1991) agreed that high anxiety was at odds with the concept of Machiavellianism, especially their detachment in situations of interpersonal conflict. More recent research has failed to resolve this paradox, with some studies finding no correlation (Allsopp, Eysenck, & Eysenck, 1991; McNamara, Durso, & Harris, 2007; Paulhus & Williams, 2002) and others finding a positive correlation (Jakobowitz & Egan, 2006; Ramanaiah, Byravan, & Detwiler, 1994).

The findings on guilt are also inconsistent: Some research indicates that Machs are more guilt prone (Drake, 1995), whereas others report that Machs are less guilt prone (Wastell & Booth, 2003). Scattered research indicates some positive correlations with other forms of psychopathology, for example, depression (Bakir, Yilmaz, & Yavas, 1996), paranoia (Christoffersen & Stamp, 1995), alexithymia (Wastell & Booth, 2003), socially prescribed perfectionism (Sherry, Hewitt, Besser, Flett, & Klein, 2006), and low self-esteem (Valentine & Fleischman, 2003; Yong, 1994). Overall links between Mach scales and psychopathology measures appear to be weak and sample-specific.

Interpersonal adjustment (Axis IV) concerns whether individuals have harmonious relations with other people. Although clearly relevant to the psychological adjustment of Machiavellians, the Axis IV diagnosis is, once again, mixed. On the one hand, Machs sometimes harm those around them, as we describe later. On the other hand, as noted, Machs can earn liking and respect under select circumstances and time frames (presumably when they deem it to be in their interest) (Hawley, 2006).

Career Issues

Career Choice

The 1992 review concluded that Machs select occupations that are more business oriented and less helping oriented. However, research shows that Machiavellianism is unrelated to specialty choice in medical students (Moore, Katz, & Holder, 1995) and nursing students (Moore & Katz, 1995). Other research on medical students finds that Machs are less likely to opt for general practice as a spe-

cialty (Diehl, Kumar, Gateley, Appleby, & O'Keefe, 2006). The latter finding is consistent with the view that, even in helping professions, career choices of high Machs are motivated by financial goals. Some commentators have raised the possibility of a reverse causal direction: Certain careers may reward manipulative behavior, thereby inducing workers to become more Machiavellian. For example, success in some professions is determined by reporting the misbehavior of coworkers (e.g., Girodo, 1998; Macrosson & Hemphill, 2001).

Career Success

We define career success as effective performance by a worker in the role assigned by the employer. The 1992 review found no overall evidence that Machiavellianism facilitates such career success. However, more recent research using behavioral outcomes indicates a clear pattern. Machs appear to have an advantage in unstructured organizations (Gable, Hollon, & Dangello, 1992; Shultz, 1993). They thrive when they have more decision power, fewer rules, and less managerial supervision. In highly structured organizations, high Machs actually perform worse than low Machs (O'Connor & Morrison, 2001; Shultz, 1993; Sparks, 1994). Our confidence in these conclusions is encouraged by the fact that concrete measures of job success were used in several of these studies. In general, the research on career success is consistent with the original notion of *latitude for improvisation*. As Christie and Geis (1970) determined in laboratory research, Machs remain cool, exploit interpersonal relationships, bend the rules, and improvise. When this flexibility is constrained, Machs are likely to incur problems.

A self-report study by Ricks and Fraedrich (1999) exemplified the tradeoff in the job success of Machiavellians: High Machs reported higher sales volume but also reported significantly lower approval rates from their supervisors. By one criterion, Machs are a success; by another criterion, they are not. Other research with self-report measures of job success has extended to a wider variety of occupations. Aziz and colleagues related success to a new measure they called the Machiavellian Behavior Scale (Mach-B). The Mach-B correlated positively with self-reports of success among stockbrokers (Aziz, May, & Crotts, 2002), car salespeople (Aziz, 2004), and real estate salespersons (Aziz, 2005). However, one wonders how much to trust self-reports of success by Machiavellians, who may be inclined to exaggerate their accomplishments.

One study investigated the question of how compatible the Machiavellian personality is with various job profiles (Macrosson & Hemphill, 2001). Fittingly, the job profile for Machs suggested that they would be ideal as spies on other employees. For such roles, organizations may find it in their interest to hire otherwise unsavory characters.

Career Satisfaction

The 1992 review concluded that Machs are generally less satisfied with their jobs. More recent research has supported this finding in retail executives (Gable & Topol, 1988), marketers (Sparks, 1994), and bank managers (Corzine, Buntzman, & Busch, 1999). Machs are more likely to feel unappreciated, to believe that they have plateaued in their careers (Corzine et al., 1999), and to leave their positions (Becker & O'Hair, 2007). Machs also report more negative feelings from coworkers (Vecchio, 2000, 2005). Indeed, hostile Machs are more likely to justify committing sabotage against a company they are upset with (Giacalone & Knouse, 1990).

Interestingly, some studies indicate that high Mach women report higher levels of promotion satisfaction (Gable & Topol, 1989; Siu & Tam, 1995). It is possible that female Machs were also satisfied in the studies reported in the previous paragraph, but the results provided no breakdown by gender. Overall, the bulk of recent research seems to confirm a general career dissatisfaction among high Machs.

Machiavellian Malevolence

Because the Mach IV scale is its most widely accepted operationalization, the construct validity of Machiavellianism rests largely on the match between high Mach IV scores and actual pragmatic manipulation. Its structural validity is clarified by evidence for the meaningfulness of the three themes measured by the Mach IV Scale: (1) belief in manipulative tactics, (2) a cynical worldview, and (3) a pragmatic morality. Accordingly, we review the evidence for these three themes, as well as overall antisocial behavior among high Machs.

Manipulation Tactics

Rather than asking respondents directly whether they manipulate others, the Mach IV poses questions about the utility of various tactics. Among other advantages, this indirect approach to measurement was designed to reduce socially desirable responding—otherwise a serious concern. Apparently successful, high Mach IV scores do predict who will and who will not engage in interpersonal manipulation.

Fehr and colleagues (1992) highlighted persuasion, self-disclosure, and ingratiation as the influence tactics most preferred by Machs. More recent research has continued to elaborate on these and other tactics. For example, Falbo's (1977) notion that Machs use more indirect persuasion strategies was supported by Kumar and Beyerlein's (1991) finding that Machs are especially inclined to use thought manipulation, deceit, and ingratiation. Machs are also more likely to use friendliness and emotional tactics, possibly because of their ability to stay emotionally detached from a situation (Grams & Rogers, 1990). High Machs are also known to use guilt induction to manipulate others (Vangelisti, Daly, & Rudnick, 1991).

Impression Management

The literature since 1992 has elaborated on the nature and degree of impression management among high Machs. Among their reported forms of self-presentation are perfectionistic self-promotion, nondisclosure of imperfection, and nondisplay of imperfection (Sherry et al., 2006). Importantly, the impression-management tactics of Machiavellians have been verified by self-reports, peer reports, and supervisor reports (Becker & O'Hair, 2007). Compared with low Machs, high Machs view impression management as a more appropriate strategy in job interview situations (Lopes & Fletcher, 2004).

As noted, the 1992 review indicated that high Machs and high self-monitors employ different impression-management strategies. Recent work has supported that conclusion (Bolino & Turnley, 2003; Corral & Calvete, 2000). Machs are more likely to use negative impression-management tactics such as supplication and intimidation (trying to be perceived as helpless or threatening, respectively), whereas high self-monitors are more likely to use more positive tactics such as exemplification (emphasizing one's moral integrity and responsibility), self-promotion (emphasizing one's competence), and ingratiation (emphasizing one's likeability).

Self-Disclosure

Recently added to the list of social influence tactics is the notion of using selective self-disclosure for manipulation (Liu, 2008). In one study, the tendency was found only among females high in Mach, suggesting that certain manipulation strategies may be sex-specific (Buss & Schmitt, 1993; Haselton, Buss, Oubaid, & Angleitner, 2005; O'Connor & Simms, 1990).

Sandbagging

One paradoxical finding concerns the willingness to "sandbag," or feign incompetence, in order to gain a competitive edge. Contrary to expectations, research indicates that low Machs are more likely to sandbag than high Machs (Shepperd & Socherman, 1997). Perhaps high Machs are too dominant and aggressive to feign incompetence. Another possible explanation is that strategies such as sandbagging are ineffective and that high Machs recognize this ineffectiveness and eschew them.

Cynical Worldview

Research confirms that Machs have a broadly negative view of other people. For example, they assume that other people are cheaters (Mudrack, 1993). They are more likely to believe that others would engage in such unethical behavior as feigning dissatisfaction with service received in order to obtain a refund (Wirtz & Kum, 2004). At the same time, high Machs report being more tolerant of unethical behavior in others (Mudrack, 1993). This finding is reminiscent of the

"projective" logic behind covert integrity tests: Workers who say they believe that others steal are the very ones who go on to steal from the company (Cunningham, Wong, & Barbee, 1994).

The original notion of Machiavellian cynicism went hand in hand with Machs' reported use of manipulative tactics, although the causal direction was ambiguous. Cynical beliefs could lead to manipulative tactics as a form of preemptive strike. Alternatively, the tendency to manipulate may require a rationalization in the form of a cynical worldview. This ambiguity has yet to be addressed empirically, presumably because it requires a complex longitudinal research design with at least two waves of data.

Morality

Understanding the moral perspective of Machiavellians continues to be a challenge. Although immorality was considered by Christie to be among the three key elements of Machiavellianism, the Morality subscale on the Mach IV comprised only two items, one favoring euthanasia and the other concerning callous bereavement. Together, they may indicate a detached pragmatism regarding emotion-laden decisions.

The 1992 review concluded that Machs behave in a less ethical manner—but only in specific circumstances. More recent research suggests a broader set of circumstances. Compared to low Machs, high Machs report having lower ethical standards (Singhapakdi & Vitell, 1991), fewer qualms about unethical behavior (Mudrack, 1995), and greater intentions to behave unethically in the future (Bass, Barnett, & Brown, 1999; Jones & Kavanagh, 1996). Specific examples include a greater acceptance of unethical consumer practices such as purchasing clothing for one night's use and returning it the following day (Shen & Dickenson, 2001). Machs are willing to accept unjustified positive benefits from an employer (Mudrach, Mason, & Stepanski, 1999). Machs also advocate the violation of privacy and intellectual property laws (Winter, Stylianou, & Giacalone, 2004). Of course, the moral perspective of Machs may be seen as either immorality or simple pragmatism (Leary, Knight, & Barnes, 1986).

A radical reinterpretation may be mandated by research indicating that low and high Machs hold qualitatively different kinds of ethical beliefs. High Machs place relatively more emphasis on competence values (i.e., valuing competence and ability to succeed), whereas low Machs report relatively more emphasis on moral values (Musser & Orke, 1992; Trapnell & Paulhus, in press). Such results can be seen as a reframing of Machiavellian morality in terms of its priorities. This reframing is consistent with Haidt's (2001) notion that people differ little in their overall moral reactions but rank the priority of moral facets (e.g., justice, integrity) rather differently.

Antisocial Behavior

Lying and Cheating

Given their manipulative tendencies, it may be surprising that Machs admit to antisocial behaviors in many self-report studies. Machs report telling more lies in daily diary studies (Kashy & DePaulo, 1996), lower intentions to honor deals that they have made (Forgas, 1998), and being more likely to withhold information that would harm them economically (e.g., not revealing a flaw in a car they are selling) (Sakalaki, Richardson, & Thepaut, 2007). In a business school simulation, Machs were also more likely to lie on tax returns (Ghosh & Crain, 1995). We contend that Machs would not report any of these antisocial inclinations if they expected that authorities might use the information against them.

The 1992 review indicated that this interaction of Machiavellianism with accountability was evident in behavioral studies of cheating. That is, high Machs cheat when the risk of detection or retaliation is low, whereas low Machs cheat when persuaded by others. Recent research indicates a similar pattern for academic cheating. High Machs were more likely to cheat on term papers (Williams, Nathanson, & Paulhus, in press) but not more likely to cheat on multiple-choice tests (Nathanson, Paulhus, & Williams, 2006). The authors explained that Machiavellians' impulse control channeled them into strategic forms of cheating (e.g., essay plagiarism) rather than opportunistic forms such as multiple-choice copying.

Revenge and Betrayal

No research on revenge or betrayal was reported in the 1992 review. Recently, Nathanson and colleagues reported a series of studies of anonymous revenge anecdotes (Nathanson & Paulhus, 2006). Although it predicts revenge reports, the Mach IV overlaps considerably with measures of subclinical psychopathy (McHoskey, Worzel, & Szyarto, 1998; Paulhus & Williams, 2002). Indeed, the association of Mach with revenge was entirely accounted for by the overlap of Machiavellianism with subclinical psychopathy (Nathanson & Paulhus, 2006).

Betrayal behavior has been studied in simulation games among college students. In a simulated sales game, Machs engaged in a variety of unethical behaviors such as kickbacks (Hegarty, 1995). In bargaining games, Meyer (1992) found that high Machs are more likely to betray another participant in a one-shot opportunistic manner. More recent research has suggested that Machs are especially likely to betray others when there is no chance for the other person to get retribution (Gunnthorsdottir, McCabe, & Smith, 2002). We suspect that Machiavellianism predicted betrayal in the simulation studies because that behavior led to success. In contrast, Machiavellianism failed to predict revenge in the Nathanson studies, where such behavior was largely maladaptive.

Aggression and Hostility

The 1992 review noted a small positive correlation between Mach and hostility but cautioned that few studies were available. As with guilt and anxiety, however, the notion that Machs are especially hostile is inconsistent with the original construct. Christie and Geis (1970) emphasized the cool detachment of Machs in conflict situations. Instead, it may be that Machs—at least in anonymous reports—are more forthright in admitting hostile feelings and behaviors (Locke & Christensen, 2007; Marusic, Bratko, & Zarevski, 1995; Wrightsman, 1991).

With regard to aggression per se, self-report data again suggest a small positive correlation with Machiavellianism (Suman, Singh, & Ashok, 2000; Watson & Morris, 1994), including verbal aggression (Martin, Anderson, &Thweatt, 1998). Machiavellian managers also report a greater willingness to use coercive power (Corzine & Hozier, 2005).

Similarly, children who report bullying (either as perpetrators or victims) score higher on Machiavellianism (Andreou, 2000, 2004). Machs may be responding strategically to being bullied by bullying others. Or they may report being bullied to garner benefits from authorities. Alternatively, Machs may be more willing to admit to the negative experiences of both bullying and being bullied.

In the one study where both self-report and behavioral measures were collected on the same children, a paradox emerged. Machiavellianism was positively correlated with misbehavior on children's self-reports but not on adult ratings (Loftus & Glenwick, 2001). It is unclear whether Machiavellian children are exaggerating their misbehavior or whether they are successful in inhibiting it when adults are present.

Summary

Machiavellian misbehavior is well documented in nonaggressive varieties, namely, cheating, lying, and betrayal. By contrast, there is no evidence for overt aggression in behavioral studies of Machiavellian adults.

New Directions

Situating Machiavellianism in Personality Space

The growing consensus on two structural models—the Big Five and the interpersonal circumplex—has helped clarify the location of Machiavellianism in broader personality space. Those two models help interpret Machiavellianism with respect to fundamental personality axes, as well as elucidating its overlap with other personality variables.

Interpersonal Circumplex

The interpersonal circumplex is framed in terms of two independent axes—agency and communion (Wiggins, 1991). Agency refers to the motivation to succeed and individuate oneself; communion refers to the motivation to merge with others and support the group. Several studies have established that Machi-

avellianism lies in quadrant 2 of the circumplex, indicating that high Machs are high on agency and low on communion (Gurtman, 1991, 1992; Wiggins & Broughton, 1991). Work by Locke and colleagues yielded a composite variable called *self-construal* that indexes a relative preference for communion over agency. As expected, self-construal falls diagonally opposite Machiavellianism in circumplex space (Locke & Christensen, 2007), confirming a key suspicion regarding Machs: They are not simply out to achieve but rather are out to achieve at the expense of (or at least without regard for) others.

The Big Five

Because it is currently the predominant personality taxonomy, relations of Machiavellianism with the Big Five "supertraits" are of interest (Costa & McCrae, 1992). The clearest correlates are low Conscientiousness and low Agreeableness (Jakobwitz & Egan, 2006; Paulhus & Williams, 2002). Interestingly, research indicates that Mach correlates more highly (and negatively) with a sixth factor of personality (Honesty–Humility) than with any of the Big Five (Lee & Ashton, 2005).

The Dark Triad

Three overlapping personality variables—Machiavellianism, narcissism, subclinical psychopathy—have come to be known as the "Dark Triad" of personality: They were so named because individuals with these traits share a tendency to be callous, selfish, and malevolent in their interpersonal dealings (Paulhus & Williams, 2002). Also overlapping is the P-scale from Eysenck's P-E-N inventory (Allsop et al., 1991), which appears to be conceptually equivalent to subclinical psychopathy (Williams & Paulhus, 2004).

The distinctiveness of the Dark Triad was disputed by McHoskey and colleagues (McHoskey, 1995, 2001a; McHoskey et al., 1998): They argued that, in nonclinical samples such as students, the three variables are equivalent. Their arguments posed a significant threat to the discriminant validity of the Mach construct. Subsequently, Paulhus and colleagues published a series of articles confirming their overlap but establishing sufficient discriminant validity to recommend measuring all three variables in Mach research (e.g., Paulhus & Williams, 2002). The authors argued that a failure to include the other two Dark Triad members renders ambiguous any research on one member alone.

Evolutionary Origins

The growing influence of evolutionary psychology has provoked discussion of the ancestral origins of Machiavellianism. Although it includes arguments for the advantages of prosocial traits (such as altruism, compassion, and cooperation), the hallmark of evolutionary theory is the notion of the "selfish gene" (Dawkins, 1989). Contrary to many observers' intuition, it is not paradoxical to include both prosocial and antisocial tendencies within the behavioral repertoire of our species (Krueger, Hicks, & McGue, 2001).

The natural selection of selfishness would naturally foster Machiavellian personalities. In ancestral times, those who exploited opportunities to cheat, steal, and manipulate others to achieve their goals would have outreproduced those who did not. Indeed, this adaptive advantage been referred to in the literature as *Machiavellian intelligence* (Byrne & Whiten, 1988): The term is often used interchangeably with terms such as *social intelligence, everyday politics, social astuteness, political intelligence, practical intelligence, emotional intelligence*, and *interpersonal intelligence*, all of which allude to cognitive abilities involving skill at adapting to social complexities. Such skills, including the ability to manipulate others, would enhance the control of resources such as food, shelter, and sex (Hawley, 2006). In sum, the term *Machiavellian intelligence* (more than the related terms) implies that the skillful manipulation of others conferred a significant evolutionary advantage.

If Machiavellianism is adaptive, it seems that all members of our species should exhibit that inclination. Instead, we see substantial variation. The explanation may be found in arguments put forth by Mealey (1995). She agreed that antisocial traits such as Machiavellianism and psychopathy may reflect an adaptive reproductive strategy but argued further that antisocial traits are frequency dependent. In other words,

not everyone in an ecology can be cooperative because the advantage of being a high Mach is too great. However, there are two reasons why not everyone in an ecology can be a high Mach. The first is that low Machs would have the advantage of building strong social relationships and cooperative alliances, and the second is that high Machs would simply be cheating each other and little would be gained. Thus there are at least two good reasons that preclude the full spread of Machiavellianism. One is that Machs have a serious disadvantage in forming cooperative alliances that depend on trust. The second reason is that Machiavellian tendencies will show marginal returns: At some point, high Machs would be trying (unsuccessfully) to cheat each other, and no advantage ensues (Mealey, 1995).

Differential Reproductive Strategies

The advantages of high and low Machiavellianism should correspond to different reproductive strategies. The opportunism ascribed to Machiavellians implies that they focus on the short term (Wilson et al., 1996). Such an opportunistic strategy is especially beneficial in unstable environments (Figueredo et al., 2005), in which repeated interactions with the same individuals are rare. In the words of Wilson and colleagues (1996), "advantages of cooperation are usually long term, whereas the advantages of exploitation are usually only short term" (p. 287).

Instead, we agree with Hawley (2006) that the behavioral repertoire of Machiavellians is "bistrategic," that is, it includes both cooperation and coercion. However, we place special emphasis on the fact that neither long-term nor short-term cooperative tactics in Machiavellians reflect true cooperation; instead, such behaviors are in the service of malevolence.

Of special concern to evolutionary psychology are sexual strategies. The data are clear that high Machiavellians tend to be more promiscuous than low Machs (Linton & Wiener, 2001; McHoskey, 2001b; Schmitt, 2004; Paulhus & Williams, 2002). Recently, more detailed analyses have partitioned promiscuous behaviors and attitudes (Webster & Bryan, 2007). Exploiting that distinction, Jones and Paulhus (2008) found that Machiavellianism correlated only with the attitude component. The lack of correlation with promiscuous behavior suggests that high Machs are no less discerning than low Machs in their actual sexual activities. Such findings are another indication that Machiavellians are not solely short term in orientation.

Sex Differences

Evolutionary psychologists emphasize the different reproductive challenges faced by men and women. Because women bear the greater parental burden, they have evolved to be more long-term-oriented in their reproductive strategies than are men (Buss & Schmitt, 1993). The short-term reproductive strategies characteristic of men should predict dismissive attachment styles and high levels of mating effort.

The research on Machiavellianism supports the gender difference in short-term reproductive strategies (Figueredo et al., 2005). Most samples show higher Mach scores in men than in women (Christie & Geis, 1970) and in young than in older adults (e.g., Rawwas & Singhapakdi, 1998). These trends suggest that Machiavellianism promotes sexual activity. Individuals who seek multiple short-term sexual opportunities (e.g., those unrestricted in sociosexuality) would benefit from manipulative tendencies and a lack of empathy.

Further research confirms that Machiavellianism confers a special reproductive advantage on men. Linton and Wiener (2001) showed that high Mach men reported higher rates of possible conceptions than low Mach men. One possible explanation is that Machiavellians are likely to deceive, coerce, and manipulate partners into sex (Jones, Harms, & Paulhus, 2008). Mach is positively associated with a variety of deceptive and self-serving tactics in romantic relationships that include feigning love, intoxicating partners, divulging intimate secrets, infidelity, and coercion (McHoskey, 2001b). The fact that these associations were more pronounced for men than for women led McHoskey (2001b) to conclude that biological sex moderates the effect of Machiavellianism on sexual behavior. Insofar as men are more likely to benefit from short-term opportunistic reproductive strategies, this interaction is predictable from evolutionary psychology (Buss & Schmitt, 1993).

These arguments rest on the assumption that manipulation is more effective for the gender that prefers promiscuity than the one that prefers investment and commitment. We dispute that assumption and suggest that female Machiavellianism manifests itself in a manner consistent with the female reproductive agenda.

Developmental Origins

Researchers have addressed how Machiavellianism develops in individual children. Christie and Geis (1970) speculated on the issue but conducted little developmental research. To encourage such research, they developed the "Kiddie Mach" Scale, which has been widely used. That version assesses Machiavellianism in children by tailoring the language to their level. For example, it includes the item "The best way to get along with people is to tell them things that make them happy" instead of the Mach IV wording, "The best way to handle people is to tell them what they want to hear."

That scale has been used in the rekindling of research on the topic of Machiavellianism in children (Repacholi & Slaughter, 2003). In McIlwain's (2003) review of that research, she concluded that the young Machiavellian is characterized by mistrust, cynicism, and affective blunting. Lack of empathy, in particular, plays a causal role in determining a young Machiavellian's behavior.

A factor analysis by Sutton and Keogh (2001) revealed three factors in the Kiddie Mach Scale: lack of faith in human nature, dishonesty, and distrust. Only lack of faith in human nature correlated with age, suggesting that cynicism increases over time. The authors also suggested that, initially, children may not differentiate manipulative from prosocial behavior. In other words, they see doing and saying things to make other people "happy" as commendable rather than dishonest or unethical.

As noted earlier, some writers had anticipated that Machiavellians would have an advanced theory of mind. Instead, the research showed no relation with theory of mind but a growing negativity among those scoring high on the Kiddie-Mach. As a result, Kiddie-Machs receive ambivalent reactions from others, even in preschool years (Repacholi et. al., 2003).

A radically different conclusion has been drawn by Hawley (2006). In her view, Machiavellian children are received well by their peers and indeed are socially competent in almost every respect. The difference in her conclusion may derive from the different methodology employed. Rather than measure children with Kiddie-Mach, she directly observed the behavior of socially competent versus socially inept children. Those who use both coercive and prosocial strategies (i.e., bistrategic controllers) were labeled Machiavellian (Hawley, 2003).

Only recently has a behavioral genetics study permitted insight into possible genetic and environmental causes. In addition to a genetic component in common with narcissism and psychopathy, Machiavellianism shows a substantial shared-environment component (Vernon, Villani, Vickers, & Harris, 2008). The latter implicates socialization mechanisms, such as parental modeling or an overreaction to harsh or unpredictable family environments.

A few other studies point to possible genetic–environment interactions. By late adolescence, Mach scores of sons correlated positively with parents' Mach scores, supporting a modeling hypothesis (Ojha, 2007). Daughters in father-absent families report higher levels of Machiavellianism, but not toward family members (Barber, 1998). Adding complexity, there is evidence that children's Mach scores initially oppose, but later come to match, parental scores (Gold, Christie, & Friedman, 1976).

Machiavellianism as a Personality Tradeoff

A repeated theme in this chapter is the notion that Machiavellianism harbors both adaptive and maladaptive qualities. Key to understanding this tradeoff is the distinction between agentic and communal notions of adaptiveness. Adaptiveness for agentic goals concerns the promotion of personal achievement, whereas adaptiveness for communal goals concerns the benefits to one's group.

Agentic Goals

A consistent theme in the literature has been that Machs thrive best in contexts that (1) afford face-to-face interaction, (2) allow latitude for improvisation, and (3) involve emotional distractions (Christie & Geis, 1970). Subsequent evidence has supported those three notions. As noted, Machs seem to thrive in business situations with a high latitude for improvisation (Shultz, 1993), but they perform worse in other situations, such as when latitude for improvisation is impeded (Sparks, 1994). Even after successful manipulations, Machs may suffer a decrement in reputation that reduces future opportunities (Wilson et al., 1996).

The source of evaluation may influence whether Machs are judged as successful or not. When evaluated by a supervisor, Machs seem to evoke negative evaluations, but they concomitantly report and record higher levels of sales in certain jobs (Ricks & Fraedrich, 1999).

Communal Goals

Surprising to the intuitions of some commentators, Machs may be just as generous and helpful as others, depending on the situation. For example, Bereczkei, Birkas, and Kerekes (2007) found that Machs volunteer less than low Machs unless their volunteering is made public, thus promoting a strong reputation (Bereczkei, Birkas, & Kerekes, 2009).

Group members may prefer high Machs for roles that help the group deal with enemies and opponents (Wilson et al., 1998). A classic example is the preference for a Machiavellian as president of the United States (Deluga, 2001; Simonton, 1986). On the other hand, Machs are less favored as friends, confidants, and business partners (Wilson et al., 1998).

Length of interaction also plays a role. As noted by Fehr and colleagues (1992), high Machs are more liked in short-term encounters (such as when participants are viewing a videotape) (Ickes, Reidhead, & Patterson, 1986). However, when individuals simulate the experience of engaging with a high Mach (such as by reading a first-person story), they judge Machs more negatively (Wilson et al., 1998).

Machiavellianism Refined: Returning to Its Roots

On the whole, our review of the literature has sustained the construct validity of Machiavellianism as measured by the Christie and Geis (1970) instruments. There is substantial confirmation of Machs' cynical worldview, pragmatic ethics, and use of duplicitous tactics. Furthermore, the apparent exceptions noted throughout this chapter fit a coherent pattern.

Disconcerting, however, are reports of positive associations of Mach IV with impulsivity (Marusic et al., 1995). Certainly, impulsive hostility may represent an evolutionarily viable strategy, but the appropriate label for that personality type is *subclinical psychopathy* (Paulhus & Williams, 2002). Psychopaths and Machiavellians do share similar antisocial tendencies (Mealey, 1995), but the original theory—from Machiavelli (1513) to Christie and Geis (1970)—specified clearly that Machs are cool and strategic rather than hostile and impulsive.

To support our case, we draw attention to a relatively unmined source regarding manipulative strategies, namely, Sun-tzu's *Art of War* (1998). His writings anticipated those of Machiavelli by nearly 2,000 years yet have been singularly overlooked. Most relevant to our current point is the special emphasis that Sun-tzu placed on the cool preparation required to effect successful political and military outcomes. In sum, the emphasis on cool strategy in all key theoretical sources is not entirely consistent with current measures of Machiavellianism (see also Hawley, 2006).

Our conclusion is that the Mach IV needs refinement to better represent this strategic element. An improved scale would confirm that (1) Machs are less impulsive than psychopaths and no more impulsive than non-Machs, (2) Machs manipulate in the long term as well as the short term, and (3) Machs engage in aggression (including revenge) only to the degree that it is deemed profitable. In short, Machs should be strategic, as well as tactical.

Strategic Machiavellians should be willing to forgo short-term benefits to achieve long-term benefits. One prediction is that Machiavellians (as opposed to psychopaths) should pay close attention to their reputations. As Machiavelli suggested, the generation and maintenance of a favorable or menacing reputation can reap benefits across a sustained period of time. Although key theoretical sources emphasize its importance, reputation propagation has been overlooked by allowing impulsive content to contaminate the Mach IV scale. To rectify this deficit,

we have begun work on a refined measure, dubbed Mach VI (Jones & Paulhus, 2008). Preliminary research indicates that the Mach VI does show the necessary properties to tap a more strategic form of Machiavellianism.

Note

1. Pronounced "mack," these labels are not to be confused with "mawk," as in Mach 4 (four times the speed of sound).

References

Allsopp, J., Eysenck, H. J., & Eysenck, S. B. G. (1991). Machiavellianism as a component in psychoticism and extraversion. *Personality and Individual Differences, 12,* 29–41.

Andreou, E. (2000). Bully/victim problems and their association with psychological constructs in 8 to 12-year-old Greek schoolchildren. *Aggressive Behavior, 26,* 49–56.

Andreou, E. (2004). Bully/victim problems and their association with Machiavellianism and self-efficacy in Greek primary school children. *British Journal of Educational Psychology, 74,* 297–309.

Austin, E. J., Farrelly, D., Black, C., & Moore, H. (2007). Emotional intelligence, Machiavellianism and emotional manipulation: Does EI have a dark side? *Personality and Individual Differences, 43,* 179–189.

Aziz, A. (2004). Machiavellianism scores and self-rated performance of automobile salespersons. *Psychological Reports, 94,* 464–466.

Aziz, A. (2005). Relationship between Machiavellianism scores and performance of real estate salespersons. *Psychological Reports, 96,* 235–238.

Aziz, A., May, K., & Crotts, J.C. (2002). Relations of Machiavellian behavior with sales performance of stockbrokers. *Psychological Reports, 90,* 451–460.

Bakir, B., Yilmaz, R., & Yavas, S. (1996). Relating depressive symptoms to Machiavellianism in a Turkish sample. *Psychological Reports, 78,* 1011–1014.

Barber, N. (1998). Sex differences in disposition towards kin, security of adult attachment, and sociosexuality as a function of parental divorce. *Evolution and Human Behavior, 19,* 125–132.

Bass, K., Barnett, T., & Brown, G. (1999). Individual difference variables, ethical judgments, and ethical behavioral intentions. *Business Ethics Quarterly, 9,* 183–205.

Becker, J. A., & O'Hair, H. D. (2007). Machiavellians' motives in organizational citizenship behavior. *Journal of Applied Communication Research, 35,* 246–267.

Bereczkei, T. Birkas, B., & Kerekes, Z. (2009). *The presence of others, prosocial traits, Machiavellianism: A personality × situation approach.* Manuscript submitted for publication.

Bereczkei, T., Birkas, B., & Kerekes, Z. (2007). Public charity offer as a proximate factor of evolved reputation-building strategy: An experimental analysis of a real-life situation. *Evolution and Human Behavior, 28*, 277–284.

Bolino, M. C., & Turnley, W. H. (2003). More than one way to make an impression: Exploring profiles of impression management. *Journal of Management, 29*, 141–160.

Buss, D. M., & Schmitt, D. P. (1993). Sexual strategies theory: An evolutionary perspective on human mating. *Psychological Review, 100*, 204–232.

Byrne, R., & Whiten, A. (Eds.). (1988). *Machiavellian intelligence: Social expertise and the evolution of intellect in monkeys, apes, and humans.* Oxford, UK: Oxford University Press.

Carnahan, T., & McFarland, S. (2007). Revisiting the Stanford Prison Experiment: Could participant self-selection have led to the cruelty? *Personality and Social Psychology Bulletin, 33*, 603–614.

Christie, R. (1991). Authoritarianism and related constructs. In J. P. Robinson, P. R. Shaver, & L. S. Wrightsman (Eds.), *Measures of personality and social psychological attitudes* (pp. 501–571). San Diego, CA: Academic Press.

Christie, R., & Geis, F. (1970). *Studies in Machiavellianism.* New York: Academic Press.

Christoffersen, D., & Stamp, C. (1995). Examining the relationship between Machiavellianism and paranoia. *Psychological Reports, 76*, 67–70.

Coie, J. D., Dodge, K. A., & Kupersmidt, J. (1990). Peer group behavior and social status. In S. R. Asher & J. D. Coie (Eds.), *Peer rejection in childhood* (pp. 17–59). New York: Cambridge University Press.

Corral, S., & Calvete, E. (2000). Machiavellianism: Dimensionality of the Mach IV and its relation to self-monitoring in a Spanish sample. *Spanish Journal of Psychology, 3*, 3–13.

Corzine, J. B., Buntzman, G. F., & Busch, E. T. (1999). Machiavellianism in U.S. bankers. *International Journal of Organizational Analysis, 7*, 72–83.

Corzine, J. B., & Hozier, G. C. (2005). Exploratory study of Machiavellianism and bases of social power in bankers. *Psychological Reports, 97*, 356–362.

Costa, P. T., & McCrae, R. R. (1992). Four ways five factors are basic. *Personality and Individual Differences, 13*, 653–665.

Cunningham, M. R., Wong, D. T., & Barbee, A. P. (1994). Self-presentation dynamics on overt integrity tests: Experimental studies of the Reid Report. *Journal of Applied Psychology, 79*, 643–658.

Davies, M., & Stone, T. (2003). Synthesis: Psychological understanding and social skills. In B. Repacholi & V. Slaughter (Eds.), *Individual differences in theory of mind* (pp. 305–353). New York: Psychology Press.

Dawkins, R. (1989). *The selfish gene* (2nd cd.). Oxford, UK: Oxford University Press.

Deluga, R. J. (2001). American presidential Machiavellianism: Implications for charismatic leadership and rated performance. *Leadership Quarterly, 12*, 339–363.

Diehl, A. K., Kumar, V., Gateley, A., Appleby, J. L., & O'Keefe, M. E. (2006). Predictors of final specialty choice by internal medicine residents. *Journal of General Internal Medicine, 21*, 1045–1049.

Drake, D. S. (1995). Assessing Machiavellianism and morality-conscience guilt. *Psychological Reports, 77*, 1355–1359.

Falbo, T. (1977). Multidimensional scaling of power strategies. *Journal of Personality and Social Psychology, 35*, 537–547.

Fehr, B., Samsom, D., & Paulhus, D. L. (1992). The construct of Machiavellianism: Twenty years later. In C. D. Spielberger & J. N. Butcher (Eds.), *Advances in personality assessment* (Vol. 9, pp. 77–116). Hillsdale, NJ: Erlbaum.

Figueredo, A. J., Vasquez, G., Brumbach, B. H., Sefcek, J. A., Kirsner, B. R., & Jacobs, W. J. (2005). The *K*-factor: Individual differences in life history strategy. *Personality and Individual Differences, 39*, 1349–1360.

Forgas, J. P. (1998). On feeling good and getting your way: Mood effects on negotiator cognition and bargaining strategies. *Journal of Personality and Social Psychology, 74*, 565–577.

Gable, M., & Dangello, F. (1994). Locus of control, Machiavellianism, and managerial job performance. *Journal of Psychology, 128*, 599–608.

Gable, M., Hollon, C., & Dangello, F. (1992). Managerial structuring of work as a moderator of the Machiavellianism and job performance relationship. *Journal of Psychology, 126*, 317–325.

Gable, M., & Topol, M. (1988). Machiavellianism and the department store executive. *Journal of Retailing, 64*, 68–84.

Gable, M., & Topol, M. (1989). Machiavellianism and job satisfaction of retailing executives in a specialty retail chain. *Psychological Reports, 64*, 107–112.

Ghosh, D., & Crain, T. L. (1995). Ethical standards, attitudes toward risk, and intentional noncompliance: An experimental investigation. *Journal of Business Ethics, 14*, 353–365.

Giacalone, R. A., & Knouse, S. B. (1990). Justifying wrongful employee behavior: The role of personality in organizational sabotage. *Journal of Business Ethics, 9*, 55–61.

Girodo, M. (1998). Machiavellian, bureaucratic, and transformational leadership styles in police managers: Preliminary findings of interpersonal ethics. *Perceptual and Motor Skills, 86*, 419–427.

Gold, A. R., Christie, R., & Friedman, L. N. (1976). *Fists and flowers: A social psychological interpretation of student dissent.* New York: Academic Press.

Grams, L. C., & Rogers, R. W. (1990). Power and personality: Effects of Machiavellianism, need for approval, and motivation on use of influence tactics. *Journal of General Psychology, 117*, 71–82.

Gunnthorsdottir, A., McCabe, K., & Smith, V. (2002). Using the Machiavellianism instrument to predict trustworthiness in a bargaining game. *Journal of Economic Psychology, 28*, 49–66.

Gurtman, M. B. (1991). Evaluating the interpersonalncss of personality scales. *Personality and Social Psychology Bulletin, 17*, 670–677.

Gurtman, M. B. (1992). Trust, distrust, and interpersonal problems: A circumplex analysis. *Journal of Personality and Social Psychology, 62*, 989–1002.

Haidt, J. (2001). The emotional dog and its rational tail: A social intuitionist approach to moral judgment. *Psychological Review, 108*, 814–834.

Haselton, M. G., Buss, D. M., Oubaid, V., & Angleitner, A. (2005). Sex, lies, and strategic interference: The psychology of deception between the sexes. *Personality and Social Psychology Bulletin, 31*, 3–23.

Hawley, P. H. (2003). Prosocial and coercive configurations of resource control in early adolescence: A case for the well-adapted Machiavellian. *Merrill–Palmer Quarterly, 49*, 279–309.

Hawley, P. H. (2006). Evolution and personality: A new look at Machiavellianism. In D. Mroczek & T. Little (Eds.), *Handbook of personality development* (pp. 147–161). Mahwah, NJ: Erlbaum.

Hegarty, H. W. (1995). Effects of group norms and learning on unethical decision behavior. *Psychological Reports, 76*, 593–594.

Ickes, W., Reidhead, S., & Patterson, M. (1986). Machiavellianism and self-monitoring: As different as "me" and "you." *Social Cognition, 4*, 58–74.

Jakobwitz, S., & Egan, V. (2006). The dark triad and normal personality traits. *Personality and Individual Differences, 40*, 331–339.

Jones, D. N., Harms, P. D., & Paulhus, D. L. (2008). *The sexual profile of the Dark Triad*. Manuscript in preparation.

Jones, D. N., & Paulhus, D. L. (2008, February). *A measure of strategic Machiavellianism: Mach VI*. Paper presented at the meeting of the Society for Personality and Social Psychology, Albuquerque, NM.

Jones, G. E., & Kavanagh, M. J. (1996). An experimental examination of the effects of individual and situational factors on unethical behavioral intentions in the workplace. *Journal of Business Ethics, 15*, 511–523.

Kashy, D. A., & DePaulo, B. M. (1996). Who lies? *Journal of Personality and Social Psychology, 70*, 1037–1051.

Krueger, R. F., Hicks, B. M., & McGue, M. (2001). Altruism and antisocial behavior: Independent tendencies, unique personality correlates, distinct etiologies. *Psychological Science, 12*, 397–402.

Kumar, K., & Beyerlein, M. (1991). Construction and validation of an instrument measuring ingratiatory behaviors in organizational settings. *Journal of Applied Psychology, 76*, 619–627.

Leary, M. R., Knight, P. D., & Barnes, B. D. (1986). Ethical ideologies of the Machiavellian. *Personality and Social Psychology Bulletin, 12*, 75–80.

Lee, K., & Ashton, M. C. (2005). Psychopathy, Machiavellianism, and narcissism in the Five-Factor Model and the HEXACO model of personality structure. *Personality and Individual Differences, 38*, 1571–1582.

Leone, C., & Corte, V. (1994). Concern for self-presentation and self-congruence: Self-monitoring, Machiavellianism and social conflicts. *Social Behavior and Personality, 22*, 305–312.

Linton, D. K., & Wiener, N. I. (2001). Personality and potential conceptions: Mating success in a modern western male sample. *Personality and Individual Differences, 31*, 675–688.

Liu, C. C. (2008). The relationship between Machiavellianism and knowledge-sharing willingness. *Journal of Business Psychology, 22*, 233–240.

Locke, K. D., & Christensen, L. (2007). Re-construing the relational-interdependent self-construal and its relationship with self-consistency. *Journal of Research in Personality, 41*, 389–402.

Loftus, S. T., & Glenwick, D. S. (2001). Machiavellianism and empathy in an adolescent residential psychiatric population. *Residential Treatment for Children and Youth, 19*, 39–57.

Lopes, J., & Fletcher, C. (2004). Fairness of impression management in employment interviews: A cross-country study of the role of equity and Machiavellianism. *Social Behavior and Personality, 32*, 747–768.

Macrosson, W. D. K., & Hemphill, D. J. (2001). Machiavellianism in Belbin team roles. *Journal of Managerial Psychology, 16*, 355–363.

Martin, M. W., Anderson, C. M., & Thweatt, K. S. (1998). Aggressive communication traits and their relationships with the cognitive flexibility scale and the communication flexibility scale. *Journal of Social Behavior and Personality, 13*, 531–540.

Marusic, I., Bratko, D., & Zarevski, P. (1995). Self-reliance and some personality traits: Sex differences. *Personality and Individual Differences, 19*, 941–943.

McHoskey, J. W. (1995). Narcissism and Machiavellianism. *Psychological Reports, 77*, 755–759.

McHoskey, J. W. (1999). Machiavellianism, intrinsic versus extrinsic goals and social interest: A self-determination theory analysis. *Motivation and Emotion, 23*, 267–283.

McHoskey, J. W. (2001a). Machiavellianism and personality dysfunction. *Personality and Individual Differences, 31*, 791–798.

McHoskey, J. W. (2001b). Machiavellianism and sexuality: On the moderating role of biological sex. *Personality and Individual Differences, 31*, 779–789.

McHoskey, J. W., Hicks, B., Betris, T., Szyarto, C., Worzel, W., Kelly, K., et al. (1999). Machiavellianism, adjustment, and ethics. *Psychological Reports, 85*, 138–142.

McHoskey, J. W., Worzel, W., & Szyarto, C. (1998). Machiavellianism and psychopathy. *Journal of Personality and Social Psychology, 74*, 192–210.

McIlwain, D. (2003). Bypassing empathy: A Machiavellian theory of mind and sneaky power. In B. Repacholi & V. Slaughter (Eds.), *Individual differences in theory of mind* (pp. 13–38). New York: Psychology Press.

McNamara, P., Durso, R., & Harris, E. (2007). "Machiavellianism" and frontal dysfunction: Evidence from Parkinson's disease. *Cognitive Neuropsychiatry, 12*, 285–300.

Mealey, L. (1995). The sociobiology of sociopathy: An integrated evolutionary model. *Behavioral and Brain Sciences, 18*, 523–599.

Meyer, H. D. (1992). Norms and self-interest in ultimatum bargaining: The prince's prudence. *Journal of Economic Psychology, 13*, 215–232.

Moore, S., & Katz, B. (1995). Machiavellianism scores of nursing faculty and students. *Psychological Reports, 77*, 383–386.

Moore, S., Katz, B., & Holder, J. (1995). Machiavellianism and medical career choices. *Psychological Reports, 76*, 803–807.

Mudrack, P. E. (1993). An investigation into the acceptability of workplace behaviors of a dubious ethical nature. *Journal of Business Ethics, 12*, 517–524.

Mudrack, P. E., & Mason, E. S. (1995). More on acceptability of workplace behaviors of a dubious ethical nature. *Psychological Reports, 76*, 639–648.

Mudrack, P. E., Mason, E. S., & Stepanski, K. M. (1999). Equity sensitivity and business ethics. *Journal of Occupational and Organizational Psychology, 72*, 539–560.

Musser, S. J., & Orke, E. A. (1992). Ethical value systems: A typology. *Journal of Applied Behavioral Science, 28,* 348–362.

Nathanson, C., & Paulhus, D. L. (2006, June). *Beyond forgiveness: Dissecting the sequence of reactions to interpersonal transgressions.* Poster presented at the meeting of the Association for Psychological Science, New York.

Nathanson, C., Paulhus, D. L., & Williams, K. M. (2006). Predictors of a behavioral measure of scholastic cheating: Personality, and competence, but not demographics. *Contemporary Educational Psychology, 31,* 97–122.

Newcomb, A. F., Bukowski, W. M., & Pattee, L. (1993). Children's peer relations: A meta-analytic review of popular, rejected, neglected, controversial, and average sociometric status. *Psychological Bulletin, 113,* 99–128.

O'Connor, E. M., & Simms, C. M. (1990). Self-revelation as manipulation: The effects of sex and Machiavellianism on self-disclosure. *Social Behavior and Personality, 18,* 95–100.

O'Connor, W. E., & Morrison, T. G. (2001). A comparison of situational and dispositional predictors of perceptions of organizational politics. *Journal of Psychology, 135,* 301–312.

Ojha, H. (2007). Parent–child interaction and Machiavellian orientation. *Journal of the Indian Academy of Applied Psychology, 33,* 285–289.

Paal, T., & Bereczkei, T. (2007). Adult theory of mind, cooperation, Machiavellianism: The effect of mindreading on social relations. *Personality and Individual Differences, 43,* 541–551.

Paulhus, D. L. (1983). Sphere-specific measures of perceived control. *Journal of Personality and Social Psychology, 44,* 1253–1265.

Paulhus, D. L., & Williams, K. M. (2002). The Dark Triad of personality: Narcissism, Machiavellianism, and psychopathy. *Journal of Research in Personality, 36,* 556–563.

Ramanaiah, N. V., Byravan, A., & Detwiler, F. R. J. (1994). Revised NEO Personality Inventory profiles of Machiavellian and non-Machiavellian people. *Psychological Reports, 75,* 937–938.

Rawwas, M. Y. A., & Singhapakdi, A. (1998). Do consumers' ethical beliefs vary with age?: A substantiation of Kohlberg's typology in marketing. *Journal of Marketing Theory and Practice, 6,* 26–38.

Repacholi, B., & Slaughter, V. (2003). *Individual differences in theory of mind.* New York: Psychology Press.

Repacholi, B., Slaughter, V., Pritchard, M., & Gibbs, V. (2003). Theory of mind, Machiavellianism, and social functioning in childhood. In B. Repacholi & V. Slaughter (Eds.), *Individual differences in theory of mind* (pp. 67–97). New York: Psychology Press.

Ricks, J., & Fraedrich, J. (1999). The paradox of Machiavellianism: Machiavellianism may make for productive sales but poor management reviews. *Journal of Business Ethics, 20,* 197–205.

Ryckman, R. M., Thornton, B., & Butler, J. C. (1994). Personality correlates of the hypercompetitive attitude scale: Validity tests of Horney's theory of neurosis. *Journal of Personality Assessment, 62,* 84–94.

Sakalaki, M., Richardson, C., & Thepaut, Y. (2007). Machiavellianism and economic opportunism. *Journal of Applied Social Psychology, 37,* 1181–1190.

Schmitt, D. P. (2004). The Big Five related to risky sexual behaviour across 10 world regions: Differential personality associations of sexual promiscuity and relationship infidelity. *European Journal of Personality, 18,* 301–319.

Shen, D., & Dickenson, M. A. (2001). Consumers' acceptance of unethical clothing consumption activities: Influence of cultural identification, ethnicity, and Machiavellianism. *Clothing and Textiles Research Journal, 19,* 76–87.

Shepperd, J. A., & Socherman, R. E. (1997). On the manipulative behavior of low Machiavellians: Feigning incompetence to "sandbag" an opponent. *Journal of Personality and Social Psychology, 73,* 1448–1459.

Sherry, S. B., Hewitt, P. L., Besser, A., Flett, G. L., & Klein, C. (2006). Machiavellianism, trait perfectionism, and perfectionistic self-presentation. *Personality and Individual Differences, 40,* 829–839.

Shultz, C. J., II. (1993). Situational and dispositional predictors of performance: A test of the hypothesized Machiavellianism × structure interaction among salespersons. *Journal of Applied Social Psychology, 23,* 478–498.

Simon, L. J., Francis, P. L., & Lombardo, J. P. (1990). Sex, sex-role, and Machiavellianism as correlates of decoding ability. *Perceptual and Motor Skills, 71,* 243–247.

Simonton, D. K. (1986). Presidential personality: Biographical use of the Gough Adjective Check List. *Journal of Personality and Social Psychology, 51,* 149–160.

Singhapakdi, A., & Vitell, S. J. (1991). Selected factors influencing marketers' deontological norms. *Journal of the Academy of Marketing Science, 19,* 37–42.

Siu, W. S., & Tam, K. C. (1995). Machiavellianism and Chinese banking executives in Hong Kong. *International Journal of Bank Marketing, 13,* 15–21.

Snyder, M. (1974). Self-monitoring of expressive behavior. *Journal of Personality and Social Psychology, 30,* 526–537.

Sparks, J. R. (1994). Machiavellianism and personal success in marketing: The moderating role of latitude for improvisation. *Journal of the Academy of Marketing Science, 22,* 393–400.

Stewart, A. E., & Stewart, E. A. (2006). The preference to excel and its relationship to selected personality variables. *Journal of Individual Psychology, 62,* 270–284.

Suman, B. J., Singh, S., & Ashok, K. (2000). Machiavellians: Their manifest need patterns. *Psycho-Lingua, 30,* 21–24.

Sun-tzu (1998). *The art of war.* (Y. Shibing & J. J. L. Duyvendak, Trans.). New York: Wordsworth.

Sutton, J., & Keogh, E. (2001). Components of Machiavellian beliefs in children: Relationships with personality. *Personality and Individual Differences, 30,* 137–148.

Trapnell, P. D., & Paulhus, D. L. (in press). Agentic and communal values. *Journal of Personality Assessment.*

Valentine, S., & Fleischman, G. (2003). The impact of self-esteem, Machiavellianism, and social capital on attorneys' traditional gender outlook. *Journal of Business Ethics, 43,* 323–335.

Vangelisti, A. L., Daly, J. A., & Rudnick, J. R. (1991). Making people feel guilty in conversations. *Human Communication Research, 18,* 3–39.

Vecchio, R. P. (2000). Negative emotion in the workplace: Employee jealousy and envy. *International Journal of Stress Management, 7,* 161–179.

Vecchio, R. P. (2005). Explorations in employee envy: Feeling envious and feeling envied. *Cognition and Emotion, 19,* 69–81.

Vernon, P. A., Villani, V. C., Vickers, L. C., & Harris, J. A. (2008). A behavioral genetic investigation of the dark triad and the Big 5. *Personality and Individual Differences, 44,* 445–452.

Wastell, C., & Booth, A. (2003). Machiavellianism: An alexithymic perspective. *Journal of Social and Clinical Psychology, 22,* 730–744.

Watson, P. J., & Morris, R. J. (1994). Communal orientation and individualism: Factors and correlations with values, social adjustment, and self-esteem. *Journal of Psychology, 128,* 289–297.

Webster, G. D., & Bryan, A. (2007). Sociosexual attitudes and behaviors: Why two factors are better than one. *Journal of Research in Personality, 41,* 917–922.

Wiggins, J. S. (1991). Agency and communion as conceptual coordinates for the understanding and measurement of interpersonal behavior. In D. Cicchetti & W. M. Grove (Eds.), *Thinking clearly about psychology. Essays in honor of Paul E. Meehl: Vol. 2. Personality and psychopathology* (pp. 89–113). Minneapolis: University of Minnesota Press.

Wiggins, J. S., & Broughton, R. (1991). A geometric taxonomy of personality scales. *European Journal of Personality, 5,* 343–365.

Williams, K. M., Nathanson, C., & Paulhus, D. L. (in press). Identifying and profiling scholastic cheaters: Their personality, cognitive ability, and motivation. *Journal of Experimental Psychology: Applied.*

Williams, K. M., & Paulhus, D. L. (2004). Factor structure of the Self-Report Psychopathy scale (SRP-II) in non-forensic samples. *Personality and Individual Differences, 37,* 765–778.

Wilson, D. S., Near, D. C., & Miller, R. R. (1996). Machiavellianism: A synthesis of the evolutionary and psychological literatures. *Psychological Bulletin, 119,* 285–299.

Wilson, D. S., Near, D. C., & Miller, R. R. (1998). Individual differences in Machiavellianism as a mix of cooperative and exploitative strategies. *Evolution and Human Behavior, 19,* 203–212.

Winter, S. J., Stylianou, A. C., & Giacalone, R. A. (2004). Individual differences in the acceptability of unethical information technology practices: The case of Machiavellianism and ethical ideology. *Journal of Business Ethics, 54,* 275–296.

Wirtz, J., & Kum, D. (2004). Consumer cheating on service guarantees. *Journal of the Academy of Marketing Science, 32,* 159–175.

Wrightsman, L. S. (1991). Interpersonal trust and attitudes towards human nature. In J. P. Robinson, P. R. Shaver, & L. S. Wrightsman (Eds.), *Measures of personality and social psychological attitudes* (pp. 373–412). San Diego, CA: Academic Press.

Yong, F. L. (1994). Self-concepts, locus of control, and Machiavellianism of ethnically diverse middle school students who are gifted. *Roeper Review, 16,* 192–194.

CHAPTER 8

■ ● ▲ ◆ ■ ● ▲ ◆

Gender Identity

WENDY WOOD
ALICE H. EAGLY

What individual differences in gender are important to study? Because gender refers to the cultural meanings ascribed to male and female social categories in societies, psychologists have focused on whether individuals define themselves in terms of these cultural meanings. We use the term *gender identity* to refer to these masculine and feminine self-definitions. Individuals differ in gender identity within each sex, and men and women differ on the average. Gender identity is only one of many possible social identities, with each identity representing one's psychological relationship to a particular social category in which one has membership (e.g., race, social class, religion; see Frable, 1997; Sherif, 1982).

Psychologists' conviction that gender identity is important has given rise to a wide range of constructs that represent culturally based masculine and feminine self-definitions. In this chapter, we organize these constructs in terms of three facets of masculinity and femininity: representations of oneself as (1) possessing gender-typed personality traits and interests, (2) having male-typical versus female-typical relationships to others, and (3) being a member of the category of women or men, as that category is defined within a given society.

From a social-role perspective, gender identity reflects the different placement of men and women into societal roles (Diekman

& Eagly, 2008; Eagly, Wood, & Diekman, 2000; Eagly, Wood, & Johannesen-Schmidt, 2004). These typical role occupancies produce gender roles, which are defined as socially shared expectations for men's and women's behavior. As gender roles are accepted by individuals, they are internalized into their self-concepts. People differ in the extent to which they accept these normative expectations about men and women as personally self-defining and thereby differ in the extent to which they incorporate cultural gender into their personal identities.

The content of gender roles reflects the characteristics that facilitate sex-typical tasks in a given society. To the extent that women more than men occupy roles that involve domestic activities and communal behavior (e.g., nurturing children, providing service to others), the psychological attributes that facilitate these role behaviors form the basis for shared gender-role expectations for women and for feminine gender identity. To the extent that men more than women occupy roles that involve economically productive activities and directive behavior (e.g., resource acquisition, managing large organizations), the psychological attributes that facilitate these role behaviors form the basis for shared gender-role expectations for men and for masculine gender identity. Yet, gender roles have origins in multiple biological and cultural factors (see Wood & Eagly,

2002, in press), and, as we explain toward the end of this chapter, gender identity arises from a similar complex of causes.

Gender identity, like gender roles, encompasses qualities that are regarded as typical or ideal of each sex in a society. Gender identity can thus refer to *descriptive* gender norms, defined as what is culturally usual for women or men in a society. In the descriptive sense, gender identity is the construal of oneself in terms of the culturally typical man or woman. Gender identity can also refer to *injunctive* (or prescriptive) gender norms, defined as what is culturally ideal for women and men. In the injunctive sense, gender identity is the construal of oneself in terms of the best of male or female qualities.

Gender identity, in referring to feminine and masculine self-definition, differs from other gender-related constructs, such as whether people hold favorable or unfavorable attitudes toward men or women or endorse gender stereotypes by believing that men have masculine attributes and women have feminine attributes. The conceptual differences between gender identity and other gender-relevant constructs are important because all of these constructs are only weakly linked within a heterogeneous, lumpy domain. Theorists of gender have repeatedly asserted this weak-link idea. Most notably, Spence (1993) proposed a *multifactorial theory* of gender constructs, and Ashmore (1990) proposed that culturally masculine and feminine traits and behaviors are held together only by *loose glue*. Other theorists borrowed the *fuzzy concept* notion from cognitive psychology, which implies not merely the multiattribute character of gender constructs but also their loose and shifting boundaries (e.g., Deaux, 1987; Helgeson, 1994b).

This multiattribute notion of gender is consistent with the weak empirical relationships generally found across separate gender constructs. For example, self-definitions on masculine and feminine traits are not consistently related to gender attitudes, masculine or feminine appearance, or sex-typed behaviors such as athletics (Spence, 1993; Spence & Buckner, 1995). Similarly, the strength of a collective identity as a man or woman is unrelated to endorsement of gender stereotypes of male superiority at math (Kiefer

& Sekaquaptewa, 2007). In general, then, facets of individuals' gender identities do not necessarily constrain their endorsement or behavioral confirmation of other gender-related distinctions.

The loose confederation among gender-related constructs should not discourage researchers from studying masculine and feminine gender identity. We urge researchers to ignore Spence and Buckner's (1995) surprising advice to abandon the concepts of masculinity and femininity. Instead, we believe that there is empirical and conceptual payoff in following the commonsense, lay persons' approach of defining masculinity and femininity as multifactorial constructs with heterogeneous content that includes interests, personality, occupations, personal appearance, sexuality, and social roles (Deaux & Lewis, 1984; Helgeson, 1994a; Myers & Gonda, 1982). As we show in this chapter, when its complexity is adequately represented conceptually and empirically, gender identity is a useful predictor of behavior.

Relating Gender Identity to Behavior

In this chapter, we consider three different types of gender identity. We first consider individual differences in self-descriptions on the personal attributes commonly associated with gender. These personal attributes include (1) personality traits, with femininity typified by communal traits and masculinity by agentic traits (Bem, 1974; Spence & Helmreich, 1978) and (2) vocational and interest self-descriptions (Lippa, 2001, 2005). We next consider gender identity as it emerges in styles of construing the self in relation to others. A feminine construal entails greater interdependence involving close relationships with significant other individuals versus a more masculine construal that might include greater independence from others (Cross & Madson, 1997) or a greater collective focus on large groupings (Gardner & Gabriel, 2004). Finally, we consider individual differences in the importance people place on defining themselves as a member of the social category of men or women (Wood, Christensen, Hebl, & Rothgerber, 1997). Given these three distinct types of gender identity constructs, a researcher's first goal should be to identify the aspect of gender identity that is relevant to the behavior under investigation.

This issue of matching gender identity constructs to relevant behaviors is crucial, above and beyond the more mundane issue faced in all individual-difference research of choosing measures to maximize reliability and validity (e.g., Marsh, 1987). To appropriately link gender identity to behavior, it is necessary to understand some elementary principles of the prediction of behavior from psychological dispositions.

The Principle of Compatibility

The choice of measures of gender identity should be guided by the *principle of compatibility* (Ajzen, 2005; Eagly & Chaiken, 1993), which stipulates that identity measures are more likely to predict responses if they are in the same content domain as the measure. This principle, initially developed for enhancing the prediction of behaviors from attitudes (Ajzen & Fishbein, 1977), also is important for predicting behaviors from personality traits (e.g., Epstein, 1980). The key insight for successful prediction of behavior from attitudes, personality, or any other disposition is that prediction is enhanced by matching the content of the behavioral measure to the content of the dispositional measure. Therefore, measures of gender identity would successfully predict behaviors in the domain of the disposition.

Based on the compatibility principle, gender identity measures that assess self-reported masculine and feminine personality traits would best predict corresponding behaviors, such as communal behaviors of taking care of others or agentic behaviors of assertiveness. Identity measures that assess gender-typed vocations and interests would best predict related behaviors, such as gender-typed hobbies and occupations. Identity measures that assess sex-typical social relational preferences would best predict the kinds of relationships that women and men form with others, including their embeddedness in dyadic pairs or larger hierarchical structures in which they relate to multiple others. Identity measures that assess membership in the socially defined categories of men and women would best predict group-related judgments such as preference for one's own sex and prejudice against the other sex.

By tailoring measures of gender identity to the domain of interest, researchers increase their chances of finding meaningful effects of gender identification.

Beyond the recommendation to match content domains across identity measures and predicted behaviors, the compatibility principle implies that good prediction follows from assessing the identity measure and the behavioral measure at the same level of generality. For example, if self-assessments on the culturally masculine trait of assertiveness were used to predict behavior, the behavioral measure ideally would include not merely a single assertive behavior such as speaking up at meetings but rather a wide range of assertive behaviors selected from a wide range of settings. A single behavior such as speaking up at a meeting is an imperfect representation of assertiveness because there are many reasons why an otherwise assertive person might not engage in this behavior, especially at a particular meeting. Because individual behaviors are multiply determined, correlations between measures of assertiveness in general and any single behavior are generally low.

When research matches dispositional and behavioral measures at the same level of generality, substantial correlations can emerge between the two measures (Epstein, 1980). However, because most research on gender identity has used general measures of identity and related these to only one or a few specific behaviors of interest, most correlations in the literature we review are relatively low. Correlations would be higher if researchers had related general identity measures to aggregated indexes of relevant behaviors. Alternatively, researchers could improve prediction by designing more specific measures of identity. For example, a narrowly defined feminine quality such as belief in one's social sensitivity could be related to relatively specific responses, such as the ability to infer others' feelings in a variety of settings.

Direct and Indirect Measures

Although most measures of gender identity involve direct self-ratings on relevant response scales, identity can be tapped through measures that are much less direct. Dual-process theories in social psychology provide a way to understand differences between these measurement approaches (see Chaiken & Trope, 1999; Smith & DeCoster, 2000). *Direct* rating scales tap propositional knowledge about oneself through verbalized judgments of gendered identity: "I am warm" or "I identify with women." Such measures require that people have some conscious awareness of their gender identity and are able and willing to report on it using the given scale format. In contrast, *indirect* measures tap spontaneous aspects of gender identity that may or may not be accessible to conscious, verbal description (see Smith & DeCoster, 2000). Furthermore, indirect measures may rely on associative processing systems that reflect the cumulation of experiences over time.

Indirect measures of gender identity often assess respondents' reaction times in making identity-relevant judgments. Such reaction times can reflect the strength of associative connections between oneself and culturally feminine and masculine traits or between oneself and male and female groups. Stronger identity, represented by closer associations between oneself and gender concepts, should produce faster reactions. For example, in a gender *priming* task, exposure to the prime of *me* or *they* is followed by the participant classifying a gendered word (e.g., *lady, fishing rod*; van Well, Kolk, & Oei, 2007) into categories of person versus object. People with a strong gender identity presumably have gender primed by the word *me* and therefore are relatively fast in making such categorizations. Another indirect measure, the Implicit Association Test (IAT), assesses the strength of association between self and aspects of gender identity through the speed of responding when categorizing the self (vs. others) as masculine or feminine (Greenwald & Banaji, 1995). The resulting IAT scores can form a bipolar dimension, reflecting the ease of associating masculine versus feminine traits with the self compared with others. IAT scores can also form unipolar scales. According to meta-analytic estimates, if direct self-ratings and IAT indirect measures are assessed in compatible ways so that both, for example, compare masculine and feminine gender identity, then correlations of around .30 consistently emerge (Hofmann, Gawronski, Gschwendner, Le, & Schmitt, 2005). Additional indirect measures include open-ended self-descriptions

(e.g., McGuire & Padawer-Singer, 1976) and content analyses of self-descriptive photographs (e.g., Clancy & Dollinger, 1993). These and other indirect measures are designed to estimate gender identity without a direct verbal report and often without participants' awareness that this identity is being assessed.

There are several reasons to expect some divergence between direct and indirect measures of gender identity. One is that direct ratings are farther *downstream* in the processes of judgment and thus subject to more deliberation than the more spontaneous, automatic associations tapped by indirect measures (Fazio & Olson, 2003). As a result, responses to direct measures can be more influenced by pressures to appear socially desirable than are responses to indirect measures (Greenwald, Poehlman, Uhlmann, & Banaji, in press). Another reason for divergence is that indirect and direct measures may not represent the same content. This occurs when researchers use different bases to select direct and indirect measures by, for example, deriving one measure but not the other from gender stereotypes. In the following sections, we consider these and other issues in analyzing the merits of direct and indirect measures of our three facets of gender identity.

Individual Differences in Self-Described Personal Traits and Attributes

Gender Identity as Bipolar Masculinity–Femininity in Heterogeneous Domains

Modern measures of gender identity originated in Terman and Miles's (1936) test of masculinity and femininity. This measure is composed of items that elicited maximally different responses from women and men. The resulting collection of items is a heterogeneous lot that includes word associations, associations to inkblots, interest items, introversion–extraversion items, and self-judgments of overall masculinity and femininity. For example, femininity scores increased with liking "nursing," "babies," and "charades," whereas masculinity increased with disliking these. This method of item selection and scoring placed masculinity and femininity as two ends of a single bipolar continuum. Other psychologists then followed this approach of selecting test items that strongly differentiated between women and men and labeling the resulting scales as measures of masculinity and femininity (see reviews by Lippa, 2001, 2005).

This tradition has been continued more recently in measures of identification that tap female-typical or male-typical interests. Favoring this approach, Lippa (1991; Lippa & Connelly, 1990) developed a method of *gender diagnosticity* in which women and men rate their preferences for occupations, hobbies, and everyday activities. These ratings then allow the computation of the pattern of preferences that maximally discriminates between the male and female raters (in terms of a weighted combination of items that constitutes a *discriminant function*). Respondents' gender identities are then determined by comparing their scores with this male-typical versus female-typical pattern of preferences.

Lippa's gender diagnosticity measure of gender identity, like the Terman and Miles (1936) measure, is based on items that maximally discriminate between women's and men's self-reports. However, it differs in its narrower focus on interests and in its calibration of what distinguishes the sexes within each sample of respondents. This method of computing a gender discriminant function has been applied to other types of items as well (e.g., Burke & Tully, 1977). As would be expected from the compatibility principle, Lippa's (1991) measure relates especially well to occupational preferences, with more masculine respondents preferring occupations that deal mainly with things and more feminine respondents preferring occupations that deal mainly with people (Lippa, 1998, 2005).

Constantinople (1973) provided an early critique of these kinds of measures of masculinity and femininity. She complained about the empirically derived selection of items, especially the motley types of content in Terman and Miles's (1936) measure and similar broad-spectrum measures. She demonstrated that statistical analyses of such items often revealed multiple dimensions, not a single bipolar dimension. Another criticism was that different versions of masculinity–femininity scales, which presumably assessed the same psychological construct, were not very strongly related to one another. Constantinople's critique and her accusation that masculinity and femininity are "among the muddiest concepts in the psychologist's vocabulary" (p. 390) catalyzed development of a different framework for assessing gender identity.

Gender Identity as Separate Masculine and Feminine Dimensions of Personality Traits

In the new framework spurred by Constantinople's (1973) and others' critiques, masculinity and femininity appear as two separate dimensions. Drawing scale items from the cultural stereotypes of the personality traits of women and men, Bem (1974) proposed the Bem Sex Role Inventory (BSRI), which represents masculinity and femininity as separate, orthogonal dimensions. These items were selected because the personality traits they represented were more stereotypical of one sex than the other and more favorably evaluated in that sex. The measure thus assesses self-defined personality traits that are either masculine (e.g., self-reliance, assertiveness, forcefulness) or feminine (e.g., affection, sympathy, warmth). Among the four quadrants that resulted, two defined respondents considered *sex typed* by Bem: (1) those high on masculinity and low on femininity, labeled *masculine*, and (2) those high on femininity and low on masculinity, labeled *feminine*. The two remaining quadrants defined respondents considered not sex typed: (1) those high on both masculinity and femininity, labeled *androgynous*, and (2) those low on both masculinity and femininity, labeled *undifferentiated*. This two-dimensional scheme decoupled gender identity from its earlier bipolar framing and thereby represented identities in all combinations of high and low masculinity and femininity.

In a related project, Spence and Helmreich (Spence & Helmreich, 1978; Spence, Helmreich, & Stapp, 1974) developed the Personal Attributes Questionnaire (PAQ), which also defined gender identity in terms of two separate dimensions of personality attributes that are stereotypical of women or of men. Spence argued that the PAQ and the BSRI are measures not of culturally defined masculinity and femininity but of constellations of socially desirable personality traits defined by either *instrumentality* (e.g., decisiveness, competitiveness, activity) or *expressiveness* (e.g., kindness, helpfulness, understanding). Alternatively, in the terminology introduced by Bakan (1966) and favored by many gender researchers, the two dimensions of the BSRI and PAQ gained the labels of *agency* and *communion*. Although some researchers have found that the items that make up the BSRI and the PAQ scales are not necessarily internally consistent (e.g., Marsh, 1987), these two-dimensional gender identity measures have remained very popular in research.

Subsequent elaborations of the PAQ included scales designed to capture negative aspects of instrumentality (e.g., being domineering, overbearing) and expressiveness (e.g., being whiny, passive) (Helmreich, Spence, & Wilhelm, 1981). Additionally, Athenstaedt (2003) extended the two dimensions to include items assessing their behavioral expressions.

These two-dimensional personality-based measures of gender identity may seem anomalous in view of modern personality theory, which has converged on a five-dimensional organization of traits known as the Big Five (Wiggins, 1996): *Extraversion, Agreeableness, Conscientiousness, Neuroticism,* and *Openness to experience*. Although the BSRI and PAQ scales correlate with some of the Big Five traits, more fine-grained analyses have revealed that each Big Five trait is made up of separate components, and sex differences are not always consistent in magnitude or direction across the components that make up the broader traits (Costa, Terracciano, & McCrae, 2001). Given such complexities, agency and communion are not readily reconfigured in terms of the Big Five. Instead, the agency–communion scheme provides an alternative organization of personality traits to the Big Five, and this two-dimensional organization is particularly useful in studying gender because of its match to gender stereotypes and roles. Attesting to the value of this two-dimensional scheme, social-psychological researchers on impression formation and stereotyping have often favored two dimensions that are construed in terms of some version of these agentic and communal families of traits (e.g., Judd, James-Hawkins, Yzerbyt, & Kashima, 2005).

Based on the compatibility principle, what behaviors are likely to be predicted by measures such as the BSRI and PAQ that represent agentic and communal traits? These measures assess only one aspect of the gender-related qualities that form the basis of people's sense of maleness or femaleness and therefore should relate to behaviors only within the relevant domain. Empirical support comes from a meta-analysis by Taylor and Hall (1982), in which people who were high on the masculine dimension of the BSRI or PAQ engaged in more agentic behaviors than those who were low, and people who were high on the feminine dimension engaged in more communal behaviors that those who were low. Furthermore, prediction from the BSRI or PAQ to behaviors in domains other than communion and agency were generally weak and inconsistent (Spence & Buckner, 1995). Despite widespread use of these measures in psychological research, investigators have only occasionally recognized that their predictive power is circumscribed to communal and agentic behaviors. Following the principle of compatibility, we expect in addition that these identity measures will have maximum impact when a study's behavioral measures are at the same level of generality. Thus identity measures defined in terms of broadly formulated personality traits, such as the BSRI and the PAQ, will more effectively predict aggregated indexes of multiple agentic and communal behaviors than any single behavior.

Indirect Measures of Personal Traits and Attributes

Indirect measures of gender identity assess more automatic and spontaneous self-descriptions. The IAT is the most popular indirect measure of traits and attributes. For example, Greenwald and Farnham's (2000) respondents categorized self-related pronouns (*me, I*) or other-related pronouns (*them, it*) with communal (*warm, tender*) or agentic (*competitive, aggressive*) attributes. The resulting IAT scores were formed into a bipolar dimension of masculinity versus femininity, reflecting the ease of associating masculine versus feminine traits with oneself compared with others. As would be expected from the compatibility principle, this bipolar measure of gender identity was positively related to the PAQ and BSRI scales when they were computed as bipolar scales. Nonetheless, the IAT also can potentially be scored to reflect separate unipolar masculinity and femininity dimensions, and in this form it should be associated with direct measures of the compatible masculinity or femininity subscale. It is unknown whether the indirect and direct forms of such masculinity and femininity measures predict behaviors differently.

Individual Differences in Interdependent Self-Construal

Gender identity also includes beliefs about oneself in social relationships, often labeled *self-construal*. This aspect of gender identity reflects the social contexts within which men and women carry out sex-typical activities in a society. To the extent that women more than men occupy roles that encourage close, interdependent relations with others, feminine gender roles are likely to include self-construals that emphasize connections to intimate others. Comparably, to the extent that men more than women in a society occupy roles that encourage independent action and/or action within larger collectives, masculine gender roles are likely to include self-construals of autonomy from others and/or positions within larger collectives. The interdependent aspects of gender identity focus not on individuals' possession of personality attributes such as communion or agency but on the ways that men and women define themselves in relationships with intimate others and with social groups.

Initial work on this aspect of gender identity focused on the degree to which men and women regard themselves as separate from or connected to other people. That is, women were thought to have a relatively *interdependent* self-definition, in which valued and important others are included in self-representations, and men to have a more *independent* self definition, in which the self is autonomous and distinct from others (Cross & Madson, 1997; Josephs, Markus, & Tafarodi, 1992; see Cross, Hardin, & Gercek Swing, Chapter 35, this volume). Sex differences would thereby align with cross-cultural differences in self-construals in the form of East Asian cultures' promotion of an interdependent sense of self that highlights relationships, group memberships, and harmony with others, as opposed to Westernized cultures' promotion of an independent sense of self that highlights individuals' unique abilities and attributes (Markus & Kitayama, 1991; but see Oyserman, Coon, & Kemmelmeier, 2002).

In a landmark article summarizing research indicating that men and women differ in such self-construals, Cross and Madson (1997) argued that women describe themselves more in terms of relationships with others, whereas men describe themselves more in terms of separateness from others. For example, women's greater interdependence is evident in their sensitivity to others' nonverbal cues, emotional empathy, and capacity to adopt others' cognitive perspectives. Furthermore, women's self-esteem tends to depend on their ability to maintain relationships with others, whereas men's depends more on maintaining independence from others. In addition, women attend more to close relationships and like to discuss them with others, whereas men prefer to discuss less personal topics such as sports and politics. Cross and Madson interpreted these (and other) findings as evidence for women's greater interdependence and men's greater independence (see also review of work on self-construals by Cross et al., Chapter 35, this volume).

Subsequent work challenged this characterization of men as less dependent on social relations than women. Reasoning that all people have a need to belong, Baumeister and Sommer (1997) argued that the sexes express this dependency differently, with women more likely to form close relationships with intimate others and men more likely to form relationships within larger collectives and groups in which they can assert power and dominance (see also Baumeister & Leary, 1995). Thus women's sense of their interdependence with others is *relational*, or oriented to committed, close relations with others, whereas men's sense of interdependence is *collective*, or oriented toward larger social groups (Gabriel & Gardner, 1999; Gardner & Gabriel, 2004).

Relational and collective gender identities align with Brewer and Gardner's (1996) analysis of the forms of interdependent selves. According to these researchers, whether people construe themselves in terms of their interpersonal relationships or in terms of larger, more interpersonal collectives determines various aspects of self-functioning (e.g., salient components of self, primary social motives). In addition, relational and collective interdependence represent not only characteristic ways of interpreting the self in relation to others but also temporarily activated states in which circumstances prime the appropriate identities and lead to perceptions of self as interlinked in relationships with intimate others or in larger groups.

Evidence that men and women differ in their chronic levels of interdependent self-construal comes from research that has compared relational and collective forms of dependence. Arguing that Cross and Madson's (1997) review had focused primarily on the relational aspect of interdependence, Gabriel and Gardner (1999) provided a variety of evidence that men are more collectively interdependent than women. For example, when asked to give spontaneous self-descriptions, men were more likely than women to list group memberships (e.g., fraternity member, black man), whereas women were more likely than men to list specific close relationships (e.g., friend, happily married; Gabriel & Gardner, 1999, Study 1). In addition, when asked to recall and describe a happy or sad emotional event, men were more likely than women to report an experience in the context of a collective (e.g., with a fraternity or sorority), whereas women were more likely than men to report an experience with a close other (e.g., friend, family member; Gabriel & Gardner, 1999, Study 3).

Direct Measures of Interdependent Self-Construal

Direct tests of the independent, relational, and collective self-concepts of women and men usually elicit self-reports on scales assessing the importance or descriptiveness of each of these self aspects. The research published thus far suggests that the sexes differ primarily in the extent to which they construe the self in relations with close others. Accordingly, relational interdependence holds most promise as a facet of gender identity.

Our review of the literature suggested that men and women do not differ consistently in their overall levels of independence. Thus few sex differences have been reported on measures assessing self-descriptions as independent as opposed to interdependent. For example, Kashima and colleagues' (1995)

investigation across five cultures revealed no sex differences in self-reported individualism as reflected in assertiveness and acting independently in group contexts. Similarly, Nario-Redmond, Biernat, Eidelman, and Palenskie (2004) found an absence of sex differences in U.S. college students' ratings of the importance of personal identity items pertaining to independence (e.g., rebelliousness, creativity). Also, Kashima and Hardie's (2000) relational, individual, and collective self-aspects scale revealed no sex differences among Australian college students in the prominence of individual aspects of the self.

In line with sex differences in the form of interdependence, women typically report higher relational dependence than men. For example, across U.S. college student samples, women consistently scored higher than men on a scale designed to assess Relationally Interdependent Self-Construal (RISC scale) with items such as, "My close relationships are an important reflection of who I am" (Cross, Bacon, & Morris, 2000; Gabriel & Gardner, 1999; Gore, Cross, & Morris, 2006). Also, across five cultures, Kashima and colleagues (1995) found that women scored consistently higher than men on measures of closeness in emotional relations with others.

Direct measures have provided less conclusive evidence of sex differences in collective interdependence. Gabriel and Gardner (1999, Study 2) found college men more collectively dependent than women on a version of the RISC designed to tap collective identity (e.g., "The groups I belong to are an important reflection of who I am"). However, other research has not obtained analogous findings (e.g., Kashima & Hardie, 2000), including studies in which respondents rated the importance of various group identities to their own self-definitions (Luhtanen & Crocker, 1992; Nario-Redmond et al., 2004). This apparent inconsistency in findings might be resolved through a comprehensive meta-analytic review of the relevant research findings.

Indirect Measures of Interdependence

Indirect measures that assess whether people spontaneously mention individual others or collectives when describing themselves also attest to women's greater relational interdependence. The best known of these measures is Kuhn and McPartland's (1954) Twenty Statements Test, which elicits open-ended self-descriptions that researchers code for self-construals. Women tend to respond with more descriptions of personal relationships and family than do men (e.g., Gabriel & Gardner, 1999, Study 1; Grace & Cramer, 2003; Kashima & Hardie, 2000; McCrae & Costa, 1988, although see Bresnahan et al., 2005). A similar spontaneous measure is the free-response assessment of "tell us about yourself" (e.g., McCrae & Costa, 1988; McGuire & Padawer-Singer, 1976).

Other researchers have invoked autophotography, or taking photos, to tell who one is. Women spontaneously included more pictures of self with others, of people touching, of groups of people, and of family, whereas men included more photos of the self alone, of physical activities, and of vehicles (Clancy & Dollinger, 1993).

Interdependent Self-Construals Predict Behavior

Based on the compatibility principle, measures of relational self-construal should predict behaviors relevant to this aspect of interdependence. In support, a growing body of evidence suggests that, for example, people who scored higher in relational interdependence on the RISC were more likely to attend to and remember information about others' relationships (Cross, Morris, & Gore, 2002). Also, more relationally interdependent individuals showed greater accuracy at judging a new roommate's values and beliefs (Cross & Morris, 2003), greater optimism about close relationships (Cross & Morris, 2003), and greater self-disclosure to others concerning emotional events and helpfulness in responding to others' needs (Cross et al., 2000; Gore et al., 2006). Furthermore, following priming of relational interdependence, people tended to treat close others' success on a task as similar to their own and did not show the classic social comparison effect of gaining esteem when outperforming others and losing esteem when outperformed by them (Gardner, Gabriel, & Hochschild, 2002).

Given the limited evidence for men's independence and collective interdependence, these attributes may have minimal utility as indicators of gender identity. Nonetheless, it may be that men adopt these identities in certain circumstances, as suggested by Maddux and Brewer's (2005) finding that, after priming with interdependence, men apparently relied on collective identity in deciding whether to trust others to allocate money in an online game, and they showed trust for ingroup but not outgroup members.

Individual Differences in Gender-Group Identification

Gender also represents a collective identity that individuals adopt when they define themselves as a member of one sex group as opposed to the other. Collective gender identity is the subjective judgment that "I identify with women" or "I identify with men." Group identity can, in addition, be defined to include the emotional significance of a group, attributes of group members, or common fate with group members (see Ashmore, Deaux, & McLaughlin-Volpe, 2004). Because such features require the initial identification of oneself as a group member, we treated these as consequences of identification and define gender-group identification as the categorization of oneself as female or male and the importance of this categorization for one's self-definition.

A central issue for social identity researchers is understanding the conditions under which people invoke one identity, such as gender, over others, such as ethnic group or musical taste. Self-categorization is flexible, and people have a repertoire of social category memberships that vary in relative importance to the self-concept (Stewart & McDermott, 2004; Turner, Hogg, Oakes, Reicher, & Wetherell, 1987). Some individuals are chronically more likely than others to identify with their gender group, as assessed by measures of collective gender identity. In addition, the tendency to define oneself as female or male varies with the salience of gender in particular social contexts (see Turner et al.'s [1987] metacontrast principle).

Measuring Collective Identity

Measures of collective gender identity can refer to typical men and women and thereby assess identification with descriptive gender categories. Alternatively, such measures can refer to ideal men and women and thereby reflect identification with injunctive categories. In addition, although some measures separately assess identification with each gender, measures often assess identification with a gender ingroup in opposition to the gender outgroup (Turner et al., 1987).

Direct Measures of Collective Gender Identity

A popular measure of identification with descriptive group categories is the *importance of identity* subscale of Luhtanen and Crocker's (1992) collective self-esteem scale. When adapted to gender groups, this measure consists of four items that assess the importance of being a woman or a man to one's self-image. Other measures elicit self-reports of how typical respondents are in their gender group (e.g., Eagan & Perry, 2001).

To capture the injunctive nature of gender categories—that is, people's beliefs about what is desirable for the sexes—measures can specify ideal or desired gender categories. For example, to assess gender ideals, Wood and colleagues (1997) assessed how important it was for respondents to be similar to the ideal man or woman and to reject the other sex ideal.

Indirect Measures of Collective Gender Identity

Reaction-time measures assess gender identity indirectly through the speed with which participants associate self (vs. others) with gender categories. The IAT assesses strength of gender identity through reaction times to differentiate self words (e.g., *me*) from nonself words (e.g., *other*) when each is paired with words indicative of gender groups (e.g., *he, female*) (Aidman & Carroll, 2003; Greenwald et al., in press). With lexical-decision measures, participants are primed or not primed with self-constructs, and then their reaction times for recognizing gender-related words are assessed (e.g., *woman, football*; van Well et al., 2007). As expected based on the principle of compatibility, the IAT and lexical-decision measures of collective gender identity are positively correlated, $r(43) = .48$ (van Well et al., 2007).

A graphic measure of spontaneous gender identity assesses the extent to which people include others in the self (Aron, Aron,

Tudor, & Nelson, 1991). It consists of a set of Venn-like diagrams with varying degrees of overlap between two circles. When it is used to assess strength of collective gender identity, respondents pick the diagram that best depicts the extent of overlap between themselves and their gender group.

Another spontaneous measure is whether people mention gender in response to an open-ended request to list self-descriptive attributes (e.g., McCrae & Costa, 1988; McGuire & Padawer-Singer, 1976). The spontaneous mention of gender categories might reflect the chronic salience of gender, as well as situationally induced salience, as indicated by the finding that children in the minority sex in a classroom mentioned their sex more often in describing their physical selves (McGuire & Padawer-Singer, 1976).

Collective Gender Identification Predicts Behavior

Given the logic of the compatibility principle, collective gender identity should predict behavior as a group member, such as valuing one's group over other groups (Tajfel, 1982). In particular, evaluative forms of group identity—that is, identification with what is good about one's gender group compatible with ingroup bias. Illustrating this effect, Wood and colleagues' (1997) participants rated their similarity to the societal ideal for their sex (e.g., the ideal woman) and their dissimilarity to the ideal for the other sex. To the extent that participants had a stronger identification with their own (vs. other) gender ideal, they experienced a boost in self-esteem when imagining themselves acting in gendered ways. Evidence for ingroup bias also has been found on measures that minimize the social desirability concerns that can limit demonstrations of outgroup prejudice, as shown by meta-analytic evidence that collective identity predicted ingroup bias better with indirect, IAT measures than with direct measures (Greenwald et al., in press).

Another group behavior associated with collective identity is *self-stereotyping*, or the ascription of group characteristics to the self (Turner et al., 1987). Given the logic of the compatibility principle, broad measures of identification with a gender group would not necessarily relate to specific behaviors such as ascription of particular gender-typed attributes to oneself. In illustration, Kiefer and Sekaquaptewa (2007) found that women with a strong gender identification were no more likely than those with a weak one to ascribe the stereotypic attribute of poor math performance to themselves. However, the predicted self-stereotyping was obtained among women with a strong gender-group identity who also believed that math is masculine and not feminine. Thus gender self-stereotyping on specific attributes can be detected in studies that assess the specific attributes that people ascribe to gender categories.

Gender self-stereotyping also is found when measures of gender identity are tailored to the specific domain of interest. For example, Witt and Wood (2008) assessed gender identity by asking respondents how important it was that they acted like a typical man or a typical woman with respect to romantic relations (e.g., dating, flirting). Experience-sampling methods revealed that highly identified students interacted with peers of the other sex in typically feminine (or masculine) ways. In general, collective gender identity relates to self-stereotyping on specific attributes primarily when the attributes are ones that respondents believe characterize their gender group or when gender identity is assessed with respect to the specific domain of interest.

Gender Identity Guides Responding

What are the mechanisms by which the three types of gender identity we have considered influence people's responses? Gender identity guides behavior through a set of biological and psychological mechanisms (see Wood & Eagly, in press). Biological processes include hormonal fluctuations that act as chemical signals that promote actions in line with gender identity. Social processes also are implicated, given that people use gender identities as self-standards against which to regulate their behavior.

Biological processes work to promote gender identities as people selectively recruit hormones and other neurochemical processes to facilitate performance of relevant behaviors. Higher levels of testosterone are associated with dominance behaviors, especially those involved in competition, risk-

taking, and aggression that may injure others (Booth, Granger, Mazur, & Kivlighan, 2006). For example, testosterone levels rise in anticipation of athletic and other competition and in response to insults. Higher levels of oxytocin are associated with behaviors that produce parental bonding, nurturance, and intimacy, especially in women (Campbell, 2008). For example, oxytocin levels rise in women during childbirth and in response to massage and sexual contact. These hormonal processes do not work in isolation but instead combine with gender identities to facilitate performance of relevant behaviors. Thus, testosterone is especially relevant for people with masculine gender identities that lead them to experience social interactions as dominance contests. Oxytocin and other neurochemical processes involved in bonding are especially relevant for people with feminine identities that lead them to define social interactions as involving bonding and affiliation with close others.

Gender identity, as a component of the self-concept, also informs self-regulation. When people self-regulate, they exercise control over their behavior to bring the self into line with valued standards. Gender identities serve as self-regulatory standards when they descriptively specify how a person of one's gender is expected to act or injunctively specify how a person of one's gender ideally would act.

According to self-regulatory theories, people guide their actions toward valued standards and goals by a matching process often likened to a cybernetic feedback loop (e.g., Carver & Scheier, 2008). With this feedback loop, the regulatory system monitors the extent to which current behavior matches self-standards. When people's behavior successfully matches their gender identity, they experience positive emotion and increased self-esteem; when their behavior deviates from their gender identity, they experience negative emotion and decreased esteem. Therefore, people with a stronger gender identity—of whatever type—would use this identity as a standard for their own behavior and experience more of a boost in positive affect and self-esteem when vicariously imagining themselves or actually behaving in ways that are consistent with this identity (Diekman & Eagly, 2008; Wood et al., 1997). Wood and her colleagues have demonstrated this mechanism with respect to collective gender identity (e.g., Witt & Wood, 2008).

Self-regulatory control proceeds not only through motivational signals of affect and self-esteem but also through enhanced attention to, processing of, and recall of information relevant to gender standards. The information processing consequences of gender identity were a cornerstone of Bem's (1981) theory that sex-typed people have a "generalized readiness to process information on the basis of the sex-linked associations" held in long-term memory (p. 355). Bem argued that gender identity provides a kind of lens for processing information relevant to the self and gender. However, only inconsistent evidence suggests that the agentic and communal forms of gender identity assessed by Bem's favored measure (i.e., BSRI) guide gender-related processing across a range of stimuli (see Kite & Deaux, 1986). Based on the compatibility principle, evidence for such processing should emerge mainly when measures of identity are in the same domain as the measures of information processing. In support, people who score higher on relational forms of gender identity are more likely to attend to and remember information about others' relationships (e.g., Cross et al., 2002).

The capacity to engage in regulatory control of gender-linked behavior appears to emerge with maturity (Bussey & Bandura, 1992). Consistent with such a developmental effect, 3-year-old children did not anticipate feeling differently about themselves after playing with same-sex or other-sex toys, whereas older children expressed more positive feelings toward playing with same-sex toys than other-sex ones. Furthermore, suggesting the developmental trajectory of regulatory mechanisms, the older but not the younger children's anticipatory affective reactions predicted their subsequent actual toy preferences.

In summary, the three facets of gender identity we address in this chapter all plausibly influence responding through a common set of biosocial mechanisms. Through self-regulatory mechanisms, people carry out behaviors that are consistent with gender identities based on gender-stereotypic traits and interests, relational closeness to others, or collective male and female groups. Hor-

monal processes include the recruitment of testosterone and oxytocin to facilitate performance in line with these identities. In support of this analysis, women high in masculinity on the BSRI, who perceived themselves as self-directed, action-oriented, and resourceful, were likely to have higher circulating testosterone (Baucom, Besch, & Callahan, 1985). Given the evidence that testosterone is recruited in the service of role performance, this pattern is consistent with the idea that agentic women are sensitive to dominance issues in daily life and recruit this hormone as they assert dominance.

Origins of Gender Identity

Gender identity is one of a variety of gender-related constructs that children develop as they mature within their society. Gender identity emerges through the interaction over time of social-cognitive learning and biological processes (see Bussey & Bandura, 1999, 2004; Ruble & Martin, 1998). These include learning to label oneself as a boy or girl and to understand gender constancy (Kohlberg, 1966). More complex learning is involved in the development of cognitive structures that link the self with gendered activities, interests, and personality traits (Martin & Ruble, 2004). Furthermore, for identity to be expressed in behavior, females and males must develop the belief that they can engage in such behavior (Bussey & Bandura, 1999).

Gender identity develops within a broader societal context in which women and men cooperate in a division of labor and thereby fill different social roles (Eagly et al., 2000). The different placement of men and women in society organizes the processes by which boys and girls come to possess a gender identity and thereby are suited to participate in sex-typical social roles. Individual differences in gender identity also reflect the unique experiences that people may have within their society.

The division of labor within a society influences gender identity because it influences the perceived costs and benefits of behaviors for each sex. Women on average perceive that communal behaviors, people-centered interests and vocations, dyadic relational styles, and a collective identity as a woman are especially rewarding. Men on average perceive that agentic behaviors, thing-centered interests and vocations, independent and/or hierarchical relational styles, and a collective identity as a man are especially rewarding. Gender identity reflects these average perceived utilities of men and women, along with the unique perceptions that each individual may develop.

Men's and women's understanding of the costs and benefits related to gender identities develops in part through the expectations held by other people. Others tend to reward behaviors consistent with gender roles because such actions validate shared beliefs about women and men and promote social interaction that is easy to follow and understand (see Wood & Eagly, in press). Others may respond with rejection to deviating behaviors that challenge gender role expectations. Through the process of responding to gender expectations, people may develop gender identities. Because people often underestimate the influence of others (Vorauer & Miller, 1997), they might observe their own expectation-consistent behavior and infer that they possess a corresponding disposition—a gender identity. Supporting this reasoning, research on gender-stereotypical expectations has yielded some of the strongest evidence of such behavioral confirmation of others' expectations (Leander, Chartrand, & Wood, 2009; see overview by Deaux & Lafrance, 1998). Further evidence that children are rewarded for acting in ways that confirm gender-role expectations comes from observations of socialization practices in nonindustrial societies (Barry, Bacon, & Child, 1957). Socialization research in industrialized nations has provided less evidence of parents' differential delivery of rewards and punishments, with the exception of certain sex-typed activities and preferences (see Lytton & Romney, 1991). Nonetheless, sex-typed expectancies also are communicated through other social channels, such as modeling of conventional family and occupational roles (Bussey & Bandura, 1999).

Biological mechanisms, especially hormonal processes, also influence the development of gender identity. The prenatal hormone environment is known to influence the development of some human behaviors that show sex differences. Perhaps best documented are the consequences of the high levels of prenatal androgen exposure of children with congenital adrenal hyperplasia (CAH) disorder. Such exposure yields increased male-typical toy, playmate, and activity preferences among girls, although it has little systematic effect for boys. Nonetheless, such exposure does not appear to have consistent effects on broader measures of gender identity (Meyer-Bahlburg et al., 2004; although see Hines, Brook, & Conway, 2004).

The general idea that biological, cognitive, and social factors interact to produce individual differences in gender identity has been embraced by evolutionary models of gender. However, evolutionary models differ in how they envision such interactions. In evolutionary psychology, contemporary gender differences are thought to originate from the successful ancestral adaptation to the different reproductive demands faced by men and women. For example, men developed attributes of aggressiveness and dominance because these facilitated mating success in competition with other men (see Buss, 2005). In such models, environmental influences reflect the contingent expression of sex-typed evolved dispositions that depends on the features of current environments that match evolutionary environments. Nonetheless, these mechanistic interactions take only limited forms given that gender identity and other psychological dispositions are thought to be preexisting in men's and women's biology and merely selected by current environments.

Proposing a more dynamic form of interaction, Wood and Eagly's (2002, 2007) biosocial model treats the psychological attributes of women and men as emergent given the evolved characteristics of the sexes, their developmental experiences, and their situated activity in society. These evolved characteristics include the physical attributes of the sexes and related behaviors, especially women's childbearing and nursing of infants and men's greater size, speed, and upper-body strength. The dispositions that characterize men and women in a given society thus are flexibly defined by the biosocial interaction. Consequently, variations in gender identity and other sex-typed attributes emerge across cultures, age cohorts, and social roles as local conditions interact with the universal framework provided by men's and women's evolved characteristics.

Conclusion

This chapter is in part a historical piece, given that the best known developments in gender identity research took place in the 1970s. Researchers' enthusiasm in that period was ignited by Bem's (1974) gender identity scale, which reflected feminist thinking at the time about the advantages of androgyny for mental health and behavioral flexibility. Bem's scale and related individual-difference measures also fit into the prevailing tendency of many feminists to regard sex differences in behavior as stemming not from causes intrinsic to women and men but from learned identity differences between the sexes.

Although interest in androgyny has waned, understanding of individual differences within gender groups has remained an important scientific agenda, and gender identity remains a viable approach. Because identities represent individuals' psychological relationships to the social categories in which they have membership, the study of identities is crucial to understanding how society infiltrates the psychology of the person. Gender identity is surely one of the most important of social identities and thus warrants psychologists' continuing attention.

Research on gender identity since the 1970s mainly has been a single-note tune, with the majority of research carried forward with Bem's (1974) BSRI scale and the related PAQ scale developed by Spence and Helmreich (1978). For example, in 2008, a search of PsycINFO turned up 1,748 total citations for the BSRI, with 266 of these during the past 5 years. The comparable figures for the PAQ are 885 overall and 218 during the past 5 years. These statistics far outpace citations to any other gender-related measure of individual differences. This continuing popularity of the PAQ and BSRI suggests that, when researchers think about explaining individual differences among women and men, their first (and often only) thought is to turn to these personality-trait-based measures of gender identity. Depending on researchers' purposes, this choice can be a mistake.

What are the consequences of the continuing popularity of the BSRI and PAQ? When researchers' main goal is not predicting agentic or communal behaviors, these measures have commonly yielded disappointing results. Because Bem's and Spence and Helmreich's scales were narrowly focused on agentic and communal personality traits, they do not predict the broad range of psychological phenomena that can flow from gender identity. The cause of the disappointing results is not in the scales themselves but in researchers' applications of them. Measures can address a variety of facets of identity, and they will be most successful at predicting responses that are compatible with the facet assessed by the gender identity scale. The classic measures of gender identity in terms of communal and agentic personality effectively predict the specific domains of communal and agentic responding, but other measures predict more satisfactorily outside of these domains.

As we have presented in this chapter, researchers can think about gender identity in ways that reach beyond traits. With these other treatments of gender identity, researchers have available to them a rich variety of measures. By bringing these other measures to researchers' attention, we hope to reinvigorate this important area of inquiry and facilitate prediction of gender-typed behavior in a wide range of domains. As we have illustrated, measures of gender identity in terms of interests predict vocations and related leisure activities. Measures of gender identity in terms of construal of oneself in intimate relationships predict reactions of men and women to close others. Finally, measures of collective gender identity predict ingroup favorability and self-ascription of gender-group attributes. The available approaches encompass a range of individual differences, and the associated measuring instruments are broadly useful to psychologists, sociologists, and other researchers interested in assessing individual differences in gender identity.

Acknowledgments

This chapter was completed while Wendy Wood was a Fellow at the Radcliffe Institute of Advanced Study, Harvard University. We thank Abigail Stewart for her helpful comments on an earlier draft of the chapter.

References

Aidman, E. V., & Carroll, S. M. (2003). Implicit individual differences: Relationships between implicit self-esteem, gender identity, and gender attitudes. *European Journal of Personality, 17*, 19–36.

Ajzen, I. (2005). *Attitudes, personality, and behavior* (2nd ed.). Milton Keynes, UK: Open University Press.

Ajzen, I., & Fishbein, M. (1977). Attitude–behavior relations: A theoretical analysis and review of empirical research. *Psychological Bulletin, 84*, 888–918.

Aron, A., Aron, E. N., Tudor, M., & Nelson, G. (1991). Close relationships as including other in the self. *Journal of Personality and Social Psychology, 60*, 241–253.

Ashmore, R. D. (1990). Sex, gender, and the individual. In L. A. Pervin (Ed.), *Handbook of personality: Theory and research* (pp. 486–526). New York: Guilford Press.

Ashmore, R. D., Deaux, K., & McLaughlin-Volpe, T. (2004). An organizing framework for collective identity: Articulation and significance of multidimensionality. *Psychological Bulletin, 130*, 80–114.

Athenstaedt, U. (2003). On the content and structure of the gender role self-concept: Including gender-stereotypical behaviors in addition to traits. *Psychology of Women Quarterly, 27*, 309–318.

Bakan, D. (1966). *The duality of human existence.* Chicago: Rand McNally.

Barry, H., III, Bacon, M. K., & Child, I. L. (1957). A cross-cultural survey of some sex differences in socialization. *Journal of Abnormal and Social Psychology, 55*, 327–332.

Baucom, D. H., Besch, P. K., & Callahan, S. (1985). Relation between testosterone concentration, sex role identity and personality among females. *Journal of Personality and Social Psychology, 48*, 1218–1226.

Baumeister, R. F., & Leary, M. R. (1995). The need to belong: Desire for interpersonal attachments as a fundamental human motivation. *Psychological Bulletin, 117*, 497–529.

Baumeister, R. F., & Sommer, K. L. (1997). What do men want? Gender differences and two spheres of belongingness: Comment on Cross and Madson (1997). *Psychological Bulletin, 112*, 38–44.

Bem, S. L. (1974). The measurement of psychological androgyny. *Journal of Consulting and Clinical Psychology, 42*, 155–162.

Bem, S. L. (1981). Gender schema theory: A cognitive account of sex typing. *Psychological Review, 88*, 354–364.

Booth, A., Granger, D. A., Mazur, A., & Kivlighan, K. T. (2006). Testosterone and social behavior. *Social Forces, 85*, 167–191.

Bresnahan, M. J., Levine, T. R., Shearman, S. M., Lee, S. Y., Park, C., & Kiyomiya, T. (2005). A multimethod multitrait validity assessment of self-construal in Japan, Korea, and the United States. *Human Communication Research, 31*, 33–59.

Brewer, M. B., & Gardner, W. (1996). Who is this "we"?: Levels of collective identity and self representations. *Journal of Personality and Social Psychology, 71*, 83–93.

Burke, P. J., & Tully, J. C. (1977). The measurement of role identity. *Social Forces, 55*, 881–897.

Buss, D. (Ed.). (2005). *Handbook of evolutionary psychology.* New York: Wiley.

Bussey, K., & Bandura, A. (1992). Self-regulatory mechanisms governing gender development. *Child Development, 63*, 1236–1250.

Bussey, K., & Bandura, A. (1999). Social-cognitive theory of gender development and differentiation. *Psychological Review, 106*, 676–713.

Bussey, K., & Bandura, A. (2004). Social cognitive theory of gender development and functioning. In A. H. Eagly, A. Beall, & R. Sternberg (Eds.), *The psychology of gender* (2nd ed., pp. 92–119). New York: Guilford Press.

Campbell, A. (2008). Attachment, aggression and affiliation: The of oxytocin in female social behavior. *Biological Psychology, 77*, 1–10.

Carver, C. S., & Scheier, M. F. (2008). Feedback processes in the simultaneous regulation of action and affect. In J. Y. Shah & W. L. Gardner (Eds.), *Handbook of motivation science* (pp. 308–324). New York: Guilford Press.

Chaiken, S., & Trope, Y. (1999). *Dual-process theories in social psychology.* New York: Guilford Press.

Clancy, S. M., & Dollinger, S. J. (1993). Photographic depictions of the self: Gender and age differences in social connectedness. *Sex Roles, 29*, 477–495.

Constantinople, A. (1973). Masculinity–femininity: An exception to a famous dictum? *Psychological Bulletin, 80*, 389–407.

Costa, P., Jr., Terracciano, A., & McCrae, R. R. (2001). Gender differences in personality traits across cultures: Robust and surprising findings. *Journal of Personality and Social Psychology, 81*, 322–331.

Cross, S. E., Bacon, P. L., & Morris, M. L. (2000). The relational-interdependent self-construal and relationships. *Journal of Personality and Social Psychology, 78*, 791–808.

Cross, S. E., & Madson, L. (1997). Models of the self: Self-construals and gender. *Psychological Bulletin, 122*, 5–37.

Cross, S. E., & Morris, M. L. (2003). Getting to know you: The relational self-construal, relational cognition, and well-being. *Personality and Social Psychology Bulletin, 29*, 512–523.

Cross, S. E., Morris, M. L., & Gore, J. S. (2002). Thinking about oneself and others: The relational-interdependent self-construal and social cognition. *Journal of Personality and Social Psychology, 82*, 399–418.

Deaux, K. (1987). Psychological constructions of masculinity and femininity. In J. M. Reinisch, L. A. Rosenblum, & S. A. Sanders (Eds.), *Masculinity–femininity: Basic perspectives* (pp. 289–303). New York: Oxford University Press.

Deaux, K., & Lafrance, M. (1998). Gender. In D. T. Gilbert, S. T. Fiske, & G. Lindzey (Eds.), *Handbook of social psychology* (4th ed., Vol. 1, pp. 788–827). New York: McGraw-Hill.

Deaux, K., & Lewis, L. L. (1984). Structure of gender stereotypes: Interrelationships among components and gender label. *Journal of Personality and Social Psychology, 46*, 991–1004.

Diekman, A. B., & Eagly, A. H. (2008). Of men, women, and motivation: A role congruity account. In J. Y. Shah & W. L. Gardner (Eds.), *Handbook of motivation science* (pp. 434–447). New York: Guilford Press.

Eagan, S. K., & Perry, D. G. (2001). Gender identity: A multidimensional analysis with implications for psychosocial adjustment. *Developmental Psychology, 37*, 451–463.

Eagly, A. H., & Chaiken, S. (1993). *The psychology of attitudes.* Orlando, FL: Harcourt Brace Jovanovich.

Eagly, A. H., Wood, W., & Diekman, A. B. (2000). Social role theory of sex differences and similarities: A current appraisal. In T. Eckes & H. M. Trautner (Eds.), *Developmental social psychology of gender* (pp. 123–174). Mahwah, NJ: Erlbaum.

Eagly, A. H., Wood, W., & Johannesen-Schmidt, M. C. (2004). Social role theory of sex differences and similarities: Implications for the partner preferences of women and men. In A. H. Eagly, A. E. Beall, & R. J. Sternberg (Eds.), *Psychology of gender* (2nd ed., pp. 269–295). New York: Guilford Press.

Epstein, S. (1980). The stability of behavior: II. Implications for psychological research. *American Psychologist, 35*, 790–806.

Fazio, R. H., & Olson, M. A. (2003). Implicit measures in social cognition research: Their meaning and uses. *Annual Review of Psychology, 54*, 297–327.

Frable, D. E. S. (1997). Gender, racial, ethnic, sexual, and class identities. *Annual Review of Psychology, 48*, 139–162.

Gabriel, S., & Gardner, W. L. (1999). Are there "his" and "hers" types of interdependence?: The implications of gender differences in collective versus relational interdependence for affect, behavior, and cognition. *Journal of Personality and Social Psychology, 77*, 642–655.

Gardner, W. L., & Gabriel, S. (2004). Gender differences in relational and collective interdependence: Implications for self-views, social behavior, and subjective well-being. In A. H. Eagly, A. E. Beall, & R. J. Sternberg (Eds.), *Psychology of gender* (2nd ed., pp. 169–191). New York: Guilford Press.

Gardner, W. L., Gabriel, S., & Hochschild, L. (2002). When you and I are "we," you are not threatening: The role of self-expansion in social comparison. *Journal of Personality and Social Psychology, 82*, 239–251.

Gore, J. S., Cross, S. E., & Morris, M. L. (2006). Let's be friends: Relational self-construal and the development of intimacy. *Personal Relationships, 13*, 83–102.

Grace, S. L., & Cramer, K. L. (2003). The elusive nature of self-measurement: The Self-Construal Scale versus the Twenty Statements Test. *Journal of Social Psychology, 143*, 649–668.

Greenwald, A. G., & Banaji, M. R. (1995). Implicit social cognition: Attitudes, self-esteem, and stereotypes. *Psychological Review, 102*, 4–27.

Greenwald, A. G., & Farnham, S. D. (2000). Using the Implicit Association Test to measure self-esteem and self-concept. *Journal of Personality and Social Psychology, 79*, 1022–1038.

Greenwald, A. G., Poehlman, T. A., Uhlmann, E. L., & Banaji, M. R. (in press). Understanding and using the Implicit Association Test: III. Meta-analysis of predictive validity. *Journal of Personality and Social Psychology.*

Helgeson, V. S. (1994a). Prototypes and dimensions of masculinity and femininity. *Sex Roles, 31*, 653–682.

Helgeson, V. S. (1994b). Relation of agency and communion to well-being: Evidence and potential explanations. *Psychological Bulletin, 116*, 412–428.

Helmreich, R. L., Spence, J. T., & Wilhelm, J. A. (1981). A psychometric analysis of the Personal Attributes Questionnaire. *Sex Roles, 7*, 1097–1108.

Hines, M., Brook, C., & Conway, G. S. (2004). Androgen and psychosexual development: Core gender identity, sexual orientation, and recalled childhood gender role behavior in women and men with congenital adrenal hyperplasia (CAH). *Journal of Sex Research, 41*, 75–81.

Hofmann, W., Gawronski, B., Gschwendner, T., Le, H., & Schmitt, M. (2005). A meta-analysis on the correlation between the Implicit Association Test and explicit self-report measures. *Personality and Social Psychology Bulletin, 31*, 1369–1385.

Josephs, R. A., Markus, H. R., & Tafarodi, R. W. (1992). Gender and self-esteem. *Journal of Personality and Social Psychology, 63*, 391–402.

Judd, C. M., James-Hawkins, L., Yzerbyt, V., & Kashima, Y. (2005). Fundamental dimensions of social judgment: Understanding the relations between judgments of competence and warmth. *Journal of Personality and Social Psychology, 89*, 899–913.

Kashima, E. S., & Hardie, E. A. (2000). The development and validation of the Relational, Individual, and Collective self-aspects (RIC) Scale. *Asian Journal of Social Psychology, 3*, 19–48.

Kashima, Y., Yamaguchi, S., Kim, U., Choi, S.-C., Gelfand, M. J., & Yuki, M. (1995). Culture, gender, and self: A perspective from individualism–collectivism research. *Journal of Personality and Social Psychology, 69*, 925–937.

Kiefer, A. K., & Sekaquaptewa, D. (2007). Implicit stereotypes, gender identification, and math-related outcomes: A prospective study of female college students. *Psychological Science, 18*, 13–18.

Kite, M. E., & Deaux, K. (1986). Gender versus category clustering in free recall: A test of gender schema theory. *Representative Research in Social Psychology, 16*, 38–43.

Kohlberg, L. A. (1966). Cognitive-developmental analysis of children's sex-role concepts and attitudes. In E. E. Maccoby (Ed.), *Development of sex differences* (pp. 82–173). Stanford, CA: Stanford University Press.

Kuhn, M. H., & McPartland, T. S. (1954). An empirical investigation of self-attitudes. *American Sociological Review, 19*, 68–76.

Leander, N. P., Chartrand, T. L., & Wood, W. (2009). *Mind your mannerisms: Eliciting stereotype conformity through behavioral mimicry.* Manuscript submitted for publication.

Lippa, R. A. (1991). Some psychometric characteristics of gender diagnosticity measures: Reliability, validity, consistency across domains, and relationship to the Big Five. *Journal of Personality and Social Psychology, 61*, 1000–1011.

Lippa, R. A. (1998). Gender-related individual differences and the structure of vocational interests: The importance of the people–things dimension. *Journal of Personality and Social Psychology, 74*, 996–1009.

Lippa, R. A. (2001). On deconstructing and reconstructing masculinity–femininity. *Journal of Research in Personality, 35*, 168–207.

Lippa, R. A. (2005). *Gender, nature, and nurture.* Mahwah, NJ: Erlbaum.

Lippa, R. A., & Connelly, S. (1990). Gender diagnosticity: A new Bayesian approach to gender-related individual differences. *Journal of Personality and Social Psychology, 59,* 1051–1065.

Luhtanen, R., & Crocker, J. (1992). A collective self-esteem scale: Self-evaluation of one's social identity. *Personality and Social Psychology Bulletin, 18,* 302–318.

Lytton, H., & Romney, D. M. (1991). Parents' differential socialization of boys and girls: A meta-analysis. *Psychological Bulletin, 109,* 267–296.

Maddux, W. W., & Brewer, M. B. (2005). Gender differences in the relational and collective bases for trust. *Group Processes and Intergroup Relations, 8,* 159–171.

Markus, H. R., & Kitayama, S. (1991). Culture and the self: Implications for cognition, emotion, and motivation. *Psychological Review, 98,* 224–253.

Marsh, H. W. (1987). The factorial invariance of responses by males and females to a multidimensional self-concept instrument: Substantive and methodological issues. *Multivariate Behavioral Research, 22,* 457–480.

Martin, C. L., & Ruble, D. (2004). Children's search for gender cues: Cognitive perspectives on gender development. *Current Directions in Psychological Science, 13,* 67–70.

McCrae, R. R., & Costa, P. T., Jr. (1988). Age, personality, and the spontaneous self-concept. *Journal of Gerontology: Social Sciences, 43,* S177–S185.

McGuire, W. J., & Padawer-Singer, A. (1976). Trait salience in the spontaneous self-concept. *Journal of Personality and Social Psychology, 33,* 743–754.

Meyer-Bahlburg, H. F. L., Dolezal, C., Baker, S. W., Carlson, A. D., Obeid, J. S., & New, M. I. (2004). Prenatal androgenization affects gender-related behavior but not gender identity in 5- to 12-year-old girls with congenital adrenal hyperplasia. *Archives of Sexual Behavior, 33,* 97–104.

Myers, A. M., & Gonda, G. (1982). Utility of the masculinity–femininity construct: Comparison of traditional and androgyny approaches. *Journal of Personality and Social Psychology, 43,* 514–522.

Nario-Redmond, M. R., Biernat, M., Eidelman, S., & Palenskie, D. J. (2004). The Social and Personal Identities scale: A measure of the differential importance ascribed to social and personal self-categorizations. *Self and Identity, 3,* 143–175.

Oyserman, D., Coon, H., & Kemmelmeier, M. (2002). Rethinking individualism and collectivism: Evaluation of theoretical assumptions and meta-analyses. *Psychological Bulletin, 128,* 3–72.

Ruble, D. N., & Martin, C. L. (1998). Gender development. In W. Damon & N. Eisenberg (Eds.), *Handbook of child psychology* (5th ed., Vol. 3, pp. 933–1016). New York: Wiley.

Sherif, C. W. (1982). Needed concepts in the study of gender identity. *Psychology of Women Quarterly, 6,* 375–395.

Smith, E. R., & DeCoster, J. (2000). Dual-process models in social and cognitive psychology: Conceptual integration and links to underlying memory systems. *Personality and Social Psychology Review, 4,* 108–131.

Spence, J. T. (1993). Gender-related traits and gender ideology: Evidence for a multifactorial theory. *Journal of Personality and Social Psychology, 64,* 624–635.

Spence, J. T., & Buckner, C. (1995). Masculinity and femininity: Defining the undefinable. In P. J. Kalbfleisch & M. Cody (Eds.), *Gender, power, and communication in human relationships* (pp. 105–138). Hillsdale, NJ: Erlbaum.

Spence, J. T., & Helmreich, R. L. (1978). *Masculinity and femininity: Their psychological dimensions, correlates, and antecedents.* Austin, TX: University of Texas Press.

Spence, J. T., Helmreich, R. L., & Stapp, J. (1974). The Personal Attributes Questionnaire: A measure of sex-role stereotypes and masculinity and femininity. *JSAS: Catalog of Selected Documents in Psychology, 4,* 43–44.

Stewart, A. J., & McDermott, C. (2004). Gender in psychology. *Annual Review of Psychology, 55,* 519–544.

Tajfel, H. (1982). Social psychology of intergroup relations. *Annual Review of Psychology, 33,* 1–39.

Taylor, M. C., & Hall, J. A. (1982). Psychological androgyny: Theories, methods, and conclusions. *Psychological Bulletin, 92,* 347–366.

Terman, L. M., & Miles, C. C. (1936). *Sex and personality: Studies in masculinity and femininity.* New York: McGraw-Hill.

Turner, J. C., Hogg, M. A., Oakes, P. J., Reicher, S. D., & Wetherell, M. S. (1987). *Rediscovering the social group: A self-categorization theory.* Oxford, UK: Blackwell.

van Well, S., Kolk, A. M., & Oei, N. Y. L. (2007). Direct and indirect assessment of gender role identification. *Sex Roles, 56,* 617–628.

Vorauer, J. D., & Miller, D. T. (1997). Failure to recognize the effect of implicit social influence on the presentation of self. *Journal of Personality and Social Psychology, 73,* 281–295.

Wiggins, J. S. (Ed.). (1996). *The five-factor model of personality: Theoretical perspectives.* New York: Guilford Press.

Witt, M. G., & Wood, W. (2009). *Self-regulation of gendered behavior in everyday life.* Manuscript submitted for publication.

Wood, W., Christensen, P. N., Hebl, M. R., & Rothgerber, H. (1997). Conformity to sex-typed norms, affect, and the self-concept. *Journal of Personality and Social Psychology, 73,* 523–535.

Wood, W., & Eagly, A. H. (2002). A cross-cultural analysis of the behavior of women and men: Implications for the origins of sex differences. *Psychological Bulletin, 128,* 699–727.

Wood, W., & Eagly, A. H. (2007). Social structural origins of sex differences in human mating. In S. W. Gangestad & J. A. Simpson (Eds.), *The evolution of mind: Fundamental questions and controversies* (pp. 383–390). New York: Guilford Press.

Wood, W., & Eagly, A. H. (in press). Gender. In S. T. Fiske, D. T. Gilbert, & G. Lindzey (Eds.), *Handbook of social psychology* (5th ed.). New York: McGraw-Hill.

PART III

■ ● ▲ ◆

EMOTIONAL DISPOSITIONS

CHAPTER 9

■ ● ▲ ◆ ■ ● ▲ ◆

Neuroticism

THOMAS A. WIDIGER

The term *neurosis* was purportedly first coined in 1769 by a Scottish doctor, William Cullen, referring to disorders resulting from a "general affection" of the nervous system. The first edition of the American Psychiatric Association's (1952) *Diagnostic and Statistical Manual: Mental Disorders* had a section devoted to "psychoneurotic disorders": "The chief characteristic of these disorders is 'anxiety' which may be directly felt and expressed or which may be unconsciously and automatically controlled by the utilization of various psychological defense mechanisms" (American Psychiatric Association, 1952, p. 31).

Neuroticism, as a fundamental trait of general personality, refers to an enduring tendency or disposition to experience negative emotional states. Individuals who score high on neuroticism are more likely than the average person to experience such feelings as anxiety, anger, guilt, and depression. They respond poorly to environmental stress, are likely to interpret ordinary situations as threatening, and can experience minor frustrations as hopelessly overwhelming. They are often self-conscious and shy, and they may have trouble controlling urges and impulses when feeling upset. Neuroticism is now recognized as one of the more reliably identified and fundamental domains of personality functioning and structure (Mc-Crae & Costa, 2003). There are few theo-

retically or empirically based models of general personality structure that fail to include a domain of neuroticism (Digman, 1990). Discussed within this chapter are alternative conceptualizations (and assessments) of neuroticism, its origins, and its important life outcomes.

Conceptualization and Assessment

In Digman's (1990) seminal review of the development of the Big Five factors of personality, he opined that "while fairly good agreement appears to be developing concerning the number of necessary dimensions, there is less accord with respect to their meaning" (p. 422). This difficulty is quite understandable, as it is unlikely that any one single word can adequately characterize such broad domains of personality functioning. Any single word places more emphasis on a particular range or aspect of the broad domain at the expense of other components or facets. Digman appeared somewhat reluctant to offer his own interpretation of this fourth factor of the Big Five, but he did indicate that "Dimension IV is usually referred to as neuroticism vs. emotional stability" (Digman, 1990, p. 422).

The term *neuroticism* has been favored by Eysenck (1967), Costa and McCrae (1992), Digman (1990), and Zuckerman (2003).

Emotional instability (or *stability*) has been favored by Guilford (1975) and Goldberg (1993). *Emotionality* is favored by Lee and Ashton (2004). *Negative emotionality* or *negative temperament* has been preferred by Watson and Tellegen (1985) and Watson and Clark (1994). Another conceptualization is *harm avoidance*, offered by Cloninger (2000). These alternative titles are similar to one another, and there is consistent empirical support to indicate that these constructs, or the instruments to assess them, are highly convergent (Watson, Clark, & Harkness, 1994; Widiger & Simonsen, 2005; Zuckerman, 2002). Nevertheless, the alternative titles do reflect somewhat different conceptualizations that become particularly evident when comparing respective assessment instruments, especially variation in facet scales.

Table 9.1 lists six alternative measures of neuroticism and how their facet scales are aligned with one another or, more accurately, how weakly they are aligned. Included within Table 9.1 are the facet scales from the NEO Personality Inventory—Revised (NEO PI-R) assessment of the five-factor model (FFM), the Multidimensional Personality Questionnaire (MPQ), the Big Five Aspects Scales (BFAS), the HEXACO Personality Inventory (HEXACO-PI), the Temperament and Character Inventory (TCI; an expansion

of the Tridimensional Personality Questionnaire, or TPQ), and the Eysenck Personality Profiler (EPP; the Eysenck Personality Questionnaire [EPQ] and the Eysenck Personality Inventory [EPI] did not include facet scales). Considered herein more closely are the facets of angry hostility and aggression, impulsivity, emotional instability, and dependency.

Angry Hostility and Aggression

Costa and McCrae (1992) suggest that "the general tendency to experience negative affects such as fear, sadness, embarrassment, anger, guilt and disgust is the core of the neuroticism domain" (p. 14). Consistent with this conceptualization, the NEO PI-R includes facet scales for angry hostility, anxiety, and depression, along with self-consciousness, vulnerability, and impulsivity (see Table 9.1). Watson and Tellegen (1985) define this domain of personality as negative emotionality, negative affectivity, or negative temperament and, when using the Positive and Negative Affect Schedule (PANAS; Watson, Clark, & Tellegen, 1988), confine its assessment to such negative affects as hostility and irritability, along with being afraid, scared, nervous, jittery, guilty, ashamed, upset, and/or distressed (surprisingly, though, no depression, sadness, or sorrow). The expanded version, the PANAS-X

TABLE 9.1. Alignment or Misalignment of Facets of Neuroticism, Negative Emotionality, Emotionality, and Harm Avoidance

NEO PI-R	EPP	MPQ	BFAS	HEXACO-PI	TCI
Anxiety	Anxiety		Withdrawal	Anxiety	Fear of uncertainty Anticipatory worry
		Alienation			
Self-Consciousness	Inferiority			Fearfulness	Shyness
				Dependency	
Depression	Unhappiness				
					Fatigability
Vulnerability Angry hostility		Stress Reaction			
		Aggression			
			Volatility		
Impulsivity					
				Sentimentality	

Note. NEO PI-R, NEO Personality Inventory—Revised (Costa & McCrae, 1992); EPP, Eysenck Personality Profiler (EPP; Eysenck et al., 1992); MPQ, Multidimensional Personality Questionnaire (Tellegen, 1982); BFAS, Big Five Aspects Scale (DeYoung et al., 2007); HEXACO-PI, HEXACO Personality Inventory (Lee & Ashton, 2006); TCI, Temperament and Character Inventory (Cloninger, 2000).

(Watson & Clark, 1994), includes subscales for each of the "basic negative emotions" of fear, sadness, and guilt, along with hostility, assessed by the trait terms *angry, hostile, irritable, scornful, disgusted*, and *loathing*.

An important distinction between the dimensional models of personality of Clark and Watson (Clark, 2005; Watson, Gamez, & Simms, 2005) and Costa and McCrae (1992) is that Clark and Watson do not include a domain of antagonism separate from negative temperament. Clark and Watson have long advocated instead a three-factor model of general personality structure, consisting of negative affect, positive affect, and constraint. Therefore, much of the antagonistic and aggressive behavior in the FFM is included within their negative affectivity domain. This is explicit within the MPQ assessment of negative emotionality (Tellegen, 1982), whose subscales include Aggression, along with Stress Reaction and Alienation (see Table 9.1). MPQ Aggression includes being physically aggressive, enjoying upsetting and frightening others, enjoying scenes of violence (e.g., fights, violent movies), and victimizing others for one's own advantage (Tellegen, 1982; Tellegen & Waller, 1987).

A conceptual rationale for including antagonistic, aggressive behavior within the domain of negative emotionality or neuroticism is that the anger could be said to be the driving force or motivating energy for aggressive behavior, just as positive emotionality can be considered to be the driving force of extraverted behavior (Watson & Clark, 1997) and anxiousness the driving force of self-conscious behavior (Costa & McCrae, 1992). "Hostile people are generally antagonistic" (Costa & McCrae, 1992, p. 45). However, a separation of antagonistic behavior from negative emotionality is supported by the factor-analytic studies of language structure (Ashton & Lee, 2001). In addition, not all antagonistic behavior will be driven by anger (e.g., manipulation, exploitation, arrogance, and deception), and even some instances of aggression can occur without significant feelings of anger (e.g., instrumental aggression).

A complementary position to shifting aggression into neuroticism is to shift angry hostility out of neuroticism and into the FFM domain of antagonism, which is precisely what is proposed by Ashton and Lee

(2005) in their HEXACO model of personality structure (HEXACO stands for Honesty, Emotionality, Extraversion, Agreeableness, Conscientiousness, and Openness). Within HEXACO Emotionality "content related to anger versus even-temper shifts from neuroticism to the new variant of low agreeableness, and content related to sensitivity, sentimentality versus toughness shifts from agreeableness to the new variant of neuroticism (which we have named emotionality to reflect this exchange of content)" (Ashton & Lee, 2005, p. 1324).

The four HEXACO-PI facets of emotionality are fear, anxiousness, dependency, and sentimentality. Ashton and Lee (2005) suggest that these four facets are more consistent with the language structure of this domain of personality (Saucier & Goldberg, 2001, suggest alternatively that the two primary lexical facets should be irritability and anxiousness/fearfulness). In this regard, the Ashton and Lee conceptualization does align more closely with Cloninger's (2000) and Eysenck's (1967) characterization and assessment of harm avoidance and neuroticism, respectively (see Table 9.1). The facet scales of Cloninger's TCI harm avoidance concern fear of uncertainty, shyness, fatigability, and anticipatory worry. The facet scales of EPP neuroticism concern anxiety, inferiority, and unhappiness. Neither includes anger (let alone aggression).

HEXACO emotionality also fails to include a facet of depressiveness. One might expect emotionality to include anger and depression. Questions have been raised as to whether such feelings as disgust and embarrassment are actually emotions, but anger does appear to be comfortably included within a domain of emotionality (Ekman, 1999; Russell, 2003) and certainly within a domain of negative emotionality, along with anxiousness and depressiveness (Watson & Tellegen, 1985).

Some of the variation in conceptualization across models can reflect simply the number of factors that are extracted. For instance, if one reduces the FFM to just three factors, it is perhaps not surprising that aggression shifts into a domain of negative affectivity (Markon, Krueger, & Watson, 2005). In this regard, one could say that the three- and five-factor models are not in conflict. They just reflect the level of a common hierarchical model in which one prefers to work and study (i.e., two-, three-, four-, five-, or six-factor models). However, even if this is the basis for the variation across models, there is still the question of which level of the hierarchy provides the optimal description of personality structure. In addition, one must remain cognizant of the substantive differences in neuroticism across the levels of the hierarchical model.

Impulsivity

Costa and McCrae (1992) suggest that neuroticism involves more than just a susceptibility to psychological distress: "Perhaps because disruptive emotions interfere with adaptation, men and women high in neuroticism are also prone to have irrational ideas [and] to be less able to control their impulses" (p. 14); hence their inclusion of a facet of impulsivity within the NEO PI-R. The NEO PI-R assessment of neuroticism is relatively unique in its inclusion of this facet. Nevertheless, studies that report correlations of NEO PI-R Impulsivity with (for instance) Zuckerman–Kuhlman Personality Questionnaire (ZKPQ) Impulsive Sensation Seeking (Zuckerman, 2002) or MPQ Constraint (Tellegen, 1982) do tend to report substantial correlations with neuroticism as well (e.g., Aluja, Garcia, & Garcie, 2004). Impulsivity itself is a rather broad trait or, at least, a variably defined construct that can refer to quite a number of different behaviors (Depue & Collins, 1999). Whiteside and Lynam (2001) have, in fact, used the NEO PI-R facet structure to distinguish between four different variants of impulsivity, one of which would be correctly placed within the domain of neuroticism: urgency. "It refers to the tendency to experience strong impulses, frequently under conditions of negative affect" (Whiteside & Lynam, 2001, p. 685).

Whiteside and Lynam (2001) suggest that additional variants of impulsivity are low premeditation, low perseverance, and sensation seeking. The disposition to refrain from acting on the spur of the moment and without regard to consequences is represented by the NEO PI-R Conscientiousness facet of deliberation, "the tendency to think carefully before acting" (Costa & McCrae, 1992, p. 18). They refer to this variant of impulsivity as a lack of premeditation: "Premedita-

tion refers to the tendency to think and reflect on the consequences of an act before engaging in that act" (Whiteside & Lynam, 2001, p. 685). NEO PI-R self-discipline refers to "the ability to begin tasks and carry them through to completion despite boredom and other distractions" (Costa & McCrae, 1992, p. 18). Whiteside and Lynam refer to this disposition as perseverance. The fourth and final variant of impulsivity is NEO PI-R excitement seeking, involving an enjoyment in taking risks and engaging in dangerous activities, which aligns closely with Zuckerman's (2002) sensation seeking. Lynam and colleagues have developed a measure of these four variants of impulsivity and have further demonstrated that the four variants have quite different correlations with existing impulsivity measures and validators (Lynam & Miller, 2004; Whiteside, Lynam, Miller, & Reynolds, 2005).

In sum, there does appear to be compelling conceptual and empirical support for including impulsivity within neuroticism, although it might not be best considered as a core trait. Perhaps it is best understood as a corollary. It might also be preferable to use the title of *urgency* when referring to this facet of the NEO PI-R rather than the more ambiguous or relatively nonspecific title of *impulsivity* (Whiteside & Lynam, 2001).

Emotional Instability

DeYoung, Quilty, and Peterson (2007), through analyses of the facet scales of the NEO PI-R (Costa & McCrae, 1992) and the Abridged Big Five Circumplex scales from the International Personality Item Pool (Goldberg, 1999), identified two facets for each domain of the FFM. They suggested that these 10 facets align well with genetic factors within the NEO PI-R identified by Jang, Livesley, Angleitner, Reimann, and Vernon (2002). "Each of the Big Five domains, therefore, appears potentially divisible into two subdomains with distinct biological sources" (DeYoung et al., 2007, p. 881). They constructed an inventory to assess these 10 facets, the Big Five Aspects Scales (BFAS). The two facets of Neuroticism are volatility and withdrawal.

The withdrawal facet is not what the name might imply, social withdrawal. Its items assess instead traditional features of neuroticism, such as feeling blue, worrying, feeling threatened, being easily discouraged, being afraid, and feeling overwhelmed. Volatility items within the BFAS include "get upset easily," "keep my emotions under control," "change my mood a lot," "am a person whose moods go up and down easily," and "get easily agitated" (DeYoung et al., 2007, p. 887). Such items are clearly referring to an emotional instability (or volatility), consistent with Goldberg's (1993) original characterization of this domain as emotional stability versus instability.

The NEO PI-R, in contrast, does not include any facet scales that represent or explicitly assess this volatility or emotionality instability. The NEO PI-R does include scales to assess anxiousness, depressiveness, and angry hostility, which are the negative emotions that would be expressed by a person who is emotionally volatile or unstable, but the NEO PI-R negative affect scales are typically interpreted as referring to a disposition to be characteristically or consistently anxious, dysphoric, or angry rather than being periodically (e.g., inconsistently) emotionally explosive, unstable, or volatile. Shedler and Westen (2004) have presented their Shedler–Westen Assessment Procedure as "an alternative to the five-factor model" (p. 1743). Factor analyses of this item pool have yielded scales that resemble four of the five domains of the FFM, but "we also identified some useful diagnostic distinctions, such as the distinction between negative affectivity and emotional dysregulation, which increasingly appear to be distinct concepts, as reflected in the difference between stable dysthymia and [the affective instability of] borderline personality disorder" (Westen & Shedler, 2007, p. 818). Further support is provided by Miller and Pilkonis (2006).

Volatility and emotional dysregulation probably should be understood as facets of neuroticism, consistent with Goldberg's (1993) characterization of this personality domain as a contrast between emotional stability and instability (DeYoung et al., 2007; Mullins-Sweatt & Widiger, 2007). Persons who are emotionally volatile, unstable, or dysregulated will characterize themselves as being higher in levels of anger, anxiety, and depressiveness than the average person. Nevertheless, there are important distinctions between being emotionally volatile and

characteristically nervous, pessimistic, or irritable (Miller & Pilkonis, 2006).

Dependency

One of the four facets of HEXACO emotionality is dependency, defined as a "need for emotional support from others" (Lee & Ashton, 2004, p. 334). Dependency is one of the personality disorders included within the *Diagnostic and Statistical Manual of Mental Disorders* (American Psychiatric Association, 2000). The essential feature of dependent personality disorder is a pervasive and excessive need to be taken care of that leads to submissive and clinging behavior and fears of separation (American Psychiatric Association, 2000). Bornstein and Cecero (2000) and Saulsman and Page (2004) conducted meta-analyses of studies correlating measures of the FFM with measures of dependency, and both reported that the highest and most consistent relationship was with the domain of neuroticism.

However, considering dependency to be a facet of neuroticism could represent a confusion of the fears, needs, and insecurities of the dependent person with his or her dependent behavior. Agreeableness, as assessed by the NEO PI-R (Costa & McCrae, 1992), is the tendency to be trusting, straightforward, altruistic, compliant, modest, and tender-minded. Well before ever considering personality disorders as maladaptive variants of the FFM, Costa and McCrae (1985) had stated that "agreeableness can also assume a pathological form, in which it is usually seen as dependency" (p. 12). Widiger, Trull, Clarkin, Sanderson, and Costa (2002) include aspects of neuroticism within their FFM conceptualization of dependency (particularly the facets of anxiousness, self-consciousness, and vulnerability) but, consistent with Costa and McCrae, they suggest that "the DSM-IV diagnostic criteria set [for dependent personality disorder] includes many explicit examples of pathological agreeableness, such as excessive compliance (difficulty expressing disagreement), altruism (volunteering to do unpleasant things), and modesty (needing advice and reassurance from others to make everyday decisions)" (p. 96). Pincus (2002) confines his conceptualization of dependency simply to interpersonal relatedness. Such trait terms as *docile, servile, self-sacrificing, modest, agreeable, compliant, clinging, obe-dient, gullible, submissive, self-effacing*, and even *dependent* have long been considered interpersonal in nature, representing various combinations of the fundamental domains of high communion and low agency that define the interpersonal circumplex (Pincus, 2002).

In sum, the self-consciousness, vulner-ability, and insecurity of neuroticism may contribute to the occurrence of dependent behavior (Miller & Pilkonis, 2006), as anx-iousness would contribute to the occurrence of self-consciousness (Costa & McCrae, 1992), as anger would contribute to the oc-currence of antagonistic behavior (Clark & Watson, 1999) and negative affects to the occurrence of urgent impulsivity (Whiteside & Lynam, 2001). This dependent behavior may perhaps be best understood as a poten-tial correlate of neuroticism or emotional-ity rather than as a fundamental or defin-ing feature of neuroticism, particularly as dependent behavior need not necessarily or always be driven by neuroticism.

In sum, there is considerable agreement as to the existence of a domain of neuroticism, emotionality, emotional instability, or nega-tive emotionality, however it may be identi-fied. And there is considerable convergence among alternative measures of this domain. Nevertheless, there is no unanimity as to its precise assessment, and this is quite evident when one considers the specific facets of respective measures of this domain of gen-eral personality functioning. This variation in how the domain is assessed can have a significant impact on research findings, as illustrated in the following section, when considering the origins, or more precisely the molecular genetics, of neuroticism.

Origins

It is not difficult to infer the reasons for a fitness advantage for emotional stability relative to instability, but there are also com-pelling arguments for the adaptivity or fit-ness value of emotional instability or, more specifically, anxiousness and depressiveness. "Normal" anxiety is an emotion that helps organisms defend against a wide variety of threats. Pain is a signal of a threat to physi-cal safety and survival; anxiety is an emo-tional pain that can be a comparable signal

of threat, either physical or social. The ab-sence of a capacity to be anxious would, in many instances, be maladaptive, as it would impair the individual's ability to anticipate or appreciate signs of threat and danger. Similarly, depression can serve as a signal to others that help is needed to overcome a loss, damage, or injury. Persons with this capac-ity to express depressed, sad, or sorrowful behavior are more likely to elicit the help and support from others that are necessary to overcome negative life events.

Given the lack of obvious clarity about the precise situations in which any such signal should or should not be emitted and the lack of certainty regarding the optimal magnitude of any signal within any particu-lar situation, it should not then be too sur-prising that there is considerable variation in individual differences in the disposition to respond with anxiety or depression (Buss, 1996; Penke, Denissen, & Miller, 2007). Evolution would favor variability in a signal expression whose adaptive value will vary across time and social, physical contexts.

There is consistent support for the heri-tability of neuroticism. The research is gen-erally consistent with the routine finding that approximately 40–60% of the vari-ance appears to be genetic, 20–30% con-cerns nonshared environmental influences, and shared environmental contribution approaches zero, with the remaining vari-ance left unexplained (Turkheimer, 2000). Yamagata and colleagues (2006) have gone beyond the univariate behavior genetic methodology to explore multivariate behav-ior genetic heritability that considers the co-variation among two or more traits. They considered NEO PI-R data obtained from three large, independent twin samples from Canada, Germany, and Japan to determine whether the facet structure of the NEO PI-R is consistent with shared genetic variance. They concluded "that the five factors are 'genetically crisp'" (Yamagata et al., 2006, p. 994). However, it should be noted that one qualification for the domain of neuroti-cism was that angry hostility, although ge-netically loading primarily on neuroticism, did also load on the genetic factor of an-tagonism within the German and Japanese samples and impulsiveness loaded as highly on the genetic factor of conscientiousness as it did for neuroticism within the Canadian and Japanese samples.

Yamagata and colleagues (2006) suggested that one implication of their findings "is that molecular genetic studies of personality seeking putative loci would clearly benefit from the use of the NEO PI-R" (p. 994). Studies of the heritability of neuroticism have gone beyond simply bivariate and multivariate genetic analyses to explore more precisely molecular genetics. The primary focus of attention has been a polymorphism of the serotonin transporter gene *5HTT-LPR*. This interest has grown from the finding that serotonergic systems are considered to be integral to emotion regulation and that drugs that are effective in reducing anxiety and depression act largely through the serotonergic system. Two meta-analyses of molecular genetic research have supported the conclusion that there is a meaningfully significant relationship (effect sizes of approximately 0.20; Cohen, 1992) between neuroticism and short versus long alleles of *5HTT-LPR*, particularly when neuroticism is assessed with the NEO PI-R (Schinka, Busch, & Robichaux-Keene, 2004; Sen, Burmeister, & Ghosh, 2004).

The specific results from and conclusions concerning these meta-analyses, however, have been disputed. A meta-analysis conducted by Munafo and colleagues (2003) also found support for the association of *5HTT-LPR* with neuroticism, although not as strong (an effect size of only 0.11; Cohen, 1992). More important, perhaps, Munafo, Clark, and Flint (2005a) subsequently explored whether the association was instrument specific and concluded on the basis of their new meta-analysis that the association was confined largely to studies using Cloninger's (2000) TCI (or TPQ) harm-avoidance scale rather than NEO PI-R neuroticism, a finding in direct contradiction to the meta-analyses of Schinka and colleagues (2004) and Sen and colleagues (2004). The inconsistency appears to reflect (in part) disagreements with regard to which studies should be included (e.g., Munafo et al., 2005a, excluded studies with psychiatric samples), how studies should be weighted, and the optimal genetic comparison group. Subsequent reanalyses have not resolved the dispute (Munafo, Clark, & Flint, 2005b; Schinka, 2005; Sen, Burmeister, & Ghosh, 2005), although when using Cohen's (1992) measure of effect size, Munafo and colleagues (2005b) replicated the findings of Schinka

(2005), showing "a strong dominant effect of *5-HTT-LPR* on NEO neuroticism, and a more modest but nevertheless significant recessive effect on TCI/TPQ harm avoidance" (pp. 895–896). This conclusion is consistent with a subsequent study by Schmitz, Hennig, Kuepper, and Reuter (2007), who reported a significant effect for neuroticism as assessed by the NEO Five-Factor Inventory (NEO FFI; Costa & McCrae, 1992) and the EPQ—Revised (EPQ-R; Eysenck, Barrett, Wilson, & Jackson, 1992; Miles & Hempel, 2004), but not by TCI harm avoidance. They further explored which specific items of the NEO FFI, EPQ-R, and TCI were most contributory, and they suggested that the significant findings are due largely to items assessing depressiveness and stress sensitivity.

Findings that the results vary in part due to the measurement instrument, though, should not be at all surprising, given the considerable variation in how each instrument assesses neuroticism (see Table 9.1). In addition, it is perhaps unrealistic to expect a very specific genetic association, or at least a strong effect size, for an endophenotype as broad as neuroticism (Flint & Munafo, 2007). And, finally, the structure of the *5HTT-LPR* gene has itself been questioned. Although most past studies considered the *5HTT-LPR* gene to have two alleles, one long and one short, there is now research to suggest that it is triallelic (Beitchman et al., 2006). It has one short allele, *s*, and two long alleles, *Lg* and *La* (Beitchman et al., 2006). The *s* and the *Lg* alleles tend to be relatively low-expressing (they are present less often), and they are associated with lower brain levels of *5HT* (Beitchman et al., 2006; Hu et al., 2007); the *La* allele is not. Research before this discovery considered only the presence of the short allele as relevant to risk; cases with the high-risk *Lg* allele were perhaps inaccurately assigned to the low-risk comparison group, thus reducing differences between the groups in gene-based risk status.

Life Outcomes

Neuroticism, as a disposition to experience negative emotional states, to respond poorly to environmental stress, and to experience even minor frustrations as hopelessly overwhelming, would, not surprisingly, be considered to contribute to the etiology of a variety of negative life outcomes. One of the more robust and heavily studied findings is the association of neuroticism with a wide variety of psychopathology. Malouff, Thorsteinsson, and Schutte (2005) conducted a meta-analysis of the relationship of neuroticism (as well as other domains of the FFM) with DSM-IV mental disorders. They reported effect sizes for the relationship of neuroticism with mood disorders to be 1.54, with anxiety disorders to be 1.04, with somatoform disorders to be 1.20, with eating disorders to be 1.29, and with schizophrenia to be 1.08 (the effective size for the relationship with substance use disorders was 0.54). An effect size of 0.80 or higher is generally understood to indicate a large effect (Cohen, 1992). Cassin and von Ranson (2005) reported comparable results in their meta-analysis of the research on neuroticism and eating disorders. Van Os and Jones (2001) reported in a prospective longitudinal study of 5,362 participants that persons with high neuroticism scores at age 16 were 1.93 times more likely to meet criteria for schizophrenia later in life. In a community sample of 2,085 young adults, Parslow, Jorm, and Christensen (2006) reported a higher likelihood of persons elevated on neuroticism to develop posttraumatic stress disorder on subsequent trauma exposure.

The robust relationship of neuroticism with various forms of psychopathology is consistent with other important life outcomes. Neuroticism is associated with the occurrence of a variety of physical illnesses, including (but not limited to) hypertension, cardiovascular disease, and diabetes, as well as reduced survival among those with the respective illnesses (Smith & MacKenzie, 2006; Suls & Bunde, 2005). The volume and robustness of the study of neuroticism and negative life outcomes is suggested simply by the number of meta-analyses that have been conducted, including meta-analyses of the relationship of neuroticism to lower subjective well-being (Steel, Schmidt, & Schultz, 2008); lower academic satisfaction (Trapmann, Hell, Hirn, & Schuler, 2007); lower job satisfaction (Judge, Heller, & Mount, 2002); lower performance motivation, such as lower self-efficacy and goal setting (Judge & Ilies, 2002); lower leadership (Judge, Bono, Ilies, & Gerhardt, 2002); higher smoking (Malouff, Thorsteinsson, &

Schutte, 2006; Munafo, Zetteler, & Clark, 2007); increased alcohol abuse (Malouff, Thorsteinsson, Rooke, & Schutte, 2007); greater unprotected sexual activity (Hoyle, Fejfar, & Miller, 2000); lower happiness (DeNeve & Cooper, (1998); higher dependency (Bornstein & Cecero, 2000); higher extrinsic religiosity (Saroglou, 2002); and higher rates of criminal arrest (Huo-Liang, 2006). Beyond these meta-analyses, neuroticism has been shown to be associated with higher existential concerns, weaker identity integration, dissatisfaction and conflict within relationships, dissolution of relationships (e.g., divorce), and financial insecurity (Ozer & Benet-Martínez, 2006). Neuroticism is clearly a very robust predictor of negative life outcomes.

These relationships between neuroticism and negative life outcomes are generally understood to be etiological, that is, neuroticism contributes to the development or occurrence of the negative life outcomes. Connor-Smith and Flachsbart (2007) conducted a meta-analysis of the relationship of personality and coping mechanisms as reported in 165 studies and reported that neuroticism was associated with problematic strategies such as wishful thinking, withdrawal, and emotion-focused coping. Of course, it is not entirely clear whether the poorer coping mechanisms were a result of neuroticism or whether poor coping strategies led to the development of anxiousness, depressiveness, vulnerability, and self-consciousness.

There are, in fact, a variety of mechanisms through which neuroticism could result in negative life outcomes. With respect to lowered physical health, neuroticism could provide a direct effect, through altered autonomic regulation of the cardiovascular system, immune suppression, and increased inflammation associated with higher levels of negative affectivity, or an indirect effect, through poorer health habits, increased exposure to daily stressors, and other life difficulties (Smith & MacKenzie, 2006; Suls & Bunde, 2005). The same can occur for the contribution of neuroticism to the etiology of psychopathology. Neuroticism can contribute both diathesis and stress (Caspi, Roberts, & Shiner, 2005), providing a vulnerability to psychopathology through both reactive and evocative person–environment transactions. The former relationship is essentially a direct effect; reacting to events with high levels of distress, anxiety, and worry provides an explicit risk for various forms of psychopathology, particularly mood and anxiety disorders. The evocative person–environment transaction may occur when one's frequent expressions of upset, worry, and vulnerability produce negative reactions from others, thus reinforcing and increasing the original distress (i.e., personality as causing stress). There is empirical support, for instance, for a relationship of neuroticism to the presence and experience of lower levels of social support (Kendler, Gardner, & Prescott, 2006). The contribution of neuroticism to the development of physical health problems, financial difficulties, and dissolution of relationships and other negative life outcomes (Ozer & Benet-Martínez, 2006) would also contribute in turn to a considerable amount of stress, which persons high in neuroticism would have an inherent difficulty emotionally surmounting.

The contribution of neuroticism to the etiology of psychopathology has also been studied at a genetic level. Munafo, Clark, Roberts, and Johnstone (2006), for instance, addressed the question of whether trait neuroticism mediates the putative association between the serotonin transporter gene polymorphism (*5HTT-LPR*) and lifetime major depression in adults. In this study, 251 participants completed the EPQ and a self-report measure of depression. The *5HTT-LPR* genotype was significantly associated with both neuroticism and lifetime major depression, as was neuroticism with lifetime major depression. Neuroticism, however, accounted for 42% of the effect of *5HTT-LPR* genotype on lifetime major depression, indicating possible mediation. Similar results have been reported by Jacobs and colleagues (2006).

The study of the etiological contribution of neuroticism to psychopathology (and other negative life outcomes) can also be hindered, or at least complicated, because of two other ways in which neuroticism and psychopathology can be associated with one another. Widiger and Smith (2008) distinguish between three fundamentally different ways in which neuroticism and psychopathology can relate to one another. In addition to a causal relationship, neuroticism and psychopathology can influence the presentation or appearance of one another

(pathoplastic relationships), and they can be associated through a common, underlying etiology (spectrum relationships). The etiological, causal relationship is the one of most interest to theorists and researchers, but any study concerned with the potential contribution of neuroticism to the development of psychopathology must be fully cognizant of the potential impact of the pathoplastic and spectrum relationships on the obtainment of significant research findings. Each of these two other forms of relationship of neuroticism to negative life outcomes are discussed in turn.

Pathoplastic Relationships

The influence of neuroticism and psychopathology on the presentation, appearance, or expression of one another is typically characterized as a pathoplastic relationship (Widiger & Smith, 2008). This pathoplastic relationship is bidirectional, as psychopathology can vary in its appearance depending on a person's premorbid level of neuroticism, and the appearance or presentation of neuroticism can similarly be affected by the presence of a current (or even recently experienced) psychopathology. Pathoplastic relationships are not confined to but are most readily understood as methodological confounds in studies on the etiological relationship of personality to negative life outcomes.

For example, a pathoplastic effect of neuroticism on the expression or appearance of ill health is the finding that persons high in neuroticism complain of more symptoms and are more likely to seek treatment (ten Have, Oldehinkel, Vollebergh, & Ormel, 2005). Objectively, they may be no more ill than the person low in neuroticism, but they are more likely to report the presence of symptoms and to seek treatment for them (Chapman, Duberstein, Sorensen, Lyness, & Emery, 2006). This does not necessarily imply that they lack a clinically significant level of actual ill health, but it is possible that the extent of the relationship of neuroticism to ill health could be due (at least in some part) to the increased reporting of symptoms in persons high in neuroticism. This concern has been primarily evident in studies of the relationship of neuroticism to physical illness (Smith & MacKenzie, 2006; Suls & Bunde, 2005), but perhaps it should be as much a concern for studies of mental illness. Duberstein and Heisel (2007) reported that neuroticism was associated with a higher level of overreporting of affective symptoms in persons with clinical depression (overreporting was suggested by higher levels of self-report relative to a clinician-based assessment of depression).

Of greater concern to researchers, however, is the pathoplastic effect of psychopathology on the self-report or perception of neuroticism (Farmer, 2000; Vitousek & Stumpf, 2005; Widiger & Samuel, 2005). Researchers will often assess patients' levels of neuroticism while they are (for instance) clinically depressed. However, persons who are very depressed will fail to provide accurate descriptions of their general personality traits (Widiger & Samuel, 2005). Distortion in self-image is a well-established symptom of a mood disorder (American Psychiatric Association, 2000), and it should not be surprising to find that persons who are depressed provide inaccurate descriptions of the levels of depressiveness, self-consciousness, or vulnerability that were present prior to or independent of their current depressed mood. Once the mood disorder is successfully treated, their levels of self-described neuroticism decrease, not because of a change in personality but simply because of a remission of the mood disorder.

Studies have consistently reported decreases in levels of the personality trait of neuroticism during the course of a psychiatric treatment, often for the presence of a mood disorder. Jorm (1989) summarized the results of 63 therapy outcome studies that included measures of trait anxiety or neuroticism. The results indicated significant reduction in neuroticism over the course of treatment (particularly by rational–emotive therapies). It is difficult not to be concerned that this change in self-reported levels of neuroticism was artifactual, reflecting to a significant extent changes in a psychiatric disorder for which the patients were seeking treatment, rather than actual changes in premorbid personality functioning.

Piedmont (2001) reported changes in FFM self-report personality assessments for 132 persons in a 6-week outpatient drug rehabilitation program. Significant changes in levels of neuroticism, agreeableness, and conscientiousness were maintained on follow-up

approximately 15 months after termination of treatment. He concluded that "personality change may be possible in the context of treatment" (p. 500). However, it is perhaps worth noting that the change in neuroticism scores was associated with changes in mental disorder symptomatology, suggesting perhaps that the original assessment of neuroticism might have been an artifact of the psychopathology.

On the other hand, to the extent that neuroticism is a disposition to experience and express negative affects, increases (and decreases) in the expression of these negative affects could be understood as expressions of (and changes to) the personality trait (Clark, Vittengl, Kraft, & Jarrett, 2003). Costa, Bagby, Herbst, and McCrae (2005) in fact argue, "rather than regard these depression-caused changes in assessed personality trait levels as a distortion, we interpret them as accurate reflections of the current condition of the individual" (p. 45). They suggest that the elevated pretreatment neuroticism scores should not be understood simply as the result of a depressed state, because these scores do correlate with other variables unrelated to depression, and they have incremental validity in the prediction of personality-relevant criteria above and beyond the effects of severity of depression. They also indicate that no significant changes occurred in the NEO PI-R profiles over the course of treatment (however, there was substantially more change in the depression and vulnerability facets of neuroticism than in any other NEO PI-R facet scores). In sum, "psychometric analyses demonstrate that the baseline NEO PI-R provides a reliable and valid assessment of personality at the time it was administered" (Costa et al., 2005, p. 52).

It is true that one should not be entirely dismissive of all personality change scores that result from brief pharmacotherapies for a mood disorder. For example, Knutson and colleagues (1998) "examined the effects of a serotonergic reuptake blockade on personality and social behavior in a double-blind protocol by randomly assigning 51 medically and psychiatrically healthy volunteers to treatment with a selective serotonin reuptake inhibitor (SSRI), paroxetine ... (N = 25), or placebo (N = 26)" (p. 374). None of the participants met current or lifetime DSM-IV diagnostic criteria for any mental disorder, as assessed with a semistructured interview. None of them had ever received a psychotropic medication, had ever abused drugs, or had ever been in treatment for a mental disorder, nor were any of them currently seeking or desiring treatment for a mental disorder. In other words, they were in many respects above normal in psychological functioning. One certainly could not attribute any subsequent changes in their personality traits to the effect of treating a co-occurring mood disorder. The paroxetine (and placebo) treatment continued for 4 weeks. Knutson and colleagues reported that the SSRI administration (relative to placebo) reduced significantly scores on a self-report measure of neuroticism. The magnitude of change even correlated with plasma levels of SSRI within the SSRI treatment group. As concluded by Knutson and colleagues, this was a clear "empirical demonstration that chronic administration of a selective serotonin reuptake blockade can have significant personality and behavioral effects in normal humans in the absence of baseline depression or other psychopathology" (p. 378). In sum, normal personality can be altered through pharmacology.

Costa and colleagues (2005) also note that it is generally accepted that Alzheimer's disease, Parkinson's disease, and traumatic brain injury can produce actual changes to personality functioning. The American Psychiatric Association's (2000) diagnostic manual does recognize the concept of personality change due to a general medical condition, including even a labile type that is characterized primarily by affective lability. In fact, the World Health Organization (WHO) recognizes within the *International Classification of Diseases* (ICD-10; WHO, 1992) the concept of personality change secondary to severe mental illness, which would include changes in levels of neuroticism secondary to a mood disorder.

However, to the extent that one considers self-report descriptions of neuroticism secondary to a mood disorder to reflect either fluctuations or actual changes in personality functioning, it becomes difficult to conduct research on the etiological contribution of neuroticism to the mood disorder. They are no longer distinguished constructs. One should at least not attempt to infer premorbid personality traits on the basis of an as-

sessment when the person is suffering from a mood (or other comparable) disorder or condition. Fluctuations in mood secondary to a mood disorder could reflect actual changes in levels of neuroticism, and mood disorders could perhaps be understood as alterations in personality functioning, but if one wishes to understand an etiological contribution of neuroticism to the onset of the mood disorder, the two conditions do need to be distinguished from one another.

Longitudinal studies that begin prior to the onset of the psychopathology are perhaps the most informative approach to controlling for pathoplastic distortions in self-description, and such studies have indeed reported strong support for the increased likelihood of future onsets of major depression in persons with elevated neuroticism, even for persons with no prior history of diagnosed mood disorder (Fanous, Neale, Aggen, & Kendler, 2007; Kendler, Gatz, Gardner, & Pederse, 2006). In cross-sectional studies, semistructured interview assessments of neuroticism may be helpful, particularly to the extent that the interviewers actively attempt to identify the level of neuroticism that predated the onset of a current psychopathology. Self-report inventories do not typically instruct participants to distinguish between their current psychopathology and their premorbid personality functioning, and some may even focus respondents' attention on their current functioning. However, there is currently only one semistructured interview for the assessment of neuroticism (Trull & Widiger, 1997), and semistructured interviews will not necessarily be immune to the pathoplastic effects of mood distortion (Widiger & Samuel, 2005).

Another approach would be to obtain assessments of neuroticism from persons who are closely familiar with the subject of the assessment. These informants (e.g., spouses, friends, or colleagues) will lack the distorting effects of the mood disorder and may even be able to clearly distinguish the target's functioning prior to versus during the onset of the current psychopathology. Agreement between self-descriptions and peer descriptions of personality traits has generally been good to excellent when sampling within nonclinical populations (McCrae, Stone, Fagan, & Costa, 1998), but agreement between self-descriptions and informant descriptions of personality within clinical samples has at times been poor to only adequate (Klonsky, Oltmanns, & Turkheimer, 2002). This disagreement may be due in part to the impact of the psychopathology on the target's self-description, but there is, as yet, inadequate research to fully understand the nature and implications of the disagreement (Ready & Clark, 2005).

Spectrum Relationships

Psychopathology is typically defined as a condition that meets the diagnostic criteria for a mental disorder currently included within DSM-IV (American Psychiatric Association, 2000). Axis I of DSM-IV includes such conditions as major depressive disorder, social phobia, eating disorders, and dysthymia. Axis II includes such conditions as borderline, avoidant, and dependent personality disorders. Neuroticism is not included as a mental disorder within this authoritative classification of psychopathology, and as a domain of personality functioning that is evident within a wide range of the general population, it is not generally considered by most theorists to be a form of psychopathology. In sum, neuroticism is considered to be a personality trait distinct from psychopathology. Hence it is meaningful to study the potential contribution of neuroticism to the etiology, course, and treatment of various forms of psychopathology.

However, an alternative perspective is that neuroticism and various forms of psychopathology may actually represent overlapping expressions of a common, underlying condition. They may exist along a common spectrum of functioning. For instance, rather than contributing to the etiology of depression, neuroticism may itself be a form of depression. Rather than its contributing to the etiology of a personality disorder, the personality disorder may itself be a variant of neuroticism. Each of these two hypotheses will be discussed in turn.

Neuroticism on a Spectrum with Axis I Psychopathology

As noted earlier, neuroticism is associated with a wide variety of Axis I mental disorders (Malouff et al., 2005). There is also considerable comorbidity (diagnostic

co-occurrence) among these Axis I mental disorders (Clark, 2005; Krueger, Markon, Patrick, & Iacono, 2005; Watson, 2005; Widiger & Clark, 2000). There are many instances in which the presence of multiple diagnoses suggests the presence of distinct yet comorbid psychopathologies; however, perhaps in just as many instances, one has instead the presence of a single, common underlying psychopathology and diathesis. "Comorbidity may be trying to show us that many current treatments are not so much treatments for transient 'state' mental disorders of affect and anxiety as they are treatments for core processes, such as negative affectivity, that span normal and abnormal variation as well as undergird multiple mental disorders" (Krueger, 2002, p. 44). Krueger and his colleagues have been particularly productive in replicating within a variety of populations the two dimensions of internalization and externalization identified by Achenbach (1966) many years ago within childhood psychopathology (Krueger & Markon, 2006a, 2006b).

The broad domain of internalization maps well onto the personality temperament of neuroticism (Clark, 2005; Krueger & Markon, 2006b; Watson, Gamez, & Simms, 2005). Kendler, Prescott, Myers, and Neale (2003) applied multivariate genetic analyses to 10 mental disorders assessed in more than 5,600 members of male–male and female–female twin pairs from a population-based registry. They concluded that "the patterns of comorbidity of these disorders (internalizing vs. externalizing, and within internalizing, anxious misery vs. fear) is driven largely by [common] genetic factors" (p. 936). Kahn, Jacobson, Gardner, Prescott, and Kendler (2005) reported large effect sizes for the association of neuroticism with depression, generalized anxiety disorder, and panic disorder in a sample of 7,588 twin pairs and found that neuroticism explained 20–45% of the comorbidity among depression and the anxiety disorders. Hettema, Neale, Myers, Prescott, and Kendler (2006) reported similarly that one-third to two-thirds of the genetic variance in mood (depressive) and anxiety disorders was shared with neuroticism.

To the extent that the relationship of neuroticism to Axis I psychopathology is due to the presence of a common diathesis, it is unclear whether it is meaningful to discuss the contribution of neuroticism to the etiology of these disorders. Smith and MacKenzie (2006) made a similar point in their review of the relationship of neuroticism to development of physical diseases: "Studies of the associations between this personality trait and later disease could involve the effects of undiagnosed mood or anxiety disorders. Similarly, prospective associations between anxiety and mood disorders with health outcomes could involve the effect of this personality trait" (Smith & MacKenzie, 2006, p. 446).

There are even some Axis I mental disorders that would be difficult to distinguish from the personality trait or temperament of neuroticism, such as generalized social phobia and early-onset dysthymia (American Psychiatric Association, 2000). Generalized social phobia is an Axis I mental disorder that is diagnosed when social anxiety goes beyond simply one specific phobic stimulus to include most every social situation. Generalized social phobia is said to have an early onset and chronic course, "emerging out of a childhood history of social inhibition or shyness" (American Psychiatric Association, 2000, p. 453). It would seem difficult to distinguish this Axis I mental disorder from being high in the anxiousness, self-consciousness, and vulnerability facets of NEO PI-R Neuroticism (Widiger, 2001). In sum, neuroticism is not currently conceptualized as a mental disorder, but it may not be long before a temperament of neuroticism is, in fact, explicitly identified as a mental disorder.

Neuroticism on a Spectrum
with Axis II Psychopathology

If neuroticism is conceptualized as a mental disorder, it would seem most natural that it be classified as a personality disorder (the existence of generalized social phobia and early-onset dysthymia notwithstanding). Each of the DSM-IV personality disorders can in fact be readily understood as a maladaptive or extreme variant of the domains and facets of the FFM (Widiger & Trull, 2007).

O'Connor and Dyce (1998) explored whether the covariation among the personality disorders reported in nine previously published studies could be explained ad-

equately by a dimensional model of general personality functioning. They conducted independent principal-axes confirmatory factor analyses of seven alternative dimensional models on 12 correlation matrices provided by the nine studies and obtained highly significant congruence coefficients for all 12 correlation matrices for two of the seven models. "The highest and most consistent levels of fit were obtained for the five-factor model and for Cloninger's [2000] seven-factor model" (O'Connor & Dyce, 1998, p. 14).

O'Connor (2005) conducted a joint factor analysis of 33 previously published personality disorder studies to yield a consensus comorbidity structure. He then conducted a comparable interbattery factor analysis to yield a consensus model for the relationship of the FFM to the personality disorders, using results reported in 20 previously published studies. He then determined empirically whether the congruence between the consensus personality disorder and consensus FFM–personality disorder structure was consistent with the theoretically based descriptions of these personality disorders provided by Widiger and colleagues (2002). He concluded that "the obtained congruences for their model are ... quite impressive, especially considering that no other ... personality disorder configuration model receives comparable degrees of support. ... The interbattery factor analytic technique used in the present study provided a more stringent test of the empirically based representation of the FFM, yet stronger support for the FFM nevertheless emerged" (O'Connor, 2005, p. 340).

Quite a few FFM studies have also been conducted on individual personality disorders (Mullins-Sweatt & Widiger, 2006; Widiger & Costa, 2002). Saulsman and Page (2004) conducted a meta-analysis of FFM personality disorder studies and concluded that "the results showed that each [personality] disorder displays a five-factor model profile that is meaningful and predictable given its unique diagnostic criteria" (p. 1055). As expressed by Clark (2007), "the five-factor model of personality is widely accepted as representing the higher-order structure of both normal and abnormal personality traits" (p. 246). Neuroticism has been the domain of the FFM consistently shown to have the strongest relationship with DSM-IV personality disorders (Saulsman & Page, 2004), particularly borderline (Widiger, 2005).

To the extent that respective DSM-IV personality disorders are extreme or maladaptive variants of the personality trait of neuroticism, it may not be particularly meaningful to study the contribution of neuroticism to the etiology of these personality disorders. How would one understand, for instance, a correlation of the HEXACO-PI (Lee & Ashton, 2006) assessment of emotionality with DSM-IV dependent personality disorder when one of the HEXACO-PI facets of emotionality is explicitly concerned with the assessment of dependency? From the perspective of Lee and Ashton (2006), dependency is not a behavior that results from neuroticism (or emotionality); it is a direct phenotypic expression or manifestation of the personality trait of neuroticism. Some of the symptomatology of a DSM-IV personality disorder can be understood as a phenotypic expression of an interaction between a temperament of negative affectivity and aversive life events (Morey & Zanarini, 2000; Widiger, 2005), but any particular assessment of neuroticism will include the assessment of this phenotypic expression, as well as the underlying temperament. In sum, neuroticism, as assessed by any existing measure of the FFM, is providing an explicit and direct assessment of the respective personality disorder.

Conclusions

It is difficult to imagine there being a personality trait on which there has been a greater amount of published research. The sheer number of meta-analyses that have been conducted on the relationship of neuroticism to other variables is itself a concrete testament as to the importance of this personality trait, or this domain of personality functioning, within existing research. Cited within this chapter alone were neuroticism meta-analyses conducted by Bornstein and Cecero (2000), Cassin and von Ranson (2005), Connor-Smith and Flachsbart (2007), DeNeve and Cooper (1998), Hoyle and colleagues (2000), Huo-Liang (2006), Jorm (1989), Judge, Bono, and colleagues (2002), Judge, Heller, and colleagues

(2002), Judge and Ilies (2002), Malouff and colleagues (2006, 2007), Markon and colleagues (2005), Munafo and colleagues (2003, 2005b, 2007), O'Connor (2005), O'Connor and Dyce (1998), Saroglou (2002), Saulsman and Page (2004), Schinka and colleagues (2004), Sen and colleagues (2004), Steel and colleagues (2008), and Trapmann and colleagues (2007); there are, of course, many additional meta-analyses beyond the focus of this chapter.

Nevertheless, it is also evident that there is not, in fact, a complete consensus as to the optimal conceptualization and assessment of neuroticism. The alternative formulations of this domain of personality functioning do appear to involve meaningful differences in conceptualization, and the respective assessment instruments do yield fundamentally different results. Further attention does appear to be needed in reaching a consensus as to the optimal facet structure of neuroticism, or at least this variation in facet structure does need to be appreciated in future neuroticism studies.

The most vibrant area of research is the contribution of neuroticism to the etiology of negative life outcomes. It is suggested herein, though, that this research will need to further consider and distinguish the alternative relationships between neuroticism and these negative life outcomes (i.e., pathoplastic, spectrum, and causal). Cross-sectional studies can and do provide quite informative results, but it is evident that the most telling findings will be obtained from longitudinal studies. Neuroticism and psychopathology, for instance, affect and alter one another over time in a complex, unfolding interaction. Many vulnerability studies have used samples of convenience (e.g., persons already in treatment for a respective disorder) in which the differentiation among pathoplastic, spectrum, and causal relationships can at times be impossible to disentangle. Any particular cross-sectional period of time may represent only an arbitrary and unrepresentative slice along a continuously interacting and mutually reaffirming sequence of events. In sum, neuroticism continues to provide a compelling understanding of the etiology of negative life events, but this relationship is complex, and it is through the dismantling of pathoplastic, spectrum, and etiological relationships that continued progress will be made.

Acknowledgment

I express my appreciation to Dr. Gregory Smith for his comments on an earlier version of this chapter.

References

Achenbach, T. M. (1966). The classification of children's psychiatric symptoms: A factor analytic study. *Psychological Monographs, 80*(615).

Aluja, A., Garcia, O., & Garcie, L. F. (2004). Replicability of the three, four, and five Zuckerman's personality super-factors: Exploratory and confirmatory factor analysis of the EQP-RS, ZKPQ, and NEO PI-R. *Personality and Individual Differences, 36*(5), 1093–1108.

American Psychiatric Association. (1952). *Diagnostic and statistical manual: Mental disorders*. Washington, DC: Author.

American Psychiatric Association. (2000). *Diagnostic and statistical manual of mental disorders* (4th ed., text rev.). Washington, DC: Author.

Ashton, M. C., & Lee, K. (2001). A theoretical basis for the major dimensions of personality. *European Journal of Personality, 15*, 327–353.

Ashton, M. C., & Lee, K. (2005). Honesty–humility, the Big Five, and the five-factor model. *Journal of Personality, 73*, 1321–1353.

Beitchman, J. H., Baldassarra L., Mik, H., De Luca, V., King, N., Bender, D., et al. (2006). Serotonin transporter polymorphisms and persistent, pervasive childhood aggression. *American Journal of Psychiatry, 163*, 1103–1105.

Bornstein, R. F., & Cecero, J. J. (2000). Deconstructing dependency in a five-factor world: A meta-analytic review. *Journal of Personality Assessment, 74*, 324–343.

Buss, D. (1996). Social adaptation and five major factors of personality. In J. S. Wiggins (Ed.), *The five-factor model of personality: Theoretical perspectives* (pp. 180–207). New York: Guilford Press.

Caspi, A., Roberts, B. W., & Shiner, R. L. (2005). Personality development: Stability and change. *Annual Review of Psychology, 56*, 453–484.

Cassin, S. E., & von Ranson, K. M. (2005). Personality and eating disorders: A decade in review. *Clinical Psychology Review, 25*, 895–916.

Chapman, B. P., Duberstein, P. R., Sorensen, S., Lyness, J. M., & Emery, L. (2006). Personality and perceived health in older adults: The five-factor model in primary care. *Journals of Gerontology: Series B. Psychological Sciences and Social Sciences, 61*, P362–P365.

Clark, L. A. (2005). Temperament as a unifying basis for personality and psychopathology. *Journal of Abnormal Psychology, 114*, 505–521.

Clark, L. A. (2007). Assessment and diagnosis of personality disorder: Perennial issues and an emerging reconceptualization. *Annual Review of Psychology, 58*, 227–257.

Clark, L. A., Vittengl, J., Kraft, D., & Jarrett, R. B. (2003). Separate personality traits from states to predict depression. *Journal of Personality Disorders, 17*, 152–172.

Clark, L. A., & Watson, D. (1999). Temperament: A new paradigm for trait psychology. In L. A. Pervin & O. P. John (Eds.), *Handbook of personality: Theory and research* (2nd ed., pp. 399–423). New York: Guilford Press.

Cloninger, C. R. (2000). A practical way to diagnose personality disorder: A proposal. *Journal of Personality Disorders, 14*, 98–108.

Cohen, J. (1992). A power primer. *Psychological Bulletin, 112*, 155–159.

Connor-Smith, J. K., & Flachsbart, C. (2007). Relations between personality and coping. *Journal of Personality and Social Psychology, 93*, 1080–1107.

Costa, P. T., Bagby, R. M., Herbst, J. F., & McCrae, R. R. (2005). Personality self-reports are concurrently reliable and valid during acute depressive episodes. *Journal of Affective Disorders, 89*, 45–55.

Costa, P. T., Jr., & McCrae, R. R. (1985). *The NEO Personality Inventory manual*. Odessa, FL: Psychological Assessment Resources.

Costa, P. T., Jr., & McCrae, R. R. (1992). *The NEO PI-R professional manual*. Odessa, FL: Psychological Assessment Resources.

DeNeve, K., & Cooper, H. (1998). The happy personality: A meta-analysis of 137 personality traits and subjective well-being. *Psychological Bulletin, 124*, 197–229.

Depue, R. A., & Collins, P. F. (1999). Neurobiology of the structure of personality: Dopamine facilitation of incentive motivation and extraversion. *Behavioral and Brain Sciences, 22*, 491–569.

DeYoung, C. G., Quilty, L. C., & Peterson, J. B. (2007). Between facets and domains: 10 aspects of the Big Five. *Journal of Personality and Social Psychology, 93*, 880–896.

Digman, J. M. (1990). Personality structure: Emergence of the five-factor model. *Annual Review of Psychology, 41*, 417–470.

Duberstein, P. R., & Heisel, M. J. (2007). Personality traits and the reporting of affective disorder symptoms in depressed patients. *Journal of Affective Disorders, 103*, 165–171.

Ekman, P. (1999). Basic emotions. In T. Dalgleish & M. Power (Eds.), *Handbook of cognition and emotion* (pp. 45–60). New York: Wiley.

Eysenck, H. J. (1967). *The biological bases of personality*. Baltimore: University Park Press.

Eysenck, H. J., Barrett, P. T., Wilson, G., & Jackson, C. (1992). Primary trait measurement of the 21 components of the P-E-N system. *European Journal of Psychological Assessment, 8*, 109–117.

Fanous, A. H., Neale, M. C., Aggen, S. H., & Kendler, K. S. (2007). A longitudinal study of personality and major depression in a population-based sample of male twins. *Psychological Medicine, 37*, 1163–1172.

Farmer, R. F. (2000). Issues in the assessment and conceptualization of personality disorders. *Clinical Psychology Review, 20*, 823–851.

Flint, J., & Munafo, M. R. (2007). The endophenotype concept in psychiatric genetics. *Psychological Medicine, 37*, 163–180.

Goldberg, L. R. (1993). The structure of phenotypic personality traits. *American Psychologist, 48*, 26–34.

Goldberg, L. R. (1999). A broad-bandwidth, public domain, personality inventory measuring the lower-level facets of several five-factor models. In I. Mervielde, I. Deary, F. DeFruyt, & F. Ostendorf

(Eds.), *Personality psychology in Europe* (Vol. 7, pp. 7–28). Tilburg, The Netherlands: Tilburg University Press.

Guilford, J. P. (1975). Factors and factors of personality. *Psychological Bulletin, 82*, 802–814.

Hettema, J. M., Neale, M. C., Myers, J. M., Prescott, C. A., & Kendler, K. S. (2006). A population-based twin study of the relationship between neuroticism and internalizing disorders. *American Journal of Psychiatry, 163*, 857–864.

Hoyle, R. H., Fejfar, M. C., & Miller, J. D. (2000). Personality and sexual risk-taking: A quantitative review. *Journal of Personality, 68*, 1203–1231.

Hu, X. Z., Rush, A. J., Charney, D., Wilson, A. F., Sorant, A. J. M., Papanicolaou, G. J., et al. (2007). Association between a functional serotonin transporter promoter polymorphism and citalopram treatment in adult outpatients with major depression. *Archives of General Psychiatry, 64*, 783–792.

Huo-Liang, G. (2006). Personality and crime: A meta-analysis of studies on criminals' personality. *Chinese Mental Health Journal, 20*, 465–468.

Jacobs, N., Kenis, G., Peeters, F., Derom, C., Vlietinck, R., & Van Os, J. (2006). Stress-related negative affectivity and genetically altered serotonin transporter function: Evidence of synergism in shaping risk for depression. *Archives of General Psychiatry, 63*, 989–996.

Jang, K. L., Livesley, W. J., Angleitner, A., Reimann, R., & Vernon, P. A. (2002). Genetic and environmental influences on the covariance of facets defining the domains of the five-factor model of personality. *Personality and Individual Differences, 33*, 83–101.

Jorm, A. F. (1989). Modifiability of trait anxiety and neuroticism: A meta-analysis of the literature. *Australian and New Zealand Journal of Psychiatry, 23*, 21–29.

Judge, T. A., Bono, J. E., Ilies, R., & Gerhardt, M. W. (2002). Personality and leadership: A qualitative and quantitative review. *Journal of Applied Psychology, 87*, 765–780.

Judge, T. A., Heller, D., & Mount, M. K. (2002). Five-factor model of personality and job satisfaction: A meta-analysis. *Journal of Applied Psychology, 87*, 530–541.

Judge, T. A., & Ilies, R. (2002). Relationship of personality to performance motivation: A meta-analytic review. *Journal of Applied Psychology, 87*, 797–807.

Kahn, A. A., Jacobson, K. C., Gardner, C. O., Prescott, C. A., & Kendler, K. S. (2005). Personality and comorbidity of common psychiatric disorders. *British Journal of Psychiatry, 186*, 190–196.

Kendler, K. S., Gardner, C. O., & Prescott, C. A. (2006). Toward a comprehensive developmental model for major depression in men. *American Journal of Psychiatry, 163*, 115–124.

Kendler, K. S., Gatz, M., Gardner, C. O., & Pederse, N. L. (2006). Personality and major depression. *Archives of General Psychiatry, 63*, 1113–1120.

Kendler, K. S., Prescott, C. A., Myers, J., & Neale, M. C. (2003). The structure of genetic and environmental risk factors for common psychiatric and substance use disorders in men and women. *Archives of General Psychiatry, 60*, 929–937.

Klonsky, E. D., Oltmanns, T. F., & Turkheimer, E. (2002). Informant reports of personality disorder: Relation to self-reports and future research directions. *Clinical Psychology: Science and Practice, 9*, 399–311.

Knutson, B., Wolkowitz, O. M., Cole, S. W., Chan, T., Moore, E. A, Johnson, R. C., et al. (1998). Selective alteration of personality and social behavior by serotonergic intervention. *American Journal of Psychiatry, 155*, 373–379.

Krueger, R. F. (2002). Psychometric perspectives on comorbidity. In J. E. Helzer & J. J. Hudziak (Eds.), *Defining psychopathology in the 21st century: DSM-V and beyond* (pp. 41–54). Washington, DC: American Psychiatric.

Krueger, R. F., & Markon, K. E. (2006a). Reinterpreting comorbidity: A model-based approach to understanding and classifying psychopathology. *Annual Review of Clinical Psychology, 2*, 111–134.

Krueger, R. F., & Markon, K. E. (2006b). Understanding psychopathology: Melding genetics, personality, and quantitative psychology to develop an empirically based model. *Current Directions in Psychological Science, 15*, 113–117.

Krueger, R. F., Markon, K. E., Patrick, C. J., & Iacono, W. G. (2005). Externalizing psychopathology in adulthood: A dimensional-spectrum conceptualization and its implications for DSM-V. *Journal of Abnormal Psychology, 114*, 537–550.

Lee, K., & Ashton, M. C. (2004). Psychometric properties of the HEXACO Personality Inventory. *Multivariate Behavioral Research, 39*, 329–358.

Lee, K., & Ashton, M. C. (2006). Further assessment of the HEXACO Personality Inventory: Two new facet scales and observer report form. *Psychological Assessment, 18*, 182–191.

Lynam, D. R., & Miller, J. D. (2004). Personality pathways to impulsive behavior and their relations to deviance: Results from three samples. *Journal of Quantitative Criminology, 20*, 319–341.

Malouff, J. M., Thorsteinsson, E. B., Rooke, S. E., & Schutte, N. S. (2007). Alcohol involvement and the five-factor model of personality: A meta-analysis. *Journal of Drug Education, 37*, 277–294.

Malouff, J. M. Thorsteinsson, E. B., & Schutte, N. S. (2005). The relationship between the five-factor model of personality and symptoms of clinical disorders: A meta-analysis. *Journal of Psychopathology and Behavioral Assessment, 27*, 101–114.

Malouff, J. M., Thorsteinsson, E. B., & Schutte, N. S. (2006). The five-factor model of personality and smoking: A meta-analysis. *Journal of Drug Education, 36*, 47–58.

Markon, K. E., Krueger, R. F., & Watson, D. (2005). Delineating the structure of normal and abnormal personality: An integrative hierarchical approach. *Journal of Personality and Social Psychology, 88*, 139–157.

McCrae, R. R., & Costa, P. T. (2003). *Personality in adulthood: A five-factor theory perspective* (2nd ed.). New York: Guilford Press.

McCrae, R. R., Stone, S. V., Fagan, P. J., & Costa, P. T. (1998). Identifying causes of disagreement between self-reports and spouse ratings of personality. *Journal of Personality, 66*, 285–313.

Miles, J., & Hempel, S. (2004). The Eysenck personality scales: The Eysenck Personality Questionnaire—

Revised (EPQ-R) and the Eysenck Personality Profiler (EPP). In M. J. Hilsenroth, D. L. Segal, & M. Hersen (Eds.), *Comprehensive handbook of psychological assessment* (Vol. 2, 99–107). New York: Wiley.

Miller, J. D., & Pilkonis, P. A. (2006). Neuroticism and affective instability: The same or different? *American Journal of Psychiatry, 163,* 839–845.

Morey, L. C., & Zanarini, M. C. (2000). Borderline personality: Traits and disorder. *Journal of Abnormal Psychology, 109,* 733–737.

Mullins-Sweatt, S. N., & Widiger, T. A. (2006). The five-factor model of personality disorder: A translation across science and practice. In R. F. Krueger & J. L. Tackett (Eds.), *Personality and psychopathology* (pp. 39–70). New York: Guilford Press.

Mullins-Sweatt, S. N., & Widiger, T. A. (2007). The Shedler–Westen Assessment Procedure from the perspective of general personality structure. *Journal of Abnormal Psychology, 116,* 618–623.

Munafo, M. R., Clark, T., & Flint, J. (2005a). Does measurement instrument moderate the association between the serotonin transporter gene and anxiety-related personality traits?: A meta-analysis. *Molecular Psychiatry, 10,* 415–419.

Munafo, M. R., Clark, T., & Flint, J. (2005b). Promise and pitfalls in the meta-analysis of genetic association studies: A response to Sen and Schinka. *Molecular Psychiatry, 10,* 895–897.

Munafo, M. R., Clark, T. G., Moore, L. R., Payne, E., Walton, R., & Flint, J. (2003). Genetic polymorphisms and personality in healthy adults: A systematic review and meta-analysis. *Molecular Psychiatry, 8,* 471–484.

Munafo, M. R., Clark, T. G., Roberts, K. H., & Johnstone, E. C. (2006). Neuroticism mediates the association of the serotonin transporter gene with lifetime major depression. *Neuropsychobiology, 53,* 1–8.

Munafo, M. R., Zetteler, J. I., & Clark, T. G. (2007). Personality and smoking status: A meta-analysis. *Nicotine and Tobacco Research, 9,* 405–413.

O'Connor, B. P. (2005). A search for consensus on the dimensional structure of personality disorders. *Journal of Clinical Psychology, 61,* 323–345.

O'Connor, B. P., & Dyce, J. A. (1998). A test of models of personality disorder configuration. *Journal of Abnormal Psychology, 107,* 3–16.

Ozer, D. J., & Benet-Martínez, V. (2006). Personality and the prediction of consequential outcomes. *Annual Review of Psychology, 57,* 401–421.

Parslow, R. A., Jorm, A. F., & Christensen, H. (2006). Associations of pre-trauma attributes and trauma exposure with screening positive for PTSD: Analysis of a community-based study of 2085 young adults. *Psychological Medicine, 36,* 387–395.

Penke, L., Denissen, J. J. A., & Miller, G. F. (2007). The evolutionary genetics of personality. *European Journal of Personality, 21,* 549–587.

Piedmont, R. L. (2001). Cracking the plaster cast: Big Five personality change during intensive outpatient counseling. *Journal of Research in Personality, 35,* 500–520.

Pincus, A. L. (2002). Constellations of dependency within the five-factor model of personality. In P. T. Costa & T. A. Widiger (Eds.), *Personality disorders and the five-factor model of personality* (pp. 203–

214). Washington, DC: American Psychological Association.

Ready, R. E., & Clark, L. A. (2005). Psychiatric patient and informant reports of patient behavior. *Journal of Personality, 73,* 1–21.

Russell, J. A. (2003). Core affect and the psychological construction of emotion. *Psychological Review, 110,* 145–172.

Saroglou, V. (2002). Religion and the five factors of personality: A meta-analytic review. *Personality and Individual Differences, 32,* 15–25.

Saucier, G., & Goldberg, L. R. (2001). Lexical studies of indigenous personality factors: Premises, products, and prospects. *Journal of Personality, 69,* 847–880.

Saulsman, L. M., & Page, A. C. (2004). The five-factor model and personality disorder empirical literature: A meta-analytic review. *Clinical Psychology Review, 23,* 1055–1085.

Schinka, J. A. (2005). Measurement scale does moderate the association between the serotonin transporter gene and trait anxiety: Comments on Munafo et al. *Molecular Psychiatry, 10,* 892–893.

Schinka, J. A., Busch, R. M., & Robichaux-Keene, N. (2004). A meta-analysis of the association between the serotonin transporter gene polymorphism (5-HTTLPR) and trait anxiety. *Molecular Psychiatry, 9,* 197–202.

Schmitz, A., Hennig, J., Kuepper, Y., & Reuter, M. (2007). The association between neuroticism and the serotonin transporter polymorphism depends on structural differences between personality measures. *Personality and Individual Differences, 42,* 789–799.

Sen, S., Burmeister, M., & Ghosh, D. (2004). Meta-analysis of the association between a serotonin transporter polymorphism (5-HTTLPR) and anxiety-related personality traits. *American Journal of Medical Genetics Part B: Neuropsychiatric Genetics, 127B,* 85–89.

Sen, S., Burmeister, M., & Ghosh, D. (2005). 5-HTTLPR and anxiety-related personality traits meta-analysis revisited: Response to Munafo and colleagues. *Molecular Psychiatry, 10,* 893–895.

Shedler, J., & Westen, D. (2004). Dimensions of personality pathology: An alternative to the five-factor model. *American Journal of Psychiatry, 161,* 1743–1754.

Smith, T. W., & MacKenzie, J. (2006). Personality and risk of physical illness. *Annual Review of Clinical Psychology, 2,* 435–467.

Steel, P., Schmidt, J., & Schultz, J. (2008). Refining the relationship between personality and subjective well-being. *Psychological Bulletin, 134,* 138–161.

Suls, J., & Bunde, J. (2005). Anger, anxiety, and depression as risk factors for cardiovascular disease: The problems and implications of overlapping affective dispositions. *Psychological Bulletin, 131,* 260–300.

Tellegen, A. (1982). *Brief manual for the Multidimensional Personality Questionnaire.* Unpublished manuscript, University of Minnesota, Minneapolis.

Tellegen, A., & Waller, N. G. (1987). *Exploring personality through test construction: Development of the Multidimensional Personality Questionnaire.* Unpublished manuscript.

ten Have, M., Oldehinkel, A., Vollebergh, W., &

Ormel, J. (2005). Does neuroticism explain variations in care service use for mental health problems in the general population?: Results from The Netherlands Mental Health Survey and Incidence Study (NEMESIS). *Social Psychiatry and Psychiatric Epidemiology, 40,* 425–431.

Trapmann, S., Hell, B., Hirn, J. O. W., & Schuler, H. (2007). Meta-analysis of the relationship between the Big Five and academic success at university. *Journal of Psychology, 215,* 132–151.

Trull, T. J., & Widiger, T. A. (1997). *Structured interview for the five-factor model of personality.* Odessa, FL: Psychological Assessment Resources.

Turkheimer, E. (2000). Three laws of behavior genetics and what they mean. *Current Directions in Psychological Science, 14,* 410–411.

Van Os, J., & Jones, P. B. (2001). Neuroticism as a risk factor for schizophrenia. *Psychological Medicine, 31,* 1129–1134.

Vitousek, K. M., & Stumpf, R. E. (2005). Difficulties in the assessment of personality traits and disorders in eating-disordered individuals. *Eating Disorders, 13,* 37–60.

Watson, D. (2005). Rethinking the mood and anxiety disorders: A quantitative hierarchical model for DSM-V. *Journal of Abnormal Psychology, 114,* 522–536.

Watson, D., & Clark, L. A. (1994). *Manual for the Positive and Negative Affect Schedule—Expanded Form.* Iowa City: University of Iowa.

Watson, D., & Clark, L. A. (1997). Extraversion and its positive emotional core. In R. Hogan, J. Johnson, & S. Briggs (Eds.), *Handbook of personality psychology* (pp. 767–793). San Diego, CA: Academic Press.

Watson, D., Clark, L. A., & Harkness, A. R. (1994). Structures of personality and their relevance to psychopathology. *Journal of Abnormal Psychology, 103,* 18–31.

Watson, D., Clark, L. A., & Tellegen, A. (1988). Development and validation of brief measures of positive and negative affect: The PANAS scales. *Journal of Personality and Social Psychology, 54,* 1063–1070.

Watson, D., Gamez, W., & Simms, L. J. (2005). Basic dimensions of temperament and their relation to anxiety and depression: A symptom-based perspective. *Journal of Research in Personality, 39,* 46–66.

Watson, D., & Tellegen, A. (1985). Toward a consensual structure of mood. *Psychological Bulletin, 98,* 219–235.

Westen, D., & Shedler, J. (2007). Personality diagnosis with the Shedler–Westen Assessment Procedure (SWAP): Integrating clinical and statistical measurement and prediction. *Journal of Abnormal Psychology, 116,* 810–822.

Whiteside, S. P., & Lynam, D. R. (2001). The five-factor model and impulsivity: Using a structural model of personality to understand impulsivity. *Personality and Individual Differences, 30,* 669–689.

Whiteside, S. P., Lynam, D. R., Miller, J. D., & Reynolds, S. K. (2005). Validation of the UPPS Impulsive Behaviour scale: A four-factor model of impulsivity. *European Journal of Personality, 19,* 559–574.

Widiger, T. A. (2001). Social anxiety, social phobia, and avoidant personality disorder. In W. R. Corzier & L. Alden (Eds.), *International handbook of social anxiety* (pp. 335–356). New York: Wiley.

Widiger, T. A. (2005). A temperament model of borderline personality disorder. In M. Zanarini (Ed.), *Borderline personality disorder* (pp. 63–81). Washington, DC: American Psychiatric Press.

Widiger, T. A., & Clark, L. A. (2000). Toward DSM-V and the classification of psychopathology. *Psychological Bulletin, 126,* 946–963.

Widiger, T. A., & Costa, P. T., Jr. (2002). Five-factor model personality disorder research. In P. T. Costa, Jr. & T. A. Widiger (Eds.), *Personality disorders and the five-factor model of personality* (2nd ed., pp. 59–87). Washington, DC: American Psychological Association.

Widiger, T. A., & Samuel, D. B. (2005). Evidence-based assessment of personality disorders. *Psychological Assessment, 17,* 278–287.

Widiger, T. A., & Simonsen, E. (2005). Alternative dimensional models of personality disorder: Finding a common ground. *Journal of Personality Disorders, 19,* 110–130.

Widiger, T. A., & Smith, G. T. (2008). Personality and psychopathology. In O. P. John, R. W. Robins, & L. A. Pervin (Eds.), *Handbook of personality: Theory and research* (3rd ed., pp. 743–769). New York: Guilford Press.

Widiger, T. A., & Trull, T. J. (2007). Plate tectonics in the classification of personality disorder: Shifting to a dimensional model. *American Psychologist, 62,* 71–83.

Widiger, T. A., Trull, T. J., Clarkin, J. F., Sanderson, C., & Costa, P. T. (2002). A description of the DSM-IV personality disorders with the five-factor model of personality. In P. T. Costa & T. A. Widiger (Eds.), *Personality disorders and the five-factor model of personality* (2nd ed., pp. 89–99). Washington, DC: American Psychological Association.

World Health Organization. (1992). *The ICD-10 classification of mental and behavioural disorders: Clinical descriptions and diagnostic guidelines.* Geneva, Switzerland: Author.

Yamagata, S., Suzuki, A., Ando, J., One, Y., Kijima, N., Yoshimura, K., et al. (2006). Is the genetic structure of human personality universal?: A cross-cultural twin study from North America, Europe, and Asia. *Journal of Personality and Social Psychology, 90,* 987–998.

Zuckerman, M. (2002). Zuckerman–Kuhlman Personality Questionnaire (ZKPQ): An alternative five-factorial model. In B. de Raad & M. Perugini (Eds.), *Big Five assessment* (pp. 377–396). Seattle, WA: Hogrefe & Huber.

Zuckerman, M. (2003). Biological bases of personality. In T. Millon, M. J. Lerner, & I. B. Weiner (Eds.), *Handbook of psychology: Vol. 5. Personality and social psychology* (pp. 85–116). New York: Wiley.

CHAPTER 10

■ ● ▲ ◆ ■ ● ▲ ◆

Happiness

ED DIENER
PELIN KESEBIR
WILLIAM TOV

Throughout the ages, many thinkers have regarded happiness as something of supreme value and observed that the pursuit of happiness underlies all sorts of other pursuits. French philosopher Blaise Pascal, for one, believed that happiness is "the motive of every act of every man, including those who go and hang themselves" (1995, p. 45). Darrin McMahon (2005), a historian of happiness, similarly concluded that countless experiments in human engineering with dreadful consequences, from Marxism to Nazism, were all part of a struggle for happiness. The inexhaustible self-help aisles of bookstores and the multibillion dollar industry revolving around psychotropic drugs are no doubt modern manifestations of the same ardent quest.

In this chapter, we aim to shed some light on the all-important question of what makes people happy, relying on the most recent research on the topic. We wish to focus not only on the question of what causes individuals to differ in their happiness levels but also on what these differences are able to predict regarding success in various life domains, such as professional achievement, health, and social relationships. However, before delving into the questions of what leads to happiness and what happiness leads to in turn, we first provide an overview of

how the notion of happiness is conceptualized and measured in current social scientific research.

Conceptualizing and Measuring Happiness

As difficult as it would be to find two lay people who agree completely on the definition of happiness, operational definitions are of crucial necessity for science to progress. Social scientists have fortunately come to a consensus regarding the conceptualization of happiness over the years. This conceptualization emphasizes the subjective nature of happiness, holding people to be the final judges of their experience of happiness (Myers & Diener, 1995).

Subjective well-being is the term employed by many happiness scholars to capture this essentially subjective quality, and it is used in this chapter interchangeably with happiness. Subjective well-being refers to people's appraisals of their lives and entails both cognitive judgments of satisfaction and affective evaluations of moods and emotions (Diener, 1984). In the past few decades, researchers have been able to identify the interconnected yet separable components of subjective well-being, which include life satisfaction

147

(global judgments of one's life), satisfaction with important life domains (e.g., marriage or work satisfaction), positive affect (prevalence of positive emotions and moods), and low levels of negative affect (prevalence of unpleasant emotions and moods). In many studies, these dimensions of subjective well-being are studied separately, and the different patterns of the predictors with various forms of subjective well-being are examined.

Prominent conceptualizations of happiness other than subjective well-being include Ryff and Singer's (1996) "psychological well-being" and Ryan and Deci's (2000) "self-determination theory." These theories exemplify a less subjective and more prescriptive approach toward happiness in that they stipulate the fulfillment of certain needs (such as autonomy, self-acceptance, or purpose in life) as a prerequisite for well-being. Whereas these theories embody valuable contributions to the definition of the good life, researchers working in the subjective well-being tradition focus their efforts on understanding people's own evaluations of their lives, believing in the meaningfulness and scientific credibility of these evaluations. It is important to emphasize at this point that individuals' appraisals of their own well-being hardly reflect empty-headed cheerfulness or raw hedonism. To the contrary, major constituents of subjective well-being, such as life satisfaction and positive affect, seem to emanate first and foremost from one's goals and values. People are most likely to experience high levels of subjective well-being when they strive for and make progress toward personal goals derived from their hallowed values, rendering feelings of meaning, purpose, and fulfillment prominent predictors of subjective well-being (Diener & Larsen, 1993).

Subjective well-being is typically assessed through self-report measures, such as the Satisfaction with Life Scale (SWLS; Pavot & Diener, 1993), the Positive and Negative Affect Schedule (PANAS; Watson, Clark, & Tellegen, 1988), or the Subjective Happiness Scale (Lyubomirsky & Lepper, 1999). The SWLS, for instance, is a five-item instrument that measures global cognitive judgments of one's life. The scale includes items such as "in most ways my life is close to my ideal" and "so far I have gotten the important things I want in life." Individuals express the degree to which they agree with these statements using a 7-point Likert scale. PANAS, unlike the SWLS, is interested in capturing directly the positive and negative affectivity components of subjective well-being. Respondents are given a list of emotion words that sample positive (e.g., *interested, excited, proud*) as well as negative (e.g., *distressed, guilty, scared*) affects and are asked to evaluate on a scale from 1–5 the extent to which they experience these emotions in general. The directions of PANAS can be rephrased to get at how the respondents have felt during the previous week, for example, or how they are feeling at the moment. The Subjective Happiness Scale, on the other hand, is an instrument measuring individuals' perceptions of how happy they are. Individuals indicate on a Likert scale from 1 to 7 how happy they consider themselves, and respond to items such as "Some people are generally not very happy. Although they are not depressed, they never seem as happy as they might be. To what extent does this characterization describe you?"

Although indispensable to the appraisal of something as private and personal as subjective well-being, self-reports of happiness suffer from the same weaknesses associated with other self-report measures; most notably, an oversensitivity to mood and context effects (Schwarz & Strack, 1999). Nevertheless, a great number of studies attest to the adequate validity of self-report subjective well-being measures by showing that they converge with friend and spousal reports of the individual's well-being (Lyubomirsky & Lepper, 1999), with recall of satisfying as opposed to unsatisfying times in one's life (Pavot, Diener, Colvin, & Sandvik, 1991), with smiling behavior (Harker & Keltner, 2001), and with greater relative left frontal activation in the brain (Tomarken, Davidson, & Henriques, 1990). Similarly, temporal stabilities for self-reports of well-being have been found to be in the range of 0.5–0.7 over a period of several years (Diener & Suh, 1997). Although multimethod measurements of subjective well-being should be undertaken whenever feasible, accumulated evidence suggests that self-report measures of well-being possess satisfactory validity and reliability to be employed in happiness research.

The Antecedents of Happiness

In this part of the chapter, we attempt to offer answers to the ever-fascinating question of how to be happy, drawing on the extant literature on happiness. A general model specifying the major sources of variation in happiness can be useful at the outset. Lyubomirsky, Sheldon, and Schkade (2005) have proposed that a person's chronic happiness level is determined by three major factors: a genetically determined set point for happiness, circumstantial factors (e.g., gender, education, culture), and the activities and practices that the person engages in. This model is remarkably similar to Seligman's happiness formula, according to which one's enduring level of happiness is the sum of (1) one's set range for happiness, (2) life circumstances, and (3) factors under one's voluntary control (Seligman, 2002). A survey of the literature suggests that whereas the genetically determined set point accounts for about 50% of variation in happiness, life circumstances account for only 10%, and intentional activities are responsible for the remaining 40% (Lyubomirsky et al., 2005). In our review of the causes and correlates of happiness, we start with the genetic determinants of happiness and move on to circumstantial and demographic factors (e.g., age, gender, intelligence, religion), finally turning to the antecedents of happiness that are relatively more amenable to individual control (e.g., social relationships, goals, leisure). Without a doubt, these three sources of happiness are not fully independent from each other, yet, in our view, they provide a fairly accurate and useful schema for understanding the antecedents of happiness.

Genes and Happiness Set Point

There is virtually no dispute among scholars that genetic inheritance plays a significant role in determining one's chronic happiness level. Studies demonstrating that identical twins are considerably more similar to each other in their happiness levels than fraternal twins (Lykken & Tellegen, 1996; Tel- legen et al., 1988) testify to the genetically determined part of subjective well-being, as do findings regarding the relative stability of happiness over the years (Costa & Mc- Crae, 1988; Magnus & Diener, 1991). It is widely believed that these genetically determined and relatively immutable differences in responding to people and events set a fixed point for individuals, around which their happiness level fluctuates. According to these set-point theories, major life events such as the birth of a child or the death of a partner have only a temporary effect on the person's happiness level, after which it reverts to the default level determined by genetic traits.

Closely affiliated with set-point theories is the "hedonic treadmill theory," which suggests that our emotional systems adjust to just about anything that happens in our lives, positive or negative, just as our noses quickly adapt to any kind of scent (Brickman & Campbell, 1971). Early studies showing that lottery winners tend to be not much happier and that paraplegics tend to be not much unhappier than a control group following an initial adjustment period (Brick- man, Coates, & Janoff-Bulman, 1978) have been broadly cited to illustrate the powerful role of adaptation in happiness. Set-point theory, in conjunction with the hedonic treadmill idea, implies that individual and societal attempts at increasing happiness are ultimately doomed to failure. In their paper documenting the high heritability coefficient of happiness, Lykken and Tellegen (1996) have indeed noted that trying to be happier may be "as futile as trying to be taller and therefore is counterproductive" (p. 189).

However, findings from longitudinal and cross-sectional studies, as well as from intervention research, fail to corroborate such pessimistic conclusions. These findings suggest that time may be ripe for a revision of the hedonic adaptation theories of well-being (Diener, Lucas, & Scollon, 2006; Easterlin, 2006). People do not rapidly and completely adapt to everything life has in store for them, and this fact is powerfully demonstrated by differences in average national happiness levels. Factors such as wealth, human rights, and societal equality significantly predict well-being in a society, which means that people do not automatically adapt to any objective life condition (Diener, Diener, & Diener, 1995). Similarly, Fujita and Diener (2005) have found in a large German sample that over a 17-year period, almost 9% of the sample changed an average of 3 or more points on a 10-point scale from the first 5 to the last 5 years of the study and that average life satisfaction in the first 5 years correlated only .51 with average life satisfaction during the last 5 years. Other studies investigating the longitudinal effects of unemployment (Lucas, Clark, Georgellis, & Diener, 2004), marriage (Lucas, Clark, Georgellis, & Diener, 2003), and even winning the lottery (Gardner & Oswald, 2007) on life satisfaction levels confirm the view that set-point and adaptation theories as they are typically conceived do not coincide with the current empirical findings and need to be modified.

In short, there seems to be a substantial genetic component to subjective well-being, which contributes to the relative stability of subjective well-being over a person's lifespan and makes some people more prone to happiness and others to unhappiness. Even so, only about half of the individual differences in happiness are accounted for by genetic influences, meaning that people are hardly doomed to miserable lives as the victims of the genetic happiness lottery. Genes affect one's happiness through their expression in dispositional patterns and personality characteristics, which is the subject we turn to next.

Personality

Among different facets of personality, extraversion and neuroticism are the ones most consistently and strongly related to happiness (Diener & Lucas, 1999; Rusting & Larsen, 1997). As expected, both of these traits are highly heritable, rooted in neurobiology, and exhibit little change over the lifespan (Lyubomirsky et al., 2005). A host of studies show that extraversion predicts positive affect moderately to strongly (e.g., Lucas & Fujita, 2000), whereas neuroticism is an exceptionally strong predictor of negative affect (e.g., Fujita, 1991). The exact processes that underlie the extraversion–happiness and neuroticism–unhappiness links have also been broadly explored. One such process seems to be the differential sensitivity of extraverts and neurotics to rewards and punishments. Specifically, extraverts are more responsive to positive mood inductions, whereas neurotics are more responsive to negative mood inductions (Derryberry & Reed, 1994; Larsen & Ketelaar, 1991). In addition to this direct effect of personality traits on happiness, studies have also uncovered an indirect route in that extraverted people experience more frequent positive objective life events and neurotic people experience more frequent negative objective events (Headey & Wearing, 1989; Magnus, Diener, Fujita, & Pavot, 1993).

Other than extraversion and neuroticism, personality traits such as dispositional optimism, trust, agreeableness, desire for control, and hardiness have been found to be positively associated with happiness (DeNeve & Cooper, 1998; Lucas, Diener, & Suh, 1996; Scheier & Carver, 1993; Watson & Clark, 1992). Another personality trait that is closely related to happiness is self-esteem. Research has consistently revealed moderate to high correlations between self-esteem and happiness (Lyubomirsky, Tkach, & DiMatteo, 2006). It is worth noting, however, that these correlations are demonstrated to be significantly stronger in individualist compared with collectivist cultures (Diener & Diener, 1995a). Furthermore, the direction of causality between the two constructs is not entirely understood (Baumeister, Campbell, Krueger, & Vohs, 2003).

Intimately related to personality characteristics that are correlated with high levels of happiness are what some have called "virtues and character strengths." Recently, a number of psychologists undertook the massive project of coming up with an exhaustive list of virtues, and their efforts culminated in a classification system made up of 24 character strengths, organized under six core virtues (Peterson & Seligman, 2004). These six core virtues are *wisdom* (e.g., love of learning, creativity), *courage* (e.g., bravery, persistence), *humanity* (e.g., kindness, social intelligence), *justice* (e.g., fairness), *temperance* (e.g., forgiveness, self-regulation), and finally, *transcendence* (e.g., gratitude, religiousness/spirituality). Research has revealed that the character strengths of hope, zest, gratitude, love, and curiosity are most strongly and robustly linked to life satisfaction. More cerebral virtues, such as love of learning, on the other hand, seem to be only weakly associated with happiness (Park, Peterson, & Seligman, 2004).

Age

Of the relation between age and happiness, Tatarkiewicz (1976) confidently wrote, "it is considered to be an elementary truth that happiness is the privilege of youth" (p. 165). Studies, however, make it plain that although young people are generally happy, happiness is hardly their exclusive privilege. Longitudinal and cross-sectional data suggest that, of the three components of well-being, positive affect slightly decreases in old age, yet so does negative affect (Charles, Reynolds, & Gatz, 2001; Mroczek & Spiro, 2005). As to life satisfaction, Mroczek and Spiro (2005) found that although there were significant individual differences, life satisfaction increased from age 40 to 65, but then declined, particularly with impending death. Though more research on the subject is required, these results alone warn against a view of old age as a wellspring of unhappiness and against oversimplified conclusions about age trends in subjective well-being.

Gender

In his famous essay "On Women," Schopenhauer (2004) argued that "the keenest sorrows and joys" are not for a woman, that "the current of her life should be more gentle, peaceful and trivial than man's, without being essentially happier or unhappier" (p. 51). Large-scale surveys dovetail with Schopenhauer's insight that women are not significantly happier or unhappier than men. When sex differences are observed in studies, it is typically women who report higher happiness levels, yet these differences tend to disappear when other demographic variables are controlled for (Diener, Suh, Lucas, & Smith, 1999). Schopenhauer's observation that women do not experience the greatest sufferings and the greatest joys, on the other hand, seems to be a poor reflection of reality. Data indicate that, quite to the contrary, women experience both negative and positive emotions more frequently and more intensely than men. In line with this observation, Fujita, Diener, and Sand-

vik (1991) have demonstrated that whereas gender accounts for less than 1% of the variance in happiness, it accounts for over 13% of the variance in the intensity of emotional experiences. In other words, women and men do not differ in their average happiness levels, though women may be overrepresented among both the extremely happy and the extremely unhappy members of society (Diener et al., 1999).

Intelligence and Education

"By all the gods above," wrote Dutch philosopher Erasmus, "is anyone happier than the sort of men who are usually called fools, dolts, simpletons, nincompoops?" (2003, p. 54). Studies, however, fail to validate this observation and point to a positive (though weak) correlation between one's level of education and happiness after controlling for other variables, explaining 1–3% of variance in happiness (Witter, Okun, Stock, & Haring, 1984). As to the effect of intelligence (as measured by IQ tests) on happiness, it seems to be very weak, if it exists at all. Emotional intelligence, on the other hand, has consistently been linked to happiness (Furnham & Petrides, 2003; Schutte, Malouff, Simunek, McKenley, & Hollander, 2002), most likely because neurotic individuals tend to score low on measures of social and emotional intelligence.

Wealth

All in all, research suggests that money has a positive, yet diminishing, effect on happiness. Although increased income contributes significantly to happiness at low levels of development across nations, the strong link between wealth and life satisfaction appears to taper off at higher levels of income (Frey & Stutzer, 2002a). Reflecting this trend, when Diener, Horowitz, and Emmons (1985) asked wealthy people chosen from the *Forbes* list of the wealthiest Americans about their happiness levels, they reported being only modestly happier than a comparable group, and 37% of them turned out to be less happy than the average American. Whereas *having* money is associated with a positive, albeit diminishing, effect on happiness, *wanting* money too much has repeatedly been shown to prove toxic to happiness. People who place a lot of importance on money and on material possessions, particularly to the expense of family and social relationships, tend to feel less satisfied with their lives and experience less positive affect and more negative affect (Kasser & Kanner, 2004).

Religion

A number of studies point to a positive yet modest effect of religion on happiness. More specifically, participation in religious services, strength of religious affiliation, relationship with God, and prayer have all been associated with greater happiness levels (e.g., Ferriss, 2002; Poloma & Pendleton, 1990; Witter, Stock, Okun, & Haring, 1985). Higher levels of religiosity have also been linked to higher life satisfaction and lower rates of suicide across nations (Diener & Seligman, 2004; Helliwell, 2007). It is believed that the beneficial effects of religion on happiness stem largely from the sense of meaning and purpose that religious beliefs provide to the individual, as well as from the social support networks associated with organized religion (e.g., churches). Importantly, it is an intrinsic as opposed to extrinsic orientation toward religion that seems to be associated positively with subjective well-being (Ardelt, 2003; Ardelt & Koenig, 2007). It is also worth noting that the positive link between religion and happiness is stronger for women, African Americans, and older adults and for Americans compared with Europeans (Argyle, 1999). Religious people in certain countries (e.g., Lithuania, Slovakia) have even reported lower levels of life satisfaction, which highlights the need for further research in order to understand the exact nature of the relationship between happiness and religion. The link of spirituality—as a concept distinct from religiousness—to subjective well-being is a similarly unstudied topic.

Societal Conditions and Culture

International surveys of happiness reveal significant mean differences across societies (Diener & Suh, 2000). These differences are substantially explained by the level of economic development in a country: Some of the unhappiest nations tend also to be among the poorest. National wealth is also highly correlated with various social indicators, such as democratic governance, human rights, and longevity (Diener & Diener, 1995b), which may partly account for its association with subjective well-being. Societies also have differing norms regarding the desirability of happiness and the appropriate expression of positive and negative emotions that contribute to cross-cultural subjective well-being differences beyond the effect of economic development. For example, relative to other cultures, Confucian cultures (such as China) regard the ideal level of life satisfaction as one of neutrality and display higher acceptance of negative emotions and lower acceptance of positive emotions. Extant norms regarding life satisfaction in a society are apparently mirrored in actual levels of life satisfaction in that society, as confirmed by the finding that the mean ideal level for life satisfaction correlates .73 with mean reported life satisfaction across nations (Diener & Suh, 1999). The variables that most influence subjective well-being are also moderated by culture. For example, as mentioned earlier, self-esteem is a stronger predictor of subjective well-being in individualistic cultures than in collectivistic cultures. In line with this finding, people in individualistic cultures tend to base their life satisfaction judgments on personal emotional experiences, whereas people from collectivistic cultures emphasize the appraisals of others (Suh, Diener, Oishi, & Triandis, 1998).

Health

Physical health inarguably affects well-being, as is evidenced by the considerably lowered happiness levels of individuals who suffer life-threatening illnesses or illnesses that interfere with their daily lives and cause pain. Given this fact, it is intriguing that researchers have reported weak and sometimes nonexistent correlations between happiness and objective health as assessed by medical personnel. Whereas associations between objective health and happiness are often weak, research documents that associations between happiness and subjective health—as it is reported by the individual—are consistently strong (Okun, Stock, Haring, & Witter, 1984). This curious phenomenon seems to be the consequence of (1) clinical error, meaning that objective health measures are sometimes not as objective as one would hope, and (2) the notion that subjective reports of health reflect emotional adjustments on the part of the individual, thus inflating the correlation between self-reported health and happiness.

Social Relationships and Friends

Having close friends and a network of social support has a distinct positive effect on happiness, to such a degree that some scholars have suggested that this could be the single most important source of happiness (Reis & Gable, 2003). Corroborating this view, Diener and Seligman (2002) found in their study of very happy people that every single one of them had excellent social relationships. Other studies document that those who enjoy close relationships are better at coping with major life stresses such as bereavement, rape, unemployment, and illness (Myers, 1999), and perceived loneliness is robustly linked to depression (Anderson & Arnoult, 1985). It is not to be forgotten, though, that happiness itself may lead to better relationships. As we show later, happy people tend to be more outgoing, empathic, and trusting than unhappy people, presumably resulting in enhanced quantity and quality of social relationships (Veenhoven, 1988).

Marriage and Children

Empirical research regarding the relationship between happiness and marriage in the last few decades has yielded the robust finding that married individuals tend to be happier than unmarried or divorced ones (e.g., Gove & Shin, 1989; White, 1992). We should again be cautioned that the arrow of causality may point both ways: A number of studies have revealed that individuals who are likely to get married and to stay married are happier long before the marriage compared with individuals who remain single (Lucas et al., 2003). Investigations about the effects of having children on one's happiness have been rarer, yet available data do not unequivocally support the conventional view that children are "the joy of life." In a well-controlled study, Kohler, Behrman, and Skytthe (2004) documented that first-born children significantly increase the happiness of their parents, whereas additional children reduce the happiness of their mothers and leave the happiness of their fathers unchanged. Another remarkable finding from their study was that having had children at one point in their lives did not have any effect on the happiness levels of men and women at ages 50–70.

Goals and Sense of Meaning

Research findings unambiguously illustrate that striving for and making progress toward meaningful, enjoyable, moderately challenging goals is an important source of happiness (Brunstein, 1993; Emmons, 1986; Little, 1989). As Myers and Diener (1995) have suggested, happiness seems to grow "less from the passive experience of desirable circumstances than from involvement in valued activities and progress toward one's goals" (p. 17). Individuals who have goals that they deem important tend to be more energetic, experience more positive affect, and feel that life is meaningful (Diener, Lucas, & Oishi, 2002). Interestingly, positive affect in itself has been found to predispose people to feel that life is meaningful (King, Hicks, Krull, & Del Gaiso, 2006).

Leisure

George Bernard Shaw once observed that the only way to avoid being miserable is not to have enough leisure time to wonder whether you're happy or not. A host of studies nonetheless document that leisure activities such as music, exercise, and reading significantly contribute to happiness (Argyle, 2002). Balatsky and Diener (1993) even reported that, among Russian students, leisure satisfaction was the single best predictor of happiness. On a related note, people who work fewer hours have been demonstrated to have higher life satisfaction (Alesina, Glaeser, & Sacerdote, 2006).

The Consequences of Happiness

In the previous section, we attempted to paint a rough picture of what causes happiness. Our assumption throughout was that happiness is something highly valuable, notwithstanding the aforementioned cultural differences in the perception of its desirability. Indeed, in a recent study conducted in 48 nations, Diener and Oishi (2006) established that respondents rated the importance of happiness 8.03 on a 9-point scale, higher than the importance of any of the other 11 attributes included in the survey, such as success, intelligence/knowledge, or material wealth. Others have found that, in America, happiness is rated as more relevant to the judgment of a good life than wealth or moral goodness, and happy people are deemed to be more likely to go to heaven (King & Napa, 1998).

Happiness indisputably feels good, and people value it greatly, yet the question that remains to be answered is whether happiness is as justifiable as it is desirable. The answer, according to happiness research, seems to be emphatically positive. A fascinating discovery made recently by happiness scholars is that happiness is not only an epiphenomenon but also plays a causal role in bringing about a plethora of individually and socially beneficial outcomes. In the next section, we provide a review of how happiness cultivates better health and achievement outcomes, better social relationships, and elevated degrees of prosocial behavior. For a more comprehensive review, the reader is advised to refer to Lyubomirsky, King, and Diener (2005).

Benefits of Happiness for Achievement Outcomes

Whereas many romanticizers of unhappiness disparage happiness for dumbing people down and praise misery for its role in sharpening one's mental faculties, the picture emerging from available data is that it is rather happiness (and not unhappiness) that leads to the development and better use of intellectual skills. Barbara Fredrickson's "broaden-and-build theory" provides a valuable framework to make sense of this phenomenon. According to this theory (Fredrickson, 1998, 2001), positive emotions allow individuals to broaden their thought–action repertoires and build their intellectual, psychological, social, and physical resources over time. Whereas negative emotions, such as fear or anger, appropriately cause the individual to focus on the immediate threat or

problem, positive emotions and general well-being produce a readiness to explore the environment and approach new goals, thereby building enduring personal resources.

The notion that happy moods render the world an easier and safer place for people to deal with is evidenced, for example, by Proffitt's (2006) finding that participants who were put in a bad mood estimated the slope of a hill dropping down in front of them to be much steeper than they did when they were put in a good mood. Individuals are hence expected to generally perform better when they are in good moods. In one test of the "sadder-but-wiser vs. happier-and-smarter" hypotheses, Staw and Barsade (1993) assessed the positive affect levels of first-year MBA students and found that positive affect significantly predicted decision-making accuracy, mastery of information, leadership, and ratings of managerial performance, after controlling for the effects of Graduate Management Admission Test (GMAT) scores, age, gender, and years of experience. These findings are further supported by data showing that individuals experimentally put in pleasant moods outperform others in various tasks, including efficient decision making (Forgas, 1989) or anagram solving (Erez & Isen, 2002), and they also persist longer at tasks that require perseverance (Kavanagh, 1987).

At the same time, however, some studies show that those experiencing elevated moods have an increased tendency to rely on heuristics. Heuristics are learned answers, or mental habits, that help people effortlessly answer problems that are frequently faced in life. When they are used in an appropriate context, they can efficiently yield accurate answers. However, high levels of positive affect might lead to inappropriate use of heuristics, possibly because good moods serve as a cue that everything is going well and that there is no need for the expenditure of extra mental energy (Schwarz, Bless, Wänke, & Winkielman, 2003). In harmony with such an interpretation, studies show that people who are in a good mood perform as well as those who are not when they are reminded that the task is important or complicated (Lyubomirsky, King, & Diener, 2005).

Happiness has also been linked to higher achievement in professional life. It has been documented, for instance, that happier individuals are more likely to graduate from college, more likely to secure jobs, more likely to have more prestigious jobs, more likely to receive favorable evaluations from their supervisors, more likely to find their jobs more meaningful, less likely to lose their jobs, quicker to be reemployed if they do, more likely to exhibit organizational citizenship behaviors, and, finally, more likely to earn higher incomes (e.g., Borman, Penner, Allen, & Motowildo, 2001; Cropanzano & Wright, 1999; Diener, Nickerson, Lucas, & Sandvik, 2002; Marks & Fleming, 1999; Roberts, Caspi, & Moffitt, 2003; Verkley & Stolk, 1989). On the whole, available data strongly suggest that happiness is not only a product of achievement but, at the same time, a producer of it. Research has yet to unveil all the mechanisms through which these effects are obtained.

Benefits of Happiness for Social Relationships and Prosocial Behavior

Whereas some have argued that only a self-centered person blind to the overwhelming suffering permeating the world could ever be happy, research fails to justify the cynicism in these beliefs. Quite to the contrary, what studies reveal is that happiness tends to bring out the best in humans, rendering them more social, cooperative, and even ethical. People with chronically high or experimentally increased positive affect have been observed to judge persons they have recently met in a more positive light, to become more interested in social interaction, and also more prone to self-disclosure (Berry & Hansen, 1996; Cunningham, 1988; Mayer, Mamberg, & Volanth, 1988). Experimentally induced positive affect also increases trust in others (Dunn & Schweitzer, 2005), which may partly help to explain the classic finding that positive moods increase helping behavior (Isen & Levin, 1972). In a similar vein, those who report higher life satisfaction exhibit more generalized trust in others (Brehm & Rahn, 1997), which in turn predicts not only individual but also societal well-being.

The view that a virtuous cycle exists between happiness and myriad socially desirable outcomes is further substantiated by the finding that not only does volunteering increase well-being but also that hap-

pier people are more likely to be community volunteers and to invest more hours in volunteer work (Thoits & Hewitt, 2001). Of great significance is the fact that happiness has also been shown to increase ethical judgments: When James and Chymis (2004) analyzed how justifiable respondents found various ethical scenarios—such as cheating on taxes if one has a chance or avoiding a fare on public transport—those with higher happiness levels responded in more ethical ways. This led the authors to conclude that improving subjective well-being may play a significant role in reducing improbity of all kinds (e.g., corruption, criminality) nationally and worldwide. Inglehart and Klingemann's (2000) similar argument that general well-being is a harbinger of democratic governance is corroborated by Tov and Diener's (2008) finding that on a national level, happier countries tend to be higher on generalized trust, volunteerism, and democratic attitudes. These findings sharply contradict a view of happiness as self-indulgent hedonism and attest to the intimate connection between a moral life and a happy life defended by many a philosopher throughout the ages.

Benefits of Happiness for Health

Accumulating evidence suggests that subjective well-being affects physical health and longevity, endorsing the Biblical notion that "a merry heart does good like a medicine" (Pressman & Cohen, 2005). Whereas it had long been established that high levels of negative emotion (e.g., stress, anger) are associated with lowered immune functioning and coronary heart disease, less was known until recently about the powerful protective influence that positive emotions exert. In a remarkable study revealing this influence, Danner, Snowdon and Friesen (2001) established that positive emotional content in handwritten autobiographies of Catholic sisters, composed when they were at the mean age of 22 years, predicted their longevity six decades later. In this study, the nuns in the highest quartile regarding the number of positive emotion words (e.g., *happy, good, fun*) lived on average 9.4 years longer than the nuns in the lowest quartile. In another study, participants were experimentally infected with a cold virus and then monitored daily in quarantine. As anticipated, individuals who reported experiencing high levels of positive emotions (i.e., those that were happy, pleased, relaxed) turned out to be much less vulnerable to the common cold (Cohen, Doyle, Turner, Alper, & Skoner, 2003) than those who reported experiencing low levels of positive emotions. Marsland, Cohen, Rabin, and Manuck (2006), interestingly, found that positive affect was a stronger predictor of immune strength than negative affect, and its predictive power persisted when demographics and body mass were controlled. Studies showing that people put into a pleasant mood exhibit greater pain tolerance compared with control participants also provide evidence for the favorable impact of positive affect on health outcomes (Zelman, Howland, Nichols, & Cleeland, 1991).

Conclusion

In this chapter we aimed to shed some light on what influences happiness and what in turn is influenced by it, based on four decades of research. These decades of accumulated research have revealed that happiness is not only universally desired, but justifiably so. We have learned that happiness is a worthwhile pursuit, because it functions as a resource that people unwittingly draw from in their endeavors toward higher levels of success, kindness, and health. Therefore, attempts at increasing happiness take on great importance, not only for individuals but also for societies. Fortunately, the science of happiness has shown and continues to show the empirically validated ways to increase happiness. We know that although some part of our capacity for happiness is inherited and simply not amenable to change, we can still choose to do certain things that will make us lastingly happier, such as counting our blessings (Emmons & McCullough, 2003) or stopping to smell the roses (Bryant & Veroff, 2006).

Our review of the literature suggests that happiness not only is a reward in itself but also brings about various individually and socially desirable outcomes. Given that happiness is functional, the optimal level of happiness becomes an essential matter for individual and societal reasons. If an extreme

lack of negative emotions can be highly dangerous, as exemplified by psychopaths, could an excessive amount of positive affect also result in suboptimal outcomes? We know, for example, that people in a good mood tend to rely more on heuristics than people in a bad or neutral mood, which also explains their more frequent use of stereotypes in person-perception tasks (Bodenhausen, Kramer, & Süsser, 1994). Intrigued by the notion of optimal happiness, Oishi, Diener, and Lucas (2007) put to test the idea that once people are moderately happy, the most effective level of happiness may depend on the life domain under question. They found those who experience the highest levels of happiness to be more successful in the domain of close relationships and volunteering. People who reported slightly lower levels of happiness, on the other hand, were the most successful ones in terms of income, education, and political participation. These findings imply that, whereas happy people in general fare much better than unhappy people, the level of most desirable happiness depends on an individual's value priorities.

As scholars of happiness, we are tremendously delighted that various knowledge disciplines, from philosophy (Haybron, 2007) to economics (Frey & Stutzer, 2002b) to neuroscience (Klein, 2006), have recently started to exhibit a serious interest in this once marginalized subject. We cannot wait to see the future of happiness studies shaped by this multidisciplinary effort, and we continue to hope for a tomorrow in which people will be optimally happy.

References

Alesina, A., Glaeser, E. L., & Sacerdote, B. (2006). Work and leisure in the U.S. and Europe: Why so different? In M. Gertler & K. Rogoff (Eds.), *NBER Macroeconomics Annual 2005* (pp. 1–64). Cambridge, MA: MIT Press.

Anderson, C. A., & Arnoult, L. H. (1985). Attributional style and everyday problems in living: Depression, loneliness, and shyness. *Social Cognition, 3*, 16–35.

Ardelt, M. (2003). Effects of religion and purpose in life on elders' subjective well-being and attitudes toward death. *Journal of Religious Gerontology, 14*, 55–77.

Ardelt, M., & Koenig, C. S. (2007). The importance of religious orientation in dying well: Evidence from three case studies. *Journal of Religion, Spirituality and Aging, 19*, 61–79.

Argyle, M. (1999). Causes and correlates of happiness. In D. Kahneman, E. Diener, & N. Schwarz (Eds.), *Well-being: The foundations of hedonic psychology* (pp. 553–373). New York: Russell Sage Foundation.

Argyle, M. (2002). *The psychology of happiness.* London: Routledge.

Balatsky, G., & Diener, E. (1993). Subjective well-being among Russian students. *Social Indicators Research, 28,* 225–243.

Baumeister, R. F., Campbell, J. D., Krueger, J. I., & Vohs, K. D. (2003). Does high self-esteem cause better performance, interpersonal success, happiness, or healthier lifestyles? *Psychological Science in the Public Interest, 4,* 1–44.

Berry, D. S., & Hansen, J. S. (1996). Positive affect, negative affect, and social interaction. *Journal of Personality and Social Psychology, 71,* 796–809.

Bodenhausen, G. V., Kramer, G. P., & Süsser, K. (1994). Happiness and stereotypic thinking in social judgment. *Journal of Personality and Social Psychology, 66,* 621–632.

Borman, W. C., Penner, L. A., Allen, T. D., & Motowildo, S. J. (2001). Personality predictors of citizenship performance. *International Journal of Selection and Assessment, 9,* 52–69.

Brehm, J., & Rahn, W. (1997). Individual-level evidence for the causes and consequences of social capital. *American Journal of Political Science, 41*(3), 999–1024.

Brickman, P., & Campbell, D. T. (1971). Hedonic relativism and planning the good society. In M. H. Appley (Ed.), *Adaptation level theory: A symposium* (pp. 287–302). New York: Academic Press.

Brickman, P., Coates, D., & Janoff-Bulman, R. (1978). Lottery winners and accident victims: Is happiness relative? *Journal of Personality and Social Psychology, 36,* 917–927.

Brunstein, J. C. (1993). Personal goals and subjective well-being: A longitudinal study. *Journal of Personality and Social Psychology, 65,* 1061–1070.

Bryant, F. B., & Veroff, J. (2006). *Savoring: A new model of positive experience.* Mahwah, NJ: Erlbaum.

Charles, S. T., Reynolds, C. A., & Gatz, M. (2001). Age-related differences and change in positive and negative affect over 23 years. *Journal of Personality and Social Psychology, 80,* 136–151.

Cohen, S., Doyle, W. J., Turner, R. B., Alper, C. M., & Skoner, D. P. (2003). Emotional style and susceptibility to the common cold. *Psychosomatic Medicine, 65,* 652–657.

Costa, P. T., & McCrae, R. R. (1988). Personality in adulthood: A six-year longitudinal study of self-reports and spouse ratings on the NEO Personality Inventory. *Journal of Personality and Social Psychology, 54,* 853–863.

Cropanzano, R., & Wright, T. A. (1999). A 5-year study of change in the relationship between well-being and job performance. *Consulting Psychology Journal: Practice and Research, 51,* 252–265.

Cunningham, M. R. (1988). Does happiness mean friendliness? Induced mood and heterosexual self-disclosure. *Personality and Social Psychology Bulletin, 14,* 283–297.

Danner, D., Snowdon D., & Friesen, W. (2001). Positive emotions in early life and longevity: Findings from the nun study. *Journal of Personality and Social Psychology, 80*(5), 804–813.

DeNeve, K. M., & Cooper, H. (1998). The happy personality: A meta-analysis of 137 personality traits and subjective well-being. *Psychological Bulletin, 124,* 197–229.

Derryberry, D., & Reed, M. A. (1994). Temperament and attention: Orienting toward and away from positive and negative signals. *Journal of Personality and Social Psychology, 66,* 1128–1139.

Diener, E. (1984). Subjective well-being. *Psychological Bulletin, 95,* 542–575.

Diener, E., & Diener, M. (1995a). Cross-cultural correlates of life satisfaction and self-esteem. *Journal of Personality and Social Psychology, 68,* 653–663.

Diener, E., & Diener, C. (1995b). The wealth of nations revisited: Income and quality of life. *Social Indicators Research, 36,* 275–228.

Diener, E., Diener, M., & Diener, C. (1995). Factors predicting the subjective well-being of nations. *Journal of Personality and Social Psychology, 69,* 851–864.

Diener, E., Horowitz, J., & Emmons, R. A. (1985). Happiness of the very wealthy. *Social Indicators Research, 16,* 263–274.

Diener, E., & Larsen, R. J. (1993). The experience of emotional well-being. In M. Lewis & J. M. Haviland (Eds.), *Handbook of emotions* (pp. 404–415). New York: Guilford Press.

Diener, E., Lucas, R., & Oishi, S. (2002). Subjective well-being: The science of happiness and life satisfaction. In C. R. Snyder & S. J. Lopez (Eds.), *The handbook of positive psychology* (pp. 63–73). New York: Oxford University Press.

Diener, E., & Lucas, R. E. (1999). Personality and subjective well-being. In D. Kahneman, E. Diener, & N. Schwarz (Eds.), *Well-being: The foundations of hedonic psychology* (pp. 213–229). New York: Russell Sage Foundation.

Diener, E., Lucas, R. E., & Scollon, C. N. (2006). Beyond the hedonic treadmill: Revisions to the adaptation theory of well-being. *American Psychologist, 61,* 305–314.

Diener, E., Nickerson, C., Lucas, R. E., & Sandvik, E. (2002). Dispositional affect and job outcomes. *Social Indicators Research, 59,* 229–259.

Diener, E., & Oishi, S. (2006). *The desirability of happiness across cultures.* Unpublished manuscript, University of Illinois, Urbana–Champaign.

Diener, E., & Seligman, M. E. P. (2002). Very happy people. *Psychological Science, 13,* 81–84.

Diener, E., & Seligman, M. E. P. (2004). Beyond money: Toward an economy of well-being. *Psychological Science in the Public Interest, 5,* 1–31.

Diener, E., & Suh, E. (1999). National differences in subjective well-being. In D. Kahneman, E. Diener, & N. Schwarz (Eds.), *Well-being: The foundations of hedonic psychology* (pp. 434–450). New York: Russell Sage Foundation.

Diener, E., & Suh, E. M. (1997). Measuring quality of life: Economic, social, and subjective indicators. *Social Indicators Research, 40,* 189–216.

Diener, E., & Suh, E. M. (Eds.). (2000). *Culture and subjective well-being.* Cambridge, MA: MIT Press.

Diener, E., Suh, E. M., Lucas, R. E., & Smith, H. L. (1999). Subjective well-being: Three decades of progress. *Psychological Bulletin, 125,* 276–302.

Dunn, J. R., & Schweitzer, M. E. (2005). Feeling and believing: The influence of emotion on trust. *Journal of Personality and Social Psychology, 88*, 736–748.

Easterlin, R. A. (2006). Life cycle happiness and its sources: Intersections of psychology, economics, and demography. *Journal of Economic Psychology, 27*, 463–482.

Emmons, R. A. (1986). Personal strivings: An approach to personality and subjective well-being. *Journal of Personality and Social Psychology, 47*, 1105–1117.

Emmons, R. A., & McCullough, M. E. (2003). Counting blessings versus burdens: An experimental investigation of gratitude and subjective well-being in daily life. *Journal of Personality and Social Psychology, 84*, 377–389.

Erasmus, D. (2003). *The praise of folly.* New Haven, CT: Yale University Press.

Erez, A., & Isen, A. M. (2002). The influence of positive affect on the components of expectancy motivation. *Journal of Applied Psychology, 87*, 1055–1067.

Ferriss, A. L. (2002). Religion and the quality of life. *Journal of Happiness Studies, 3*, 199–215.

Forgas, J. P. (1989). Mood effects on decision making strategies. *Australian Journal of Psychology, 41*, 197–214.

Fredrickson, B. L. (1998). What good are positive emotions? *Review of General Psychology, 2*, 300–319.

Fredrickson, B. L. (2001). The role of positive emotions in positive psychology: The broaden-and-build theory of positive emotions. *American Psychologist, 56*, 218–226.

Frey, B. S., & Stutzer, A. (2002a). *Happiness and economics: How the economy and institutions affect human well-being.* Princeton, NJ: Princeton University Press.

Frey, B. S., & Stutzer, A. (2002b). What can economists learn from happiness research? *Journal of Economic Literature, 40*, 402–435.

Fujita, F. (1991). *An investigation of the relation between extraversion, neuroticism, positive affect, and negative affect.* Unpublished master's thesis, University of Illinois, Urbana–Champaign.

Fujita, F., & Diener, E. (2005) Life satisfaction set point: Stability and change. *Journal of Personality and Social Psychology, 88*(1), 158–164.

Fujita, F., Diener, E., & Sandvik, E. (1991). Gender differences in negative affect and well-being: The case for emotional intensity. *Journal of Personality and Social Psychology, 61*, 427–434.

Furnham, A., & Petrides, K. V. (2003). Trait emotional intelligence and happiness. *Social Behavior and Personality, 31*, 815–824.

Gardner, J., & Oswald, A. J. (2007). Money and mental well-being: A longitudinal study of medium-sized lottery wins. *Journal of Health Economics, 26*, 49–60.

Gove, W. R., & Shin, H. (1989). The psychological well-being of divorced and widowed men and women. *Journal of Family Issues, 10*, 122–144.

Harker, L., & Keltner, D. (2001). Expressions of positive emotion in women's college yearbook pictures and their relationship to personality and life outcomes across adulthood. *Journal of Personality and Social Psychology, 80*, 112–124.

Haybron, D. M. (2007). Philosophy and the science of subjective well-being. In M. Eid & R. J. Larsen (Eds.), *The science of subjective well-being* (pp. 17–43). New York: Guilford Press.

Headey, B., & Wearing, A. (1989). Personality, life events, and subjective well-being: Toward a dynamic equilibrium model. *Journal of Personality and Social Psychology, 57*, 731–739.

Helliwell, J. F. (2007). Well-being and social capital: Does suicide pose a puzzle? *Social Indicators Research, 81*, 455–496.

Inglehart, R., & Klingemann, H.-D. (2000). Genes, culture, democracy, and happiness. In E. Diener & E. M. Suh (Eds.), *Culture and subjective well-being* (pp. 165–184). Cambridge, MA: MIT Press.

Isen, A. M., & Levin, P. F. (1972). Effect of feeling good on helping: Cookies and kindness. *Journal of Personality and Social Psychology, 21*, 384–388.

James, H. S., & Chymis, A. (2004). *Are happy people ethical people?: Evidence from North America and Europe.* (Working Paper No. AEWP 2004-8). Columbia: University of Missouri, Department of Agricultural Economics

Kasser, T., & Kanner, A. D. (Eds.). (2004). *Psychology and consumer culture: The struggle for a good life in a materialistic world.* Washington, DC: American Psychological Association.

Kavanagh, D. J. (1987). Mood, persistence, and success. *Australian Journal of Psychology, 39*, 307–318.

King, L. A., Hicks, J. A., Krull, J., & Del Gaiso, A. K. (2006). Positive affect and the experience of meaning in life. *Journal of Personality and Social Psychology, 90*, 179–196.

King, L. A., & Napa, C. K. (1998). What makes a life good? *Journal of Personality and Social Psychology, 75*, 156–165.

Klein, S. (2006). *The science of happiness: How our brains make us happy and what we can do to get happier.* New York: Marlowe.

Kohler, H. P., Behrman, J. R., & Skythe, A. (2005). Partner + children = happiness?: The effect of fertility and partnerships on subjective well-being. *Population and Development Review, 31*(3), 407–445.

Larsen, R. J., & Ketelaar, T. (1991). Personality and susceptibility to positive and negative emotional states. *Journal of Personality and Social Psychology, 61*, 132–140.

Little, B. R. (1989). Personal projects analysis: Trivial pursuits, magnificent obsessions, and the search for coherence. In D. M. Buss & N. Cantor (Eds.), *Personality psychology: Recent trends and emerging directions* (pp. 15–31). New York: Springer.

Lucas, R. E., Clark, A. E., Georgellis, Y., & Diener, E. (2003). Reexamining adaptation and the set point model of happiness: Reactions to changes in marital status. *Journal of Personality and Social Psychology, 84*, 527–539.

Lucas, R. E., Clark, A. E., Georgellis, Y., & Diener, E. (2004). Unemployment alters the set point for life satisfaction. *Psychological Science, 15*(1), 8–13.

Lucas, R. E., Diener, E., & Suh, E. (1996). Discriminant validity of well-being measures. *Journal of Personality and Social Psychology, 71*, 616–628.

Lucas, R. E., & Fujita, F. (2000). Factors influencing the relation between extraversion and pleasant affect. *Journal of Personality and Social Psychology, 79*, 1039–1056.

Lykken, D., & Tellegen, A. (1996). Happiness is a

stochastic phenomenon. *Psychological Science, 7,* 186–189.

Lyubomirsky, S., King, L., & Diener, E. (2005). The benefits of frequent positive affect: Does happiness lead to success? *Psychological Bulletin, 131,* 803–855.

Lyubomirsky, S., & Lepper, H. (1999). A measure of subjective happiness: Preliminary reliability and construct validation. *Social Indicators Research, 46,* 137–155.

Lyubomirsky, S., Sheldon, K. M., & Schkade, D. (2005). Pursuing happiness: The architecture of sustainable change. *Review of General Psychology, 9,* 111–131.

Lyubomirsky, S., Tkach, C., & DiMatteo, M. R. (2006). What are the differences between happiness and self-esteem? *Social Indicators Research, 78,* 363–404.

Magnus, K., & Diener, E. (1991, May). *A longitudinal analysis of personality, life events, and subjective well-being.* Paper presented at the annual meeting of the Midwestern Psychological Association, Chicago.

Magnus, K., Diener, E., Fujita, F., & Pavot, W. (1993). Extraversion and neuroticism as predictors of objective life events: A longitudinal analysis. *Journal of Personality and Social Psychology, 65,* 1046–1053.

Marks, G. N., & Fleming, N. (1999). Influences and consequences of well-being among Australian young people: 1980–1995. *Social Indicators Research, 46,* 301–323.

Marsland, A. L., Cohen, S., Rabin, B. S., & Manuck, S. B. (2006). Trait positive affect and antibody response to hepatitis B vaccination. *Brain Behavior and Immunity, 20,* 261–269.

Mayer, J. D., Mamberg, M. H., & Volanth, A. J. (1988). Cognitive domains of the mood system. *Journal of Personality, 56,* 453–486.

McMahon, D. M. (2005). *Happiness: A history.* New York: Atlantic Monthly Press.

Mroczek, D. K., & Spiro, A., III. (2005). Change in life satisfaction during adulthood: Findings from the Veterans Affairs Normative Aging Study. *Journal of Personality and Social Psychology, 88,* 189–202.

Myers, D. G. (1999). Close relationships and the quality of life. In D. Kahneman, E. Diener, & N. Schwartz (Eds.), *Well-being: The foundations of hedonic psychology* (pp. 374–380). New York: Russell Sage Foundation.

Myers, D. G., & Diener, E. (1995). Who is happy? *Psychological Science, 6,* 10–19.

Oishi, S., Diener, E., & Lucas, R. E. (2007). The optimal level of well-being: Can we be too happy? *Perspectives on Psychological Science, 2,* 346–360.

Okun, M. A., Stock, W. A., Haring, M. J., & Witter, R.A. (1984). Health and subjective well-being: A meta-analysis. *International Journal of Aging and Human Development, 19,* 111–131.

Park, N., Peterson, C., & Seligman, M. E. P. (2004). Strengths of character and well-being. *Journal of Social and Clinical Psychology, 23,* 603–619.

Pascal, B. (1995). *Pensées* (A. J. Krailsheimer, Trans.). London: Penguin Books.

Pavot, W., & Diener, E. (1993). Review of the Satisfaction with Life Scale. *Psychological Assessment, 5,* 164–172.

Pavot, W., Diener, E., Colvin, C. R., & Sandvik, E.

(1991). Further validation of the Satisfaction with Life Scale: Evidence for the cross-method convergence of well-being measures. *Journal of Personality Assessment, 57,* 149–161.

Peterson, C., & Seligman, M. E. P. (2004). *Character strengths and virtues: A classification and handbook.* Washington, DC: American Psychological Association.

Poloma, M. M., & Pendleton, B. F. (1990). Religious domains and general well-being. *Social Indicators Research, 22,* 255–276.

Pressman, S. D., & Cohen, S. (2005). Does positive affect influence health? *Psychological Bulletin, 131,* 925–971.

Proffitt, D. R. (2006). Distance perception. *Current Directions in Psychological Research, 15,* 131–135.

Reis, H. T., & Gable, S. L. (2003). Toward a positive psychology of relationships. In C. L. Keyes & J. Haidt (Eds.), *Flourishing: The positive person and the good life* (pp. 129–159). Washington, DC: American Psychological Association.

Roberts, B. W., Caspi, A., & Moffitt, T. E. (2003). Work experiences and personality development in young adulthood. *Journal of Personality and Social Psychology, 84,* 582–593.

Rusting, C. L., & Larsen, R. J. (1997). Extraversion, neuroticism, and susceptibility to positive and negative affect: A test of two theoretical models. *Personality and Individual Differences, 22,* 607–612.

Ryan, R. M., & Deci, E. L. (2000). Self-determination theory and the facilitation of intrinsic motivation, social development and well-being. *American Psychologist, 55,* 68–78.

Ryff, C. D., & Singer, B. (1996). Psychological well-being: Meaning, measurement, and implications for psychotherapy research. *Psychotherapy and Psychosomatics, 65,* 14–23.

Scheier, M. F., & Carver, C. S. (1993). On the power of positive thinking: The benefits of being optimistic. *Current Directions in Psychological Science, 2,* 26–30.

Schopenhauer, A. (2004). *Studies in pessimism: The essays of Arthur Schopenhauer* (T. B. Saunders, Trans.). Whitefish, MT: Kessinger.

Schutte, N. S., Malouff, J. M., Simunek, M., McKenley, J., & Hollander, S. (2002). Characteristic emotional intelligence and emotional well-being. *Cognition and Emotion, 16,* 769–785.

Schwarz, N., Bless, H., Wänke, M., & Winkielman, P. (2003). Accessibility revisited. In G. V. Bodenhausen & A. J. Lambert (Eds.), *Foundations of social cognition: A festschrift in honor of Robert S. Wyer, Jr.* (pp. 51–78). Mahwah, NJ: Erlbaum.

Schwarz, N., & Strack, F. (1999). Reports of subjective well-being: Judgmental processes and their methodological implications. In D. Kahneman, E. Diener, & N. Schwarz (Eds.), *Well-being: The foundations of hedonic psychology* (pp. 61–84). New York: Russell Sage Foundation.

Seligman, M. E. P. (2002). *Authentic happiness.* New York: Free Press.

Staw, B. M., & Barsade, S. G. (1993). Affect and managerial performance: A test of the sadder-but-wiser vs. happier-and-smarter hypotheses. *Administrative Science Quarterly, 38,* 304–331.

Suh, E., Diener, E., Oishi, S., & Triandis, H. C. (1998). The shifting basis of life satisfaction judgments across cultures: Emotions versus norms. *Journal of Personality and Social Psychology, 74,* 482–493.

Tatarkiewicz, W. (1976). *Analysis of happiness.* Warsaw, Poland: Polish Scientific.

Tellegen, A., Lykken, D. T., Bouchard, T. J., Wilcox, K. J., Segal, N. L., & Rich, S. (1988). Personality similarity in twins reared apart and together. *Journal of Personality and Social Psychology, 54,* 1031–1039.

Thoits, P. A., & Hewitt, L. N. (2001). Volunteer work and well-being. *Journal of Health and Social Behavior, 42,* 115–131.

Tomarken, A. J., Davidson, R. J., & Henriques, J. B. (1990). Resting frontal brain asymmetry predicts affective responses to films. *Journal of Personality and Social Psychology, 59,* 791–801.

Tov, W., & Diener, E. (2008). The well-being of nations: Linking together trust, cooperation, and democracy. In B. A. Sullivan, M. Snyder, & J. L. Sullivan (Eds.), *Cooperation: The political psychology of effective human interaction* (pp. 323–342). Malden, MA: Blackwell.

Veenhoven, R. (1988). The utility of happiness. *Social Indicators Research, 20,* 333–354.

Verkley, H., & Stolk, J. (1989). Does happiness lead into idleness? In R. Veenhoven (Ed.), *How harmful is happiness?* (pp. 79–93). Rotterdam, The Netherlands: University of Rotterdam.

Watson, D., & Clark, L. A. (1992). On traits and temperament: General and specific factors of emotional experience and their relation to the five-factor model. *Journal of Personality, 60,* 441–476.

Watson, D., Clark, L. A., & Tellegen, A. (1988). Development and validation of brief measures of positive and negative affect: The PANAS scales. *Journal of Personality and Social Psychology, 54,* 1063–1070.

White, J. M. (1992). Marital status and well-being in Canada. *Journal of Family Issues, 13,* 390–409.

Witter, R. A., Okun, M. A., Stock, W. A., & Haring, M. J. (1984). Education and subjective well-being: A meta-analysis. *Education Evaluation and Policy Analysis, 6,* 165–173.

Witter, R. A., Stock, W. A., Okun, M. A., & Haring, M. J. (1985). Religion and subjective well-being in adulthood: A quantitative synthesis. *Review of Religious Research, 26,* 332–342.

Zelman, D. C., Howland, E. W., Nichols, S. N., & Cleeland, C. S. (1991). The effects of induced mood on laboratory pain. *Pain, 46,* 105–111.

CHAPTER 11

■ ● ▲ ◆ ■ ● ▲ ◆

Depression

PATRICK H. FINAN
HOWARD TENNEN
ALEX J. ZAUTRA

Psychological theories of depression have broadened our understanding of the various situational contexts and individual vulnerabilities that appear to precipitate depressive episodes. Yet the factors involved in the development of depression and its maintenance long after the original impetus has passed are a source of continued debate. As we discuss in this chapter, research has been able to pinpoint certain attributional styles, environmental contexts, and physical conditions that give rise to depressive symptoms. Despite these advances, the primary conundrum of research on depression remains the pursuit of explanations of why depression initially develops, why it continues for some, and why others are resilient in the face of life stress.

A key issue in the psychological literature on depression is its operationalization in research studies, the methods available for measuring depression, and how these measurement approaches have been implemented in empirical studies. We begin this chapter, then, by presenting an overview of the methods found to be most useful in identifying and diagnosing depression. Next, we highlight several of the most prominent psychological theories of depression that, we hope, capture the essence of how depression both differentiates people and, in turn, is differentiated by social, cognitive, and psy-

chophysiological factors. Finally, we discuss recent research on resilience factors that distinguish people with little to no history of depression from individuals who become recurrently or chronically depressed.

Measuring Depression

Two of the most widely used types of depression measures are diagnostic classification measures and depressive symptom severity scales (Nezu, Nezu, McClure, & Zwick, 2002). Measures used for diagnostic classification involve semistructured or structured diagnostic interviews. The three most widely used diagnostic interviews are the Schedule for Affective Disorders and Schizophrenia (SADS; Endicott & Spitzer, 1978), the Diagnostic Interview Schedule—IV (DIS-IV; Compton & Cottler, 2004) and the Structured Clinical Interview for DSM-IV: Axis I Disorders (SCID-I; First, Spitzer, Gibbon, & Williams, 1997). Although time-intensive, these interview-based assessments, when applied to depression, offer the investigator the opportunity to obtain a diagnosis of major depression (including subtypes), minor depression, and dysthymic disorder consistent with the *Diagnostic and Statistical Manual of Mental Disorders* (DSM-IV; American Psychiatric Association, 2000).

A long-standing controversy in the psychology literature is whether depression severity scales are adequate in identifying individuals who are then classified as "depressed." Although depression severity scales continue to be widely used in social psychological studies of depression, critics of this approach have argued that clinician- (or highly trained interviewer-) administered structured diagnostic interviews establish diagnoses reliably (Pepper & Nieuwsma, 2006). This argument is based on evidence suggesting that such interviews distinguish symptoms of depression from symptoms resulting from physical illness, medications, drug or alcohol use, or bereavement (Tennen, Hall, & Affleck, 1995) and that the items on most depression severity scales capture global psychological distress (Coyne, 1994) or general psychopathology (Gotlib, 1984; but see Flett, Vredenburg, & Krames, 1997) rather than depression per se. Several authors have suggested combining structured interviews and symptom severity measures (e.g., Joiner, Walker, Pettit, Perez, & Cukrowicz, 2005), though in the psychological literature this is the exception rather than the rule.

Santor, Gregus, and Welch (2006) identified more than 280 published depression diagnosis and severity scales. Remarkably, only a handful of these measures—the Beck Depression Inventory (BDI-II; Beck, Steer, & Brown, 1996), Center for Epidemiologic Studies of Depression Scale (CES-D; Radloff, 1977), Montgomery–Asberg Depression Rating Scale (MADRS; Montgomery & Asberg, 1979), Hamilton Rating Scale for Depression (HRSD; Hamilton, 1960) and the Depression subscale of the Symptom Checklist—90R (SCL-90R D-scale; Derogatis, 1977) have appeared in the literature sufficiently often to be mentioned explicitly in Santor et al's review. Three other equally remarkable conclusions can be derived from this review. First, one of the two most widely used measures, the HRSD, is rarely seen in the vast social-psychological literature on depression. Second, the two most widely used measures, the HRSD and the BDI, share only 25–50% of their variance (varying across studies). Third, two of the five most widely used measures, the HRSD and the CES-D, differ from measures in general in *all* of the domains assessed, including mood, concentration, and behavioral, somatic, and

cognitive symptoms. That different depression measures seem to tap different aspects of depression is a problem in its own right. This problem is complicated further by the fact that different samples endorse different types of depression symptoms (Pepper & Nieuwsma, 2006), and these differences cannot be explained by varying symptom levels across samples (Santor & Coyne, 2001). Depression severity measures designed for certain age groups, such as the Children's Depression Inventory (CDI; Kovacs, 1992) and the Geriatric Depression Scale (Yesavage et al., 1983), have comparable problems.

Nearly all depression severity scales were developed using classical test theory. A recent exception is Watson and colleagues' Inventory of Depression and Anxiety Symptoms (IDAS; 2007), which is based on modern psychometric principles and appears to capture various dimensions of depressive symptoms across samples. However, as documented by Santor and colleagues (2006) (see also Simms, 2006), *all* of the most widely used depression severity measures were developed more than 25 years ago, and new measures are employed only rarely, with investigators relying nearly exclusively on the usual suspects.

In response to the publication of DSM-III and DSM-IV, the BDI-II (Beck et al., 1996), the Inventory to Diagnose Depression (IDD; Zimmerman & Coryell, 1987), the Hamilton Depression Inventory (HDI; Reynolds & Kobak, 1998), and, more recently, the Inventory of Depressive Symptomatology (IDS; Rush, Carmody & Reimitz, 2000) have been developed to be consistent with DSM criteria for major depression. These and comparable measures are now being endorsed frequently for use in clinical trials (e.g., Thase, 2007). Remarkably, despite their content correspondence to DSM criteria, these measures, with the exception of the BDI, are employed relatively rarely in basic science depression studies (Santor et al., 2006). Moreover, many investigators who use the BDI continue to rely on the original version that is not tied to DSM-IV (Nezu et al., 2002).

Subclinical Depression

Although several recent depression severity scales have been developed or revised so as to capture DSM-IV symptoms of major depression, most investigators use depression severity scales to study some aspect of subclinical depression, which is a "state in which depressive symptoms are present, but with too few symptoms or symptoms with insufficient severity to warrant a diagnosis of major depressive episode" (Ingram & Siegle, 2002). Tennen, Eberhart, and Affleck (1999) reviewed a wide-ranging literature to demonstrate that subclinical depression—and its assessment with depression severity scales—predicts morbidity, mortality, and health service utilization. Since Tennen and colleagues' review, converging evidence reveals that depressive symptoms anticipate the development of heart disease, and even minimal depressive symptoms appear to increase mortality risk after a myocardial infarction (see Stanton, Revenson, & Tennen, 2007). The limitations of these scales notwithstanding, there is thus good reason to continue to study subclinical depression using depression severity scales.

Depression History: An Area of Relative Neglect

Depression is typically a recurrent disorder, which means that many individuals with a current major depression have been depressed previously. Despite repeated calls for greater attention to the assessment of depression history, studies in the psychological literature—especially in personality and social psychology—have given depression history scant attention. Yet many research participants with subclinical depression have had a depressive episode in the preceding year (Shelbourne et al., 1994), and previously depressed individuals manifest coping vulnerabilities when compared with their never-depressed counterparts (Conner et al., 2006). Moreover, individuals with more than one previous depressive episode can be distinguished from those with only one previous episode in several areas of considerable interest to psychological investigators, including greater sleep disturbance, lower levels of perceived support, and more self-generated stressful life events (see Zautra, Parrish, et al., 2007). It is therefore disquieting that so few studies in the psychological literature have assessed depression history and that fewer still have addressed the difficulties associated with requiring research

participants to accurately recall the details of an episode of depression that may have occurred years before the assessment. We conclude our overview of depression measurement with a brief discussion of what is known about the recall of emotional experiences and implications for the assessment of depression.

Can People Accurately Recall Symptoms and Emotional Experiences?

Even if depression severity scales captured DSM symptoms with great precision and if these scales demonstrated perfect item overlap, they would still require research participants to recall their recent symptoms and emotional experiences. Tennen (2006) questioned whether people can, in fact, accurately recall their sadness, general satisfaction, guilt, sleep, and related symptoms over the previous week or two as required by both self-report and interview-administered depression measures. Extensive evidence demonstrates that people do not actually recall such experiences when asked to do so. Instead, they reconstruct their past experience by using implicit theories and various cognitive heuristics (Kahneman, 1999; Ross & Wilson, 2003). Robinson and Clore (2002) demonstrated that people provide very different answers depending on whether mood is assessed in real time or retrospectively. As Tennen notes, because belief-based recollections of emotional experience rely on narrative coherence, recalled emotional states—the currency of all structured diagnostic depression interviews and questionnaires—easily become dissociated from actual emotional experience (see Robinson & Clore, 2002). Overall, depression researchers have been lulled into concluding that because people are able to respond to their depression severity scales and interviews without difficulty, their responses are accurate reflections of recent experience. The social and personality psychology literature indicates that such conclusions may be misguided.

Cognitive Vulnerability to Depression

Perhaps the most dominant etiological conceptualization of depression today lies in diathesis–stress theory, in which the development of depression is precipitated by the activation of a dormant vulnerability by a stressor (Monroe & Simons, 1991). Years of research have been devoted to the identification of stressors (e.g., negative life events; Kessler, 1997), diatheses (e.g., cognitive vulnerability; Abramson, Metalsky, & Alloy, 1989), and the contexts in which the two interact (e.g., interpersonal interactions; Coyne & Wiffen, 1995). Beck (1967, 1987) provided a framework through which depression came to be viewed as a dysfunction in cognitive processing and, through this work, gave the diathesis–stress model traction as an explanatory tool for the development of depression (Monroe & Simons, 1991). Beck's theory asserts that for people who develop depression, a cognitive vulnerability imperceptible to the individual must have existed prior to the development of symptoms and that this vulnerability was necessary but not sufficient to bring about the onset of illness. For the pathogenesis of depression to commence, ultimately a negative event must activate the cognitive vulnerability by triggering what Beck (1967) termed a negative "self-schema." These negative schemas typically promote a cascade of dysfunctional thoughts about one's self-worth, the world, and the future, known collectively as the "negative cognitive triad." Beck contended that the cognitive processing that leads to the automatic depressogenic thoughts that constitute the negative cognitive triad is necessarily distorted and thus represents a key moment in the etiology of depression. Consequently, subsequent efforts by Beck (1976) and colleagues identified therapeutic methods to target changes in thought processes that, under the volition of the patient, could reverse some of the maladaptive automatic behaviors originally brought about by distorted cognition.

In a similar vein, Abramson and colleagues (1989) developed the hopelessness theory of depression in an effort to identify a specific cognitive vulnerability (i.e., hopelessness) that could account for the development of certain depressions. Hopelessness has been identified as a key factor in the exacerbation of suicidality among depressed patients (Beck, Kovacs, & Weissman, 1975; Minkoff, Bergman, Beck, & Beck, 1973). In accordance with the principles of the

diathesis–stress model, hopelessness theory holds that individual differences in cognitive and attributional style determine how people respond to negative life events (Abramson et al., 2002). Specifically, hopelessness and depression arise when attributions for negative events imply that the cause of the event is stable over time, global in its influence, a forebearer of future negative events, and indicative of a personal flaw (Abramson et al., 1989). Abramson and colleagues' (2002) negative cognitive style can be considered akin to Beck's negative cognitive schema in that they are both considered necessary precursors to the development of depression and, when combined with negative life events, often produce that outcome. In the absence of negative events, the mere possession of a cognitive vulnerability is insufficient to bring about depressive symptoms (Abramson et al., 2002). Rather, it is the interaction of distorted cognition with a sufficiently negative occurrence that proves affectively toxic for the vulnerable individual.

Critics of the cognitive vulnerability approach to understanding depression have been skeptical that the mechanisms by which dysfunctional cognition is proposed to causally precede the development of depression truly represent the clinical etiology of depression (Coyne & Gotlib, 1983). For example, many studies proposed to have provided validation for hopelessness theory have been criticized for using subclinical populations and retrospective designs while drawing inferences about a feed-forward pathway of diatheses, stressors, and clinical outcomes (for review, see Henkel, Bussfeld, Moller, & Hegerl, 2002). Researchers, however, have responded to the critics' call for more rigorous designs by implementing the behavioral high-risk design (Abramson et al., 2002). Such a prospective design allows depressive symptoms or disorders that develop in the sample throughout the time course of the study to be attributed to trait factors measured earlier. Indeed, prospective studies have collectively provided the most compelling evidence for a cognitive vulnerability to depression (Abramson et al., 2002)

Although the Beck and hopelessness theories of depression are considered the "gold standard" when it comes to delineating specific attributional styles and cognitive distortions that lead to depressive symptoms, they leave room for speculation regarding why some people display symptoms of depression yet remain free of clinical illness, why some people experience major depression yet are able to rebound and live largely depression-free, and why others develop a depressive episode and are catapulted into a lifelong cycle of chronic and recurrent depression. Additionally, these theories are largely silent on the extent to which varying levels of life stress affect the development of both first-onset and recurrent depression. Understanding the various profiles of stable beliefs that make up a cognitive vulnerability is a necessary first step in the conceptualization of depression, but individual differences in the ability to respond to stress requires a life-stress perspective, as well.

Life Stress in the Development and Maintenance of Depression

Making the claim that life stress influences the development of depression requires an explanation of the meaning of the term *life stress*. Life stress typically applies to single events and/or accumulated disruptions that severely tax an individual's coping resources. The severity of a stressful event also contributes to variability in how individuals respond to it (Brown & Harris, 1989). A review by Mazure (1998) concluded that stressful experiences classified as major and undesirable life events are reliably associated with onset of major depression. Events that involve the loss of a loved one and events that are perceived as uncontrollable by the individual are indeed more prevalent among clinical populations (Mazure, 1998). Within depressed populations, individuals who have experienced a high number of severe life-stress events exhibit more intense depressive symptoms than depressed patients with relatively few severe negative life experiences (Monroe & Hadjiyannakis, 2002).

Chronic stressors are conceptually different from major life stressors in the ways in which they are thought to affect the individual and contribute to the development of depressive symptoms. Chronic stress takes many forms, including caring for a sick or disabled loved one, having a chronic medical illness oneself, living in poverty, or undergoing marital strife (Hammen, 2005). The etiological connection of chronic stress to depression, however, is unclear. Some evidence implicates chronic stressors, such as financial strains and loss of social support, as mediators in the pathway from major life events to depression (Kessler, 1997). However, inconsistencies in the operationalization of chronic stress and methodological difficulties in the identification of the temporal location of chronic stress in the causal chain that produces depression have led major reviews to conclude that the precise role of chronic stress in depression remains ambiguous (Hammen, 2005; Kessler, 1997). Chronic pain represents a primary target for research on the relation of chronic stress to depression in that it provides a context in which stressful daily life events can exacerbate both the perception of pain associated with a pain condition and the affective state reported by the individual. Furthermore, chronic pain itself can be considered a constant threat. Conditions such as fibromyalgia (FM) and rheumatoid arthritis (RA) are commonly associated with the onset and maintenance of depression (Dickens, McGowan, Clark-Carter, & Creed, 2002), as individuals with these disorders often endure uncertainties in medical diagnoses, erosion of social resources, and deterioration of physical capabilities. Loss of control and personal mastery are commonly reported in these patient populations as factors leading to dysfunction in affective regulation (Reich, Johnson, Zautra, & Davis, 2006).

Intensive repeated-measure designs have examined pain, stress, and mood relations in chronic pain populations without concern for the inferential bias typically produced by aggregate analysis, in which extremely painful or extremely stressful days can skew the overall effect size. In a study of patients with RA, Zautra and Smith (2001) found that elevated levels of weekly stress and weekly negative life events, as well as greater stress reactivity, resulted in elevated weekly depressive symptoms.

These results tell us that chronic stressors that challenge the individual's adaptive capacity to respond to physical, psychological, and social threats on a daily basis evidence a link to depressive symptoms. We do not know, however, what levels and duration of chronic stress are required to initiate a bout of major depression. Furthermore, there is much to learn regarding the interaction of major life events and minor everyday stressors in predicting the onset and maintenance of depression. For example, Zautra, Schultz, and Reich (2000) found that the type of major life stressor one experiences differentially affects the influence of small life events on depression. In this study, small undesirable events served to maintain depressive symptoms for older adults who had recently become disabled, but not for older adults who had recently grieved the loss of a spouse. Clearly, future efforts to identify specific types of stressors and how they interact with each other would produce dividends, not only for the clinical understanding of targets for cognitive-behavioral treatment of depression but also for the social-psychological understanding of depression as a variable that identifies individual differences in adaptive capacity.

The diathesis–stress model provides a parsimonious account of how the loss of a parent can send one sibling with a global and stable attributional style into a major depression whereas another sibling lacking an attributional risk profile can endure the loss without a significant detriment to his or her affective-regulatory abilities. But life is rarely as simple and deterministic as an interaction between a cognitive profile and a major adverse event. Chronic stressors, such as chronic illness or social isolation (Symister & Friend, 2003), provide an additional burden on individuals both with and without cognitive vulnerabilities to depression. So it should be expected that they are associated with depressive states. The manner in which this association manifests itself is up for debate. McEwen (1998) introduced the concept of allostatic load to describe the neurobiological phenomenon of hormonal and cognitive dysregulation that results after prolonged exposure to a variety of stressors. The catch-22 of allostasis, or the maintenance of homeostasis through change, is that the hormones (e.g., glucocorticoids) employed for short-term benefit that aid the body in adaptation often have deleterious consequences if they are overused and constantly needed to combat a chronic stressor. Although this topic remains controversial, it highlights the need to study prospectively the propensity of chronic stressors, accumulated over time, to contribute to the development of depression. Behavioral high-risk designs similar to those employed by cognitive vulnerability researchers should be adapted for prospective studies of chronic stressors, with individuals separated into groups according to their exposure to chronic stressors and followed longitudinally to determine whether there is variability by group in the incidence of depression. Such designs would serve to clarify the role of chronic stress in the time course and maintenance of depression where existing diathesis–stress theories fail.

Depression in the Development and Maintenance of Life Stress

Thus far, we have introduced the concepts of cognitive vulnerabilities and life stress and discussed how their interaction provides fertile ground for the development of depression. We now shift gears to discuss how depression itself is implicated in the generation of life stress. The bidirectional relationship between stress and depression has major implications for the methodology associated with diathesis–stress models. Consider this example: A researcher proposes a simple hypothesis that a hopeless attributional style interacts with work stress to produce depression. A longitudinal design is implemented to test this hypothesis, in which individuals are identified at Time 1 as having a hopeless disposition and report at Time 2 levels of depressive symptoms. Between Time 1 and Time 2, participants report the prevalence of work stress. If hopelessness and work stress interact to predict depressive symptoms at Time 2, and if work stress does not predict depressive symptoms alone, the researcher may feel confident concluding that work stress activated the latent construct of hopelessness to produce depressive symptoms. Depending on the analysis, the researcher may go so far as to conclude that as work stress increases, so, too, does the likelihood of onset of depressive symptoms.

Research on stress generation tells us to be more cautious with our design and interpretation of effects when measuring stress and depression. Specifically, the investigator's design fails to take into account the influence depressive symptoms may have had between Time 1 and Time 2 in generating work stress. A pre–post prediction of depression from the interaction of a dispositional cognitive vulnerability and a prospective experience with multiple stressors must take into account when, specifically, depression started and how, if at all, it influenced the generation of additional stressors that may have contributed to its maintenance over time.

Hammen (1991) proposed that depressed people often provoke stressful events by their own actions and reactions to everyday life problems. Interpersonal difficulties are common in the lives of depressed individuals and are typically associated with negative appraisals of others and critical opinions about themselves. Although these negative appraisals may be a result of depressive biases in interpersonal perception, just as frequently they reflect an accurate judgment of the exasperated response of a relationship partner. States of mind commonly found in the midst of depression, such as self-loathing and fatalism, negatively influence the quality of existing relationships by inciting both avoidance and overtly negative confrontation from friends, family, and coworkers (Joiner, 2002). Findings in support of the stress-generation hypothesis have been reported for community samples (Daley et al., 1997), including both men and women (Joiner, Wingate, Gencoz, & Gencoz, 2005), and these adverse effects appear to be even greater when depression coexists with other disorders, such as anxiety (Daley et al., 1997).

A prospective study by Safford, Alloy, Abramson, and Crossfield (2007) calls into question the temporal parameters within which depression contributes to stress generation. Undergraduates with a prior history of depression did not report more stressful events over a 6-month period than their never-depressed counterparts. In this study, however, stress reports were, on average, several years removed from any previous depressive episode. The authors speculate that the dysphoria of a recent depressive episode, rather than the presence of depression history per se, may account for the generation of stress that has typically been associated with depression history. Furthermore, Safford and colleagues found that although past depression did not predict future stressful experiences, cognitive vulnerability to hopelessness did. This finding comes on the heels of a report by Joiner and colleagues (2005)

that hopelessness mediates the prediction of stressful events from depression. Taken together, these findings add to the complex mural of the diathesis–stress approach to understanding depression by emphasizing that cognitive style, stress, and depression interact in myriad ways that depend on factors such as type of cognitive vulnerability, type of stressor, timing of stressor, and timing of depression. Clearly, the literature on stress generation highlights the need to consider the types of stressful events that occur during or following depression as meaningful indicators of peripheral factors such as personality type, social context, and comorbidity.

Interpersonal Antecedents of Depression

As mentioned earlier, interpersonal life stress is a particularly potent trigger of depressive episodes. Indeed, the roots of cognitive theories of depression contain interpersonal elements (i.e., negative cognitive schemas about the world). Individual perceptions of the quality of relationships with others can influence one's mood. For example, when there is a discrepancy between an individual's notion of an ideal interpersonal relationship and the actual state of that relationship, the individual may lose motivation to pursue self-regulatory goals, such as the promotion of positive interpersonal relations and the prevention of harm. When such a failure in self-regulation becomes chronic, vulnerability to depression may increase substantially (Strauman, 2002). Research on peer rejection has shown that adolescents who have been rejected or ostracized by their peers are more likely to report depressive symptoms than their socially integrated counterparts (Patterson & Stoolmiller, 1991). Moreover, some studies have shown that peer-rejected adolescents are at greater risk for future clinical depression diagnoses (Lewinsohn, Hops, Roberts, Seeley, & Andrews, 1993; Windle, 1992). Peer rejection appears to be more influential for adolescents than adults and is particularly influential for adolescent girls (Stice, Ragan, & Randall, 2004). As Hammen (2003) notes, "These years of emerging adulthood are fraught with challenges and stressors, and they mark a period during which young women in effect create the environments with which they will interact for years to come. For many young women these environments are depression-inducing, and contribute to a social context in which depression and stress influence each other in a dismally recurring pattern" (p. 49).

The parent–child relationship has been consistently associated with children's subsequent vulnerability to depression. Brown and his colleagues (Bifulco, Brown, & Harris, 1987; Brown, Harris, & Copeland, 1977) have demonstrated the significance of parental loss in the development of depression. Specifically, they have shown that (1) parental loss is a stronger predictor of future depression when the deceased parent is the mother; (2) girls are disproportionately vulnerable to future depression after enduring the loss of a mother; and (3) the quality of parental care following the loss of one parent may mediate the subsequent development of depression postloss.

Goodman and Gotlib (1999) concluded that breakdowns in communication between parent and child, as well as the transmission of negative cognitions through maladaptive behaviors in depressed mothers, both serve as significant predictors of future depression among adolescents. The intimate social dynamic between a depressed mother and child, in which negative cognitions shared by each party can create and maintain communication problems, further elevate a child's risk for depression (Hammen, 2003; Hammen, Burge, & Adrian, 1991). In the absence of parental support, through either the parent's death or his or her emotional unavailability, the child's coping resources are threatened, just as they are among adults who lack adequate social support (Coyne & DeLongis, 1986). The antecedents of depression are thus closely tied to the dynamics of social relationships. Indeed, a critical task for studies of depression vulnerabilities and precipitants is the distinction between interpersonal and noninterpersonal forms of life stress.

Depression History: Past Events as Kindling

If depression and a depressogenic style contribute to the generation of new stressors, and if stressors contribute to the onset of depression, it follows that new depressive episodes are likely to arise from previous episodes. The numbers support this assumption, with a significant proportion of people who have experienced a depressive episode reporting at least one more in the future (American Psychiatric Association, 2000; Rao, Hammen, & Daley, 1999). Thus a therapist's work is rarely complete when a client is in remission from depression. The cognitive vulnerability model provides only a partial explanation of why people continue to experience episodes of depression: A high-risk cognitive style is stable over time, and major adverse life events, such as loss and trauma, are bound to happen more than once in an individual's lifetime. According to the cognitive vulnerability model, then, each interaction of a major adverse life event with a stable latent cognitive vulnerability should be just as likely to produce a depressive episode as the initial depression-producing interaction. Yet we know that the likelihood of experiencing a new depressive episode increases as the number of past episodes experienced increases.

The differential activation hypothesis (Teasdale, 1983) provides an alternative conceptualization of vulnerability to recurrent depression. In this view, dysfunctional thinking akin to the cognitive distortions described by Beck (1987) interacts with dysphoric mood to produce depression. Individuals who have already experienced depression are hypothesized to be at greater risk for new onsets of depression than those who have never had a depressive episode, because they are more prone to heightened dysfunctional thinking and, consequently, dysphoric mood (Teasdale, 1983). Recent studies support the differential activation hypothesis with prospective designs demonstrating increased risk of major depression among people with a history of depression identified as high risk according to Teasdale's criteria (Lewinsohn, Allen, Seeley, & Gotlib, 1999).

The role of stressful events in provoking depression may change as a consequence of repeated episodes. Post (1992) proposed the kindling hypothesis, which contends that life stressors play a less important role in the onset of recurrent depression than they do in the onset of first-episode depression. As stressors become less influential in the onset of recurrent depression, biological factors may become more influential. Mazure (1998) found mixed support for the kindling hypothesis and cautiously concluded that the phenomenon appears to be real for people with unipolar depression but not for those with bipolar depression. Monroe and Harkness (2005) provide less equivocal evidence that the association of life stress and depression diminishes as a function of episode recurrence. In their review of eight empirical studies testing the kindling hypothesis for unipolar depression, they concluded that the presence of depression history contributes to a *changed*, but not necessarily a weakened, relationship between life stressors and prospective onset of recurrent depression, independent of any person or environmental factors that may exist.

According to Monroe and Harkness (2005), the interpretations made to date from empirical tests of the kindling hypothesis have largely taken the view of "stress autonomy," stipulating that the effects observed occurred as a result of recurrent depression growing increasingly autonomous from life stressors. In the place of stress, it is presumed that a "quasi-independent process" (p. 427), perhaps biological and endogenous, assumes the role of depression provocateur. Monroe and Harkness offer instead a "stress sensitization" explanation. In this framework, chronically depressed people, rather than becoming less reactive to life stress, become increasingly sensitive to the effects of stress, such that even minor stressors (not typically measured in the study of life stress) are capable of provoking a depressive episode. For the stress-sensitized individual, the impact of both major and minor life events on the experience of the depressive episode increases. However, due to the increase in the likelihood of minor life events to precipitate depression, major life events will be associated with recurrent episodes of depression with a reduced frequency. Thus, the stress-sensitized individual will continue to detect stressors at a similar rate, but with each new depression, minor stressors have increasingly greater impact.

Implications of Depression History for Chronic Pain

Depression history is of particular interest in the study of chronic pain. Depression and chronic pain have been well documented as concomitant disorders (Romano & Turner,

1985). Conceptualizing pain as both a physical and psychosocial stressor, it becomes clear that chronic pain, like life stress, is not an epiphenomenon secondary to depression but an interactive participant in the development and maintenance of depression. Romano and Turner (1985) provided a sweeping review of the literature on the relationship of chronic pain and depression and concluded that the available data at the time did not support a single, unifying etiological pathway for pain and depression. Subsequent research has validated their interpretation by revealing a mutually influential relationship between pain and depression (Williamson & Schulz, 1992). Not until recently, however, have researchers begun to question the relation of depression history to the experience of chronic pain. Due to the sensitivity of certain pain-related syndromes, such as rheumatoid arthritis (RA) and fibromyalgia syndrome (FMS), to psychosocial influences, there is a strong clinical imperative that the lingering residual mood effects, changes in social support dynamics, and adjustments in coping strategies associated with prior depressive episodes be explored—even, perhaps especially, among individuals who are not currently reporting depressive symptoms.

A recent series of studies have attempted to evaluate how a history of depression affects the experience of pain, and vice versa. Fifield, Tennen, Reisine, and McQuillan (1998) provided the first account of how a previous depression could residually affect current pain ratings in patients with RA under current mood-priming conditions (i.e., dysphoria). Using DSM-III-R (American Psychiatric Association, 1987) criteria, they found that patients who were not currently depressed but had experienced at least one past episode of depression *and* had reported elevated current dysphoria reported more severe pain than both patients with RA who had a history of depression but were not experiencing elevated negative mood and never-depressed individuals who were currently dysphoric. It seems that the residual effects of previous depressive episodes act as a latent vulnerability (Lewinsohn, Hoberman, & Rosenbaum, 1989) that can be primed under certain circumstances, such as dysphoric mood, and exacerbate pain levels in the absence of current depression. This finding speaks to the importance of identifying a variety of physical and psychosocial stressors that can be used to extend previous research on the multifarious manifestations of depression. Hammen and colleagues' (1991) work on stress generation may offer clues regarding what in the experience of a prior depression contributes to a greater susceptibility to current pain.

In an effort to extend the work of Fifield and colleagues (1998), Tennen, Affleck, and Zautra (2006) utilized an electronic diary method and daily process analysis to reveal both between- and within-person relations of depression history and pain. In a sample of women with FMS, participants who had experienced at least one previous episode of major depression but were not currently depressed reported increases in emotion-focused coping and decreases in perceived coping efficacy on high-pain days. Additionally, current depressive symptoms moderated the relation between daily pain and pleasant mood for the formerly depressed, such that higher levels of daily depressive symptoms resulted in a reduction in pleasant mood on high-pain days. The pleasant mood of participants who had never been depressed was not affected by depressive symptoms on high-pain days. Again we see evidence for a priming effect, whereby maladaptive coping strategies are stoked when depressive symptoms prime a latent vulnerability conferred by past depression status. In a similar daily process study with patients with RA, Conner and colleagues (2006) found that depression history was associated with greater reactivity to daily pain, as well as with the employment of more emotion-based pain coping strategies when problem-focused strategies might have been appropriate. Depression history, even episodes that occurred years earlier, seems to narrow the field of coping resources that are crucial to successful navigation of high-pain days when they occur throughout the course of chronic illness.

The studies just described operationalized depression history as an all-or-nothing phenomenon in which group assignment did not differ depending on whether a person had one prior depressive episode or several. There is evidence, however, that individuals with recurrent, multiple-episode depression exhibit unique cognitive and behavioral deficits (Basso & Bornstein, 1999) and increased stress reactivity (i.e., "kindling"; Post, 1992)

compared with individuals who have experienced only a single episode. To that end, Zautra, Parrish, and colleagues (2007) found that recurrently depressed patients with RA reported higher levels of pain than never-depressed patients and those who had experienced only a single episode. Perhaps more important, increases in perceived stress *and* pain and decreases in positive affect in response to an experimentally induced interpersonal stressor were greater among the recurrently depressed than among the never- or once-depressed patients with RA. Providing further support for the notion that recurrent depression is implicated in the emotion-regulation abilities of people with chronic pain, Zautra, Davis, and colleagues (2007) found that a mindfulness-based emotion-regulation intervention resulted in decreased daily negative affect and increased daily positive affect and decreased physician-assessed tenderness and swelling among patients with RA with two or more prior episodes of depression compared with those with one or no prior depressive episodes.

Taken together, these studies provide several key insights regarding depression's influence on the experience of chronic pain. First, they show that depression history negatively affects people's subsequent pain and perceived stress and does so in the absence of current depression diagnosis (Zautra, Parrish, et al., 2007). However, current dysphoric mood may serve as a moderator in this relationship (Fifield et al., 1998). Second, they show that depression history may serve as a latent vulnerability to maladaptive coping strategies and poor affective regulation when adaptive regulatory abilities are needed most: in the face of high levels of pain (Conner et al., 2006; Tennen et al., 2006). Finally, they reveal the importance of distinguishing between recurrent, multiple-episode depression and single-episode depression when evaluating the emotion-regulatory capacities and stress reactivity of people with a chronic pain condition (Zautra, Davis, et al., 2007; Zautra, Parrish, et al., 2007). Critics of the depression history perspective might argue that the vulnerability to pain, stress, and affective regulation conferred by a past history of the illness could instead be explained by factors that actually predate the onset of the first depressive episode. The studies just described, however, are well suited to answer such a critique, as they avoid confounding depression history with a preexisting vulnerability by controlling for such "nuisance" variables as neuroticism.

Chronicity may reflect differences in the resources available to the person to ward off future bouts of depression. It may also reflect qualitative differences in the type of depression and/or in the nature of genetic contributions to the onset of and recovery from an episode. Individual differences in resilience, to which we now turn, may also contribute to depression recurrence vulnerability.

Finding Resilience on the Road from Risk to Depression

Thus far in this chapter, we have highlighted social, cognitive, and psychophysiological research on the vulnerability to and development of depression. In focusing on vulnerability, we have omitted a discussion of resilience. Indeed, until recently, most research in this area has focused on vulnerability and pathology. However, the field has now begun to pay attention to the other side of the coin, and so, too, do we in concluding this chapter. Now, the question is being asked, "What makes an individual resilient?" There are several intriguing new findings in the literature on resilience to depression but at this point no clear conclusions.

As we have noted, the literature has identified the occurrence of a major adverse life event as a primary culprit in the onset of depression. Yet nearly every living person will at some point encounter what, by common standards, is a major adverse event. Often, this is the death of a close loved one. Less often, it is a traumatic event related to war, assault, or sexual abuse. Despite this, most people are able to navigate their way through life without experiencing the disabling effects of chronic depression (Masten, 2001).

Resilience is often discussed in terms of either the outcomes associated with it or the trajectories it assumes. Regarding outcomes, some theorists have defined resilience as the absence of psychopathological symptoms and the situations in which those symptoms are fostered (Conrad & Hammen, 1993; Haeffel & Grigorenko, 2007). An alternative conceptualization incorporates both the absence of psychopathology and the pres-

ence of positive resources that can be used to combat major and daily stressors. Regarding trajectories, one prominent conceptualization of the etiological path that resilience takes is that of recovery, whereby an individual "bounces back" or "rebounds" from a decrease in functioning following an aversive event (Tugade, Fredrickson, & Feldman-Barrett, 2004). Bonanno (2004) defines resilience as "the ability of adults in otherwise normal circumstances who are exposed to an isolated and potentially highly disruptive event ... to maintain relatively stable, healthy levels of psychological and physical functioning ... as well as the capacity for generative experiences and positive emotions" (pp. 20–21). For Bonanno, resilience is distinguished from a trajectory of recovery in that resilient individuals never experience clinically significant emotional disruptions throughout the process of coping with an adverse event. With these definitions in mind, we examine evidence related to the trajectory of resilience following a major adverse event and the personal resources that have been linked to resilience in relation to depression.

Longitudinal and prospective findings now offer evidence for the prevalence of distinct grieving trajectories, including a resilient trajectory, following loss. In a longitudinal study following bereaved spouses 18 months after the loss, a resilient pattern of bereavement, in which the bereaved spouse experienced only minor perturbations in depressive symptoms over time, was the predominant bereavement pattern observed (Bonanno et al., 2002). This resilience to depression pattern is in stark contrast to the inevitability of depression postulated in stage theories of loss and grief (e.g., Maciejewski, Zhang, Block, & Prigerson, 2007). The resilient response was observed more frequently than either a chronic grief response or a pattern of depression followed by recovery. Bonanno, Moskowitz, Papa, and Folkman (2005) replicated this dominant resilient pattern of responding to loss and extended the explanatory power of a resilient trajectory in showing that even HIV-positive caregivers who carried with them the burden of an incurable illness were highly resilient in the months following the loss of a partner to AIDS. Longitudinal studies such as these provide convincing evidence for the prevalence of resilient coping. In our work examining resilience in everyday life, we have found evidence that daily positive interpersonal experiences fortify patients with chronic pain by reducing their negative affective reactions to episodic pain and everyday interpersonal stress (Zautra, Johnson, & Davis, 2005). Ong, Bergeman, Bisconti, and Wallace (2006) have investigated the role of resilience resources in the daily lives of older adults. These resilient responses in daily life and the resilient responses identified by Bonanno and colleagues warrant further examination. Although Bonanno and colleagues were able to replicate their obtained prevalence rates for resilient bereavement, a recent study using a hierarchical clustering analytic technique to identify bereavement patterns, rather than a priori theoretical identification, discovered that among bereaved spouses, a trajectory of depression followed by recovery occurred with greater frequency than a trajectory of resilience (Ott, Lueger, Kelber, & Prigerson, 2007).

What promotes the resilience that protects some people from risk of depression? Laughter, positive emotional disclosure, problem-focused coping, optimism, and positive affect have all been linked to better physical and psychological health among people at risk for negative health outcomes (Tugade et al., 2004). For example, caregivers of recently deceased AIDS patients who express positive emotion more than negative emotion for up to a year after the loss report fewer depressive symptoms than caregivers with a propensity for negative emotional expression (Stein, Folkman, Trabasso, & Richards, 1997). In addition to positive emotional expression, sense making and benefit finding have been identified as two key resources thought to confer resilience in response to loss or trauma. In a longitudinal study of bereaved spouses, making sense of a loss conferred less distress at 1 year after the loss, and construing some personal benefit from the loss resulted in less distress, including fewer depressive symptoms, 18 months after the loss (Davis, Nolen-Hoeksema, & Larson, 1998).

The field, it seems, is moving toward a fuller understanding of depression through the exploration of psychological markers of resilience. In this effort, we hope to grow beyond our knowledge of the pathological im-plications of depression to learn how people adapt in the face of stress. Such an undertaking can only serve to benefit and inform the parallel exploration of dysfunction in the course of depression.

References

Abramson, L. Y., Alloy, L. B., Hankin, B. L., Haeffel, G. J., MacCoon, D. G., & Gibb, B. E. (2002). Cognitive vulnerability–stress models of depression in a self-regulatory and sociobiological context. In I. H. Gotlib & C. L. Hammen (Eds.), Handbook of depression (pp. 268–294). New York: Guilford Press.

Abramson, L. Y., Metalsky, G. I., & Alloy, L. B. (1989). Hopelessness depression: A theory-based subtype of depression. Psychological Review, 96, 358–372.

American Psychiatric Association. (1987). Diagnostic and statistical manual of mental disorders (3rd ed., text rev.). Washington, DC: Author.

American Psychiatric Association. (2000). Diagnostic and statistical manual of mental disorders (4th ed., text rev.). Washington, DC: Author.

Basso, M. R., & Bornstein, R. A. (1999). Relative memory deficits in recurrent versus first-episode depression on a word-list learning task. Neuropsychology, 13, 557–563.

Beck, A. T. (1967). Depression: Causes and treatment. Philadelphia: University of Pennsylvania Press.

Beck, A. T. (1976). Cognitive therapy and the emotional disorders. New York: International Universities Press.

Beck, A. T. (1987). Cognitive models of depression. Journal of Cognitive Psychotherapy: An International Quarterly, 1, 5–37.

Beck, A. T., Kovacs, M., & Weissman, A. (1975). Hopelessness and suicidal behavior: An overview. Journal of the American Medical Association, 234, 1146–1149.

Beck, A. T., Steer, R. A., & Brown, G. K. (1996). Manual for the Beck Depression Inventory: II. San Antonio, TX: Psychological Corporation.

Bifulco, A. T., Brown, G. W., & Harris, T. O. (1987). Childhood loss of parent, lack of adequate parental care and adult depression: A replication. Journal of Affective Disorders, 12, 115–128.

Bonanno, G. (2004). Loss, trauma, and human resilience. American Psychologist, 59, 20–28.

Bonanno, G. A., Moskowitz, J. T., Papa, A., & Folkman, S. (2005). Resilience to loss in bereaved spouses, bereaved parents, and bereaved gay men. Journal of Personality and Social Psychology, 88, 827–843.

Bonanno, G. A., Wortman, C. B., Lehman, D. R., Tweed, R. G., Haring, M., Sonnega, J., et al. (2002). Resilience to loss and chronic grief: A prospective study from preloss to 18 months' postloss. Journal of Personality and Social Psychology, 83, 1150–1164.

Brown, G. W., & Harris, T. O. (1989). Life events and illness. New York: Guilford Press.

Brown, G. W., Harris, T. O., & Copeland, J. (1977). Depression and loss. British Journal of Psychiatry, 130, 1–18.

Compton, W. M., & Cottler, L. B. (2004). The Diagnostic Interview Schedule (DIS). In M. J. Hilsenroth & D. L. Segal (Eds.), *The comprehensive handbook of psychological assessment: Vol. 2. Personality assessment* (pp. 153–162). Hoboken, NJ: Wiley.

Conner, T. S., Tennen, H., Zautra, A. J., Affleck, G., Armeli, S., & Fifield, J. (2006). Coping with rheumatoid arthritis pain in daily life: Within-person analyses reveal hidden vulnerability for the formerly depressed. *Pain, 126,* 198–209.

Conrad, M., & Hammen, C. (1993). Protective and resource factors in high- and low-risk children: A comparison of unipolar, bipolar, medically ill, and normal mothers. *Development and Psychopathology, 5,* 593.

Coyne, J. C. (1994). Self-reported distress: Analog or ersatz depression? *Psychological Bulletin, 116,* 29–45.

Coyne, J. C., & DeLongis, A. (1986). Going beyond social support: The role of social relationships in adaptation. *Journal of Consulting and Clinical Psychology, 54,* 454–460.

Coyne, J. C., & Gotlib, I. H. (1983). The role of cognition in depression: A critical appraisal. *Psychological Bulletin, 94,* 472–505.

Coyne, J. C., & Wiffen, V. E. (1995). Issues in personality as diathesis for depression: The case of sociotropy–dependency and autonomy–self-criticism. *Psychological Bulletin, 118,* 358–378.

Daley, S. E., Hammen, C., Burge, D., Davila, J., Paley, B., Lindberg, N., et al. (1997). Predictors of the generation of episodic stress: A longitudinal study of late adolescent women. *Journal of Abnormal Psychology, 106*(2), 251–259.

Davis, C. G., Nolen-Hoeksema, S., & Larson, J. (1998). Making sense of loss and benefiting from the experience: Two construals of meaning. *Journal of Personality and Social Psychology, 75,* 561–574.

Derogatis, L. R. (1977). *SCL-90-R: Administration, scoring, procedures. Manual I for the revised version.* Baltimore: John Hopkins University School of Medicine.

Dickens, C., McGowan, L., Clark-Carter, D., & Creed, F. (2002). Depression in rheumatoid arthritis: A systematic review of the literature with meta-analysis. *Psychosomatic Medicine, 64,* 52–60.

Endicott, J., & Spitzer, R. L. (1978). A diagnostic interview: The Schedule for Affective Disorders and Schizophrenia. *Archives of General Psychiatry, 35,* 237–244.

Fifield, J., Tennen, H., Reisine, S., & McQuillan, J. (1998). Depression and the long-term risk of pain, fatigue, and disability in patients with rheumatoid arthritis. *Arthritis and Rheumatism, 41,* 1851–1857.

First, M. B., Spitzer, R. L., Gibbon, M., & Williams, J. B. W. (1997). *Structured Clinical Interview for DSM-IV Axis I Disorders—Patient edition.* New York: New York State Psychiatric Institute.

Flett, G. L., Vredenburg, K., & Krames, L. (1997). The continuity of depression in clinical and nonclinical samples. *Psychological Bulletin, 121,* 395–416.

Goodman, S., & Gotlib, I. (1999). Risk for psychopathology in the children of depressed mothers: A developmental model for understanding mechanisms of transmission. *Psychological Review, 106,* 458–490.

Gotlib, I. H. (1984). Depression and general psychopathology in university students. *Journal of Abnormal Psychology, 93,* 19–30.

Haeffel, G. J., & Grigorenko, E. L. (2007). Cognitive vulnerability to depression: Exploring risk and resilience. *Child and Adolescent Psychiatric Clinics of North America, 16,* 435–448.

Hamilton, M. (1960). A rating scale for depression. *Journal of Neurology, Neurosurgery, and Psychiatry, 23,* 56–62.

Hammen, C. (1991). Generation of stress in the course of unipolar depression. *Journal of Abnormal Psychology, 100,* 555–561.

Hammen, C. (2003). Interpersonal stress and depression in women. *Journal of Affective Disorders, 74,* 49–57.

Hammen, C. (2005). Stress and depression. *Annual Review of Clinical Psychology, 1,* 293–319.

Hammen, C., Burge, D., & Adrian, C. (1991). Timing of mother and child depression in a longitudinal study of children at risk. *Journal of Consulting and Clinical Psychology, 59,* 341–345.

Henkel, V., Bussfeld, P., Moller, H. J., & Hegerl, U. (2002). Cognitive-behavioural theories of helplessness/hopelessness: Valid models of depression? *European Archives of Psychiatry and Clinical Neuroscience, 252,* 240–249.

Ingram, R. E., & Siegle, G. J. (2002). Contemporary methodological issues in the study of depression: Not your father's Oldsmobile. In I. H. Gotlib & C. L. Hammen (Eds.), *Handbook of depression* (pp. 86–113). New York: Guilford Press.

Joiner, T. E. (2002). Depression in its interpersonal context. In I. H. Gotlib & C. L. Hammen (Eds.), *Handbook of depression* (pp. 295–313). New York: Guilford Press.

Joiner, T. E., Walker, R. L., Pettit, J. W., Perez, M., & Cukrowicz, K. C. (2005). Evidence-based assessment of depression in adults. *Psychological Assessment, 17,* 267–277.

Joiner, T. E., Wingate, L. R., Gencoz, T., & Gencoz, F. (2005). Stress generation in depression: Three studies on its resilience, possible mechanism, and symptom specificity. *Journal of Social and Clinical Psychology, 24,* 236–253.

Kahneman, D. (1999). Objective happiness. In D. Kahneman, E. Diener, & N. Schwarz (Eds.), *Well-being: The foundations of hedonic psychology* (pp. 85–105). New York: Russell Sage Foundation.

Kessler, R. C. (1997). The effects of stressful life events on depression. *Annual Review of Psychology, 48,* 191–214.

Kovacs, M. (1992). *Children's Depression Inventory manual.* North Tonawanda, NY: Multi-Health Systems.

Lewinsohn, P. M., Allen, N. B., Seeley, J. R., & Gotlib, I. H. (1999). First onset versus recurrence of depression: Differential processes of psychosocial risk. *Journal of Abnormal Psychology, 108,* 483–489.

Lewinsohn, P. M., Hoberman, H. M., & Rosenbaum, M. (1989). Probability of relapse after recovery from an episode of depression. *Journal of Abnormal Psychology, 97,* 251–264.

Lewinsohn, P. M., Hops, H., Roberts, R. E., Seeley, J. R., & Andrews, J. A. (1993). Adolescent psychopathology: 1. Prevalence and incidence of depression and other DSM-III-R disorders in high school students. *Journal of Abnormal Psychology, 102,* 133–144.

Maciejewski, P. K., Zhang, B., Block, S. D., & Prigerson, H. G. (2007). An empirical examination of the stage theory of grief. *Journal of the American Medical Association, 297,* 716–723.

Masten, A. S. (2001). Ordinary magic: Resilience processes in development. *American Psychologist, 56,* 227–238.

Mazure, C. M. (1998). Life stressors as risk factors in depression. *Clinical Psychology: Science and Practice, 5,* 291–313.

McEwen, B. S. (1998). Stress, adaptation and disease: Allostasis and allostatic load. *Annals of the New York Academy of Sciences, 840,* 33–44.

Minkoff, K., Bergman, E., Beck, A. T., & Beck, R. (1973). Hopelessness, depression, and attempted suicide. *American Journal of Psychiatry, 130,* 455–459.

Monroe, S. M., & Hadjiyannakis, K. (2002). The social environment and depression: Focusing on severe life events. In I. H. Gotlib & C. L. Hammen (Eds.), *Handbook of depression* (pp. 314–340). New York: Guilford Press.

Monroe, S. M., & Harkness, K. L. (2005). Life stress, the "kindling" hypothesis, and the recurrence of depression: Considerations from a life stress perspective. *Psychological Review, 112,* 417–445.

Monroe, S. M., & Simons, A. D. (1991). Diathesis–stress theories in the context of life-stress research: Implications for depressive disorders. *Psychological Bulletin, 110,* 406–425.

Montgomery, S. A., & Asberg, M. (1979). A new depression scale designed to be sensitive to change. *British Journal of Psychiatry, 134,* 382–389.

Nezu, A. M., Nezu, C. M., McClure, K. S., & Zwick, M. L. (2002). Assessment of depression. In I. H. Gotlib & C. L. Hammen (Eds.), *Handbook of depression* (pp. 61–85). New York: Guilford Press.

Ong, A. D., Bergeman, C. S., Bisconti, T. L., & Wallace, K. A. (2006). Psychological resilience, positive emotions, and successful adaptation to stress in later life. *Journal of Personality and Social Psychology, 91,* 730–749.

Ott, C. H., Lueger, R. J., Kelber, S. T., & Prigerson, H. G. (2007). Spousal bereavement in older adults: Common, resilient, and chronic grief with defining characteristics. *Journal of Nervous and Mental Disease, 195,* 332–341.

Patterson, G. R., & Stoolmiller, M. (1991). Replications of a dual failure model for boys' depressed mood. *Journal of Consulting and Clinical Psychology, 59,* 491–498.

Pepper, C. M., & Nieuwsma, J. A. (2006). Issues in the measurement of depression: Purpose, population, and interpretation. *Measurement, 4,* 165–169.

Post, R. M. (1992). Transduction of psychosocial stress into the neurobiology of recurrent affective disorder. *American Journal of Psychiatry, 149,* 999–1010.

Radloff, L. S. (1977). The CES-D scale: A self-report depression scale for research in the general population. *Applied Psychological Measurement, 1,* 385–401.

Rao, U., Hammen, C., & Daley, S. E. (1999). Continuity of depression during the transition to adulthood.

Journal of the American Academy of Child and Adolescent Psychiatry, 38, 908–915.

Reich, J. W., Johnson, L. M., Zautra, A. J., & Davis, M. C. (2006). Uncertainty of illness relationships with mental health and coping processes in fibromyalgia patients. *Journal of Behavioral Medicine, 29,* 307–316.

Reynolds, W. M., & Kobak, K. A. (1998). *Hamilton Depression Inventory (HDI): Professional manual.* Odessa, FL: Psychological Assessment Resources.

Robinson, M. D., & Clore, G. L. (2002). Belief and feeling: Evidence for an accessibility model of emotional self-report. *Psychological Bulletin, 128,* 934–960.

Romano, J. M., & Turner, J. A. (1985). Chronic pain and depression: Does the evidence support a relationship? *Psychological Bulletin, 97,* 17–34.

Ross, M., & Wilson, A. E. (2003). Autobiographical memory and conceptions of self: Getting better all the time. *Current Directions in Psychological Science, 12,* 66–69.

Rush, A. J., Carmody, T., & Reimitz, P. E. (2000). The Inventory of Depressive Symptomatology (IDS): Clinician (IDS-C) and self-report (IDS-SR) ratings of depressive symptoms. *International Journal of Methods in Psychiatric Research, 9,* 45–59.

Safford, S. M., Alloy, L. B., Abramson, L. Y., & Crossfield, A. G. (2007). Negative cognitive style as a predictor of negative life events in depression-prone individuals: A test of the stress generation hypothesis. *Journal of Affective Disorders, 99,* 147–154.

Santor, D. A., & Coyne, J. C. (2001). Evaluating the continuity of symptomatology between depressed and nondepressed individuals. *Journal of Abnormal Psychology, 110,* 216–225.

Santor, D. A., Gregus, M., & Welch, A. (2006). Eight decades of measurement in depression. *Measurement, 4,* 135–155.

Shelbourne, C. D., Wells, K. B., Hays, R. D., Rogers, W., Burnham, M., & Judd, L. L. (1994). Subthreshold depression and depressive disorder: Clinical characteristics of general medical and mental health specialty outpatients. *American Journal of Psychiatry, 151,* 1777–1784.

Simms, L. J. (2006). The future of depression measurement research. *Measurement, 4,* 169–174.

Stanton, A. L., Revenson, T. A., & Tennen, H. (2007). Health psychology: Psychological adjustment to chronic disease. *Annual Review of Psychology, 58,* 565–592.

Stein, N., Folkman, S., Trabasso, T., & Richards, T. A. (1997). Appraisal and goal processes as predictors of well-being in bereaved caregivers. *Journal of Personality and Social Psychology, 72,* 872–884.

Stice, E., Ragan, J., & Randall, P. (2004). Prospective relations between social support and depression: Differential direction of effects for parental and peer support? *Journal of Abnormal Psychology, 113,* 155–159.

Strauman, T. J. (2002). Self-regulation and depression. *Self and Identity, 1,* 151–157.

Symister, P., & Friend, R. (2003). The influence of social support and problematic support on optimism and depression in chronic illness: A prospective study evaluating self-esteem as a mediator. *Health Psychology, 22,* 123–129.

Teasdale, J. D. (1983). Negative thinking in depression: Cause, effect, or reciprocal relationship? *Advances in Behaviour Research and Therapy, 5,* 3–25.

Tennen, H. (2006). Accuracy of recalled experience: Depression measurement's enduring illusion. *Measurement, 4,* 180–187.

Tennen, H., Affleck, G., & Zautra, A. J. (2006). Depression history and coping with chronic pain: A daily process analysis. *Health Psychology, 25,* 370–379.

Tennen, H., Eberhart, T., & Affleck, G. (1999). Depression research methodologies at the social-clinical interface: Still hazy after all these years. *Journal of Social and Clinical Psychology, 18,* 121–159.

Tennen, H., Hall, J. A., & Affleck, G. (1995). Depression research methodologies in the *Journal of Personality and Social Psychology:* A review and critique. *Journal of Personality and Social Psychology, 68,* 870–884.

Thase, M. E. (2007, June). *Depression rating scales: History and current status.* Paper presented at the Consensus Conference on Advancing Signal Strength in Proof of Concept Studies in Major Depression, Bethesda, MD.

Tugade, M. M., Fredrickson, B. L., & Feldman-Barrett, L. (2004). Psychological resilience and positive emotion granularity: Examining the benefit of positive emotions on coping and health. *Journal of Personality, 72,* 1161–1190.

Watson, D., O'Hara, M. W., Simms, L. J., Kotov, R., Chmielewski, M., & McDade-Montez, E. A. (2007). Development and validation of the Inventory of Depression and Anxiety Symptoms (IDAS). *Psychological Assessment, 19,* 253–268.

Williamson, G. M., & Schulz, R. (1992). Pain, activity restriction, and symptoms of depression among community-residing elderly adults. *Journal of Gerontology, 47,* 367–372.

Windle, M. (1992). A longitudinal study of stress buffering for adolescent problems. *Developmental Psychology, 28,* 522–530.

Yesavage, J. A., Brink, T. L., Rose, T. L., Lum, O., Huang, V., Adey, M., et al. (1983). Development and validation of a geriatric depression screening scale: A preliminary report. *Journal of Psychiatric Research, 17,* 37–49.

Zautra, A. J., Davis, M. C., Nicassio, P., Tennen, H., Finan, P. H., Parrish, B. P., et al. (2007). *Comparison of cognitive-behavioral and mindfulness meditation interventions on adaptation to rheumatoid arthritis for patients with and without history of recurrent depression.* Manuscript submitted for publication.

Zautra, A. J., Johnson, L. M., & Davis, M. C. (2005). Positive affect as a source of resilience for women in chronic pain. *Journal of Consulting and Clinical Psychology, 73,* 212–220.

Zautra, A. J., Parrish, B. P., Van Puymbroeck, C. M., Tennen, H., Davis, M. C., Reich, J. W., et al. (2007). Depression history, stress, and pain in rheumatoid arthritis patients. *Journal of Behavioral Medicine, 30*(3), 187–197.

Zautra, A. J., Schultz, A. S., & Reich, J. W. (2000). The role of everyday events in depressive symptoms for older adults. In G. M. Williamson, D. R. Shaffer, & P. A. Parmalee (Eds.), *Physical illness and depression in older adults: A handbook of theory, research, and practice* (pp. 65–91). New York: Plenum Press.

Zautra, A. J., & Smith, B. W. (2001). Depression and reactivity to stress in older women with rheumatoid arthritis and osteoarthritis. *Psychosomatic Medicine, 63,* 687–696.

Zimmerman, M., & Coryell, W. (1987). The Inventory to Diagnose Depression (IDD): A self-report scale to diagnose major depressive disorder. *Journal of Consulting and Clinical Psychology, 55,* 55–59.

CHAPTER 12

■ ● ▲ ◆ ■ ● ▲ ◆

Social Anxiousness, Shyness, and Embarrassability

ROWLAND S. MILLER

Envision a large group of people at a wedding reception. If they realize that they have maladroitly greeted the groom using the name of the bride's prior boyfriend, they are very likely to become abashed; almost everyone is (at least somewhat) susceptible to embarrassment. Even if nothing goes wrong, the social setting will cause many of them to experience discomfort that may range from mild unease to outright dread; merely being surrounded by others can evoke social anxiety. And a sizable number of them will interact with others in a cautious manner, being timidly reluctant to strike up a conversation with strangers because they are chronically shy.

The states of embarrassment, social anxiety, and shyness can have profound influence on the interactions in which they occur. They engender potent motives and may elicit strong feelings, and behavior typically changes as a result. However, they also emerge from dispositions that vary substantially from person to person, so they occur more frequently and with greater intensity in some people than in others. This chapter considers the traits of embarrassability, shyness, and social anxiousness. I ponder their origins and detail their interactive effects, but I begin by comparing and contrasting the states they educe.

The Nature of the States

Embarrassment is the state of mortification, abashment, and chagrin that washes over us when social life takes an awkward turn and we suddenly face the prospect of undesired evaluations from others. It typically strikes without warning and causes startled, self-conscious feelings of ungainliness, conspicuousness, and befuddlement. Embarrassment is usually sudden, automatic, and brief (rather than gradual and prolonged; Miller, 1996); it hinges on the realization that one has made some misstep or that an interaction has gone awry, but such appraisals occur without deliberation or reflection, and embarrassment can be in full flower before one ever thinks things through. It also has a distinctive physiological signature involving autonomic and adrenal arousal (Gerlach, Wilhelm, & Roth, 2003) that is accompanied by a singular response: blushing that results from the dilation of facial veins that brings blood closer to the surface of the cheeks (Edelmann, 2001). These physical changes are usually accompanied by a recognizable pattern of nonverbal behavior that unfolds over 5–6 seconds (Keltner & Buswell, 1997). When embarrassment strikes, people avert their gazes, lower their heads, touch their faces, and try (but normally fail) to suppress goofy grins of chagrin that are noticeably different from smiles of genuine amusement (Asendorpf, 1990). Speech errors and exaggerated movements may also occur (Edelmann & Hampson, 1979). Only a few of these various cues need to be present for a person's embarrassment to be obvious and unmistakable, so, ordinarily, observers are aware of embarrassment in their midst (Marcus & Miller, 1999). And because it is detectable and transparent, embarrassment has different effects on our interactions than social anxiety and shyness do, as I discuss.

In contrast, social anxiety is fretful disquiet that stems from the prospect of evaluations from others in the absence of any predicament. It occurs when we believe ourselves to be subject to real, implied, or imagined social evaluation, and it takes the form of nervous concern for what others may be thinking, even when nothing has gone wrong (Leary, 2001a). Unlike embarrassment, social anxiety often occurs over long periods of time, gradually waxing and waning. It depends on contemplation of social settings that portrays them as daunting and intimidating, so it is usually gradual, prolonged, and mindful (rather than automatic; Miller, 2001a). Physically, social anxiety resembles other fears; it involves activation of the "fight or flight" responses of the sympathetic nervous system—causing higher heart rates, faster, shallower breathing, and increased blood pressure (Borkovec, Stone, O'Brien, & Kaloupek, 1974)—but it is not accompanied by a characteristic pattern of coherent behavior that signals its presence to other people. Outwardly, then, it may take various forms, but inwardly, it is experienced as aversive arousal that involves tension, apprehension, and unease.

Shyness occurs when social anxiety is paired with reticent, cautious, and guarded social behavior (Leary, 2001a). Shy behavior may range from mild inhibition, involving bashful timidity or wary watchfulness, to stronger distancing behavior that can include total withdrawal from social settings. That is a broad range, and no one pattern of behavior reliably distinguishes shyness from cooler, calmer states (such as those associated with introversion) that lead one to be quiet and reserved in the absence of any anxiety (Henderson & Zimbardo, 2001). Shy behavior may thus seem ambiguous to observers; it is obviously not gregarious and convivial, but whether it derives from shy trepidation, a mild manner, dullness, or unfriendly lack of interest may be hard to judge. In any case, because it involves anxious affect that is paired with inhibited behavior, shyness is best considered a *syndrome*, rather than an emotion or mood per se (Leary, 1986a).

Social-Evaluative Siblings

Social anxiety, shyness, and embarrassment are clearly separable, distinct states, but they share a common foundation. All of them spring from a person's attentive concern for interpersonal evaluation. Each emerges from situations in which one is subject to real or imagined inspection by others, and each is unlikely when one's actions are genuinely private and will not become known to anyone else. Consider social anxiety. A classic formulation posits that social anxiety arises when we wish to portray ourselves to others in a particular, desired fashion, but we doubt that we can do so successfully (Schlenker & Leary, 1982); the combination of desire and doubt is thought to trigger the aversive arousal of social anxiety. In this model, without some motivation to construct a preferred image for others—that is, if we really do not care what a particular audience thinks of us—social anxiety will not occur.[1] Leary (2001b) has since revised this formulation, suggesting that the fundamental motivation at work is not merely to succeed at impression management but, instead, to maintain our level of inclusion and acceptance by others. Self-presentational challenges fuel social anxiety, Leary asserted, when they engender the threatening possibility that others will come to devalue their associations with us (because they think of us less favorably). Nevertheless, the key role of social evaluation in social anxiety, it should be recognized, remains the same in the revised model: Absent the wish to be accepted by others, social anxiety is unlikely to occur.

Indeed, circumstances that make the threat of rejection less imposing reduce the social anxiety of those who encounter them. Leary (1986b) provided a clever demonstration of this when he placed young adults with chronic social anxiety in a noisy room with a stranger. The noise, which was supposed to mimic the ambience of a lively tavern, was supplied by an audiotape that was always played at a constant volume—but it was explained in two different ways. Some participants were told that the noise was not loud enough to interfere with their conversation, whereas others were told that the noise was likely to be a hindrance. Participants in this latter condition were given an explicit excuse for their interactions to go poorly, and it was evidently a comforting rationale: Whereas those in the "soft" noise condition became anxious and behaved shyly, those in the "loud" environment stayed calm and did not appear to be shy at all. Clearly, social anxiety in these situations depended on the amount of evaluative threat perceived to be present; it was unrelated to the objective setting.

Embarrassment is also tied to our marvelous human ability to comprehend—and to care—what others are thinking of us. For instance, people with autism who do not possess a normal "theory of mind" (a typical awareness of the likely content of others' thoughts) do not recognize and understand embarrassment as readily as do people who do not have autism (Heerey, Keltner, & Capps, 2003). Embarrassment is difficult to produce when one cannot take others' points of view and see oneself as they do. Furthermore, the ability to infer others' thoughts is tied to the medial regions of the prefrontal cortex; when those areas are damaged, understanding of others' thoughts and feelings is impaired (Beer, Heerey, Keltner, Scabini, & Knight, 2003). Remarkably, the same region becomes active when people encounter violations of social norms (Berthoz, Armony, Blair, & Dolan, 2002), and children who suffer damage to the region never fully learn ordinary social graces and rules of appropriate conduct (Anderson, Bechara, Damasio, Tranel, & Damasio, 1999). Most important, adults who develop orbitofrontal lesions may become incapable of experiencing embarrassment at all (Beer et al., 2003); they can commit the most glaring improprieties with unruffled aplomb, being heedless of their social peril. The converging evidence seems conclusive: Embarrassment quite clearly depends on the ability to imagine others' perceptions of us. When this ability is lacking, embarrassment does not occur.

Moreover, unlike other self-conscious emotions such as shame and guilt (Tangney, Miller, Flicker, & Barlow, 1996), embarrassment rarely occurs when we are alone (Miller, 1992). The missteps and misbehavior that give rise to embarrassment cause us chagrin either because others are present or because they are about to be. Inadvertently entering a restroom for the other sex can cause a flash of embarrassment even when the room is unoccupied (and no one else knows of the mistake) if one envisions a witness arriving. Similarly, most of us sometimes contentedly engage in private actions that suddenly gain embarrassing potential when anyone else shows up. Like social anxiety and shyness, embarrassment *can* occur when one is entirely alone—but all three states occur in such circumstances only when we imagine the likely future reactions of others to our present conduct.

Thus they are discrete states, but social anxiety, shyness, and embarrassment are all close cousins, or perhaps step-siblings, with the same mother but different fathers (Miller, 2001b). Embarrassment is an unbidden, emotional response to actual predicaments, whereas social anxiety and shyness emerge from more deliberate contemplation of one's situation that influences interaction even when nothing has (yet) gone wrong. Each is also influenced by its own moderators, so that, as I discuss, shyness is more affected by insecure doubts about one's social skills than embarrassment is (Miller, 1995). Still, they all emerge from the same parent, the same core ingredient: Each depends on an awareness of, sensitivity to, and concern for the evaluations of us by others, and any dispositional characteristic that makes these components more potent will make these states more frequent and more intense.

A Brief History of Assessment

Modern studies of social anxiety, shyness, and embarrassment have become quite sophisticated, involving cutting-edge technology. Neuroimaging methodologies such as electroencephalography and functional magnetic resonance imaging (Schmidt & Tasker, 2000), various cardiovascular, neuroendocrine, and electrodermal measures (Marshall & Stevenson-Hinde, 2001), and behavior genetics (Saudino, 2001) are all now routinely used to assess individual differences associated with the three states. Indeed, studies of social anxiety, shyness, and embarrassment have become robust, vibrant areas of investigation—but it has not always been so. Systematic inquiry began with the creation of self-report scales that allowed convenient assessment of our chronic susceptibilities to experience social anxiety, shyness, and embarrassment—termed *social anxiousness*, *trait shyness*, and *embarrassability*, respectively.

Two measures jump-started studies of social anxiousness. In psychology, Watson and Friend (1969) created the Social Avoidance and Distress Scale, and in communication studies, McCroskey (1970) developed a Personal Report of Communication Apprehension. Watson and Friend's measure contained two subscales that addressed the tendency to feel anxious in social interactions (e.g., "I often find social occasions upsetting") and to withdraw from them altogether (e.g., "I often think up excuses in order to avoid social engagements"). McCroskey's scale focused more broadly on anxiety associated with public speaking in larger groups, as well as in dyadic conversations. The two measures thus had different emphases, but both were influential, stimulating new programs of research in their respective disciplines.

Since then, a variety of other inventories have been developed to assess social anxiety in particular domains. These include measures of physique anxiety (i.e., unease about others' evaluations of one's body; Hart, Leary, & Rejeski, 1989), anxiety associated with public physical activity and sports participation (Norton, Hope, & Weeks, 2004), and performance anxiety, or stage fright (e.g., Osborne, Kenny, & Holsomback, 2005). Other measures have been designed specifically for children (e.g., Storch et al., 2006), and still others have targeted the stronger fears and more profound disruption of social life associated with social anxiety disorder (e.g., Johnson, Inderbitzen-Nolan, & Anderson, 2006) or "social phobia" (Turner, Beidel, Dancu, & Stanley, 1989). However, like Watson and Friend's (1969) Social Avoidance and Distress Scale, many of these measures conflate items that tap anxious phenomenology with other items

that describe avoidant and inhibited behavior that often—but not always—occurs in anxious episodes. Arguably, accurate assessment of social anxiety should not be confounded with measurement of shy behavior, a point averred by Leary (1983b), who developed separate measures of interaction anxiousness (e.g., "Parties often make me feel anxious and uncomfortable") and audience anxiousness (which pertains to nervous dread of audiences, e.g., "I usually get nervous when I speak in front of a group") that exclude any references to specific social behaviors.

The gold standard for assessing social anxiety that *is* accompanied by reticent, inhibited behavior is the Shyness Scale created by Cheek and Buss in 1981 (and later expanded to a slightly longer form; see Hopko, Stowell, Jones, Armento, & Cheek, 2005). It contains both affective (e.g., "I feel tense when I'm with people I don't know well") and behavioral (e.g., "I have trouble looking someone right in the eye") items that appear to comprise three different factors (Hopko et al., 2005): (1) nervous distress in social situations, (2) wary awkwardness around strangers, and (3) difficulty with forthright behavior. Systematic study of shyness began when Zimbardo (1977) created the Stanford Shyness Survey, and other useful scales, such as the Social Reticence Scale (Jones, Briggs, & Smith, 1986), have since been created, but the revised Cheek and Buss Shyness Scale is the measure most widely used in current research.

Interest in embarrassment was rare, and studies of embarrassability did not exist until Modigliani created an Embarrassability Scale in 1968.[2] The measure asks respondents to imagine themselves in a variety of awkward situations and to rate the amount of embarrassment they would feel in each case. The situations range widely, from innocent conspicuousness (e.g., "Suppose a group of friends were singing 'Happy Birthday' to you") to inelegant interactions (e.g., "Suppose you were talking to a stranger who stuttered badly due to a speech impediment") and on to situations in which others are at risk and empathic embarrassment is possible (Miller, 1987; e.g., "Suppose you were watching an amateur show and one of the performers was trying to do a comedy act but was unable to make anyone laugh").

Also included, of course, are several personal pratfalls and faux pas. Notably, these diverse scenarios encompass all of the diverse types of situations that cause us actual embarrassments (Miller, 1992), so the scale has substantial content validity. Kelly and Jones (1997) have since developed a Susceptibility to Embarrassment Scale that performs quite well, and Sabini, Siepmann, Stein, and Meyerowitz (2000) created a scale that assesses sensitivity to three different classes of embarrassing situations; still, the Embarrassability Scale remains better known. Measures that assess one's chronic tendencies to blush in social situations have also been developed by Leary and Meadows (1991) and Bögels and Reith (1999).

Finally, studies of social anxiousness, trait shyness, and embarrassability have been aided and abetted by several other self-report measures that are meaningfully correlated with all three traits. Foremost among these are the Fear of Negative Evaluation Scale created by Watson and Friend (1969; and revised into a shorter, handier measure by Leary, 1983a), and the Self-Consciousness Scale (SCS) developed by Fenigstein, Scheier, and Buss (1975; and revised for use with the lay public by Scheier & Carver, 1985). The SCS contains items that assess one's chronic awareness of and attention to one's public image (e.g., "I'm concerned about what other people think of me"), and people who are high in such self-consciousness are more embarrassable and more prone to social anxiety (Miller, 1995). Fear of negative evaluation refers to chronic dread of disapproval from others (e.g., "I am afraid that others will not approve of me"), and it, too, is positively related to social anxiousness, shyness, and embarrassability (Miller, 1995). *Any* evaluation from others may be threatening to some people, and new scales that will refine our assessment and understanding of the social-evaluative siblings continue to be produced (e.g., Weeks, Heimberg, & Rodebaugh, 2008). However, much has obviously already been learned.

The Nature of the Traits

To varying degrees, people who are prone to social anxiety, shyness, and embarrassment live social lives that are different from those managed by others who are less anxious, shy, or embarrassable. Their higher chronic concern over social evaluation appears to result in patterns of cognition, motivation and emotion, and behavior that are recognizably different from the thoughts, feelings, and actions of those with weaker social-evaluative worries. This section of the chapter surveys these patterns. It begins with combined consideration of social anxiousness and shyness, which share the same cognitive underpinnings.

Social Anxiousness and Shyness

Social Cognition

One of the most distinguishing characteristics of those who are high in social anxiousness and trait shyness is the nature of their thoughts in social situations (Clark & Wells, 1995). They are prone to *worry* about their interactions with others, and this nervous apprehension is manifested in three facets of their mental lives: biased *attention, interpretation*, and *rumination*.

Attention. People with high social anxiousness appear to be edgily alert to stimuli that signal the approach of social threats (Ledley & Heimberg, 2006). Studies using an emotional Stroop test—which asks participants to name the color in which a provocative word is printed while ignoring the meaning of the word—routinely find that it is relatively difficult for people high in social anxiousness to divert their attention from words denoting social threats (e.g., *mocked, rejected, disgraced*) (e.g., Amir, Freshman, & Foa, 2002); they take longer to identify the colors of such words than of neutral words (e.g., *house*) or positive words (e.g., *admired, accepted*). In contrast, people low in social anxiousness are not differentially attentive to semantic cues of social peril (Maidenberg, Chen, Craske, Bohn, & Bystritsky, 1996).

Words are relatively pallid stimuli, and several studies have now confronted participants with richer threat cues—angry facial expressions—using a method that arguably provides a purer measure of attention, the dot-probe paradigm. In this computerized procedure, participants are asked to designate as quickly as possible the position of a dot that flashes onscreen after the simultaneous presentation of two facial images; shorter latencies in locating the dot are thought to indicate greater attention to the face that appeared in the same place as the dot. Investigations using this technique have demonstrated that social anxiousness seems to be associated with a preconscious vigilance for evaluative faces that is absent in those who are less often anxious. Compared with those who are less prone to social anxiety, socially anxious people are more attentive to faces depicting positive (i.e., happy) or negative (i.e., anger, disgust, fear, or sadness) emotions than to neutral faces when they face a daunting public performance (a speech about a controversial topic; Mansell, Clark, Ehlers, & Chen, 1999). They are also more attentive to angry faces than to happy or neutral expressions, but only when the faces are presented too quickly—a duration of one-half second—to allow deliberate consideration of the images; when longer inspection is allowed—for 1¼ seconds—the greater attention paid to angry faces disappears (Mogg, Philippot, & Bradley, 2004).

Socially anxious people are thus attuned to emotive faces, and their attention is instantly drawn to faces that denote hostility or rejection. Thereafter, given a chance to consciously consider their options, people with high social anxiousness are relatively *in*attentive to evaluative stimuli. When they can take their time to react to their surroundings, people high in social anxiousness avoid emotional facial expressions, paying both smiling and angry faces less heed than they give to neutral stimuli; they also attend less to them than less anxious people do (Heuer, Rinck, & Becker, 2007). This temporal pattern is consistent with a *vigilance–avoidance* model that suggests that social anxiousness leads people to be constantly watchful for signs of social evaluation—and, preconsciously, particularly alert for anger and antagonism—that are then ducked and dodged once they are noticed (Mogg, Bradley, de Bono, & Painter, 1997). In ordinary social interactions, both reactions may be counterproductive. High levels of relentless, automatic vigilance are probably needless and wearing, leaving socially anxious people jittery and depleted. Then, their wish to evade the feedback they do encounter may rob them of the opportunity to learn over time that rejection from others is actually quite rare.

When they do assay the responses they are receiving from others, those with high social anxiousness more accurately detect disapproving or bored reactions than accepting and approving ones. Two studies have placed participants of high or low social anxiousness in a threatening setting, asking them to give brief speeches to evaluative audiences that provided mixed reactions to the talk. In Veljaca and Rapee (1998), participants were face-to-face with the experimenter and two confederates who provided distinctly different nonverbal feedback; one of them leaned forward, smiled, and nodded, while the other looked sleepy, yawned, and looked at a watch. In Perowne and Mansell (2002), participants gave their talks looking at a video screen that showed six people who were obviously interested, bored, or neutral while they ostensibly watched the speech from the next room. In both studies, socially anxious speakers were clearly attuned to the negative reactions they encountered; compared with their less anxious counterparts, they noticed bored responses more often and enthusiastic responses less often (Veljaca & Rapee, 1998), and they knew who had disliked, but not who had liked, their talks (Perowne & Mansell, 2002).

These results are consistent with those from visual search procedures that have demonstrated that social anxiousness is positively associated with the speed with which people can pick an angry face out of a neutral crowd (e.g., Gilboa-Schechtman, Foa, & Amir, 1999). In general, then, when people with high social anxiousness scan their social environments, they evidently do so attuned to disregard. They are more alert than others are for signs of antagonism or rejection, but they defensively work to withdraw from such signals when they are encountered. This is a pattern of attentiveness that, rather than gradually promoting calmer, cooler reactions to social evaluation, is likely instead to perpetuate groundless, misplaced trepidation in social settings (Bögels & Mansell, 2004).

Compared with those who are less anxious, those with high social anxiousness are also more attentive to internal physiological cues regarding their arousal in public places. Indeed, they are even more attentive to information about their internal states (such as heart rate feedback) than to threatening external cues (such as angry faces; Pineles

& Mineka, 2005), especially when they are placed in evaluative social situations (such as giving a speech on a controversial topic; Mansell, Clark, & Ehlers, 2003). Thus people with high social anxiousness are particularly likely to be distracted by, and then preoccupied with, the sensations of their physical activation in social situations. The presence of others is stimulating, and some arousal is normal; people with high social anxiousness do not necessarily become more aroused than anyone else in social situations—but they *think* they do (Edelmann & Baker, 2002). Then the self-focused attention that accompanies social anxiousness makes one's unease seem even more intense, making anxiety even worse (Zou, Hudson, & Rapee, 2007).

Moreover, people with high social anxiousness think differently about upcoming social interactions before they even begin. Their *anticipatory processing* is characterized by recurrent and intrusive thoughts regarding their physical nervousness, past failures, and fantasies of escape from the current threat that are more frequent and compelling than those experienced by those with less anxiousness (Vassilopoulos, 2004). This train of thought is disadvantageous, both interfering with their preparation for the event and intensifying their anxiety (Vassilopoulos, 2005). In particular, when people who are not socially anxious are instructed to adopt this outlook before an upcoming speech—"think of a particular social situation that you felt did not go well; try to anticipate the worst thing that could happen while you are giving the speech"—they get more nervous, both before and during the performance (Hinrichsen & Clark, 2003). Furthermore, when people with high social anxiousness are distracted by another task and their usual fearful anticipation is interrupted, an imminent threat causes them less concern (Hinrichsen & Clark, 2003; Vassilopoulos, 2005).

Altogether, then, the greater attention chronically paid by those who are socially anxious to cues of rejection, internal arousal, and worst-possible outcomes appears to leave them continually ill at ease in social settings. Indeed, through their eyes, the social environments they encounter probably seem more routinely menacing than those same situations seem to others with lower social anxiousness.

Interpretation. Higher levels of social anxiousness also lead people to imagine the worst in innocuous stimuli that do not seem worrisome to those who are less routinely anxious (Hirsch & Clark, 2004). They attach pejorative interpretations to ambiguous actions from others, and they perceive disapproval where it does not objectively exist—and the higher their levels of social anxiousness, the more pronounced these tendencies become (Huppert, Foa, Furr, Filip, & Matthews, 2003).

In one study, for instance, people with high or low social anxiousness read a scenario describing a blind date (Constans, Penn, Ihen, & Hope, 1999). At several junctures in the story, ambiguous statements were made (e.g., "When meeting her date, Lisa said 'You're certainly not what I expected'"), and the participants were asked to consider the plausibility of various interpretations of each ambiguity (e.g., "When Lisa said to Steve, 'You're certainly not what I expected,' she was impressed"). When the ambiguity involved an interpersonal evaluation, people with high social anxiousness judged positive possibilities to be less likely than less anxious people did; they were not more pessimistic, however, about impersonal judgments (such as a first impression of a restaurant).

In a subsequent investigation (Voncken, Bögels, & de Vries, 2003), the participants were themselves the targets of brief scenarios that involved a variety of outcomes ranging from favorable (e.g., "someone makes a compliment about your looks") through ambiguous (e.g., "somebody you know looks in your direction") to profoundly negative (e.g., "a friend tells you that a colleague dislikes you"). People with high levels of social anxiousness made more negative interpretations of all of these events than did those with lower anxiousness, but they did not differ from their less anxious counterparts in judgments of nonsocial events.

Evidently, social anxiousness does not lead people to be generally gloomy, but it does lead them to have pessimistic perceptions of social situations that are most apparent in uncertain interactions in which others' evaluations are indistinct (Amir, Beard, & Bower, 2005). When they complete ambiguous sentences involving social evaluations (e.g., "As you give a speech, you see a person in the crowd smiling, which means that your speech is _____"), people with high social anxiousness provide more fretful and derogatory responses than less anxious people do (Huppert, Pasupuleti, Foa, & Matthews, 2007). Social anxiousness makes social interactions seem more costly and dangerous than they would appear to be were one less anxious (Schofield, Coles, & Gibb, 2007).

People with high social anxiousness also judge themselves more harshly. They underestimate their physical attractiveness, tend to blame themselves for disappointing outcomes, and tend to doubt the accuracy of the praise they receive (Cheek & Briggs, 1990). Because they are usually nervous and uneasy, socially anxious people do make relatively poor impressions on their audiences when they give public presentations; nevertheless, their self-evaluations of their poise and preparation are more damning than the appraisals they actually receive from others. Social anxiousness is unrelated to judgments of others' performances, but it does seem to make people unduly hard on themselves (Ashbaugh, Antony, McCabe, Schmidt, & Swinson, 2005).

Rumination. Finally, socially anxious people ponder their problems more persistently than others do. In particular, they brood after a public presentation, replaying the event in their minds and fussing over their (perceived) imperfections (Edwards, Rapee, & Franklin, 2003). They may also be beset by the fear that their nervous disarray caused discomfort to others (Rector, Kocovski, & Ryder, 2006). This pejorative style of *postevent processing* is even more pronounced after one-on-one interactions than after solo performances, and among people with high social anxiousness, it is specific to social-evaluative situations as opposed to impersonal threats (Fehm, Schneider, & Hoyer, 2007). Thus the peril posed by social settings does not end when an interaction is done; self-criticism and self-censure persevere, often for days thereafter (Dannahy & Stopa, 2007).

Motivation and Emotion

Burdened with excessive self-focus and a pessimistic outlook, people with high social anxiousness approach social life more cautiously than do those who are less anxious. Arguably, they do not seek approval from others so much as they defensively strive to avoid disapproval (Shepperd & Arkin, 1990). This leads them to interact with others in a manner that is self-protective rather than acquisitive, and their interpersonal behavior is intentionally innocuous: They sit on the sides or in the back of classrooms, they express neutral opinions, and they conform readily (see Shepperd & Arkin, 1990). There is only a modest negative correlation ($r = -.30$) between shyness and sociability, so people with high social anxiousness do not necessarily wish to be left alone; indeed, some shy people are quite sociable (Cheek & Buss, 1981). They generally do not much like to interact with anyone they do not already know, however, because they are averse to social risk (Brown, Silvia, Myin-Germeys, & Kwapil, 2007). Their motivation to minimize the chances of disapproval from others seems to leave them wary, watchful, and relatively unwilling to take advantage of social opportunities that are attractive and pleasurable to those with lower anxiousness.

Indeed, people with high social anxiousness are less curious about new ideas and experiences than less anxious people are (Kashdan, 2007). Curiosity is a "pleasant, appetitive state," and "when people feel curious, they thrive on novel and challenging interactions with the world, with exploratory behavior inevitably leading to an expansion of knowledge, skills, and resources" (Kashdan, 2007, p. 350). Being relatively lacking in curiosity, socially anxious people would rather stay close to home.

However, this preference may be costly. When respondents describe their feelings several times a day in experience-sampling studies, social anxiousness is associated with higher negative affect (Brown et al., 2007), less positive affect, and the enjoyment of fewer positive events (Kashdan & Steger, 2006) day by day. As we have seen, bouts of social anxiety cause autonomic arousal, nervousness, and disquiet; these unhappy sensations are disagreeable enough, but chronic susceptibility to such states is also linked to fewer positive emotions and more unpleasant feelings in one's daily routine. Social anxiousness is no fun.

Behavior

The fretful, fearful orientation to social life described here is unpleasant, but—of course—the actual distress socially anxious people experience varies widely from person to person. Social anxiousness ranges from a tendency to feel mild nervousness in interactions with strangers, a common propensity, to more profound, pervasive fears that afflict and impair most of one's relationships with others (Schneier, Blanco, Antia, & Liebowitz, 2002). Some of us are prone to social anxiety in delimited situations, such as public speaking or first dates, whereas others of us are uneasy whenever we are out in public. When it is extreme, social anxiousness becomes *social anxiety disorder* (also known as *social phobia*), in which one's fears of social evaluation are marked, persistent, and unremitting, interfering with ordinary activity and sometimes severely limiting one's social life (Beidel & Turner, 2007). Intense social anxiousness of this sort occurs at some point in 7–13% of us over the course of our lives (Furmark, 2002), and the worrying and negative affect described earlier are clearly more potent and formidable in such cases than in the lower levels of social anxiousness that are more commonplace (Beidel & Turner, 2007).

And so it is with the interpersonal behavior that stems from social anxiousness. People may be anxious in a particular interaction but give no visible sign of their unease. Alternatively, their anxiety may be conspicuously manifested in inhibited, guarded behavior in which they shrink from perceived threats. Social anxiousness is typically, but not always, accompanied by shyness (which is why I distinguished them), and shyness itself may be mild or intense. The depiction of shy behavior that follows describes patterns that, given the extent and strength of one's shyness, will apply to individual cases with variable precision.

Conversational Behavior. Nevertheless, with that caveat in place, it is clear that shy people generally interact with others in an impoverished manner that makes a relatively poor impression on their partners (Leary & Buckley, 2000). They tend to be reserved and tentative rather than enthusiastic and animated. There is little zest in their nonverbal behavior; they make fewer gestures (Baker & Edelmann, 2002), lean away more, and nod and smile less (Heerey & Kring, 2007) than do those who are less shy. Men who are shy frequently look at women to whom they are talking, but they avert their gazes if the women look back; thus lower levels of eye contact occur (Garcia, Stinson, Ickes, Bissonnette, & Briggs, 1991).

Their speech is less fluent (Baker & Edelmann, 2002) and their conversations rather bleak: They ask bland questions of others but are slow to respond to the answers they receive, and they speak less overall than those who are less shy (Asendorpf, 1990). They tend not to reciprocate others' self-disclosures (Papsdorf & Alden, 1998), and what they do say about themselves tends to be short and superficial (DePaulo, Epstein, & LeMay, 1990), so more long, awkward silences occur (Alden & Taylor, 2004). They also tend to suppress their emotions and to be unassertive (Davila & Beck, 2002).

Small talk with people they do not know well is quite clearly hard for people who are shy (Kashdan & Roberts, 2006). They are more relaxed among closer companions, but when they are dealing with strangers, shy people conduct interactions that are less deft and less fulfilling than those enjoyed by people who are less shy (Heerey & Kring, 2007). This is undoubtedly due in part to their excessive sensitivity to social evaluation. Like others who are socially anxious, shy people tend to be high in fear of negative evaluation (Miller, 1995)—but, as we have seen, when they have an excuse for small talk to go badly, they stay more relaxed and interact with strangers with comfort and grace (Leary, 1986b). They also interact more contentedly when they are online rather than face-to-face with new acquaintances (Stritzke, Nguyen, & Durkin, 2004); they are more self-disclosing and they form new relationships more easily online (though still less readily than do those who are less shy; Ward & Tracey, 2004).

However, on average, people who are high in shyness also possess poorer social skills than those who are less inhibited (Stravynski & Amado, 2001). They lack self-confidence in social situations, and perhaps with good reason; they feel less adept at decoding others' nonverbal behavior, they describe themselves as relatively clumsy at conversation, and they think that they have less dexterity in social situations than others do (Miller, 1995). The behavioral inhibition that defines shyness is tied both to nervous dread of what others are thinking and to doubts about one's social competence that magnify one's unease.

Interactive and Relational Effects. None of this escapes the notice of those with whom shy people interact. The reticence of shy people can make them seem detached and unfriendly, and they make poorer impressions on conversation partners than do those who are less shy (Heerey & Kring, 2007). This is regrettably ironic: Concern about others' judgments leads shy people to behave in a timid, cautious, and clumsy manner that engenders the disregard they hoped to avoid (see Curtis & Miller, 1986); this confirms their fears, conceivably leading to stronger shyness and further withdrawal.

These unhappy outcomes may add up over time. In school, the hesitance and diffidence of shy adolescents may be mistaken for a lack of intelligence (Evans, 2001) and lead to victimization by their peers (Blöte & Westenberg, 2007). Compared with those who are less shy, teenagers with higher levels of trait shyness have fewer friends, with whom they share weaker emotional ties and who provide them less support, so their friendships are less satisfying and of lower quality (Rubin, Wojslawowicz, Rose-Krasnor, Booth-LaForce, & Burgess, 2006). They develop attachment styles that tend to be characterized by anxiety over abandonment, and they are relatively unlikely to enjoy secure attachments (Darcy, Davila, & Beck, 2005).

When they go to college, shy people make friends more slowly than others do, and they are less likely to start a new romance (Asendorpf, 2000). They have fewer sex partners (Leary & Dobbins, 1983), and the sex they have is of poorer quality (Bradshaw, 2006). Shyness is probably associated with these outcomes not only because it makes one's interactions less rewarding but also because it reduces one's *opportunities* to make new friends and to find new loves (Leary & Buckley, 2000). Being less socially dexterous than others, shy people initiate fewer conversations, interact with fewer people, and go on fewer dates (Asendorpf, 2000),

and this may cumulatively be quite disadvantageous. Down the road, shy men marry 3 years later, on average, than men who are not shy, and they take longer to establish their careers (Caspi, Bem, & Elder, 1988). Shy people of both sexes also suffer more health problems, such as sleep disturbances and nausea (Langston & Cantor, 1989); the greater stress they encounter in social situations may take a toll over time.

This all sounds rather grim, but shyness is not all bad. The intimate partners of shy people describe them as modest, sensitive, and tactful (Gough & Thorne, 1986), so shy diffidence may play well in close quarters once a partner's love is won. Moreover, it is entirely sensible to be cautious and reserved when one is in unfamiliar territory, governed by unknown norms. On the whole, however, the patterns of cognition, motivation and emotion, and behavior that emerge from social anxiousness and shyness operate as anticipatory preparation for social rejection that rarely occurs—unless the pessimistic outlook and inhibited behavior of anxious and shy people make their fears come true. In this sense, then, social anxiousness and shyness are maladaptive. They are costly, and their benefits are few. Are the social-evaluative siblings undesirable, then? Not entirely.

Embarrassability

With their common roots in social-evaluative concern, social anxiousness, shyness, and embarrassability have much in common. As you might expect, socially anxious and/or shy people respond to social predicaments with more intense embarrassment than do those who are less anxious or shy (Hofmann, Moscovitch, & Kim, 2006). They are clearly more embarrassable (Miller, 1995). However, the traits are far from being synonymous; the correlation between embarrassability and social anxiousness is 0.48—sizable, but not enormous—and shyness is even more distinct (being correlated with embarrassability, $r = .37$; Miller, 1995). Stemming from alert sensitivity to impropriety that is coupled with a dread of disapproval, embarrassability leads to pessimistic vigilance, much like the other traits. Nevertheless, within its normal range, it has fewer adverse effects on daily life.

Social Cognition

One of the best predictors of embarrassability is *social sensitivity*, or attentiveness to the normative appropriateness of behavior (Miller, 1995; Riggio, 1986). Highly embarrassable people take note of social rules, and they are more likely than those who are less embarrassable to detect improprieties that (they think) are violations of them. They are probably thin-skinned in this regard, because they are embarrassed by the same types of events as anyone else, but they encounter more of them and then react more intensely to them (Miller, 1992). They become discombobulated by events that go unnoticed or are shrugged off by others.

Highly embarrassable people also experience stronger worries than those who are less embarrassable. They fear negative evaluation from others (Miller, 1995), are prone to stage fright and anxiety over abandonment (Withers & Vernon, 2006), and fret overmuch about hurting others' feelings (Sharkey & Kim, 2000). Embarrassability is also associated with a specific social concern, a fear of blushing. Highly embarrassable people think that they blush more frequently and more conspicuously than others do (Leary & Meadows, 1991), and the belief that others have noticed their blushes causes them more discomfort (Drummond et al., 2003). For the most part, these concerns are overwrought; people who fear blushing do not actually blush more intensely than others, on average (Chen & Drummond, 2008). However, they *think* they do; they perceive physiological responses that are really no stronger than those experienced by others to be more compelling and forceful (Chen & Drummond, 2008).

These patterns resemble the self-focus and worries associated with social anxiousness, and they may be mostly due to the higher social anxiousness typically found in highly embarrassable people. In particular, excessive fear of blushing appears to be more closely associated with the exaggerated fears of social anxiousness than with embarrassability per se (Edelmann, 2001). However, highly embarrassable people are thin-skinned about social propriety, whether or not they are prone to social anxiety (Miller, 1995). Thus, regardless of their other social concerns, embarrassable people are espe-cially alert for violations of social norms and quick to be flustered when such disturbances occur.

Motivation and Emotion

In the throes of embarrassment, people sometimes become so perturbed that they abandon the situation and simply flee the scene. More often, however, they respond in an agreeable, conciliatory manner; they poke fun at themselves or, if they have inconvenienced others, they apologize and offer reparations (Miller, 1996). These are actions that are likely to forestall rejection by others. Indeed, people are especially helpful, generous, and eager to please after embarrassment strikes (Apsler, 1975). Some of this may be chronic in those who are prone to embarrassment; highly embarrassable people are highly motivated to gain acceptance from others (Miller, 1995), and they are more likely than others to issue apologies when they become embarrassed (Tarr, Kim, & Sharkey, 2005).

Their interest in being socially accepted is also reflected in their attachment styles: Embarrassability is associated with anxiety over abandonment (Withers & Vernon, 2006), so highly embarrassable people tend to be nervously preoccupied with the quality of their relations with others. In general, then, embarrassability is characterized by vigilance with respect to propriety that is coupled with fretfulness regarding the consequences if social predicaments occur.

Behavior

Unlike shyness, embarrassability is not related to one's global level of social skill (Miller, 1995). People do not seem to be prone to embarrassment because they are blind to others' feelings or clumsy at small talk. However, embarrassable people *are* less deft at flexibly tailoring their behavior to adapt to new situations—a component of social skill termed *social control* (Riggio, 1986)—so they are less nimble and adroit in their interactions than are those who are less embarrassable (Miller, 1995).

Moreover, embarrassability can make a bad impression on observers if it leads people to respond to minor peccadilloes with levels of emotion that seem disproportionate to the circumstances (Miller, 2007). In one study bearing on perils of this sort, a young woman requesting help from a college class dropped a stack of forms and responded with evident chagrin in one of two ways (Levin & Arluke, 1982): she either yelped, "Oh, my God, I can't continue," and ran from the room, or she stayed put and seemed obviously embarrassed as she made her request. She received more assistance from her peers when her embarrassment was apparent but not excessive. Indeed, embarrassment that is calibrated to its circumstances is usually met with sympathy and support by the others present; oddly extreme reactions, however, are not (Miller, 1996, 2007).

The most important influence of embarrassability on behavior, however, may be the manner in which it may lead people to avoid situations that promise to be embarrassing, even if such situations will be good for them (Miller, 2007). In particular, people too often put off or avoid medical treatment for such conditions as sexually transmitted infections (Hook & Sharma, 2005), colorectal cancer (Hou, 2005), and urinary incontinence (Horrocks, Somerset, Stoddart, & Peters, 2004) because of misplaced concern about others' opinions of them. Despite having good intentions, they may also fail to buy and use condoms (Moore, Dahl, Gorn, & Weinberg, 2006). In these cases, social sensitivity that at more appropriate levels would promote decorous, genteel behavior is actually disadvantageous.

Conclusion

If they are so often distressing and detrimental, why are social anxiousness, shyness, and embarrassability so prevalent? Most theorists agree that ours is a social species with evolved mechanisms that help us maintain congenial relations with our fellows (Miller, 2004). The social-evaluative siblings presumably arose because they were beneficial in some way—and, in moderation, keeping track of others' opinions of us is undoubtedly of service to our survival. In particular, mechanisms that alert us when rejection is imminent provide invaluable feedback that interrupts undesirable behavior and promotes remedial action (Leary & Baumeister, 2000).

Too often, however, people are *too* concerned about what others are thinking of them (Leary, 2004), and this is frequently the case with social anxiousness, shyness, and embarrassability. Social *awareness* is undoubtedly almost always valuable, but the fretful concerns of social anxiety are only rarely useful. Beyond modest levels, social anxiousness has people edgily fearing threats that never arrive. Or worse, as in the case of shyness, it leads people to behave in ineffective ways that produce the outcomes they fear.

Within their normal ranges of operation, embarrassability seems the most desirable of these three traits, because a person completely without it would be impaired, being implacably unruffled in outrageous situations and seeming to observers to lack a conscience. In contrast, were the fretful anticipation of unlikely rejection that characterizes social anxiousness and the usually misplaced timidity and inhibition of shyness entirely absent from our lives, most of us would be better off. Still, the social-evaluative siblings exist for good reason; there are occasions that *are* socially risky, and the caution that the siblings promote is sometimes beneficial. We might not wish to be without some measure of social anxiousness, shyness, and embarrassability, even if they could be avoided. They are inevitable influences, then, on our transactions with others. The trick lies in keeping them in check so that they operate within beneficial limits.

Notes

1. The accuracy of this point was driven home to me when, as a favor to a friend, I gave a brief talk on "What Professors Do" to an audience of 3- and 4-year-olds at a day care facility. The talk did not go well. I was met with the most profound uninterest I have ever encountered, and my audience's boredom was palpable. This would have been distressing had my friend or any other adult been present, but I was alone with the preschoolers, all of them strangers. I was relieved to find that I seemed to be immune to their indifference. It was enough that my friend was grateful for my help; I would never see these kids again, and it simply didn't matter whether they liked me or not. Being accepted by them was of no importance to me. Given that, I could be frustrated by my failure to entertain them, but I was incapable of being anxious about the prospect of their rejection. It was rather a freeing experience.

2. The Embarrassability Scale was originally written using only masculine pronouns. A version appropriate for use for both sexes, adapted by me with Modigliani's permission, appears in Miller (1996).

References

Alden, L. E., & Taylor, C. T. (2004). Interpersonal processes in social phobia. *Clinical Psychology Review, 24,* 857–882.

Amir, N., Beard, C., & Bower, E. (2005). Interpretation bias and social anxiety. *Cognitive Therapy and Research, 29,* 433–443.

Amir, N., Freshman, M., & Foa, E. (2002). Enhanced Stroop interference for threat in social phobia. *Journal of Anxiety Disorders, 16,* 1–9.

Anderson, S. W., Bechara, A., Damasio, H., Tranel, D., & Damasio, A. R. (1999). Impairment of social and moral behavior related to early damage in human prefrontal cortex. *Nature Neuroscience, 2,* 1032–1037.

Apsler, R. (1975). Effects of embarrassment on behavior toward others. *Journal of Personality and Social Psychology, 32,* 145–153.

Asendorpf, J. (1990). The expression of shyness and embarrassment. In W. R. Crozier (Ed.), *Shyness and embarrassment: Perspectives from social psychology* (pp. 87–118). Cambridge, UK: Cambridge University Press.

Asendorpf, J. B. (2000). Shyness and adaptation to the social world of university. In W. R. Crozier (Ed.), *Shyness: Development, consolidation and change* (pp. 103–120). New York: Routledge.

Ashbaugh, A. R., Antony, M. M., McCabe, R. E., Schmidt, L. A., & Swinson, R. P. (2005). Self-evaluative biases in social anxiety. *Cognitive Therapy and Research, 29,* 387–398.

Baker, S. R., & Edelmann, R. J. (2002). Is social phobia related to lack of social skills?: Duration of skill-related behaviours and ratings of behavioural adequacy. *British Journal of Clinical Psychology, 41,* 243–257.

Beer, J. S., Heerey, E. A., Keltner, D., Scabini, D., & Knight, R. T. (2003). The regulatory function of self-conscious emotion: Insights from patients with orbitofrontal damage. *Journal of Personality and Social Psychology, 85,* 594–604.

Beidel, D. C., & Turner, S. M. (2007). *Shy children, phobic adults: Nature and treatment of social anxiety disorder* (2nd ed.). Washington, DC: American Psychological Association.

Berthoz, S., Armony, J. L., Blair, R. J. R., & Dolan, R. J. (2002). An fMRI study of intentional and unintentional (embarrassing) violations of social norms. *Brain, 125,* 1696–1708.

Blöte, A., & Westenberg, P. M. (2007). Socially anxious adolescents' perceptions of treatment by classmates. *Behaviour Research and Therapy, 45,* 189–198.

Bögels, S. M., & Mansell, W. (2004). Attention processes in the maintenance and treatment of social phobia: Hypervigilance, avoidance and self-focused attention. *Clinical Psychology Review, 24,* 827–856.

Bögels, S. M., & Reith, W. (1999). Validity of two questionnaires to assess social fears: The Dutch Social Phobia and Anxiety Inventory and the Blushing, Trembling and Sweating Questionnaire. *Journal of Psychopathology and Behavioral Assessment, 21,* 51–66.

Borkovec, T. D., Stone, N., O'Brien, G., & Kaloupek, D. (1974). Identification and measurement of anxiety in an analogue social situation. *Journal of Consulting and Clinical Psychology, 44,* 143–153.

Bradshaw, S. D. (2006). Shyness and difficult relationships: Formation is just the beginning. In D. C. Kirkpatrick, S. Duck, & M. K. Foley (Eds.), *Relating difficulty: The processes of constructing and maintaining difficult interaction* (pp. 15–41). Mahwah, NJ: Erlbaum.

Brown, L. H., Silvia, P. J., Myin-Germeys, I., & Kwapil, T. R. (2007). When the need to belong goes wrong: The expression of social anhedonia and social anxiety in daily life. *Psychological Science, 18,* 778–782.

Caspi, A., Bem, D. J., & Elder, D. J. (1988). Continuities and consequences of interactional styles across the life course. *Journal of Personality, 57,* 375–406.

Cheek, J. M., & Briggs, S. R. (1990). Shyness as a personality trait. In W. R. Crozier (Ed.), *Shyness and embarrassment: Perspectives from social psychology* (pp. 315–337). Cambridge, UK: Cambridge University Press.

Cheek, J. M., & Buss, A. H. (1981). Shyness and sociability. *Journal of Personality and Social Psychology, 41,* 330–339.

Chen, V., & Drummond, P. (2008). Fear of negative evaluation augments negative affect and somatic symptoms in social-evaluative situations. *Cognition and Emotion, 22,* 21–43.

Clark, D. M., & Wells, A. (1995). The cognitive model of social phobia. In R. G. Heimberg, M. R. Liebowitz, D. A. Hope, & F. R. Schneier (Eds.), *Social phobia: Diagnosis, assessment, and treatment* (pp. 69–93). New York: Guilford Press.

Constans, J. I., Penn, D. L., Ihen, G. H., & Hope, D. A. (1999). Interpretive biases for ambiguous stimuli in social anxiety. *Behaviour Research and Therapy, 37,* 643–651.

Curtis, R. C., & Miller, L. (1986). Believing another likes or dislikes you: Behaviors making the beliefs come true. *Journal of Personality and Social Psychology, 51,* 284–290.

Dannahy, L., & Stopa, L. (2007). Post-event processing in social anxiety. *Behaviour Research and Therapy, 45,* 1207–1219.

Darcy, K., Davila, J., & Beck, J. G. (2005). Is social anxiety associated with both interpersonal avoidance and interpersonal dependence? *Cognitive Therapy and Research, 29,* 171–186.

Davila, J., & Beck, J. G. (2002). Is social anxiety associated with impairment in close relationships?: A preliminary investigation. *Behavior Therapy, 33,* 427–446.

DePaulo, B. M., Epstein, J. A., & LeMay, C. S. (1990). Responses of the socially anxious to the prospect of interpersonal evaluation. *Journal of Personality, 58,* 623–640.

Drummond, P. D., Camacho, L., Formentin, N., Heffernan, T. D., Williams, F., & Zekas, T. E. (2003). The impact of verbal feedback about blushing on social discomfort and facial blood flow during embarrassing tasks. *Behaviour Research and Therapy, 41*, 413–425.

Edelmann, R. J. (2001). Blushing. In W. R. Crozier & L. E. Alden (Eds.), *International handbook of social anxiety: Concepts, research and interventions relating to the self and shyness* (pp. 301–323). Chichester, UK: Wiley.

Edelmann, R. J., & Baker, S. R. (2002). Self-reported and actual physiological responses in social phobia. *British Journal of Clinical Psychology, 41*, 1–14.

Edelmann, R. J., & Hampson, R. J. (1979). Changes in non-verbal behaviour during embarrassment. *British Journal of Social and Clinical Psychology, 18*, 385–390.

Edwards, S. L., Rapee, R. M., & Franklin, J. (2003). Postevent rumination and recall bias for a social performance event in high and low socially anxious individuals. *Cognitive Therapy and Research, 27*, 603–617.

Evans, M. A. (2001). Shyness in the classroom and home. In W. R. Crozier & L. E. Alden (Eds.), *International handbook of social anxiety: Concepts, research and interventions relating to the self and shyness* (pp. 159–183). Chichester, UK: Wiley.

Fehm, L., Schneider, G., & Hoyer, J. (2007). Is postevent processing specific for social anxiety? *Journal of Behavior Therapy and Experimental Psychiatry, 38*, 11–22.

Fenigstein, A., Scheier, M. F., & Buss, A. H. (1975). Public and private self-consciousness: Assessment and theory. *Journal of Consulting and Clinical Psychology, 43*, 522–527.

Furmark, T. (2002). Social phobia: Overview of community surveys. *Acta Psychiatrica Scandinavica, 105*, 84–93.

Garcia, S., Stinson, L., Ickes, W., Bissonnette, V., & Briggs, S. R. (1991). Shyness and physical attractiveness in mixed-sex dyads. *Journal of Personality and Social Psychology, 61*, 35–49.

Gerlach, A. L., Wilhelm, F. H., & Roth, W. T. (2003). Embarrassment and social phobia: The role of parasympathetic activation. *Journal of Anxiety Disorders, 17*, 197–210.

Gilboa-Schechtman, E., Foa, E. B., & Amir, N. (1999). Attentional biases for facial expressions in social phobia: The face-in-the-crowd paradigm. *Cognition and Emotion, 13*, 305–318.

Gough, H. G., & Thorne, A. (1986). Positive, negative, and balanced shyness: Self-definitions and the reactions of others. In W. H. Jones, J. M. Cheek, & S. R. Briggs (Eds.), *Shyness: Perspectives on research and treatment* (pp. 205–226). New York: Plenum Press.

Hart, E. A., Leary, M. R., & Rejeski, W. J. (1989). The measurement of social physique anxiety. *Journal of Sport and Exercise Psychology, 11*, 94–104.

Heerey, E. A., Keltner, D., & Capps, L. M. (2003). Making sense of self-conscious emotion: Linking theory of mind and emotion in children with autism. *Emotion, 3*, 394–400.

Heerey, E. A., & Kring, A. M. (2007). Interpersonal consequences of social anxiety. *Journal of Abnormal Psychology, 116*, 125–134.

Henderson, L., & Zimbardo, P. (2001). Shyness as a clinical condition: The Stanford model. In W. R. Crozier & L. E. Alden (Eds.), *International handbook of social anxiety: Concepts, research*

and interventions relating to the self and shyness (pp. 431–447). Chichester, UK: Wiley.

Heuer, K., Rinck, M., & Becker, E. S. (2007). Avoidance of emotional facial expressions in social anxiety: The Approach–Avoidance Task. *Behaviour Research and Therapy, 45*, 2990–3001.

Hinrichsen, H., & Clark, D. M. (2003). Anticipatory processing in social anxiety: Two pilot studies. *Journal of Behavior Therapy and Experimental Psychiatry, 34*, 205–218.

Hirsch, C. R., & Clark, D. M. (2004). Information-processing bias in social phobia. *Clinical Psychology Review, 24*, 799–825.

Hofmann, S. G., Moscovitch, D. A., & Kim, H. (2006). Autonomic correlates of social anxiety and embarrassment in shy and non-shy individuals. *International Journal of Psychophysiology, 61*, 134–142.

Hopko, D. R., Stowell, J., Jones, W. H., Armento, M. E. A., & Cheek, J. M. (2005). Psychometric properties of the Revised Cheek and Buss Shyness Scale. *Journal of Personality Assessment, 84*, 185–192.

Hook, E. W., III, & Sharma, A. K. (2005). Public tolerance, private pain: Stigma and sexually transmitted infections in the American Deep South. *Culture, Health, and Sexuality, 7*, 43–57.

Horrocks, S., Somerset, M., Stoddart, H., & Peters, T. J. (2004). What prevents older people from seeking treatment for urinary incontinence?: A qualitative exploration of barriers to the use of community continence services. *Family Practice, 21*, 689–696.

Hou, S. (2005). Factors associated with intentions for colorectal cancer screenings in a Chinese sample. *Psychological Reports, 96*, 159–162.

Huppert, J. D., Foa, E. B., Furr, J. M., Filip, J. C., & Matthews, A. (2003). Interpretation bias in social anxiety: A dimensional perspective. *Cognitive Therapy and Research, 27*, 569–577.

Huppert, J. D., Pasupuleti, R. V., Foa, E. B., & Matthews, A. (2007). Interpretation biases in social anxiety: Response generation, response selection, and self-appraisals. *Behaviour Research and Therapy, 45*, 1505–1515.

Johnson, H. S., Inderbitzen-Nolan, H. M., & Anderson, E. R. (2006). The Social Phobia Inventory: Validity and reliability in an adolescent community sample. *Psychological Assessment, 18*, 269–277.

Jones, W. H., Briggs, S. R., & Smith, T. G. (1986). Shyness: Conceptualization and measurement. *Journal of Personality and Social Psychology, 51*, 629–639.

Kashdan, T. B. (2007). Social anxiety spectrum and diminished positive experiences: Theoretical synthesis and meta-analysis. *Clinical Psychology Review, 27*, 348–365.

Kashdan, T. B., & Roberts, J. E. (2006). Affective outcomes in superficial and intimate interactions: Roles of social anxiety and curiosity. *Journal of Research in Personality, 40*, 140–167.

Kashdan, T. B., & Steger, M. F. (2006). Expanding the topography of social anxiety: An experience-sampling assessment of positive emotions, positive events, and emotion suppression. *Psychological Science, 17*, 120–128.

Kelly, K. M., & Jones, W. H. (1997). Assessment of dispositional embarrassability. *Anxiety, Stress and Coping: An International Journal, 10*, 307–333.

Keltner, D., & Buswell, B. N. (1997). Embarrassment:

Its distinct form and appeasement function. *Psychological Bulletin, 122,* 250–270.

Langston, C. A., & Cantor, N. (1989). Social anxiety and social constraint: When making friends is hard. *Journal of Personality and Social Psychology, 56,* 649–661.

Leary, M. R. (1983a). Brief version of the Fear of Negative Evaluation Scale. *Personality and Social Psychology Bulletin, 9,* 371–375.

Leary, M. R. (1983b). Social anxiousness: The construct and its measurement. *Journal of Personality Assessment, 47,* 66–75.

Leary, M. R. (1986a). Affective and behavioral components of shyness: Implications for theory, measurement, and research. In W. H. Jones, J. M. Cheek, & S. R. Briggs (Eds.), *Shyness: Perspectives on research and treatment* (pp. 27–38). New York: Plenum Press.

Leary, M. R. (1986b). The impact of interactional impediments on social anxiety and self-presentation. *Journal of Experimental Social Psychology, 22,* 122–135.

Leary, M. R. (2001a). Shyness and the self: Attentional, motivational, and cognitive self-processes in social anxiety and inhibition. In W. R. Crozier & L. E. Alden (Eds.), *International handbook of social anxiety: Concepts, research and interventions relating to the self and shyness* (pp. 217–234). Chichester, UK: Wiley.

Leary, M. R. (2001b). Social anxiety as an early warning system: A refinement and extension of the self-presentation theory of social anxiety. In S. G. Hofmann & P. M. DiBartolo (Eds.), *From social anxiety to social phobia: Multiple perspectives* (pp. 321–334). Boston: Allyn & Bacon.

Leary, M. R. (2004). *The curse of the self: Self-awareness, egotism, and the quality of human life.* New York: Oxford University Press.

Leary, M. R., & Baumeister, R. F. (2000). The nature and function of self-esteem: Sociometer theory. In M. Zanna (Ed.), *Advances in experimental social psychology* (Vol. 32, pp. 1–62). San Diego, CA: Academic Press.

Leary, M. R., & Buckley, K. E. (2000). Shyness and the pursuit of social acceptance. In W. R. Crozier (Ed.), *Shyness: Development, consolidation and change* (pp. 139–153). New York: Routledge.

Leary, M. R., & Dobbins, S. E. (1983). Social anxiety, sexual behavior, and contraceptive use. *Journal of Personality and Social Psychology, 45,* 1347–1354.

Leary, M. R., & Meadows, S. (1991). Predictors, elicitors, and concomitants of social blushing. *Journal of Personality and Social Psychology, 60,* 254–262.

Ledley, D. R., & Heimberg, R. G. (2006). Cognitive vulnerability to social anxiety. *Journal of Social and Clinical Psychology 25,* 755–778.

Levin, J., & Arluke, A. (1982). Embarrassment and helping behavior. *Psychological Reports, 51,* 999–1002.

Maidenberg, E., Chen, E., Craske, M., Bohn, P., & Bystritsky, A. (1996). Specificity of attentional bias in panic disorder and social phobia. *Journal of Anxiety Disorders, 10,* 529–541.

Mansell, W., Clark, D. M., & Ehlers, A. (2003). Internal versus external attention in social anxiety: An investigation using a novel paradigm. *Behaviour Research and Therapy, 41,* 555–572.

Mansell, W., Clark, D. M., Ehlers, A., & Chen, Y. (1999). Social anxiety and attention away from angry faces. *Cognition and Emotion, 13,* 673–690.

Marcus, D. K., & Miller, R. S. (1999). The perception of "live" embarrassment: A social relations analysis of class presentations. *Cognition and Emotion, 13,* 105–117.

Marshall, P. J., & Stevenson-Hinde, J. (2001). Behavioral inhibition: Physiological correlates. In W. R. Crozier & L. E. Alden (Eds.), *International handbook of social anxiety: Concepts, research and interventions relating to the self and shyness* (pp. 53–76). Chichester, UK: Wiley.

McCroskey, J. C. (1970). Measures of communication-bound anxiety. *Speech Monographs, 37,* 269–277.

Miller, R. S. (1987). Empathic embarrassment: Situational and personal determinants of reactions to the embarrassment of another. *Journal of Personality and Social Psychology, 53,* 1061–1069.

Miller, R. S. (1992). The nature and severity of self-reported embarrassing circumstances. *Personality and Social Psychology Bulletin, 18,* 190–198.

Miller, R. S. (1995). On the nature of embarrassability: Shyness, social evaluation, and social skill. *Journal of Personality, 63,* 315–339.

Miller, R. S. (1996). *Embarrassment: Poise and peril in everyday life.* New York: Guilford Press.

Miller, R. S. (2001a). Embarrassment and social phobia: Distant cousins or close kin? In S. G. Hofmann & P. M. DiBartolo (Eds.), *From social anxiety to social phobia: Multiple perspectives* (pp. 65–85). Boston: Allyn & Bacon.

Miller, R. S. (2001b). Shyness and embarrassment compared: Siblings in the service of social evaluation. In W. R. Crozier & L. E. Alden (Eds.), *International handbook of social anxiety: Concepts, research and interventions relating to the self and shyness* (pp. 281–300). Chichester, UK: Wiley.

Miller, R. S. (2004). Emotion as adaptive interpersonal communication: The case of embarrassment. In L. Z. Tiedens & C. W. Leach (Eds.), *The social life of emotions* (pp. 87–104). Cambridge, UK: Cambridge University Press.

Miller, R. S. (2007). Is embarrassment a blessing or a curse? In J. L. Tracy, R. W. Robins, & J. P. Tangney (Eds.), *Self-conscious emotions* (pp. 245–262). New York: Oxford University Press.

Modigliani, A. (1968). Embarrassment and embarrassability. *Sociometry, 31,* 313–326.

Mogg, K., Bradley, B. P., de Bono, J., & Painter, M. (1997). Time course of attentional bias for threat information in non-clinical anxiety. *Behaviour Research and Therapy, 35,* 297–303.

Mogg, K., Philippot, P., & Bradley, B. P. (2004). Selective attention to angry faces in clinical social phobia. *Journal of Abnormal Psychology, 113,* 160–165.

Moore, S. G., Dahl, D. W., Gorn, G. J., & Weinberg, C. B. (2006). Coping with condom embarrassment. *Psychology, Health and Medicine, 11,* 70–79.

Norton, P. J., Hope, D. A., & Weeks, J. W. (2004). The Physical Activity and Sport Anxiety Scale (PASAS): Scale development and psychometric analysis. *Anxiety, Stress and Coping: An International Journal, 17,* 363–382.

Osborne, M. S., Kenny, D. T., & Holsomback, R. (2005). Assessment of music performance anxiety in late childhood: A validation study of the Music Performance Anxiety Inventory for Adolescents (MPAI-A). *International Journal of Stress Management, 12,* 312–330.

Papsdorf, M., & Alden, L. (1998). Mediators of social rejection in social anxiety: Similarity, self-disclosure, and overt signs of anxiety. *Journal of Research in Personality, 32,* 351–369.

Perowne, S., & Mansell, W. (2002). Social anxiety, self-focused attention, and the discrimination of negative, neutral and positive audience members by their non-verbal behaviours. *Behavioural and Cognitive Psychotherapy, 30,* 11–23.

Pineles, S. L., & Mineka, S. (2005). Attentional biases to internal and external sources of potential threat in social anxiety. *Journal of Abnormal Psychology, 114,* 314–318.

Rector, N. A., Kocovski, N. L., & Ryder, A. G. (2006). Social anxiety and the fear of causing discomfort to others: Conceptualization and treatment. *Journal of Social and Clinical Psychology, 25,* 906–918.

Riggio, R. E. (1986). Assessment of basic social skills. *Journal of Personality and Social Psychology, 51,* 649–660.

Rubin, K. H., Wojslawowicz, J. C., Rose-Krasnor, L., Booth-LaForce, C., & Burgess, K. B. (2006). The best friendships of shy/withdrawn children: Prevalence, stability, and relationship quality. *Journal of Abnormal Child Psychology, 34,* 143–157.

Sabini, J., Siepmann, M., Stein, J., & Meyerowitz, M. (2000). Who is embarrassed by what? *Cognition and Emotion, 14,* 213–240.

Saudino, K. J. (2001). Behavioral genetics, social phobia, social fears, and related temperaments. In S. G. Hofmann & P. M. DiBartolo (Eds.), *From social anxiety to social phobia: Multiple perspectives* (pp. 200–215). Boston: Allyn & Bacon.

Scheier, M. F., & Carver, C. S. (1985). The Self-Consciousness Scale: A revised version for use with general populations. *Journal of Applied Social Psychology, 15,* 687–699.

Schlenker, B. R., & Leary, M. R. (1982). Social anxiety and self-presentation: A conceptualization and model. *Psychological Bulletin, 92,* 641–669.

Schmidt, L. A., & Tasker, S. L. (2000). Childhood shyness: Determinants, development and "depathology." In W. R. Crozier (Ed.), *Shyness: Development, consolidation and change* (pp. 30–46). New York: Routledge.

Schneier, F. R., Blanco, C., Antia, S. X., & Liebowitz, M. R. (2002). The social anxiety spectrum. *Psychiatric Clinics of North America, 25,* 757–774.

Schofield, C. A., Coles, M. E., & Gibb, B. E. (2007). Social anxiety and interpretation biases for facial displays of emotion: Emotion detection and ratings of social cost. *Behaviour Research and Therapy, 45,* 2950–2963.

Sharkey, W. F., & Kim, M. (2000). The effect of embarrassability on perceived importance of conversational constraints. *Human Communication, 3,* 27–40.

Shepperd, J. A., & Arkin, R. M. (1990). Shyness and self-presentation. In W. R. Crozier (Ed.), *Shyness and embarrassment: Perspectives from social psychology* (pp. 286–314). Cambridge, UK: Cambridge University Press.

Storch, E. A., Masia-Warner, C., Heidgerken, A. D., Fisher, P. H., Pincus, D. B., & Liebowitz, M. R. (2006). Factor structure of the Liebowitz Social Anxiety Scale for Children and Adolescents. *Child Psychiatry and Human Development, 37,* 25–37.

Stravynski, A., & Amado, D. (2001). Social phobia as a deficit in social skills. In S. G. Hofmann & P. M. DiBartolo (Eds.), *From social anxiety to social phobia: Multiple perspectives* (pp. 107–129). Boston: Allyn & Bacon.

Stritzke, W. G. K., Nguyen, A., & Durkin, K. (2004). Shyness and computer-mediated communication: A self-presentational theory perspective. *Media Psychology, 6,* 1–22.

Tangney, J. P., Miller, R. S., Flicker, L., & Barlow, D. H. (1996). Are shame, guilt, and embarrassment distinct emotions? *Journal of Personality and Social Psychology, 70,* 1256–1264.

Tarr, N. D., Kim, M., & Sharkey, W. F. (2005). The effects of self-construals and embarrassability on predicament response strategies. *International Journal of Intercultural Relations, 29,* 497–520.

Turner, S. M., Beidel, D. C., Dancu, C. V., & Stanley, M. A. (1989). An empirically derived inventory to measure social fears and anxiety. *Psychological Assessment, 1,* 35–40.

Vassilopoulos, S. P. (2004). Anticipatory processing in social anxiety. *Behavioural and Cognitive Psychotherapy, 32,* 303–311.

Vassilopoulos, S. P. (2005). Anticipatory processing plays a role in maintaining social anxiety. *Anxiety, Stress, and Coping, 18,* 321–332.

Veljaca, K., & Rapee, R. M. (1998). Detection of negative and positive audience behaviours by socially anxious subjects. *Behaviour Research and Therapy, 36,* 311–321.

Voncken, M. J., Bögels, S. M., & de Vries, K. (2003). Interpretation and judgmental biases in social phobia. *Behaviour Research and Therapy, 41,* 1481–1488.

Ward, C. C., & Tracey, T. J. G. (2004). Relation of shyness with aspects of online relationship involvement. *Journal of Social and Personal Relationships, 21,* 611–623.

Watson, D., & Friend, R. (1969). Measurement of social-evaluative anxiety. *Journal of Consulting and Clinical Psychology, 33,* 448–457.

Weeks, J. W., Heimberg, R. G., & Rodebaugh, T. L. (2008). The Fear of Positive Evaluation Scale: Assessing a proposed cognitive component of social anxiety. *Journal of Anxiety Disorders, 22,* 44–55.

Withers, L. A., & Vernon, L. L. (2006). To err is human: Embarrassment, attachment, and communication apprehension. *Personality and Individual Differences, 40,* 99–110.

Zimbardo, P. G. (1977). *Shyness: What it is and what to do about it.* Reading, MA: Addison-Wesley.

Zou, J. B., Hudson, J. L., & Rapee, R. M. (2007). The effect of attentional focus on social anxiety. *Behaviour Research and Therapy, 45,* 2326–2333.

CHAPTER 13

■ ● ▲ ◆ ■ ● ▲ ◆

Proneness to Shame and Proneness to Guilt

JUNE PRICE TANGNEY
KERSTIN YOUMAN
JEFFREY STUEWIG

An important but understudied component of personality is how people react to their own failures and transgressions. To err is human, to occasionally sin is … inevitable. People vary considerably in how they feel when they recognize that they have failed or behaved badly. For example, given the same event—say, hurting a friend's feelings—an individual prone to guilt would be likely to respond by ruminating about the offensive remark, feeling bad about hurting a friend, and being compelled to apologize and make up for it. A shame-prone individual, instead, is likely to see the event as proof that he or she is a bad friend—indeed, a bad person. Feeling small and worthless, the shame-prone person may be inclined to slink away and avoid the friend for fear of further shame.

Shame and guilt are siblings (together with pride and embarrassment) in the family of "self-conscious emotions" that are evoked by self-reflection and self-evaluation. This self-reflection is not always engaged in purposefully, and the emotional response does not always reach the conscious level of awareness. Nonetheless, as people reflect on themselves, these emotions provide immediate punishment (or reinforcement) of behavior and, importantly, a countervailing force to the reward structure based on more immediate, selfish, id-like desires. In effect, shame and guilt can be considered moral emotions that function as an emotional moral barometer, providing immediate and salient feedback on our social and moral acceptability. When we fall short of important standards, aversive feelings of shame, guilt, or both are likely to ensue.

This chapter summarizes recent theory and empirical work on individual differences in proneness to shame and guilt. Shame proneness and guilt proneness are stable personality dispositions representing the propensity to experience these moral emotions across time and situations.

The Difference between Shame and Guilt

The terms *shame* and *guilt* are inextricably linked in the minds of most people, but a number of attempts have been made to differentiate between them. The three major approaches to differentiating between shame and guilt involve distinctions based on: (1) the types of events that evoke the emotions, (2) the public-versus-private nature of the emotion-eliciting situation, and

(3) the degree to which the person construes the emotion-eliciting event as a failure of self or of behavior.

There is surprisingly little empirical evidence that shame and guilt differ reliably in terms of the types of situations that elicit them. Analyses of personal shame and guilt experiences provided by children and adults revealed few, if any, reliably shame-inducing or guilt-inducing situations (Keltner & Buswell, 1996; Tangney, 1992; Tangney, Marschall, Rosenberg, Barlow, & Wagner, 1994; Tracy & Robins, 2006). Researchers agree that guilt is more narrowly linked to moral transgressions, whereas shame is evoked by a broader range of situations, including both "moral" and "nonmoral" failures (Ferguson, Stegge, & Damhuis, 1991; Sabini & Silver, 1997; Smith, Webster, Parrott, & Eyre, 2002), but most types of events (e.g., lying, cheating, stealing, failing to help another, disobeying parents, etc.) are sometimes cited by people in connection with feelings of shame and sometimes in connection with guilt.

A frequently cited distinction between shame and guilt highlights the public-versus-private nature of the emotion-eliciting situation (e.g., Benedict, 1946). From this point of view, shame is the more "public" emotion, arising from exposure to disapproving others, whereas guilt is a more "private" experience that arises from internal pangs of conscience. However, empirical tests have not supported this distinction (Tangney et al., 1994; Tangney, Miller, Flicker, & Barlow, 1996). For example, a systematic analysis of shame and guilt events described by several hundred children and adults (Tangney et al., 1994) indicated that both emotions were typically experienced in the presence of others. "Solitary" shame experiences were no less common than "solitary" guilt experiences. Moreover, the frequency with which others were aware of the respondents' behavior did not vary as a function of shame or guilt. Similarly, although achievement and personal events are each more private than relational and familial events, the former were more likely to elicit shame rather than guilt in a study of personal emotion narratives (Tracy & Robins, 2006). Several other studies (Smith et al., 2002) provide ample evidence that actual public exposure is no more likely to evoke shame than guilt.

The most widely used basis for distinguishing between shame and guilt—focus on self versus behavior—was first proposed by Helen Block Lewis (1971) and more recently elaborated by Tracy and Robins (2004) in their appraisal-based model of self-conscious emotions. According to Lewis, shame involves a negative evaluation of the global self, whereas guilt involves a negative evaluation of a specific behavior. Although the self–behavior distinction may, at first glance, appear subtle, research supports that this differential emphasis on self ("*I* did that horrible thing") versus behavior ("I *did* that horrible *thing*") sets the stage for different emotional experiences and different patterns of motivations and subsequent behavior.

Shame is typically the more painful, disruptive emotion because the self, not simply one's behavior, is the object of judgment. When people feel shame about the self, they feel "small," worthless, powerless, and exposed. Even though an actual observing audience need not be present, they often imagine how one's defective self would appear to others. Lewis (1971) described a split in self-functioning in which the self is both agent and object of observation and disapproval. Regarding motivations or "action tendencies," shame is apt to prompt efforts to hide and defend the diminished, defective self and to escape the shame-inducing situation (Ketelaar & Au, 2003; Lewis, 1971; Lindsay-Hartz, 1984; Tangney, Miller, et al., 1996; Wallbott & Scherer, 1995; Wicker, Payne, & Morgan, 1983).

Guilt, on the other hand, typically wreaks less havoc. Although painful, guilt is less overwhelming because the object of condemnation is a specific behavior, somewhat apart from the self. Instead of feeling compelled to defend the naked core of one's identity, people stricken with guilt are drawn to consider their *behavior* and its consequences. People feeling guilt often ruminate over the misdeed, feeling the pain of remorse and regret. Regarding action tendencies, whereas shame often motivates hiding, guilt often motivates reparative action (e.g., confession, apology, efforts to make amends for the wrongdoing) (de Hooge, 2008; de Hooge, Zeelenberg, &

Breugelmans, 2007; Lindsay-Hartz, 1984; Tangney, Miller, et al., 1996; Wallbott & Scherer, 1995; Wicker et al., 1983).

There is broad empirical support for Lewis's (1971) distinction between shame and guilt from a range of experimental and correlational studies utilizing diverse methodologies, including qualitative case studies, content analyses of shame and guilt narratives, participants' quantitative ratings of personal shame and guilt experiences, analyses of attributions associated with shame and guilt, and analyses of participants' counterfactual thinking (for reviews, see Tangney & Dearing, 2002; Tangney, Stuewig, & Mashek, 2007a). For example, Tracy and Robins (2006) employed both experimental and correlational methods that revealed that, although both shame and guilt were positively related to internal attributions for failure, they differed with respect to attributions on the dimensions of stability and controllability. Whereas guilt was related to unstable, controllable attributions for failure (e.g., a behavior), shame was related to stable and uncontrollable attributions (e.g., the self).

Why is the notion that shame is a more "public" emotion so pervasive and persistent? Research shows that when experiencing shame, people may *feel* more exposed and more aware of others' disapproval (Tangney et al., 1994). It is a short leap from thinking what a horrible person one is to thinking that others are probably noticing this, too. The reality is that situations causing both shame and guilt are typically social in nature. But people are more aware of themselves and the possibility of negative social approval when experiencing shame. From this perspective, shame is the more "egocentric" and selfish emotion. In contrast, a person experiencing guilt focuses not on the self but rather on a specific harmful behavior, thinking specifically about its impact on others. In this sense, guilt is a more "other-oriented" emotion. Far from private, guilt is as social an emotion as shame. But a key consequence of the focus on self versus behavior is the nature of interpersonal concerns that ensue. With shame, it's all about oneself and what others might be thinking about oneself. With guilt, it's about one's behavior and the effect of that behavior on others.

Emotion States versus Emotion Dispositions

The research summarized thus far has focused on emotion *states*—situation-specific experiences of shame and guilt. Importantly, there are two types of moral emotional states: anticipatory and consequential (Tangney, Stuewig, & Mashek, 2007b). Shame and guilt can influence people even before they engage in a negative behavior. People can *anticipate* their likely emotional reactions (e.g., guilt, shame, pride) as they consider behavioral alternatives. Thus shame and guilt can exert a strong influence on moral choice and behavior by providing critical feedback regarding anticipated behavior (feedback in the form of *anticipatory* shame or guilt) and actual behavior (feedback in the form of *consequential* shame or guilt). Moreover, anticipatory and consequential emotional reactions work together in a recursive feedback loop. Anticipated or "forecasted" affective responses to behavior not yet enacted are inferred from past consequential emotions to similar behaviors and events.

In the realm of moral emotions, researchers are also interested in *dispositional* tendencies to experience shame and guilt in the face of failure or transgression. By definition, shame-prone (or guilt-prone) individuals are more susceptible to both anticipatory and consequential experiences of shame (or guilt) relative to their peers. Guilt-prone people are inclined to anticipate guilt in response to a range of *potential* behaviors and outcomes, as well as inclined to experience guilt as a consequence of *actual* failures and transgressions.

Notably, shame-prone and guilt-prone people do not walk through life in a constant state of shame or guilt. Rather, when they encounter emotion-relevant situations (e.g., failure or transgression), shame-prone people are inclined to respond with shame, and guilt-prone people are inclined to respond with guilt. In this way, shame proneness is conceptually distinct from "internalized shame" defined by Cook (1988) as an "enduring, chronic shame that has become internalized as part of one's identity and which can be most succinctly characterized as a deep sense of inferiority, inadequacy, or deficiency." Internalized shame is thus akin to low self-esteem, whereas proneness to shame is the propensity to experience episodic shame states in response to failures or transgressions.

Assessing Individual Differences in Proneness to Shame and Guilt

How are shame and guilt proneness measured at the dispositional or trait level? Often researchers look to people's self-reports to assess dimensions of personality or affective style, but in the case of guilt and shame, self-reports can be problematic because most people have difficulty recognizing the distinction between them. Research indicates that feelings of shame and guilt frequently co-occur, that it is difficult for people to verbalize the difference between the two, and that, in Western contexts at least, people are apt to avoid the term *shame* altogether, using *guilt* to refer to either or both emotions. Thus simply asking a person, "In general, do you feel guilt rarely, sometimes, often, or very often?" may tell us something about his or her propensity to experience guilt, shame, or both. Fortunately, a number of researchers have tackled this measurement challenge, although much more work needs to be done at the trait level and especially at the state level.[1] Here, we focus on measures at the level of trait or emotion disposition—proneness to shame and proneness to guilt.

Measures Assessing Only One Disposition

Much of the pioneering work on moral emotions, and thus the early measures, focused exclusively on the propensity to experience guilt without consideration of shame (Buss & Durkee, 1957; Klass, 1987; Kugler & Jones, 1992; Mosher, 1966; Zahn-Waxler, Kochanska, Krupnick, & Mayfield, 1988). These measures utilized a range of formats—selection of a single adjective, ratings of descriptive statements, forced-choice alternatives, ratings of emotional responses to specific situations, and qualitative analysis of narratives. Because these measures do not take into account the difference between shame and guilt, the assessment is apt to confound the propensity to experience guilt with the propensity to experience shame

and is thus of little use in examining shame and guilt proneness in psychological and social functioning. Moreover, because correlates of shame proneness and guilt proneness sometimes differ in sign, measures that confound shame and guilt may produce null results, as the differential relationships cancel each other out, leading to erroneous conclusions (e.g., that guilt is not important to the context under study). For this reason, researchers are advised to use caution when considering measures that purport to assess the propensity to experience guilt without explicitly considering shame.

Fewer measures assess shame proneness without reference to guilt proneness. The most widely used measure of this type is the Internalized Shame Scale (ISS; Cook, 1988). Ironically, the potential conceptual confound here is not with guilt but rather with its strong conceptual and operational similarity to low self-esteem. Many of the items composing the ISS were drawn from Rosenberg's (1965) Self-Esteem Scale. Consequently, the ISS correlates very highly with self-esteem (Cook, 1991), raising concerns about its discriminant validity.

Measures Assessing (and Distinguishing between) Shame Proneness and Guilt Proneness

Measures designed to distinguish between shame proneness and guilt proneness vary substantially in structure or format due to different conceptual distinctions between shame and guilt and to the unique challenges posed by the assessment of these two emotions in particular (e.g., people don't always use the emotion terms precisely; there is no identifiable facial expression for guilt). In selecting a measure, it is important to consider the measure's suitability for the population to be studied and the match between empirically supported distinctions between shame and guilt and the way in which they are operationalized.

Shame- versus Guilt-Inducing Situations

An approach first introduced by Perlman (1958) assesses emotional reactivity to "shame-inducing" versus "guilt-inducing" situations, under the assumption that different kinds of situations induce shame versus guilt. Measures by Crouppen (1976), Johnson and colleagues (1987), and Cheek and Hogan (1983) were designed under this assumption. In light of research showing no reliably shame-specific or guilt-specific eliciting situations, discussed earlier, researchers should consider the rationale for using such an approach.

Global Adjective Checklists

This approach draws on a list of shame- and guilt-related adjectives for which people are asked to make overall ratings of how much they experience each affective term or how well each term describes them. Examples of such measures include Hoblitzelle's (1987) Revised Shame–Guilt Scale (RSGS) and Harder and colleagues' (Harder, Cutler, & Rockart, 1992; Harder & Lewis, 1987) Personal Feelings Questionnaire (PFQ) and revised PFQ-2.

These measures have the advantages of high face validity and ease of administration. There are some limitations, however, that may outweigh the advantages. First, extended adjective checklists require advanced verbal skills. The RSGS, for example, includes vocabulary that is challenging for most college students. The PFQ measures utilize somewhat less sophisticated vocabulary. A second limitation is that adjective checklists rely heavily on respondents' ability to accurately distinguish between "shame" and "guilt" in an abstract context, which is questionable. Even among well-educated adults, providing meaningful definitions of shame and guilt is difficult (Lindsay-Hartz, 1984; Tangney & Dearing, 2002). As a consequence, the correlation between shame proneness and guilt proneness assessed via global adjective checklists is typically in the .70s, raising concerns about multicollinearity and discriminant validity. Not surprisingly, research using measures such as the RSGS and PFQ-2 rarely identifies unique variance in proneness to shame and guilt that is differentially related to other theoretically relevant constructs. For instance, using the PFQ-2, Sherry (2007) found that secure attachment was negatively correlated with both shame and guilt proneness, whereas fearful and preoccupied

attachment were positively related to both emotional dispositions among lesbian, gay, or bisexual adults. The correlation between PFQ-2 shame and guilt was .73, affording little discriminant validity. A third, and perhaps most problematic, aspect of global checklists is that the process of filling them out is essentially a shame-like task—making global ratings about oneself (or one's general affective state) in the absence of any specific situational context (Tangney, 1995). Whereas this approach may be appropriate for the assessment of shame, which involves rather global negative assessments of the entire self, it is a problem when attempting to assess the tendency to experience guilt about specific behaviors apart from the global self.

Scenario-Based Measures

A third method for assessing shame proneness and guilt proneness is the scenario-based approach exemplified by the Test of Self-Conscious Affect (TOSCA) measures (Tangney, Wagner, & Gramzow, 1989) and the Adolescent Shame Measure (ASM; Reimer, 1995). In these measures, people rate how they would respond to a series of common hypothetical situations (e.g., "You make a mistake at work and find out a coworker is blamed for the error"). Importantly, the terms *shame* and *guilt* are not used, thereby avoiding confusion common among laypersons. Instead, responses reflect brief phenomenological descriptions of shame and guilt reactions (as described in the theoretical, phenomenological, and empirical literature). For the scenario described, the shame response is "You would keep quiet and avoid the coworker." The guilt response is "You would feel unhappy and eager to correct the situation." People rate their likelihood of responding in each manner indicated. Thus people may endorse both shame and guilt, which can co-occur in a given situation. Although scenario based, the distinction between shame and guilt here is not in the content of the situation but rather in the phenomenological reaction of the respondent.

The primary strength of this approach is that the structure of scenario-based measures is conceptually consistent with our current understanding of guilt as a behavior-specific negative appraisal within a given situational context. Scenario-based measures provide a vehicle for assessing tendencies to experience guilt about specific behaviors, distinct from shame about the self, by avoiding the global nature of adjective rating scales that are more apt to tap into the characteristics of shame. A second advantage of the scenario-based approach is that the situation-specific phenomenological descriptions of shame and guilt do not require the respondent to distinguish between the terms *shame* and *guilt*. Third, the likelihood of a defensive response bias is lower than with adjective checklist-type measures. As Lewis (1971) and others have noted, repression or denial of shame experiences are not uncommon. Scenario-based measures may partly circumvent people's defensiveness because they are not directly asked to acknowledge tendencies to experience "shame" and "guilt" but rather to rate phenomenological descriptions of shame and guilt experiences with respect to specific situations that avoid use of the emotionally charged words *shame* and *guilt*.

Scenario-based measures are easily adapted for use with younger participants. There are TOSCAs for adolescents and for children ages 8–12 (see Tangney & Dearing, 2002), and Stegge and Ferguson (1990) have developed the Child Attribution and Reaction Survey—Child Version (C-CARS) for children as young as 5 years. Common to these measures is a range of age-appropriate situations (sampling from home, work/school, peer, and other domains) that are likely to elicit shame and/or guilt responses.

Of course, scenario-based measures have limitations. In general, they yield somewhat lower internal consistency estimates of reliability than adjective checklists, with Cronbach's alphas ranging from .71 to .86 for checklists versus .61 to .83 for scenario-based measures (Tangney & Dearing, 2002). Coefficient alphas, however, are apt to underestimate reliability due to the variability introduced by the use of different scenarios. In contrast, test–retest estimates of reliability for scenario-based measures tend to be higher than internal consistencies, equivalent to those observed for global adjective checklist measures.

A second limitation is the necessary constraint on the types of shame- and guilt-eliciting situations that can be used. Efforts are generally made to include scenarios from diverse settings (e.g., home, work/school, peer, and significant others) and to focus on diverse behaviors (e.g., missing an appointment, breaking something, hurting another person's feelings, failing a test). Nonetheless, such measures cover only a small subset of possible transgressions or failures. In particular, preference is given to situations and behaviors likely to be encountered by most respondents at some point in their day-to-day lives—ones that people can relate to easily and can readily imagine themselves. What is missing are less common, more idiosyncratic events (e.g., eating your roommate's food, behaving insensitively with a mentally ill family member) and more serious transgressions (e.g., hitting a child with a car, losing the family fortune in an ill-advised business deal) or events for which no reparation seems possible (e.g., involuntary manslaughter) that are irrelevant to most respondents but may dominate a specific person's emotional life. These events may lead individuals to experience "maladaptive" levels of guilt (Luyten, Fontaine, & Corveleyn, 2002). Stated another way, measures such as the TOSCA are less apt to capture intense but more circumscribed shame and guilt experiences focused in a specific domain (e.g., failures at dieting, marital infidelity, mistreating a vulnerable or stigmatized family member).[2]

A third concern is whether scenario-based measures such as the TOSCA assess emotional response tendencies (shame and guilt) as opposed to emotion-prompted behavior (hiding vs. amending). Some researchers have raised the possibility that in eschewing the use of the terms *shame* and *guilt* in favor of phenomenological descriptions, scenario-based proponents may have thrown out the emotional baby with the linguistic bathwater, as it were (Eisenberg, 2000; Ferguson, Brugman, White, & Eyre, 2007). A close analysis, however, reveals that only 25% (4 of 16) of guilt responses on the TOSCA-3 describe actual behavior (hiding for shame, amending for guilt). The rest refer to thoughts and feelings about what one should have done in the past or what one should do in the future. Only 2 of the 16 shame items describe behavioral responses. More important, the shame items, such as "feel incompetent," "feel inadequate," "feel immature," "think: 'I'm terrible'" and the guilt items, such as "think: 'this is making me anxious. I need to either fix it or get someone else to'," "feel unhappy and eager to correct the situation" are anything but affectively barren. The TOSCA-C and TOSCA-A also hold up well under this same scrutiny. The TOSCA-SD, developed for inmates, however, is heavily weighted toward behavior, based on initial assumptions about the need to use concrete responses with this population. Based on several years of research with jail inmates, we believe it is feasible to employ language and concepts similar to those employed on the other versions of the TOSCA. Thus, the TOSCA-SD is currently under revision.

In summary, global adjective checklists and scenario-based measures each have pros and cons. Both approaches yield reasonably valid indices of proneness to shame, but scenario-based measures seem uniquely able to capture proneness to guilt about behaviors, independent of shame about the self.

Shame Proneness and Guilt Proneness Are Not at Opposite Ends of a Single Continuum

Just as people may experience shame, guilt, or some combination of the two in response to a single event, at the dispositional level some people are prone to shame, some to guilt, and some to both. The correlation between shame proneness and guilt proneness is positive—about .42 for the TOSCA-3, higher among children using the TOSCA-C (about .6), and lower among inmates using the TOSCA-SD (about .2). We believe these two moderately correlated measures represent unipolar as opposed to bipolar dimensions (see Russell & Carroll, 1999). Specifically, high scores on shame proneness and guilt proneness carry meaning, but low scores are less informative, particularly for shame. There is no polar opposite to shame proneness. The unipolar, as opposed to bipolar, nature of these scales was underscored in our longitudinal study of jail inmates (Tangney, Mashek, & Stuewig, 2007). In a sample of 500 male and female inmates, psychopathy, a serious form of antisocial personality disorder (assessed by the Psychopathy Check-

list: Screening Version; Hare, Cox, & Hare, 1995), was unrelated to proneness to shame and only weakly negatively correlated with proneness to guilt ($r = -.16$), showing that psychopaths are not prone to either shame or guilt. But low scores on the TOSCA do not imply a pathological *absence* of shame and guilt. Stated another way, it is meaningful for someone to score (1) higher than his or her peers on shame but not guilt, (2) higher than his or her peers on both shame and guilt, and (3) higher than his or her peers on guilt but not shame. Low scores on both are not terribly informative.

What Is Shame-Free Guilt?

Theoretically, the adaptive features of guilt should be most evident when unaccompanied by the painful feelings of shame (Tangney & Dearing, 2002). Similarly, shame unaccompanied by guilt may have unique negative consequences. To model this important unique variance, it is common to calculate semipartial (part) correlations that reflect "shame-free" guilt and "guilt-free" shame. For example, in one study the relationship of parental rejection to shame proneness ($r = .15$) and guilt proneness ($r = -.09$) changed substantially once the semipartial correlation was used ($rs = .27$ and $-.24$) (Stuewig & McCloskey, 2005). Another way to think about the relationship of shame and guilt to constructs is as suppressors (Paulhus, Robins, Trzesniewski, & Tracy, 2004). As with self-esteem and narcissism, for instance, differential relationships of shame proneness and guilt proneness become evident once each is residualized on the other. These differential patterns of results have been found in many samples (Dearing, Stuewig, & Tangney, 2005; Paulhus et al., 2004; Tangney, 1991; Tangney, Wagner, Fletcher, & Gramzow, 1992) and are theoretically consistent with the notion that it is the capacity to experience guilt about behaviors without the interference of shame about the self that leads to more adaptive intrapersonal and interpersonal outcomes. For this reason, interpretation of the correlates of shame-free guilt (and sometimes guilt-free shame) may be necessary to identify relationships that might otherwise be obscured by suppressor effects.[3]

Psychological and Social Correlates of Proneness to Shame and Proneness to Guilt

Proneness to shame and proneness to guilt are stable individual differences that have different implications for social behavior and adjustment. In brief, empirical research suggests that shame-prone individuals are vulnerable to a range of interpersonal and intrapersonal problems, when considering both zero order and residualized analyses. In contrast, proneness to shame-free guilt is unrelated to such vulnerabilities. Rather, guilt-prone individuals (and others in their social circle) are likely to benefit from this prosocial emotional disposition (Baumeister, Stillwell, & Heatherton, 1994; Tangney, 1991; Tangney & Dearing, 2002). Here we summarize several lines of research indicating that guilt proneness is the more adaptive moral emotional style.

Other-Oriented Empathy versus Self-Oriented Distress

Empathy serves crucial functions in interpersonal relationships (Eisenberg, Valiente, & Champion, 2004). Research has repeatedly shown that the capacity for other-oriented empathy is differentially related to proneness to shame versus proneness to guilt. Specifically, guilt proneness goes hand in hand with perspective taking and other-oriented empathy. Shame proneness, in contrast, has been negatively or negligibly related to individual differences in perspective taking and empathic concern. For example, in a study of delinquent and nondelinquent adolescents (Robinson, Roberts, Strayer, & Koopman, 2007), guilt proneness was positively associated with five measures of dispositional empathy, whereas no relationship between shame proneness and empathy was found. Shame was, however, positively correlated with problematic self-oriented personal distress. The same pattern of findings has been observed in studies of children, adolescents, college students, and adults from all walks of life (for a review, see Tangney et al., 2007a), consistent with the notion that the self-focus of shame is apt to inhibit empathic connectedness, whereas the behavioral focus of guilt facilitates other-oriented empathy. In fact, the differential relationship of shame

and guilt to empathy is apparent at both the dispositional and emotional state levels (Joireman, 2004; Leith & Baumeister, 1998; Tangney, 1991, 1995; Tangney & Dearing, 2002; Tangney et al., 1994).

Psychological Symptoms

A wealth of research employing diverse measurement methods, age groups, and populations consistently links proneness to shame to a wide range of psychological symptoms, including low self-esteem, depression, anxiety, eating-disorder symptoms, posttraumatic stress disorder, and suicidal ideation (for a review, see Tangney et al., 2007a). Because guilt is also a negative self-conscious emotion, it has traditionally been thought to play a similar role in psychological symptoms. Empirical support for this assumption, however, has not been strong or clear-cut. Tangney (1996) argued that when one considers the distinction between shame about the self and guilt about a behavior, guilt should not necessarily be associated with poor psychological adjustment. It is much easier to repair or make amends for a specific behavior than for a flawed self. Feelings of guilt, however, may become problematic when fused with shame. Consistent with this conceptual analysis, studies utilizing measures that insufficiently distinguish between shame and guilt typically find that guilt proneness is associated with psychological symptoms (e.g., Harder & Lewis, 1987). On the other hand, measures sensitive to Lewis's (1971) distinction (shame about self vs. guilt about behavior) allow the examination of shame-free guilt. Such studies show that guilt is essentially unrelated to psychological symptoms. For instance, proneness to guilt and proneness to shame were both seemingly positively related to depression among college students; however, shame-free guilt was unrelated to depression, whereas guilt-free shame remained a significant positive correlate of depression (Webb, Heisler, Call, Chickering, & Colburn, 2007). In cases in which people have an exaggerated or distorted sense of responsibility for events, psychological problems associated with guilt may emerge (Tangney & Dearing, 2002; Zahn-Waxler & Robinson, 1995), but psychological problems are generally unrelated to the propensity to experience shame-free guilt when one legitimately takes the responsibility for one's failures and transgressions. A recent study comparing two clinical populations suggested that guilt proneness might be related to psychopathology. Rusch and colleagues (2007) reported that guilt proneness was higher in women with comorbid borderline personality disorder (BPD) and posttraumatic stress disorder as compared with women with only a BPD diagnosis. Furthermore, shame had an analogous though nonsignificant positive relationship with comorbidity. Because shame and guilt were not partialled out, however, interpretation of these results should be made with caution. It is unclear whether shame-free guilt would be stronger among those women with comorbid diagnoses.

Shaming, Blaming, and Maiming

One robust empirical finding involves the differential link of shame and guilt to blame and anger. In addition to assessing proneness to shame and guilt, the TOSCA measures assess externalization of blame, initially included as filler items. Externalization of Blame (blaming the situation or other people for one's failure or transgression) has emerged as a reliable, valid scale in its own right. As expected, guilt-prone individuals are inclined to take responsibility for their blunders; externalization of blame has been consistently negatively correlated with proneness to guilt. But, whereas attribution theory would predict that shame-prone individuals would be inclined to blame themselves for their failures, studies consistently show a *positive* link between shame proneness and blaming others. How is it that shame-prone people (in attributional terms, people who make internal, stable, and global attributions for failures and transgression; see Tangney, 1990; Tracy & Robins, 2006) are also inclined to blame others? People suffering from the pain and self-diminishment of shame may become defensive and angry and attempt to deflect blame outward. Lewis (1971) described the "humiliated fury" unleashed by clients' shame in clinical practice, and Scheff's (1987) qualitative research describes a "shame–rage spiral" that can lead to blame, rage, and occasionally aggression.

In fact, research with individuals of all ages consistently demonstrates a link between shame proneness and externalization of blame, hostility, anger, and unconstructive expression of anger (Ahmed & Braithwaite, 2004; Andrews, Brewin, Rose, & Kirk, 2000; Bennett, Sullivan, & Lewis, 2005; Harper & Arias, 2004; Harper, Cercone, & Arias, 2005; Lutwak, Panish, Ferrari, & Razzino, 2001; Robinson et al., 2007). Shame-prone individuals may also express verbal or physical aggression, although the pathways and circumstances leading to such behavior are unclear (Stuewig & Tangney, 2007). Perhaps feelings of shame prompt a strong tendency to become defensive, shift blame, and attack others (verbally or physically) in order to escape the pain of shame. This proclivity to lash out may satisfy the short-term goal of regaining a sense of control and moral superiority, but at what cost? It is difficult to maintain healthy relations when friends, coworkers, and loved ones are frequently exposed to outbursts of anger. In contrast, guilt proneness is unrelated to anger—that is, guilt-prone people are as prone to anger as anyone else. But when angered, guilt-prone individuals are inclined to manage their anger constructively (e.g., through nonhostile discussion or direct corrective action), and they are *disinclined* toward aggression (Ahmed & Braithwaite, 2004; Lutwak et al., 2001; Paulhus et al., 2004; Tangney, Wagner, Hill-Barlow, Marschall, & Gramzow, 1996).

Risky, Illegal, and/or Immoral Behavior

Because shame and guilt are painful emotions providing negative feedback for wrongdoing, it is often assumed that both motivate individuals to do the right thing. But research tells a different story. There is stronger empirical support for the moral function of guilt as opposed to shame (Stuewig & Tangney, 2007). Among all age groups, guilt proneness is associated with low levels of consensually immoral behavior, but there is little evidence for the presumed moral inhibitory functions of shame. If anything, shame-prone individuals have difficulty following the straight and narrow. In one study of incarcerated adolescent offenders and a comparison group from the community, shame-free guilt proneness was negatively related to anger and antiauthority and distrustful attitudes, whereas shame proneness was positively related to anger and distrustful attitudes across groups (Robinson et al., 2007). Contrary to expectations, however, shame proneness and guilt proneness only marginally differentiated between the two groups. Using a sample of incarcerated individuals, Hosser, Windzio, and Greve (2008) found that shame was related to higher recidivism rates, whereas guilt was related to less recidivism. In a study of college students, Tibbetts (2003) entered a number of shame and guilt measures simultaneously into a regression analysis; the TOSCA Shame scale was unrelated to illegal behaviors, whereas guilt was negatively related to illegal acts. Similarly, in a longitudinal study, Stuewig and McCloskey (2005) found a negative relationship between guilt proneness and delinquency; shame proneness was unrelated to delinquency.

Shame proneness and guilt proneness are also related to substance use and abuse. Compared with individuals in community settings, adults in recovery programs had lower guilt-prone scores and higher shame-prone scores (Meehan et al., 1996; O'Connor, Berry, Inaba, Weiss, & Morrison, 1994). Among college students and jail inmates, shame proneness was consistently positively related to alcohol and drug problems. There was also evidence for a negative relationship between substance use problems and guilt proneness (Dearing et al., 2005). In a longitudinal study, shame and guilt proneness in the fifth grade predicted alcohol and drug use as reported at 18 years of age (Tangney, Stuewig, Kendall, Reinsmith, & Dearing, 2006). Children high in shame tended to start drinking earlier than those low in shame and were more likely to later use heroin, "uppers," and hallucinogens. Those high in guilt started drinking at a later age than those low in guilt and were less likely to use heroin, with similar trends for marijuana and "uppers."

Very few studies have examined the relationship of the moral emotions to other risky behaviors, such as needle use or risky sexual behavior, although one study of college students reported little relationship between reports of previous high-risk sexual behaviors and current state shame or guilt (Murray, Ciarrocchi, & Murray-Swank, 2007). In another study of recently incarcerated inmates, shame proneness and guilt proneness were unrelated to risky intravenous-drug use during the year prior to incarceration, but guilt was negatively related to number of sexual partners and to an index of risky sexual behavior (Stuewig, Tangney, Mashek, Forkner, & Dearing, in press).

Understanding Adaptive and Maladaptive Effects of Shame and Guilt: Mediational Models

Much evidence shows that shame and guilt are differentially related to a number of psychological and behavioral constructs. Research has begun to delve deeper by examining the mediational pathways that underlie these relationships. A number of studies show support for several hypothesized processes that may explain how shame and guilt influence social behavior. Notably, anger and externalization of blame appear to mediate the relationship between shame and aggression. Specifically, men's anger has been found to mediate the relationship between shame proneness and perpetration of psychological abuse in dating relationships (Harper et al., 2005). Stuewig, Tangney, Heigel, and Harty (2006) found that across four diverse samples (early adolescents, at-risk older adolescents, college students, and incarcerated adults), externalization of blame mediated the relationship between shame proneness and both verbal and physical aggression. Guilt proneness had the opposite effect in that proneness to guilt was negatively related to aggression in three of the four samples, partially mediated through other-oriented empathy and accepting responsibility.

Ashby, Rice, and Martin (2006) identified shame as a mediator of the effects of maladaptive perfectionism on depression in a sample of college students. Among men, internalized shame fully mediated the relationship. Among women, maladaptive perfectionism directly predicted depression, but there was also partial mediation through shame and low self-esteem. This finding is consistent with earlier empirical support of the relationship between negative perfectionism and both state and trait shame and the negative relationship between adaptive perfectionism and state shame (Fedewa, Burns, & Gomez, 2005).

In a sample of several hundred undergraduates, Williamson, Sandage, and Lee (2007) evaluated several mediational models to examine the implications of social connectedness for guilt proneness, shame proneness, differentiation of self, and hope. At the bivariate level, proneness to shame-free guilt was positively related to social connectedness and hope, whereas proneness to (guilt-free) shame was negatively associated with social connectedness, hope, and differentiation of self. Support was found for two of three alternative models. In one, social connectedness positively predicted guilt and negatively predicted shame. In turn, guilt proneness positively predicted both hope and differentiation of the self; shame negatively predicted both hope and differentiation of the self. In an alternative model, dependent variables (hope and differentiation of self) were switched with mediating variables (shame and guilt); this second model, with shame and guilt as dependent variables, fit equally well.

In sum, the bivariate correlates of proneness to shame and guilt have been pretty well mapped out. Research that examines more complex models involving mediation and moderation has just begun. We anticipate that future research will expand on this work considerably, clarifying the functional nature of the relationship of shame proneness and guilt proneness to a range of personality factors, psychological symptoms, and patterns of interpersonal behavior.

Where Do Shame–Prone and Guilt–Prone Styles Come From?

Given the implications of shame proneness and guilt proneness described thus far, it is clear that these individual differences matter. How does one become shame or guilt prone? This remains largely a mystery. Few prospective studies have examined the development of shame and guilt proneness, especially starting in early childhood (Mills, 2005; Reimer, 1996). Whereas a large number of possible mechanisms have been proposed—including genetic/temperament factors (e.g., Dienstbier, 1984; Kochanska, 1993; Zahn-Waxler & Robinson, 1995) and socialization factors, especially parenting style (e.g., Barrett, 1995; Ferguson & Steg-

ge, 1995; Kochanska, 1993; Kochanska & Aksan, 2006; Lewis, 1992; Miyake & Yamazaki, 1995; Potter-Efron, 1989; Rosenberg, 1997; Zahn-Waxler & Robinson, 1995)—the research and measurement lags far behind theory (Eisenberg, 2000).

In the developmental literature, similarities between parents and offspring have been found for a number of attributes and behaviors (Serbin & Stack, 1998). There is good reason to expect intergenerational continuity for shame proneness and guilt proneness, as well. There may be a direct link between parents' affective styles and those of their children through behavioral modeling. Children observe how their parents react to negative events and may learn, via direct modeling, that a certain pattern of emotional, cognitive, and behavioral responses is appropriate in certain kinds of situations. To the degree that direct modeling occurs, one would expect a direct link between parents' affective styles and those of their children.

Little research has examined whether shame proneness and guilt proneness show continuities across generations. In one longitudinal study of fifth-grade children with follow-up in seventh grade, measures of shame proneness and guilt proneness were collected from children, parents, and grandparents. Children were interviewed a third time when they were 18. There was only very modest evidence of transmission of shame and guilt, with a weighted mean correlation of .09 across generations (Stuewig, Kendall, & Tangney, 2004). Although the direct relationship between parent and child was minimal, there may be important moderators of intergenerational continuity in shame-prone and guilt-prone styles. For example, age may play a role, such that the similarity between parent and child may be strongest at a similar developmental stage for each.

Perhaps families play other roles in the development of shame-prone and guilt-prone styles. Tendencies toward shame proneness may be perpetuated through family dynamics shaped by family members' affective styles that in turn reinforce individual members' characteristic emotional responses. The literatures on family systems and on codependence describe, for example, a *shame-based* family system that is characterized by maladaptive patterns of communication and extremes of family conflict or enmeshment

(Bradshaw, 1988; Fossum & Mason, 1986). However, little empirical research has been conducted in this area.

Another possibility is that parents' child-rearing practices are most important to the development of children's moral affective styles. In general, studies provide support for parental practices as a component in the socialization of moral emotions. In a study of 5- to 12-year-old children, Ferguson and Stegge (1995) found that children's guilt was associated with parents' reports of induction and parental anger in negative situations, whereas children's shame was associated with parental hostility, little recognition of positive outcomes, and a lack of discipline. Alessandri and Lewis (1993) reported that parents' specific (but not global) negative comments were associated with children's displays of shame, an unexpected result. Gilbert, Allan, and Goss (1996) found that recalled put-downs and shaming from childhood were associated with shame proneness in adulthood. Finally, evidence suggests that children of depressed mothers may be at risk for developing "maladaptive" patterns of guilt (Zahn-Waxler & Robinson, 1995).

Child maltreatment in its different forms (physical abuse, sexual abuse, harsh parenting, neglect) may leave children vulnerable to the development of a shame-prone disposition and less likely to acquire an adaptive guilt-prone style. Research indicates a link between retrospective reports of abuse and shame (Andrews, 1995; Andrews & Hunter, 1997; Hoglund & Nicholas, 1995; Webb et al., 2007). Alessandri and Lewis (1996) observed that mothers' negative behaviors were correlated with children's shame reactions during laboratory tasks and that girls with a history of maltreatment showed higher non-verbal shame than did girls with no history of abuse. Moreover, longitudinal research shows that negative or harsh parenting is associated with shame proneness (Bennett et al., 2005; Mills, 2003; Stuewig & McCloskey, 2005).

Taken together, evidence supports a link between emotional or physical abuse and proneness to shame. Surprisingly, evidence for the relationship between sexual abuse and shame is less clear-cut, with some studies finding positive results and others finding null results (Alessandri & Lewis, 1996; Andrews, 1995; Andrews et al., 2000; Stuewig & McCloskey, 2005). There are a number of possible reasons for these inconsistent findings, including small sample sizes and differences in operational definitions. An interesting hypothesis is that the specific findings may depend on the coping style and recovery process of the individual (Bonanno, Keltner, & Noll, 2002; Negrao, Bonanno, Noll, Putnam, & Trickett, 2005).

Finally, temperament may play a role in the development of proneness to shame and to guilt. The strongest support for a temperamental perspective on children's development of conscience has been reported by Kochanska and colleagues (Kochanska, DeVet, Goldman, Murray, & Putnam, 1994; Kochanska, Gross, Lin, & Nichols, 2002), who found that expression of behavioral and affective discomfort subsequent to misbehaving was related to temperamental qualities of fearfulness and reactivity. In one study, Kochanska and colleagues (2002) found that fearfulness at 22, 33, and 45 months of age was related concurrently to guilt (measured as observed discomfort after misbehaving) at each time. Furthermore, this measure of guilt (a composite from all three previous waves) mediated the relationship between fearfulness and a tendency to violate rules at 56 months. Toddlers who responded fearfully to risky activities were more likely to show discomfort after transgressing, which in turn led to lower likelihood of violating rules. These studies did not differentiate between shame and guilt, however.

Gender and Culture

A consistent empirical finding is that women have higher levels than men of both shame proneness and guilt proneness. This gender difference has been observed, without exception, in studies involving over 3,000 individuals from early childhood through the elder years and from all walks of life (Tangney & Dearing, 2002). Females' higher scores on both shame and guilt proneness could be due to a number of factors: Females may, in fact, experience shame and guilt more often and more intensely, females may be more willing and/or able to report on emotional experiences, females may be more self-reflective and hence more inclined to experience self-conscious emotions, and females may be more attuned to issues of morality, especially those involving interpersonal relationships (Gilligan, 1982). In short, multiple features of these self-reflective, moral emotions may account for higher shame proneness and guilt proneness among girls and women. Tangney and Dearing (2002) cautioned that females' higher propensity to "moral" emotions does not necessarily imply that they are more moral, as the moral benefits of proneness to guilt may be negated to some degree by the negative consequences of proneness to shame.

Theory and research presented thus far has been grounded in traditional Western cultural norms that emphasize ideals of individualism and responsibility for one's own actions, but non-Western cultures embrace more collectivist ideals of interdependence and group responsibility. Cross-cultural research highlights how culture may influence the intensity and frequency of moral emotions, as well as their causes and consequences (Lagattuta & Thompson, 2007). For example, Furukawa, Tangney, Higashihara, and Pak (2008) examined differences in proneness to shame, guilt, and pride among children residing in Japan, Korea, and the United States. Significant group differences were observed in children's propensity to experience self-conscious emotions. Specifically, Japanese children were more shame prone than children in the United States and Korea. In this sense, Japan may represent a "shame" culture (Benedict, 1946; Hogan & Sussner, 2001) in a way that is distinct from another Asian culture, Korea. Korean children were more prone to guilt than Japanese and American children (results inconsistent with the notion of a Western "guilt culture"). Regarding the correlates of shame proneness, it was hypothesized that shame would be less problematic among Japanese children relative to those raised in Korea and the United States, owing to the fact that shame is more normative and would therefore be less painful in the self-critical Japanese culture. There were, however, surprisingly few cross-cultural differences in the relationship of shame to aggression-related cognitions, emotions, and behavior. In the face of failure or transgression, shame-prone children in Japan, Korea, and the United States were all more inclined to blame oth-

ers and to feel anger relative to their less shame-prone peers. Notably, in no case did shame seem to inhibit aggression-relevant cognitions, emotion, or behavior. In short, although there were significant cultural differences in children's propensity to experience self-conscious emotions, the correlates of individual differences in shame and guilt were remarkably similar across these three cultures in at least one important domain—anger and aggression.

Psychobiological Correlates

A recent focus of moral-emotions research is the identification of psychobiological markers of shame and guilt in response to laboratory manipulations designed to threaten the social self (Dickerson, Kemeny, Aziz, Kim, & Fahey, 2004; Gruenewald, Kemeny, Aziz, & Fahey, 2004; see Dickerson, Gruenewald, & Kemeny, 2004, for a review). Participants who wrote about incidents involving heavy doses of self-blame, compared with those who wrote about more mundane daily activities, evidenced increased levels of self-reported shame (and guilt) from pretest to posttest. Importantly, increases in shame (but not guilt or general negative affect) coincided with increased proinflammatory cytokine activity (Dickerson, Kemeny, et al., 2004).

Other immunological research is equally suggestive: Among HIV positive individuals, persistent feelings of shame (but not other negative emotions) were positively related to prospective T-cell decline, an indicator of compromised immune function (Weitzman, Kemeny, & Fahey, 2004). Experiences of shame have also been linked to elevated cortisol in studies of adults (Gruenewald et al., 2004) and children (Lewis & Ramsay, 2002). Importantly, Dickerson, Gruenewald, and colleagues (2004) noted that shame, cortisol, and proinflammatory cytokine system activation increased specifically in response to social-evaluative threat (negative social evaluation and rejection) but not in response to more general negative affect or distress. They hypothesized that individual differences in shame proneness may be correlated with individual differences in immunosystem responsivity and that state experiences of shame and related emotions may be the mediating mechanism for biological response to social threat.

Such physiological markers may prove useful as a measurement tool of situation-specific states of shame. Physiological markers may also be useful as a means of objectively assessing individual differences in proneness to shame and guilt. Developmental research would be useful to shed light on whether shame proneness or guilt proneness leads to biological reactivity or vice versa.

Conclusions

Life is full of daily negotiations between situational demands, our personal codes of ethics, and our interpretations of societal proscriptions for behavior. Shame and guilt are closely related yet distinct emotions that affect our perception of ourselves, that influence our social interactions, and that ultimately guide our moral behavior. This chapter reviewed the theoretical and empirical literature on shame proneness and guilt proneness and described the relative strengths and weaknesses of several assessment methods. Across multiple domains of social behavior and psychological adjustment, guilt proneness emerges as the more adaptive moral emotional style, and there is little evidence that proneness to shame helps people inhibit harmful impulses. Despite decades of research, we know little about the origins of individual differences in proneness to shame and proneness to guilt. It appears that parents do not directly transmit these emotional styles via genes or modeling. There is some evidence that harsh, abusive parenting can lead to the propensity to experience shame and that frequent use of "induction" (coaching children to be aware of others' emotions) may foster a guilt-prone style, but much work remains. In particular, the field would benefit from longitudinal studies, tests of more complex models involving theoretically derived mediators and moderators, and additional work on measurement. Perhaps the most exciting development in recent years is the work on biological correlates of shame. This line of work may add importantly to our ability to more accurately measure shame and guilt and to our understanding of the roots of shame proneness and guilt proneness.

Notes

1. For an in-depth review of the literature on the emotions of shame and guilt, including information on state measures of these emotions, see Robins, Noftle, and Tracy (2007) and Tangney and Dearing (2002).
2. Recently, researchers have begun to develop measures of proneness to shame and proneness to guilt with respect to *specific domains*. For example, researchers concerned with the psychology of eating disorders have assessed feelings of shame specifically in reference to one's body (Andrews, 1995). Trauma-related guilt cognitions, such as false beliefs about responsibility or preoutcome knowledge, are assessed by the Trauma-Related Guilt Inventory (TRGI; Kubany, Haynes, & Abueg, 1996).
3. It should be noted that the reliability of residualized scores is necessarily lower than the reliabilities of the scales themselves (because only systematic variance has been removed). Moreover, to the extent that shame and guilt legitimately share features (e.g., self-awareness, negative affect), the residuals may not reflect all features of guilt or shame. The emphasis here is on their unique characteristics.

References

Ahmed, E., & Braithwaite, V. (2004). "What, me ashamed?": Shame management and school bullying. *Journal of Research in Crime and Delinquency, 41,* 269–294.
Alessandri, S., & Lewis, M. (1993). Parental evaluation and its relation to shame and pride in young children. *Sex Roles, 29,* 335–343.
Alessandri, S., & Lewis, M. (1996). Differences in pride and shame in maltreated and nonmaltreated preschoolers. *Child Development, 67,* 1857–1869.
Andrews, B. (1995). Bodily shame as a mediator between abusive experiences and depression. *Journal of Abnormal Psychology, 104,* 277–285.
Andrews, B., Brewin, C. R., Rose, S., & Kirk, M. (2000). Predicting PTSD symptoms in victims of violent crime: The role of shame, anger, and childhood abuse. *Journal of Abnormal Psychology, 109,* 69–73.
Andrews, B., & Hunter, E. (1997). Shame, early abuse and course of depression in a clinical sample: A preliminary study. *Cognition and Emotions, 11,* 373–381.
Ashby, J. S., Rice, K. G., & Martin, J. L. (2006). Perfectionism, shame and depressive symptoms. *Journal of Counseling and Development, 84,* 148–156.
Barrett, K. C. (1995). A functionalist approach to shame and guilt. In J. P. Tangney & K. W. Fischer (Eds.), *Self-conscious emotions: The psychology of shame, guilt, embarrassment, and pride* (pp. 25–63). New York: Guilford Press.
Baumeister, R. F., Stillwell, A. M., & Heatherton, T. F. (1994). Guilt: An interpersonal approach. *Psychological Bulletin, 115,* 243–267.

Benedict, R. (1946). *The chrysanthemum and the sword*. Boston: Houghton Mifflin.

Bennett, D. S., Sullivan, M. W., & Lewis, M. (2005). Young children's adjustment as a function of maltreatment, shame, and anger. *Child Maltreatment, 10*(4), 311–323.

Bonanno, G., Keltner, D., & Noll, J. (2002). When the face reveals what words do not: Facial expressions of emotions, smiling, and the willingness to disclose childhood sexual abuse. *Journal of Personality and Social Psychology, 83*(1), 94–110.

Bradshaw, J. (1988). *Healing the shame that binds you*. Deerfield Beach, FL: Health Communications.

Buss, A., & Durkee, A. (1957). An inventory for assessing different kinds of hostility. *Journal of Consulting Psychology, 21*(4), 343–349.

Cheek, J. M., & Hogan, R. (1983). Self-concepts, self-presentations, and moral judgments. In J. Suls & A. G. Greenwald (Eds.), *Psychological perspectives on the self* (Vol. 2, pp. 249–273). Hillsdale, NJ: Erlbaum.

Cook, D. R. (1988, August). *The measurement of shame: The Internalized Shame Scale*. Paper presented at the annual meeting of the American Psychological Association, Atlanta, GA.

Cook, D. R. (1991). Shame, attachment, and addictions: Implications for family therapists. *Contemporary Family Therapy, 13*, 405–419.

Crouppen, G. A. (1976). Field dependence–independence in depressive and "normal" males as an indicator of relative proneness to shame or guilt and ego-functioning. *Dissertation Abstracts International, 37*, 4669B–4670B. (UMI No. 77-6292)

de Hooge, I. E. (2008). *Moral emotions in decision making: Towards a better understanding of shame and guilt*. Unpublished doctoral dissertation, University of Tilburg, The Netherlands.

de Hooge, I. E., Zeelenberg, M., & Breugelmans, S. M. (2007). Moral sentiments and cooperation: Differential influences of shame and guilt. *Cognition and Emotion, 21*, 1025–1042.

Dearing, R. L., Stuewig, J., & Tangney, J. P. (2005). On the importance of distinguishing shame from guilt: Relations to problematic alcohol and drug use. *Addictive Behaviors, 30*(7), 1392–1404.

Dickerson, S. S., Gruenewald, T. L., & Kemeny, M. E. (2004). When the social self is threatened: Shame, physiology, and health. *Journal of Personality, 72*, 1191–1216.

Dickerson, S. S., Kemeny, M. E., Aziz, N., Kim, K. H., & Fahey, J. L. (2004). Immunological effects of induced shame and guilt. *Psychosomatic Medicine, 66*, 124–131.

Dienstbier, R. A. (1984). The role of emotion in moral socialization. In C. Izard, J. Kagan, & R. B. Zajonc (Eds.), *Emotions, cognitions, and behaviors* (pp. 484–513). New York: Cambridge University Press.

Eisenberg, N. (2000). Emotion, regulation, and moral development. *Annual Review of Psychology, 51*, 665–697.

Eisenberg, N., Valiente, C., & Champion, C. (2004). Empathy-related responding: Moral, social, and socialization correlates. In A. G. Miller (Ed.), *The social psychology of good and evil* (pp. 386–415). New York: Guilford Press.

Fedewa, B. A., Burns, L. R., & Gomez, A. A. (2005). Positive and negative perfectionism and the shame/guilt distinction: Adaptive and maladaptive characteristics. *Personality and Individual Differences, 38*, 1609–1619.

Ferguson, T. J., Brugman, D., White, J., & Eyre, H. L. (2007). Shame and guilt as morally warranted experiences. In J. L. Tracy, R. W. Robins, & J. P. Tangney (Eds.), *The self-conscious emotions: Theory and research* (pp. 330–348). New York: Guilford Press.

Ferguson, T. J., & Stegge, H. (1995). Emotional states and traits in children: The case of guilt and shame. In J. P. Tangney & K. W. Fischer (Eds.), *Self-conscious emotions: The psychology of shame, guilt, embarrassment, and pride* (pp. 174–197). New York: Guilford Press.

Ferguson, T. J., Stegge, H., & Damhuis, I. (1991). Children's understanding of guilt and shame. *Child Development, 62*, 827–839.

Fossum, M. A., & Mason, M. J. (1986). *Facing shame: Families in recovery*. New York: Norton.

Furukawa, E., Tangney, J. P., Higashihara, F., & Pak, H. (2008). *Cross-cultural continuities and discontinuities in shame, guilt, and pride: A study of children in Japan, Korea, and the United States*. Manuscript under review.

Gilbert, P., Allan, S., & Goss, K. (1996). Parental representations, shame, interpersonal problems, and vulnerability to psychopathology. *Clinical Psychology and Psychotherapy, 3*, 23–34.

Gilligan, C. (1982). *In a different voice: Psychological theory and women's development*. Cambridge, MA: Harvard University Press.

Gruenewald, T. L., Kemeny, M. E., Aziz, N., & Fahey, J. L. (2004). Acute threat to the social self: Shame, social self-esteem, and cortisol activity. *Psychosomatic Medicine, 66*, 915–924.

Harder, D. W., Cutler, L., & Rockart, L. (1992). Assessment of shame and guilt and their relationship to psychopathology. *Journal of Personality Assessment, 59*, 584–604.

Harder, D. W., & Lewis, S. J. (1987). The assessment of shame and guilt. In J. N. Butcher & C. D. Spielberger (Eds.), *Advances in personality assessment* (Vol. 6, pp. 89–114). Hillsdale, NJ: Erlbaum.

Hare, S. D., Cox, D. N., & Hare, R. D. (1995). *The Hare Psychopathy Checklist: Screening Version (PCL:SV)*. Toronto, Ontario, Canada: Multi-Health Systems.

Harper, F. W. K., & Arias, I. (2004). The role of shame in predicting adult anger and depressive symptoms among victims of child psychological maltreatment. *Journal of Family Violence, 19*(6), 367–375.

Harper, F. W. K., Cercone, J., & Arias, I. (2005). The role of shame, anger, and affect regulation in men's perpetration of psychological abuse in dating relationships. *Journal of Interpersonal Violence, 20*, 1648–1662.

Hoblitzelle, W. (1987). *The measurement of shame and guilt and the role of shame in depression*. Unpublished doctoral dissertation, Yale University.

Hogan, J. D., & Sussner, B. D. (2001). Cross-cultural psychology in historical perspective. In L. L. Adler & U. P. Gielen (Eds.), *Cross-cultural topics in psychology* (pp. 15–28). Westport, CT: Praeger.

Hoglund, C. L., & Nicholas, K. B. (1995). Shame, guilt, and anger in college students exposed to abusive family environments. *Journal of Family Violence, 10*, 141–157.

Hosser, D., Windzio, M., & Greve, W. (2008). Guilt and shame as predictors of recidivism: A longitudinal study with young prisoners. *Criminal Justice and Behavior, 35*, 138–152.

Johnson, R. C., Danko, G. P., Huang, Y. H., Park, J. Y., Johnson, S. B., & Nagoshi, C. T. (1987). Guilt, shame and adjustment in three cultures. *Personality and Individual differences, 8*, 357–364.

Joireman, J. (2004). Empathy and the self-absorption paradox: II. Self-rumination and self-reflection as mediators between shame, guilt, and empathy. *Self and Identity, 3*, 225–238.

Keltner, D., & Buswell, B. N. (1996). Evidence for the distinctness of embarrassment, shame, and guilt: A study of recalled antecedents and facial expressions of emotion. *Cognition and Emotion, 10*, 155–171.

Ketelaar, T., & Au, W. T. (2003). The effects of feelings of guilt on the behavior of uncooperative individuals in repeated social bargaining games: An affect-as-information interpretation of the role of emotion in social interaction. *Cognition and Emotion, 17*, 429–453.

Klass, E. T. (1987). Situational approach to the assessment of guilt: Development and validation of a self-report measure. *Journal of Psychopathology and Behavioral Assessment, 9*, 35–48.

Kochanska, G. (1993). Toward a synthesis of parental socialization and child temperament in early development of conscience. *Child Development, 64*, 325–347.

Kochanska, G., & Aksan, N. (2006). Children's conscience and self-regulation. *Journal of Personality, 74*, 1587–1617.

Kochanska, G., DeVet, K., Goldman, M., Murray, K., & Putnam, S. P. (1994). Maternal reports of conscience development and temperament in young children. *Child Development, 65*, 852–868.

Kochanska, G., Gross, J. N., Lin, M.-H., & Nichols, K. E. (2002). Guilt in young children: Development, determinants, and relations with a broader system of standards. *Child Development, 73*, 461–482.

Kubany, E. S., Haynes, S. N., & Abueg, F. R. (1996). Development and validation of the Trauma-Related Guilt Inventory (TRGI). *Psychological Assessment, 8*(4), 428–444.

Kugler, K., & Jones, W. H. (1992). On conceptualizing and assessing guilt. *Journal of Personality and Social Psychology, 62*, 318–327.

Lagattuta, K. H., & Thompson, R. A. (2007). The development of self-conscious emotions: Cognitive processes and social influences. In J. L. Tracy, R. W. Robins, & J. P. Tangney (Eds.), *The self-conscious emotions: Theory and research* (pp. 91–113). New York: Guilford Press.

Leith, K. P., & Baumeister, R. F. (1998). Empathy, shame, guilt, and narratives of interpersonal conflicts: Guilt-prone people are better at perspective taking. *Journal of Personality, 66*, 1–37.

Lewis, H. B. (1971). *Shame and guilt in neurosis.* New York: International Universities Press.

Lewis, M. (1992). *Shame: The exposed self.* New York: Free Press.

Lewis, M., & Ramsay, D. (2002). Cortisol response to embarrassment and shame. *Child Development, 73*, 1034–1045.

Lindsay-Hartz, J. (1984). Contrasting experiences of shame and guilt. *American Behavioral Scientist, 27*, 689–704.

Lutwak, N., Panish, J. B., Ferrari, J. R., & Razzino, B. E. (2001). Shame and guilt and their relationship to positive expectations and anger expressiveness. *Adolescence, 36*, 641–653.

Luyten, P., Fontaine, J. R. J., & Corveleyn, J. (2002). Does the Test of Self-Conscious Affect (TOSCA) measure maladaptive aspects of guilt and adaptive aspects of shame?: An empirical investigation. *Personality and Individual Differences, 33*, 1373–1387.

Meehan, M. A., O'Connor, L. E., Berry, J. W., Weiss, J., Morrison, A., & Acampora, A. (1996). Guilt, shame, and depression in clients in recovery from addiction. *Journal of Psychoactive Drugs, 28*, 125–134.

Mills, R. S. (2003). Possible antecedents and developmental implications of shame in young girls. *Infant and Child Development, 12*, 329–349.

Mills, R. S. (2005). Taking stock of the developmental literature on shame. *Developmental Review, 25*, 26–63.

Miyake, K., & Yamazaki, K. (1995). Self-conscious emotions, child rearing, and child psychopathology in Japanese culture. In J. P. Tangney & K. W. Fischer (Eds.), *Self-conscious emotions: Shame, guilt, embarrassment, and pride* (pp. 488–504). New York: Guilford Press.

Mosher, D. L. (1966). The development and multitrait-multimethod matrix analysis of three measures of three aspects of guilt. *Journal of Consulting and Clinical Psychology, 30*, 25–29.

Murray, K. M., Ciarrocchi, J. W., & Murray-Swank, N. A. (2007). Spirituality, religiosity, shame and guilt as predictors of sexual attitudes and experiences. *Journal of Psychology and Theology, 35*, 222–234.

Negrao, C., Bonanno, G. A., Noll, J. G., Putnam, F. W., & Trickett, P. K. (2005). Shame, humiliation, and childhood sexual abuse: Distinct contributions and emotional coherence. *Child Maltreatment, 10*(4), 350–363.

O'Connor, L. E., Berry, J. W., Inaba, D., Weiss, J., & Morrison, A. (1994). Shame, guilt, and depression in men and women in recovery from addiction. *Journal of Substance Abuse Treatment, 11*, 503–510.

Paulhus, D. L., Robins, R. W., Trzesniewski, K. H., & Tracy, J. L. (2004). Two replicable suppressor situations in personality research. *Multivariate Behavioral Research, 39*, 303–328.

Perlman, M. (1958). An investigation of anxiety as related to guilt and shame. *Archives of Neurology and Psychiatry, 80*, 752–759.

Potter-Efron, R. T. (1989). *Shame, guilt and alcoholism: Treatment issues in clinical practice.* New York: Haworth Press.

Reimer, M. (1995). *The Adolescent Shame Measure (ASM).* Philadelphia: Temple University Press.

Reimer, M. S. (1996). "Sinking into the ground": The development and consequences of shame in adolescence. *Developmental Review, 16*, 321–363.

Robins, R. W., Noftle, E. E., & Tracy, J. L. (2007). Assessing self-conscious emotions: A review of self-report and nonverbal measures. In J. L. Tracy, R. W.

Robins, & J. P. Tangney (Eds.), *Self-conscious emotions: Theory and research* (pp. 443–467). New York: Guilford Press.

Robinson, R., Roberts, W. L., Strayer, J., & Koopman, R. (2007). Empathy and emotional responsiveness in delinquent and non-delinquent adolescents. *Social Development, 16*, 555–579.

Rosenberg, K. L. (1997) *The socialization of shame and guilt.* Unpublished doctoral dissertation, George Mason University.

Rosenberg, M. (1965). *Society and the adolescent self-image.* Princeton, NJ: Princeton University Press.

Rusch, N., Corrigan, P. W., Bohus, M., Kuhler, T., Jacob, G. A., & Lieb, K. (2007). The impact of post-traumatic stress disorder on dysfunctional implicit and explicit emotions among women with borderline personality disorder. *Journal of Nervous and Mental Disease, 195*, 537–539.

Russell, J. A., & Carroll, J. M. (1999). On the bipolarity of positive and negative affect. *Psychological Bulletin, 125*, 3–30.

Sabini, J., & Silver, M. (1997). In defense of shame: Shame in the context of guilt and embarrassment. *Journal for the Theory of Social Behaviour, 27*, 1–15.

Scheff, T. J. (1987). The shame–rage spiral: A case study of an interminable quarrel. In H. B. Lewis (Ed.), *The role of shame in symptom formation* (pp. 109–149). Hillsdale, NJ: Erlbaum.

Serbin, L. A., & Stack, D. M. (1998). Introduction to the special section: Studying inter-generational continuity and the transfer of risk. *Developmental Psychology, 34*, 1159–1161.

Sherry, A. (2007). Internalized homophobia and adult attachment: Implications for clinical practice. *Psychotherapy: Theory, Research, Practice, Training, 44*, 219–225.

Smith, R. H., Webster, J. M., Parrot, W. G., & Eyre, H. L. (2002). The role of public exposure in moral and nonmoral shame and guilt. *Journal of Personality and Social Psychology, 83*, 138–159.

Stegge, H., & Ferguson, T. J. (1990). *Child–Child Attribution and Reaction Survey (C-CARS).* Unpublished manuscript, Utah State University.

Stuewig, J., Kendall, S., & Tangney, J. (2004, April). *Intergenerational transmission of moral emotional style: How valid is the myth of the guilt-inducing mother?* Poster presented at the Conference on Human Development, Washington, DC.

Stuewig, J., & McCloskey, L. (2005). The impact of maltreatment on adolescent shame and guilt: Psychological routes to depression and delinquency. *Child Maltreatment, 10*, 324–336.

Stuewig, J., & Tangney, J. P. (2007). Shame and guilt in antisocial and risky behaviors. In J. L. Tracy, R. W. Robins, & J. P. Tangney (Eds.), *The self-conscious emotions: Theory and research* (pp. 371–388). New York: Guilford Press.

Stuewig, J., Tangney, J. P., Heigel, C., & Harty, L. (2006, August). *The moral emotions, externalization of blame, and aggression.* Paper presented at the meeting of the American Psychological Association, New Orleans, LA.

Stuewig, J., Tangney, J. P., Mashek, D., Forkner, P., & Dearing, R. L. (in press). The moral emotions, alcohol dependence, and HIV risk behavior in an incarcerated sample. *Substance Use and Misuse.*

Tangney, J. P. (1990). Assessing individual differences in proneness to shame and guilt: Development of the Self-Conscious Affect and Attribution Inventory. *Journal of Personality and Social Psychology, 59*, 102–111.

Tangney, J. P. (1991). Moral affect: The good, the bad, and the ugly. *Journal of Personality and Social Psychology, 61*, 598–607.

Tangney, J. P. (1992). Situational determinants of shame and guilt in young adulthood. *Personality and Social Psychology Bulletin, 18*, 199–206.

Tangney, J. P. (1995). Shame and guilt in interpersonal relationships. In J. P. Tangney & K. W. Fischer (Eds.), *Self-conscious emotions: The psychology of shame, guilt, embarrassment, and pride* (pp. 114–139). New York: Guilford Press.

Tangney, J. P. (1996). Conceptual and methodological issues in the assessment of shame and guilt. *Behaviour Research and Therapy, 34*, 741–754.

Tangney, J. P., & Dearing, R. (2002). *Shame and guilt.* New York: Guilford Press.

Tangney, J. P., Marschall, D. E., Rosenberg, K., Barlow, D. H., & Wagner, P. E. (1994). *Children's and adults autobiographical accounts of shame, guilt and pride experiences: An analysis of situational determinants and interpersonal concerns.* Unpublished manuscript.

Tangney, J. P., Mashek, D., & Stuewig, J. (2007). Working at the social–clinical–community–criminology interface: The GMU inmate study. *Journal of Social and Clinical Psychology, 26*, 1–21.

Tangney, J. P., Miller, R. S., Flicker, L., & Barlow, D. H. (1996). Are shame, guilt and embarrassment distinct emotions?: An analysis of participant ratings. *Journal of Personality and Social Psychology, 70*, 1256–1269.

Tangney, J. P., Stuewig, J., Kendall, S., Reinsmith, C., & Dearing, R. (2006). *Implications of childhood shame and guilt for risky and illegal behaviors in young adulthood.* Unpublished manuscript.

Tangney, J. P., Stuewig, J., & Mashek, D. J. (2007a). Moral emotions and moral behavior. *Annual Review of Psychology, 58*, 345–372.

Tangney, J. P., Stuewig, J., & Mashek, D. J. (2007b). What's moral about the self-conscious emotions? In J. L. Tracy, R. W. Robins, & J. P. Tangney (Eds.), *The self-conscious emotions: Theory and research* (pp. 21–37). New York: Guilford Press.

Tangney, J. P., Wagner, P., & Gramzow, R. (1989). *The test of self-conscious affect.* Unpublished manuscript, George Mason University.

Tangney, J. P., Wagner, P. E., Fletcher, C., & Gramzow, R. (1992). Shamed into anger?: The relation of shame and guilt to anger and self-reported aggression. *Journal of Personality and Social Psychology, 62*, 669–675.

Tangney, J. P., Wagner, P. E., Hill-Barlow, D. H., Marschall, D., & Gramzow, R. (1996). The relation of shame and guilt to constructive vs. destructive responses to anger across the lifespan. *Journal of Personality and Social Psychology, 70*, 797–809.

Tibbetts, S. G. (2003). Self-conscious emotions and criminal offending. *Psychological Reports, 93*, 101–126.

Tracy, J. L., & Robins, R. W. (2004). Putting the self into self-conscious emotions: A theoretical model. *Psychological Inquiry, 15*(2), 103–125.

Tracy, J. L., & Robins, R. W. (2006). Appraisal antecedents of shame and guilt: Support for a theoretical model. *Personality and Social Psychology Bulletin, 32*(10), 1339–1351.

Wallbott, H. G., & Scherer, K. R. (1995). Cultural determinants in experiencing shame and guilt. In J. P. Tangney & K. W. Fischer (Eds.), *Self-conscious emotions: The psychology of shame, guilt, embarrassment, and pride* (pp. 465–487). New York: Guilford Press.

Webb, M., Heisler, D., Call, S., Chickering, S. A., & Colburn, T. A. (2007). Shame, guilt, symptoms of depression, and reported history of psychological maltreatment. *Child Abuse and Neglect, 31,* 1143–1153.

Weitzman, O., Kemeny, M. E., & Fahey, J. L. (2004). *HIV-related shame and guilt predict CD4 decline.* Manuscript submitted for publication.

Wicker, F. W., Payne, G. C., & Morgan, R. D. (1983). Participant descriptions of guilt and shame. *Motivation and Emotion, 7,* 25–39.

Williamson, I., Sandage, S. J., & Lee, R. M. (2007). How social connectedness affects guilt and shame: Mediation by hope and differentiation of self. *Personality and Individual Differences, 43,* 2159–2170.

Zahn-Waxler, C., Kochanska, G., Krupnick, J., & Mayfield, A. (1988). *Coding manual for children's interpretations of interpersonal distress and conflict.* Bethesda, MD: National Institutes of Mental Health, Laboratory of Developmental Psychology.

Zahn-Waxler, C., & Robinson, J. (1995). Empathy and guilt: Early origins of feelings of responsibility. In J. P. Tangney & K. W. Fischer (Eds.), *Self-conscious emotions: Shame, guilt, embarrassment, and pride* (pp. 143–173). New York: Guilford Press.

CHAPTER 14

■ ● ▲ ◆ ■ ● ▲ ◆

Hostility and Proneness to Anger

JOHN C. BAREFOOT
STEPHEN H. BOYLE

Hostile behavior clearly plays an important role in social life and has a major influence on the nature and course of relationships. Much of the variance in antagonism is the product of situations, yet there are clearly reliable individual differences in tendencies to experience and express negative interpersonal feelings. Test–retest correlations on most hostility measures are high, even across extended time periods. This consistency in social orientation has implications for a person's social life, psychological well-being, and physical health.

The study of hostility and anger has been pursued from many viewpoints, including studies of social pathology, marital functioning, emotion theory, and intergroup relations. This chapter is not comprehensive in its treatment of them. For example, we do not deal with extreme or abnormal manifestations such as habitual violence or paranoia, which may operate under different principles and have different origins than does hostility as usually seen in normal social life. Instead, the emphasis is on those aspects of hostility that most commonly affect social relationships and health. The tradition most relevant to this chapter is social perception, because the focus of the chapter is on the predisposition of some people to evaluate their social interactions negatively and the consequences of that tendency.

This chapter concentrates on hostility phenomena from the perspective of current health research, much of which emphasizes cognitive predispositions. The role of hostility in health has received extensive attention in recent years and has several advantages as a focus. It illustrates the significance of this psychological dimension for important outcomes. Health-related physiological reactions also provide a convenient and meaningful way to gauge the impact of an event on an individual. Furthermore, the hostility and health literature illustrates the interdependence of one's psychological, social, and physical well-being.

Conceptual Approaches

Stable negative interpersonal orientations have been given a variety of names, and they are not always used consistently, which increases the potential for confusion. For example, the term *hostility* is sometimes used to refer specifically to beliefs about others. At other times it more broadly encompasses negative emotional reactions and aggressive actions as well. The approach used here is to rely on established distinctions between cognition, affect, and behavior and to treat the hostility complex in the broad sense, incorporating all three.

Various theoretical traditions have attempted to place the hostility components in their broader view of personality. Others have emphasized particular components and distinctions.

Trait Taxonomies

The factor-analytic approach to describing the interrelationships of personality traits has an extensive history in personality psychology (e.g., Cattell, 1946; Eysenck & Eysenck, 1985). The five-factor model (FFM; McCrae & Costa, 1985) has been the most prominent trait taxonomy in hostility research. The FFM divides personality into the domains of Extraversion, Neuroticism, Openness, Agreeableness, and Conscientiousness, each of which has subscales, or facets, in the system of Costa and McCrae (1992). Hostility is most closely related to facets of the Neuroticism and Agreeableness domains. The Neuroticism dimension, which emphasizes negative emotional experiences, contains the Angry Hostility facet, and the Agreeableness domain emphasizes altruistic and friendly tendencies versus predispositions toward egocentrism and argumentativeness.

Circumplex Model

Smith, Glazer, Ruiz, and Gallo (2004) have outlined the applicability of the Circumplex model (Wiggins & Trapnell, 1996) for the study and description of hostile personality characteristics as they relate to interpersonal phenomena. This model contains two orthogonal dimensions that describe a person's approach to interpersonal relationships. One dimension is based on affective tone and ranges from antagonism and coldness to friendliness and warmth. The other dimension is based on power or control and ranges from dominance to submissiveness. These dimensions also describe interpersonal motivations of communion (desire for affiliation and intimacy) and agency (desire for achievement and status). Anger is certainly related to the friendliness dimension, and ambitious behavior defines one extreme of dominance orientations. Particular characteristics can be located in the two-dimensional space formed by these orthogonal dimensions. For example, aggression can be seen as a blend of high dominance and low friendliness, whereas withdrawal would be characterized as low dominance and low friendliness.

The inclusion of the dominance dimension sets the Circumplex model somewhat apart from other approaches to the hostility complex in that many of the behaviors that compose it (e.g., desire to influence or gain status) need not be motivated by feelings of ill will or anger. Therefore, this broadens the concept, and the fact that studies of dominance (e.g., Houston, Babyak, Chesney, Black, & Ragland, 1997; Siegman, Kubzansky, et al., 2000; Smith et al., 2004) have observed health effects that are similar to those seen in hostility studies supports this extension.

Component Model

The widely accepted division of experience into cognition, affect, and behavior underlies many of the conceptualizations of hostility phenomena and guides the presentation in this chapter. The cognitive component of hostility is generally thought to be primarily composed of negative beliefs about the nature of other people (cynicism) and suspicion regarding their intent (mistrust). This should lead to a vigilant and protective tone in one's interactions. Research on the affective component often focuses on angry feelings, but there are other important related emotions, such as disgust and resentment, that are often neglected. Likewise, the hallmark of the behavioral component is verbal and physical aggression, but these can be suppressed or expressed indirectly, a phenomenon that is sometimes underemphasized.

The three-component model highlights some important distinctions. If hostility is treated as a unitary construct it overlooks the fact that the cognitive, affective, and behavioral components are differentially associated with other variables, such as age and socioeconomic position (Barefoot, Beckham, Haney, Siegler, & Lipkus, 1993; Haukkala, 2002), and may behave somewhat independently depending on the setting. Furthermore, studies of the associations between multiple hostility measures have found three factors that correspond to the dimensions of the component model (Barefoot et al., 1993; Martin, Watson, & Wan, 2000). Much of the literature and much of this chapter treat the three components as part of the same complex without stressing their potential differential effects. That point should be kept in mind when reading the literature and conducting future research.

Anger Regulation

Many of the social and personal consequences of the experience of anger depend on the way that a person copes with it. Research in this area has identified multiple anger-regulation strategies, including rumination, avoidance, assertion, reflective coping, discussion, aggression, suppression, and various forms of repression (Deffenbacher, Oetting, Lynch, & Morris, 1996; Garssen, 2007; Linden et al., 2003). These strategies can be thought of as attempts to regulate anger at different points in the emotion-generative process through situation selection (e.g., avoidance), modification of the situation (e.g., problem-focused coping), deployment of attention (e.g., rumination), change in cognitions (reflective coping), and selection of behavioral responses (e.g., expression and suppression) (John & Gross, 2004).

The focus of much of this work has been the congruity between negative emotional experiences of animosity and the overt behavioral expression of those feelings. The most widely used approach has contrasted Anger-Out, involving overt behavior that displays the negative feelings in a verbally or physically aggressive manner, and Anger-In, involving efforts to conceal negative feelings and to avoid direct confrontation (Speilberger et al., 1985). This dichotomy was originally thought to represent extremes of one dimension, but it is clear that this is an oversimplification. Measures of these tendencies load on separate dimensions: Neuroticism and Agreeableness in the FFM (Martin et al., 2000) as well as the affective and behavioral factors of the component model of hostility (Barefoot et al., 1993). In addition, recent work has identified other anger response styles such as those mentioned earlier, as well as multiple modes of overt expression (e.g., anger discussion, assertion, and reciprocal communication) that reflect a desire to communicate one's feelings of anger in non-aggressive ways.

Anger-regulation styles can have implications for social relations and one's own physiology. For example, openly expressing one's anger in an aggressive manner often elicits reciprocal aggressive behavior and acrimony, escalating conflicts, impeding successful problem resolution, and eroding important relationships. It is also associated with elevated indicators of cardiovascular reactivity that have important implications for health (Siegman, 1994). On the other hand, researchers have also noted deleterious social and physiological effects of the failure to express emotion. Accurately communicating emotional states is important to interpersonal functioning, and suppression of emotion can impair communication, making it more difficult to form and maintain close relationships (Butler et al., 2003; Gross, 2002). In addition, some forms of covert coping with anger are associated with delayed physiological recovery after anger-producing episodes (Brosschot & Thayer, 1998; Hogan & Linden, 2004).

As these findings suggest, research on anger-regulation styles has resulted in a picture clouded by findings that appear to be contradictory on the surface and by somewhat conflicting theoretical approaches. This state of affairs calls for theoretical approaches that better recognize the complexities of potential anger-regulation styles and their appropriateness for particular social settings.

Questionnaire Measures

One approach to hostility measurement has been based on dimensions from omnibus personality inventories. The most prominent example is the use of the NEO Personality Inventory (NEO PI; Costa & McCrae, 1992), which operationalizes the FFM. It is available in forms that allow for both self-reports and peer reports. Congruence between self-reports and peer reports has been reported to be good and supportive of the division of traits into these dimensions (McCrae & Costa, 1987).

Another tactic is the derivation of scales specifically designed to evaluate hostile tendencies. These measures can be divided according to the three hostility components. A large number of instruments have been devised to assess aspects of hostility. Therefore, we do not attempt to be comprehensive in the following descriptions, which concentrate on the most frequently used scales that are relevant to the health psychology literature.

Cognitive Aspects

The most widely used measure of hostility in the health psychology literature is the Cook–Medley Hostility Scale (Ho; Cook & Medley, 1954). The popularity of this measure is certainly not based on its psychometric properties, which have repeatedly been found to be mediocre (Barefoot & Lipkus, 1994; Contrada & Jussim, 1992) even though its reported test–retest reliabilities and internal consistency have been quite high (Barefoot, Dodge, Peterson, Dahlstrom, & Williams, 1989; Shekelle, Gale, Ostfeld, & Paul, 1983). In fact, the instrument was not even originally devised to be a measure of hostility per se but was empirically derived to identify items that discriminated between teachers who had good or bad rapport with their students. The resulting items appeared to reflect a hostile interpersonal orientation, so the scale was classified as a hostility measure. The frequent use of the Ho scale stems from its ability to predict important outcomes, including interpersonal stress and conflict (Smith, Pope, Sanders, Allred, & O'Keefe, 1998), mental well-being (Mao, Bardwell, Major, & Dimsdale, 2003), and health outcomes such as coronary heart disease and mortality (Smith et al., 2004).

The original Ho scale contains 50 items. However, a rational analysis identified 11 items that did not appear to reflect hostility and divided the remaining ones into four subsets reflecting cognition (cynicism and hostile attributions), affect (hostile affect), and behavioral tendencies (aggressive responding) (Barefoot et al., 1989). The bulk of the scale represents cynicism and mistrust (Smith & Frohm, 1985). The full 50 Ho items are often administered, but several briefer versions have been used to predict health outcomes (e.g., Boyle et al., 2005; Julkunen, Salonen, Kaplan, Chesney, & Salonen, 1994; Surwit et al., 2002).

Two other measures focusing on trust should be noted, although they are not used as widely as the Ho scale in health research.

The Rotter Interpersonal Trust Scale (Rotter, 1967) consists of 19 items designed to reflect the belief that one can rely on the promises and intent of others. It correlates highly with the Ho scale (Barefoot et al., 1993) and has been used in a variety of studies to explore the implications of trust for interpersonal relationships (e.g., Rotter, 1980).

Another trust measure is Factor L from the Sixteen Personality Factor (16PF) Personality Inventory, which is derived from Cattell's (1946) theory of personality, an early product of the use of factor analysis to derive personality dimensions from trait adjectives. Factor L is described as a measure of vigilance ranging from the extremes of suspicious to trusting. The 16PF has been widely used, and its inclusion in important longitudinal studies has permitted the exploration of multiple consequences of suspicious tendencies compared to trusting ones.

Affective Aspects

A variety of affects may be associated with hostility, but most of the self-report instruments have focused on anger. The most prominent measure has been from the Spielberger State–Trait Personality Inventory (Spielberger, Jacobs, Russell, & Crane, 1983). The trait component of the scale asks respondents to rate the frequency with which they experience anger and annoyance. The State Anger scale asks similar questions about the respondent's feelings at the moment.

The issue of the direction of anger expression is most frequently assessed via the Spielberger Anger Expression Scale (Spielberger et al., 1985). It directly asks the respondents to report their tendencies to direct anger inward and suppress it or express it outwardly toward others by arguing or other overt actions.

Aggression

The Buss–Durkee Hostility Inventory (Buss & Durkee, 1957) has traditionally been one of the most widely used measures of aggressive tendencies. It contains seven subscales that tend to fall into two dimensions (Bushman, Cooper, & Lemke, 1991). One represents components of anger-related affect that correlate with Neuroticism in the FFM, and it is most strongly related to the Resentment and Suspicion subscales. The other reflects aggressive tendencies and is composed of the Assault and Verbal Aggression subscales.

Buss and Perry (1992) noted that the factor structure of the Buss–Durkee measure was somewhat inconsistent across studies and that some of the item interpretations were ambiguous. Therefore they developed a new version, the Aggression Questionnaire. It contains four subscales: Anger and Hostility, which correlate with the Neuroticism dimension of the FFM, in addition to Physical Aggression and Verbal Aggression, which correlate with Agreeableness (Gallo & Smith, 1998).

Another measure that combines assessment of anger arousal and expression style is the Multidimensional Anger Inventory (Siegel, 1986). It differentiates between five dimensions: ease of anger arousal; range of anger-eliciting situations; hostile outlook; anger-in, which has items indicative of rumination; and anger-out.

Measures Based on Behavioral Observations

In addition to standard self-report measures, there is a tradition in this line of research to base assessments purely on observations of the target person's overt behaviors. There are reasons to believe that this strategy will capture information that is not obtained from more traditional questionnaire methods (Barefoot & Lipkus, 1994). One obvious barrier to effective self-report measures is the possibility that respondents, especially those who are not trusting, may be reluctant to openly admit their hostile tendencies given the socially undesirable status of those traits. Another is that many of those who have a hostile or combative interaction style appear to be unaware of this aspect of behavior, and therefore they may not describe themselves as hostile on a questionnaire. It is as if they see their behavior to be a justifiable reaction to a provoking interaction partner or situation rather than a product of their own personalities. Some investigators (e.g., Ketterer et al., 1998) have noticed frequent discrepancies between self- and spouse rat-

ings in heart patients and have conceptualized this as a form of denial. This work has shown that men are more likely than women to underestimate their own hostility. In addition, there are sizable individual differences in self-awareness, which should also lower the congruence between overt behavior and self-reports in some people.

One class of behavioral measures employs coding of interactions during standardized interviews or laboratory tasks. The impetus for the development of these methods came from the Western Collaborative Group Study (WCGS; Rosenman, Swan, & Carmilli, 1988), which administered structured interviews dealing with daily habits and coded responses based on vocal characteristics (e.g., speech rate, loudness) and interaction style, as well as content. This procedure was used to categorize participants on the basis of their Type A behavior, a predictor of later coronary disease in this sample. Later scoring schemes separately scored the hostility reflected in the respondent's behavior and made the scoring procedures more explicit. The most recent system, the Interpersonal Hostility Assessment Technique (IHAT; Haney et al., 1996), extends the method devised by Chesney, Hecker, and Black (1989), concentrating on four categories of hostility-related behaviors. Direct Challenges involve open verbal aggression directed toward the interviewer. A more common behavior is an Indirect Challenge, which is a more subtle implication of hostility that is judged from voice stylistics. For example, the statement "of course" can be said in an agreeable fashion or in a tone implying that the answer is obvious and the question is stupid. The category of Irritation is based on indicators of negative emotional arousal as judged from vocal stylistics. The final category, Hostile Withhold-Evade, is coded when the respondent fails to answer a question and does so in an antagonistic manner. The sum of scores from these four categories has been shown to correlate with nonverbal expressions of negative affect (Brummett et al., 1998). More important, it has been shown to be associated with the extent of coronary disease in patient samples (Haney et al., 1996; Siegman, Townsend, Civelek, & Blumenthal, 2000) and to predict coronary mortality in a population sample of men at high risk (Matthews, Gump, Harris, Haney, & Barefoot, 2004).

Interview-based measures have also been devised for the direct study of dominance, a primary component of the Circumplex model and a behavioral dimension shown to be important in laboratory studies of cardiovascular reactivity (Smith et al., 2004; see the section on social interactions). Houston and colleagues (1997) performed cluster analyses of speech characteristics observed during structured interviews from the WCGS. People whose vocal styles could be characterized by attempted dominance (e.g., verbally competitive, with fast speaking rates and immediate responses) had higher mortality rates over the ensuing 22 years of follow-up. Siegman, Townsend, and colleagues (2000) found that a rating of dominance behavior was associated with coronary disease in patients undergoing thallium scan testing independent of their IHAT scores.

Another behavioral observation measurement strategy is to utilize judgments made by the target person's peers and family. The ratings are obviously less standardized and structured than interview or laboratory-based systems and are subject to some biases (Barefoot & Lipkus, 1994), but they can capitalize on the extensive experience the informant has had with the target in a variety of settings. In health research, spouse ratings of hostility have been better than self-ratings in identifying those with coronary disease (Ketterer et al., 2004; Kneip et al., 2004; Smith et al., 2007), especially in men.

Origins of Hostile Tendencies

Biological Underpinnings

There has been a considerable amount of work on possible physiological bases of hostility, anger, and, particularly, aggression. A good deal of this effort has focused on the processes that influence the levels of the neurotransmitter serotonin in the brain (Carver & Miller, 2006). Experimental manipulations of central nervous system serotonin have demonstrated decreases in aggressive tendencies with serotonin enhancement. Serotonin depletion leads to increases in aggression, especially in those with preexisting aggressive tendencies (Dougherty, Bjork,

Marsh, & Moeller, 1999). Consistent with this, low levels of serotonin function have been linked to measures of aggressive behavior and impulsivity in clinical and normal samples (Carver & Miller, 2006; Manuck, Flory, Muldoon, & Ferrell, 2002). Most evidence regarding serotonin shows effects on measures of overt behavior affected by impulse control, with less support for links to more subtle manifestations of hostility seen in normal interactions.

The role of testosterone in facilitating aggressive behavior has also received a great deal of attention (Archer, 2006). Positive associations between levels of testosterone and trait aggression have been reported in many studies, and these associations appear to be strongest for measures of aggressive dominance. Testosterone levels are also associated with higher levels of aggressive behavior in response to tasks involving competition or interpersonal challenge. There is also evidence that testosterone influences how people assess physical and psychological threats to their status, a potential mediator for those associations. Although the focus of much of this research has been men, there is evidence that similar associations are present in women.

There have been multiple investigations and frequent speculation regarding the possible genetic origins of hostility and anger. The plausibility of this line of inquiry is bolstered by family studies showing that genetic influences are likely to account for a substantial amount of the variance in hostility scores (Weidner et al., 2000). Searches for specific genes associated with hostile tendencies have been conducted, but the findings are complex. As with the studies of serotonin manipulation, the clearest findings have come from studies dealing with genetic influences on overt aggression and violent behavior (Manuck et al., 2002). The strategy of searching for meaningful interactions between genes and environmental factors promises to be the most promising course to pursue in the future (Moffitt, Caspi, & Rutter, 2005).

Developmental History

Learning based on childhood environment plays a significant role in the acquisition of hostile tendencies. Several studies have emphasized family experiences as a source of later hostile tendencies in offspring. An important perspective on this literature comes from the social-cognitive approach of Dodge (2006). The initial tenet is that aggression is a universal and natural response to perceived threat. One task of socialization is the development of benign attributional schemas to counteract the tendency to make hostile attributions to explain the actions of others. These schemas are fostered in children by secure attachments with a caregiver, modeling of benign attribution habits from others, success experiences, and living in a culture that values cooperation. Without these experiences, it is more likely that the child will develop a defensive attitude that is the precursor to aggressiveness and problem behavior.

These principles can be seen in the voluminous literature on childhood environments and hostile tendencies. For example, children who have been abused at home or have experienced other significant stressors are more likely to have hostile attributional tendencies toward others, including peers (Price & Glad, 2003; Turner, Russell, Glover, & Hutto, 2007). However, much of the literature on family environment and hostility development uses retrospective and/or subjective measures of family environment, which carry a large potential for bias. Methods that circumvent those problems have also been employed. For example, Matthews, Woodall, Kenyon, and Jacob (1996) coded the interactions between fathers and their adolescent sons while they discussed a disagreement in a laboratory setting. The observed levels of hostile behavior on the part of both fathers and sons predicted the sons' scores on multiple hostility measures 3 years later after controlling for initial levels.

Dodge's (2006) approach also predicts that supportive family environments can be protective against the effects of trauma in children. Luecken (2000) compared university students who had experienced the loss of a parent with students from intact families. Those who had experienced loss reported more hostility and depression if they had poor family relationships. No difference between loss groups was present for those with supportive families. Simons and colleagues (2006) report that supportive parenting successfully reduces hostile attribution and aggressive tendencies in African American adolescents who are subject to discrimination. This appears to reduce their likelihood of delinquency and similar problems.

Trauma

Aside from childhood stressors that can affect developmental processes, trauma experienced in adulthood can also result in high levels of mistrust and other aspects of hostility. It is one of the hallmark symptoms of posttraumatic stress disorder (PTSD) resulting from many types of severe stress (Orth & Wieland, 2006), although the association between anger and PTSD is somewhat larger in those exposed to military stressors. Even combat veterans who only have subclinical levels of PTSD symptoms show evidence of heightened anger and hostility (Jakupcak et al., 2007). Women with PTSD also report high levels of hostility (Beckham, Calhoun, Glenn, & Barefoot, 2002). In the general population, PTSD is more prevalent in women than in men and is most frequently associated with a history of sexual assault (Kessler, Sonnega, Bromet, Hughes, & Nelson, 1995).

Demographic Distributions of Hostility

Differences in hostility between various demographic groups reflect many of the influences discussed earlier. Most of the data for these comparisons are based on the Ho scale because it is the most widely administered measure in community samples.

Gender

One of the strongest consistent demographic differences is the tendency for women to have lower scores on measures of cynicism and aggression. For example, they have lower Ho scores in every age group of a U.S. national sample (Barefoot et al., 1991). This pattern is seen as an integral part of the female gender role, consistent with its emphasis on communion and positive interpersonal relationships (Helgeson, 1994). Therefore, social learning and developmental experiences should influence these tendencies. However, women do not consistently have lower scores on measures of anger or anger expression, indicating that they acknowledge anger experiences but tend to employ less aggressive modes of expression (Stoney & Engebretson, 1994).

Age

A second common trend is a curvilinear association between hostility and age (Barefoot et al., 1991; Swenson, Pearson, & Osbourne, 1973). There are large reductions in scores between adolescence and adulthood, with levels rising slightly among those above 60. The elevation in older respondents was investigated more thoroughly in a sample of 125 middle-aged and older community volunteers using multiple hostility measures (Barefoot et al., 1993). The positive association with age was seen most clearly in the cognitive measures reflecting cynicism and mistrust, although it was also present in the interview-based behavioral assessment. In contrast, self-report measures of aggressiveness showed a weak inverse relationship with age, and there was no significant effect for self-reports of more covert experiential aspects of hostility.

Ethnicity

There are clear differences in Ho scores across ethnic groups, with minorities having higher scores (Barefoot et al., 1991). This difference is consistently seen across studies and may be due to an environment filled with discrimination and economic challenges that hinder the development of benign attributional styles. Hostile attributions can be seen as a potentially adaptive response to a threatening and objectively hostile environment.

Socioeconomic Position

Multiple studies (e.g., Barefoot et al., 1991; Scherwitz, Perkins, Chesney, & Hughes, 1991; Haukkala, 2002) have demonstrated inverse associations of hostility with income and education. As with ethnicity, it could be argued that cynicism is an understandable response to the harsher living conditions experienced by those groups. Childhood socioeconomic status appears to be an especially

potent predictor of hostility scores (Harper et al., 2002), perhaps reflecting the importance of that life stage for personality development.

Most of the studies cited previously have used versions of the Ho scale. Although this establishes an inverse association between socioeconomic position and cognitive aspects of hostility, other associations have been found with measures of anger expression. Lower status groups actually report lower scores on the Anger-Out measure, indicating a reluctance to express these feelings overtly (Haukkala, 2002). This is hypothesized to indicate that a position of power or prestige provides the conditions for acceptable anger expression.

Culture

Culture influences hostile tendencies through shared childrearing practices, modeling, and cultural experiences. Thus differences in hostile tendencies are not confined to the level of the individual. For example, there are notable differences in emotional responding between Western European–based and Asian-based cultures. In American samples, suppression of emotions can have a number of negative social outcomes, such as weaker social attachments and relationship closeness (Gross, 2002). In contrast, emotional expression is more often suppressed in Asian cultures, and these negative consequences are not seen in interactions among individuals sharing Asian values (Butler, Lee, & Gross, 2007). Consequences of cultural differences in expressiveness can be seen in studies from multicultural societies that compare anger-related physiological reactions of individuals varying in ethnicity. For example, both laboratory and ambulatory monitoring studies of Singapore residents have found ethnic variations in blood pressure responses during daily life and in response to laboratory stressors (Bishop & Robinson, 2000; Enkleman et al., 2005). Although there have been some variations across studies, the general finding is that hostile ethnic Indians have more cardiovascular reactivity to stressors than do Chinese and Malay study participants who are otherwise similar. These findings are consistent with the higher rates of cardiovascular disease found in the Indian subpopulation.

Social Capital

Large sociodemographic and cultural differences in levels of hostility should translate into between-group differences in behavior. These are thought to be more meaningful than mere mean differences in that forces operating at the group or population level can influence important outcomes, so the study of group-level variables is needed to fully understand social phenomena. In this approach, groups differ in the collective resources, such as cohesion, constructive atmospheres, and capacity for mutual aid, that will facilitate or hinder the achievement of goals. These resources have been given the label *social capital* (Kawachi & Berkman, 2000). One of the key ingredients in social capital is the level of interpersonal trust, a prime element of the cognitive component of hostility. Interpersonal trust correlates substantially with trust in public institutions (Brehm & Rahn, 1997), so those who live in societies with ample social capital will be more involved and contribute more to the group, thereby improving its functioning. Those in areas of high social capital will also receive benefits, such as lower stress and resources, to apply to the achievement of their personal goals. This should translate into better health habits and healthier social environments. One of the primary applications of the social capital approach has been in the study of societal-level predictors of population health. A good example of this is the work of Kopp and her colleagues (Kopp, Skrabski, Szántó, & Siegrist, 2006), who have investigated possible explanations for the dramatic rise of death rates in Eastern Europe during the past two decades, despite improvements in living standards and health care. They have argued that societal changes during that period have undermined social resources, and they have demonstrated that psychosocial indicators are powerful predictors of mortality rates measured on a macro level. Over 12,500 Hungarians from 150 subregions were administered extensive interviews that included a large number of psychosocial measures. Premature cardiovascular death rates in those geographic areas were predicted by average hostility scores, as well as by other indicators of social stress, especially support from friends, depression, anomie, working conditions, and related health habits such as smoking and alcohol consumption.

Hostility, Anger, and Social Interactions

The transactional model of Smith and colleagues (2004) posits a multistage process in which a person's hostile tendencies partially determine the course of their social interactions that, in turn, have an important impact on the person. This reciprocal process might be broken down into several stages. Social cognition plays a role in the initiation of this process. The cynical and mistrusting component of the hostility complex affects the way a person interprets the actions of others. This has been demonstrated on a subtle level in studies of the perception of nonverbal behavior. Those who score high on hostility were less accurate in identifying affects portrayed in standard facial affect photographs, with men and high hostiles showing a bias toward attributions of negative affect (Larkin, Martin, & McClain, 2002). This perceptual bias has also been demonstrated in impressions formed of a confederate during laboratory interactions (Allred & Smith, 1991). Participants interacted with a confederate who behaved in either a neutral or negative manner. High scorers on the Ho scale rated the confederates as more hostile and later recalled more hostile adjectives when describing the unfriendly confederate. Similarly, it has been shown that those who behave in an antagonistic fashion during an interview perceive more hostility in the interviewer than is seen by independent observers (Hall & Davidson, 1996). Effects can also be seen on the processing of adjectives describing liked and disliked acquaintances. Those with higher scores on the Buss–Perry Aggression Questionnaire more readily associate negative adjectives with disliked targets (Guyll & Madon, 2003). Thus hostile individuals appear to be vigilant regarding threatening or unfriendly actions by others, and this affects their social perceptions.

There are several potential consequences of this predisposition. The first is the arousal of negative affects such as anger or disgust. Studies of physiological reactivity during social interactions show that hostile individuals have greater blood pressure changes during social interactions (Smith et al., 2004). This not only shows the level of emotional arousal, but it also makes up part of the explanation for the impaired cardiovascular health of hostile people (see the following section).

A related consequence of this perceptual bias is that hostile individuals will tend to see others as less supportive. Indeed, they tend to report lower levels of social support (Benotsch, Christensen, & McKelvey, 1997) and report more social negativity in their work environments (McCann, Russo, Benjamin, & Andrew, 1997). Even when available, social support may have less psychological and physiological impact as well, somewhat negating its normally beneficial effects. Lepore (1995) had participants who varied on cynicism perform a stressful speaking task with or without the presence of a supportive confederate. Those who were low in cynicism showed more benefit from the support, both in ratings of stress and blood pressure levels during the task. These effects on perceived social support constitute another potential pathway to the mental and physical health problems associated with high hostility.

The transactional model identifies yet another important consequence of this process. The ill intent that is perceived and that leads to anger or other negative affects can ultimately lead to the activation of the behavioral component: aggression or related negative actions. Of course, this can elicit reciprocal negative responses from others, resulting in interactions that are more filled with animosity. The end product is a social environment that is both objectively and subjectively less supportive and more stressful. This process was demonstrated in a laboratory study (Smith, Sanders, & Alexander, 1990) that paired married participants of varying hostility for a series of discussion tasks (a low-conflict topic followed by a conflict-inducing topic and then another low conflict topic) and coded the amount of negative interpersonal behavior that occurred. The initial discussion did not elicit much conflict behavior, regardless of the composition of the couple. Couples composed of two hostile people reacted to the high-conflict topic with more frequent negative interpersonal behaviors, and the negative interaction tone was maintained into discussion of the subsequent low-conflict topic. Couples composed

of two members with low hostility were not argumentative regardless of the discussion task. Of most interest was the behavior of the couples with one member high and one low in hostility. Their behaviors resembled those of the couples composed of two people high in hostility, showing an increase in antagonistic behavior in response to the high-conflict topic and maintaining it during the final discussion. Therefore the member of the mixed pair with high hostility evidently elicited conflict behavior from the normally nonaggressive partner. Thus the transactional theory illustrates a process in which people's own hostility not only affects their interpretations of their social experiences but also initiates a scenario of potential reciprocal escalation that enhances the level of stressful encounters.

Components of this process have been documented in questionnaire and laboratory studies, but its consequences can be seen best by examining the naturally occurring social interactions in the daily lives of people who vary in hostility. For example, Brissette and Cohen (2002) interviewed community volunteers on 7 consecutive days about their social experiences and their sleep patterns during the previous 24 hours. Those high in hostility reported more negative affect associated with conflict experiences, and their sleep was more disturbed on nights following days with high levels of conflict. This may indicate a tendency for them to ruminate about those conflicts. It is also important because of the significance of adequate sleep for both physical and mental well-being.

Even more detailed pictures of the effects of hostility on experience can be obtained with ambulatory monitoring of cardiovascular reactions during the person's regular daily activities accompanied by diaries that ask the participant to describe the nature of the activity that is going on at the time of the physiological reading. Several studies of hostility and ambulatory monitoring have been conducted. Brondolo and colleagues (2003) monitored 104 volunteers, taking blood pressure and heart rate readings every 20 minutes during the day. Diaries indicated whether the person was engaging in social interaction and his or her affective reactions at the time of the reading. Those high in hostility reported fewer social interactions, suggesting that they might have a tendency to avoid others or that they are being avoided by others. The interactions they did have were more likely to be negative, and the ratings of negativity were more intense. Positively toned interactions were rated as less intense when they did occur. Some, but not all, of these trends were reflected in blood pressure readings, with larger diastolic readings for highly hostile participants during intense negative interactions. Findings from other ambulatory studies generally agree with these results (e.g., Benotsch et al., 1997), but some found slight differences. For example, Jamner, Shapiro, Goldstein, and Hug (1991) studied the blood pressures of paramedics. Those with high Ho scores had higher cardiovascular activity levels during working hours, especially in contexts that were likely to involve interpersonal conflicts. This effect was strongest in those with a defensive coping style, a tendency to deny or minimize negative affect. Guyll and Contrada (1998) compared cardiovascular activity in participants varying in hostility during social and nonsocial activities, finding a positive association during social encounters primarily in men.

Another way to illustrate the naturally occurring consequences of hostility in daily life can be found in the literature on marital relationships, which are obviously an important component of a person's well-being. Trust is an essential component of successful close relationships (Rempel, Holmes, & Zanna, 1985), and the existence of frequent anger and aggression in a relationship is likely to be especially detrimental. The overall importance of hostility can be demonstrated in longitudinal studies of hostility scores in married couples and the course of their marital satisfaction. Miller, Marksides, Chiriboga, and Ray (1995) found that the Irritability subscale of the Buss–Durkee Hostility Inventory, a measure of anger proneness, was predictive of marital dissolution in a large sample of Mexican Americans over an 11-year follow-up. A study of 53 newlywed couples followed for 3 years found that men's hostility, assessed with the Ho scale, was associated with decreases in both their own and their wives' marital satisfaction (Newton & Kiecolt-Glaser, 1995). No such effect was found for the women's hostility scores. Support for this gender difference has been obtained from other cross-sectional studies (Houston & Kelly, 1989; Smith et al., 1988). In contrast, Baron and colleagues (2007) examined hostility components measured by the Buss–Perry scale to predict marital adjustment trends over 18 months in 122 couples. The cognitive and anger components were both negatively correlated with adjustment in cross-sectional analyses, but temporal trends were most closely related to anger, especially the wives' anger.

The findings relating to the differential roles of hostility in marital adjustment of men and women are complex. This issue is potentially important for understanding the nature of close relationships and for dealing with the mental and physical health consequences of marital problems. In general, marital relationships have been shown to play a larger role in the physical health and psychological well-being of men (Kiecolt-Glaser & Newton, 2001; Shumaker & Hill, 1991). More detailed insight into the roles of hostility in close relationships can be found in the literature on physiological reactivity during marital interactions in laboratory settings (Kiecolt-Glaser & Newton, 2001). Results from studies using this paradigm are not only useful for understanding emotional arousal in the marital context and its potential implications for health, but they have also been found to predict subsequent marital dissolution or marital success. Discussions of topics that are the basis of problems in the marriage or experimentally induced disagreements result in elevated physiological indicators of stress, effects that are present in samples of both newlyweds and long-term married couples. Most studies find that these effects are more pronounced in women. Hostility of the participants also plays a role, and the nature of the effect appears to be dependent on the nature of the experimental task. When placed in a setting that emphasizes dominance or agency (e.g., convincing the spouse to accept a position on an issue), men high but not low in hostility show heightened physiological reactivity (Smith & Brown, 1991; Smith & Gallo, 1999). Women's hostility did not seem to have an impact on their own reactivity, but they did tend to have greater physiological reactions during the high-conflict discussions if they were married to men with high hostility scores. This picture is further complicated by the recent suggestion that trait anger scores may be more predictive than hostility scores of women's physiological responses (Smith et al., 2004). One plausible explanation is that men tend to react to challenges related to the dimension of agency, whereas women respond to disturbances in communion (Smith, Gallo, Goble, Ngu, & Stark, 1998).

Hostility and Physical Health

The link between components of hostility and health has been hypothesized for many decades, but interest in the topic was accelerated by studies of the Type A behavior pattern as a predictor of heart disease (Rosenman et al., 1988) and the identification of hostility as its critical component (Williams & Barefoot, 1988). Subsequently, a large number of epidemiological, clinical, and laboratory studies have explored the health consequences of hostile components and their mechanisms of action. Much of this work has focused on coronary heart disease (Smith et al., 2004), but hostility measures have also been associated with other health outcomes, such as stroke, disability, and total mortality (e.g., Adams, 1994; Kivimaki, Vahtera, Koskenvuo, Uutela, & Pentti, 1998; Williams, Nieto, Sanford, Couper, & Tyroler, 2002). The Ho scale has been most frequently used in this work, but other measures, such as anger indicators (e.g., Williams et al., 2002) and interview ratings (e.g., Matthews et al., 2004), have also been successful predictors. There are a number of plausible explanations that could account for these phenomena.

Research cited earlier regarding transactional processes has shown that the perceptions and behaviors of hostile people tend to create more stressful environments. This produces higher cardiovascular reactivity in both laboratory and natural settings, resulting in elevated coronary disease risk. Other physiological systems that are responsive to stressors are also affected. For example, high hostiles show enhanced activation of the sympathetic nervous system and hypothalamic–pituitary–adrenal cortex system in response to interpersonal stress (Suarez, Kuhn, Schanberg, Williams, & Zimmerman, 1998). The resulting hemodynamic and hormonal changes can contribute

to alterations in lipids, glucose metabolism, inflammation, and blood pressure (Golden, 2007; Steptoe, Hamer, & Chida, 2007).

Health behaviors constitute another potential set of pathways (Bunde & Suls, 2006). For example, smoking has been associated with hostility measures in several population studies (e.g., Scherwitz et al., 1992; Shekelle et al., 1983). Part of this association appears to be due to the difficulties hostile people face when trying to quit smoking (Lipkus, Barefoot, Williams, & Siegler, 1994), perhaps because of the role that nicotine can play in affect regulation and the negative affects aroused during cessation attempts. Jamner, Shapiro, and Jarvik (1999) found that nicotine patches were especially effective in reducing anger among more hostile people, whether or not they were smokers.

Elevated alcohol consumption among highly hostile individuals has also been noted in multiple studies (e.g., Scherwitz et al., 1992; Shekelle et al., 1983). Boyle, Mortensen, Grønbæk, and Barefoot (2008) observed a high prevalence of an unhealthy pattern of heavy episodic drinking in those with high Ho scores in addition to higher total alcohol intake. One possible contributing factor is that alcohol consumption appears to be a more effective stress reducer in hostile drinkers (Zeichner, Giancola, & Allen, 1995).

Another relevant lifestyle indicator is body mass index (BMI). Bunde and Suls (2006) note a "fairly robust" positive relationship between BMI and hostility across studies. Haukkala and Uutela (2000) found that the effect was stronger among women with low education. Related phenomena with even more significant health implications are the associations of hostile characteristics with central adiposity, insulin resistance, abnormal glucose, and lipid functioning, as well as hypertension, although racial and gender differences in the associations have been noted (Goldbacher & Matthews, 2007; Surwit et al., 2002). These physiological indicators are important risk factors for cardiovascular disease.

Conclusions and Future Directions

The research based on the transactional model demonstrates the reciprocal interchanges between personality, social life, and personal well-being. Social experiences shape hostile predispositions, which, in turn, influence the person's social environment through selection, perception, and their impact on the behavior of others. These social experiences help determine a person's experience of stress or tranquility and, coupled with coping behaviors, his or her health and psychological well-being.

One of the most prominent trends in this work has been the demonstration of the relevance of the hostility concept for topics such as marital relationships, social capital, and physical health. These extensions into areas with potential practical applications can continue to fuel the interests of researchers in related fields that will provide new perspectives. Another direction of recent work that should be pursued is the growing emphasis on more complex hypotheses evaluating interactions with demographic variables, other personality characteristics, and situations. The person–situation interaction issue is particularly noteworthy. Much of the literature, including this chapter, has focused on the consistencies in hostile predispositions, perhaps underestimating the significance of situational factors (e.g., Porter, Stone, & Schwartz, 1999). Their influence should not be neglected, and a more complex interactional approach could help remedy that. Such investigations can yield a better understanding of the detailed impact of hostile predispositions and lead to more useful sophisticated theoretical explanations.

A caveat is in order. The research presented here and the literature in general tend to emphasize the negative consequences of hostile predispositions. However, it should be remembered that positive functions are also served by hostility, at least in its milder forms. Oppositional behavior is often necessary for the benefit of society, and the absence of hostility and extreme or unmitigated communion is also dysfunctional (Helgeson, 1994). The appropriate balance is needed for psychological, social, and physical health.

Acknowledgments

This work was supported in part by Grant No. R01 HL54780 from the National Heart, Lung, and Blood Institute with cofunding from the National Institute on Aging and Grant No. PO1HL37687 from the National Heart, Lung, and Blood Institute.

References

Adams, S. H. (1994). The role of hostility in women's health during midlife: A longitudinal study. Health Psychology, 13, 488–495.

Allred, K. D., & Smith, T. W. (1991). Social cognition in cynical hostility. Cognitive Therapy and Research, 15, 399–412.

Archer, J. (2006). Testosterone and human aggression: An evaluation of the challenge hypothesis. Neuroscience and Biobehavioral Reviews, 30, 319–412.

Barefoot, J. C., Beckham, J. C., Haney, T. L., Siegler, I. C., & Lipkus, I. M. (1993). Age differences in hostility among middle-aged and older adults. Psychology and Aging, 8, 3–9.

Barefoot, J. C., Dodge, K. A., Peterson, B. L., Dahlstrom, W. G., & Williams, R. B. (1989). The Cook–Medley Hostility Scale: Item content and ability to predict survival. Psychosomatic Medicine, 51, 46–57.

Barefoot, J. C., & Lipkus, I. M. (1994). Assessment of anger–hostility. In A. W. Siegman & T. W. Smith (Eds.), Anger, hostility and the heart (pp. 43–66). Hillsdale, NJ: Erlbaum.

Barefoot, J. C., Peterson, B. L., Dahlstrom, W. G., Siegler, I. C., Anderson, N. B., & Williams, R. B. (1991). Hostility patterns and health implications: Correlates of Cook–Medley scores in a national survey. Health Psychology, 10, 18–24.

Baron, K. G., Smith, T. W., Butler, J., Nealy-Moore, J., Hawkins, M. W., & Uchino, B. M. (2007). Hostility, anger, and marital adjustment: Concurrent associations with psychosocial vulnerability. Journal of Behavioral Medicine, 30, 1–10.

Beckham, J. C., Calhoun, P. S., Glenn, D. M., & Barefoot, J. C. (2002). Posttraumatic stress disorder, hostility, and health in women: A review of current research. Annals of Behavioral Medicine, 24, 219–228.

Benotsch, E. G., Christensen, A. J., & McKelvey, L. (1997). Hostility, social support, and ambulatory cardiovascular activity. Journal of Behavioral Medicine, 20, 163–176.

Bishop, G. D., & Robinson, G. (2000). Anger, harassment, and cardiovascular reactivity among Chinese and Indian men in Singapore. Psychosomatic Medicine, 62, 684–692.

Boyle, S. H., Mortensen, L., Grønbæk, M., & Barefoot, J. C. (2008). Hostility, drinking pattern, and mortality. Addiction, 163, 54–59.

Boyle, S. H., Williams, R. B., Mark, D. B., Brummett, B. H., Siegler, I. C., & Barefoot, J. C. (2005). Hostility, age, and mortality in a sample of cardiac patients. American Journal of Cardiology, 96, 64–66.

Brehm, J., & Rahn, W. (1997). Individual-level evidence for the causes and consequences of social capital. American Journal of Political Science, 41, 999–1023.

Brissette, I., & Cohen, S. (2002). The contribution of individual differences in hostility to the associations between daily interpersonal conflict, affect, and sleep. *Personality and Social Psychology Bulletin, 28,* 1265–1274.

Brondolo, E., Rieppi, R., Erickson, S. A., Bagiella, E., Shapiro, P. A., McKinley, P., et al. (2003). Hostility, interpersonal interactions, and ambulatory blood pressure. *Psychosomatic Medicine, 65,* 1003–1011.

Brosschot, J. F., & Thayer, J. F. (1998). Anger inhibition, cardiovascular recovery, and vagal function: A model of the link between hostility and cardiovascular disease. *Annals of Behavioral Medicine, 20,* 326–332.

Brummett, B. H., Maynard, K. E., Babyak, M. A., Haney, T. L., Siegler, I. C., Helms, M. J., et al. (1998). Measures of hostility as predictors of facial affect during social interaction: Evidence for construct validity. *Annals of Behavioral Medicine, 20,* 168–173.

Bunde, J., & Suls, J. (2006). A quantitative analysis of the relationship between the Cook–Medley Hostility Scale and traditional coronary artery disease risk factors. *Health Psychology, 25,* 493–500.

Bushman, B. J., Cooper, H. M., & Lemke, K. M. (1991). Meta-analysis of factor analyses: An illustration using the Buss–Durkee Hostility Inventory. *Personality and Social Psychology Bulletin, 17,* 344–349.

Buss, A. H., & Durkee, A. (1957). An inventory for assessing different kinds of hostility. *Journal of Consulting Psychology, 21,* 343–349.

Buss, A. H., & Perry, M. (1992). The aggression questionnaire. *Journal of Personality and Social Psychology, 63,* 452–459.

Butler, E. A., Egloff, B., Wilhelm, F. H., Smith, N. C., Erickson, E. A., & Gross, J. J. (2003). The social consequences of expressive suppression. *Emotion, 3,* 48–67.

Butler, E. A., Lee, T. L., & Gross, J. J. (2007). Emotion regulation and culture: Are the social consequences of emotion suppression culture specific? *Emotion, 7,* 30–48.

Carver, C. S., & Miller, C. J. (2006). Relations of serotonin function to personality: Current views and a key methodological issue. *Psychiatry Research, 144,* 1–15.

Cattell, R. B. (1946). *Description and measurement of personality.* Yonkers on Hudson, NY: World Book.

Chesney, M. A., Hecker, M., & Black, G. A. (1989). Coronary-prone components of Type A behavior in the WCGS: A new methodology. In B. K. Houston & C. R. Snyder (Eds.), *Type A behavior pattern: Research, theory, and intervention* (pp. 168–188). New York: Wiley.

Contrada, R. J., & Jussim, L. (1992). What does the Cook–Medley Hostility Scale measure?: In search of an adequate measurement model. *Journal of Applied Social Psychology, 22,* 615–627.

Cook, W. W., & Medley, D. M. (1954). Proposed hostility and pharisaic virtue scales for the MMPI. *Journal of Applied Psychology, 38,* 414–418.

Costa, P. T., Jr., & McCrae, R. R. (1992). *NEO PI-R Professional Manual.* Odessa, FL: Psychological Assessment Resources.

Deffenbacher, J. L., Oetting, E. R., Lynch, R. S., & Morris, C. D. (1996). The expression of anger and its consequences. *Behavior Research and Therapy, 34,* 575–590.

Dodge, K. A. (2006). Translational science in action: Hostile attributional style and the development of aggressive behavior problems. *Development and Psychopathology, 18,* 791–814.

Dougherty, D. M., Bjork, J. M., Marsh, D., & Moeller, F. G. (1999). Influence of trait hostility on tryptophan depletion-induced laboratory aggression. *Psychiatry Research, 88,* 227–232.

Enkleman, H. C., Bishop, G. D., Tong, E. M. W., Diong, S. M., Why, V. P., Khader, M., et al. (2005). The relationship of hostility, negative affect, and ethnicity to cardiovascular responses: An ambulatory study in Singapore. *International Journal of Psychophysiology, 56,* 185–197.

Eysenck, H., & Eysenck, M. (1985). *Personality and individual differences: A natural science approach.* New York: Plenum Press.

Gallo, L. C., & Smith, T. W. (1998). Construct validation of health-relevant personality traits: Interpersonal circumplex and five-factor model analyses of the Aggression Questionnaire. *International Journal of Behavioral Medicine, 5,* 129–147.

Garssen, B. (2007). Repression: Finding our way in the maze of concepts. *Journal of Behavioral Medicine, 30,* 471–481.

Goldbacher, E. M., & Matthews, K. A. (2007). Are psychological characteristics related to risk of the metabolic syndrome?: A review of the literature. *Annals of Behavioral Medicine, 34,* 240–252.

Golden, S. H. (2007). A review of the evidence for a neuroendocrine link between stress, depression and diabetes. *Current Diabetes Review, 3,* 252–259.

Gross, J. J. (2002). Emotion regulation: Affective, cognitive, and social consequences. *Psychophysiology, 39,* 281–291.

Guyll, M., & Contrada, R. (1998). Trait hostility and ambulatory cardiovascular activity: Responses to social interaction. *Health Psychology, 17,* 30–39.

Guyll, M., & Madon, S. J. (2003). Trait hostility: The breadth and specificity of schema effects. *Personality and Individual Differences, 34,* 681–693.

Hall, P., & Davidson, K. (1996). The misperception of aggression in behaviorally hostile men. *Cognitive Therapy and Research, 20,* 377–389.

Haney, T. L., Maynard, K. E., Houseworth, S. J., Scherwitz, L. W., Williams, R. B., & Barefoot, J. C. (1996). Interpersonal Hostility Assessment Technique: Description and validation against the criterion of coronary artery disease. *Journal of Personality Assessment, 66,* 386–401.

Harper, S., Lynch, J., Hsu, W. L., Everson, S. A., Hillemeier, M. M., Raghunathan, T. E., et al. (2002). Life course socioeconomic conditions and adult psychosocial functioning. *International Journal of Epidemiology, 31,* 391–403.

Haukkala, A. (2002). Socio-economic differences in hostility measures: A population-based study. *Psychology and Health, 17,* 191–202.

Haukkala, A., & Uutela, A. (2000). Cynical hostility, depression, and obesity: The moderating role of education and gender. *International Journal of Eating Disorders, 27,* 106–109.

Helgeson, V. S. (1994). Relation of agency and communion to well-being: Evidence and potential explanations. *Psychological Bulletin, 116,* 412–428.

Hogan, B. E., & Linden, W. (2004). Anger response styles and blood pressure: At least don't ruminate about it! *Annals of Behavioral Medicine, 27*, 38–49.

Houston, B. K., Babyak, M. A., Chesney, M. A., Black, G., & Ragland, D. R. (1997). Social dominance and 22-year all-cause mortality in men. *Psychosomatic Medicine, 59*, 5–12.

Houston, B. K., & Kelly, K. E. (1989). Hostility in employed women: Relation to work and marital experiences, social support, stress, and anger expression. *Personality and Social Psychology Bulletin, 15*, 175–182.

Jakupcak, M., Conybeare, D., Phelps, L., Hunt, S., Holmes, H. A., Felker, B., et al. (2007). Anger, hostility, and aggression among Iraq and Afghanistan War veterans reporting PTSD and subthreshold PTSD. *Journal of Traumatic Stress, 20*, 945–954.

Jamner, L. D., Shapiro, D., Goldstein, I. B., & Hug, R. (1991). Ambulatory blood pressure and heart rate in paramedics: Effects of cynical hostility and defensiveness. *Psychosomatic Medicine, 53*, 393–406.

Jamner, L. D., Shapiro, D., & Jarvik, M. E. (1999). Nicotine reduces the frequency of anger reports in smokers and nonsmokers with high but not low hostility: An ambulatory study. *Experimental and Clinical Psychopharmacology, 7*, 454–463.

John, O. P., & Gross, J. J. (2004). Healthy and unhealthy emotional regulation: Personality processes, individual differences, and life span development. *Journal of Personality, 72*, 1301–1333.

Julkunen, J., Salonen, R., Kaplan, G. A., Chesney, M. A., & Salonen, J. T. (1994). Hostility and the progression of carotid atherosclerosis. *Psychosomatic Medicine, 56*, 519–525.

Kawachi, I., & Berkman, L. (2000). Social cohesion, social capital, and health. In L. F. Berkman & I. Kawachi (Eds.), *Social epidemiology* (pp. 174–190). New York: Oxford University Press.

Kessler, R. C., Sonnega, A., Bromet, E., Hughes, M., & Nelson, C. B. (1995). Posttraumatic stress disorder in the National Comorbidity Survey. *Archives of General Psychiatry, 52*, 1048–1060.

Ketterer, M. W., Denollet, J., Chapp, J., Thayer, B., Keteyian, S., Clark, V., et al. (2004). Men deny and women cry, but who dies?: Do the wages of "denial" include early ischemic coronary heart disease? *Journal of Psychosomatic Research, 56*, 119–123.

Ketterer, M. W., Huffman, J., Lumley, M. A., Wassef, S., Gray, L., Kenyon, L., et al. (1998). Five-year follow-up for adverse outcomes in males with at least minimally positive angiograms: Importance of "denial" in assessing psychosocial risk factors. *Journal of Psychosomatic Research, 44*, 241–250.

Kiecolt-Glaser, J. K., & Newton, T. L. (2001). Marriage and health: His and hers. *Psychological Bulletin, 27*, 472–503.

Kivimaki, M., Vahtera, J., Koskenvuo, M., Uutela, A., & Pentti, J. (1998). Response of hostile individuals to stressful changes in their working lives: Test of a psychosocial vulnerability model. *Psychological Medicine, 28*, 903–913.

Kneip, R. C., Delamater, A. M., Ismond, T., Milford, C., Salvia, L., & Schwartz, D. (1993). Self and spouse ratings of anger and hostility as predictors of coronary heart disease. *Health Psychology, 12*, 301–307.

Kopp, M., Skrabski, A., Szántó, Z., & Siegrist, J. (2006). Psychosocial determinants of premature cardiovascular mortality differences within Hungary. *Journal of Epidemiology and Community Health, 60*, 782–788.

Larkin, K. T., Martin, R. R., & McClain, S. E. (2002). Cynical hostility and the accuracy of decoding facial expressions of emotions. *Journal of Behavioral Medicine, 25*, 286–292.

Lepore, S. (1995). Cynicism, social support, and cardiovascular reactivity. *Health Psychology, 14*, 210–216.

Linden, W., Hogan, B. E., Rutledge, T., Chawla, A., Lenz, J. W., & Leung, D. (2003). There is more to anger coping than "in" or "out." *Emotion, 3*, 12–29.

Lipkus, I. M., Barefoot, J. C., Williams, R. B., & Siegler, I. C. (1994). Personality measures as predictors of smoking initiation and cessation. *Health Psychology, 13*, 149–155.

Luecken, L. J. (2000). Attachment and loss experiences during childhood are associated with adult hostility, depression, and social support. *Journal of Psychosomatic Research, 49*, 85–91.

Manuck, S. B., Flory, J. D., Muldoon, M. F., & Ferrell, R. E. (2002). Central nervous system serotonergic responsivity and aggressive disposition in men. *Physiology and Behavior, 77*, 705–709.

Mao, W., Bardwell, W. A., Major, J. M., & Dimsdale, J. E. (2003). Coping strategies, hostility, and depressive symptoms: A path model. *International Journal of Behavioral Medicine, 10*, 331–342.

Martin, R., Watson, D., & Wan, C. K. (2000). A three-factor model of trait anger: Dimensions of affect, behavior, and cognition. *Journal of Personality, 68*, 869–897.

Matthews, K. A., Gump, B. B., Harris, K. F., Haney, T. L., & Barefoot, J. C. (2004). Hostile behaviors predict cardiovascular mortality among men enrolled in the Multiple Risk Factor Intervention Trial. *Circulation, 109*, 66–70.

Matthews, K. A., Woodall, K. L., Kenyon, K., & Jacob, T. (1996). Negative family environment as a predictor of boys' future status on measures of hostile attitudes, interview behavior, and anger expression. *Health Psychology, 15*, 30–37.

McCann, B. S., Russo, J., Benjamin, G., & Andrew, H. (1997). Hostility, social support, and perceptions of work. *Journal of Occupational Health Psychology, 2*, 175–185.

McCrae, R. R., & Costa, P. T., Jr. (1985). Updating Norman's "adequate taxonomy": Intelligence and personality dimensions in natural language and in questionnaires. *Journal of Personality and Social Psychology, 49*, 110–121.

McCrae, R. R., & Costa, P. T., Jr. (1987). Validation of the five-factor model of personality across instruments and observers. *Journal of Personality and Social Psychology, 52*, 81–90.

Miller, T. Q., Marksides, K. S., Chiriboga, D. A., & Ray, L. A. (1995). A test of the psychosocial vulnerability and health behavior models of hostility: Results from an 11-year follow-up study of Mexican Americans. *Psychosomatic Medicine, 57*, 572–581.

Moffitt, T. E., Caspi, A., & Rutter, M. (2005). Strategies for investigating interactions between measured genes and measured environments. *Archives of General Psychiatry, 62,* 473–481.

Newton, T. L., & Kiecolt-Glaser, J. K. (1995). Hostility and the erosion of marriage quality during early marriage. *Journal of Behavioral Medicine, 18,* 601–619.

Orth, U., & Wieland, E. (2006). Anger, hostility, and posttraumatic stress disorder in trauma-exposed adults: A meta-analysis. *Journal of Consulting and Clinical Psychology, 74,* 698–706.

Porter, L. S., Stone, A. A., & Schwartz, J. E. (1999). Anger expression and ambulatory blood pressure: A comparison of state and trait measures. *Psychosomatic Medicine, 61,* 454–463.

Price, J. M., & Glad, K. (2003). Hostile attributional tendencies in maltreated children. *Journal of Abnormal Child Psychology, 31,* 329–343.

Rempel, J. K., Holmes, J. G., & Zanna, M. P. (1985). Trust in close relationships. *Journal of Personality and Social Psychology, 49,* 95–112.

Rosenman, R. H., Swan, G. E., & Carmilli, D. (1988). Definition, assessment, and evolution of the Type A behavior pattern. In B. K. Houston & C. R. Snyder (Eds.), *Type A behavior pattern: Research, theory, and intervention* (pp. 8–31). New York: Wiley.

Rotter, J. (1967). A new scale for the measurement of interpersonal trust. *Journal of Personality, 35,* 651–665.

Rotter, J. (1980). Interpersonal trust, trustworthiness, and gullibility. *American Psychologist, 35,* 1–7.

Scherwitz, L., Perkins, L., Chesney, M., & Hughes, G. (1991). Cook–Medley Hostility Scale and subsets: Relationship to demographic and psychosocial characteristics in young adults in the CARDIA Study. *Psychosomatic Medicine, 53,* 36–49.

Scherwitz, L., Perkins, L., Chesney, M., Hughes, G., Sidney, S., & Manolio, T. A. (1992). Hostility and health behaviors in young adults: The CARDIA Study. *American Journal of Epidemiology, 136,* 136–145.

Shekelle, R. B., Gale, M., Ostfeld, A. M., & Paul, O. (1983). Hostility, risk of coronary heart disease, and mortality. *Psychosomatic Medicine, 45,* 109–114.

Shumaker, S. A., & Hill, D. R. (1991). Gender differences in social support and physical health. *Health Psychology, 10,* 102–111.

Siegel, J. M. (1986). The Multidimensional Anger Inventory. *Journal of Personality and Social Psychology, 51,* 191–200.

Siegman, A. W. (1994). Cardiovascular consequences of expressing and repressing anger. In A. W. Siegman & T. W. Smith (Eds.), *Anger, hostility, and the heart* (pp. 173–198) Hillsdale, NJ: Erlbaum.

Siegman, A. W., Kubzansky, L. D., Kawachi, I., Boyle, S., Vokonas, P. S., & Sparrow, D. (2000). A prospective study of dominance and coronary heart disease in the Normative Aging Study. *American Journal of Cardiology, 86,* 145–149.

Siegman, A. W., Townsend, S. T., Civelek, A. C., & Blumenthal, R. S. (2000). Antagonistic behavior, dominance, hostility, and coronary heart disease. *Psychosomatic Medicine, 62,* 248–257.

Simons, R. L., Simons, L. G., Burt, C. H., Drummund, H., Stewart, E., Brody, G. H., et al. (2006). Supportive parenting moderates the effect of discrimination upon anger, hostile view of relationships, and violence among African American boys. *Journal of Health and Social Behavior, 47,* 373–389.

Smith, T. W., & Brown, P. W. (1991). Cynical hostility, attempts to exert social control, and cardiovascular reactivity in married couples. *Journal of Behavioral Medicine, 14,* 581–592.

Smith, T. W., & Frohm, K. D. (1985). What's so unhealthy about hostility?: Construct validity and psychosocial correlates of the Cook and Medley Ho scale. *Health Psychology, 4,* 503–520.

Smith, T. W., & Gallo, L. C. (1999). Hostility and cardiovascular reactivity during marital interaction. *Psychosomatic Medicine, 61,* 436–445.

Smith, T. W., Gallo, L. C., Goble, L., Ngu, L. Q., & Stark, K. A. (1998). Agency, communion, and cardiovascular reactivity during marital interaction. *Health Psychology, 17,* 537–545.

Smith, T. W., Glazer, K., Ruiz, J. M., & Gallo, L. C. (2004). Hostility, anger, aggressiveness, and coronary heart disease: An interpersonal perspective on personality, emotion, and health. *Journal of Personality, 72,* 1217–1270.

Smith, T. W., Pope, M. K., Sanders, J. D., Allred, K. D., & O'Keefe, J. L. (1988). Cynical hostility at home and work: Psychosocial vulnerability across domains. *Journal of Research in Personality, 22,* 525–548.

Smith, T. W., Sanders, J. D., & Alexander, J. F. (1990). What does the Cook and Medley Hostility Scale measure?: Affect, behavior, and attributions in the marital context. *Journal of Personality and Social Psychology, 58,* 699–708.

Smith, T. W., Uchino, B. N., Berg, C. A., Florsheim, P., Gale, G., Hawkins, M., et al. (2007). Hostile personality traits and coronary artery calcification in middle-aged and older married couples: Different effects for self-reports versus spouse ratings. *Psychosomatic Medicine, 69,* 441–448.

Spielberger, C. D., Jacobs, G., Russell, S. F., & Crane, R. J. (1983). Assessment of anger: The State–Trait Anger Scale. In J. N. Butcher & C. D. Spielberger (Eds.), *Advances in personality assessment* (Vol. 2, pp. 159–187). Hillsdale, NJ: Erlbaum.

Spielberger, C. D., Johnson, E. H., Russell, S. F., Crane, R. J., Jacobs, G. A., & Worden, T. J. (1985). The experience and expression of anger: Construction and validation of an anger expression scale. In M. A. Chesney & R. H. Rosenman (Eds.), *Anger and hostility in cardiovascular and behavioral disorders* (pp. 5–30). New York: McGraw-Hill.

Steptoe, A., Hamer, M., & Chida, Y. (2007). The effects of acute psychological stress on circulating inflammatory factors in humans: A review and meta-analysis. *Brain Behavior and Immunity, 21,* 901–912.

Stoney, C. M., & Engebretson, T. O. (1994). Anger and hostility: Potential mediators of the gender difference in cardiovascular disease. In A. W. Siegman & T. W. Smith (Eds.), *Anger, hostility, and the heart* (pp. 215–238). Hillsdale, NJ: Erlbaum.

Suarez, E. C., Kuhn, C. M., Schanberg, S. M., Williams, R. B., & Zimmerman, E. A. (1998). Neuroendocrine, cardiovascular, and emotional responses of hostile men: The role of interpersonal challenge. *Psychosomatic Medicine, 60,* 78–88.

Surwit, R. S., Williams, R. B., Siegler, I. C., Lane, J. D., Helms, M. J., Applegate, K. L., et al. (2002). Hostility, race, and glucose metabolism in nondiabetic individuals. *Diabetes Care, 25,* 835–839.

Swenson, W. M., Pearson, J. S., & Osbourne, D. (1973). *An MMPI sourcebook: Basic item, scale, and pattern data on 50,000 medical patients.* Minneapolis: University of Minnesota Press.

Turner, R. J., Russell, D., Glover, R., & Hutto, P. (2007). The social antecedents of anger proneness in young adulthood. *Journal of Health and Social Behavior, 48,* 68–83.

Weidner, G., Rice, T., Knox, S. S., Ellison, R. C., Province, M. A., Rao, D. C., et al. (2000). Familial resemblance for hostility: The National Heart, Lung, and Blood Institute Family Heart Study. *Psychosomatic Medicine, 62,* 197–204.

Wiggins, J. S., & Trapnell, P. D. (1996). A dyadic interactional perspective on the five-factor model. In J. S. Wiggins (Ed.), *The five-factor model of personality: Theoretical perspectives* (pp. 88–162). New York: Guilford Press.

Williams, J. E., Nieto, F. J., Sanford, C. P., Couper, D. J., & Tyroler, H. A. (2002). The association between trait anger and incident stroke risk: The Atherosclerosis Risk in Communities (ARIC) study. *Stroke, 33,* 13–20.

Williams, R. B., & Barefoot, J. C. (1988). The emerging role of the hostility complex. In B. K. Houston & C. R. Snyder (Eds.), *Type A behavior pattern: Research, theory, and intervention* (pp. 189–211). New York: Wiley.

Zeichner, A., Giancola, P. R., & Allen, J. D. (1995). Effects of hostility on alcohol stress-response dampening. *Alcoholism: Clinical and Experimental Research, 19,* 977–983.

CHAPTER 15

■ ● ▲ ◆ ■ ● ▲ ◆

Loneliness

JOHN T. CACIOPPO
LOUISE C. HAWKLEY

Conceptualization of Loneliness

Although the nature and purpose of loneliness have long been discussed in philosophy, theology, and literature, the scientific study of loneliness has a relatively short history. The first scientific paper on loneliness can be traced back just five decades to the now-classic psychoanalytic treatise by Frieda Fromm-Reichman (1959), and phenomenological and existential perspectives followed soon afterward (Moustakas, 1961; Rogers, 1961). The work of John Bowlby on attachment bonds (Bowlby, 1973) heralds the beginning of theoretical conceptualizations of loneliness. Robert S. Weiss (1973) delineated an attachment theory of loneliness in which deficiencies in social relationships serving specific functions (e.g., attachment, social integration, nurturance) were posited to contribute to feelings of loneliness. Weiss described loneliness as "a chronic distress without redeeming features" (p. 15), and he further distinguished between social loneliness (e.g., lack of social integration) and emotional loneliness (e.g., absence of a reliable attachment figure). This theoretical perspective, also called the "social needs" approach, continues to motivate loneliness research (Dykstra & Fokkema, 2007).

A second conceptual approach to loneliness has focused on social skill deficits and personality traits that impair the formation and maintenance of social relationships. Research in the social skills area has shown that loneliness is associated with more self-focus, poorer partner attention skills, a lack of self-disclosure to friends, especially among females, and less participation in organized groups, especially among males (reviewed in Marangoni & Ickes, 1989). Personality research has shown that loneliness is associated with depressive symptoms, shyness, and neuroticism and low self-esteem, optimism, conscientiousness, and agreeableness (Marangoni & Ickes, 1989). Early studies suggested that behavioral and personality correlates of loneliness tend to be true only for chronically lonely individuals, not for "state-lonely" individuals whose loneliness is adequately explained by potent situational factors (e.g., widowhood, geographical relocation) (reviewed in Marangoni & Ickes, 1989). More recently, however, loneliness has been observed to operate like a trait even when induced in an acute fashion. Under hypnotic suggestion, young adults were made to feel lonely and then socially connected (or vice versa, in a counterbalanced order) by recalling a time when they felt either rejected and as though they did not belong or accepted and that they belonged. Measures of affect, social factors, and even personality traits mirrored and tracked the acute changes in loneliness induced by the hypnotic manipulation. Relative to their baseline levels of loneliness, individuals made to feel lonely reported significantly more negative mood and lower self-esteem, optimism, social skills, social support, sociability, extraversion, and agreeableness and greater shyness, anxiety, anger, fear of negative evaluation, and neuroticism (Cacioppo, Hawkley, et al., 2006). These results identify loneliness as a potential causal factor in characteristics such as self-esteem, depressive symptomatology, shyness, and so forth.

A third conceptual approach to loneliness is represented by cognitive discrepancy theory, which specifies loneliness as the consequence of altered social perceptions and attributions. Specifically, loneliness is defined as the distress that occurs when one's social relationships are perceived as being less satisfying than what is desired (Peplau & Perlman, 1982). From a cognitive discrepancy perspective, it is clear that loneliness is not synonymous with being alone, nor does being with others guarantee protection from feelings of loneliness (Peplau & Perlman, 1982). Rather, discrepancies between ideal and perceived interpersonal relationships produce and maintain feelings of loneliness.

A fourth approach derives from an evolutionary analysis of loneliness, with an emphasis on inclusive fitness (Cacioppo, Hawkley, et al., 2006). This approach calls into question the conceptualization of loneliness as an aversive condition without redeeming features and instead conceptualizes loneliness as an aversive condition that promotes inclusive fitness by signaling ruptures in social connections to motivate the repair or replacement of these connections. For many species, offspring need little or no parenting to survive and reproduce. *Homo sapiens*, however, are born to the longest period of abject dependency of any species. Simple reproduction, therefore, is not sufficient to ensure that one's genes make it into the gene pool. For one's genes to make it to the gene pool, the offspring must survive to reproduce. Moreover, social connections and the behaviors they engender (e.g., cooperation, altruism, alliances) enhance the survival and reproduction of those involved, increasing inclusive fitness.

Humans walked the earth as hunter–gatherers for tens of thousands of years, often under conditions of privation. Hunter–gatherers who chose not to return to share their food and offer protection to mother and child (i.e., who felt no loss severing social/family bonds) may have survived to reproduce again, but their offspring and, with them their genes, would have been unlikely to survive to reproduce. In contrast, hunter–gatherers whose genetic predisposition inclined them to share food with their families may have lowered their own chances of survival but increased the survival odds of their offspring, thereby propagating their genes. Of course, a hunter–gatherer who survives a famine may then live to have another family another day, suggesting that no single strategy is necessarily best. Such an evolutionary scenario suggests that humans might inherit differing tendencies to experience loneliness. Adoption and twin studies among children and adults have confirmed that loneliness has a sizeable heritable component (Boomsma, Willemsen, Dolan, Hawkley, & Cacioppio, 2005; McGuire & Clifford, 2000).

Measures of Loneliness

Individual differences in loneliness are typically measured using paper-and-pencil questionnaires, a number of which are reviewed in Cramer and Barry (1999). Among the multidimensional scales tapping emotional and social loneliness are the De Jong Gierveld Loneliness Scale (De Jong Gierveld & Kamphuis, 1985) and the Social and Emotional Loneliness Scale for Adults (SELSA; DiTommaso & Spinner, 1993). These two scales probe social relational deficits with items such as "I have friends to whom I can talk about the pressures in my life" and "There are plenty of people I can rely on when I have problems." The De Jong Gierveld Loneliness Scale probes emotional relational deficits with items such as "I experience a general sense of emptiness," whereas the SELSA distinguishes between relational deficits in family relationships (e.g., "I feel close to my family") and romantic relationships (e.g., "I have someone who fulfills my needs for intimacy").

The most frequently used instrument is the UCLA Loneliness Scale developed at the University of California at Los Angeles (version 3; Russell, 1996). Items probe the frequency and intensity of loneliness-related experiences (e.g., "How often do you feel alone?" "How often do you feel part of a group of friends?" and "How often do you feel that there are people who really understand you?"). To avoid response bias, the terms *lonely* and *loneliness* do not appear in any of the items. Although conceptualized as a unidimensional scale, factor analyses of the UCLA Loneliness Scale have revealed anywhere from two to five dimensions. Second-order factor analyses, however, have shown a single overarching loneliness construct (Hawkley, Browne, & Cacioppo, 2005; Russell, 1996) that supports its use as a unidimensional bipolar measure of loneliness. An abbreviated three-item version of this scale has been validated for use in large population surveys (Hughes, Waite, Hawkley, & Cacioppo, 2004).

Stability

Temporal stability of loneliness scores is relatively high, with test–retest reliabilities of .69, .57, and .51 across 2, 3, and 5 years, respectively, in children between 7 and 12 years of age (Bartels, Cacioppo, Hudziak, & Boomsma, 2008); .74 across a 2-week to 2-month time period in young adults (Cacioppo, Hawkley, et al., 2006); and from .73 to .84 across 1–2 years in middle-aged and older adults (Cacioppo, Hughes, Waite, Hawkley, & Thisted, 2006; Russell, 1996).

Antecedents of Loneliness

Heritability

If the motivation to form and maintain social bonds has evolutionary origins, one might expect significant genetic contributions to loneliness. In a study of adoptive families, loneliness data were obtained from 69 biologically related sibling pairs and 64 unrelated pairs when the children were 9, 10, 11, and 12 years of age. In a second study, 22 monozygotic (MZ) twins, 40 dizygotic (DZ) twins, and 80 full siblings 8–14 years of age completed a 16-item scale to assess loneliness in relation to their schoolmates. Results revealed significant genetic (h^2 = 55 and 48%, respectively, in Studies 1 and 2) and unshared environmental contributions to individual differences in loneliness (McGuire & Clifford, 2000).

Heritability estimates of complex traits such as loneliness may also change across the lifespan, as the frequency, duration, and range of exposure to environmental influences accrues. To address this question, data from young adult and adult Dutch twins (average age 24 years) in the Netherlands Twin Register Study were analyzed with genetic structural equation models, which provide estimates of the shared environmental and unique environmental contributions, as well as the genetic contributions (Boomsma, Willemsen, Dolan, Hawkley, & Cacioppo, 2005). The estimate of genetic contributions to variation in loneliness in adults was 48%, with the remaining variance explained by unique environmental factors. Thus the heritability estimates in adults were similar to those found previously in children. Moreover, no evidence was found for sex or age differences in genetic architecture or for nonadditive genetic effects.

A follow-up longitudinal study of young Dutch twins at ages 7, 10, and 12 years found that the influence of shared family environment increased from .06 and .08 at ages 7 and 10 to .35 at age 12, paralleling a reduction in heritability estimates from .58 and .56 at ages 7 and 10 to .26 at age 12 (Bartels et al., 2008). As these children move through adolescence and adapt to new biological and social challenges, environmental influences are expected to decline and heritable dispositions to reemerge to levels observed in the young adult and adult twins.

Predictors

Research on the predictors of loneliness is predominantly cross-sectional, and longitudinal studies have tended to focus on older adults. These limitations notwithstanding, a sizeable body of research indicates that sociodemographic factors, social roles, quantity and quality of social contact, health, and dispositions contribute to individual differences in feelings of loneliness.

Sociodemographics

Structural factors such as age, gender, race/ethnicity, education, and income constrain opportunities for integration into meaningful groups and social roles, and these factors contribute to individual differences in loneliness. Age has been associated with loneliness, but the shape of that association is a flattened U, not linear as conventional wisdom might suggest. Prevalence and intensity of lonely feelings are greater in adolescence and young adulthood (i.e., 16–25 years of age) than in any other age group except the oldest old (i.e., >80 years) (Pinquart & Sörensen, 2003). Findings in longitudinal studies are consistent with those in cross-sectional studies, and cohort effects have been largely ruled out as an explanation for age effects (Pinquart & Sörensen, 2003). Indeed, in the Americans' Changing Lives study of adults 24 years of age and older, age was inversely associated with loneliness even when the loneliness-augmenting effect of lost social roles (e.g., marriage, work) was held constant (Schnittker, 2007).

Females tend to report slightly greater loneliness than males, but only when the measure includes terms such as *lonely* or *loneliness* (Pinquart & Sörensen, 2003). When examined as a function of marital status, however, nonmarried men are lonelier than nonmarried women (Pinquart, 2003).

In the United States, African Americans tend to be lonelier than whites (Barg et al., 2006), although single African American women were less lonely than Latina and white women in the Southern California Social Survey (Tucker & Mitchell-Kernan, 1998). Cultural differences in loneliness levels have also been observed. Chinese students at an American university reported greater loneliness than their U.S. counterparts (Anderson, 1999), an effect that some have argued is attributable to the Asian collectivist perspective in the context of an individualistic American society (Goodwin, Cook, & Yung, 2001).

Greater educational attainment and higher income are associated with less loneliness (Pinquart & Sörensen, 2003), but this effect is predominantly indirect and has been attributed to larger social networks (Dykstra & De Jong Gierveld, 1999; Lauder, Mummery, & Sharkey, 2006). Holding social network size constant, however, the attainment of a high school diploma continued to protect against loneliness in our population-based sample of middle-aged adults in the Chicago Health, Aging, and Social Relations Study (CHASRS), possibly indicating the relationship-enhancing benefit of higher social status and self-esteem associated with this accomplishment (Hawkley, Hughes, et al., 2007).

Social Roles

Marriage is well known to protect against loneliness, and loneliness is greater among those who are divorced or never married (Dykstra & Fokkema, 2007; Pinquart, 2003). Retirement and unemployment also represent loss of social roles, and both groups are lonelier than the employed (Hansson, Briggs, & Rule, 1990; Viney, 1985). Voluntary group membership (e.g., social club, athletic team) (Cattan, White, Bond, & Learmouth, 2005) and religious/church membership (Johnson & Mullins, 1989) are other roles that have been observed to protect against loneliness.

Social Contact Quantity and Quality

Smaller social networks and less frequent interactions with friends and family promote loneliness (Dykstra, van Tilburg, & De Jong Gierveld, 2005; Pinquart & Sörensen, 2003). Accordingly, situational factors that influence the availability of social opportunities have also been associated with loneliness. For instance, geographical relocation predicts loneliness in first-year university students (Shaver, Furman, & Buhrmester, 1985). Conversely, participation in senior center activities protects against loneliness in older adults living alone (Aday, Kehoe, & Farney, 2006). Contact with friends is more important than contact with adult children and other family members in preventing loneliness (Pinquart & Sörensen, 2003), and the chronic unavailability of social partners with whom to enjoy social activities has been associated with greater loneliness (Rook, 1984).

Social relationship quality is a more potent predictor of loneliness than quantity of social contacts, and this is true of relationships with friends, family, and adult children (Pinquart & Sörensen, 2003). In addition, although marriage is generally protective, only marriages that are close and satisfy a need for a confidant serve to reduce loneliness (Olson & Wong, 2001).

Health

Health-related factors impose another constraint on quantity and quality of social contact. For instance, sensory impairment, particularly the challenge to effective communication posed by impaired hearing, contributes to loneliness (Savikko, Routasalo, Tilvis, Strandberg, & Pitkälä, 2005; Wallhagen, Strawbridge, Shema, Kurata, & Kaplan, 2001). In addition, loneliness is associated with impaired mobility as evident in greater functional limitations and restrictions in the activities of daily life (Bondevik & Skogstad, 1998; Dykstra & De Jong Gierveld, 1999), and with physical symptoms of chronic health conditions (Pinquart & Sörensen, 2003). In late life, institutionalized adults are lonelier than their community-dwelling counterparts (Pinquart & Sörensen, 2003), but loneliness also influences the likelihood of institutionalization (Russell, Cutrona, de la Mora, & Wallace, 1997), suggesting a bidirectional causal association.

Dispositions

Personality characteristics related to loneliness include traits from the "Big Five" such as greater neuroticism, less conscientiousness, and less agreeableness, as well as lower self-esteem and greater shyness, hostility, insecure attachment styles, anxiety, pessimism, and fear of negative evaluation. Loneliness, however, is distinct stochastically and functionally from these dispositions (Cacioppo, Hawkley, et al., 2006; DiTommaso, Brannen-McNulty, Ross, & Burgess, 2003; Ernst & Cacioppo, 1998; Marangoni & Ickes, 1989; Shaver & Brennan, 1991).

Loneliness is sometimes confused with depressed affect and poor social support, a confusion that exists despite theoretical and empirical distinctions among these related constructs (Cacioppo, Hawkley, et al., 2006; Russell, 1996). For instance, empirical work has shown that companionship is a stronger predictor of loneliness than social support (Rook, 1987). These distinctions highlight the difficulty of finding the language to speak about the core experience of human sociality (Dunbar & Shultz, 2007). Just as there are no single terms for the opposite of pain and thirst, there is no simple, precise term that means the opposite of loneliness. We have used "social connection" and "social contentment," and "social bondedness" has recently been suggested (Dunbar & Shultz, 2007), but all fall short for lack of precision. The absence of a term for "not lonely" suggests that this is the normal or default state required to maintain a healthy and balanced life and that loneliness is the problematic state. Indeed, people's mental representations of their sociality conform to the importance of social bonds at every level of human endeavor.

Social Cognition

Mental Representations

Theories of the self have underscored the importance of individual, relational, and collective aspects (Brewer & Gardner, 1996). To the extent that we define ourselves in terms of our interactions with and relationships to others, the mental representation of these connections may similarly be characterized by individual intimate, relational, and collective dimensions. Factor-analytic studies of items from the UCLA Loneliness Scale in young and middle-aged adults and replications using items from other scales designed to gauge oneself in relation to others (Hawkley et al., 2005) provided support for this reasoning. Moreover, in our CHASRS sample of middle-aged men and women, marital status predicted intimate connectedness, frequency of contact with friends and family predicted relational connectedness, and voluntary group membership predicted collective connectedness (Hawkley et al., 2005). This three-dimensional representation of loneliness held in young adults and across gender and racial/ethnic lines in middle-aged adults, suggesting a universality to this representational structure of the social self (Hawkley et al., 2005).

Mental Processes

Chronic loneliness is the result of an interaction between a genetic bias and life circumstances that are in part beyond our control. However, once loneliness is triggered, the defensive form of thinking that it generates—a "lonely" social cognition— can make every social molehill look like a mountain. The lonely not only react more intensely to the negatives but also experience less of a soothing uplift from the positives (Hawkley, Preacher, & Cacioppo, 2007). Even when they succeed in eliciting nurturing support from a friend or loved one, they tend to perceive the exchange as less fulfilling (Hawkley, Burleson, Berntson, & Cacioppo, 2003).

The lonely are aware that their social needs are not being met, but they perceive that they do not have a great deal of control over their ability to fulfill those needs (Solano, 1987). Tending to be more anxious, pessimistic, and fearful of negative evaluation than people who feel good about their social lives, lonely people are more likely to act and relate to others in ways that are anxious, negative, and self-protective, which leads paradoxically to self-defeating behaviors (Cacioppo & Hawkley, 2005). For instance, Rotenberg (1994) found that lonely and nonlonely individuals were equally likely to cooperate with a stranger at the outset and during the early trials of a prisoner's dilemma game in which the stranger was playing a tit-for-tat strategy. As play continued and they betrayed their partners, only to find that their partners then betrayed them, the lonely individuals were especially likely to escalate the betrayals than nonlonely individuals.

Not only do the lonely contribute to their own negative reality, but others also begin to view them more negatively and begin to act accordingly (Lau & Gruen, 1992). One study showed that individuals who were told that an opposite-gender partner they were about to meet was lonely subsequently rated that partner as being less sociable. The individuals primed to have these expectations also behaved toward their partners in a less sociable manner than they did toward partners whom they expected to be nonlonely (Rotenberg, Gruman, & Ariganello, 2002). Once this negative feedback loop starts rolling, the cycle of defensive behavior and negative social results spins even further downhill. In essence, lonely individuals inhabit an inhospitable social orbit that repels others or elicits their negative responses.

Expecting social rejection, the lonely are keenly attuned to cues of social acceptance in their environment. In a test of social monitoring, lonely participants remembered a greater proportion of information related to interpersonal or collective social ties than did nonlonely participants. It made no difference whether the detail, which was presented in diary format, was emotionally positive or negative (Gardner, Pickett, Jeffries, & Knowles, 2005). In another study, participants who were asked to "relive" a rejection experience showed greater attention to vocal tone in a vocal Stroop task than did participants asked to relive an academic failure experience or a neutral experience (the walk to campus that morning) (Pickett, Gardner, & Knowles, 2004).

Greater attention to social cues does not ensure greater social sensitivity, however. We have noted that lonely individuals are less accurate at decoding facial and postural expressions of emotion (Pickett & Gardner, 2005; Pitterman & Nowicki, 2004). In addition, the participants who relived a rejection experience were less accurate in decoding the meaning of the words in the vocal Stroop task (Pickett et al., 2004).

A lack of correspondence between attention and accuracy in responses to social cues has also been demonstrated in a brain imaging study of lonely and nonlonely young adults. When presented with equally arousing positive and negative pictures of scenes and objects (nonsocial stimuli) and people (social stimuli), a set of brain regions often associated with visual attention and perspective taking varied in response to negative social (in contrast to matched nonsocial) pictures. Relative to the nonlonely, lonely individuals showed greater visual cortical activation (consistent with greater attention to the negative social than nonsocial pictures) and less activation of the temporo-parietal junction (consistent with less attention devoted to the other person's perspective). Another set of brain regions, associated with reward systems (i.e., ventral striatum), was found to be down-regulated in lonely, compared with nonlonely, individuals when viewing positive social (in contrast to matched nonsocial) pictures—results consistent with the finding that lonely individuals derive less pleasure from viewing positive social circumstances than nonlonely individuals (Cacioppo, Norris, Decety, Monteleone, & Nusbaum, 2009). This latter finding may bear on the finding that lonely individuals find positive social interactions during the course of a normal day less satisfying than do nonlonely individuals (Hawkley, Preacher, & Cacioppo, 2007).

One might expect that a lonely person, hungry to fulfill unmet social needs, would be very accepting of a new acquaintance, just as a famished person might take pleasure in food that was not as tasty as their usual fare. Indeed, experimentally increasing individuals' feelings of social isolation leads to an increase in anthropomorphism that reflects increased efforts to reconnect (Epley, Waytz, & Cacioppo, 2007). However, when confronted with an opportunity to form a social connection, studies show that the lonely are actually far less accepting of potential new friends than are the nonlonely (Rotenberg & Kmill, 1992). Similarly, lonely students were less responsive to their classmates during class discussions and provided less appropriate and less effective feedback than nonlonely students (Anderson & Martin, 1995). Lonely undergraduates also held more negative perceptions of their roommates than did the nonlonely (Wittenberg & Reis, 1986), and this perceptual divide widened as one moved from roommates to suite mates to floor mates to dorm mates (Cacioppo & Hawkley, 2005).

Time also plays a role in constructing these negative "realities." Researchers asked participants to interact with a friend and to rate the quality of the relationship and the communication immediately; after watching a videotape of the same social exchange; a few weeks later, after being reminded of the interaction; and after again watching the videotape. At all four measurement points, lonely individuals rated relationship quality more negatively than did nonlonely individuals. Interestingly, the further in time they were removed from the social exchange, the more negatively they rated it. They were especially negative after the second videotape viewing (Duck, Pond, & Leatham, 1994). When lonely individuals rated the interaction soon after it happened, it appears that their negative social cognition was reined in by a better understanding of the reasons for their friend's behavior. The more time that passed, the more the objective reality succumbed to the "reality" constructed by the lonely individual's negative social cognition.

In sum, lonely individuals are more likely to construe their world as threatening, to hold more negative expectations, and to interpret and respond to ambiguous social behavior in a more negative, off-putting fashion, thereby confirming their construal of the world as threatening and beyond their control. These cognitions, in turn, activate neurobiological mechanisms that, with time, take a toll on health.

Consequences of Loneliness

Self-Regulation

Self-regulation refers to the capacity to change one's cognitions, emotions, and/or behavior to better meet social standards and personal goals. Evidence from young adults who performed a dichotic listening task indicates that self-regulatory processes are impaired in lonely individuals (Cacioppo et al., 2000). In the dichotic listening task, participants are asked to identify the consonant–vowel pair presented in the left or right ear. Typically, performance shows a right-ear advantage. In addition, performance is generally better for the ear to which participants have been instructed to attend. In our study of lonely and nonlonely young adults, we observed a right-ear advantage and an attentional instruction advantage, but an interaction between these effects revealed that, although lonely and nonlonely individuals showed a large attentional shift to the right ear when so instructed, lonely but not nonlonely participants failed to show a left-ear advantage when instructed to attend to this ear (Cacioppo et al., 2000).

Experimental manipulations that lead people to believe they face a future in social isolation also increases the challenge of self-regulation (Baumeister & DeWall, 2005), and this impaired self-regulation has consequences for mental functioning. Undergraduate volunteers were provided with feedback to induce in them the possibility that they would experience a future alone (e.g., "You're the type who probably will end up alone. Relationships just won't last for you ... "), a future belonging (e.g., "You're the type who'll have rewarding relationships throughout your life. Most likely you'll have lifelong friendships and a long and happy marriage ... "), a future of misfortunes (e.g., "You're inherently accident prone. Even if this has not manifested itself in your life so far, you can count on breaking an arm or a leg fairly often ... "), or no feedback at all. The future-alone group showed significantly greater impairment in both speed and accuracy on the subsequent Reading Comprehension Test of the Graduate Record Exam than either the future-belonging group or the misfortune control group. Bad news itself, then, was not enough to cause the disruption, only bad news about social connection. In addition, the mood measure for the future-alone group showed no indication of emotional distress, suggesting that any decline in cognitive ability was not a simple matter of being flustered (Baumeister, Twenge, & Nuss, 2002).

Stress-Related Processes and Outcomes

Stress Exposure

Surveys of undergraduate students showed that lonely and nonlonely young adults do not differ in their exposure to major life stressors or in the number of major changes they endured in the previous 12 months (Cacioppo et al., 2000). A "beeper study," in which these students were asked to sit down and record their thoughts and experiences at various times during the day, also showed that there was no difference in the reported frequency of hassles or uplifts they experience on an average day, nor in the number of minor irritants they were confronting when their beeping wristwatch randomly interrupted them (Hawkley, Burleson, Berntson, & Cacioppo, 2003). At least for young adults, then, there was no evidence that loneliness increased exposure to objective causes of stress. However, the number of objective stressors described as "current" had indeed increased among the middle-aged adults in CHASRS, and the lives of chronically lonely adults involved more objective chronic stressors than the lives of the nonlonely (Hawkley et al., 2008). Moreover, the increasing stress load over the course of a lifetime is aggravated by having fewer meaningful relationships to provide relief. Loneliness is an "added" stress.

Stress Perceptions and Coping

Even setting aside the greater number of objective stressors in their lives, the lonely express proportionately greater feelings of helplessness and threat. The lonely, both young and old, perceived the hassles and stresses of everyday life to be more severe than did their nonlonely counterparts. Compounding the problem, the lonely found the small, social uplifts of everyday life to be less intense and less gratifying (Hawkley et al., 2003). The presence of and interaction with other people did not lessen their ratings of the severity of their everyday stressors.

Stress is not uniformly "bad" but can foster growth and motivate better performance. Lonely individuals, however, are far less likely than nonlonely individuals to see any given stressor as an invigorating challenge. Instead of responding with optimism and active engagement, they tend to respond with pessimism and avoidance, a passive coping strategy that carries its own costs. Among young adults, the greater the degree of loneliness, the more the individual withdrew when faced with stressors. Similarly, the greater the loneliness, the less the individual sought out emotional support, as well as instrumental (practical) support (Cacioppo, Hawkley, Crawford, et al., 2002). Behavioral withdrawal and failure to seek emotional support are common among lonely older adults, as well (Hawkley & Cacioppo, 2007).

Health Behaviors

Poor health behaviors are appealing mechanistic candidates for associations between loneliness and health. High-calorie, high-fat diets and sedentary lifestyles, for example, contribute to being overweight or obese, major risk factors for disease in Western society. In a large cross-sectional survey of 1,289 adults 18 years and older (mean age = 46.3 years), the lonely group had a higher mean BMI and a greater proportion of overweight/obese individuals than the nonlonely group did (Lauder, Mummery, Jones, & Caperchione, 2006).

Loneliness differences in physical activity have not been observed in studies of young adults (Hawkley et al., 2003) or in samples that cover a wide age range from young to older adults (Lauder et al., 2006). However, in our CHASRS sample of middle-aged adults, loneliness was associated with significantly reduced odds of physical activity (OR = 0.65 per SD of loneliness) (Hawkley,

Thisted, & Cacioppo, 2007). This association was independent of sociodemographic variables (age, gender, ethnicity, education, income), psychosocial variables (depressive symptoms, perceived stress, hostility, social support), and self-rated health. Moreover, deficits in self-regulation, in this case the diminished tendency of lonely individuals to optimize positive emotions (i.e., poor hedonic emotion regulation), explained the association between loneliness and physical activity likelihood. Longitudinal analyses revealed that loneliness also predicted diminished odds of physical activity in the subsequent 2 years (OR = 0.61) and greater likelihood of transitioning from physical activity to inactivity (OR = 1.58). These data suggest that age-related decreases in physical activity among the lonely may exacerbate risk for cardiovascular disease onset and progression and contribute to an accelerated physiological decline.

Physiological Functioning

Cardiovascular Functioning

Blood pressure is a function of cardiac output (CO) and total peripheral resistance (TPR). In young adults, we found that loneliness was related to differential regulation of systolic blood pressure (SBP). Although lonely and nonlonely individuals did not differ in blood pressure levels, maintenance of blood pressure was attributable to higher vascular resistance and lower cardiac output among lonely relative to nonlonely individuals (Cacioppo, Hawkley, Crawford, et al., 2002; Hawkley et al., 2003). Results from the Framingham Heart Study indicate that changes in TPR play a dominant role in determining SBP from age 30 until approximately age 50 (Franklin et al., 1997). Given the temporal stability of loneliness and its substantial heritable component, it is plausible that loneliness-related elevations in TPR in early to middle adulthood may lead to higher blood pressure in middle and older age. Consistent with this hypothesis, loneliness was associated with elevated SBP in a population-based sample of older adults in the CHASRS. Moreover, the association between loneliness and elevated SBP was exaggerated in older relative to younger lonely adults in this sample (Hawkley, Masi, Berry,

& Cacioppo, 2006), consistent with our hypothesis of accelerated physiological decline in lonely relative to nonlonely individuals.

Neuroendocrine Functioning

Activity of the hypothalamic–pituitary–adrenocortical (HPA) axis is critical to immune functioning and inflammatory processes, and dysregulation of HPA activity has been associated with loneliness and related psychosocial variables (Hawkley, Bosch, Engeland, Marucha, & Cacioppo, 2007). Evidence for a loneliness difference in activity of the HPA axis was first reported by Kiecolt-Glaser and colleagues (1984), who observed that lonely nonpsychotic psychiatric inpatients excreted significantly greater amounts of urinary cortisol than did nonlonely inpatients. More recently, Steptoe, Owen, Kunz-Ebrecht, and Brydon (2004) found that lonely individuals showed a greater 30-minute postawakening increase in salivary cortisol, and Pressman and colleagues (2005) found that loneliness was associated with higher early-morning and late-night levels of circulating cortisol in young adult university students.

In our study of young adults, we measured catecholamines, adrenocorticotropic hormone (ACTH), and cortisol in blood samples collected in the morning and again in the late afternoon. Analyses revealed that only morning levels of ACTH were significantly higher among lonely than nonlonely students (Cacioppo et al., 2000). We found no loneliness differences in the diurnal pattern of cortisol secretion or in mean daily levels of salivary cortisol, nor did we find differences in HPA reactivity to acute stressors in lonely and nonlonely individuals (Cacioppo et al., 2000).

Among older adults in CHASRS, however, HPA activity across a 3-day period in participants' everyday lives showed an effect consistent with a causal role for loneliness. Diary reports of daily psychosocial, emotional, and physical states were completed at bedtime on each of 3 consecutive days. Salivary cortisol levels were measured at awakening, 30 minutes after awakening, and at bedtime each day. Multilevel models revealed that prior day feelings of loneliness and related feelings of sadness, threat, and lack of control were associated with a higher cortisol awakening response the next day, but morning cortisol awakening responses did not predict experiences of these psychosocial states later the same day (Adam, Hawkley, Kudielka, & Cacioppo, 2006). The relevance of this association is particularly noteworthy given recent evidence that loneliness-related alterations in HPA activity may occur at the level of the gene.

DNA Transcription Regulation

Cortisol can regulate a wide variety of physiological processes via nuclear hormone receptor-mediated control of gene transcription. Cortisol activation of the glucocorticoid receptor (GR) exerts broad anti-inflammatory effects by inhibiting proinflammatory signaling pathways.

Social isolation, however, is associated with increased risk of inflammation-mediated diseases. One possible explanation for inflammation-related disease in individuals with high cortisol levels involves impaired GR-mediated signal transduction that prevents the cellular genome from effectively "hearing" the anti-inflammatory signal sent by circulating glucocorticoids (Cole et al., 2007). Consistent with this hypothesis, a systematic examination of genome-wide transcriptional alterations in circulating leukocytes showed increased expression of genes carrying proinflammatory elements and decreased expression of genes carrying anti-inflammatory glucocorticoid response elements in lonely relative to nonlonely middle-aged adults (Cole et al., 2007). Impaired transcription of glucocorticoid response genes and increased activity of proinflammatory transcription control pathways provide a functional genomic explanation for elevated risk of inflammatory disease in individuals who experience chronically high levels of loneliness.

Cognitive Functioning and Depression

Cognitive Functioning

Social isolation increases the risk of developing dementia, and this risk extends to those who perceive themselves to be socially isolated or lonely. In a 4-year prospective study of initially dementia-free older adults (mean age = 80.7 years), the risk of Alzheimer's disease was more than twice as great in lonely as in nonlonely individuals (RR scores of 3.2 vs. 1.4, respectively), and this effect was independent of functional physical impairments and vascular risk factors and conditions (Wilson et al., 2007). In addition, loneliness was associated with lower cognitive ability at baseline and with a more rapid decline in cognition during the 4-year follow-up (Wilson et al., 2007). Loneliness has been associated with poorer self-reported memory among older black adults (Bazargan & Barbre, 1992) and predicted more rapid cognitive decline over a 10-year period in a Finnish sample of adults 75 years of age and older (Tilvis et al., 2004).

Depression

We have noted that loneliness and depressive symptoms are conceptually and empirically distinct (Cacioppo, Hawkley, et al., 2006). Nevertheless, levels of loneliness and depressive symptoms covary across the lifespan. Moreover, despite age-group differences in loneliness, the association between loneliness and depressive symptoms appears stable (i.e., moderately and equivalently positive) across age (Nolen-Hoeksema & Ahrens, 2002).

Loneliness has been identified as a risk factor for depressive symptoms in longitudinal studies of older adults (Heikkinen & Kauppinen, 2004). However, as has been noted, loneliness is associated with a constellation of demographic and psychosocial risk factors (e.g., hostility, low social support, perceived stress) for depressive symptoms that could explain the association between loneliness and depressive symptoms (e.g., Cacioppo, Hawkley, et al., 2006). Recent evidence from a nationally representative sample of adults 54 years old and older revealed that loneliness was associated with more depressive symptoms independent of demographic factors (age, gender, ethnicity, socioeconomic status, marital status) and related feelings of hostility, perceived stress, and poor social support (Cacioppo, Hughes, et al., 2006). Extending these findings, longitudinal data from a population-based sample of 50- to 67-year-old adults in CHASRS showed reciprocal influences between loneliness and depressive symptoms over a 3-year period that again were independent of demographic and psychosocial risk factors (Cacioppo, Hughes, et al., 2006). The mutually synergistic effects of loneliness and depressive symptoms are consistent with a downward spiral of negativity in lonely and depressed individuals and suggest that interventions at either or both fronts could reduce emotional suffering and improve well-being.

Sleep Salubrity

Sleep deprivation has been associated with reduced glucose tolerance, elevated evening cortisol levels, and increased sympathetic nervous system activity (Spiegel, Leproult, & Van Cauter, 1999). However, sleep quality is as at least as important as sleep duration in accomplishing its restorative effects. Nonrestorative sleep (i.e., sleep that is nonrefreshing despite normal sleep duration) results in daytime impairments such as physical and intellectual fatigue, role impairments, irritability, and cognitive and memory problems (Ohayon, 2005).

Prior research has shown that poor social relations and loneliness are associated with poor sleep quality and daytime dysfunction (Cacioppo, Hawkley, Crawford, et al., 2002; Friedman et al., 2005). Prior research also has shown that the greater daytime dysfunction reported by lonely young adults is accompanied by more nightly micro awakenings and not by differential sleep duration (Cacioppo, Hawkley, Berntson, et al., 2002). In an extension of these findings, loneliness was associated with greater daytime dysfunction in a 3-day diary study completed by the CHASRS sample of middle-aged adults, an association that was independent of age, gender, race/ethnicity, household income, health behaviors, BMI, chronic health conditions, daily illness symptom severity, and related feelings of stress, hostility, poor social support, and depressive symptoms. Moreover, cross-lagged panel analyses supported a causal role for loneliness: Lonely feelings predicted daytime dysfunction the following day, but daytime dysfunction was not a significant predictor of lonely feelings the following day (Hawkley, Preacher, Waite, & Cacioppo, 2007). These results were independent of sleep duration and suggest that the same amount of sleep is less salubrious in individuals who feel more socially isolated.

Conclusion

In sum, loneliness used to be characterized as an aversive state with no redeeming features, and as a state barely different from general negativity or depressed mood. Recent research suggests a very different depiction of loneliness. Early in our history as a species, humans survived and prospered only by banding together—in couples, in families, in tribes—to provide mutual protection and assistance. In this context, disconnection from others was a life-threatening circumstance, and loneliness evolved as a signal to change behavior—very much like hunger, thirst, or physical pain—that serves to help one avoid damage and promote the transmission of genes to the gene pool. In the case of loneliness, the signal is a prompt to renew the connections we need to survive and prosper. The evocation of loneliness disrupts executive functioning, increases vascular resistance, and decreases the salubrity of sleep. Left unresolved, loneliness not only disrupts social relationships, it also leads to increased depressive symptomatology and increases organismic wear and tear.

Acknowledgments

This research was supported by National Institute on Aging Program Project Grant No. PO1 AG18911 and by an award from the Templeton Foundation.

References

Adam, E. K., Hawkley, L. C., Kudielka, B. M., & Cacioppo, J. T. (2006). Day-to-day dynamics of experience–cortisol associations in a population-based sample of older adults. *Proceedings of the National Academy of Sciences of the USA, 103,* 17058–17063.

Aday, R. H., Kehoe, G. C., & Farney, L. A. (2006). Impact of senior center friendships on aging women who live alone. *Journal of Women and Aging, 18,* 57–73.

Anderson, C. A. (1999). Attributional style, depression, and loneliness: A cross-cultural comparison of American and Chinese students. *Personality and Social Psychology Bulletin, 25,* 482–499.

Anderson, C. M., & Martin, M. M. (1995). The effects of communication motives, interaction involvement, and loneliness on satisfaction. *Small Group Research, 26,* 118–137.

Barg, F. K., Huss-Ashmore, R., Wittink, M. N., Murray, G. F., Bogner, H. R., & Gallo, J. J. (2006). A mixed-methods approach to understanding loneliness and depression in older adults. *Journals of Gerontology: Psychological Sciences and Social Sciences, 61B*, S329–S339.

Bartels, M., Cacioppo, J. T., Hudziak, J. J., & Boomsma, D. I. (2008). Genetic and environmental contributions to stability in loneliness throughout childhood. *American Journal of Medical Genetics: Part B. Neuropsychiatric Genetics, 147B*, 385–391.

Baumeister, R. F., & DeWall, C. N. (2005). The inner dimension of social exclusion: Intelligent thought and self-regulation among rejected persons. In K. D. Williams, J. P. Forgas, & W. von Hippel (Eds.), *The social outcast: Ostracism, social exclusion, rejection, and bullying* (pp. 53–73). New York: Psychology Press.

Baumeister, R. F., Twenge, J. M., & Nuss, C. K. (2002). Effects of social exclusion on cognitive processes: Anticipated aloneness reduces intelligent thought. *Journal of Personality and Social Psychology, 83*, 817–827.

Bazargan, M., & Barbre, A. R. (1992). Self-reported memory problems among the black elderly. *Educational Gerontology, 18*, 71–82.

Bondevik, M., & Skogstad, A. (1998). The oldest old, ADL, social network, and loneliness. *Western Journal of Nursing Research, 20*, 325–343.

Boomsma, D. I., Willemsen, G., Dolan, C. V., Hawkley, L. C., & Cacioppo, J. T. (2005). Genetic and environmental contributions to loneliness in adults: The Netherlands Twin Register Study. *Behavior Genetics, 35*, 745–752.

Bowlby, J. (1973). *Attachment and loss: Vol. 2. Separation.* New York: Basic Books.

Brewer, M. B., & Gardner, W. (1996). Who is this "we"?: Levels of collective identity and self representations. *Journal of Personality and Social Psychology, 71*, 83–93.

Cacioppo, J. T., Ernst, J. M., Burleson, M. H., McClintock, M. K., Malarkey, W. B., Hawkley, L. C., et al. (2000). Lonely traits and concomitant physiological processes: The MacArthur Social Neuroscience Studies. *International Journal of Psychophysiology, 35*, 143–154.

Cacioppo, J. T., & Hawkley, L. C. (2005). People thinking about people: The vicious cycle of being a social outcast in one's own mind. In K. D. Williams, J. P. Forgas, & W. von Hippel (Eds.), *The social outcast: Ostracism, social exclusion, rejection, and bullying* (pp. 91–108). New York: Psychology Press.

Cacioppo, J. T., Hawkley, L. C., Berntson, G. G., Ernst, J. M., Gibbs, A. C., Stickgold, R., et al. (2002). Do lonely days invade the nights?: Potential social modulation of sleep efficiency. *Psychological Science, 13*, 385–388.

Cacioppo, J. T., Hawkley, L. C., Crawford, L. E., Ernst, J. M., Burleson, M. H., Kowalewski, R. B., et al. (2002). Loneliness and health: Potential mechanisms. *Psychosomatic Medicine, 64*, 407–417.

Cacioppo, J. T., Hawkley, L. C., Ernst, J. M., Burleson, M. H., Berntson, G. G., Nouriani, B., et al. (2006). Loneliness within a nomological net: An evolutionary perspective. *Journal of Research in Personality, 40*, 1054–1085.

Cacioppo, J. T., Hughes, M. E., Waite, L. J., Hawkley, L. C., & Thisted, R. (2006). Loneliness as a specific risk factor for depressive symptoms in older adults: Cross-sectional and longitudinal analyses. *Psychology and Aging, 21*, 140–151.

Cacioppo, J. T., Norris, C. J., Decety, J., Monteleone, G., & Nusbaum, H. (2009). In the eye of the beholder: Individual differences in perceived social isolation predict regional brain activation to social stimuli. *Journal of Cognitive Neuroscience, 21*, 83–92.

Cattan, M., White, M., Bond, J., & Learmouth, A. (2005). Preventing social isolation and loneliness among older people: A systematic review of health promotion interventions. *Ageing and Society, 25*, 41–67.

Cole, S. W., Hawkley, L. C., Arevalo, J. M., Sung, C. Y., Rose, R. M., & Cacioppo, J. T. (2007). Social regulation of gene expression in humans: Glucocorticoid resistance in the leukocyte transcriptome. *Genome Biology, 8*, R189.1–R189.13.

Cramer, K. M., & Barry, J. E. (1999). Conceptualizations and measures of loneliness: A comparison of subscales. *Personality and Individual Differences, 27*, 491–502.

De Jong Gierveld, J., & Kamphuis, F. (1985). The development of a Rasch-type loneliness scale. *Applied Psychological Measurement, 9*, 289–299.

DiTommaso, E., Brannen-McNulty, C., Ross, L., & Burgess, M. (2003). Attachment styles, social skills and loneliness in young adults. *Personality and Individual Differences, 35*, 303–312.

DiTommaso, E., & Spinner, B. (1993). The development and initial validation of the Social and Emotional Loneliness Scale for Adults (SELSA). *Personality and Individual Differences, 14*, 127–134.

Duck, S., Pond, K., & Leatham, G. (1994). Loneliness and the evaluation of relational events. *Journal of Social and Personal Relationships, 11*, 253–276.

Dunbar, R. I. M., & Shultz, S. (2007). Evolution in the social brain. *Science, 317*, 1344–1347.

Dykstra, P. A., & De Jong Gierveld, J. (1999). Loneliness differentials among older adults: The importance of type of partner, partner history, health, socioeconomic position, and social relationships. *Tijdschrift voor Gerontologie en Geriatrie, 30*, 212–225.

Dykstra, P. A., & Fokkema, T. (2007). Social and emotional loneliness among divorced and married men and women: Comparing the deficit and cognitive perspectives. *Basic and Applied Social Psychology, 29*, 1–12.

Dykstra, P. A., van Tilburg, T., & De Jong Gierveld, J. (2005). Changes in older adult loneliness: Results from a seven-year longitudinal study. *Research on Aging, 27*, 725–747.

Epley, N., Waytz, A., & Cacioppo, J. T. (2007). On seeing human: A three-factor theory of anthropomorphism. *Psychological Bulletin, 114*, 864–886.

Ernst, J. M., & Cacioppo, J. T. (1998). Lonely hearts: Psychological perspectives on loneliness. *Applied and Preventive Psychology, 8*, 1–22.

Franklin, S. S., Gustin, W. I., Wong, N. D., Larson, M. G., Weber, M. A., Kannel, W. B., et al. (1997). Hemodynamic patterns of age-related changes in blood pressure: The Framingham Heart Study. *Circulation, 96*, 308–315.

Friedman, E. M., Hayney, M. S., Love, G. D., Urry, H. L., Rosenkranz, M. A., Davidson, R. J., et al. (2005). Social relationships, sleep quality, and interleukin-6 in aging women. *Proceedings of the National Academy of Sciences of the USA, 102*, 18757–18762.

Fromm-Reichman, F. (1959). Loneliness. *Psychiatry, 22*, 1–15.

Gardner, W. L., Pickett, C. L., Jeffries, V., & Knowles, M. (2005). On the outside looking in: Loneliness and social monitoring. *Personality and Social Psychology Bulletin, 31*, 1549–1560.

Goodwin, R., Cook, O., & Yung, Y. (2001). Loneliness and life satisfaction among three cultural groups. *Personal Relationships, 8*, 225–230.

Hansson, R. O., Briggs, S. R., & Rule, B. L. (1990). Old age and unemployment: Predictors of perceived control, depression, and loneliness. *Journal of Applied Gerontology, 9*, 230–240.

Hawkley, L. C., Bosch, J. A., Engeland, C. G., Marucha, P. T., & Cacioppo, J. T. (2007). Loneliness, dysphoria, stress and immunity: A role for cytokines. In N. Plotnikoff, R. Faith, A. Murgo, & R. Good (Eds.), *Cytokines: Stress and immunity* (2nd ed., pp. 67–85). Boca Raton, FL: CRC Press.

Hawkley, L. C., Browne, M. W., & Cacioppo, J. T. (2005). How can I connect with thee?: Let me count the ways. *Psychological Science, 16*, 798–804.

Hawkley, L. C., Burleson, M. H., Berntson, G. G., & Cacioppo, J. T. (2003). Loneliness in everyday life: Cardiovascular activity, psychosocial context, and health behaviors. *Journal of Personality and Social Psychology, 85*, 105–120.

Hawkley, L. C., & Cacioppo, J. T. (2007). Aging and loneliness: Downhill quickly? *Current Directions in Psychological Science, 16*, 187–191.

Hawkley, L. C., Hughes, M. E., Waite, L. J., Masi, C. M., Thisted, R. A., & Cacioppo, J. T. (2008). From social structure factors to perceptions of relationship quality and loneliness: The Chicago Health, Aging, and Social Relations Study. *Journal of Gerontoloy: Social Sciences, 63B*, S375–S384.

Hawkley, L. C., Masi, C. M., Berry, J. D., & Cacioppo, J. T. (2006). Loneliness is a unique predictor of age-related differences in systolic blood pressure. *Psychology and Aging, 21*, 152–164.

Hawkley, L. C., Preacher, K. J., & Cacioppo, J. T. (2007). Multilevel modeling of social interactions and mood in lonely and socially connected individuals: The MacArthur Social Neuroscience Studies. In A. D. Ong & M. H. M. van Dulmen (Eds.), *Oxford handbook of methods in positive psychology* (pp. 559–575). New York: Oxford University Press.

Hawkley, L. C., Preacher, K., J., Waite, L. J., & Cacioppo, J. T. (2007). *Perceived loneliness and the salubrity of sleep.* Manuscript submitted for publication.

Hawkley, L. C., Thisted, R. A., & Cacioppo, J. T. (in press). Loneliness predicts reduced physical activity: Cross-sectional and longitudinal analyses. *Health Psychology.*

Heikkinen, R., & Kauppinen, M. (2004). Depressive symptoms in late life: A 10-year follow-up. *Archives of Gerontology and Geriatrics, 38*, 239–250.

Hughes, M. E., Waite, L. J., Hawkley, L. C., & Cacioppo, J. T. (2004). A short scale for measuring loneliness in large surveys: Results from two population-based studies. *Research on Aging, 26*, 655–672.

Johnson, D. P., & Mullins, L. C. (1989). Religiosity and loneliness among the elderly. *Journal of Applied Gerontology, 8*, 110–131.

Kiecolt-Glaser, J. K., Ricker, D., George, J., Messick, G., Speicher, C. E., Garner, W., et al. (1984). Urinary cortisol levels, cellular immunocompetency and loneliness in psychiatric inpatients. *Psychosomatic Medicine, 46*, 15–23.

Lau, S., & Gruen, G. E. (1992). The social stigma of loneliness: Effect of target person's and perceiver's sex. *Personality and Social Psychology Bulletin, 18*, 182–189.

Lauder, W., Mummery, K., Jones, M., & Caperchione, C. (2006). A comparison of health behaviours in lonely and non-lonely populations. *Psychology, Health, and Medicine, 11*, 233–245.

Lauder, W., Mummery, K., & Sharkey, S. (2006). Social capital, age and religiosity in people who are lonely. *Journal of Clinical Nursing, 15*, 334–339.

Marangoni, C., & Ickes, W. (1989). Loneliness: A theoretical review with implications for measurement. *Journal of Social and Personal Relationships, 6*, 93–128.

McGuire, S., & Clifford, J. (2000). Genetic and environmental contributions to loneliness in children. *Psychological Science, 11*, 487–491.

Moustakas, C. E. (1961). *Loneliness.* Englewood Cliffs, NJ: Prentice-Hall.

Nolen-Hoeksema, S., & Ahrens, C. (2002). Age differences and similarities in the correlates of depressive symptoms. *Psychology and Aging, 17*, 116–124.

Ohayon, M. M. (2005). Prevalence and correlates of nonrestorative sleep complaints. *Archives of Internal Medicine, 165*, 35–41.

Olson, K. L., & Wong, E. H. (2001). Loneliness in marriage. *Family Therapy, 28*, 105–112.

Peplau, L. A., & Perlman, D. (1982). Perspectives on loneliness. In L. A. Peplau & D. Perlman (Eds.), *Loneliness: A sourcebook of current theory, research and therapy* (pp. 1–20). New York: Wiley.

Pickett, C. L., & Gardner, W. L. (2005). The social monitoring system: Enhanced sensitivity to social cues as an adaptive response to social exclusion. In K. D. Williams, J. P. Forgas, & W. von Hippel (Eds.), *The social outcast: Ostracism, social exclusion, rejection, and bullying* (pp. 213–226). New York: Psychology Press.

Pickett, C. L., Gardner, W. L., & Knowles, M. (2004). Getting a cue: The need to belong and enhanced sensitivity to social cues. *Personality and Social Psychology Bulletin, 30*, 1095–1107.

Pinquart, M. (2003). Loneliness in married, widowed, divorced, and never-married older adults. *Journal of Social and Personal Relationships, 20*, 31–53.

Pinquart, M., & Sörensen, S. (2003). Risk factor for loneliness in adulthood and old age: A meta-analysis. In S. P. Shohov (Ed.), *Advances in psychology research* (Vol. 19, pp. 111–143). Hauppauge, NY: Nova Science.

Pitterman, H., & Nowicki, S. (2004). A test of the ability to identify emotion in human standing and sitting postures: The Diagnostic Analysis of Nonverbal Accuracy—2 Posture Test (DANVA2-POS). *Genetic, Social, and General Psychology Monographs, 130*, 146–162.

Pressman, S. D., Cohen, S., Miller, G. E., Barkin, A., Rabin, B. S., & Treanor, J. J. (2005). Loneliness, social network size, and immune response to influenza vaccination in college freshmen. *Health Psychology, 24*, 297–306.

Rogers, C. R. (1961). Ellen West—and loneliness. *Review of Existential Psychology and Psychiatry, 1,* 94–101.

Rook, K. S. (1984). Promoting social bonding: Strategies for helping the lonely and socially isolated. *American Psychologist, 39,* 1389–1407.

Rook, K. S. (1987). Social support versus companionship: Effects on life stress, loneliness, and evaluations by others. *Journal of Personality and Social Psychology, 52,* 1132–1147.

Rotenberg, K. (1994). Loneliness and interpersonal trust. *Journal of Social and Clinical Psychology, 13,* 152–173.

Rotenberg, K. J., Gruman, J. A., & Ariganello, M. (2002). Behavioral confirmation of the loneliness stereotype. *Basic and Applied Social Psychology, 24,* 81–89.

Rotenberg, K. J., & Kmill, J. (1992). Perception of lonely and non-lonely persons as a function of individual differences in loneliness. *Journal of Social and Personal Relationships, 9,* 325–330.

Russell, D. W. (1996). UCLA Loneliness Scale (Version 3): Reliability, validity, and factor structure. *Journal of Personality Assessment, 66,* 20–40.

Russell, D. W., Cutrona, C. E., de la Mora, A., & Wallace, R. B. (1997). Loneliness and nursing home admission among rural older adults. *Psychology and Aging, 12,* 574–589.

Savikko, N., Routasalo, P., Tilvis, R. S., Strandberg, T. E., & Pitkälä, K. H. (2005). Predictors and subjective causes of loneliness in an aged population. *Archives of Gerontology and Geriatrics, 41,* 223–233.

Schnittker, J. (2007). Look (closely) at all the lonely people: Age and social psychology of social support. *Journal of Aging and Health, 19,* 659–682.

Shaver, P., & Brennan, K. A. (1991). Measures of depression and loneliness. In J. P. Robinson, P. R. Shaver, & L. S. Wrightsman (Eds.), *Measures of personality and social psychological attitudes* (pp. 195–289). San Diego, CA: Academic Press.

Shaver, P., Furman, W., & Buhrmester, D. (1985). Transition to college: Network changes, social skills, and loneliness. In S. Duck & D. Perlman (Eds.), *Understanding personal relationships: An interdisciplinary approach* (pp. 193–219). Thousand Oaks, CA: Sage.

Solano, C. H. (1987). Loneliness and perceptions of control: General traits versus specific attributions. *Journal of Social Behavior and Personality, 2*(2), 201–214.

Spiegel, K., Leproult, R., & Van Cauter, E. (1999). Impact of sleep debt on metabolic and endocrine function. *Lancet, 354,* 1435–1439.

Steptoe, A., Owen, N., Kunz-Ebrecht, S. R., & Brydon, L. (2004). Loneliness and neuroendocrine, cardiovascular, and inflammatory stress responses in middle-aged men and women. *Psychoneuroendocrinology, 29,* 593–611.

Tilvis, R. J., Kähönen-Väre, M. H., Jolkkonen, J., Valvanne, J., Pitkala, K. H., & Strandberg, T. E. (2004). Predictors of cognitive decline and mortality of aged people over a 10-year period. *Journals of Gerontology Series A: Biological Sciences and Medical Sciences, 59,* M268–M274.

Tucker, M. B., & Mitchell-Kernan, C. (1998). Psychological well-being and perceived marital opportunity among single African American, Latina and white women. *Journal of Comparative Family Studies, 29,* 57–72.

Viney, L. L. (1985). "They call you a dole bludger": Some experiences of unemployment. *Journal of Community Psychology, 13,* 31–45.

Wallhagen, M. I., Strawbridge, W. J., Shema, S. J., Kurata, J., & Kaplan, G. A. (2001). Comparative impact of hearing and vision impairment on subsequent functioning. *Journal of the American Geriatrics Society, 49,* 1086–1092.

Weiss, R. S. (1973). *Loneliness: The experience of emotional and social isolation.* Cambridge, MA: MIT Press.

Wilson, R. S., Krueger, K. R., Arnold, S. E., Schneider, J. A., Kelly, J. F., Barnes, L. L., et al. (2007). Loneliness and risk of Alzheimer's disease. *Archives of General Psychiatry, 64,* 234–240.

Wittenberg, M. T., & Reis, H. T. (1986). Loneliness, social skills, and social perception. *Personality and Social Psychology Bulletin, 12*(1), 121–130.

CHAPTER 16

■ ● ▲ ◆ ■ ● ▲ ◆

Affect Intensity

RANDY J. LARSEN

History of Affect Intensity

Affect intensity refers to individual differences in the typical intensity with which people experience their emotional responses (Larsen & Diener, 1987). The construct also includes affective variability, such that not only are persons high on affect intensity more emotionally reactive but also, over time, their emotional states vary more widely as they react to ongoing life events. The construct generalizes over emotions, such that, for example, people who experience their positive emotions more strongly will, over time, generally experience their negative emotions more strongly as well. The characteristic highlights that folk notion that "the higher you go up when you are up, the lower you go down when you are down."

Research on affect intensity began in the mid-1980s, when Larsen and colleagues (e.g., Larsen & Diener, 1985) began conducting daily studies of mood and emotion using the experience-sampling method (ESM). When examining global daily mood plotted for individuals over several months, they noticed that participants who exhibited wide swings upward in positive mood on good days also showed wide swings downward in negative mood on bad days. In fact, when they calculated the mean positive mood on positive days and mean negative mood on negative

days, these two measures of daily mood intensity correlated .60 to .77 across persons in their samples. Moreover, a mean daily emotional intensity score could be calculated (by averaging positive and negative intensity scores) that in turn exhibited high test–retest reliability and that correlated in interesting ways with peer reports of emotionality, with parental ratings, and with various other criterion variables. It appeared to be a meaningful individual-difference characteristic and one not clearly identified as such in existing taxonomies of personality.

Only a few prior studies had examined individual differences in constructs related to intensity of emotional response. One important study was that published by Weissman and Ricks (1966), which examined the daily moods of Harvard and Radcliff students using ESM. They identified two aspects of individual differences in daily affect; mean mood level over time and mean variability over time. A person's amount of mood variability, indexed by a within-subject standard deviation on mood measures over time, would be a natural consequence of having an intense emotional response system. A second important paper was written by Underwood and Froming (1980), who were interested in trait-like characteristics of mood and who developed a questionnaire measure of mood level and mood reactivity. However, the mood reactivity scale was never validated against daily mood measures or laboratory or field measures of emotional reactivity and so remains rarely used or cited.

Larsen and Diener's (1987) early work assessed emotional intensity using ESM, calculating affect intensity scores based on the average distance each participant's daily moods deviated from the expected values. Several important observations were made based on these data, including the fact that the frequency with which people experienced their positive and negative emotions was independent of their intensity (Diener, Larsen, Levine, & Emmons, 1985). Affect intensity also correlated with a cluster of other variables, including ratings of the importance of life events and life goals (Emmons & King, 1989; Larsen, Diener, & Emmons, 1986). However, using ESM to assess affect intensity has drawbacks. Primary among these is the inordinate amount of time and effort it takes to obtain repeated measures of mood on enough occasions to calculate a reliable estimate of mean affect intensity for each participant.

Measurement of Affect Intensity

Because of the need for an efficient and economical measure of trait affect intensity, Larsen (1984) constructed and validated a questionnaire measure called the Affect Intensity Measure (AIM). The scale construction strategy, including item generation, selection, and refinement into a final 40-item measure, is described in Larsen and Diener (1987). That report also includes preliminary reliability and validity information as well, some of which I review later.

Since the AIM was originally published (Larsen, 1984), at least four other measures of affect intensity have been developed. The Emotional Intensity Scale (EIS; Bachorowski & Braaten, 1994) has 30 items that each ask the participant to imagine him- or herself in a specific emotionally evocative situation, then to indicate which of several responses (which vary on intensity) they are most likely to have in that scenario. This scale correlates .45 with the AIM (Bachorowski & Braaten, 1994) and exhibits a pattern of correlations with third variables that is very similar to the AIM. Incremental validity of the EIS over the AIM has not been documented, and validity evidence for the EIS is sparser than it is for the AIM. Another scale, the Affect Intensity Questionnaire (EIQ—Elliot, Sherwin, Harkins, & Marmarosh, 1995; Harkins, Gramling, & Elliot, 1990) is a visual analog scale with 18 items that asks the participants to rate the relative intensities of distinct affects that they experience. This scale seems most useful for assessing state, rather than trait, affect. Two other drawbacks of the EIQ are that the psychometrics of this measure are influenced by the ipsatizing effects of the instructions to rate emotions *relative to each other*. In addition, this scale remains unpublished.

A third measure is the Intensity and Time Affect Survey (ITAS—Diener, Fujita, & Seidlitz, 1991; Lucas, Diener, & Larsen, 2003; Schimmack & Diener, 1997), which was developed in tandem with another affect intensity measure called the Scenario Rating Task (SRT; Schimmack & Diener, 1997). The ITAS is an adjective-rating task, employing 24 emotion terms, in which the participant is asked: "How intensely do you typically experience X, if you experience X?" (where X is one of the 24 emotions). In examining the predictive validity correlates of several affect intensity measures, the ITAS showed lower validity coefficients than either the AIM or the SRT (Schimmack & Diener, 1997). The SRT presents participants with 20 standardized scenarios and asks them to imagine being in each of these situations, much like the EIS. However, for each of the SRT scenarios, the participant rates 10 emotions on how much of each he or she thinks will be evoked by the imaginary scenarios. The SRT is thus a long and repetitive instrument (requiring 200 ratings) and is based on respondents' hypothetical responses to imagined situations. It does, however, exhibit validity correlations that are comparable to the much shorter and more economical AIM (Schimmack & Diener, 1997). Whereas the SRT has not been published, the ITAS is reproduced in Lucas and colleagues (2003).

Because the predominant measure of affect intensity remains the AIM, this chapter focuses primarily on this measure. The AIM has been translated into several languages (e.g., German, Spanish, Portuguese, Italian, Swedish, Croatian), has been shortened, has had its reading level lowered, and has been widely used in research. The two papers in which the AIM has been published (Larsen & Diener, 1987; Larsen, Diener, & Emmons, 1986) have been widely cited. The original item set for the AIM was written based on a construct definition derived from prior empirical work (e.g., Larsen & Diener, 1985). The construct definition emphasizes a distinction between frequency and intensity of emotional experience such that intensity applies to all emotions regardless of their specific hedonic tone and that individual differences in affect intensity would be evident in a variety of channels, including felt affect, bodily responses, and certain aspects of cognitive performance.

Larsen and Diener (1987) provide details on construction and validation of the AIM. The 40-item total score exhibits an acceptable level of internal consistency, with a coefficient alpha ranging from .90 to .94 across four samples (Larsen & Diener, 1987), with split-half correlations ranging from .73 to .82, and with the mean corrected item-total correlations ranging from .41 to .51. In terms of temporal stability, the AIM obtains 1-, 2-, and 3-month test–retest correlations of .80, .81, and .81, respectively. The AIM is not related to extreme response style or to social desirability response set.

The original report (Larsen, 1984) describes five interpretable yet highly intercorrelated factors, which break out as two positive intensity factors, two negative intensity factors, and a method factor. Several researchers have published factor analyses of the AIM item set, with several reporting four factors (Goldsmith & Walters, 1989; Weinfurt, Bryant, & Yarnold, 1994) and several others reporting three factors (Bryant, Yarnold, & Grimm, 1996; Geuens & de Pelsmacker, 2002; Simonsson-Sarnecki, Lundh, & Törestad, 2000). The most useful conclusion to come out of this factor-analytic work is that, in some situations, it may be appropriate to consider subscales within the 40-item AIM. In testing various theories, it may be useful to make a distinction between positive affect intensity and negative affect intensity, which, although highly correlated with each other, can differentially correlate with third variables.

Research on Affect Intensity

Construct Validity

Because the AIM was developed as a convenient replacement measure for the ESM approach to assessing affect intensity, an important validity consideration is the correlation between these two very different forms of measuring affect intensity. Larsen and Diener (1987) report that average daily affect intensity, calculated with ESM data, correlated with the AIM at .61 ($n = 62$, $p < .01$) in one sample, .53 ($n = 74$, $p < .01$) in another, and .49 ($n = 54$, $p < .01$) in a third sample. In addition, Larsen and Diener (1985) found that self-reports of affect intensity assessed with the AIM correlated .50 with parental reports of their children's affect intensity and .41 with peer reports of affect intensity.

Because the construct of affect intensity also refers to emotional reactivity to life events, it should correlate with measures of emotional variability. Larsen (1987) used spectral analysis to quantify the frequency of daily mood changes and found that the affect intensity correlated with a significantly faster frequency of daily mood change. In addition, affect intensity correlated with a measure of being at risk for cyclothymia and bipolar affective disorder (Diener, Sandvik, & Larsen, 1985).

In another important validity study, Larsen, Diener, and Emmons (1986) had 62 participants in an ESM study write down the most significant good event and bad event each day for 8 consecutive weeks, resulting in 3,064 good-event descriptions and 2,907 bad-event descriptions. Participants also rated their moods each day of the study. The event descriptions were rated by a team of raters for "how good or bad would this event be for the average person," essentially norming the events for objective emotional impact. Larsen and colleagues found that, at each level of objective event severity, participants high on affect intensity reported more extreme emotions than participants low on affect intensity. This finding was also replicated using a scenario task in Study 2 in Larsen and colleagues. Moreover, there was no correlation between the AIM and the average objective severity of life events. Thus, although the life events of participants with high and low affect intensity appear to be about the same, the participants with high affect intensity report stronger emotional reactions to those events than participants with low affect intensity.

To examine how individuals with high affect intensity come to react so differently to the same kinds of events compared with individuals with low affect intensity, Larsen, Diener, and Cropanzano (1987) conducted a thought-sampling study while exposing participants to emotionally evocative images. They proposed that affect intensity would be associated with a distinct pattern of cognitive operations that would be present while viewing the emotional images. The theoretical notion was that these cognitive operations would lead individuals to interpret or construe emotion-provoking stimuli in a manner that intensifies the affective response to those stimuli. Larsen and colleagues found that individuals with high affect intensity engaged in significantly more personalizing cognition and more generalizing cognition than those with low affect intensity. *Personalizing cognition* refers to the tendency to relate to an event by seeing it as self-relevant or focusing on the personal meanings for oneself. So a person might see an image of a child wounded in a war and start thinking about a time when he or she was hurt as a child. *Generalizing cognition* refers to abstracting from a single event to arrive at broad conclusions that are not warranted. For example, seeing an image of a child wounded in war, a person might start thinking about how war is horrible and that human nature at its core is dark and destructive. People high in affect intensity, relative to those low in it, tended to both personalize and generalize more often, and they did this to both positive and negative emotional images (relative to neutral). These findings were replicated in a study by Dritschel and Teasdale (1991) using a sample of middle-aged British women. Larsen, Billings, and Cutler (1996) conceptually replicated these effects by having participants generate informative descriptions of life events, finding that the descriptions of participants with high affect intensity contained significantly more generalizing and more references to arousal and personal feeling states than the descriptions of participants with low affect intensity.

The cognitive style of personalizing and generalizing most likely intensifies affective responses by increasing the perceived importance of events. Schimmack and Diener (1997) demonstrate that affect intensity is correlated with the importance ratings of life events, and they argue that the attribution of importance to events is a likely cause of affect intensity. Diener, Colvin, Pavot, and Allman (1991) also demonstrate, across five studies, that the importance one attaches to an event strongly influences the intensity of emotional reactions to that event.

Correlates and Consequences of Affect Intensity

Physiology

Emotional experience depends in part on perceived physiological changes. Several researchers have therefore examined affect intensity in relation to perceptions of physiological activity. One interesting study reported by Chwalisz, Diener, and Gallagher (1988) examined affective reactions in persons with spinal cord injuries, who have limited perception of their bodily states. Participants with greater autonomic feedback (i.e., lower spinal cord injury) reported more intense emotions than participants with weaker autonomic feedback. However, participants with very high lesions, who had almost no autonomic feedback, still reported the experience of emotions, but at a lower intensity level. Such findings suggest that the perception of autonomic arousal may not be necessary for emotional experience. However, increased perception of autonomic arousal may enhance the felt intensity of emotional experience.

Blascovich and colleagues (1992) provide another perspective on the perception of physiological arousal in relation to trait affect intensity. The authors report three separate studies of individual differences in visceral self-perception assessed using a standard heartbeat detection paradigm. Although the AIM was unrelated to actual cardiac arousal, it was negatively related to perceived cardiac arousal in all three studies. These findings suggest that individuals with high affect intensity have relatively diminished visceral awareness of their own cardiac activity. These results are discussed in terms of how individuals with high affect intensity may not become aware of their emotional reactions until those reactions become quite strong. As such, these individuals would require stronger emotional stimulation before they engaged in self-regulation to dampen their emotional reactions. Larsen (2000; Larsen et al., 1996) presents a control-theory model of emotion regulation, with individual differences in the self-perception of physiological arousal playing an important role.

Vanman, Dawson, and Brennan (1998) report similar findings of diminished physiological reactivity on the part of participants with high affect intensity. This study examined the eyeblink startle reflex to affect-laden images. Loud auditory tones were presented quasi-randomly while participants viewed a series of affective images. The standard finding is that, when viewing negative slides, the eyeblink reaction to the auditory startle probe tends to be stronger than it is to positive or neutral images. However, this eyeblink startle effect was significantly diminished for participants high in affect intensity, suggesting that individuals high in affect intensity are less easily aroused by the startle probe.

Larsen, Diener, and Emmons (1986) also report negative correlations between affect intensity and measures of peripheral physiology. Both resting galvanic skin response (the number of spontaneous spikes in a 1-minute interval) and resting heart rate were found to correlate negatively with the AIM ($r = -.31$ and $-.26$, respectively). These negative associations suggest that individuals high in affect intensity, when placed in a quiet, stimulus-reduced environment, are physiologically less aroused relative to the participants low in affect intensity. These findings, and those in the preceding paragraph, are consistent with basic notions of arousal regulation theory, which I now briefly describe.

An Arousal Regulation Theory of Affect Intensity

This theory has a few basic postulates. The first is that, for any given task, there exists an optimal level of arousal for completing the task; the second is that individuals will seek a common optimal level of arousal in a given situation (Hebb, 1955). A third postulate is that individuals differ with respect to baseline arousal and/or their reactivity to stimulation. Consequently, the fourth postulate is that some individuals will need more stimulation than others to reach their optimal levels and some will need less stimulation. The theory predicts individual differences in stimulation-seeking behavior, mainly to compensate for underreactivity and/or lower levels of baseline arousal. This homeostatic theory of arousal regulation has existed in personality theory in various forms for some time (e.g., Eysenck, 1967; Gale, 1986; Geen, 1983; Zuckermann, 1979).

Most of the research on arousal regulation has focused on two sources of stimulation that are sought out to compensate for underreactivity. One source is behavior: either socializing, heightened activity level, or sensation seeking. In fact, both Eysenck's theory of extraversion and Zuckerman's early theory of sensation seeking were based on the notion of individual differences in baseline arousal and the management of arousal level through the regulation of behavioral activities (Eysenck, 1967; Zuckermann, 1979). Extraverted behavior is seen as an attempt to maximize stimulation input through social activity in order to compensate for a relatively underaroused condition at baseline. Introverts, on the other hand, avoid social stimulation (as well as intense stimulation in general) in order to avoid increasing their already relatively overaroused condition at baseline.

A second mechanism of arousal regulation is through sensory stimulation. Some individuals exhibit dampened reactivity to sensory stimulation. Theories of this individual difference have variously been called stimulus intensity modulation theory (Barnes, 1976; Petrie, 1967), reducer–augmenter theory (Herzog, Williams, & Weintraub, 1985; Sales, 1971, 1972), and strength of the nervous system theory (Pavlov, 1957; Strelau, 1982, 1985). All refer to the tendency of some people to react less strongly to sensory stimuli, as, for example, in individual differences in pain tolerance. Low-reactive persons should be motivated to seek out stronger forms of stimulation, whereas high-reactive persons, those who are more sensitive, should seek to avoid strong sensory stimulation. Research testing these predictions generally find support in that low-sensory-reactive persons do exhibit a greater need for stimulation (Herzog et al., 1985; Mishara & Baker, 1981), are bored easily and are motivated to seek out stronger forms of stimulation (Larsen & Baggs, 1986), and have higher levels of activity and socializing (Petrie, 1967; Sales, 1971) and a tendency to abuse illicit stimulant and consciousness-altering drugs (Kohn, Barnes, & Hoffman, 1979).

Larsen (1984; Larsen & Diener, 1987) suggested that emotion might be a third source of stimulation that could play a role in arousal regulation. If this is true, then individuals with high affect intensity should display diminished physiological reactivity, a hypothesis consistent with the findings described in the previous section. Moreover, if the regular experience of intense emotions is a compensatory strategy for overcoming low levels of baseline arousal or diminished reactivity, then affect intensity should correlate with other individual differences related to arousal regulation, such as extraversion, sensation seeking, and sensory reducing. Such correlations have been reported in the literature (e.g., Dritschel & Teasdale, 1991; Larsen & Diener, 1987; Larsen, Diener, & Emmons, 1986; Maio & Esses, 2001; Ruch, Angleitner, & Strelau, 1991). Also, both questionnaire and psychophysical measures of sensory reducing have been found to correlate negatively with the AIM (Larsen & Zarate, 1991). The study by Larsen and Zarate (1991) also demonstrated that people use emotions to compensate for diminished arousal. In this study we induced boredom in participants for 35 minutes, then offered them the choice of participating in an emotion manipulation study or a questionnaire study. Participants who chose to undergo the emotion manipulation experience scored significantly more in the reducing direction on a measure of sensory reducing–augmenting.

In a study of desired affect, Rusting and Larsen (1995) showed that most people desire more pleasant and positive emotions, though affect intensity correlated significantly with the desire for stronger felt arousal. The arousal regulation theory of affect intensity generates a variety of interesting predictions concerning the behavioral and experiential implications of emotion-provoking situations for individuals high versus low in affect intensity. For example, in one study we examined the effects of high sensory stimu-

lation (85 dB intermittent white noise and bright flashing lights) on the proofreading performance of participants who scored high or low on the affect intensity dimension (Larsen, Zarate, & Dare, 1986). We found that strong sensory stimulation actually improved the performance of participants high on the affect intensity dimension, whereas participants low in affect intensity showed a decline in performance when going from normal to high stimulation conditions. In another study participants were asked how they would perform in a situation while they were emotionally aroused (e.g., being angry when having to do homework, feeling nervous while taking a test, feeling jealous while having to work on a term paper). We found that participants low in affect intensity reported that the emotion would interfere with or disrupt their performance, whereas persons high in affect intensity thought that having the emotional stimulation would actually facilitate their performance. Further research on how emotions can facilitate or impair performance, as well as individual differences in these kinds of effects, is an important topic for future research. One interesting observation I have made over the years is that persons high on affect intensity, while acknowledging that their emotions sometimes get them into trouble, nevertheless like their intense emotional lifestyle and generally do not want to change.

Emotion Regulation

Whereas arousal regulation refers to felt levels of energy and activation, emotion regulation refers to self-control attempts to modulate hedonic tone or specific emotional reactions. By up-regulating felt arousal through strong emotions, persons with high affect intensity may appear low on emotion regulation. Moreover, due to its relation to emotional reactivity and variability, affect intensity likely is related to low levels of emotional control. Several researchers (e.g., Hunt, 1993; Goldsmith & Walters, 1989) have found that persons high in affect intensity express their emotions more and are more socially expressive and sensitive (Flett, Blankstein, Bator, & Pliner, 1989). When people high in affect intensity engage in suppression as a coping style, they are especially likely to experience distress or depression (Lynch, Robins, Morse, & MorKrause, 2001). Cheavens and colleagues (2005) have argued that attempts to suppress emotions can actually backfire, resulting in stronger emotions that are even more difficult to regulate.

Other researchers have examined beliefs and expectancies about the self-regulation of emotion. For negative emotions, affect intensity is associated with the expectation of diminished ability to regulate negative moods (Flett, Blankstein, & Obertynski, 1996). Affect intensity correlates negatively with perceived emotional self-control, though it is unrelated to perceived self-control in other areas of life or to generalized self-control expectancies (Flett et al., 1989). Research suggests that such beliefs in diminished self-control of emotions are veridical. Eisenberg and Okun (1996) showed that, in stressful circumstances, individuals with high negative affect intensity engage in fewer emotion regulation behaviors and experience more personal distress. An exploratory yet interesting report on rapid eye movement (REM) sleep and affect intensity (Nofzinger et al., 1994) reported a positive correlation between affect intensity and the amount and density of REM sleep patterns. They argue that the intense experience of emotions in the daytime is carried over into sleep, resulting in elevated phasic REM sleep, which they see as an indicator of autonomic instability.

Several researchers have shown that affect intensity is unrelated to overall happiness or life satisfaction (e.g., Chamberlain, 1988; Diener, Colvin, et al., 1991; Larsen & Diener, 1987). Although counterintuitive given the preceding discussion, there may be several reasons for this finding. First, the experience of intense emotions may be a compensatory mechanism in providing desired levels of heightened arousal. Although high affect intensity comes with the cost of wear and tear on the autonomic nervous system and distress when things do not go well, it may satisfy a more basic need to up-regulate felt arousal. A second reason affect intensity may be unrelated to happiness is that, because happiness is the ratio of long-term positive to negative affect (Larsen & Prizmic, 2008) and because persons with high affect intensity do have strong positive emotional reactions when good events happen (along with strong negative reactions when bad events

happen), the net effect on long-term happiness is nil.

Psychopathology

The connection between affect intensity and various forms of psychopathology has been an active area of research. One disorder receiving much attention is borderline personality disorder (BPD), which is characterized, in part, by extreme emotional instability. Bland, Williams, Scharer, and Manning (2004) showed that women with BPD scored higher on affect intensity, though the effect was particularly strong for the Negative Intensity subscale (consistent with the idea that BPD is related to deficient anger management). A relationship between BPD and affect intensity has also been found by other researchers (e.g., Yen, Zlotnick, & Costello, 2002). Henry and colleagues (2001) provides a strong test of this relationship by examining affect intensity in BPD compared with other disorders of affect, including bipolar disorder. They report that affect intensity is elevated in BPD relative to other disorders. In terms of etiological factors, Rosenthal, Cheavens, Lejuez, and Lynch (2005) showed that elevated affect intensity also was related to a (self-reported) history of childhood abuse among persons with BPD.

BPD is also related to self-harm, and at least one study (Gratz, 2006) has shown that, in a nonclinical sample of adult women, the AIM subscales discriminated women with a history of self-harming behavior from women with no history of self-harm. In particular, high negative affect intensity and low positive affect intensity distinguished women high in self-harm (illustrating the utility of considering subscales, in addition to the total score, when using the AIM). Others studies have found elevated affect intensity among persons with a history of suicidal behavior (Iancu et al., 1999). Lynch, Cheavens, Morse, and Rosenthal (2004) found that, although affect intensity was elevated in persons with a suicidal history, this relationship was moderated by emotional suppression, such that persons with high affect intensity were more likely to be at risk for suicide when they also chronically inhibit their emotional reactions.

Flett and Hewitt (1995) took a broadband approach to personality disorders by administering the Millon Clinical Multi-axial Inventory (Millon, 1983), along with the AIM, in a sample of adult psychiatric patients. Affect intensity was found to correlate positively with indices of BPD, as well as with passive–aggressive personality, and negatively with compulsive–conforming personality. Affect intensity also correlated with symptom measures of poor adjustment, somatization, hypomania, alcohol abuse, and psychotic thinking. The authors conclude that affect intensity may contribute to a variety of forms of psychopathology, primarily through diminished self-control of emotion and poor inhibition (Flett & Hewitt, 1995).

A variety of other forms of psychopathology have also been related to affect intensity. For example, Day and Wong (1996) found that persons high in psychopathy (or antisocial character traits) have lower affect intensity and exhibit less intense emotional reactions to everyday life events than persons low in psychopathy. Also, not surprisingly, affect intensity is associated with being at risk for anxiety and panic disorder. At least one study has shown that persons high in affect intensity are at risk for substance abuse, most likely in attempts to self-medicate for emotional suppression (Thorberg & Lyvers, 2006). And finally, as might be imagined, extremely low affect intensity is associated with alexithymia, a characteristic deficiency in understanding, processing, or describing emotions (Iancu et al., 1999; Jacob & Hautekeete, 1999; Ritz, 1994). Alexithymia is characterized by difficulty in identifying and describing feelings, constricted imagination and paucity of fantasy, and an externally oriented cognitive style (Taylor, Bagby, & Parker, 1997). Although not classified as a mental disorder, alexithymia is a trait that places people at risk for developing disorders, as well as making people less responsive to various psychological treatments.

Cognition and Emotion

Because cognitive and emotional processes are linked, it is likely that individual differences in one are related to, or perhaps even driven by, individual differences in the other. As mentioned earlier, Larsen and colleagues (Larsen et al., 1987, 1996) reported that affect intensity is associated with a cognitive style of personalizing events and overgeneralizing from events. They also found that this cognitive style was stable over time and consistent across situations and that it operated similarly for men and women.

A study by Sheldon (1994) found that affect intensity discriminated between art and science graduate students, with art students scoring significantly higher on affect intensity than science students. Affect intensity was assessed at the start of their training, so it is likely that affect intensity differences existed prior to exposure to training in these respective fields. Sheldon suggests that the cognitive style associated with affect intensity lends itself to an interest in art more than in science. Moreover, he suggests that artists and scientists face different social norms regarding the expression of emotion, with artists being encouraged to exaggerate, dwell on, and express their emotional reactions and scientists encouraged to downplay theirs. His findings suggest that individual differences in such temperamental factors as affect intensity, and their associated cognitive styles, may underlie vocational choices.

Another cognitive style concerns event appraisal. If an event is appraised as very important, then affective reactions to the outcome of that event will be more intense than if the event were viewed as less important. Indeed, if you want to know what is important to a person, you might proceed by inquiring about the kinds of events that provoke the strongest emotions. Along these lines, Emmons and King (1989) reported that the importance ratings attached to life goals and strivings were associated with individual differences in affect intensity. Moreover, individuals high in affect intensity had more differentiated goals, that is, more strivings that were unrelated to each other. Individuals with high affect intensity want all sorts of things out of life, even though their goals may be in conflict (e.g., to have a high-powered career, a loving and committed marriage, lots of interesting hobbies, and a large family). Moreover, individuals with high affect intensity had fewer discrete plans for how they might achieve their goals. In other words, their goal structure was relatively shallow, with many discrete goals but fewer concrete plans for ways they might realize those goals. Similarly, a study by Dance, Kuiper, and Martin (1990) demonstrated that affect intensity is associated with a higher number of distinct self-relevant roles, as assessed in a role-sorting task. It may be that affect intensity is related to high self-concept complexity (Linville, 1985).

Personality and Demographic Correlates

Far and away the personality variables most frequently found to correlate with affect intensity are extraversion and neuroticism (e.g., Dritschel & Teasdale, 1991; Kardum, 1999; Larsen & Diener, 1987; McFatter, 1998). Both of these personality variables correlate positively and moderately with affect intensity. The reason most likely is that extraversion (E) is related to a disposition to respond with stronger positive emotional reactivity and neuroticism (N) with a disposition to respond with negative emotional reactivity (as found in experimental studies of laboratory mood induction procedures; see Larsen & Ketelaar, 1989, 1991; Rusting & Larsen, 1997, 1998, 1999; Zelenski & Larsen, 1999, 2002). If personality space is defined by the orthogonal dimensions of E and N, then affect intensity is a vector that is located halfway between them. The incremental validity of affect intensity over E and N concerns the focus on affective reactions for these two constructs. Whereas the construct definition of N has always contained reference to affect, particularly anxiety and fear, the construct definition of E has not, until very recently, made much reference at all to the affective associates of this trait. Moreover, because E and N are unrelated, the distribution of persons in the two-dimensional space defined by these constructs is normally distributed around any vector passing through the origin of the space. This means that the affect intensity dimension represents, at the high end, persons who are high on *both* positive and negative emotional reactivity—or, in other words, persons who have *both* high approach motivation *and* high avoidance motivation (Larsen & Augustine, 2008) or are highly sensitive to *both* cues of reward *and* cues of punishment (Zelenski & Larsen, 1999).

Other personality variables have also been studied in relation to affect intensity, including self-esteem variability (Oosterwegel, Field, Hart, & Anderson, 2001), public and private self-consciousness and the social-stimulation facet of affiliation motivation (Blankstein, Flett, Koledin, & Bortolotto, 1989), and trait arousability (Mehrabian, 1995). One study examined emotional intelligence in relation to affect intensity (Engelberg & Sjöberg, 2004), wherein the Mayer–Salovey–Caruso Emotional Intelligence Test (MSCEIT; Mayer, Salovey, & Caruso, 2001), which has been highly criticized in the literature (e.g., Larsen & Lerner, 2006), showed no correlations with affect intensity or with the criterion behavior of accuracy in the assessment of mood experienced by others.

In terms of demographics, a consistent finding is that women score higher than men, at least among young adult samples (Fujita, Diener, & Sandvik, 1991; Goldsmith & Walters, 1989; Seidlitz & Diener, 1998; Williams & Barry, 2003). The gender difference tends to get smaller with age, such that, by late middle age, men and women are no longer significantly different (Diener, Sandvik, & Larsen, 1985). Although men and women both decline on affect intensity with age, women decline faster. Looking at gender roles, Jakupcak, Salters, Gratz, and Roemer (2003) found that stereotypically masculine men report even lower levels of affect intensity than men with more modern gender-role attributes. The stereotype of women as the more emotional gender appears to have a kernel of truth, at least when it comes to self-report measures of affect intensity among young adult women. The constructive aspect of this gender difference is that women also report more intense positive emotions, such as enthusiasm and joy, compared with men (Fujita et al., 1991).

In terms of age trends, after it peaks in adolescence, affect intensity appears to drop with age (Diener, Sandvik, & Larsen, 1985). Many others have also shown that subjective emotional experiences go down with age, particularly for negative emotions (e.g., Carstensen, Pasupathi, Mayr, & Nesselroade, 2000; Gross et al., 1997). Studies of aging and emotion have also examined physiological measures of emotional reactivity, and these studies have also documented decreased reactivity to emotional stimuli among older adults (e.g., Levenson, Carstensen, Friesen, & Ekman, 1991; Levenson, Carstensen, & Gottman, 1994). A recent study by Mather and colleagues (2004) examined amygdala activation during exposure to positive and negative images, with older participants showing diminished amygdala activation to negative, relative to positive, stimuli.

Applications of Research on Affect Intensity

One applied aspect receiving some attention concerns individual differences in response to advertising appeals. Some advertisers target emotional reactions, whereas others appeal to facts in their advertisements. Chang (2006) reviews the literature on affect intensity within consumer research and discusses several mechanisms whereby individual differences in affect intensity might influence how people respond to advertising materials—for example, persons with high affect intensity might be more likely to elaborate on positive emotional appeals, more likely to respond to appeals that promise to relieve negative affect, and so forth. Moore, Harris, and Chen (1995) present empirical data from two experiments showing that participants high, compared with low, in affect intensity are more responsive to emotional advertising appeals and showed no differences in response to nonemotional appeals. In a later study, Moore and Homer (2000) showed that participants with high affect intensity responded with significantly stronger emotions in response to affectively charged advertising appeals and that affect intensity predicts arousing lifestyle activity preferences. Moore and Harris (1996) also demonstrated that the effects of emotional advertising appeals, both positive and negative, were stronger for participants high in affect intensity than for those low in it. They argue that the relation between affect intensity and responding to advertising appeals, as well as attitudes toward the ads, are mediated by emotional responses.

Weiss, Nicholas, and Daus (1999) discuss affective variables in organizational behavior contexts. They report a study of affect in the workplace that found that affect intensity predicted heightened variability in mood on the job, consistent with other studies of affect intensity and mood variability. Rhoades, Arnold, and Jay (2001) examined affective traits during episodes of organizational conflict in an experience sampling study of business employees. Conflict management was related to affective traits, including affect intensity, though the effects of these traits on conflict behaviors were fully mediated by state affect on the day of the conflict. Given that other people are a frequent source of emotion, understanding the implications of individual differences in affect intensity for social relations and within social organizations is an important topic for further research.

Social justice research often examines how people react to the behaviors of others that are perceived as fair or unfair. Given that such reactions often contain a strong affective component, van den Bos, Maas, Waldring, and Semin (2003) hypothesized that affect intensity would be related to an exaggerated response to unfairness. In two studies, they found that people high in affect intensity show strong affective reactions following the experience of outcome and procedural unfairness. Participants with low affect intensity exhibited weak to no unfairness effects, leading the authors to suggest that, for them, actual fairness may not be an important aspect of social justice concerns.

Conclusions

Affect intensity is a construct that refers to individual differences in the characteristic magnitude of emotion reactions. It generalizes to both positive and negative affect, as well as to specific emotions. It implies emotional variability over time, as individuals react strongly to various hedonic events in their lives. Several measures of affect intensity have been developed, though the one with the most validity evidence and the longest research track record is the AIM. The AIM exhibits desirable psychometric properties, has been translated into a number of languages, and exists in a short form.

The broad theoretical appeal of the affect intensity construct is likely due to several things. One is the existence of a sound measure with good validity evidence. Another is the explosion of research on affect and emotion that occurred in the 1990s and early 2000s. A third reason has to do with using individual-differences measures to test various theories. For example, if some phenomenon is theorized to be driven by affect, or if affect is the underlying mechanism, then individual differences in the phenomenon might be related to individual differences in affect intensity. For example, a researcher might theorize that a certain attitude effect relies on affect for its impact. If this is true, then individual differences in affective reactivity should predict individual differences in the attitude effect. As a different example, a researcher might hypothesize that affect produces a narrowing of attention. If this is true, then individual differences in affect intensity should predict individual differences in the narrowing of attention. In this way, affect intensity can be a useful tool for testing broad theories that posit an important role for affect in producing some main-effect phenomenon.

Similarly, if there is a theory about some causal mechanism involved in affect, then that mechanism might relate to individual differences in affect intensity. For example, if personalizing cognitions are thought to produce stronger affective responses, then persons with characteristically stronger affective responses (i.e., those high in trait affect intensity) should display more personalizing cognitions. If the mechanism is truly causal, then manipulating the mechanism should diminish affect intensity such that a person high in affect intensity would begin to react more like a person low in affect intensity. The idea of testing general theories with individual-difference measures is an interesting and effective application of personality psychology to the broader questions of psychology in general.

A final question about the nature of individual differences in affect is implicit in the material covered earlier. The question concerns the locus and interpretation of individual differences in affect intensity. Most experimental studies of affect intensity involve the manipulation or measurement of some stimulus, typically a mood induction or the hedonic value of some life event. Then emotional responses are assessed and examined for predictable individual differences. This can be displayed in the typical stimulus–organism–response model:

$$S \rightarrow O \rightarrow R$$

This simple formulation suggests that the locus of individual differences in affective response could originate from two different processes. One process concerns the link on the right side between organism and response and implies that the individual difference is in the response magnitude or the response output side of the equation. Throughout most this chapter, I have been treating affect intensity as though it were due to this part of the formulation. However, another possibility is that the individual difference is due to the link on the left side, between the stimulus and the organism. This component refers to the stimulus sensitivity, or threshold-for-activation side of the formulation. In a few places in this chapter I have treated affect intensity as though this process might also be involved, for example, when talking about affect intensity as reactivity to life events. Distinguishing these component parts of the affect system is important for understanding the mechanisms of affect and will also contribute to our understanding of the nature of affect intensity as an individual difference.

Acknowledgment

Preparation of this chapter was supported in part by Grant No. RO1-AG028419 from the National Institute on Aging.

References

Bachorowski, J., & Braaten, E. B. (1994). Emotional intensity: Measurement and theoretical implications. *Personality and Individual Differences, 17,* 191–199.

Barnes, G. E. (1976). Individual differences in perceptual reactance: A review of the stimulus intensity modulation individual difference dimension. *Canadian Psychological Review, 17,* 29–52.

Bland, A. R., Williams, C. A., Scharer, K., & Manning, S. (2004). Emotion processing in borderline personality disorders. *Issues in Mental Health Nursing, 25,* 655–672.

Blankstein, K. R., Flett, G. L., Koledin, S., & Bortolotto, R. (1989). Affect intensity and dimensions of affiliation motivation. *Personality and Individual Differences, 10,* 1201–1203.

Blascovich, J., Adlin, R., Brennan, K., Coad, M. L., Hughes, P., Kelsey, R. M., et al. (1992). Affect intensity and cardiac arousal. *Journal of Personality and Social Psychology, 63,* 164–174.

Bryant, F. B., Yarnold, P. R., & Grimm, L. G. (1996). Toward a measurement model of the Affect Intensity Measure: A three-factor structure. *Journal of Research in Personality, 30,* 223–247.

Carstensen, L. L., Pasupathi, M., Mayr, U., & Nesselroade, J. R. (2000). Emotional experience in everyday life across the adult life span. *Journal of Personality and Social Psychology, 79,* 644–655.

Chamberlain, K. (1988). On the structure of subjective well-being. *Social Indicators Research, 20,* 581–604.

Chang, C. (2006). Context-induced and ad-induced affect: Individual differences as moderators. *Psychology and Marketing, 23,* 757–782.

Cheavens, J. S., Daughters, S. B., Kosson, D., Lejuez, C. W., Lynch, T. R., Nowak, J., et al. (2005). An analogue investigation of the relationships among perceived parental criticism, negative affect, and borderline personality disorder features the role of thought suppression. *Behaviour Research and Therapy, 43,* 257–268.

Chwalisz K., Diener, E., & Gallagher, D. (1988). Autonomic arousal feedback and emotional experience: Evidence from the spinal cord injured. *Journal of Personality and Social Psychology, 54,* 820–828.

Dance, K., Kuiper, N. A., & Martin, R. (1990). Intensity of affect, role self-concept, and self-evaluative judgments. *Psychological Reports, 67,* 347–350.

Day, R., & Wong, S. (1996). Anomalous perceptual asymmetries for negative emotional stimuli in the psychopath. *Journal of Abnormal Psychology, 105,* 648–652.

Diener, E., Colvin, C. R., Pavot, W. G., & Allman, A. (1991). The psychic costs of intense positive affect. *Journal of Personality and Social Psychology, 61,* 492–503.

Diener, E., Fujita, F., & Seidlitz, L. (1991). *Manual for the Intensity and Time Affect Survey (ITAS).* Unpublished manuscript, University of Illinois at Urbana–Champaign.

Diener, E., Larsen, R. J., Levine, S., & Emmons, R. A. (1985). Intensity and frequency: Dimensions underlying positive and negative affect. *Journal of Personality and Social Psychology, 48,* 1253–1265.

Diener, E., Sandvik, E., & Larsen, R. J. (1985). Age and sex effects for emotional intensity. *Developmental Psychology, 21,* 542–546.

Dritschel, B. H., & Teasdale, J. D. (1991). Individual differences in affect-related cognitive operations elicited by experimental stimuli. *British Journal of Clinical Psychology, 30,* 151–160.

Eisenberg, N., & Okun, M. S. (1996). The relations of dispositional regulation and emotionality to elders' empathy-related responding and affect while volunteering. *Journal of Personality, 64,* 157–183.

Elliott, T. R., Sherwin, E., Harkins, S. W., & Marmarosh, C. (1995). Self-appraised problem-solving ability, affective states, and psychological distress. *Journal of Counseling Psychology, 42,* 105–115.

Emmons, R. A., & King, L. A. (1989). Personal striving differentiation and affective reactivity. *Journal of Personality and Social Psychology, 56,* 478–484.

Engelberg, E., & Sjöberg, L. (2004). Emotional intelligence, affect intensity, and social adjustment. *Personality and Individual Differences, 37,* 533–542.

Eysenck, H. J. (1967). *The biological basis of personality.* Springfield, IL: Thomas.

Flett, G. L., Blankstein, K. R., & Obertynski, M. (1996). Affect intensity, coping styles, mood regulation expectancies and depressive symptoms. *Personality and Individual Differences, 20,* 221–228.

Flett, G. L., Blankstein, K. R., Bator, C., & Pliner, P. (1989). Affect intensity and self-control of emotional behaviour. *Personality and Individual Differences, 10,* 1–5.

Flett, G. L., & Hewitt, P. L. (1995). Criterion validity and psychometric properties of the Affect Intensity Measure in a psychiatric sample. *Personality and Individual Differences, 19,* 585–591.

Fujita, F., Diener, E., & Sandvik, E. (1991). Gender differences in negative affect and well-being: The case for emotional intensity. *Journal of Personality and Social Psychology, 61,* 427–434.

Gale, A. (1986). Extraversion–introversion and spontaneous rhythms of the brain: Retrospect and prospect. In J. Strelau, F. Fareley, & A. Gale (Eds.), *The biological bases of personality and behavior* (pp. 25–42). Washington, DC: Hemisphere.

Geen, R. G. (1983). The psychophysiology of extraversion–introversion. In J. T. Cacioppo & R. E. Petty (Eds.), *Social psychophysiology* (pp. 391–416). New York: Guilford Press.

Geuens, M., & de Pelsmacker, P. (2002). Developing a short Affect Intensity Scale. *Psychological Reports, 91,* 657–670.

Goldsmith, R. E., & Walters, H. (1989). A validity study of the Affect Intensity Measure. *Journal of Social Behavior and Personality, 4,* 133–140.

Gratz, K. L. (2006). Risk factors for deliberate self-harm among female college students: The role and interaction of childhood maltreatment, emotional inexpressivity, and affect intensity/reactivity. *American Journal of Orthopsychiatry, 76,* 238–250.

Gross, J. J., Carstensen, L. L., Pasupathi, M., Tsai, J., Skorpen, C. G., & Hsu, A. Y. C. (1997). Emotion and aging: Experience, expression, and control. *Psychology and Aging, 12,* 590–599.

Harkins, S. W., Gramling, S., & Elliott, T. (1990). *The Affect Intensity Questionnaire.* Unpublished manuscript, Virginia Commonwealth University.

Hebb, D. O. (1955). Drives and the CNS (conceptual nervous system). *Psychological Review, 62,* 243–254.

Henry, C., Mitropoulou, V., New, A. S., Koenigsberg, H. W., Silverman, J., & Siever, L. J. (2001). Affective instability and impulsivity in borderline personality and bipolar II disorders: Similarities and differences. *Journal of Psychiatric Research, 35,* 307–312.

Herzog, T., Williams, D. M., & Weintraub, D. J. (1985). Meanwhile, back at personality ranch: The augmenters and reducers ride again. *Journal of Personality and Social Psychology, 48,* 1342–1352.

Hunt, M. G. (1993). Expressiveness does predict well-being. *Sex Roles, 29,* 147–169.

Iancu, I., Horesh, N., Offer, D., Dannon, P. N., Lepkifker, E., & Kotler, M. (1999). Alexithymia, affect intensity and emotional range in suicidal patients. *Psychotherapy and Psychosomatics, 68,* 276–280.

Jacob, S., & Hautekeete, M. (1999). Alexithymia is associated with a low self-estimated affective intensity. *Personality and Individual Differences, 27,* 125–133.

Jakupcak, M., Salters, K., Gratz, K. L., & Roemer, L. (2003). Masculinity and emotionality: An investigation of men's primary and secondary emotional responding. *Sex Roles, 49,* 111–120.

Kardum, I. (1999). Affect intensity and frequency: Their relation to mean level and variability of positive and negative affect and Eysenck's personality traits. *Personality and Individual Differences, 26,* 33–47.

Kohn, P. M., Barnes, G. E., & Hoffman, F. M. (1979). Drug-use history and experience seeking among adult male correctional inmates. *Journal of Consulting and Clinical Psychology, 47,* 708–715.

Larsen, R. J. (1984). Theory and measurement of affect intensity as an individual difference characteristic. *Dissertation Abstracts International, 85,* 2297B. (UMI No. 84-22112).

Larsen, R. J. (1987). The stability of mood variability: A spectral analytic approach to daily mood assessments. *Journal of Personality and Social Psychology, 52,* 1195–1204.

Larsen, R. J. (2000). Toward a science of mood regulation. *Psychological Inquiry, 11,* 129–141.

Larsen, R. J., & Augustine, A. A. (2008). Basic personality dispositions related to approach and avoidance: Extraversion/neuroticism, BIS/BAS, and positive/negative affect. In A. J. Elliot (Ed.), *Handbook of approach and avoidance motivation* (pp. 151–164). Mahwah, NJ: Erlbaum.

Larsen, R. J., & Baggs, D. W. (1986). Some psychophysical and personality correlates of the Strelau Temperament Inventory. *Personality and Individual Differences, 7,* 561–565.

Larsen, R. J., Billings, D. W., & Cutler, S. E. (1996). Affect intensity and individual differences in informational style. *Journal of Personality, 64,* 185–207.

Larsen, R. J., & Diener, E. (1985). A multitrait–multimethod examination of affect structure: Hedonic level and emotional intensity. *Personality and Individual Differences, 6,* 631–636.

Larsen, R. J., & Diener, E. (1987). Affect intensity as an individual difference characteristic: A review. *Journal of Research in Personality, 21,* 1–39.

Larsen, R. J., Diener, E., & Cropanzano, R. S. (1987). Cognitive operations associated with individual differences in affect intensity. *Journal of Personality and Social Psychology, 53,* 767–774.

Larsen, R. J., Diener, E., & Emmons, R. A. (1986). Affect intensity and reactions to daily life events. *Journal of Personality and Social Psychology, 51,* 803–814.

Larsen, R. J., & Ketelaar, T. (1989). Extraversion, neuroticism, and susceptibility to positive and negative mood induction procedures. *Personality and Individual Differences, 10,* 1221–1228.

Larsen, R. J., & Ketelaar, T. (1991). Personality and susceptibility to positive and negative emotional states. *Journal of Personality and Social Psychology, 61,* 132–140.

Larsen, R. J., & Lerner, C. (2006). Emotional intelligence and mood regulation following the attack of September 11. In A. Delle Fave (Ed.), *Dimensions of well-being: Research and intervention* (pp. 489–511). Milano, Italy: FrancoAngeli.

Larsen, R. J., & Prizmic, Z. (2008). Regulation of emotional well-being: Overcoming the hedonic treadmill. In M. Eid & R. J. Larsen (Eds.), *The science of subjective well-being* (pp. 258–289). New York: Guilford Press.

Larsen, R. J., & Zarate, M. A. (1991). Extending reducer/augmenter theory into the emotion domain: The role of affect in regulating stimulation level. *Personality and Individual Differences, 12,* 713–723.

Larsen, R. J., Zarate, M. A., & Dare, T. (1986, May). *Individual differences in emotional reactivity and performance under stress.* Paper presented at the annual meeting of the Midwestern Psychological Association, Chicago.

Levenson, R. W., Carstensen, L. L., Friesen, W. V., & Ekman, P. (1991). Emotion, physiology, and expression in old age. *Psychology and Aging, 6,* 28–35.

Levenson, R. W., Carstensen, L. L., & Gottman, J. M. (1994). The influence of age and gender on affect, physiology, and their interrelations: A study of long-term marriages. *Journal of Personality and Social Psychology, 67,* 56–68.

Linville, P. W. (1985). Self-complexity and affective extremity: Don't put all of your eggs in one cognitive basket. *Social Cognition, 3*(1), 94–120.

Lucas, R. E., Diener, E., & Larsen, R. J. (2003). Measuring positive emotions. In S. J. Lopez & C. R. Snyder (Eds.), *Positive psychological assessment: A handbook of models and measures* (pp. 201–218). Washington, DC: American Psychological Association.

Lynch, T. R., Cheavens, J. S., Morse, J. Q., & Rosenthal, M. Z. (2004). A model predicting suicidal ideation and hopelessness in depressed older adults: The impact of emotion inhibition and affect intensity. *Aging and Mental Health, 8,* 486–497.

Lynch, T. R., Robins, C. J., Morse, J. Q., & MorKrause, E. D. (2001). A mediational model relating affect intensity, emotion inhibition, and psychological distress. *Behavior Therapy, 32,* 519–536.

Maio, G. R., & Esses, V. M. (2001). The need for affect: Individual differences in the motivation to approach or avoid emotions. *Journal of Personality, 69,* 583–615.

Mather, M., Canli, T., English, T., Whitfield, S. L., Wais, P., Ochsner, K. N., et al. (2004). Amygdala activity in response to emotional pictures in older adults. *Psychological Science, 15,* 259–263.

Mayer, J. D., Salovey, P., & Caruso, D. R. (2001). *Technical manual for the Mayer–Salovey–Caruso Emotional Intelligence Test V.2.0.* Toronto, Ontario, Canada: MHS.

McFatter, R. M. (1998). Emotional intensity: Some components and their relations to extraversion and neuroticism. *Personality and Individual Differences, 24,* 747–758.

Mehrabian, A. (1995). Theory and evidence bearing on a scale of trait arousability. *Current Psychology: Developmental, Learning, Personality, Social, 14,* 3–28.

Millon, T. (1983). *The Millon Clinical Multiaxial Inventory manual* (3rd ed.). Minneapolis, MN: National Computer Systems.

Mishara, B. L., & Baker, A. H. (1981). Individual differences in stimulus intensity modulation in the elderly. *International Journal of Aging and Human Development, 13,* 285–295.

Moore, D. J., & Harris, W. D. (1996). Affect intensity and the consumer's attitude toward high impact emotional advertising appeals. *Journal of Advertising, 25,* 37–50.

Moore, D. J., Harris, W. D., & Chen, H. C. (1995). Affect intensity: An individual difference response to advertising appeals. *Journal of Consumer Research, 22,* 154–164.

Moore, D. J., & Homer, P. M. (2000). Dimensions of temperament: Affect intensity and consumer lifestyles. *Journal of Consumer Psychology, 9,* 231–242.

Nofzinger, E. A., Fasiczka, A. L., Frank, E., Garamoni, G. L., Jennings, J. R., Kupfer, D. J., et al. (1994). Affect intensity and phasic REM sleep in depressed men before and after treatment with cognitive-behavioral therapy. *Journal of Consulting and Clinical Psychology, 62,* 83–91.

Oosterwegel, A., Field, N., Hart, D., & Anderson, K. (2001). The relation of self-esteem variability to emotion variability, mood, personality traits, and depressive tendencies. *Journal of Personality, 69,* 689–708.

Pavlov, I. P. (1957). *Experimental psychology and other essays.* New York: Philosophical Library.

Petrie, A. (1967). *Individuality in pain and suffering.* Chicago: University of Chicago Press.

Rhoades, J. A., Arnold, J., & Jay, C. (2001). The role of affective traits and affective states in disputants' motivation and behavior during episodes of organizational conflict. *Journal of Organizational Behavior, 22,* 329–345.

Ritz, T. (1994). Alexithymic characteristics and affective intensity: Adaptation and relationship between two self-report instruments. *Zeitschrift für Differentielle und Diagnostische Psychologie, 15,* 23–39.

Rosenthal, M. Z., Cheavens, J. S., Lejuez, C. W., & Lynch, T. R. (2005). Thought suppression mediates the relationship between negative affect and borderline personality disorder symptoms. *Behavior Research and Therapy, 43,* 1173–1185.

Ruch, W., Angleitner, A., & Strelau, J. (1991). The Strelau Temperament Inventory—Revised (STI-R): Validity studies. *European Journal of Personality, 5,* 287–308.

Rusting, C. L., & Larsen, R. J. (1995). Moods as sources of stimulation: Relationships between personality and desired mood states. *Personality and Individual Differences, 19,* 321–329.

Rusting, C. L., & Larsen, R. J. (1997). Extraversion, neuroticism, and susceptibility to positive and negative affect: A test of two theoretical models. *Personality and Individual Differences, 22,* 607–612.

Rusting, C. L., & Larsen, R. J. (1998). Personality and cognitive processing of affective information. *Personality and Social Psychology Bulletin, 24,* 200–213.

Rusting, C. L., & Larsen, R. J. (1999). Clarifying Gray's theory of personality: A response to Pickering, Corr and Gray. *Personality and Individual Differences, 26,* 367–372.

Sales, S. M. (1971). Need for stimulation as a factor in social behavior. *Journal of Personality and Social Psychology, 19,* 124–134.

Sales, S. M. (1972). Need for stimulation as a factor in preferences for different stimuli. *Journal of Personality and Social Psychology, 36,* 55–61.

Schimmack, U., & Diener, E. (1997). Affect intensity: Separating intensity and frequency in repeatedly measured affect. *Journal of Personality and Social Psychology, 73,* 1313–1329.

Seidlitz, L., & Diener, E. (1998). Sex differences in the recall of affective experiences. *Journal of Personality and Social Psychology, 74,* 262–271.

Sheldon, K. M. (1994). Emotionality differences between artists and scientists. *Journal of Research in Personality, 28,* 481–491.

Simonsson-Sarnecki, M., Lundh, L., & Törestad, B. (2000). Factor structure and validity of the Affect Intensity Measure in a Swedish sample. *Personality and Individual Differences, 29,* 337–350.

Strelau, J. (1982). Biologically determined dimensions of personality or temperament? *Personality and Individual Differences, 3,* 355–360.

Strelau, J. (1985). Temperament and personality: Pavlov and beyond. In J. Strelau, F. Farely, & A. Gale (Eds.), *Biological foundations of personality and behavior* (pp. 25–43). New York: Hemisphere.

Taylor, G. J., Bagby, R. M., & Parker, J. D. A. (1997). *Disorders of affect regulation: Alexithymia in medical and psychiatric illness.* Cambridge, UK: Cambridge University Press.

Thorberg, F. A., & Lyvers, M. (2006). Negative mood regulation (NMR) expectancies, mood, and affect intensity among clients in substance disorder treatment facilities. *Addictive Behaviors, 31,* 811–820.

Underwood, B., & Froming, W. J. (1980). The Mood Survey: A personality measure of happy and sad moods. *Journal of Personality Assessment, 44,* 404–414.

van den Bos, K., Maas, M., Waldring, I. E., & Semin, G. R. (2003). Toward understanding the psychology of reactions to perceived fairness: The role of affect intensity. *Social Justice Research, 16*(2), 151–168.

Vanman, E. J., Dawson, M. E., & Brennan, P. A. (1998). Affective reactions in the blink of an eye: Individual differences in subjective experience and physiological responses to emotional stimuli. *Personality and Social Psychology Bulletin, 24,* 994–1005.

Weinfurt, K. P., Bryant, F. B., & Yarnold, P. R. (1994). The factor structure of the Affect Intensity Measure: In search of a measurement model. *Journal of Research in Personality, 28,* 314–331.

Weiss, H. M., Nicholas, J. P., & Daus, C. S. (1999). An examination of the joint effects of affective experiences and job beliefs on job satisfaction and variations in affective experiences over time. *Organizational Behavior and Human Decision Processes, 78,* 1–24.

Weissman, A. E., & Ricks, D. F. (1966). *Mood and personality.* New York: Holt, Rinehart & Winston.

Williams, L. M., & Barry, J. (2003). Do sex differences in emotionality mediate sex differences in traits of psychosis-proneness? *Cognition and Emotion, 17,* 747–758.

Yen, S., Zlotnick, C., & Costello, E. (2002). Affect regulation in women with borderline personality disorder traits. *Journal of Nervous and Mental Disease, 190,* 693–696.

Zelenski, J. M., & Larsen, R. J. (1999). Susceptibility to affect: A comparison of three personality taxonomies. *Journal of Personality, 67,* 761–791.

Zelenski, J. M., & Larsen, R. J. (2002). Predicting the future: How affect-related personality traits influence likelihood judgments of future events. *Personality and Social Psychology Bulletin, 28*(7), 1000–1010.

Zuckermann, M. (1979). *Sensation seeking: Beyond the optimal level of arousal.* Hillsdale, NJ: Erlbaum.

PART IV

■ ● ▲ ◆

COGNITIVE DISPOSITIONS

CHAPTER 17

■ ◎ ▲ ◆ ■ ◎ ▲ ◆

Openness to Experience

ROBERT R. MCCRAE
ANGELINA R. SUTIN

Confronted with the choice, the American people would choose
the policeman's truncheon over the anarchist's bomb.
—ATTRIBUTED TO SPIRO T. AGNEW

Their *ethics* are a short summary of police ordinances; for them
the most important thing is to be a useful member of the state,
and to air their opinions in the club of an evening; they have
never felt homesickness for something unknown and far away. ...
—SØREN KIERKEGAARD (1936)

An intellectual is a man who doesn't know how to park a bike.
—ATTRIBUTED TO SPIRO T. AGNEW

This chapter is arguably misplaced. It was assigned to a section on cognition in a book on individual differences in social behavior. Yet Openness to Experience is not a cognitive disposition, nor is it a dimension of social behavior. McCrae and Costa (1997) argued that Openness must be understood "in both structural and motivational terms. Openness is seen in the breadth, depth, and permeability of consciousness, and in the recurrent need to enlarge and examine experience" (p. 826). This description makes Openness fundamentally an intrapsychic variable, associated with such esoteric phenomena as chills in response to sudden beauty (McCrae, 2007), the experience of *déjà vu* (McCrae, 1994), and homesickness for the unknown.

Yet, as the editors understand, these characteristics of mind have profound consequences for social behavior at all levels, much of it mediated by cognitive processes. Openness affects social perceptions and the formation of social attitudes, the choice of friends and spouses, political activity, and cultural innovation. All these connections were pointed out in an earlier review (McCrae, 1996); this chapter can be seen as an update.

Openness: An Orientation

Openness is one of the dimensions of the Five-Factor Model (FFM; Digman, 1990) of personality traits. As such, it is a very broad construct that is often difficult to grasp. The component traits or facets of Openness are the most loosely related of any of the five factors and thus the weakest in replication studies (McCrae et al., 2005a). Piedmont and Aycock (2007) showed that terms for Openness entered the English language centuries after terms for Extraversion and Agreeableness, and McCrae (1990) noted that many O-related traits, such as aesthetic sensitivity, are still not represented by single trait adjectives in English. Lay conceptions of Openness are often confounded with interpersonal openness (Sneed, McCrae, & Funder, 1998). It is therefore understandable that there are different conceptualizations of Openness among experts (De Raad & Van Heck, 1994).

In this chapter we adopt the view of Openness operationalized in the Revised NEO Personality Inventory (NEO-PI-R; Costa & McCrae, 1992a), but in general there are substantial correlations among different measures of Openness, including the Openness scale of the Big Five Inventory (BFI; Benet-Martínez & John, 1998), and Goldberg's (1990) adjective-based Intellect scales. (However, the fifth factor in the Five-Factor Personality Inventory [Hendriks, Hofstee, & De Raad, 1999] is called Autonomy and is only modestly related to Openness; De Fruyt, McCrae, Szirmák, & Nagy, 2004.)

The NEO-PI-R has facet scales for Openness to Fantasy, Aesthetics, Feelings, Actions, Ideas, and Values. Highly open people are thus seen as imaginative, sensitive to art and beauty, emotionally differentiated, behaviorally flexible, intellectually curious, and liberal in values. Closed people are down-to-earth, uninterested in art, shallow in affect, set in their ways, lacking curiosity, and traditional in values.[1] Most psychologists would judge the high pole of this dimension to be desirable, because most psychologists are themselves high in Openness (Staudinger, Maciel, Smith, & Baltes, 1998), but among laypeople there is a strong correlation between their social desirability ratings of Openness and their own self-reports (Konstabel, 2007): Open people admire openness, closed people despise it.

Like the other basic factors, Openness is strongly heritable, and the covariation of Openness facets to define the factor appears at the genetic level as well as the phenotypic level (Yamagata et al., 2006)—that is, people who are intellectually curious also tend to be imaginative and artistically sensitive in part because the same genes help shape these three traits. Like the other basic factors, Openness shows high levels of differential stability across the adult lifespan (Terracciano, Costa, & McCrae, 2006), but it shows a distinctive pattern of maturational trends, increasing from early adolescence until some time in the 20s and then gradually declining (e.g., McCrae et al., 2005a).

It is useful to distinguish Openness from constructs with which it might be confused, particularly intelligence.[2] Although adjective Intellect scales include such terms as *perceptive*, *analytical*, and *intelligent*, and although they correlate well with Openness, the association of Openness with measured intelligence is modest and specific. Correlations around .40 are found with measures of divergent thinking, which is often thought to underlie creativity (McCrae, 1987). Openness scores were associated ($rs \approx .30$) with performance on verbal and facial emotion recognition tasks for both Caucasians and African Americans (Terracciano, Merritt, Zonderman, & Evans, 2003). Noftle and Robins (2007) reported an overall correlation of .26 between Openness and the verbal score on the Scholastic Aptitude Test, but only .05 with the math score. Higher verbal scores may reflect more and broader reading among students high in Openness rather than greater native ability.

Finally, it will be useful to discuss the relation of Openness to some of the other constructs discussed in this book. Openness is inversely, and rather strongly, related to Authoritarianism/Dogmatism: Trapnell (1994) reported correlations of from −.29 to −.63 between NEO-PI-R Openness facet scales and Right Wing Authoritarianism, with the largest correlation unsurprisingly with Openness to Values. To the extent that aggression is related to authoritarianism (weakly; see Carnahan & McFarland, 2007), we would expect authoritarians to be antagonistic as well as closed.

Need for Closure (Webster & Kruglanski, 1994), the desire for definite and final answers, is also related to low Openness ($r = −.42$, $N = 84$, $p < .001$; Costa & McCrae, 1998) but is unrelated to Agreeableness ($r = −.08$, n.s.). Instead, this construct includes a preference for order and predictability that gives it an association with Conscientiousness ($r = .42$, $p < .001$). Thus people prone to seizing on the first idea offered and then freezing on this solution (Kruglanski & Webster, 1996) are in general uninterested in exploring alternative possibilities, keeping their views simple and uncluttered.

Other people pursue ideas vigorously, being high on both Openness and Conscientiousness. Such people score high on Need for Cognition (Cacioppo & Petty, 1982; Sadowski & Cogburn, 1997; P. D. Trapnell, personal communication, November 9, 2007). Need for Cognition is most directly relevant to O5: Ideas,[3] but it is related to most facets of Openness (Berzonsky & Sullivan, 1992). Remarkably, a PsycINFO search found 474 entries for "Need for Cognition" and 1,032 for "Openness to Experience," but only 6 that included both terms. The Need for Cognition scale was created by social psychologists and has been used widely in experimental studies, whereas Openness is employed in correlational studies in the personality literature. Petty, Briñol, Loersch, and McCaslin (Chapter 21, this volume) should give readers an idea of how Openness might function if it were included as a moderator variable in social-psychological experiments. For example, research by D'Agostino and Fincher-Kiefer (1992) suggests that highly open people would be less susceptible to the correspondence bias, that is, to misattribute behavior to dispositional rather than situational causes

Tetlock, Peterson, and Berry (1993) reported that Integrative Complexity (a form of cognitive complexity in which people tend to consider a range of possibilities before coming to a conclusion) showed positive associations with Myers–Briggs Type Indicator Intuition, Adjective Check List Creative Personality, and California Psychological Inventory Flexibility—all known correlates of Openness (McCrae & Costa, 1997). Kensinger (1996) scored Thought Complexity from definitions given in response to 11 words (see Kreitler & Kreitler, 1990) and found that it was associated with total Openness ($r = .36$, $N = 60$, $p < .05$) and with O2: Aesthetics ($r = .30$) and especially O5: Ideas ($r = .51$, $p < .01$).

Given the association of Openness with emotion recognition (Terracciano et al., 2003), one might guess that it would also be related to emotional intelligence, and there are some data supporting a modest association (Schulte, Ree, & Carretta, 2004). Finally, one of the variables classified as a motivational disposition, Sensation Seeking, has an Experience Seeking subscale that is clearly related to Openness (Zuckerman, Kuhlman, Joireman, Teta, & Kraft, 1993).

We do not mean to suggest that these constructs are equivalent to O; they differ both in their associations with other factors and in their specific content that gives each a unique focus of convenience. However, if measures of all of them were factored together, it is likely that a first general factor would be defined chiefly by Openness. The social consequences of Openness, to some degree, include the social consequences of Authoritarianism, Need for Closure, and so on.

Individual Social Interactions

Person Presentation and Perception

Do open people express their Openness in ways that other people can detect? Are others able to recognize these cues accurately, or do lay observers have intuitive ideas about what behaviors reflect Openness that may not be diagnostic of the individual's actual level of Openness? Can multiple observers come to consensus on whether another is open? And are they accurate? The person-perception literature addresses each of these questions and paints a broad picture of how Openness is manifested in daily living and interpersonal interactions and how others perceive these cues.

Open individuals express their creativity, intellectual curiosity, and need for variety in characteristic ways across a variety of mediums. They are verbally fluent, humorous, and expressive in interpersonal interactions (Sneed, McCrae, & Funder, 1998). When going about their daily lives, these individuals use fewer third-person pronouns and past-tense verbs and spend more of their time in restaurants, bars, and coffee shops (Mehl, Gosling, & Pennebaker, 2006). Given that open individuals have both artistic and intellectual proclivities, it is not surprising that these interests are expressed in how they present themselves to the world. For example, on their personal Web pages, open individuals choose to highlight their own creative and work projects and present information that expresses their emotions and personal opinions (Marcus, Machilek, & Schütz, 2006). These same proclivities are manifested in their working and living spaces. Their love of novelty and originality is evident here: Open individuals decorate both their offices and bedrooms in distinctive and unconventional ways, and, consistent with their intellectual interests, own and display varied books and magazines (Gosling, Ko, Mannarelli, & Morris, 2002).

Observers are fairly good at picking up on these behavioral indicators of Openness. For example, perceivers judge individuals who speak fluently, initiate humor, and are expressive to be high on Openness (Sneed et al., 1998). Individuals who use fewer past-tense verbs and who frequent restaurants, bars, and coffee shops are perceived as being open (Mehl et al., 2006), as are individuals with websites that have links to work/ personal projects and that express personal opinions (Marcus et al., 2006). Likewise, perceivers use the distinctiveness of both office space and bedrooms to judge the inhabitant's level of Openness (Gosling et al., 2002). Observers appear relatively adept at recognizing many behavioral cues diagnostic of Openness.

Yet lay perceivers also have their own ideas about what behaviors are indicative of Openness that are not necessarily diagnostic; that is, lay conceptions can be inaccurate. For example, observers judge individuals who have highly decorated, cheerful, and colorful offices to be open, whereas these office characteristics are largely unrelated to the individual's actual level of Openness (Gosling et al., 2002). Likewise, using big words in everyday speech is perceived to be a sign of Openness, when in fact Openness is unrelated to this speech characteristic. On personal Web pages, perceivers judge individuals who post many pictures and reveal much personal information to be open (Marcus et al., 2006), and in chatrooms, the number of topics discussed and number of self-deprecating remarks are taken as signs of Openness, whereas Openness is unrelated to these behaviors (Rouse & Haas, 2003).

This discrepancy, of course, raises the question of how accurately others can infer Openness. Multiple judges do agree with each other on the individual's level of Openness, which suggests that lay conceptions of Openness are not idiosyncratic. Although early research addressing this question found little consensus among observers at zero acquaintance (Kenny, Albright, Malloy, & Kashy, 1994), more recent research, perhaps because of better conceptualizations of

Openness coupled with more reliable measures, has found considerable consensus. This is true across a variety of sources of zero-acquaintance information: Observers agree on Openness when judging personal websites (Vazire & Gosling, 2004), top-10 song lists (Rentfrow & Gosling, 2006), and offices and bedrooms (Gosling et al., 2002). Compared with the other traits in the FFM, Openness and Extraversion typically show similar levels of consensus, and consensus on both remains high as acquaintanceship increases (Borkenau, Mauer, Riemann, Spinath, & Angleitner, 2004). A slightly different pattern emerges for virtual acquaintanceships. In chatrooms, there is moderate consensus on Openness for one-on-one chats—albeit lower than consensus on Extraversion and Agreeableness—but this consensus disappears when chatting in a group rather than one on one (Markey & Wells, 2002). Although there were no differences in the amount of text written in the two conditions, consensus may have decreased because the content of the text may have been more superficial during group interactions and thus less diagnostic.

Across these varied contexts, consensus among observers tends to be higher than accuracy: Others can agree on whether they believe a person is open, but they may not be right (perhaps because shared lay conceptions of the cues of Openness are not always correct). Accuracy also depends on the task observed; some tasks are more diagnostic of Openness than others. Open individuals are imaginative and creative people, and observers are more accurate when judging Openness from tasks that allow these qualities to be expressed rather than from highly structured tasks (Borkenau et al., 2004).

Finally, perceivers in laboratory studies form an impression of Openness very quickly that is resistant to change. From observing as little as 5 seconds of a getting-to-know-you conversation, perceivers can make attributions about Openness. Although accuracy ratings are generally lower for Openness than for the other traits in this context, accuracy does not vary as a function of slice length—it takes a very narrow sliver of time for a perceiver to form a judgment of Openness (Carney, Colvin, & Hall, 2007). And once this impression is formed, it is not easily changed. Openness is a low-maintenance trait (Kammrath, Ames, & Scholer, 2007). That is, initial impressions can be resistant to reevaluation. In contrast to traits such as Agreeableness and Conscientiousness, which require frequent confirmatory evidence to maintain the judgment, impressions of Openness are relatively impervious to disconfirming evidence; information that contradicts the initial Openness impression tends to be disregarded. Once an individual is tagged as being open (or closed), regardless of the amount of evidence to the contrary, the impression sticks. Kammrath and colleagues (2007) suggested that lay conceptions of both Openness and ability may contribute to stable impressions of Openness. Specifically, people equate Openness with ability and perceive ability as stable; thus people are less sensitive to disconfirming evidence.

These laboratory studies of person perception are complemented by correlational studies, in which agreement among observer ratings and between ratings and self-reports can be studied among people who have known each other, not for seconds or minutes, but for up to 70 years (Costa & McCrae, 1992b). Such studies typically show that length of acquaintance increases cross-observer agreement over the course of weeks or months (Kurtz & Sherker, 2003). Among long-term acquaintances, cross-observer correlations for Openness, typically .40 to .60, are similar to those found for other factors (Connolly, Kavanagh, & Viswesvaran, 2007). This level of agreement is seen in studies around the world (McCrae et al., 2004).

Marriage and Family

In any relationship, dynamics of the interaction are shaped, in part, by the personalities of the individuals involved. Although true for any dyadic interaction, most evidence comes from research on romantic relationships and married couples. At each stage, from deciding whether to get married to parenting, Openness shapes these choices, interactions, and consequences.

Marriage is a normative and expected event; there is often considerable social pressure to "find someone, settle down, and start a family." Yet, despite this pressure, some choose to remain single and never marry.

These men and women tend to be high on Absorption and low on Traditionalism, two scales from the Multidimensional Personality Questionnaire (MPQ) closely related to Openness (Johnson, McGue, Krueger, & Bouchard, 2004). They may find fulfillment in other types of relationships and activities and, without a strong internal need to conform to the expectations of society, pursue these interests instead of potential mates.

Whether single, dating, or married, people have a good idea of what they want in their ideal partners—often someone like themselves, particularly on Openness. When contemplating the ideal mate, single individuals prefer partners who strongly resemble them on Openness, with Agreeableness and Extraversion coming in a distant second and third, respectively (Figueredo, Sefcek, & Jones, 2006). A similar pattern holds for both dating couples and newlyweds, although at the stage of marriage, similarity on Conscientiousness becomes slightly more important than a match on Openness (Botwin, Buss, & Shackelford, 1997). And regardless of their own personalities, women in particular value mates who are open and dominant (Botwin et al., 1997). Taking an evolutionary perspective, Botwin and colleagues (1997) suggested that women prefer these qualities because they are the most strongly associated with resource acquisition.

Despite these clear preferences, most people settle for much less. Some studies find no correlation between ratings of an ideal partner and ratings of an actual partner (Figueredo et al., 2006); others find a moderate correlation at best (Botwin et al., 1997). Although we can build the ideal mate in our minds, the constraints of reality typically force compromise. In the end, other factors, such as physical attractiveness, proximity, or availability, may be more important than the ideal personality.

But people do want a partner with a similar personality, and it is important to ask to what extent individuals succeed in finding such a match. This question is of considerable interest to behavioral geneticists, who typically assume no assortative mating in calculating estimates of heritability. That is, they presume that an open man would be just as likely to marry a closed woman as an open woman. Researchers have now documented couples' similarity on a variety of attributes, from intelligence to social attitudes to personality. In one large-scale study of newlyweds, Watson and colleagues (2004) found the highest similarity correlations for age, religiousness, and political conservatism (mean r = .71), lower correlations for education and intelligence (mean r = .43), and virtually no correlation for any of the FFM personality traits (mean r = –.03).

But given that Openness is strongly related to political conservatism, religiosity, and education, one would expect some evidence of assortative mating for this trait. And indeed, despite somewhat mixed findings, similarity on Openness emerges more often than not. Neyer and Voigt (2004), for example, found significant correlations for both Openness (r = .25) and Conscientiousness (r = .39), but not for Neuroticism, Extraversion, or Agreeableness. Similar findings are summarized in McCrae (1996). Biases such as age, gender, education, and assessment method may contribute to these inconsistent findings.

Recently, McCrae and colleagues (2008) analyzed trait similarity using both self-reports and spouse ratings of personality in married couples across four cultures, controlling for these potential biases. Consistent with previous research, similarity correlations for the broad domains were generally modest, and Openness had the largest correlation (mean r for Openness across the three cultures = .22). Facet-level analyses revealed that couples were drawn together on some aspects of Openness more than others. Across the different cultures, Openness to Values consistently showed the most evidence for trait similarity: liberals seek out other liberals, whereas conservatives seek out other conservatives. Part of this pairing is likely a matter of convenience; these two types of people inhabit very different social worlds. In addition, their differing ideologies would likely be a continued source of argument and conflict within the relationship.

Although lower in magnitude, individuals also tend to marry partners who are similar to themselves on O2: Aesthetics (McCrae et al., 2008). In the early stages of dating, to get to know each other, couples may engage in shared interests, such as going to art museums or the symphony. If one partner adores the arts, whereas the other one is bored stiff, the relationship may last only one or two dates. This trait similarity among married couples appears to come from initial choice rather than convergence over time. People with the same values and intellectual pursuits seek each other out rather than mold each other into their likenesses over time.

Openness not only influences mate selection, but it also shapes relationship quality, conflict interactions, and daily life within the family. Although people maintain that they want someone similar to themselves on Openness and are somewhat successful in finding a similar mate on this trait, similarity does not necessarily imply relationship satisfaction. Nemechek and Olson (1999), for example, found that partners who were similarly conscientious had higher levels of marital adjustment but that similarity on Openness was unrelated to adjustment. Even discrepancies between ideal partner personality and actual partner personality do not predict dissatisfaction (Botwin et al., 1997).

In contrast, degree of Openness, rather than similarity, is associated with satisfaction in both serious dating relationships (e.g., Neyer & Voigt, 2004) and among married couples (e.g., Donnellan, Conger, & Bryant, 2004). Interestingly, husbands' and wives' Openness contributes to different aspects of relationship satisfaction. For both husbands and wives, husbands' level of Openness is related to satisfying relationships overall (Botwin et al., 1997; Neyer & Voigt, 2004) and well-adjusted marriages (Bouchard, Lussier, & Sabourin, 1999). Wives' level of Openness, however, is unrelated to marital adjustment (Neyer & Voigt, 2004). On the flip side, wives', but not husbands', level of Openness is related to the couple's sexual satisfaction (Donnellan et al., 2004). Donnellan and colleagues speculated that Openness is related to sexual satisfaction because open individuals are motivated to seek out new and varied experiences; open wives may be more willing to explore new and varied sexual experiences, which may translate into greater sexual satisfaction for both partners.

Conflict between two people, however, is inevitable, and communication is often touted as the key to maintaining a healthy, satisfying relationship. How individuals approach (or avoid), work through, and resolve conflict has major implications for the health of the relationship. The flexibility, perspective-taking ability, and willingness to tolerate differences of opinion of open people may facilitate communication and reduce conflict. Open men and women have a constructive communicative style in which they actively negotiate conflicts while recognizing the other's perspective. That is, both members of the couple face the conflict, freely express their feelings, and work together toward resolution. In contrast, closed women prefer to avoid discussion or change activities when conflict occurs. And, regardless of their own Openness, men perceive conflict interactions with closed wives as characterized by demand–withdraw: The wife criticizes, complains, and demands change, and in response the husband avoids the conflict by being silent or walking away (Heaven, Smith, Prabhakar, Abraham, & Mete, 2006). With these types of interaction styles, it is hardly surprising that closed individuals typically have less satisfying relationships.

In addition to communication, effective coping is also important to the health of the relationship. When faced with marital difficulties, both husbands and wives high in Openness engage in problem-focused coping (Bouchard, 2003). That is, they try to identify the cause of the relationship stress and then actively work to change the identified elicitor. Open individuals may be comfortable with this strategy because of their natural ability to find novel solutions to problems and their willingness to try new approaches when old ones fail. In contrast, when faced with interpersonal stress, closed individuals employ distancing coping strategies, such as ignoring the problem or refusing to become emotionally involved (Lee-Baggley, Preece, & DeLongis, 2005). These individuals are uncomfortable with strong emotional reactions and may employ distancing techniques as a preemptive strategy against such experiences. These strategies are not without consequence, however, and their relative effectiveness may be observable by others. Donnellan and colleagues (2004), for example, found that independent observers judged open men and women to have interactions that were less negative while discussing their relationships.

In some contexts, however, low Openness may be related to more beneficial outcomes. Following therapy, for example, couples who score higher on conventionalism report less marital distress (Snyder, Mangrum, & Wills, 1993). Furthermore, among middle-aged women, divorce is associated with a more liberal/radical political orientation (Fahs, 2007). Both conventionalism and political ideology have been associated with Openness, and these findings suggest that the relation between Openness and relationship satisfaction and length may be a complex one.

Finally, Openness shapes daily life within the family, particularly when it comes to parenting. Closed individuals value obedience and deference to authority without question, whereas open individuals are more open-minded, tolerant, and willing to listen to opposing arguments. These characteristics are readily apparent in their different parenting philosophies. In interactions with their children, open parents are emotionally expressive and warm, and they encourage children to voice their opinions. In contrast, closed parents demand obedience, expect their children to follow their rules without question, and limit their children's autonomy (Metsäpelto & Pulkkinen, 2003). The consequence of these different parenting styles may be evident in their children's behavior: Open parents are less likely to report child misbehavior as a major daily stressor (Lee-Baggley et al., 2005). It is possible, however, that open parents are more tolerant of child misbehavior rather than actually having more well-behaved children.

Strangers and Friends

The social consequences of Openness for interpersonal interactions are not limited to romantic relationships and the family. Open and closed individuals have different styles of interacting with the world that influence how they interact with strangers, the types of friends they seek out, and how those relationships are maintained. Open and closed individuals differ in their political orientations, beliefs about religion, and intellectual interests. These characteristics may influence friendships for at least two reasons. First, people tend to meet each other when enjoying shared interests; thus a foreign-film buff and a NASCAR fanatic are not likely to cross paths often. Second, politics and religion are often sources of great conflict when strongly held convictions differ. Constant argument does not make a good basis for friendship.

Across the five factors, correlations between friends tend to be modest at best (Berry, Willingham, & Thayer, 2000). Similarity correlations for Openness, however, are clearly the largest ($r = .35$). Similar to romantic partners, individuals tend to seek out friends who share similar interests. As McCrae (1996) pointed out, "open people are bored by the predictable and intellectually undemanding amusements of closed people; closed people are bored by what they perceive to be the difficult and pretentious culture of the open" (p. 331). Given these different orientations to the world, open and closed individuals are unlikely to voluntarily spend enough time with each other to develop a lasting friendship.

In addition to studying the basis for friendship, it is also of interest to ask how Openness shapes casual interactions among strangers and its role in interpersonal interactions between friends. When getting acquainted, open individuals spend more time looking at their interaction partners and less time talking about themselves. Observers to these conversations mistake this greater visual attention as an indication of relationship quality (Berry & Hansen, 2000). Yet Openness is unrelated to perceived interaction quality in either spontaneous interactions in same-sex dyads (Berry & Hansen, 2000) or in getting-to-know-you conversations in opposite-sex interactions (Berry & Miller, 2001). Open individuals are curious and attentive to the world around them and, in the process of getting to know somebody new, their curiosity may lead them to look more intently at their interaction partners as they take them in and try to figure them out. This nonverbal cue, however, does not facilitate high-quality interactions.

Closed individuals are sensitive to appropriate social interactions between strangers and react strongly when norm expectations are violated. In one study, for example, compared with the control condition, closed participants became less friendly after being teased by a confederate, and their narratives of the interaction with the confederate were less positive. For open participants, in contrast, being teased did not influence their interaction with the teaser (Bollmer, Har-

ris, Milich, & Georgesen, 2003). Teasing a stranger, even if playfully, violates norm expectations and may create a novel situation that closed people find uncomfortable.

Low Openness has likewise been associated with other problems in interpersonal functioning. In evaluating their interpersonal interactions, these individuals endorse items related to difficulty in perspective taking, being easily persuaded by others (presumably those in positions of authority), and losing their sense of self when interacting with strong-minded others (Gurtman, 1995). And just as these characteristics influence conflict and communication in couples' interactions, they also affect interactions between friends. In a diary study, for example, closed individuals had more conflicts with a close friend over a 4-week period than did open individuals. In response to the conflict, closed friends were more likely to engage in passive–aggressive strategies, whereas open friends adopted a forgive-and-forget strategy. Also similar to couples, these strategies do not go unnoticed; friends get more irritated with closed friends than with open ones (Berry et al., 2000).

The relation between Openness and conflict, however, takes a different course among college roommates than between friends; in this case, open individuals are more likely to have conflict with their roommates (Bono, Boles, Judge, & Lauver, 2002). Unlike friendships, students typically have little choice in their roommates, and a mismatch on Openness may be one source of conflict. And, indeed, conflict was unrelated to Openness when roommates had similar mean levels and conflict was marginally related to mean-level differences in Openness between roommates. At both ends of the continuum, like-minded individuals may understand each other better and feel more comfortable as roommates. Roommates mismatched on Openness, in contrast, may be likely to butt heads if one is unconventional and emotional and the other conservative and stoic. In addition, what might be fun argumentativeness for an open individual may amount to a serious conflict for a closed individual. For both reasons, there may be less conflict when roommates are matched on Openness.

Finally, one great benefit of a close relationship is the support that can be provided by the other during times of great stress. Openness is associated with both the type and frequency of support offered to others. Open individuals reciprocate emotional support, whereas closed individuals reciprocate instrumental support (Knoll, Burkert, & Schwarzer, 2006). Once open individuals receive emotional support from a friend, they easily return the favor, which likely deepens the emotional bond between them. In contrast, instrumental support is more concrete and costly; perhaps closed individuals feel indebted and thus more compelled to reciprocate. Instrumental support, although costly for the individual, is often more beneficial for the recipient due to the practical application of the support. Thus, in times of distress, when concrete solutions are needed, closed individuals may provide more useful support. These different approaches to support likely affect the nature and closeness of the friendship over time.

Taken together, these findings demonstrate how Openness shapes interpersonal interactions, from casual interactions to long-term committed relationships. Open and closed individuals tend to develop lasting relationships with like-minded individuals, and subsequently these pairings have implications for a variety of outcomes, from relationship satisfaction to conflict resolution to parenting to social support. Clearly, an individual's experiential orientation to the world profoundly affects his or her interaction with the people in it.

Openness in Work Groups

In the past decade, industrial/organizational psychologists have taken an interest in the effects of personality traits on team performance. Although teams with high mean levels of Conscientiousness tend to perform well in many situations, results are much more mixed for Openness. High team-level Openness is generally advantageous, but often only for certain kinds of tasks or within certain contexts. And in some respects, Openness interferes with the work of the group.

An early study of team personality elevation (mean level) and variability (within-team variance) examined customer service and task completion ratings for 82 teams of retail assistants. Higher elevations of Openness (as well as Agreeableness and Conscientiousness) were associated with better performance (Neuman, Wagner, & Christiansen, 1999). Taggar (2000) analyzed data from 94 teams at both individual and team levels and found that Openness had no effect at the individual level but that the greater the proportion of team members high in Openness was, the better the performance was. An analysis of the specific behaviors responsible for good performance suggested that open members contributed by generating ideas, promoting free discussion, and synthesizing team efforts. Openness has also been found to promote emergent leadership—the ability to take charge of a leaderless group (Kickul & Neuman, 2000).

A meta-analysis of job performance and team personality found advantages for teams higher in Openness, but only in field studies, not laboratory studies (Bell, 2007), suggesting that it is the long-term effects of Openness that are noticeable. Another meta-analysis sorted studies by the kind of task involved, using Holland's (1985) vocational typology. Predictably, team-level Openness predicted success in Investigative tasks (Anderson, 2006) but was unrelated to success in Social, Conventional, or Enterprising tasks. LePine (2003) examined the effect of introducing an unforeseen change—a breakdown of communication—in a simulated military "command and control" task. Teams high in Openness (and low in C2: Order, C3: Dutifulness, and C6: Deliberation) adapted to the new situation more readily and successfully. Bing and Lounsbury (2000) studied performance of managers of Japanese companies operating in the United States; presumably because they could handle the complexities of cross-cultural interactions, managers high in Openness were rated higher in performance.

However, high Openness also presents problems for groups. For example, G. H. Kickul (2000) found that Openness was negatively related to goal clarity (presumably because people high in Openness kept generating new ideas), and Lun and Bond (2006) found that it interfered with achieving relationship harmony in a work group (perhaps because members high in Openness were too individualistic). A study of 220 individuals in 45 teams also found that Openness (like low Agreeableness) was inversely related to peer-rated social role behavior—that is, how well group members got along (Stewart, Fulmer, & Barrick, 2005). In another study, employees high in Openness were low in organizational loyalty, especially if they lacked resources (Moss, McFarland, Ngu, & Kijowska, 2006).

At least one finding relates to the team variability in Openness. Given the frequent antagonism between individuals high and low in Openness and their very different working styles and goals, it is perhaps not surprising that a meta-analysis found that homogeneity with respect to Openness led to better group performance, at least among professional teams. Presumably the best results—and the highest levels of morale—would be obtained by choosing teams uniformly high in Openness to deal with changeable situations and investigative tasks and teams uniformly low in Openness to deal with well-structured, conventional tasks.

Social and Political Effects

The quotations from Agnew and Kierkegaard that open this chapter illustrate not only the substantive differences between closed and open people in social attitudes but also the affective tone: Both sides hold the other in contempt. Agnew famously declared that so-called intellectuals were "an effete corps of impudent snobs," whereas Kierkegaard clearly regarded his fellow citizens as Philistines. There is, however, a subtle asymmetry in these characterizations. Agnew, spokesman for the Silent Majority, assures us that Americans, preferring order to freedom, share his values. By contrast, the Danish existentialist emphasizes his isolation, distinguishing himself from "them." Open people prize uniqueness and individuality (Dollinger, Ross, & Preston, 2002) at the cost of some social alienation; closed people are loyal and patriotic, strongly identified with their own kind. Open people root for the underdog; closed people support favorites (Wilkinson, 2007).

The dark side of closed people's in-group loyalty is their intolerance for out-groups, characterized by Agnew as "Yippies, Hippies, Yahoos, Black Panthers, lions and tigers ... the whole damn zoo." In a Swedish sample, Ekehammar and Akrami (2007) examined correlations of generalized prejudice (a composite of ethnic prejudice, sexism, homophobia, and prejudice against people with mental disabilities) with NEO-PI-R scales. At the domain level, the strongest correlations (both −.49) were with Openness and Agreeableness; at the facet level, the strongest were A6: Tender-Mindedness (−.61) and O6: Values (−.55), which are considered attitudinal facet scales. However, prejudice was also inversely related to Openness to Fantasy, Aesthetics, Feelings, and Actions, $rs = −.25$ to $−.49$, $N = 170$, $p < .05$.

Flynn (2005), in studies of white Americans, found that Openness is associated with lower racial prejudice, more favorable judgments of a fictional black character, and more favorable assessments of black interviewees, and attributed this in part to the willingness of people high in Openness to consider stereotype-disconfirming information. Duriez and Soenens (2006) found that racism was related to low Openness (and low Agreeableness) among Belgian adolescents. Given the strong, consistent, and theoretically expectable associations of low Openness with prejudice and racism, it is extraordinary that, of 11,015 items found in a PsycINFO search on "prejudice or racism," only 10 involved Openness. Social psychologists have overlooked one of the key determinants of one of their most-studied phenomena.

There has been much less research on reverse prejudice, but Lecci and Johnson (2008) reported the intriguing finding that, among American blacks, in addition to the expectable inverse association with Agreeableness, there is a small ($r = .15$) but significant positive correlation between Openness and antiwhite attitudes. Perhaps it was Openness that led the Black Panthers to challenge the racist status quo in mid-20th-century America.

There is ample evidence that Openness is inversely related to authoritarianism, as well as to other, less extreme forms of social conservativism. Van Hiel, Kossowska, and Mervielde (2000) examined left–right political ideology in Belgium and Poland. A right-wing ideology score was defined in part by preference for nationalist parties over socialist and green parties, as well as by general conservative political beliefs. This index was inversely related to O6: Values in each of four samples (*r*s = −.37 to −.64, *p* < .001), but it was also more modestly related to each of the other facets in one or more of the samples. For example, O1: Fantasy, which shares no obvious content with measures of ideology, showed correlations ranging from −.20 to −.39, all *p* < .05, in the Belgian samples.

In a later study, Van Hiel and Mervielde (2004) related Openness to separate measures of cultural and economic conservatism. Cultural conservatism was related to Openness and all its facets, but economic conservatism was unrelated to total Openness and only weakly related to O2: Aesthetics (*r* = −.19) and O6: Values (*r* = −.15). The strongest personality predictor of economic conservatism was low Agreeableness (*r* = −.23, *p* < .001). Economic conservatives may be mean, but they are not necessarily closed. Economic conservatism is presumably based on ideology and self-interest; cultural conservatism is psychological rather than ideological (cf. Van Hiel & Mervielde, 2004) and seems to reflect the preference of closed individuals for simple, stable, and familiar beliefs and values. In a Polish study, cultural but not economic conservatism was found to be heritable (Oniszczenko & Jakubowska, 2005).

Aggregate Openness and Culture

Cross-Cultural Analyses

Within the past few years, cross-cultural studies have suggested that nations differ systematically in mean levels of personality traits (but see Poortinga, van de Vijver, & van Hemert, 2002, for a critical view of that claim). McCrae (2002) assembled self-report NEO-PI-R data from 36 cultures, and McCrae and colleagues (2005b) gathered observer-rating NEO-PI-R data from 51 cultures. Mean aggregate personality scores were calculated for each culture. Across the two datasets, convergent culture-level correlations were significant for 4 of the 5 factors and 26 of the 30 facets. In particular, correlations for Openness facets ranged from .44 for O4: Actions to .75 for O6: Values, with a correlation of .50 for total Openness. Thus different samples using different methods of measurement generally concurred in describ-

ing the citizens of some cultures as being, in general, more open than others—although differences between cultures were generally small compared with the ubiquitous individual differences within cultures.

Which cultures are most open? Of the 28 cultures with both self-report and observer-rating data, the highest mean Openness scores were found for French-speaking Switzerland, Serbia, Austria, Germany, and German-speaking Switzerland, with *T*-scores of 53 to 59. The lowest-scoring countries were Croatia, Spain, Hong Kong, Malaysia, and India, with *T*-scores of 46 to 49. It is surely puzzling that Serbia scores so much higher than Croatia, but the other findings make a certain sense: Modern, progressive, well-educated countries are higher in Openness than are traditional cultures. The United States was near average on aggregate Openness.

It is possible to move past simple impressions about these sets of cultures by conducting culture-level analyses, relating aggregate Openness levels to other features of nations. McCrae (2002) showed that Openness was significantly related to three of Hofstede's (2001) dimensions of culture: low Power Distance, high Individualism, and high Masculinity. The first two of these associations were replicated in the observer-rating study (McCrae et al., 2005b). Thus people from cultures with high mean levels of Openness prefer egalitarian to hierarchical social structures and focus on themselves as individuals rather than on the groups to which they belong. McCrae and colleagues (2005b) examined country scores on Schwartz's (1994) values survey and found positive correlations of Openness with Affective Autonomy, Intellectual Autonomy, and Egalitarian Commitment values and a negative correlation with Conservatism.

Based on data from the World Values Survey, Inglehart and Norris (2003) identified two broad dimensions: Survival versus Self-Expression and Traditional versus Secular–Rational. Openness was significantly related to Secular–Rational values (*r* = .34, *N* = 42, *p* < .05) and showed a trend toward a positive association with Self-Expression (*r* = .29, *N* = 42, *p* < .10). Traditional cultures are guided by religion and tend to reject abortion, divorce, and euthanasia—values shared by closed individuals. Survival values are generally found in poorer countries, where material prosperity is a major concern. Cultures with a history of high economic development have citizens more concerned about tolerance, imagination, and personal fulfillment—goals more congenial to open individuals.

In general, these are sensible correlates and suggest that associations found on the individual level may also be found on the culture level. This is by no means always the case. Cultures high in O6: Values show higher use of the drug Ecstasy (McCrae & Terracciano, 2008), but a study at the individual level in the Netherlands found no difference in Openness levels between those who did and did not use the drug (instead, Ecstasy users were higher on Extraversion and lower on Conscientiousness; ter Bogt, Engels, & Dubas, 2006). The widespread use of Ecstasy is presumably limited to wealthy nations, and Openness is correlated with per-capita gross domestic product. Thus effects of aggregated personality traits may be inflated or masked by other culture-level variables.

However, one association that unfortunately seems to hold on both levels is that between low Openness and HIV stigmatization. In Russia and the United States, stigmatization was associated with low Openness and especially low O6: Values (McCrae et al., 2007). In the self-report study, black South African, Zimbabwean, Indian, and Malay cultures scored lowest on O6: Values (McCrae, 2002). In both South Africa and Zimbabwe, the AIDS epidemic has been fueled by indifference or denial on the part of the governments. In India, where at least 2 million people are living with HIV infection, "the HIV epidemic is misunderstood and stigmatised among the Indian public. People living with HIV have faced violent attacks; been rejected by families, spouses and communities; been refused medical treatment; and even, in some reported cases, denied the last rites before they die" (AVERT, 2007). Fortunately, having learned from the experience in Africa, both Malaysia and India have programs in place to educate the public about HIV infection risks. Given the public's perceptions, anonymous testing and confidential treatment ought to be emphasized.

Critics of this line of research (e.g., Poortinga et al., 2002) have argued that apparent differences in mean levels of traits in different cultures might be due to artifacts, such as problems in the translation, culture-specific response styles, or inadequacies in sampling. But a demonstration of the validity of aggregate personality scores has recently been provided by Rentfrow, Gosling, and Potter (2008), who used Internet data on the BFI collected from over 600,000 respondents to compare mean personality trait levels in the 50 U. S. states and the District of Columbia. Here language and national culture were held constant, and Rentfrow and colleagues argued that their sample was broadly representative. Yet mean-level differences still appeared and, in general, made sense. They found the highest aggregate level of Openness in Washington, D.C.—which joined only Massachusetts in favoring McGovern and Shriver over Nixon and Agnew in the 1972 presidential election—followed by New York, Oregon, and Massachusetts. Lowest in Openness were Alabama, Alaska, Wyoming, and North Dakota. Rentfrow and colleagues correlated these scores with state-level indicators and showed that Openness was positively related to favorable aggregate attitudes toward legalizing marijuana, abortion, and same-sex marriage; to the proportion of the state population employed in occupations related to the arts and entertainment and to computers and mathematics; and, unexpectedly, to the per-capita robbery and murder rates. Openness was negatively related to spending time in a bar or tavern and to attending church. Especially in a democracy, personality traits can have a dramatic effect on collective behavior: Oregon was the first state to decriminalize marijuana, and Massachusetts recognizes same-sex marriages.

The chief question remaining is how traits come to be associated with features of culture. Do cultural practices promote the development of certain traits, or do common traits stimulate the evolution of cultural institutions? Until quite recently, anthropologists and psychologists would have reflexively presumed that culture shapes personality. But the strong evidence of predominant genetic influence on individual differences within cultures makes it reasonable to suppose that the distribution of personality-related trait alleles may differ across nations and give rise to different mean personality profiles. Over the course of centuries, these collective personality differences may have been one influence on culture (McCrae, 2004). Both sides have been argued as an explanation for the links between aggregate traits and Hofstede dimensions (Hofstede & McCrae, 2004), but there is very little empirical evidence. Some support for environmental influences comes from the changes in values that accompany changes in economic development (Inglehart & Norris, 2003). Some evidence for genetic effects comes from studies of isolated populations (Ciani, Capiluppi, Veronese, & Sartori, 2007). Perhaps the most informative designs are acculturation studies, in which members of an ethnic group move from one culture to another. Do they retain their ethnic profile or come to resemble the citizens of the host culture? One such study has been reported (McCrae, Yik, Trapnell, Bond, & Paulhus, 1998); it found that Chinese born in Hong Kong scored about one-half standard deviation lower in Openness than ethnic Chinese born in Canada (an acculturation effect), but that these Canadian-born Chinese Canadians still scored significantly lower than European Canadians on O3: Feelings and O6: Values (ethnicity effects). Both ethnicity and acculturation may affect mean trait levels for Openness. As Rentfrow, Gosling, and Potter (2008) pointed out, genetic and environmental influences are likely to be mutually reinforcing: Open people may be inclined to move to Massachusetts, and the cultural and academic opportunities it provides may encourage greater openness.

Conclusion

Concepts related to Openness—such as Authoritarianism, Need for Closure, and Integrative Complexity—have long been employed by social psychologists, but usually without a good grasp of their relation to basic personality traits. There is considerable advantage to construing such scales as indicators of Openness, because a great deal is known about the origins, development, and correlates of that factor. For example, there appear to be no studies on the heritability of Need for Cognition, but there are many that show that Openness to Experience, and in particular Openness to Ideas, have a strong genetic basis (e.g., Jang, McCrae, Angleitner,

Riemann, & Livesley, 1998); the large correlation between Need for Cognition and O5: Ideas ($r = .78$; Berzonsky & Sullivan, 1992) virtually guarantees that Need for Cognition must be substantially heritable. Again, we know that Openness reaches it highest mean level during the early 20s—a fact that surely affects the generalizability of findings from experiments on college students. Social psychologists are not accustomed to thinking about the long-term implications of their findings, but the longitudinal stability of Openness suggests that patterns of behavior observed in students may persevere for decades. How might awareness of that fact reshape theories of social behavior?

This volume is dedicated to integrating the topics of individual differences, most often studied by personality psychologists, and the social behavior that is the focus of social psychology. Because of its deep intrapsychic basis and its widespread social consequences, Openness to Experience may be a particularly useful construct on which to center a dialogue between these two fields.

Acknowledgments

Preparation of this chapter was supported by the Intramural Research Program, National Institutes of Health, National Institute on Aging. Robert R. McCrae receives royalties from the Revised NEO Personality Inventory.

Notes

1. Recall that the facets of Openness are only loosely related and thus that individuals may be high in some facets and low in others. As a group, the people of India are high in Openness to Aesthetics and low in Openness to Values (McCrae, 2002), as were, perhaps, T. S. Eliot and Ezra Pound. Those pioneers of modern poetry ended up, respectively, as an orthodox Anglican and a propagandist for Mussolini. Or perhaps their Openness to Values was so high that they questioned and rejected the tenets of conventional liberalism.
2. Spiro Agnew studied chemistry at Johns Hopkins University before obtaining a law degree.
3. By convention, the 30 facet scales of the NEO-PI-R are designated by the factor initial, a facet number from 1 to 6, and the facet name. The names of facets of Openness are understood to include "Openness to," so that O5: Ideas is read "Openness to Ideas."

References

Anderson, M. G. (2006). The team personality–outcomes relationship moderated by task type: A meta-analytic investigation. *Dissertation Abstracts International, 67*(3B), 1737.

AVERT. (2007, October 31). *Overview of HIV and AIDS in India.* Retrieved November 15, 2007, from *www.avert.org/aidsindia.htm.*

Bell, S. T. (2007). Deep-level composition variables as predictors of team performance: A meta-analysis. *Journal of Applied Psychology, 92,* 595–615.

Benet-Martínez, V., & John, O. P. (1998). *Los cinco Grandes* across cultures and ethnic groups: Multitrait multimethod analyses of the Big Five in Spanish and English. *Journal of Personality and Social Psychology, 75,* 729–750.

Berry, D. S., & Hansen, J. S. (2000). Personality, nonverbal behavior, and interaction quality in female dyads. *Personality and Social Psychology Bulletin, 26,* 278–292.

Berry, D. S., & Miller, K. M. (2001). When boy meets girl: Attractiveness and the five-factor model in opposite-sex interactions. *Journal of Research in Personality, 35,* 62–77.

Berry, D. S., Willingham, J. K., & Thayer, C. A. (2000). Affect and personality as predictors of conflict and closeness in young adults' friendships. *Journal of Research in Personality, 34,* 84–107.

Berzonsky, M. D., & Sullivan, C. (1992). Social-cognitive aspects of identity style: Need for cognition, experiential openness, and introspection. *Journal of Adolescent Research, 7,* 140–155.

Bing, M. N., & Lounsbury, J. W. (2000). Openness and job performance in U.S.-based Japanese manufacturing companies. *Journal of Business and Psychology, 14,* 515–522.

Bollmer, J. M., Harris, M. J., Milich, R., & Georgesen, J. C. (2003). Taking offense: Effects of personality and teasing history on behavioral and emotional reactions to teasing. *Journal of Personality, 71,* 557–603.

Bono, J. E., Boles, T. L., Judge, T. A., & Lauver, K. J. (2002). The role of personality in task and relationship conflict. *Journal of Personality, 70,* 311–344.

Borkenau, P., Mauer, N., Riemann, R., Spinath, F. M., & Angleitner, A. (2004). Thin slices of behavior as cues of personality and intelligence. *Journal of Personality and Social Psychology, 86,* 599–614.

Botwin, M. D., Buss, D. M., & Shackelford, T. K. (1997). Personality and mate preferences: Five factors in mate selection and marital satisfaction. *Journal of Personality, 65,* 106–136.

Bouchard, G. (2003). Cognitive appraisals, neuroticism, and openness as correlates of coping strategies: An integrative model of adaptation to marital difficulties. *Canadian Journal of Behavioural Science, 35,* 1–12.

Bouchard, G., Lussier, Y., & Sabourin, S. (1999). Personality and marital adjustment: Utility of the Five-Factor Model of personality. *Journal of Marriage and Family, 61,* 651–660.

Cacioppo, J. T., & Petty, R. E. (1982). The need for cognition. *Journal of Personality and Social Psychology, 42,* 116–131.

Carnahan, T., & McFarland, S. (2007). Revisiting the Stanford Prison Experiment: Could participant self-selection have led to the cruelty? *Personality and Social Psychology Bulletin, 33,* 603–614.

Carney, D. R., Colvin, C. R., & Hall, J. A. (2007). A thin slice perspective on the accuracy of first impressions. *Journal of Research in Personality, 41,* 1054–1072.

Ciani, A. S. C., Capiluppi, C., Veronese, A., & Sartori, G. (2007). The adaptive value of personality differences revealed by small island population dynamics. *European Journal of Personality, 21,* 3–22.

Connolly, J. J., Kavanagh, E. J., & Viswesvaran, C. (2007). The convergent validity between self- and observer ratings of personality: A meta-analytic review. *International Journal of Selection and Assessment, 15,* 110–117.

Costa, P. T., Jr., & McCrae, R. R. (1992a). *Revised NEO Personality Inventory (NEO-PI-R) and NEO Five-Factor Inventory (NEO-FFI) professional manual.* Odessa, FL: Psychological Assessment Resources.

Costa, P. T., Jr., & McCrae, R. R. (1992b). Trait psychology comes of age. In T. B. Sonderegger (Ed.), *Nebraska Symposium on Motivation: Psychology and aging* (pp. 169–204). Lincoln: University of Nebraska Press.

Costa, P. T., Jr., & McCrae, R. R. (1998). Trait theories of personality. In D. F. Barone, M. Hersen, & V. B. VanHasselt (Eds.), *Advanced personality* (pp. 103–121). New York: Plenum Press.

D'Agostino, P. R., & Fincher-Kiefer, R. (1992). Need for cognition and the correspondence bias. *Social Cognition, 10,* 151–163.

De Fruyt, F., McCrae, R. R., Szirmák, Z., & Nagy, J. (2004). The Five-Factor Personality Inventory as a measure of the Five-Factor Model: Belgian, American, and Hungarian comparisons with the NEO-PI-R. *Assessment, 11,* 207–215.

De Raad, B., & Van Heck, G. L. (Eds.). (1994). The fifth of the Big Five [Special issue]. *European Journal of Personality, 84*(4).

Digman, J. M. (1990). Personality structure: Emergence of the Five-Factor Model. *Annual Review of Psychology, 41,* 417–440.

Dollinger, S. J., Ross, V. J., & Preston, L. A. (2002). Intellect and individuality. *Creativity Research Journal, 14,* 213–226.

Donnellan, M. B., Conger, R. D., & Bryant, C. M. (2004). The Big Five and enduring marriages. *Journal of Research in Personality, 38,* 481–504.

Duriez, B., & Soenens, B. (2006). Personality, identity styles, and authoritarianism: An integrative study among late adolescents. *European Journal of Personality, 20,* 397–417.

Ekehammar, B., & Akrami, N. (2007). Personality and prejudice: From Big Five personality factors to facets. *Journal of Personality, 75,* 899–925.

Fahs, B. (2007). Second shifts and political awakenings: Divorce and the political socialization of middle-aged women. *Journal of Divorce and Remarriage, 47,* 43–66.

Figueredo, A. J., Sefcek, J. A., & Jones, D. N. (2006). The ideal romantic partner personality. *Personality and Individual Differences, 41,* 431–441.

Flynn, F. J. (2005). Having an open mind: The impact of Openness to Experience on interracial attitudes and impression formation. *Journal of Personality and Social Psychology, 88,* 816–826.

Goldberg, L. R. (1990). An alternative "description of personality": The Big Five factor structure. *Journal of Personality and Social Psychology, 59*, 1216–1229.

Gosling, S. D., Ko, S., Mannarelli, T., & Morris, M. E. (2002). A room with a cue: Personality judgments based on offices and bedrooms. *Journal of Personality and Social Psychology, 82*, 379–398.

Gurtman, M. B. (1995). Personality structure and interpersonal problems: A theoretically guided item analysis of the Inventory of Interpersonal Problems. *Assessment, 2*, 343–361.

Heaven, P. C. L., Smith, L., Prabhakar, S. M., Abraham, J., & Mete, M. E. (2006). Personality and conflict communication patterns in cohabiting couples. *Journal of Research in Personality, 40*, 829–840.

Hendriks, A. A. J., Hofstee, W. K. B., & De Raad, B. (1999). The Five-Factor Personality Inventory (FFPI). *Personality and Individual Differences, 27*(2), 307–325.

Hofstede, G. (2001). *Culture's consequences: Comparing values, behaviors, institutions, and organizations across nations* (2nd ed.). Thousand Oaks, CA: Sage.

Hofstede, G., & McCrae, R. R. (2004). Personality and culture revisited: Linking traits and dimensions of culture. *Cross-Cultural Research, 38*, 52–88.

Holland, J. L. (1985). *Making vocational choices: A theory of vocational personalities and work environments*. Englewood Cliffs, NJ: Prentice-Hall.

Inglehart, R., & Norris, P. (2003). *Rising tide: Gender equality and cultural change around the world*. New York: Cambridge University Press.

Jang, K. L., McCrae, R. R., Angleitner, A., Riemann, R., & Livesley, W. J. (1998). Heritability of facet-level traits in a cross-cultural twin sample: Support for a hierarchical model of personality. *Journal of Personality and Social Psychology, 74*, 1556–1565.

Johnson, W., McGue, M., Krueger, R. F., & Bouchard, T. J., Jr. (2004). Marriage and personality: A genetic analysis. *Journal of Personality and Social Psychology, 86*, 285–294.

Kammrath, L. K., Ames, D. R., & Scholer, A. A. (2007). Keeping up impressions: Inferential rules for impression change across the Big Five. *Journal of Experimental Social Psychology, 43*, 450–457.

Kenny, D. A., Albright, L., Malloy, T. E., & Kashy, D. A. (1994). Consensus in interpersonal perception: Acquaintance and the Big Five. *Psychological Bulletin, 116*, 245–258.

Kensinger, E. A. (1996). *Openness to Experience and the communication of meaning*. Unpublished manuscript, Gerontology Research Center, Baltimore, MD.

Kickul, G. H. (2000). Antecedents of self-managed work team performance in a computerized business simulation: Personality and group interaction. *Dissertation Abstracts International, 61*(6A), 2270.

Kickul, J., & Neuman, G. (2000). Emergent leadership behaviors: The function of personality and cognitive ability in determining teamwork performance and KSAs. *Journal of Business and Psychology, 15*, 27–51.

Kierkegaard, S. (1936). The journals (A. Dru, Trans.). In R. Bretall (Ed.), *A Kierkegaard anthology* (pp. 1–18). New York: Random House.

Knoll, N., Burkert, S., & Schwarzer, R. (2006). Reciprocal support provision: Personality as a moderator? *European Journal of Personality, 20*, 217–236.

Konstabel, K. (2007). *"The more like me, the better": Individual differences in social desirability ratings of personality items*. Unpublished manuscript, University of Tartu, Estonia.

Kreitler, S., & Kreitler, H. (1990). *The cognitive foundations of personality traits*. New York: Plenum Press.

Kruglanski, A. W., & Webster, D. M. (1996). Motivated closing of the mind: "Seizing" and "freezing." *Psychological Review, 103*, 263–283.

Kurtz, J. E., & Sherker, J. L. (2003). Relationship quality, trait similarity, and self–other agreement on personality traits in college roommates. *Journal of Personality, 71*, 21–48.

Lecci, L., & Johnson, J. D. (2008). Black anti-white attitudes: The influence of racial identity and the Big Five. *Personality and Individual Differences, 44*, 182–192.

Lee-Baggley, D., Preece, M., & DeLongis, A. (2005). Coping with interpersonal stress: Role of Big Five traits. *Journal of Personality, 73*, 1141–1180.

LePine, J. A. (2003). Team adaptation and postchange performance: Effects of team composition in terms of members' cognitive ability and personality. *Journal of Applied Psychology, 88*, 27–39.

Lun, V. M.-C., & Bond, M. H. (2006). Achieving relationship harmony in groups and its consequence for group performance. *Asian Journal of Social Psychology, 9*, 195–202.

Marcus, B., Machilek, F., & Schütz, A. (2006). Personality in cyberspace: Personal Web sites as media for personality expressions and impressions. *Journal of Personality and Social Psychology, 90*, 1014–1031.

Markey, P. M., & Wells, S. M. (2002). Interpersonal perception in Internet chat rooms. *Journal of Research in Personality, 36*, 134–146.

McCrae, R. R. (1987). Creativity, divergent thinking, and Openness to Experience. *Journal of Personality and Social Psychology, 52*, 1258–1265.

McCrae, R. R. (1990). Traits and trait names: How well is Openness represented in natural languages? *European Journal of Personality, 4*, 119–129.

McCrae, R. R. (1994). Openness to Experience: Expanding the boundaries of Factor V. *European Journal of Personality, 8*, 251–272.

McCrae, R. R. (1996). Social consequences of experiential openness. *Psychological Bulletin, 120*, 323–337.

McCrae, R. R. (2002). NEO-PI-R data from 36 cultures: Further intercultural comparisons. In R. R. McCrae & J. Allik (Eds.), *The Five-Factor Model of personality across cultures* (pp. 105–125). New York: Kluwer Academic/Plenum.

McCrae, R. R. (2004). Human nature and culture: A trait perspective. *Journal of Research in Personality, 38*, 3–14.

McCrae, R. R. (2007). Aesthetic chills as a universal marker of Openness to Experience. *Motivation and Emotion, 31*, 5–11.

McCrae, R. R., & Costa, P. T., Jr. (1997). Conceptions and correlates of Openness to Experience. In R. Hogan, J. A. Johnson, & S. R. Briggs (Eds.), *Handbook of personality psychology* (pp. 825–847). Orlando, FL: Academic Press.

McCrae, R. R., Costa, P. T., Jr., Martin, T. A., Oryol,

V. E., Rukavishnikov, A. A., Senin, I. G., et al. (2004). Consensual validation of personality traits across cultures. *Journal of Research in Personality, 38,* 179–201.

McCrae, R. R., Costa, P. T., Jr., Martin, T. A., Oryol, V. E., Senin, I. G., & O'Cleirigh, C. (2007). Personality correlates of HIV stigmitization in Russia and the United States. *Journal of Research in Personality, 41,* 190–196.

McCrae, R. R., Martin, T. A., Hřebíčková, M., Urbánek, T., Boomsma, D. I., Willemsen, G., et al. (2008). Personality trait similarity between spouses in four cultures. *Journal of Personality, 76(5),* 1137–1164.

McCrae, R. R., & Terracciano, A. (2008). The Five-Factor Model and its correlates in individuals and cultures. In F. J. R. Van de Vijver, D. A. van Hemert, & Y. H. Poortinga (Eds.), *Multilevel analyses of individual and culture* (pp. 249–283). Mahwah, NJ: Erlbaum.

McCrae, R. R., Terracciano, A., & 79 Members of the Personality Profiles of Cultures Project. (2005a). Personality profiles of cultures: Aggregate personality traits. *Journal of Personality and Social Psychology, 89,* 407–425.

McCrae, R. R., Terracciano, A., & 79 Members of the Personality Profiles of Cultures Project. (2005b). Universal features of personality traits from the observer's perspective: Data from 50 cultures. *Journal of Personality and Social Psychology, 88,* 547–561.

McCrae, R. R., Yik, M. S. M., Trapnell, P. D., Bond, M. H., & Paulhus, D. L. (1998). Interpreting personality profiles across cultures: Bilingual, acculturation, and peer rating studies of Chinese undergraduates. *Journal of Personality and Social Psychology, 74,* 1041–1055.

Mehl, M. R., Gosling, S. D., & Pennebaker, J. W. (2006). Personality in its natural habitat: Manifestations and implicit folk theories of personality in daily life. *Journal of Personality and Social Psychology, 90,* 862–877.

Metsäpelto, R. L., & Pulkkinen, L. (2003). Personality traits and parenting: Neuroticism, Extraversion, and Openness to Experience as discriminative factors. *European Journal of Personality, 17,* 59–78.

Moss, S. A., McFarland, J., Ngu, S., & Kijowska, A. (2006). Maintaining an open mind to closed individuals: The effect of resource availability and leadership style on the association between Openness to Experience and organizational commitment. *Journal of Research in Personality, 41,* 259–275.

Nemechek, S., & Olson, K. R. (1999). Five-factor personality similarity and marital adjustment. *Social Behavior and Personality, 27,* 309–318.

Neuman, G. A., Wagner, S. H., & Christiansen, N. D. (1999). The relationship between work-team personality composition and the job performance of teams. *Group and Organization Management, 24,* 28–45.

Neyer, F. J., & Voigt, D. (2004). Personality and social network effects on romantic relationships: A dyadic approach. *European Journal of Personality, 18,* 279–299.

Noftle, E. E., & Robins, R. W. (2007). Personality predictors of academic outcomes: Big Five correlates of GPA and SAT scores. *Journal of Personality and Social Psychology, 93,* 116–130.

Oniszczenko, W., & Jakubowska, U. (2005). Genetic determinants and personality correlates of sociopolitical attitudes in a Polish sample. *Twin Research, 8,* 47–52.

Piedmont, R. L., & Aycock, W. (2007). An historical analysis of the lexical emergence of the Big Five personality adjective descriptors. *Personality and Individual Differences, 42,* 1059–1068.

Poortinga, Y. H., van de Vijver, F., & van Hemert, D. A. (2002). Cross-cultural equivalence of the Big Five: A tentative interpretation of the evidence. In R. R. McCrae & J. Allik (Eds.), *The Five-Factor Model of personality across cultures* (pp. 273–294). New York: Kluwer Academic/Plenum.

Rentfrow, P. J., & Gosling, S. D. (2006). Message in a ballad: The role of music preferences in interpersonal perception. *Psychological Science, 17,* 236–242.

Rentfrow, P. J., Gosling, S. D., & Potter, J. (2008). A theory of the emergence, persistence, and expression of geographical variation in psychological characteristics. *Perspectives on Psychological Science, 3,* 339–369.

Rouse, S. V., & Haas, H. A. (2003). Exploring the accuracies and inaccuracies of personality perception following Internet-mediated communication. *Journal of Research in Personality, 37,* 446–467.

Sadowski, C. J., & Cogburn, H. E. (1997). Need for Cognition in the Big Five structure. *Journal of Psychology: Interdisciplinary and Applied, 131,* 307–312.

Schulte, M. J., Ree, M. J., & Carretta, T. R. (2004). Emotional intelligence: Not much more than g and personality. *Personality and Individual Differences, 37,* 1059–1068.

Schwartz, S. H. (1994). Beyond individualism/collectivism: New cultural dimensions of values. In U. Kim, H. C. Triandis, C. Kagitcibasi, S.-C. Choi, & G. Yoon (Eds.), *Individualism and collectivism: Theory, method, and applications* (pp. 85–119). Thousand Oaks, CA: Sage.

Sneed, C. D., McCrae, R. R., & Funder, D. C. (1998). Lay conceptions of the Five-Factor Model and its indicators. *Personality and Social Psychology Bulletin, 24,* 115–126.

Snyder, D. K., Mangrum, L. F., & Wills, R. M. (1993). Predicting couples' response to marital therapy: A comparison of short- and long-term predictors. *Journal of Consulting and Clinical Psychology, 61,* 61–69.

Staudinger, U. M., Maciel, A. G., Smith, J., & Baltes, P. B. (1998). What predicts wisdom-related performance?: A first look at personality, intelligence, and facilitative contexts. *European Journal of Personality, 12,* 1–17.

Stewart, G. L., Fulmer, I. S., & Barrick, M. R. (2005). An exploration of member roles as a multilevel linking mechanism for individual traits and team outcomes. *Personnel Psychology, 58,* 343–365.

Taggar, S. (2000). Personality, cognitive ability and behaviour: The antecedents of effective autonomous work teams. *Dissertation Abstracts International, 60(9A),* 3438.

ter Bogt, T. F. M., Engels, R. C. M. E., & Dubas, J. S. (2006). Party people: Personality and MDMA use of house party visitors. *Addictive Behaviors, 31,* 1240–1244.

Terracciano, A., Costa, P. T., Jr., & McCrae, R. R.

(2006). Personality plasticity after age 30. *Personality and Social Psychology Bulletin, 32*, 999–1009.

Terracciano, A., Merritt, M., Zonderman, A. B., & Evans, M. K. (2003). Personality traits and sex differences in emotion recognition among African Americans and Caucasians. *Annals of the New York Academy of Sciences, 1000*, 309–312.

Tetlock, P. E., Peterson, R. S., & Berry, J. M. (1993). Flattering and unflattering personality portraits of integratively simple and complex managers. *Journal of Personality and Social Psychology, 64*, 500–511.

Trapnell, P. D. (1994). Openness versus intellect: A lexical left turn. *European Journal of Personality, 8*, 273–290.

Van Hiel, A., Kossowska, M., & Mervielde, I. (2000). The relationship between Openness to Experience and political ideology. *Personality and Individual Differences, 28*, 741–751.

Van Hiel, A., & Mervielde, I. (2004). Openness to Experience and boundaries in the mind: Relationships with cultural and economic conservative beliefs. *Journal of Personality, 72*, 659–686.

Vazire, S., & Gosling, S. D. (2004). e-Perceptions: Personality impressions based on personal websites. *Journal of Personality and Social Psychology, 87*, 123–132.

Watson, D., Klohnen, E. C., Casillas, A., Simms, E. N., Haig, J., & Berry, D. S. (2004). Match makers and deal breakers: Analyses of assortative mating in newlywed couples. *Journal of Personality, 72*, 1029–1068.

Webster, D. M., & Kruglanski, A. W. (1994). Individual differences in need for cognitive closure. *Journal of Personality and Social Psychology, 67*, 1049–1062.

Wilkinson, T. J. (2007). Individual difference and sport fans: Who roots for the underdog? *Dissertation Abstracts International, 67*(8B), 4750.

Yamagata, S., Suzuki, A., Ando, J., Ono, Y., Kijima, N., Yoshimura, K., et al. (2006). Is the genetic structure of human personality universal?: A cross-cultural twin study from North America, Europe, and Asia. *Journal of Personality and Social Psychology, 90*, 987–998.

Zuckerman, M., Kuhlman, D. M., Joireman, J., Teta, P., & Kraft, M. (1993). A comparison of three structural models for personality: The Big Three, the Big Five, and the Alternative Five. *Journal of Personality and Social Psychology, 65*, 757–768.

CHAPTER 18

■ ● ▲ ◆ ■ ● ▲ ◆

Locus of Control and Attribution Style

Adrian Furnham

Locus of control and attributional style are closely related cognitive dispositions involving beliefs that are relatively stable over time but changeable. Although both constructs have been correlated with traditional traits, such as the Eysenckian "Giant Three" or Costa and McCrae's "Big Five," trait psychologists have not generally attempted to integrate cognitive individual differences into their models or to plot cognitive personality concepts in personality factor space. Yet there is a vast interdisciplinary literature on locus of control and attribution style in clinical, social, educational, health, and organizational psychology that attests to the importance of these variables in understanding individual differences. By the end of 2007, there were nearly 2,500 citations to Rotter (1966) and more than 750 citations to Rotter (1975); seminal articles on locus of control. Similarly, articles on attributional style have shown similar figures attesting to their influence: Abramson, Seligman, and Teasdale (1978) has more than 2,750 citations, Maier and Seligman (1976) more than 800 citations, and Peterson and colleagues (1982) more than 750 citations.

According to Weiner (1980), the popularity of his work on locus on control took Rotter by surprise: "Alluding to the widespread use of this scale, Rotter once confided, 'I was walking in the wood, lit my pipe and threw away the match and when I looked behind me there was a forest fire'" (p. 237). Rotter (1990) later attempted to explain the "enormous and somewhat surprising popularity" of the internal versus external control of reinforcement construct. He attributed the heuristic value of the variable to four factors: The variable was precisely defined; the variable construct was imbedded in a broader theory (namely social learning theory); the scale developed to measure this variable was derived from psychological theory (providing the best assurance of construct validity); and the construct was widely disseminated in a research monograph. The same factors could not be said to have contributed to the popularity of attributional style, but, even so, the concept of attribution/explanatory style has remained a popular research topic for more than 30 years.

This chapter is divided into two major sections, one dealing with locus of control and the other with attributional style. In each section the concept is defined and relevant research described. Critiques and revisions of each concept are also dealt with. Along the way, the chapter examines three basic issues that mark this research endeavor: the robustness of the theoretical issues underlying the various concepts in this area, the effort to develop context- or content-specific measures that aim to test highly specific control beliefs, and the application of the attribution theory and measures, particularly in the areas of clinical, health, work/vocational, and sport psychology. The chapter also describes many of the scales that have been developed to measure these concepts.

Locus of Control

Locus of control refers to the belief that a behavioral response will or will not influence the attainment of reinforcement. Rotter (1966) defined locus of control as follows:

> When a reinforcement is perceived by the subject as ... not being entirely contingent upon his action, then, in our culture, it is typically perceived as the result of luck, chance, fate, as under the control of powerful others, or as unpredictable because of the great complexity of the forces surrounding him. When the event is interpreted in this way by an individual, we have labelled this a belief in external control. If the person perceived that the event is contingent upon his own behaviour or his own relatively permanent characteristics, we have termed this a belief in internal control. (p. 1)

Rotter's (1966) locus-of-control concept was initially assessed with a 29-item self-report inventory, the Internal–External Control Scale (I–E Scale). Each item has a forced-choice format with an internal belief pitted against an external belief that is classifiable into one of six subcategories: academic recognition, social recognition, love and affection, dominance, social-political beliefs, and life philosophy. Rotter (1975) indicated that the scale "was developed not as an instrument ... to allow for a very high prediction of some specific situation, such as achievement or political behaviour, but rather to allow for a low degree of prediction of behaviour across a wide range of potential situations" (p. 62). Although situational cues in a setting were seen as the most potent influences on people's expectancy of reinforcement, generalized beliefs about control were also presumed to affect the expectancy of success across a wide array of environments. This instrument remains one of the most widely used scales in psychology. Indeed, the easy use of the test may in part account for the popularity of the concept.

Conceptual Issues

Many questions have arisen regarding the concept of locus of control, many of which have not been resolved. Rotter (1975) pointed out some of the conceptual and measurement problems associated with the internal–external concept, many of which remain crucially important yet frequently ignored.

Reinforcement Valence

First, Rotter pointed out that investigators often fail to treat reinforcement value (valence) as a separate variable. Behavioral outcomes and perceptions based on these outcomes are a function of both generalized expectancies and outcome value. Most assessments of locus of control, however, are concerned only with expectancies. Valence can be easily measured with a single scale that assesses the degree to which an outcome is salient, valuable, or important to the person, but researchers generally do not do this.

Specificity–Generality

Rotter (1975) noted confusion in the literature regarding specificity versus generality of locus-of-control beliefs. Researchers have often tried to predict specific behavior (often academic performance) by using scales that were designed to measure generalized expectancies for internal and external control. However, a scale designed to assess locus-of-control beliefs in the specific situation is required if accurate prediction of actions in specific situations is wanted (Rotter, 1975). Researchers have responded by developing many new locus-of-control scales for particular behaviors and domains.

Defensive Externality

Rotter (1975) described the phenomenon of defensive externality, in which people may verbally express what appear to be external locus-of-control beliefs as a defense against expected failure but act in an internal locus-of-control fashion in competitive situations. Defensive externality must be addressed to avoid confounding locus of control with other variables, such as performance or outcome anxiety. This is usually done by studying separate groups of low-anxiety externals and high-anxiety externals (Dawkins & Furnham, 1989).

Another approach to the problem of defensive externality may be to include questionnaire items that have been shown to elicit a fairly uniform internal attribution. If the experimental participant makes an external attribution on such an item, there may be good reason to infer that this response is defensively motivated. The possibility that defensive processes may influence locus-of-control judgments should also be considered in connection with the preceding discussion of reinforcement valence. That is, a person may verbally indicate that a certain reinforcement or outcome is not important as a defense against expected failure. Such a reaction might be described as "defensive undervaluation." This tendency goes hand in hand with the tendency toward defensive externality.

Healthy–Unhealthy Dichotomy

Much research starts with the assumption that having an internal locus of control is good, adaptive, and healthy, but that it is bad or maladaptive to have an external locus of control. Indeed, an overwhelming body of evidence suggests that internality is generally associated with more desirable characteristics and behaviors than externality. For example, internals are more likely to display many sorts of healthy and adaptive behaviors at school, work, and play (Lefcourt, 1991). However, it is questionable to assume that only positive attributes and actions are associated with internality. As people with an internal locus of control tend to take responsibility for the consequences of their actions more readily than externals, they are more likely to experience lower self-esteem when faced with failure. They may also respond to uncontrollable events less well than externals. Therefore, externality may sometimes be associated with altruism and collectivist attitudes and internality with selfish and ruggedly individualistic modes of action.

Not all conceptualizations of locus of control involve only the internal and external dimensions. More complex conceptualizations provide a means of exploring the interrelationships of different varieties of internal and external locus-of-control beliefs (Wall-

ston & Wallston, 1981). Tremendous situation specificity and intraindividual variation may exist across domains of activity and settings. In this sense, a person may be internal with regard to one set of activities or actions and external with regard to another. This seeming contradiction may be both perfectly explicable in terms of the person's life experiences and highly adaptable.

Self versus Other

People may maintain different locus-of-control belief systems for themselves and for others (Furnham & Steele, 1993; Gurin, Gurin, Lao, & Beattie, 1969). For example, an individual's profile of expectancy beliefs may show that he or she has an internal locus of control when assessing other people's behavior but an external locus of control with respect to him- or herself. Or a person may be an instrumentalist with regard to his or her own beliefs and behaviors but react to others as if they were fatalists or at least at the mercy of forces beyond their control. Furthermore, people may hold person-specific as well as situation-specific locus-of-control beliefs, constituting multiple sets of beliefs that may overlap in differing degrees. Thus they may hold internal locus-of-control beliefs about themselves but external locus-of-control beliefs about their families or vice versa. The picture takes on added complexity when we consider that some of these beliefs are more or less defensively motivated.

Attributions of Cause, Responsibility, and Blame

The locus-of-control and attribution-of-cause literatures clearly overlap. The major difference between these concepts is that whereas attributional measures are concerned with the *causes of past events*, locus of control measures are concerned mainly with the *expectation of future events*. Hence the paradox that although an *external* ascription can be made about the physical or psychological *cause* of an event—for example, failure to achieve a goal—an internal attribution may be made concerning responsibility if the consequence could have been foreseen. Causation and responsibility should therefore be treated as separate but related concepts. Locus of control is frequently associated with perceived cause but not responsibility (for future events), and the two operate quite differently. Locus-of-control beliefs are partially the product of causal attributional beliefs about past events and should be distinguished conceptually from both causal beliefs and responsibility beliefs.

Stability and Temporality

People may hold more internal beliefs for outcomes that are temporally distant because they are separated from present actions by various intervening or confounding events. Thus locus-of-control beliefs for events imminent in the short term may differ from beliefs for events expected to occur only in the long term. This possibility may affect the stability of the locus of control patterns, which may be stable or unstable depending on what is being predicted. This issue has not been addressed in the use of the locus-of-control scales.

Cause, Effect, and Reciprocity

To what extent do locus-of-control beliefs determine attributional style, or to what extent are locus-of-control beliefs determined by experiences that shape attributions? Various cycles of influence have been proposed such that pessimistic or optimistic attributional styles are likely to become self-perpetuating. Positive successful life experiences probably increase internal locus-of-control beliefs through optimistic attributions that, in turn, may increase confidence, initiative, and motivation and lead to more successful experiences. The opposite may occur with negative, unsuccessful life experiences that leave people feeling at the mercy of powerful and hostile forces beyond their control, thereby increasing external locus of control.

Methodological Issues

Three primary methodological issues apply to both the locus-of-control and attribution literatures.

Dimensionality

A major issue concerns whether the locus-of-control measure is uni- or multidimensional (Ashkanasy, 1985). Both Rotter (1966) and Franklin (1963) reported that the Rotter Internal–External Locus of Control Scale was unidimensional, but a number of later studies did not replicate their results. Gurin and colleagues (1969) and Sanger and Walker (1972) reported two factors involving personal control and control ideology, whereas Mirels (1970) and Cherlin and Bourque (1974) found two different factors (general control and political control). Collins (1974), who separated item pairs for the analysis, reported four factors, and Schneider and Parsons (1970) isolated five.

Empirical and theoretical analyses by Levenson (1981) suggested that the inconsistencies and inadequacies of the I–E Scale would be improved by making a distinction in the external scale between believing in powerful others who control the world and believing that the world is merely unordered and unpredictable. In the former case, a potential for control exists, whereas in the latter it does not. On this basis, Levenson developed the Internal, Powerful Others, Chance (IPC) Scales, which have been extensively used. Similarly, Wallston, Wallston, and De Vellis (1978) used these dimensions in their revised multidimensional health locus-of-control scale (Marshall, Collins, & Crooks, 1990).

O'Brien (1981) attempted to clarify the issue further by introducing two positions between internal and external locus-of-control beliefs. He proposed four dimensions: *internals* (who believe in internal control across all situations), *realists* (whose internal and external beliefs vary as a function of the domain or situation they consider), *structuralists* (whose external beliefs stress societal determinants of behavior), and *fatalists* (who see all outcomes as dependent on luck, fate, or chance).

Although several efforts have been made to distinguish different varieties of external locus-of-control beliefs, few researchers have attempted to subdivide the internal belief pattern—Bradley, Brewin, Gamsu, and Moses (1984) and Furnham, Sadka, and Brewin (1991) being exceptions. Internality (or instrumentality) may result from either effort or ability. That is, by exercising sufficient salient effort, one may control outcomes; or, simply by virtue of one's ability, certain outcomes can be controlled.

Outcome Valence

Many researchers have pointed out that locus-of-control beliefs include both positive (successful) and negative (unsuccessful) outcomes. Brewin and Shapiro (1984) provided support for Gregory's (1978) finding that locus-of-control beliefs for positive outcomes can be viewed as two separate dimensions. They found that beliefs about responsibility for positive outcomes predicted exam performance, whereas responsibility for negative outcomes predicted self-esteem more than performance itself. Unlike Gregory, though, Brewin and Shapiro found that the Rotter I–E Scale correlated with responsibility for positive outcomes and not with responsibility for negative outcomes.

Domain Specificity

Researchers have known for some time that attitudes predict behavior more strongly when both attitudes and behavior are measured at the same level of specificity. Along the same lines, scales that measure locus-of-control beliefs in specific domains predict behavior better than scales that measure general locus of control. However, there have been three quite distinct approaches to domain specificity. The *first approach* divides perceived control into different behavioral spheres, as when Paulhus and Christie (1981) distinguished four domains involving personal achievement (personal efficacy), interactions with other people in dyads and group situations (interpersonal control), the political and social system (sociopolitical control), and instances in which the person tries to control him- or herself (as in conflicts of self-discipline and self-actualization). Paulhus and Christie developed a measure that entails a systematic positioning of the individual's control expectancy in these specific spheres or activities.

A *second approach* is typified by Rothbaum, Weisz, and Snyder (1982), who redefined control in terms of four types of control (predictive, illusory, vicarious, and interpretive) and two processes—primary control (bringing the environment into line with one's wishes) and secondary control (bringing themselves into line with environmental forces). They believed that when perceived control is recognized in both its primary and secondary forms, a broad range of inward behaviors can be seen as efforts to sustain rather than relinquish control (Weisz, Rothbaum, & Blackburn, 1984).

The *third approach* is to devise a questionnaire that measures behavior in a specific domain, such as work-related or health-related domains. For example, in the health psychology literature, one sees measures such as the Australian Health Locus of Control Scale (Roberts & Ho, 1996) and the New Disease-Specific Health Locus of Control Scale (Dahnke, Garlick, & Kazoleas, 1994). These highly specific scales often relate to a very narrow range of behaviors, such as drinking of alcoholic beverages (Donovan & O'Leary, 1978) or trying to prevent accidents at work (Jones & Wuebker, 1985). This approach, which appears to have caused the proliferation of so many new locus-of-control scales, is motivated much more by practical issues specific to the domain of inquiry than by theoretical issues concerning the locus-of-control concept.

Review of Locus-of-Control Measures

Lefcourt (1991) reviewed 16 locus-of-control scales, providing evidence and a commentary on their psychometric validity, and Furnham and Steele (1993) reviewed nearly 25 years of scale development. They separated the 56 different measures into general locus-of-control scales (7), health locus-of-control scales (28), children and adolescent locus-of-control scales (10), the Nowicki–Strickland Life Span scales (5), and work locus-of-control scales. Since these reviews appeared, even more scales have been developed, refined, and tested, such as the Strategic Locus-of-Control Scale (Hodgkinson, 1992), the Vocational Locus-of-Control Scale (Fournier & Jeanrie, 1999), and the improbably named Alcohol-Related God Locus-of-Control Scale for Adolescents (Goggin, Murray, Malcarne, Brown, & Wallston, 2007). One area that has drawn scale construction efforts over the past decade is religion with respect to health. Hence, we now have the Spiritual Health Locus-of-Control Scale (Holt, Clark, Kreuter, & Rubio, 2003) and the God Locus of Health Control Scale (Wallston et al., 1999). There has also been a renewed interest in locus-of-control beliefs with respect to the environment (Schmidt & Gifford, 1989).

In their review of the extant locus-of-control measures, Furnham and Steele (1993) noted the ongoing proliferations of measures that often correlate only modestly with one another. They also raised the fundamental question of whether new scales show incremental validity beyond that provided by existing scales. Furthermore, many of the measures have not considered some of the theoretical distinctions, such as locus versus controllability and positive versus negative outcomes, that have been demonstrated to be important to people's beliefs about control. Researchers who have recognized the importance of these issues have tended to move toward attributional style instruments based on the work of Seligman (Abramson et al., 1978) rather than the relatively simple unidimensional structure found in Rotter's (1966) scale.

A second, more practical issue concerns whether locus-of-control beliefs can be altered by educational or therapeutic interventions. Many researchers assume that the purpose of designing locus-of-control scales is to identify people whose beliefs are maladaptive so that they can be helped. Yet few researchers have discussed the issue of whether locus-of-control beliefs can be targeted by different treatments or how effective such interventions are. An extensive literature in cognitive therapy addresses this issue, but it appears to have been ignored by those who have designed locus-of-control measures.

Whereas the locus-of-control enterprise has been primarily psychometric, the attributional-style literature has been primarily clinical. Locus-of-control researchers have been more interested in measurement, and attributional-style researchers more concerned with cognitive change. Thus, whereas research interest on locus of control appears to have peaked, the same is not true of attribution or explanatory style.

Attribution and Explanatory Style

The concepts of attribution style and explanatory style are used interchangably in the literature. During the 1980s a great deal of research inspired by attribution theory focused on the processes that underlie how people explain the events (particularly successes and failures) in their lives (Hewstone, 1989). At the same time, clinical psychologists, inspired by cognitive theories of depression, developed and extended learned helplessness theory (Abramson et al., 1978), which suggested that people develop a specific, pervasive, and highly consequential attributional or explanatory style for making sense of what happens to them. The theory asserted that these styles could be efficiently measured and, more important, changed through cognitive behavior therapy.

Attribution or explanatory style is concerned with how people explain or attribute the causes of success and failure, happiness and unhappiness, and other positive and negative experiences in a fairly consistent way. Early researchers tended to distinguish two styles that may reflect opposite ends of the same dimension, namely optimistic versus pessimistic attribution styles (sometimes called healthy vs. unhealthy). The early literature (from about 1980 to 2000) was mainly concerned with pessimistic attribution styles and the causes and consequences of attributing negative outcomes in a particular way. Nearly all the original work was in clinical psychology and was concerned with the cause and alleviation of depression. However, since the turn of the century, the interest has swung to positive emotions, happiness, and well-being.

The Concept of Style

This literature deals with attribution and explanatory *style*. The world *style* has different implications from terms such as *trait*, *temperament*, or *ability*, all of which imply greater stability and perhaps biological or genetic determinants. Furnham (2008) pointed out a number of unanswered problems with the concept of style. First, the question arises as to whether styles are biologically based, the result of early learning, neither, or both. Aetiology determines both how, and how much, a style may be changed and therefore developed. Second is the issue of variance accounted for. Specifically, is the amount of variance accounted for by style factors so small as to be trivial, or are these factors strongly related to people's emotions and actions? Do styles have incremental validity over ability, personality, and value measures? Third is the nature of style as a variable. If attribution style is a moderator variable between personality and mental health, the precise nature of this relationship needs to be spelled out. Fourth, little is known about a style's underlying mechanism. Most research in this field has been descriptive and taxonomic, aimed at identifying various styles and their correlates and consequences. Less work has gone into describing the mechanism or process whereby the style operates. In another critique of style constructs, Messick (1994) noted that "the literature of cognitive and learning styles is peppered with unstable and inconsistent findings, whereas style theory seems either vague in glossing over inconsistencies or confused in stressing differentiated features selectively" (p. 131). The question is to what extent this charge is true of the attribution-style literature as well.

Sternberg and Grigorenko (1997), however, defended the style concept. They stressed that:

> styles have a great deal of promise for the future. *First*, they have provided and continue to provide a much-needed interface between research on cognition and personality. *Second*, unlike some psychological constructs, they have lent themselves to operationalization and direct empirical tests. *Third*, they show promise for helping psychologists understand some of the variation in school and job performance that cannot be accounted for by individual differences in abilities. For example they predict school performance significantly and add to the prediction provided by ability tests. Finally they can truly tell something about environments as well as individuals' interactions with these environments, as shown by the fact that correlations of styles with performance that are significantly positive in one environment are significantly negative in another environment. (p. 710)

Measures and Research Domains

The most commonly used general measures of attributional style include the Causal Dimension Scale (McAuley, Duncan, & Russell, 1992), the Attribution Style Assessment Test (Anderson & Arnoult, 1985), the Context Analysis of Verbatim Explanations Technique (Peterson et al., 1982), and the Balanced Attributional Style Questionnaire (Feather, 1983). These scales assess people's

general tendency to make certain kinds of attributions across a variety of situations. In addition, several context-specific measures have been developed to assess attributional style in particular domains. For example, the Academic Attribution Style Questionnaire (Peterson & Barrett, 1987) assesses attributional style with respect to one's academic outcomes. In contrast, the Occupational Attribution Style Questionnaire (Furnham et al., 1991), Organizational Attributional Style Questionnaire (Kent & Martinko, 1995), and Work Attributional Style Questionnaire (Ashforth & Fugate, 2006) measure people's attributions for outcomes that occur in the workplace. There are also scales that measure attributional style for sport performance (the Sport Attributional Style Scale; Hanrahan, Grove & Hattie, 1989) and for events that occur in romantic relationships (the Relationship Attribution measure; Fincham & Bradbury, 1992).

Attributional-style research using these measures has shown the utility of the construct in many domains, including achievement, education, sport, and work, as well as in areas of therapy and training. Sometimes the research was stimulated by early researchers showing the relevance of attribution style to a particular type of behavior in a particular context. This is usually followed by the development of context-specific measures.

Classic attribution style relies on three fundamental dimensions. The *internal–external* dimension is essentially identical to the well-established locus-of-control dimension covered earlier. The second dimension is *stable–unstable*, referring to how changeable or malleable a cause was perceived to be. For example, lack of ability and physical size are relatively stable causes, whereas mood and education are less so. Luck, change, and fate are usually viewed as unstable causes, although they can also be regarded as stable in some instances (e.g., I am an unlucky person). The third dimension is *global-specific*, which involves how pervasive the effect of a cause is. Some perceived causes, such as an inability to communicate, may have widespread global consequences, whereas being color blind has much less overall effect. According to this system every attribution or explanation for an event can be categorized as shown in Figure 18.1.

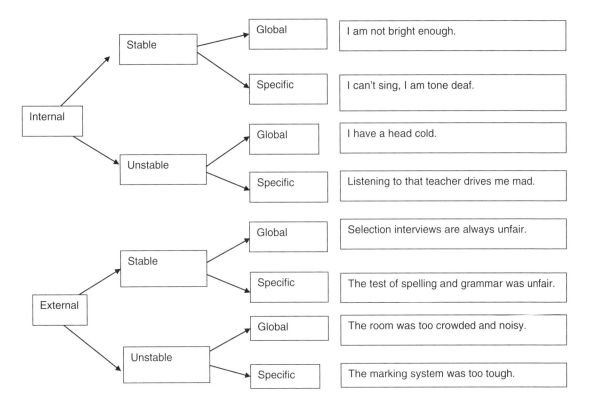

FIGURE 18.1. Examples of attributions based on the basic three dimensions.

Although people's attributions for a particular event are influenced by many factors, people tend to have a habitual pattern or style of attribution. The initial system suggested that there is an optimally healthy and adaptive versus unhealthy and maladaptive style. In this view, a maladaptive attributional style involves consistently or habitually attributing negative events in one's life (such as academic failure, divorce, job termination, or underachievement) to events that are internal, stable, and global while attributing positive events to external, unstable, and global causes.

Attributional Style: Depression, Work, Sport, and Loneliness

Three distinct literatures have arisen around the concept of attribution style. The "experimental academic" literature is most concerned with the measurement of style, as well as the theory behind it. The "applied" literature focuses on testing attribution-style ideas in settings such as education, work, and sport. The "clinical" literature is mainly concerned with links between attributional style and psychological problems, as well as the efficacy of attribution-based treatments.

Depression

A vast literature has arisen on attribution style and depression. Studies have sought to show that the relationship between a pessimistic attributional or explanatory style and depression is cross-culturally consistent (Anderson, 1999), as well as present in a wide range of different groups (Kneebone & Dunmore, 2004). Longitudinal studies have shown that attribution style may lead to particular behaviors (e.g., teenage pregnancy) but may change as a result of particular experiences (motherhood) (Wagner, Berenson, Harding, & Joiner, 1998). Some studies have shown that attribution style is more clearly linked with some types of depression (hopelessness) rather than others (endogenous) (Joiner, 2001). Overall, the results clearly and consistently show that attribution style is one of the vulnerability factors for depression. The tendency to make internal, stable, and global attributions for negative events predisposes people to experience the symptoms associated with depression, such as passivity, negative affect, psychosomatic problems associated with sleep and eating, and low self-esteem.

Furthermore, changing attribution style is a (short-term) successful treatment for depression. Indeed, the great popularity and widespread influence of cognitive therapy and cognitive-behavioral therapy could be seen as the direct application of attribution-style therapy to a range of conditions. What is not clear, however, is how easy it is to maintain an optimistic as opposed to a pessimistic attribution style and how style interacts with other vulnerability factors.

Studies have shown genetic influence on attribution style that has been thought to mediate genetic influences on depression (Lau, Rijsdijk, & Eley, 2006). Other studies have pointed to the instability of attribution style. Indeed, Ball, McGuffin, and Farmer (2008) suggested that attribution style is really little more than a mood state that does not reflect a risk factor for depression. They noted that "the way in which individuals attribute their experiences may be less of a risk factor and more of a symptom of depression than previously thought. Past episodes of depression may produce long-lasting negative attributions relating to the self, in addition to other pessimistic attributions that are linked to both observed and self reported current depression. It is therefore important to look out for and address these pessimistic attributions in people with recurrent depression." (p. 278).

Academic Performance

Peterson and Barrett (1987) published a longitudinal study that demonstrated that students' academic explanatory styles (i.e., why they performed as they did in college) measured 2 weeks into the academic year predicted their grades at the end of the year. Efforts to replicate this finding have been mixed, however. Some researchers suggest that the effect does not always replicate because of sample differences, range restrictions, or the low reliability of dependent variables. Others have suggested that other factors need to be taken into consideration. Academic success is influenced by students' ability (intelligence), personality, and learning style, as well as their attribution styles (Furnham, 2008). Indeed, researchers have demonstrated clear and predictable relationships between these variables (Cheng & Furnham, 2000).

Work Settings

A good example of applied psychological interest involves attribution style in work settings. In a seminal and often-cited paper, Seligman and Schulman (1986) studied 94 experienced life insurance sales agents who as a result of their jobs repeatedly encounter failure, rejection, and indifference from prospective clients. In testing the link between explanatory style and work productivity and quitting, they found that, as predicted, agents who saw failure as caused by internal, stable, and global factors initiated fewer sales attempts, were less persistent, produced less, and quit more frequently than those with a more optimistic explanatory style. The results also showed that agents who had optimistic explanatory styles sold 37% more insurance in their first 2 years of service than those with pessimistic styles. More strikingly, agents in the top decile sold 88% more insurance than those in the bottom decile. In a prospective 1-year study of 103 newly hired agents, individuals who had optimistic explanatory styles when hired remained in their jobs twice as long and sold more insurance than agents with more pessimistic explanatory styles (Seligman & Shulman, 1986). Corr and Gray (1996) replicated this finding, and Furnham and colleagues (1991) showed that attribution style was linked, as predicted, to job satisfaction and motivation. Furthermore, Furnham, Brewin, and O'Kelly (1994) found that it also predicted job involvement and organizational commitment. More recently, Ashforth and Fugate (2006) showed a link between attributional style and work adjustment. In light of such findings, organizational psychologists have been particularly interested in the attributional-style concept, although measuring it has sometimes proved problematic.

Sports Behavior and Performance

Another example is taken from the world of sports. A study by McAuley and Gross (1983) involving college table tennis players found that the attributions of winning players tended to be more internal, stable, and global than those of losing players. In another imaginative experiment, Seligman (1990) showed how attribution style affected sports performance. Swimmers were asked to swim their best events and were subsequently informed that their times were slightly slower than they actually were. After an appropriate rest period, the simmers reswam their events. The resulting performances showed that swimmers with a pessimistic explanatory style swam significantly slower than their initial times, whereas those with an optimistic explanatory style did not differ from their initial races. This finding suggests that a pessimistic explanatory style may reduce motivation and response initiation after a defeat, whereas an optimistic style facilitates a consistent level of motivation and performance. Along the same lines, Gordon (2008) found that soccer and basketball players who had optimistic attributional styles performed better than those with pessimistic styles.

Problems in Living

Another application of the attributional-style literature has been to what one might call "problems in living" (Anderson, 1999). Certainly the prototype of a lonely person (and that of a depressed individual) suggests that they habitually attribute social failure to characterological defects in themselves. That is, they believe that they fail to get social invitations and maintain and initiate social relationships because of unchangeable trait-like deficits in themselves. Anderson demonstrated this pattern in range of important studies (Anderson, Miller, Riger, Dill, & Sedikides, 1994). Furthermore, in a 2-year longitudinal study, Toner and Heaven (2005) found that attributional style predicted both depression and loneliness over a 2-year period.

Measurement Issues

Researchers concur that it is difficult to measure attributional style. In most questionnaires, respondents read vignettes of events that are important to their lives. Typically, these stories involve either success or failure in the sense that the event leads to positive or negative outcomes. Participants are encouraged to imagine themselves in these situations vividly and to write down the most likely cause for that particular outcome. They then rate the cause on a number of dimensions. The example from Furnham and colleagues (1991) in Figure 18.2 is a good, comprehensive example.

Attribution-style measures minimally assess ratings of internality, controllability, and globality for positive and negative events that may be aggregated into scores for optimistic and pessimistic attribution styles. However, aggregate scales often show unacceptable levels of internal reliability (Xenikou, Furnham, & McCarrey, 1997), even though locus-of-control measures often have very good reliability (Cronbach's alpha > .7).

Researchers have been puzzled and frustrated by the psychometric weakness of many of these scales, and various writers have tried to offer solutions to the dilemma. Xenikou and colleagues (1997) maintained that the evidence points to the fact that internal and external attributions for positive events are not opposites but rather are orthogonal. Thus, to improve the internal reliability of measures of internality, one must distinguish between various dimensions of internality. Kinderman and Bentall (1997) also made suggestions for measurement that were followed up by Day and Maltby (2000). Their studies showed that low reliability is due to aggregating attributional dimensions into higher level categories.

Conclusion

Few areas of individual psychology have seen such an enthusiastic conceptual uptake and measurement development as the related topics of locus of control and attribution style. Even though psychometricians and theoreticians have been frustrated with

1.	To what extent was the cause due to something about you?							
Totally due to me		6	5	4	3	2	1	Not all due to me
2.	In the future, at work, will this cause again influence what happens?							
Will never again influence what happens		6	5	4	3	2	1	Will always influence what happens
3.	Is the cause something that just affects problem solving or does it influence other areas of your life?							
Influence just this situation		6	5	4	3	2	1	Influences all areas of my life
4.	To what extent was the cause to do with other people or circumstances?							
Totally due to other people or circumstances		6	5	4	3	2	1	Not at all due to other people or circumstances
5.	To what extent was the cause due to chance?							
Totally due to chance		6	5	4	3	2	1	Not at all due to chance
6.	To what extent was the cause controllable by you?							
Totally controllable by me		6	5	4	3	2	1	Not at all controllable by me
7.	To what extent was the cause controllable by your colleagues?							
Totally controllable by my colleagues		6	5	4	3	2	1	Not at all controllable by my colleagues
8.	To what extent do you think you could have foreseen the cause?							
Totally foreseeable by me		6	5	4	3	2	1	Not at all foreseeable by me
9.	How important would the situation be if it happened to you?							
Not at all important		6	5	4	3	2	1	Extremely important

FIGURE 18.2. A rating scale for each cause given by a participant for an event.

some aspects of theoretical clarity and measurement, clinical practitioners have embraced the ideas and developed training and therapeutic interventions that build on these concepts. On the whole, differential psychologists interested in one of the two worlds of ability and personality have shown less interest in the other concept. This is not to imply that there have not been efforts to locate locus of control in "five factor space" or at Carroll's (1993) level II of intelligence but rather that trait psychologists have not been as interested in these concepts. There may be many reasons for this. For example, both constructs originate from social learning theory, which, at least traditionally, did not favor ideas of stable individual differences. In addition, there have been few attempts to look at biological markers of locus of control or attributional style. Indeed, both are seen as learned individual differences that can and sometimes should be unlearned. There is still a discomfort at the heart of the locus-of-control and attribution-style literatures about the conceptualization of style as stable and sometimes resistant to change.

The psychometrician looking at this literature may be disturbed by scale proliferation that has been fueled by the belief that domain-specific measures perform better than general ones. Dozens of scales have appeared and then disappeared after one or two studies that were in some senses little more than pilot studies of a new questionnaire. Although it is easy to demonstrate face and concurrent validity, the development of a reliable and robust measure needs to demonstrate predictive and incremental validity. Unfortunately, few of these studies have sufficiently established predictive and incremental validity, so it remains an open question whether specific measures tailored to a particular domain achieve better results than general measures. Perhaps it would be wise to call a moratorium on the development of new scales until the nature of existing scales is better understood.

Psychometricians would also, no doubt, be displeased with the psychometric quality of many attribution-style questionnaires, which often show poor internal reliability and weak concurrent validity. Paradoxically, these style measures even have difficulty measuring the control dimension of locus of control, namely the internal–external dimension that is most central to the construct.

Practicing psychologists in counseling, clinical, educational, industrial–organizational, and sports psychology have done the most not only to keep alive and proselytize the locus-of-control and attribution-style concepts but also to implement treatment programs aimed at changing people's styles when they become dysfunctional. Indeed, one could argue that the most popular of all therapies, cognitive-behavioral therapy, is the "applied child" of attribution-style theory. With the growth of positive psychology, locus-of-control and attribution-style theories and concepts may become even more popular, although the focus may switch from beliefs that promote dysfunction to those that enhance well-being.

References

Abramson, L., Seligman, M., & Teasdale, J. (1978). Learned helplessness in humans: Critique and reformulation. *Journal of Abnormal Psychology, 87,* 32–40.

Anderson, C. (1999). Attribution style, depression, and loneliness. *Personality and Social Psychology Bulletin, 25,* 482–499.

Anderson, C., Miller, R., Riger, A., Dill, J., & Sedikides, C. (1994). Behavioural and characterological attribution styles as predictors of depression and loneliness. *Journal of Personality and Social Psychology, 66,* 549–558.

Anderson, C. A., & Arnoult, L. H. (1985). Attributional style and everyday problems in living: Depression, loneliness and shyness. *Social Cognition, 3,* 16–35.

Ashforth, B., & Fugate, M. (2006). Attribution style in work settings: Development of a measure. *Journal of Leadership and Organizational Studies, 12,* 12–29.

Ashkanasy, N. (1985). Rotter's internal–external scale: Confirmatory factor analysis and correlation with social desirability for alternative scale formats. *Journal of Personality and Social Psychology, 48,* 1328–1341.

Ball, H., McGuffin, P., & Farmer, A. (2008). Attribution style and depression. *British Journal of Psychiatry, 192,* 275–278.

Bradley, C., Brewin, C. R., Gamsu, D., & Moses, J. (1984). Development of scales to measure perceived control of diabetes mellitus and diabetes-related health beliefs. *Diabetic Medicine, 1,* 213–218.

Brewin, C., & Shapiro, D. (1984). Beyond locus of control: Attribution of responsibility for positive and negative outcomes. *British Journal of Psychology, 15,* 43–50.

Carroll, J. (1993). *Human cognitive abilities.* New York: Cambridge University Press.

Cheng, H., & Furnham, A. (2000). Attribution style and personality as predictors of happiness and mental health. *Journal of Happiness Studies, 2,* 307–327.

Cherlin, A., & Bourque, L. (1974). Dimensionality and reliability of the Rotter I–E scale. *Sociometry, 37,* 565–582.

Collins, B. (1974). Four components of the Rotter internal–external scale. *Journal of Personality and Social Psychology, 29,* 381–391.

Corr, P., & Gray, J. A. (1996). Attributional style as a personality factor in insurance sales performance in the UK. *Journal of Occupational and Organisational Psychology, 69,* 83–87.

Dahnke, G., Garlick, R., & Kazoleas, D. (1994). Testing a new disease-specific health locus of control among cancer and aplastic anaemia patients. *Health Communication, 6,* 37–53.

Dawkins, K., & Furnham, A. (1989). The colour naming of emotional words. *British Journal of Psychology, 80,* 383–389.

Day, L., & Maltby, J. (2000). Can Kinderman and Bentall's suggestions for a personal and situational attributions questionnaire be used to examine all aspects of attribution style? *Personality and Individual Differences, 29,* 1047–1053.

Donovan, D., & O'Leary, M. (1978). The drinking-related locus of control scale: Reliability, factor structure and validity. *Journal of Studies on Alcohol, 39,* 759–784.

Feather, N. (1983). Causal attributions for good and bad outcomes in achievement and affiliation situations. *Australian Journal of Psychology, 35,* 37–48.

Fincham, F. D., & Bradbury, T. N. (1992). Assessing attributions in marriage: The Relational Attribution Measure. *Journal of Personality and Social Psychology, 62,* 457–468.

Fournier, G., & Jeanrie, C. (1999). Validation of a five-level locus of control scale. *Journal of Career Assessment, 7,* 63–89.

Franklin, R. (1963). *Youth's expectancies about internal vs. external control reinforcement related to N variables.* Unpublished doctoral dissertation, Purdue University.

Furnham, A. (2008). *Personality and intelligence at work.* London: Routledge.

Furnham, A., Brewin, C., & O'Kelly, H. (1994). Cognitive style and attitudes to work. *Human Relations, 47,* 1509–1521.

Furnham, A., Sadka, V., & Brewin, C. (1991). The development of an occupational attributional style questionnaire. *Journal of Organisational Behaviour, 13*, 27–39.

Furnham, A., & Steele, H. (1993). Measuring locus of control. *British Journal of Psychology, 84*, 443–479.

Goggin, K., Murray, T., Malcarne, V., Brown, S., & Wallston, K. (2007). Do religious and control cognitions predict risky behaviour?: I. Development and validation of the Alcohol-Related God Locus-of-Control Scale for Adolescents (AGLOC-A). *Cognitive Research and Therapy, 31*, 111–122.

Gordon, R. (2008). Attribution style and athletic performance. *Psychology of Sport and Exercise, 9*, 336–350.

Gregory, W. (1978). Locus of control for positive and negative outcomes. *Journal of Personality and Social Psychology, 36*, 840–849.

Gurin, P., Gurin, G., Lao, R., & Beattie, M. (1969). Internal–external control in the motivation dynamics of Negro youth. *Journal of Social Issues, 25*, 29–53.

Hanrahan, S., Grove, J. R., & Hattie, J. A. (1989). Development of a questionnaire measure of sport-related attributional style. *International Journal of Sport Psychology, 20*, 144–134.

Hewstone, M. (1989). *Causal attribution*. Oxford, UK: Blackwell.

Hodgkinson, G. (1992). Research notes and communications development and validation of the strategic locus of control scale. *Management Journal, 13*, 311–317.

Holt, C., Clark, E., Kreuter, M., & Rubio, D. (2003). Spiritual health locus of control and breast cancer beliefs among African American women. *Health Psychology, 22*, 294–299.

Joiner, T. (2001). Negative attribution style, hopelessness, depression and endogenous depression. *Behavioural Research and Therapy, 39*, 139–149.

Jones, J., & Wuebker, L. (1985). Development and validation of the safety locus of control scale. *Perceptual and Motor Skills, 61*, 151–161.

Kent, R. L., & Martinko, M. J. (1995). The development and evaluation of a scale to measure organizational attributional style. In M. J. Martinko (Ed.), *Attribution theory: An organizational perspective* (pp. 53–75). Delray Beach, FL: St. Lucie Press.

Kinderman, P., & Bentall, R. (1997). Causal attributions in paranoia: Internal, personal, and situational attributions for negative events. *Journal of Abnormal Psychology, 106*, 341–345.

Kneebone, I., & Dunmore, E. (2004). Attribution style and symptoms of depression in persons with multiple sclerosis. *International Journal of Behavioural Medicine, 11*, 110–115.

Lau, J., Rijsdijk, F., & Eley, T. (2006). I think therefore I am: A twin study of attributional style in adolescents. *Journal of Child Psychology and Psychiatry, 47*, 696–703.

Lefcourt, H. (1991). Locus of control. In J. Robinson, P. Shaver, & L. Wrightsman (Eds.), *Measures of personality and social psychological attitudes* (Vol. 1, pp. 413–499). New York: Academic Press.

Levenson, H. (1981). Differentiating among internally powerful others and chance. In H. M. Lefcourt (Ed.), *Research with the locus of control construct* (Vol. 1, pp. 15–63). New York: Academic Press.

McAuley, E., Duncan, T. E., & Russell, D. W. (1992). Measuring causal attributions: The Revised Causal Dimension Scale (CDSII). *Personality and Social Psychology Bulletin, 18*, 566–573.

McAuley, E., & Gross, J. (1983). Perceptions of causality in sport. *Journal of Sport Psychology, 5*, 72–76.

Maier, S., & Seligman, M. (1976). Learned helplessness: Theory and evidence. *Journal of Experimental Psychology, 105*, 3–46.

Marshall, G., Collins, B., & Crooks, V. (1990). A comparison of two multidimensional health locus of control instruments. *Journal of Personality Assessment, 54*, 181–190.

Messick, S. (1994). The matter of style: Manifestations of personality in cognition, learning and teaching. *Educational Psychologist, 29*, 121–136.

Mirels, H. (1970). Dimensions of internal vs. external control. *Journal of Consulting and Clinical Psychology, 34*, 226–228.

O'Brien, G. (1981). Locus of control, work, and retirement. In H. Lefcourt (Ed.), *Research with the locus of control construct* (Vol. 3, pp. 7–71). London: Academic Press.

Paulhus, D., & Christie, R. (1981). Spheres of control: An interactionist approach to assessment of perceived control. In H. Lefcourt (Ed.), *Research with the locus of control construct* (Vol. 1, pp. 161–188). New York: Academic Press.

Peterson, C., & Barrett, L. C. (1987). Explanatory style and academic performance among university freshmen. *Journal of Personality and Social Psychology, 53*, 603–607.

Peterson, C., Semmel, A., Von Baeyer, C., Abramson, L., Metalsky, G., & Seligman, M. (1982). The Attributional Style Questionnaire. *Cognitive Therapy and Research, 6*, 281–300.

Roberts, L., & Ho, R. (1996). Development of an Australian health locus of control scale. *Personality and Individual Differences, 20*, 629–639.

Rothbaum, F., Weisz, J., & Snyder, R. (1982). Changing the world and changing the self: A two process model of perceived control. *Journal of Personality and Social Psychology, 42*, 5–37.

Rotter, J. (1966). Generalised expectancies for internal versus external control of reinforcement. *Psychological Monographs, 80*(1), Whole No. 609.

Rotter, J. (1975). Some problems and misconceptions related to the construct of internal versus external control of reinforcement. *Journal of Consulting and Clinical Psychology, 43*, 56–67.

Rotter, J. (1990). Internal versus external control of reinforcement: A case history of a variable. *American Psychologist, 45*, 489–493.

Sanger, S., & Walker, H. (1972). Dimensions of internal–external control and the women's liberation movement. *Journal of Social Issues, 28*, 115–129.

Schmidt, F., & Gifford, R. (1989). A dispositional approach to hazard perception. *Journal of Environmental Psychology, 9*, 57–67.

Schneider, J., & Parsons, O. (1970). Categories on the locus of control scale and cross-cultural comparisons in Denmark and the United States. *Journal of Cross-Cultural Psychology, 2*, 131–138.

Seligman, M. (1990). *Learned optimism*. New York: Pocket Books.

Seligman, M., & Schulman, P. (1986). Exploratory

style as a predictor of productivity and quitting among life insurance sales agents. *Journal of Personality and Social Psychology, 50*, 832–830.

Sternberg, R., & Grigorenko, E. (1997). Are cognitive styles still in style? *American Psychologist, 52*, 700–712.

Toner, M., & Heaven, P. (2005). Peer social attributional predictors of socio-economic adjustment in early adolescence. *Personality and Individual Differences, 38*, 579–590.

Wagner, K., Berenson, A., Harding, O., & Joiner, T. (1998). Attribution style and depression in pregnant teenagers. *American Journal of Psychiatry, 155*, 1227–1233.

Wallston, K., & Wallston, B. (1981). Health locus of control scales. In H. Lefcourt (Ed.), *Research with the locus of control construct* (Vol. 1, pp. 189–241). New York: Academic Press.

Wallston, K., Wallston, B., & De Vellis, R. (1978). Development of the multidimensional health locus of control (MHLC) scales. *Health Education Monographs, 6*, 160–169.

Wallston, K. A., Malcarne, V. L., Flores, L., Hansdottir, I., Smith, C. A., Stein, M. J., et al. (1999). Does God determine your health?: The God Locus of Health Control Scale. *Cognitive Therapy and Research, 23*, 131–142.

Weiner, B. (1980). *Human motivation.* New York: Holt, Rinehart & Winston.

Weisz, J., Rothbaum, F., & Blackburn, T. (1984). Standing out and standing in: The psychology of control in America and Japan. *American Psychologist, 39*, 955–956.

Xenikou, A., Furnham, A., & McCarrey, M. (1997). Attribution style for negative events. *British Journal of Psychology, 88*, 53–69.

CHAPTER 19

■ ● ▲ ◆ ■ ● ▲ ◆

Belief in a Just World

CLAUDIA DALBERT

Conceptualization of the Belief in a Just World

Societies are full of inequalities and injustices—the disproportionate distribution of wealth and inequality of access to health care and education, to name just a few. Individuals react differently to observed or experienced injustice. Some feel moral outrage and seek to restore justice (e.g., Montada, Schmitt, & Dalbert, 1986). Others show disdain for the victims (for a review, see Lerner & Miller, 1978) or adopt belief systems that serve to justify existing social, economic, and political arrangements (Jost, Banaji, & Nosek, 2004). In other words, people confronted with injustices that are difficult to redress in reality may try to restore justice cognitively by blaming the victim or justifying the status quo.

The Just-World Hypothesis

Several psychological theories propose explanations for justice-driven reactions. One of the most influential is the just-world hypothesis introduced by Lerner (1965, 1980). The just-world hypothesis states that people need to believe in a just world in which everyone gets what they deserve and deserves what they get. This belief enables them to deal with their social environment as though it were stable and orderly and thus serves

important adaptive functions. As a result, people are motivated to defend their belief in a just world when it is threatened by injustices, either experienced or observed. If possible, justice is restored in reality (e.g., by compensating victims). If the injustice seems unlikely to be resolved in reality, however, people restore justice cognitively by reevaluating the situation in line with their belief in a just world. This cognitive process is called the *assimilation of injustice*.

This just-world dynamic was first evidenced by Lerner and Simmons (1966). These researchers confronted their participants with an "innocent victim," a young women participating in a learning task who was punished for each mistake by being administered seemingly painful electric shocks. When led to believe that the experiment would continue in the same way, the participants showed disdain for the victim on an adjective measure; when led to believe that the victim would be compensated for the pain of the electric shocks by receiving money for each correct answer in a second part of the experiment, they stopped showing disdain. Finally, nearly all participants who were given the choice between continuing the shock condition and switching to the compensation condition voted for the latter. Note, however, that merely voting to award the victim compensation did not stop participants from derogating the victim. It was only when they were certain that compensation would be given that the injustice was no longer assimilated. This innocent-victim paradigm remains the most influential in modern experimental just-world research; it is only the type of innocent victim that has changed (e.g., Correia, Vala, & Aguiar, 2007).

The Belief in a Just World as a Disposition

A substantial amount of research on belief in a just world has been experimental in nature (for a review, see Hafer & Bègue, 2005), focusing primarily on the maladaptive functions of the belief in a just world, such as disdain for the victim. Since the 1970s, however, another strand of research has examined individual differences in the belief in a just world and found that it also serves important adaptive functions (for a review, see Furnham, 2003). This research agenda was triggered by the introduction of the first Belief in a Just World Scale by Rubin and Peplau (1973, 1975), which assessed individual differences in the belief that the world is generally a just place. This approach allowed the role of the belief in a just world to be investigated within the framework of personality dispositions, and positive associations were found particularly with authoritarianism and internal locus of control (for a review, see Furnham & Procter, 1989).

Justice Motive versus Justice Motivation

In the context of just-world research and theory, scholars often speak of the justice motive (e.g., Ross & Miller, 2002). The shift from the experimental to the individual-differences approach to the belief in a just world made it necessary to differentiate between a justice motive and justice motivation. Motives are individual dispositions reflecting individual differences in the tendency to strive for a specific goal. A justice motive is thus an individual disposition to strive for justice as an end in itself. According to Lerner (1977), the individual belief in a just world can be interpreted as an indicator of such a justice motive. The belief in a just world indicates a personal contract; the more people want to rely on being treated justly by others, the more obligated they should feel to behave justly themselves.

Thus, the stronger the belief in a just world, the stronger the justice motive. Experimental just-world research typically does not assess individual differences, however, but interprets experimental reactions in the light of just-world reasoning. Such research thus addresses justice motivation, and not the justice motive as an individual-differences disposition. Motivation can be defined as a person's orientation toward a specific goal in a specific situational state; thus justice motivation means the orientation toward justice in a given situation. Justice motivation is triggered by specific situational circumstances in interaction with personal dispositions. In the case of justice motivation, that personal disposition may be the justice motive or other dispositions (e.g., Lind & van den Bos, 2002; Miller, 1999).

Differentiation of the Belief in a Just-World Disposition

Since the 1990s, more studies have investigated the positive as well as the negative social consequences of the belief in a just world, and the focus of these investigations has been extended to cover the consequences of holding a belief in a just world for the believers. Based on suggestions originating from earlier research (Furnham & Procter, 1989; Lerner & Miller, 1978), these studies have shown that it is necessary to distinguish the belief in a personal just world, in which one is usually treated fairly, from the belief in a general just world, or the belief in a just world for others in which people in general get what they deserve (Dalbert, 1999; Lipkus, Dalbert, & Siegler, 1996). In line with the self-serving bias in general (Taylor, Wright, Moghaddam, & Lalonde, 1990) and with fairness reasoning in particular (Messick, Bloom, Boldizar, & Samuelson, 1985), research evidenced that people tend to endorse the personal more strongly than the general belief in a just world and that the two constructs have a different meaning. The personal belief in a just world is a better predictor of adaptive outcomes (e.g., subjective well-being), and the belief in a just world for others or in general is a better predictor, for example, of harsh social attitudes (e.g., Bègue & Muller, 2006).

Of course, other differentiations of the just-world construct have also been proposed. To give just two examples for the general just-world belief: A general belief in immanent justice has been distinguished from a general belief in ultimate justice (Maes & Kals, 2002), and a general belief in distributive justice has been distinguished from a general belief in procedural justice (Lucas, Alexander, Firestone, & LeBreton, 2007). Finally, the general belief in a just world has been differentiated from the general belief in an *un*just world (Dalbert, Lipkus, Sallay, & Goch, 2001; Loo, 2002). This research showed that general belief in a just world should not be seen as a bipolar construct but as a two-dimensional one. Because the differentiation between a more general and a more personal just-world belief thus far seems to be the most widespread and well-examined distinction, however, this summary focuses on research on general and personal just-world beliefs.

Measures of the Belief in a Just World

The starting point for individual-differences research on the belief in a just world was Rubin and Peplau's (1975) 20-item Belief in a Just World Scale (sample items: "Basically, the world is a just place"; "Men who keep in shape have little chance of suffering a heart attack"; "Good deeds often go unnoticed and unrewarded"). This scale was later criticized as being heterogeneous in content (e.g., Furnham & Procter, 1989): It included both general and domain-specific items, as well as items on the belief in an unjust world and items tapping other constructs, such as authoritarianism (e.g., "When parents punish their children it is almost always for good reasons"). Consequently, some researchers used a subsample of the general items to assess general just-world belief (e.g., Steensma & van Dijke, 2006). In the light of these criticisms, two homogenous general just-world scales were developed. Dalbert, Montada, and Schmitt (1987) constructed a homogenous six-item scale tapping general belief in a just world (sample item: "I think people try to be fair when making important decisions"), which shows convergent validity with the Rubin and Peplau scale, is independent of social desirability (Loo, 2002), and has been used in numerous studies (e.g., Allen, Ng, & Leiser, 2005). In addition, Lipkus (1991) constructed a seven-item Global Belief in a Just World Scale that is positively associated with the Rubin and Peplau scale and has also been successfully implemented in several studies (e.g., Hafer, 2000). All three general just-world scales are positively correlated with each other (Lipkus et al., 1996). Surprisingly, however, although there are at least two homogenous, short, and valid measures of general just-world belief, the 20-item Rubin and Peplau scale is still in use (e.g., Edlund, Sagarin, & Johnson, 2007). Finally, in line with the differentiation of the just-world construct, Lipkus and colleagues (1996) and Dalbert (1999) introduced reliable scales differentiating the belief in a just world for others or, in general, from the belief in a personal just world.

Belief in a Just World and Other Personality Dispositions

One of the first associations observed between the belief in a just world and other personality dispositions was the positive correlation between general just-world belief and *religiosity* (Dalbert & Katona-Sallay, 1996; Rubin & Peplau, 1973). Research on the differences between the two has confirmed that they are distinct dispositions (e.g., Hui, Chan, & Chan, 1989), and cross-cultural research has found few differences in the just-world belief across cultures with contrasting religious and political backgrounds (e.g., Furnham, 1993). A positive and sometimes substantial association has also been found between *authoritarianism* and general just-world belief (for a review, see Furnham & Procter, 1989). Analyses of the common factor structure of the two constructs support the two-factor hypothesis and their differential meaning, with the belief in a just world providing a more positive outlook than authoritarianism (Dalbert, 1992; Lerner, 1978). The positive associations repeatedly observed between just-world belief and *internal locus of control* have prompted speculation about an overlap between these two constructs as well (for a review, see Furnham & Procter, 1989). The two constructs should be distinct from a theoretical perspective, however. The belief in personal agency is consistent with the belief in a just world as long as the justice principle endorsed is the equity norm. Other ideas of justice (e.g., the equality or the need principle of justice or the belief in a just God) are not consistent with the belief in internal control.

Finally, there is some evidence to suggest that the belief in a just world as a personality trait is correlated with *global personality dimensions*. In particular, empirical findings indicate a negative relationship between personal just-world belief and neuroticism, consistent with the positive outlook that the belief in a just world provides (e.g., Lipkus et al., 1996). Nevertheless, studies controlling for neuroticism evidenced the incremental validity of the personal just-world belief (e.g., Dalbert & Dzuka, 2004). Taken collectively, research supports the differential validity of the belief in a just world within the network of personality dispositions.

Functions of the Belief in a Just World

In the past decade, research has shown that the belief in a just world as a personality disposition serves at least three primarily adaptive functions and can thus be seen as a resource that sustains subjective well-being (Dalbert, 2001). This research is summarized in the following subsections.

Belief in a Just World and the Assimilation of Injustice

When individuals with a strong just-world belief experience an injustice that they do not believe can be resolved in reality, they try to assimilate the experience to their just-world belief. This can be done, for example, by justifying the experienced unfairness as being at least partly self-inflicted (e.g., Bulman & Wortman, 1977), by playing down the unfairness (Lipkus & Siegler, 1993), by avoiding self-focused rumination (Dalbert, 1997), or by forgiving (Strelan, 2007). As a result of these mechanisms, positive relationships have been observed between the belief in a just world and justice judgments in various domains of life. Most research into the assimilation function of the just-world belief have dealt with blaming the victim and justice judgments.

Blaming the Victim

A wealth of evidence from traditional research into the just-world construct shows that individuals confronted by unfairness are motivated to defend their just-world belief. When observers are given the opportunity to adequately compensate an "innocent" victim (e.g., Berscheid & Walster, 1967) and thus restore justice in reality, nearly all choose to do so (Lerner & Simmons, 1966). If they are not in a position to secure compensation for the victim, observers tend to defend their belief in a just world by psychological means. Two of these means have been examined in detail in just-world research. Observers can either show disdain for victims, reasoning that their fate is a deserved punishment for a bad character (characterological attribution), or they can blame victims for having inflicted their fate upon themselves—after all, a self-inflicted fate is not unfair (behavioral attribution). Just-world research has shown that observers prefer to blame the victim rather than to show disdain (e.g., Lerner, 1965). The more a fate is seen as self-inflicted, the less disdain is observed (e.g., Lerner & Matthews, 1967). In sum, when people are confronted with the victim of an unjust fate, blaming the victim seems to be a crucial element in the defense of their belief in a just world.

Similar mechanisms can be assumed to operate for the victims of injustice themselves. Comer and Laird (1975) have shown experimentally that internal attributions seem to be a way of reevaluating one's fate as just. The significance of causal attributions, and especially of internal attributions, has thus been a subject of much discussion in the context of the just-world hypothesis (e.g., Lerner & Miller, 1978). People with a strong just-world belief are expected to be motivated to defend their belief by making internal attributions of negative outcomes, thus maintaining their subjective well-being. Although some research evidenced the hypothesized positive association between just-world belief and internal attributions of the victims themselves (e.g., Hafer & Correy, 1999; Kiecolt-Glaser & Williams, 1987), other studies found no association between them (e.g., Agrawal & Dalal, 1993; Fetchenhauer, Jacobs, & Belschak (2005). Overall, then, the pattern of results for the belief in a just world and victims' internal attributions is rather mixed.

Justice Judgments

As a consequence of the assimilation process, individuals with a strong just-world belief are expected to evaluate observed events and events in their own lives as being more just. For example, school students with a strong belief in a personal just world have been found to be more likely to evaluate their school grades and their teachers', peers', and parents' behavior toward them as just (Correia & Dalbert, 2007; Dalbert & Stoeber, 2006). Similarly, prisoners with strong personal just-world beliefs are more likely to evaluate the justice of the legal proceedings leading to their conviction, the treatment by their prison officers, and decisions on prison affairs as more just (Dalbert & Filke, 2007; Otto & Dalbert, 2005).

The personal just-world belief is usually seen as a personal disposition, but results indicating a causal effect of justice experiences on the belief in a just world qualify this assumption. Research has shown that justice experiences in the school and the family modify the personal just-world belief (Dalbert & Stoeber, 2006) and that factors such as length of imprisonment (Otto & Dalbert, 2005), monotony at work, and mobbing experiences at work (Cubela Adoric & Kvartuc, 2007; Dzuka & Dalbert, 2007; Otto & Schmidt, 2007) are negatively related to the personal just-world belief. Thus the belief in a personal just world must be seen as a partly experiential construct (Maes & Schmitt, 2004). Nevertheless, an unambiguous pattern of results clearly indicates that a strong personal just-world belief leads to events being evaluated as just. Cubela Adoric and Kvartuc (2007) have suggested that injustice experiences only affect the belief in a just world when they reach a specific degree of adversity. Further studies are needed to determine under which conditions the just-world belief fosters the assimilation of injustice and under which conditions injustice can no longer be assimilated but instead undermines the belief in a just world.

Belief in a Just World and the Trust in Justice

People with a strong belief in a just world are thought to be confident in being treated justly by others, and it is this trust in particular that is hypothesized to give the just-world belief the character of a resource in everyday life. Assuming that people get what they deserve, they will be punished for deceiving others. Accordingly, in a just world, people are expected to be honest with one another, and people who have been deceived may conclude that they deserved it in some way. It can thus be hypothesized that people with a strong just-world belief prefer not to think they have been deceived or taken advantage of. Research has shown the expected positive association of just-world belief with general interpersonal trust (e.g., Bègue, 2002; Zuckerman & Gerbasi, 1977), trust in societal institutions (Correia & Vala, 2004), and young adolescents' trust in the justice of their future workplace (Sallay, 2004). This trust in future justice has a number of implications.

Risk Perception

Individuals with a strong just-world belief are convinced that good things happen to good people and that bad things happen to bad people. Because individuals tend to think of themselves as good people (e.g., Brown, 1986; Messick et al., 1985), the belief in a just world can be expected to give them an optimistic outlook on the future. This buffering effect is expected to be particularly evident when people are threatened by unfairness. Lambert, Burroughs, and Nguyen (1999) were the first to study the meaning of the belief in a just world for risk perception and showed that the just-world belief seems to enable fearful individuals (i.e., those high in authoritarianism) to be confident of avoiding an unjust fate. It is particularly important for individuals exposed to *external* risks (i.e., those perceived to be controlled by others or by fate; e.g., robbery) rather than to *internal* risks (i.e., those that are under their personal control; e.g., suicide) to be able to rely on the environment being fair. Indeed, Dalbert (2001) found that the buffering effect of the general just-world belief for fearful individuals held only for external risks, not for internal risks. Finally, Hafer, Bogaert, and McMullen (2001) found that individuals with strong general just-world beliefs but low in interpersonal control seem to put themselves at greater risk, presumably as a consequence of a lowered risk perception. In sum, the general just-world belief appears to function as a buffer against the perception of external risk for those who tend to need such a buffer, but this mechanism may result in higher exposure to risks in reality.

Investment in One's Future

The belief in a just world enables individuals to rely on their good deeds being rewarded at some point in the future. The certitude that everyone will ultimately get what they deserve encourages individuals to invest in their futures. In contrast, those who do not believe in a just world doubt the value of such an investment because the return on it is uncertain. Zuckerman (1975) was the first to observe that people with a strong just-world belief may choose to invest in their futures when in a state of need to trust in the fairness of their own futures. Hafer (2000) corroborated these findings and demonstrated experimentally that individuals with a particular need to believe in a bright future defended their just-world beliefs more strongly in the face of threat. In the same vein, questionnaire studies with samples of students facing the school-to-work transition (Dette, Stöber, & Dalbert, 2004), young male prisoners (Otto & Dalbert, 2005), and young adults living in assisted accommodation (Sutton & Winnard, 2007) have shown that the personal just-world belief is positively associated with confidence that personal goals will be attained.

Achievement Behavior

Individuals with strong beliefs in a just world show more trust in their future and in others' behavior toward them. It is thus hypothesized that they expect to be confronted with fair tasks in achievement situations and their efforts to be fairly rewarded. They can thus be hypothesized to feel less threatened and more challenged by the need to achieve, to experience fewer negative emotions, and to achieve better results. Tomaka and Blascovich (1994) conducted a laboratory study to test the basic hypotheses outlined herein and confronted their participants with two rapid serial subtraction tasks. Participants with strong general just-world beliefs felt more challenged and less threatened and performed better than those with weak beliefs. Extending this laboratory research to the school and work setting, studies have revealed a positive correlation between the personal just-world belief and school achievement (Dalbert, 2001; Dalbert & Stoeber, 2005, 2006) and self-rated per-

formance at work (Otto & Schmidt, 2007). Finally, Allen et al. (2005) have observed that nations whose citizens have stronger general just-world beliefs show a faster pace of workforce modernization and gross national product and per-capita growth.

Belief in a Just World as a Justice Motive Indicator

In a just world, a positive future is not the gift of a benevolent world but a reward for the individual's behavior and character. Consequently, the more individuals believe in a just world, the more compelled they should feel to strive for justice themselves. The just-world belief is thus indicative of a personal contract (Lerner, 1977), the terms of which oblige the individual to behave justly. Therefore, strong just-world believers are more likely to help people in need (Bierhoff, Klein, & Kramp, 1991), at least as long as the victims are seen as "innocent" (DePalma, Madey, Tillman, & Wheeler, 1999) or as members of the ingroup (Correia et al., 2007). In addition, the belief in a just world has been shown to be one of the important correlates of social responsibility (Bierhoff, 1994), commitment to just means (Cohn & Modecki, 2007; Hafer, 2000; Sutton & Winnard, 2007), and, inversely, rule-breaking behavior (Correia & Dalbert, 2008; Otto & Dalbert, 2005). Moreover, the obligation of reciprocity has been found to be stronger among individuals with a strong general just-world belief (Edlund et al., 2007). Finally, a laboratory study revealed that one's own unjust behavior is censured by a decrease in self-esteem only for those with a strong belief in a personal just world (Dalbert, 1999).

Belief in a Just World and Subjective Well-Being

Because the main properties of the belief in a just world—indicating commitment to a personal contract, endowing trust in the fairness of the world, and providing a framework for the interpretation of the events in one's life—have a variety of adaptive implications, the belief in a just world can be expected to positively affect subjective well-being, either directly or indirectly, mediated by these implications. There is ample evidence of a positive relationship between just-world beliefs and subjective well-being. Moreover, research has shown that the belief in a personal just world is more important than the general just-world belief in explaining well-being (Dalbert, 1999; Lipkus et al., 1996; Otto, Boos, Dalbert, Schöps, & Hoyer, 2006; Sutton & Douglas, 2005) and that this positive association between just-world belief and well-being is true for nonvictims (e.g., Dzuka & Dalbert, 2006; Otto & Schmidt, 2007; Ritter, Benson, & Snyder, 1990) and for various groups of victims (e.g., Agrawal & Dalal, 1993; Bulman & Wortman, 1977; Otto et al., 2006). In addition, Dzuka and Dalbert (2007) demonstrated that teachers' well-being was positively associated with their beliefs in a personal just world and that this relationship held when exposure to student violence was controlled. This study is one of the few to have found evidence for a buffering effect of the just-world belief: It was only among teachers with weak personal just-world beliefs that exposure to violence was associated with more negative affect; exposure to violence did not explain negative affect among those with strong personal just-world beliefs.

A personal resource can be defined as a personal disposition that helps people to cope with the events of their daily lives. The stronger the resource, the better equipped they are to cope. A personal resource thus implies a main-effect hypothesis. A personal buffer, in contrast, is usually seen as a resource that takes effect only under specific adverse conditions. A buffer thus implies a moderator hypothesis; the buffer moderates the association between strain and outcome. Overall, research findings are very much in line with the resource hypothesis and do not support the buffer hypothesis. The belief in a personal just world should thus be seen as a personal resource helping to sustain the well-being of people of all ages in diverse situations, victims and nonvictims alike.

The Developmental Trajectories of Belief in a Just World

Until the age of 7 or 8, children typically believe in immanent justice, and they are convinced that wrongdoings are automatically punished (Piaget, 1932/1997). As they grow older, however, they slowly abandon this belief in immanent justice. As a result of cognitive development, older children and

adults have no difficulty in identifying random events. Nevertheless, they sense that a random fate is unjust, and when given the possibility to justify a random fate, they will do so (e.g., Jose, 1990; Weisz, 1980). Children thus develop a belief in a just world—which can be interpreted as a more mature version of the belief in immanent justice—the belief that people generally deserve their fate accompanied by the cognitive ability to identify causality and randomness (Raman & Winer, 2004).

During adolescence, personal and general just-world beliefs emerge as two distinct beliefs. The strength of both beliefs seems to decrease slightly during adolescence and young adulthood. Both of these developmental changes—differentiation and decline—can be interpreted as consequences of increasing cognitive maturity. Even after its initial decline, the belief in a personal just world tends to be rather strong. The strength of just-world belief seems to increase again slightly in late adulthood and old age (e.g., Dalbert, 2001; Maes & Schmitt, 2004).

The meaning of the just-world belief also seems to differ systematically across the lifespan (Maes & Schmitt, 2004). In adolescence and young adulthood, especially, the just-world belief's main function seems to be to provide trust in the fairness of the world, thus enabling people to master challenges in school and at the workplace and to invest in their personal goals. In old age, when the remaining lifetime is shorter, the just-world belief's primary function seems to be to provide a framework to help people interpret the events of their lives in a meaningful way. A strong just-world belief allows older adults to see themselves as having been less discriminated against during the course of their lives, prevents them from ruminating about the negative aspects of their lives, and instead enables them to find meaning in them.

To explore the development of individual differences in the just-world belief, studies have investigated the impact of parenting on the just-world belief. In adolescence, at least (cf. Schönpflug & Bilz, 2004), there does not seem to be direct transmission from parent to child; however, parenting styles have proved to be positively associated with the children's just-world belief (e.g., Dalbert & Radant, 2004). Nurture, as reflected by a harmonious family climate with a low rate

of conflict and manipulation, and the experience of a just family climate are positively
associated with a strong belief in a personal
just world. Restriction, defined as a family orientation toward strict rules and rule
reinforcement in which breaking rules has
aversive consequences, is not. These findings indicate that the belief in a just world
is fostered by the trust in justice and is not
learned by adopting social rules.

Conclusion

Just-world research has shown that people
need to believe in justice and that they strive
for justice in order to maintain their basic
belief in a just world (e.g., Lerner & Miller,
1978). This justice motive is reflected by an
interindividually varying just-world disposition and explains the differences in people's
striving for justice as an end in itself, including their own behavior and assimilation of
observed or experienced injustices. In return, the justice motive endows trust in the
fairness of the world and in being treated
justly by others.

The basic idea of the just-world hypothesis is that people confronted with injustices
suffer and feel the unconscious need to restore justice (e.g., Lerner, 1980). As a consequence, the belief in a just world particularly
affects intuitive justice-driven reactions such
as, for example, the assimilation of injustice.
Thus research suggests that the belief in a
just world is an essential but unconscious
source of responses to injustice, in line
with the role of other implicit human motives (McClelland, Koestner, & Weinberger,
1989). Justice motive theory (Dalbert, 2001)
thus interprets the belief in a just world as
indicating an implicit justice motive. Lerner
and Goldberg (1999) argue that conscious
and intuitive justice-driven reactions coex-
ist and may be elicited simultaneously in the
same situation. The belief in a just world
seems to operate on an unconscious level and
can thus be expected to better explain intuitive than conscious reactions to injustice.
Important challenges for future research on
the just-world construct include integrating
just-world research within such a broader
framework and differentiating between the
explanations of more controlled versus more
intuitive justice-driven reactions in the light
of just-world reasoning.

References

Agrawal, M., & Dalal, A. K. (1993). Beliefs about the
world and recovery from myocardial infarction.
Journal of Social Psychology, 133, 385–394.
Allen, M. W., Ng, S. G., & Leiser, D. (2005). Adult
economic model and values survey: Cross-national
differences in economic beliefs. *Journal of Economic Psychology, 26*, 159–185.
Bègue, L. (2002). Beliefs in justice and faith in people:
Just world, religiosity and interpersonal trust. *Personality and Individual Differences, 32*, 375–382.
Bègue, L., & Muller, D. (2006). Belief in a just world
as moderator of hostile attributional bias. *British
Journal of Social Psychology, 45*, 117–126.
Berscheid, E., & Walster, E. (1967). When does a
harm-doer compensate a victim? *Journal of Personality and Social Psychology, 6*, 435–441.
Bierhoff, H. W. (1994). Verantwortung und altruis-
tische Persönlichkeit [Responsibility and altruistic
personality]. *Zeitschrift für Sozialpsychologie, 25*,
217–226.
Bierhoff, H. W., Klein, R., & Kramp, P. (1991). Evidence for the altruistic personality from data on
accident research. *Journal of Personality, 59*, 263–
280.
Brown, Y. D. (1986). Evaluations of self and others:
Self-enhancement biases in social judgements. *Social Cognition, 4*, 353–376.
Bulman, R. J., & Wortman, C. B. (1977). Attributions
of blame and coping in the "real world": Severe accident victims react to their lot. *Journal of Personality and Social Psychology, 35*, 351–363.
Cohn, E. S., & Modecki, K. L. (2007). Gender differences in predicting delinquent behavior: Do individual differences matter? *Social Behavior and
Personality, 35*, 359–374.
Comer, R., & Laird, J. D. (1975). Choosing to suffer
as a consequence of expecting to suffer: Why do
people do it? *Journal of Personality and Social Psychology, 32*, 92–101.
Correia, I., & Dalbert, C. (2007). Belief in a just
world, justice concerns, and well-being at Portuguese schools. *European Journal of Psychology in
Education, 22*, 421–437.
Correia, I., & Dalbert, C. (2008). School bullying: Belief in a personal just world of bullies, victims and
defenders. *European Psychologist, 13*, 249–254.
Correia, I., & Vala, J. (2004). Belief in a just world,
subjective well-being and trust of young adults. In
C. Dalbert & H. Sallay (Eds.), *The justice motive
in adolescence and young adulthood: Origins and
consequences* (pp. 85–100). London: Routledge.
Correia, I., Vala, J., & Aguiar, O. (2007). Victim's innocence, social categorization, and the threat to the
belief in a just world. *Journal of Experimental Social Psychology, 43*, 31–38.
Cubela Adoric, V., & Kvartuc, T. (2007). Effects of
mobbing on justice beliefs and adjustment. *European Psychologist, 12*, 261–271.
Dalbert, C. (1992). Der Glaube an die gerechte Welt:
Differenzierung und Validierung eines Konstruk-
ts [The belief in a just world: Differentiation and
validation of a construct]. *Zeitschrift für Sozialpsychologie, 23*, 268–276.
Dalbert, C. (1997). Coping with an unjust fate: The
case of structural unemployment. *Social Justice Research, 10*, 175–189.

Dalbert, C. (1999). The world is more just for me than generally: About the Personal Belief in a Just World Scale's validity. *Social Justice Research, 12,* 79–98.

Dalbert, C. (2001). *The justice motive as a personal resource: Dealing with challenges and critical life events.* New York: Kluwer Academic/Plenum.

Dalbert, C., & Dzuka, J. (2004). Belief in a just world, personality, and well-being of adolescents. In C. Dalbert & H. Sallay (Eds.), *The justice motive in adolescence and young adulthood: Origins and consequences* (pp. 101–116). London: Routledge.

Dalbert, C., & Filke, E. (2007). Belief in a just world, justice judgments, and their functions for prisoners. *Criminal Justice and Behavior, 34,* 1516–1527.

Dalbert, C., & Katona-Sallay, H. (1996). The "belief in a just world" construct in Hungary. *Journal of Cross-Cultural Psychology, 27,* 293–314.

Dalbert, C., Lipkus, I. M., Sallay, H., & Goch, I. (2001). A just and an unjust world: Structure and validity of different world beliefs. *Personality and Individual Differences, 30,* 561–577.

Dalbert, C., Montada, L., & Schmitt, M. (1987). Glaube an eine gerechte Welt als Motiv: Validierungskorrelate zweier Skalen [The belief in a just world as a motive: Validity correlates of two scales]. *Psychologische Beiträge, 29,* 596–615.

Dalbert, C., & Radant, M. (2004). Parenting and young adolescents' belief in a just world. In C. Dalbert & H. Sallay (Eds.), *The justice motive in adolescence and young adulthood: Origins and consequences* (pp. 11–25). London: Routledge.

Dalbert, C., & Stoeber, J. (2005). The belief in a just world and distress at school. *Social Psychology of Education, 8,* 123–135.

Dalbert, C., & Stoeber, J. (2006). The personal belief in a just world and domain-specific beliefs about justice at school and in the family: A longitudinal study with adolescents. *International Journal of Behavioral Development, 30,* 200–207.

DePalma, M., Madey, S. F., Tillman, T. C., & Wheeler, J. (1999). Perceived patient responsibility and belief in a just world affect helping. *Basic and Applied Social Psychology, 21,* 131–137.

Dette, D., Stöber, J., & Dalbert, C. (2004). Belief in a just world and adolescents' vocational and social goals. In C. Dalbert & H. Sallay (Eds.), *The justice motive in adolescence and young adulthood: Origins and consequences* (pp. 11–25). London: Routledge.

Dzuka, J., & Dalbert, C. (2006). The belief in a just world's impact on subjective well-being in old age. *Aging and Mental Health, 10,* 439–444.

Dzuka, J., & Dalbert, C. (2007). Student violence against teachers: Teachers' well-being and the belief in a just world. *European Psychologist, 12,* 253–260.

Edlund, J. E., Sagarin, B. J., & Johnson, B. S. (2007). Reciprocity and the belief in a just world. *Personality and Individual Differences, 43,* 589–596.

Fetchenhauer, D., Jacobs, G., & Belschak, F. (2005). Belief in a just world, causal attributions, and adjustment to sexual violence. *Social Justice Research, 18,* 25–42.

Furnham, A. (1993). Just world beliefs in twelve societies. *Journal of Social Psychology, 133,* 317–329.

Furnham, A. (2003). Belief in a just world: Research progress over the past decade. *Personality and Individual Differences, 34,* 795–817.

Furnham, A., & Procter, E. (1989). Belief in a just world: Review and critique of the individual difference literature. *British Journal of Social Psychology, 28,* 365–384.

Hafer, C. L. (2000). Investment in long-term goals and commitment to just means drive the need to believe in a just world. *Personality and Social Psychology Bulletin, 26,* 1059–1073.

Hafer, C. L., & Bègue, L. (2005). Experimental research on just-world theory: Problems, development, and future challenges. *Psychological Bulletin, 131,* 128–167.

Hafer, C. L., Bogaert, A. F., & McMullen, S. L. (2001). Belief in a just world and condom use in a sample of gay and bisexual men. *Journal of Applied Social Psychology, 31,* 1892–1910.

Hafer, C. L., & Correy, B. L. (1999). Mediators of the relation of beliefs in a just world and emotional responses to negative outcomes. *Social Justice Research, 12,* 189–204.

Hui, C. H., Chan, I. S. Y., & Chan, J. (1989). Death cognition among Chinese teenagers: Beliefs about consequences of death. *Journal of Research in Personality, 23,* 99–117.

Jose, P. E. (1990). Just world reasoning in children's immanent justice judgements. *Child Development, 61,* 1024–1033.

Jost, J. T., Banaji, M. R., & Nosek, B. A. (2004). A decade of system justification theory: Accumulated evidence of conscious and unconscious bolstering of the status quo. *Political Psychology, 25,* 881–919.

Kiecolt-Glaser, J. K., & Williams, D. A. (1987). Self-blame, compliance, and distress among burn patients. *Journal of Personality and Social Psychology, 53,* 187–193.

Lambert, A. J., Burroughs, T., & Nguyen, T. (1999). Perceptions of risk and the buffering hypothesis: The role of just world beliefs and right-wing authoritarianism. *Personality and Social Psychology Bulletin, 25,* 643–656.

Lerner, M. J. (1965). Evaluation of performance as a function of performer's reward and attractiveness. *Journal of Personality and Social Psychology, 1,* 355–360.

Lerner, M. J. (1977). The justice motive: Some hypotheses as to its origins and forms. *Journal of Personality, 45,* 1–52.

Lerner, M. J. (1978). "Belief in a just world" versus the "authoritarianism" syndrome … but nobody liked the Indians. *Ethnicity, 5,* 229–237.

Lerner, M. J. (1980). *The belief in a just world: A fundamental delusion.* New York: Plenum Press.

Lerner, M. J., & Goldberg, J. H. (1999). When do decent people blame victims?: The differing effects of the explicit/rational and implicit/experiential cognitive systems. In S. Chaiken & Y. Trope (Eds.), *Dual-process theories in social psychology* (pp. 627–640). New York: Guilford Press.

Lerner, M. J., & Matthews, J. (1967). Reactions to suffering of others under conditions of indirect responsibility. *Journal of Personality and Social Psychology, 5,* 319–325.

Lerner, M. J., & Miller, D. T. (1978). Just world research and the attribution process: Looking back and ahead. *Psychological Bulletin, 85,* 1030–1051.

Lerner, M. J., & Simmons, C. H. (1966). The observer's reaction to the "innocent victim": Compassion or rejection? *Journal of Personality and Social Psychology, 4*, 203–210.

Lind, E. A., & van den Bos, K. (2002). When fairness works: Toward a general theory of uncertainty management. *Research in Organizational Behavior, 24*, 181–223.

Lipkus, I. (1991). The construction and preliminary validation of a Global Belief in a Just World Scale and the exploratory analysis of the Multidimensional Belief in a Just World Scale. *Personality and Individual Differences, 12*, 1171–1178.

Lipkus, I. M., Dalbert, C., & Siegler, I. C. (1996). The importance of distinguishing the belief in a just world for self versus for others: Implications for psychological well-being. *Personality and Social Psychology Bulletin, 22*, 666–677.

Lipkus, I. M., & Siegler, I. C. (1993). The belief in a just world and perceptions of discrimination. *Journal of Psychology, 127*, 465–474.

Loo, R. (2002). Belief in a just world: Support for independent just-world and unjust-world dimensions. *Personality and Individual Differences, 33*, 703–711.

Lucas, T., Alexander, S., Firestone, I., & LeBreton, J. (2007). Development and initial validation of a procedural and distributive just world measure. *Personality and Individual Differences, 43*, 71–82.

Maes, J., & Kals, E. (2002). Justice beliefs in school: Distinguishing ultimate and immanent justice. *Social Justice Research, 15*, 227–244.

Maes, J., & Schmitt, M. (2004). Belief in a just world and its correlates in different age groups. In C. Dalbert & H. Sallay (Eds.), *The justice motive in adolescence and young adulthood: Origins and consequences* (pp. 11–25). London: Routledge.

McClelland, D. C., Koestner, R., & Weinberger, J. (1989). How do self-attributed and implicit motives differ? *Psychological Review, 96*, 680–702.

Messick, D. M., Bloom, S., Boldizar, J. P., & Samuelson, C. D. (1985). Why are we fairer than others? *Journal of Experimental Social Psychology, 21*, 480–500.

Miller, D. T. (1999). The norm of self-interest. *American Psychologist, 54*, 1053–1060.

Montada, L., Schmitt, M., & Dalbert, C. (1986). Thinking about justice and dealing with one's own privileges: A study of existential guilt. In H. W. Bierhoff, R. L. Cohen, & J. Greenberg (Eds.), *Justice in social relations* (pp. 125–143). New York: Plenum Press.

Otto, K., Boos, A., Dalbert, C., Schöps, D., & Hoyer, J. (2006). Posttraumatic symptoms, depression, and anxiety of flood victims: The impact of the belief in a just world. *Personality and Individual Differences, 40*, 1075–1084.

Otto, K., & Dalbert, C. (2005). Belief in a just world and its functions for young prisoners. *Journal of Research in Personality, 39*, 559–573.

Otto, K., & Schmidt, S. (2007). Dealing with stress in the workplace: Compensatory effects of belief in a just world. *European Psychologist, 12*, 253–260.

Piaget, J. (1997). *The moral judgment of the child.* Glencoe, IL: Free Press. (Original work published 1932)

Raman, L., & Winer, G. A. (2004). Evidence of more immanent justice responding in adults than children: A challenge to traditional developmental theories. *British Journal of Developmental Psychology, 22*, 255–274.

Ritter, C., Benson, D. E., & Snyder, C. (1990). Belief in a just world and depression. *Sociological Perspectives, 33*, 235–252.

Ross, M., & Miller, D. T. (Eds.). (2002). *The justice motive in everyday life.* Cambridge, UK: Cambridge University Press.

Rubin, Z., & Peplau, L. A. (1973). Belief in a just world and reaction to another's lot: A study of participants in the national draft lottery. *Journal of Social Issues, 29*(4), 73–93.

Rubin, Z., & Peplau, L. A. (1975). Who believes in a just world? *Journal of Social Issues, 31*(3), 65–89.

Sallay, H. (2004). Entering the job market: Belief in a just world, fairness and well-being of graduating students. In C. Dalbert & H. Sallay (Eds.), *The justice motive in adolescence and young adulthood: Origins and consequences* (pp. 215–230). London: Routledge.

Schönpflug, U., & Bilz, L. (2004). Transmission of the belief in a just world in the family. In C. Dalbert & H. Sallay (Eds.), *The justice motive in adolescence and young adulthood: Origins and consequences* (pp. 153–171). London: Routledge.

Steensma, H., & van Dijke, R. (2006). Attributional styles, self-esteem, and just world belief of victims of bullying in Dutch organizations. *International Quarterly of Community Health Education, 25*, 381–392.

Strelan, P. (2007). The prosocial, adaptive qualities of just world beliefs: Implications for the relationship between justice and forgiveness. *Personality and Individual Differences, 43*, 881–890.

Sutton, R. M., & Douglas, K. M. (2005). Justice for all, or just for me?: More evidence of the importance of the self–other distinction in just-world beliefs. *Personality and Individual Differences, 39*, 637–645.

Sutton, R. M., & Winnard, E. J. (2007). Looking ahead through lenses of justice: The relevance of just-world beliefs to intentions and confidence in the future. *British Journal of Social Psychology, 46*, 649–666.

Taylor, D. M., Wright, G. C., Moghaddam, F. M., & Lalonde, R. N. (1990). The personal/group discrimination discrepancy: Perceiving my group, but not myself, to be a target for discrimination. *Personality and Social Psychology Bulletin, 16*, 254–262.

Tomaka, J., & Blascovich, J. (1994). Effects of justice beliefs on cognitive, psychological, and behavioral responses to potential stress. *Journal of Personality and Social Psychology, 67*, 732–740.

Weisz, J. R. (1980). Developmental change in perceived control: Recognizing noncontingency in the laboratory and perceiving it in the world. *Developmental Psychology, 16*, 385–390.

Zuckerman, M. (1975). Belief in a just world and altruistic behavior. *Journal of Personality and Social Psychology, 31*, 972–976.

Zuckerman, M., & Gerbasi, K. C. (1977). Belief in a just world and trust. *Journal of Research in Personality, 11*, 306–317.

CHAPTER 20

■ ● ▲ ◆ ■ ● ▲ ◆

Authoritarianism and Dogmatism

JOHN DUCKITT

An important discovery from early social-psychological research was that prejudice or outgroup dislike was not directed just against specific outgroups or minorities but that it tended to be generalized over outgroups. Thus there was a stable pattern of individual differences in prejudice, with some people tending to be generally prejudiced and others generally tolerant. Moreover, this pattern formed part of a broader patterning in social attitudes, with persons high in prejudice and ethnocentrism also being more socially conservative, nationalistic, and politically right wing, preferring strict laws and rules, and supporting tough, punitive social control and authority. Persons low in prejudice, on the other hand, tended to be tolerant and liberal, favoring individual liberties, high levels of personal freedom, self-expression, individual self-regulation, and democracy.

This systematic patterning in social, political, economic, and intergroup attitudes and beliefs gave rise to the widely accepted idea that a basic individual-difference dimension, which has typically been labeled *authoritarianism*, underlies and produces this coherence. Since being first proposed in the 1930s and 1940s, largely to explain the appeal of German Nazism and anti-Semitism, authoritarianism has become an important construct in social psychology. The concept of dogmatism has been much less prominent. It

emerged as an alternative, rival construct to authoritarianism, but strong initial interest in dogmatism waned as it became apparent that its conceptualization and measurement were flawed.

Authoritarianism as an individual-difference construct has had a somewhat checkered history, and three issues in particular have generated disagreement and controversy. One has been that of conceptualization, involving questions of whether authoritarianism is a personality characteristic or a social attitude and value dimension, how broad or narrow this construct might be, the core meaning of the construct, and whether it consists of one or two dimensions. The second issue has involved psychometric measurement of the construct, and the third issue involves theory or explanation. These issues have had different influences on research and theory at different historical times so that the study of authoritarianism divides fairly naturally into four distinct periods or stages.

The first stage was during the 1930s and 1940s, when social scientists first proposed the construct of authoritarianism as a personality dimension to explain the mass appeal of fascism and anti-Semitism. The concept of an authoritarian personality was to be enormously influential and dominated research and thinking on authoritarianism to the end of the 20th century. The 1950s and 1960s form a second stage, beginning with the publication of Adorno, Frenkel-Brunswik, Levinson, and Sanford's *The Authoritarian Personality* (1950), which presented the first systematic theory of the authoritarian personality and the first attempt to measure it psychometrically by means of their F Scale. This period was dominated by controversies over the methodological and measurement problems of their research and problems with alternative conceptualizations and measures, such as Rokeach's (1954) dogmatism, that emerged in response to critiques of their work. The failure of these alternatives to resolve these problems led to a general loss of interest and confidence in the validity and utility of the construct.

A third stage opened in 1981, with the publication of Altemeyer's research on his Right-Wing Authoritarianism (RWA) Scale, which for the first time seemed to provide a reliable and unidimensional measure of authoritarianism. This was followed by a great deal of research validating the construct and exploring its correlates, with most of the research reflecting Altemeyer's conceptualization of authoritarianism as a personality dimension, and validating his RWA Scale as a measure of this authoritarian personality dimension. The period continued with the discovery of the concept of social dominance orientation (SDO), viewed by Altemeyer (1998) as a second authoritarian personality dimension, and research delineating the differences between these two "authoritarian personality" dimensions.

Today, this third stage still continues, but, together with it, a new, fourth stage emerged during the past decade. This new stage is characterized by a very different conceptualization of authoritarianism that no longer views it, or SDO, as personality dimensions but as social attitude or value dimensions. This perspective has raised a number of research and theoretical questions that were previously obscured or neglected, most notably the role of situational factors in influencing authoritarian attitudes and in moderating and mediating their impact.

This chapter reviews the way in which the constructs of authoritarianism and dogmatism have been conceptualized and measured over these four stages. It shows how these shifts have influenced research and theory,

culminating with a detailed outline and discussion of new theories and directions that have emerged during the past decade.

First Stage: Emergence of the Construct

The rise of fascism and virulent anti-Semitism in Europe during the 1930s stimulated attempts to understand the psychological appeal of these ideologies. These speculative theories were strongly influenced by psychoanalysis and Marxism, as well as by the culture and personality approach that was widely held in the social sciences at the time. Thus they typically argued that the family structures characteristic of Western, capitalist societies would produce a particular kind personality that would make people emotionally and cognitively susceptible to right-wing, fascist, nationalist ideologies and to hostility and aggression against vulnerable, culturally deviant minorities, particularly under stressful social circumstances.

Reich (1975), for example, argued that capitalist social structures generated authoritarian families, which used childrearing practices involving extensive sexual repression to create authoritarian personalities, who would be unlikely to rebel against exploitative social conditions. This authoritarian character structure was described as conservative, afraid of freedom, submissive to authority, obedient, yet with "natural aggression distorted into brutal sadism" (p. 66). Maslow (1943) and Fromm (1941) produced very similar descriptions of an authoritarian personality.

An interesting question is why these theorists and those who followed them ignored situational factors and focused so completely on personality-based explanations. Historically, the rise of German fascism was clearly linked to social factors such as the social, economic, and political consequences of Germany's defeat in World War I, the Great Depression, and profound political instability. Some early theorists, notably Fromm (1941), did discuss the role that social factors, and particularly social threat, might play in causing people to support fascist movements and adopt antidemocratic and prejudiced attitudes. However, theorists largely ignored the role of social factors in favor of personality-based explanations. There seem to be several reasons for this.

First, research had begun to show stable individual differences in peoples' social attitudes, with some persons being generally prejudiced, ethnocentric, nationalistic, conservative, and inclined to agree with profascist sentiments, whereas others were generally tolerant, liberal, and opposed to fascism. These findings suggested that these attitudes were caused by some stable characteristic, and personality seemed a likely possibility. Second, the liberal and radical political sympathies of these early theorists led them to see racism, prejudice, and fascism as profoundly irrational and unjustified attitudes and ideologies, so explanations in terms of underlying problems within the personality seemed plausible. And third, Marxist ideas, such as that of false consciousness, which were very influential at the time, rejected the view that ordinary working people could accept ideologies such as fascism out of any realistic appraisal of their social circumstances. These considerations made an explanation in terms of authoritarian personality dynamics generated by the socialization practices typical of authoritarian families and social systems seem particularly plausible.

These early speculative approaches were not based on systematic empirical research and did not develop empirically based measures of the construct. As a result, they had relatively little influence on social scientists and generated little research. However, their core theoretical idea that social and ideological beliefs are a direct expression of basic needs in the personality was enormously influential and dominated the way in which authoritarianism has been conceptualized up to the end of the 20th century.

Second Stage: First Theories and Measures

Adorno and Colleagues' Authoritarian Personality and the F Scale

The publication of Adorno and colleagues' classic volume in 1950 introduced the construct of an authoritarian personality to mainstream social science. Unlike its speculative predecessors, Adorno et al.'s approach, along with their measure of this authoritarian personality dimension (the F Scale), were based on extensive empirical research. Their initial research demonstrated that individuals' prejudiced attitudes were generalized over outgroups, with some people being generally prejudiced and others generally tolerant. Moreover, generalized prejudice seemed to be strongly associated with other social, political, and economic attitudes and beliefs, that is, broadly ideological beliefs. People who were generally prejudiced were also characterized by nationalism, ethnocentrism, social and economic conservatism, antiegalitarianism, and proauthority attitudes. Adorno and colleagues followed Maslow, Reich, and Fromm in assuming that these covarying social and ideological attitudes must be an expression of needs in the personality, that is, an authoritarian personality dimension.

Their F Scale was developed to measure this authoritarian personality dimension. The F Scale was always controversial as a measure of authoritarianism and ultimately did not survive. However, it was very important because it powerfully influenced later measures of authoritarianism, such as the most widely used measure today, the RWA Scale, by providing the broad pool of items from which later measures were developed. Thus it delineated and defined the initial bounds of the construct.

Where, then, did these items come from? They did not come from any explicit construct definition or any clearly defined construct domain. They were collected and written more or less ad hoc, with their primary sources being fascist writings, the speeches of anti-Semitic agitators, and persistent themes in the interview protocols and Thematic Apperception Test (TAT) stories of the participants classified high in ethnocentrism in Adorno and colleagues' research (Brown, 1965). All of the items were statements of opinion that seemed to the researchers to express attitudes and beliefs that were implicitly antidemocratic and involved a potentiality for fascism. They were explicitly selected not to express antiminority attitudes and political or economic conservatism, because these attitudes were assessed in their research by the Ethnocentrism and Politico-Economic Conservatism scales. The items of the F Scale, therefore, covered a broad range of relatively indirect expressions of socially conservative, antiliberal, and antiegalitarian attitudes and beliefs of a broadly ideological nature. None of its items measured personality in the sense of being self-descriptive statements indicating behavioral consistencies or behavioral traits.

Adorno and colleagues (1950) organized their F Scale items into the following nine content categories:

- *Conventionalism* (rigid adherence to conventional middle-class values).
- *Authoritarian submission* (a submissive, uncritical attitude toward authorities).
- *Authoritarian aggression* (tendency to condemn, reject, and punish people who violate conventional values).
- *Anti-intraception* (opposition to the subjective, imaginative, and tender-minded).
- *Superstition and stereotypy* (belief in mystical determinants of the individual's fate; disposition to think in rigid categories).
- *Power and toughness* (preoccupation with the dominance–submission, strong–weak, leader–follower dimension; identification with power, strength, toughness).
- *Destructiveness and cynicism* (generalized hostility; vilification of the human).
- *Projectivity* (disposition to believe that wild and dangerous things go on in the world; the projection outward of unconscious emotional impulses).
- *Sex* (an exaggerated concern with sexual "goings-on").

Although these content categories were defined in largely attitudinal terms, they came to be seen by the researchers as a set of traits that covaried to form the authoritarian personality syndrome. Their theory of this personality suggested that these surface traits arose from underlying psychodynamic conflicts originating in harsh, punitive parental socialization in childhood. This parental style was presumed to create underlying feelings of resentment and anger toward parental authority, later generalized to all authority, which were repressed and replaced by deference and idealization of authority. The underlying repressed anger and aggression were then displaced in the form of hostility toward deviant persons, outgroups, and minorities.

Initially, Adorno and colleagues' (1950) theory and the F Scale elicited a great deal

of interest and enthusiasm. In the first decade after the publication of their book, the F Scale was used in hundreds of studies. However, their theory and research, and the F Scale itself, soon generated a great deal of criticism and controversy (see Christie & Jahoda, 1954). First, research did not support the psychodynamic propositions of their theory, and much of their research validating their F Scale, which compared participants high and low in prejudice, seemed seriously compromised because of their failure to use blind ratings and to control for sociodemographic and other group differences. Second, the construct of authoritarianism seemed to explain only authoritarianism of the political right and ignored authoritarianism of the left. And, third, the F Scale became a particular focus of controversy because all of its items were positively worded. As a result, acquiescence might have inflated the internal consistency reliability of the F Scale, and its apparent unidimensionality might therefore be spurious.

A great deal of research, therefore, focused on trying to develop a balanced F Scale with equal numbers of protrait and contrait items to control acquiescence. None of these attempts succeeded, however, with balanced F Scales typically having very low internal consistency. At the time it was thought that the nature of the original F Scale items made it difficult to psychologically reverse their meaning. The alternative possibility that the F Scale might simply cover a range of item content that was not unidimensional was not seriously investigated until much later when Altemeyer (1981) showed that this was the case.

The many criticisms of Adorno and colleagues' (1950) theory and their F Scale resulted in a number of attempts to develop alternative conceptualizations and measures of the construct, with the most prominent being those of Allport (1954), Rokeach (1954), and Wilson (1973). All three shared the basic assumption that the social attitudes being measured either by the F Scale or, in the case of Rokeach and Wilson, by new measures, were expressions of an underlying personality dimension. All three, however, refined and simplified the conceptualization of this dimension by narrowing the core meaning of the construct and discarding Adorno and colleagues' complex psychodynamic explanation.

Allport's Concept of the Authoritarian Personality

Allport (1954), in *The Nature of Prejudice*, published shortly after Adorno and colleagues' (1950) volume, described an authoritarian personality that would be generally prejudiced, with a list of characteristics very similar to the nine "traits" listed by Adorno and colleagues. Allport, however, suggested that the core of this personality did not reside in psychodynamic conflicts but rather was characterized by insecurity and fearfulness, or "ego weakness." As a result of their basic insecurity, authoritarian personalities find it difficult to cope with inner psychological conflict and uncertainty or external social environmental change, uncertainty, and novelty. Their insecurity and fearfulness would cause these authoritarian personalities to need structure, order, and control in their social environments and to react with punitive hostility to unconventionality, novelty, and change. Allport's simplified conceptualization, rather than Adorno and colleagues' more complex theory of psychodynamic inner conflicts, most influenced later theorists, notably Wilson (1973), Jost, Glaser, Kruglanski, and Sulloway (2003), and Altemeyer (1981). However, Allport did not develop a measure of his concept of the authoritarian personality, so his ideas never acquired the prominence of those of Adorno and colleagues or later theorists.

Rockeach's Dogmatism and the D Scale

Rokeach (1954) also produced a simplified conceptualization of an "authoritarian" personality, which he termed *dogmatism*. Dogmatism was conceptualized as "a relatively closed cognitive organization of beliefs and disbeliefs about reality" (p. 195). According to Rokeach, this cognitive organization makes it difficult for dogmatic people to deal with new information that would change their existing beliefs and predisposes them to authoritarianism in general, rather than only to authoritarianism of the right. It also causes them to dislike and reject people and outgroups with dissimilar beliefs and values to their own. Rokeach developed his Dogmatism, or D, Scale to measure this construct.

However, the D Scale proved to be extremely problematic. Instead of using items that were directly and clearly derived from his conceptualization, Rokeach used items that were broad, vague statements of opinion or social attitude. Many had ideological implications, and some overlapped with items of the F Scale (e.g., "In this complicated world of ours, the only way we can know what's going on is to rely on leaders or experts who can be trusted").

Moreover, like the F Scale, all of the items of the D Scale were formulated in the protrait direction, with agreement always indicating high dogmatism. Critics pointed out that its internal consistency reliability was relatively low and that most of the internal consistency that it did show seemed to derive from acquiescence (Altemeyer, 1996). Factor-analytic studies suggested that the scale did not measure a unidimensional construct, and this was confirmed when studies that tried to balance the D Scale with equal numbers of protrait and contrait items found that its internal consistency virtually disappeared. And, finally, research found that the D Scale typically correlated very highly with the F Scale, so that there seemed to be little differentiation in what the F and D scales were measuring.

As a result of these criticisms, research on the D Scale and interest in Rokeach's concept of dogmatism largely collapsed during the 1960s. Like the concept of authoritarianism, it would be revived several decades later, when Altemeyer (1996) developed a more psychometrically satisfactory measure and when other theorists developed a set of distinct, though possibly related, cognitive style constructs, some of which are dealt with in other chapters in this volume (e.g., need for cognitive closure; see Kruglanski & Fishman, Chapter 23, this volume).

Wilson's Conservatism and the C Scale

The third alternative conceptualization of authoritarianism was Wilson's (1973) conservatism. Wilson also proposed a basic personality dimension that, unlike Adorno and colleagues, he specified very clearly as a "generalized susceptibility to experiencing threat or anxiety in the face of uncertainty" (p. 259). This conception was therefore similar to Allport's (1954) idea that the core of the authoritarian personality was fearfulness and insecurity. Like Adorno and colleagues (1950), Wilson viewed this personality dimension as being directly expressed in conservative social attitudes. The Conservatism, or C, Scale that he developed therefore consisted entirely of social attitude items, which covered a wide range of content but had as their core themes dislike for and resistance to change, novelty, and diversity and a preference for order, structure, the traditional, and the established. The items, therefore, covered a similar range of content to the F and D Scales, with which it correlated very highly, suggesting that it measured essentially the same construct.

As Altemeyer (1981) noted, the C Scale was a major improvement in one important respect: By using items on which a high conservatism score required both agreement and disagreement, it controlled for acquiescent responding. Unfortunately, it also shared its predecessors' weaknesses of having extremely low internal consistency. The mean interitem correlation obtained in Altemeyer's own research with the C Scale was a fairly typical $r = .05$, indicating that, like the F and D Scales, the C Scale did not measure a unidimensional construct. Moreover, factor-analytic studies of the C Scale also did not reveal a meaningful factor structure that enabled the extraction of a unidimensional core of items. Wilson's theory and his C Scale had very little impact subsequent to the publication of his edited volume on the topic in 1973. This was partly due to the weaknesses of the C Scale and partly due to disenchantment with individual-difference approaches to explaining ideological beliefs and prejudice that derived from the failure of a succession of approaches to the issue.

Conclusion: A Failure of Measurement

The theories of authoritarian personality that emerged in the 1950s and 1960s differed markedly in their nomenclature, but less so in how they conceptualized this personality construct, with Allport (1954), Rokeach (1954), and Wilson (1973) refining the complex psychodynamics initially proposed by Adorno and colleagues (1950) in a similar manner. These theories and measures also

shared two important, and more problematic, assumptions.

One assumption, which went unchallenged at the time, was that the relatively stable individual differences in people's social and ideological attitudes seemingly shown by early empirical research were direct expressions of a particular personality dimension. Thus measures consisting entirely of these social attitudes were seen as directly measuring and fully determined by that underlying personality dimension.

A further, even more problematic assumption was that these social and ideological attitudes used to measure the authoritarian personality dimension were unidimensional. There seem to be several reasons for this. First, if these social attitudes were direct expressions of a particular personality disposition, then they should be unidimensional. Second, early research such as that by Adorno and colleagues (1950) suggested that social and ideological attitudes were strongly correlated. However, much of this research used scales that were not balanced so that acquiescence could have spuriously inflated these correlations. And third, although theorists had focused on conceptualizing the presumed underlying authoritarian (or dogmatic, or conservative) personality dimension, they generally did not try to clarify the core meaning of the social attitudes they were using to measure this personality and so left its boundaries and domain broad, vague, and unclear.

Third Stage: RWA and SDO

Altemeyer's RWA Scale and His Authoritarian Personality

Interest in authoritarianism revived in the 1980s with the development and validation of a new and psychometrically sound measure by Altemeyer (1981, 1988, 1996)—the Right-Wing Authoritarianism (RWA) Scale. The development of the RWA Scale did not proceed from any theoretical conceptualization or construct definition but rather was purely inductive. Altemeyer began with a large pool of items comprising those used to develop the F Scale, items from other previous authoritarianism scales, and items he had written. This item pool was then subjected to repeated item analyses to produce a core set of items that intercorrelated highly enough to form a unidimensional scale that was balanced against acquiescence. This produced the initial version of the RWA Scale, which showed high internal consistency reliability. Its unidimensionality was confirmed by factor analyses that typically produced only two factors—one comprising most protrait items and the other most contratrait items (Altemeyer, 1981, 1988, 1996). In addition, research showed high levels of stability over time, with test–retest correlations being .85 over 6 months, .75 over 4 years, .62 over 12 years, and .59 over 18 years (Altemeyer, 1996). All of the items included in the RWA Scale were statements of social attitude and belief of a broadly ideological nature, as had been the case for other authoritarianism measures. Altemeyer (1981) followed earlier authoritarianism theorists in assuming that these social attitudes and beliefs were expressions of an authoritarian personality dimension and that his RWA Scale was therefore a measure of personality.

Altemeyer's (1981) inspection of the content of the RWA Scale suggested that it expressed only three of Adorno and colleagues' (1950) nine content categories—authoritarian submission, authoritarian aggression, and conventionalism. He interpreted these as covarying *traits* and defined their covariation as constituting the core of the authoritarian personality dimension (e.g., Altemeyer, 1981, p. 19). He suggested that his RWA Scale was unidimensional precisely because his successive item analyses had stripped away all items and facets included in the F Scale and other earlier measures that had been peripheral to these core traits of the authoritarian personality dimension.

The development of the RWA Scale stimulated a great deal of research and interest in the construct. Most of this research was guided by Altemeyer's theoretical assumption that authoritarianism was a personality dimension comprising three covarying traits. Indeed, in comprehensively reviewing RWA research, Altemeyer (1996) treated much of it as directly validating RWA as a measure of the three traits of authoritarian submission, authoritarian aggression, and conventionalism. This "validational" RWA research on these three traits is described

and discussed later, but for virtually all the studies reviewed, the "validity" indices are actually attitudinal self-ratings that overlap with RWA item content rather than independent behavioral indices of the three "traits."

Altemeyer's "Validational" RWA Research on Authoritarian Submission

Altemeyer (1996) cited a number of research findings as supporting the validity of the RWA Scale as a measure of a "trait" of authoritarian submission. Thus RWA scores correlated powerfully (i.e., >.50) with ratings of how justified or unjustified illegal, unfair acts by government officials were perceived to be (i.e., vignette descriptions of illegal wiretaps, illegal searches, denial of right to protest, and use of agent provocateurs), particularly when these targeted unconventional groups (Altemeyer, 1981). RWA scores also correlated moderately to strongly with American students' reports of how long they had continued to believe in Richard Nixon's innocence during the Watergate crisis (Altemeyer, 1981) and with the way Canadian and U.S. students rated bogus letters attacking the Canadian Charter of Rights and Freedoms and the American Bill of Rights, respectively (Altemeyer, 1988, 1996). Moghaddam and Vuksanovic (1990) also found that the RWA Scale correlated moderately to strongly with lower support for human rights, and McFarland, Ageyev, and Abalakina (1990) found that RWA correlated powerfully with lower support for democracy in the U.S.S.R. in the late 1980s.

These findings clearly show an association between RWA and positive attitudes toward and greater support for established authorities and less positive attitudes and lower support for individual rights and liberties. They do not, however, as Altemeyer (1996) suggested, support a link between RWA and a personality trait, or behaviors, indicative of authoritarian submission.

Altemeyer's "Validational" RWA Research on Authoritarian Aggression

Altemeyer's (1996) review also suggested that research findings supported the validity of the RWA Scale as a measure of a "trait" of authoritarian aggression. RWA scores correlated strongly with length of sentences recommended for lawbreakers (Altemeyer, 1981, 1988; Wylie & Forest, 1992). However, the correlation was not found in cases in which the lawbreakers were government officials and was reversed if the victims of the government officials who broke the law were unconventional or deviant, with higher RWA then associated with more lenient sentences (Altemeyer, 1981, 1988). In addition, RWA was correlated with selecting more severe shock levels to punish a learner for mistakes on a task. However, although these studies seem to deal with a kind of behavioral aggression, the interpretation that they support a direct link between RWA and authoritarian aggression seems questionable. In the sentencing studies, for example, the general levels of sentences recommended were typically low, so the responses seem unlikely to reflect aggression as such and seem more parsimoniously interpreted as reflecting greater favorability to the authorities and lower favorability to persons challenging or violating authority. In the learning task, the levels of shocks selected were also extremely weak, so the finding may simply reflect an association between RWA and a belief in the efficacy of punishment in learning situations rather than indicating a trait of authoritarian aggression. These interpretations seem to be supported by Altemeyer's (1988, pp. 186–187) finding that general levels of aggression irrespective of target were uncorrelated with RWA.

A great deal of research has shown moderate to strong correlations between RWA and prejudice, assessed as less favorable attitudes toward a variety of ethnic minority or deviant social groups. Targets have included gay people (Altemeyer, 1988; Whitley & Lee, 2000), Jews and ethnic minorities in the U.S.S.R. (McFarland et al., 1990), AIDS victims in the United States (Peterson, Doty, & Winter, 1993), blacks among South African whites (Duckitt, 1992), homeless people (Peterson et al., 1993), atheists, drug users, and welfare recipients (Leak & Randall, 1995). Correlations have also been shown with indices of generalized prejudice (i.e., aggregated attitudes to blacks, women, homosexuals, and patriotism) in the United States and Canada (Altemeyer, 1998; McFarland, 1998; McFarland & Adelson, 1996) and with ethnocentrism scales targeting attitudes to a number of minorities and outgroups in Canada and the United States (Altemeyer, 1996). In a series of "posse" studies, Altemeyer (1988, 1996) also found that RWA scores were associated with lower opposition to the government's proscribing and persecuting a variety of radical or deviant groups, even when they were right-wing groups. RWA scores were also associated with being less condemning of gay bashing (Altemeyer, 1996).

These findings replicate earlier research using measures such as the F Scale (Meloen, 1983) in indicating a relationship between RWA and less favorable attitudes toward outgroups, minorities, and deviant social groups and, in some cases, less opposition to measures harming such groups. However, the inference that these attitudes indicate a trait of authoritarian aggression seems doubtful. In all the research reviewed, only one finding involved actual behavior, and that study found a very weak relationship between RWA and sexual aggression among men toward women (Walker, Rowe, & Quinsey, 1993). The finding was not replicated in other, larger scale research (Altemeyer, 1996).

Altemeyer's "Validational" RWA Research on Conventionalism

Altemeyer's (1996) review cited a number of findings to support the empirical validity of the RWA Scale as a measure of a "trait" of conventionalism. First, RWA scores correlated powerfully with religiosity, particularly fundamentalist religiosity, whether Christian, Jewish, or Muslim (Altemeyer, 1996). Indeed, the correlations were so powerful that Altemeyer (1996) concluded that fundamentalism was simply the "religious manifestation of right-wing authoritarianism" (p. 166). Second, RWA correlated consistently and generally powerfully with support for traditional sex roles in a variety of samples and cultures (Altemeyer, 1996; Leak & Randall, 1995; McFarland et al., 1990). Third, RWA correlated with agreement with traditional norms of distributive justice in different societies, correlating negatively with belief in equality in the United States and positively in the Soviet Union. Fourth, the RWA Scale correlated very strongly with measures of conservatism, traditionalism, and acceptance of the rules and norms of society (McFarland et al., 1990; Tarr & Lorr, 1991; Trappnell, 1992, cited in Altemeyer, 1996). And fifth, the RWA Scale showed consistent, though only weak to moderate, correlations with support for right-wing political parties in a number of countries, with the effects stronger for persons who were more interested in politics (Altemeyer, 1996).

Altemeyer (1996) argued that these relationships supported the validity of the RWA Scale as measuring a "trait" of conventionalism, which he defined as "a high degree of adherence to conventions that are perceived to be endorsed by society and established authorities" (Altemeyer, 1981, p. 148). However, virtually all the research reported pertained to conventionalism, conservatism, and traditionalism in attitudes, beliefs, or values, rather than to the expressions of any kind of behavioral trait.

Although Altemeyer (1996) viewed certain other correlates of the RWA Scale as not pertaining to the three presumed "traits," they do seem broadly classifiable as indicative of conventionalism or traditionalism in social attitudes. Thus RWA scores had weak to moderate negative correlations with proenvironmental attitudes (Peterson et al., 1993; Schultz & Stone, 1994). They also correlated with unfavorable attitudes toward drug use (Peterson et al., 1993), though there was no correlation with actual drug use (Cormer, 1993, cited in Altemeyer, 1996), and were moderately correlated with antiabortion attitudes (Altemeyer, 1996; Moghaddam & Vuksanovic, 1990).

Conclusions from Altemeyer's Review of "Validational" RWA Research

Virtually all Altemeyer's research validating RWA as a measure of three authoritarian personality traits used attitudinal rather than behavioral indictors. Most of these indicators also involved content overlap with items included in the RWA scale that express attitudes and beliefs about homosexuals, fundamentalist religiosity, governmental and other authorities, deviant people, people challenging authority, right- and left-wing political issues, traditional gender roles, the importance of conforming to group norms

and traditional social practices, and the efficacy and appropriateness of punishment in various situations. This research therefore seems more reasonably interpreted as showing concurrent validity for the RWA scale as assessing a broad social attitudinal dimension without really elucidating the crucial issue of what lies at the core of these attitudes and gives them their coherence.

Research on the Origins of RWA

Research on the origins or determinants of RWA by Altemeyer (1996) and others during this period focused primarily on social learning, parental attitudes, family environment, and personal experiences. Interestingly, given their assumption that RWA measured a personality dimension, they showed little interest in genetic or biological inheritance as a possible causal factor. However, during this period other researchers reported important findings bearing on the role of both genetic and environmental factors in authoritarianism.

Genetic Influences

During the past few decades two major sets of studies, the Minnesota and Jena twin studies, have reported on the correlation between monozygotic and dizygotic twins reared apart or together for RWA and closely related measures such as traditionalism, conservatism, and religiosity (McCourt, Bouchard, Lykken, Tellegen, & Keyes, 1999; Stößell, Kämpfe, & Riemann, 2006). These findings have shown consistently powerful correlations between RWA scores of monozygotic twins reared apart that have been much higher than the correlations for dizygotic twins reared apart. Thus findings from both sets of studies have concurred in finding strong genetic effects (accounting for 40–60% of phenotypic variance) on these social-attitude measures similar in magnitude to those found for standard personality measures, such as the Big Five. These studies also found strong environmental effects accounting for approximately 50% of variance in RWA that were almost entirely due to unshared environmental sources (i.e., unique individual experiences as opposed to shared family environmental influences).

Social-Environmental Influences

Two theoretical approaches to the social-environmental origins of authoritarianism have dominated in the research literature. The first was that of Adorno and colleagues (1950) and other early theorists, who located the origins of authoritarianism in childhood, and the second that of Altemeyer (1991, 1996), who has seen adolescence as the critical formative period for authoritarianism. Both approaches saw parents as having important though different roles in the socialization of authoritarianism.

For Adorno and colleagues (1950), the primary influences were exposure to a particular family structure, parental roles, and socialization practices, particularly strict and punitive parenting during early and middle childhood. Allport (1954) and Wilson (1973), though not as specific, also saw their authoritarian syndrome of "ego weakness" as influenced by such early experiences. A great deal of research, however, has investigated the relationship between strict and punitive parenting and found little association with offspring authoritarianism, particularly when other relevant variables, such as parental authoritarianism, were controlled (Altemeyer, 1981; Duckitt, 1992; Duriez, Soenens, & Vansteenkiste, 2007).

According to Altemeyer (1996), RWA is acquired through social learning, with these attitudes established primarily during adolescence and early adulthood but also modified throughout the lifespan. Interestingly, this explanation does not seem particularly consistent with Altemeyer's insistence that RWA is a personality dimension, but seems more consistent with RWA being an attitude or value dimension. In his research, Altemeyer has systematically investigated a number of social influences, specifically parental RWA, parental religious socialization, personal experiences, education, having children, and social threat.

Parental RWA and parental religious socialization have each shown consistent and moderately strong correlations with offspring RWA. However, the findings for parental RWA average about .40 (Altemeyer, 1988, 1996), and the findings from the twin studies noted earlier suggest that the effect might be due to the heritability factor influencing RWA rather than to social learning. The effect for parental religious socialization, though consistent, is eliminated when parental RWA is controlled (Altemeyer, 1996), suggesting that the effect may also be plausibly accounted for by the effect of heritability. Altemeyer (1988) did find very powerful correlations between an inventory of personal experiences and RWA. However, the items of this personal experiences inventory were very similar to those of the RWA Scale, and the effect seems therefore likely to have been due to content overlap between the measures.

Altemeyer's (1996) impressive longitudinal research on the effects of education and having children, as well as his and others' research on the effects of social threat, have generated more compelling findings. Altemeyer found significant decreases in RWA scores over 4 years of college, with very substantial decreases (close to 1 standard deviation) for liberal arts majors and smaller decreases for nursing and commerce majors. Farnen and Meloen (2000) found similar differential effects for different kinds of educational experiences in their cross-national surveys. Altemeyer's research also showed that the decreases for persons initially high in RWA were approximately double those for persons initially low in RWA. These longitudinal findings are very similar to those from Newcomb and colleagues' classic Bennington College studies conducted in the early 1930s, which showed that students responded to the liberal education and atmosphere of Bennington College with substantial shifts from initially conservative to markedly more liberal social attitudes at college, with a follow-up 30 years later showing substantial postcollege stability in these liberal attitudes (Newcomb, Koenig, Flacks, & Warwick, 1967).

Altemeyer's (1996) longitudinal studies also showed important and powerful effects of parental roles on RWA. Ex-students who had been followed up over 12- and 18-year periods who had not become parents maintained the decreases in RWA that had occurred in their university years, whereas those who had become parents increased markedly in RWA, with approximately two-thirds of the decrease due to their university years reversed.

Finally, experimental research by Altemeyer (1988) and experimental and longitudinal research by others (Doty, Peterson, & Winter, 1991; Duckitt & Fisher, 2003; McCann, 1999; Sales, 1973; Sales & Friend, 1973) has shown that social threats—such as crime, political and economic crises, and insecurity—increased RWA and other indices of authoritarianism or conservatism. These effects were sometimes substantial, with Altemeyer's crisis scenarios producing increases in RWA of approximately two-thirds of a standard deviation. Consistent with this, many other studies have shown moderate to strong correlations of RWA with the degree to which people perceive their social environments as dangerous and threatening (Altemeyer, 1988; Duckitt, 2001), and longitudinal research has shown that these perceptions have causal effects on RWA (Sibley, Wilson, & Duckitt, 2007).

Overall, although much of the research on environmental influences on RWA is inconclusive or unclear, the findings of strong effects for liberal educational experiences, becoming a parent, and exposure to social threat support Altemeyer's contention that personal experiences are important in the formation and change of RWA. These findings also seem consistent with his idea that RWA is not formed in early childhood, as Adorno and colleagues (1950) had thought, but that adolescence and early adulthood may be particularly important periods and that important changes might occur throughout the lifespan. Interestingly, these conclusions seem more consistent with the idea that RWA is an attitude or value dimension than a personality dimension.

General Conclusions from Origins of RWA Research

Although much is still unclear about RWA and its origins, certain findings seem well established. First, there seems to be a powerful genetic influence. This, together with the high degree of unidimensionality for the relatively diverse content of the RWA Scale and its high level of stability over extended periods, could be consistent with the idea that the attitudinal items of the RWA Scale measure a personality trait dimension. However, the findings that certain experiences—such as liberal education, exposure

to social threat, and parental roles—cause major changes in RWA that can occur at any stage in the lifespan, with adolescence and early adulthood seemingly particularly critical, seem to militate against the personality interpretation.

RWA and Cognition

Adorno and colleagues (1950) and other early theorists assumed that authoritarian personalities are characterized by particular cognitive styles, ways of processing information, and making judgments. Allport (1954), for example, suggested that the authoritarian person's weak ego and general fearfulness would express itself in dichotomization (engaging in simplistic categorical thinking) and a need for definiteness (being intolerant of ambiguity, preferring structure, and avoiding and disliking uncertainty). For Rokeach (1954), pervasive rigidity and closed-mindedness of thought and belief were direct expressions of dogmatism.

Altemeyer's (1996) research has provided the most extensive effort to demonstrate an association between RWA and a variety of deficits and limitations in reasoning, processing information, and making decisions. He found that after reading essays on socialized medicine or corporal punishment, higher RWA was associated with remembering less about the material and being less able to recognize false inferences about it. High RWA was associated with greater inconsistency in responses on social-attitude questionnaires and a greater tendency to agree with contradictory statements on such issues. People high in RWA were uncritical about religious messages and made more fundamental attribution errors about pro- or antihomosexual essays, but particularly when the essay was antihomosexual (i.e., when they themselves agreed with it). People high in RWA were also more ready to believe a political message that they liked, even though the source seemed likely to be insincere. Those high in RWA showed greater double standards, first, by supporting the right of a majority to impose their religion in public schools when it was their religion but opposing it when it was a different religion and, second, by opposing the right to secession for nationalities they disliked but supporting it for nationalities they liked.

People high in RWA were also less ready to want further information about a test they believed they had done badly on and were less receptive to negative information about themselves.

Martin (2001), however, argued that virtually all of this research involved issues and values that are ego involving for persons higher in RWA (e.g., religion, national identity and cohesion, intergroup attitudes, homosexuality) and that ego involvement, rather than any general cognitive differences, might account for the effects obtained. This possibility was supported by an important program of research that investigated liberal–conservative differences in dispositional versus situational attributions across a range of situations (Skitka, Mullen, Griffin, Hutchinson, & Chamberlin, 2002). Skitka and colleagues (2002) found that liberals and conservatives made the same kinds of attributions in social-issue situations but then adjusted these attributions to fit with their liberal or conservative values. This finding suggests that the biased and deficient reasoning, judgment, and decisions associated with RWA in Altemeyer's (1996) research might have motivational rather than cognitive bases.

Dogmatism and Authoritarianism

Interest in dogmatism had languished since Rokeach's research during the 1960s for two primary reasons. First, although Rokeach's (1960) conceptualization of dogmatism as closed-mindedness seemed conceptually distinguishable from authoritarianism, his D Scale correlated so powerfully with the F Scale and other measures of authoritarianism that it seemed to be measuring essentially the same dimension. Second, the D Scale, like the earlier measures of authoritarianism, proved to be a psychometrically very poor measure.

After his success in developing the RWA Scale, Altemeyer (1996) turned his attention to dogmatism and its measurement. He began by clarifying Rokeach's idea of dogmatism by defining it as a "relatively unchangeable, unjustified certainty" (p. 201) in one's beliefs and produced a balanced, 20-item scale with the items having an impressively high level of face validity ("My opinions are right and will stand the test of time" and "Flexibility is a real virtue in thinking, since you

may well be wrong"). Preliminary research showed that this DOG Scale was highly reliable and the mean interitem correlation high enough to suggest unidimensionality (.28 for a student sample, .30 for a parent sample; Altemeyer, 1996), comprehensively outperforming the Rokeach (1960) D Scale in these respects.

However, validational research on the DOG Scale has been limited. Altemeyer (1996) reported that the DOG Scale significantly predicted positive changes in homophobic attitudes and readiness to shift pro- or antireligious beliefs. The DOG Scale was also significantly correlated with denial of contradictions and inconsistencies in the Bible (Altemeyer, 2002) and with lower flexibility and openness in religious attitudes, whereas the older Rokeach D Scale was not (Altemeyer, 1996).

The DOG Scale correlated strongly with RWA (.52 for students, .53 for parents), but these correlations were below the reliabilities of the two scales and so compatible with their being empirically distinct constructs (Altemeyer, 1996). This suggests that RWA is strongly associated with generally dogmatic inflexibility and rigidity in holding beliefs. However, there is a problem with this interpretation, which bears on a major unresolved question about the validity of the DOG Scale. The DOG Scale correlates highly with Religious Fundamentalism (.57 students, .60 parents) (Altemeyer, 1996), and all the studies supporting the validity of the DOG Scale thus far pertain to religious beliefs or beliefs closely related to religion (e.g., attitudes to homosexuals). This raises the possibility that the items of the DOG Scale assess religious dogmatism specifically and not dogmatism in other spheres of belief. Thus the correlation between the DOG Scale and RWA might be due to the religiosity of people high in RWA rather than to any tendency for them to be generally rigid or inflexible in their beliefs. Indeed, with religious fundamentalism controlled, the strong and significant correlations between RWA and DOG in Altemeyer's research seem likely to largely disappear.

In conclusion, Altemeyer's (1996) new Dogmatism Scale seems a promising development but still needs validation. A particular issue that needs to be clarified is its capacity to assess and detect dogmatism in nonreligious belief domains or only in the way religious beliefs are held.

Social Dominance Orientation: A Second Authoritarian Personality?

During the 1990s an important new individual-difference construct and measure, social dominance orientation (SDO), was proposed (Pratto, Sidanius, Stallworth, & Malle, 1994; Sidanius & Pratto, 1999). The SDO Scale taps a "general attitudinal orientation toward intergroup relations, reflecting whether one generally prefers such relations to be equal, versus hierarchical" (Pratto et al., 1994, p. 742). Research has shown that the SDO Scale predicts a range of "authoritarian" sociopolitical and intergroup phenomena similar to those predicted by the RWA Scale, such as generalized prejudice, intolerance, right-wing political party preference, nationalism, patriotism, militarism, support for capital punishment, and generally punitive attitudes (Pratto, Sidanius, & Levin, 2006; Sidanius & Pratto, 1999). However, a great deal of evidence indicates that the SDO and RWA scales are different and relatively independent dimensions (Altemeyer, 1998; Duckitt, 2001).

First, the item content of the two scales is clearly different. RWA items express beliefs in coercive social control, obedience and respect for existing authorities, and conforming to traditional moral and religious norms and values. SDO items, on the other hand, pertain to beliefs in social and economic inequality as opposed to equality and the right of powerful groups to dominate weaker ones.

Second, the RWA and SDO scales correlate differently with other variables (Altemeyer, 1998; Duckitt, 2001; Ekehammar & Akrami, 2003; McFarland, 2006; Van Hiel & Mervielde, 2002). RWA is powerfully associated with religiosity and valuing order, structure, conformity, and tradition, whereas SDO is not. SDO, on the other hand, is strongly associated with valuing power, achievement, and hedonism and with being male, whereas RWA is not. RWA is influenced by social threat and correlated with a view of the social world as dangerous and threatening, whereas SDO is not. SDO is correlated with a social Darwinist view of the world as a ruthlessly competitive jungle

in which the strong win and the weak lose, whereas RWA is not.

Third, the correlations between the RWA and SDO scales suggest that they are substantially independent dimensions. Although some studies, notably in Western European countries, have reported strong positive correlations (e.g., Duriez & Van Hiel, 2002; Van Hiel & Mervielde, 2002), most research, particularly in North America, has found weak or nonsignificant correlations (see reviews and meta-analyses by Duckitt, 2001, and Roccato & Ricolfi, 2005). Some studies, notably in East European countries, have even found negative correlations between RWA and SDO (Krauss, 2002; Van Hiel, Duriez, & Kossowska, 2006).

These findings indicate that although SDO and RWA both predict "authoritarian" phenomena such as prejudice, intolerance, nationalism, punitive attitudes, and right-wing politics, they seem to be independent dimensions or syndromes. Altemeyer (1998) noted that the RWA and SDO scales relate to different sets of the original nine "trait" clusters listed by Adorno and colleagues (1950). He therefore concluded that these scales measure two different kinds of authoritarian personality dimensions: the "submissive" and the "dominant."

The idea that there are two authoritarian dimensions helps to explain the checkered history of the authoritarian personality and the difficulties of the early theorists. It seems that Adorno and colleagues' (1950) original conceptualization of the authoritarian personality and their F Scale combined these two dimensions and syndromes, resulting in a lack of unidimensionality. Allport (1954), Rokeach (1960), and Wilson (1973) had attempted to simplify the conceptualization of this personality by focusing on the "submissive" authoritarian, but they failed to narrow their measures correspondingly, and they remained multidimensional. The success of Altemeyer's (1981) RWA Scale thus seems largely due to its having stripped off those items that tapped the factorially different "authoritarian dominance" syndrome in his item development studies.

Altemeyer (1998, 2004) also proposed two new hypotheses suggesting different kinds of interaction between the presumed personality dimensions of RWA and SDO. First, a "double high" hypothesis suggests that persons who are high in both RWA and SDO may "combine the worst elements of each kind of personality" (Altemeyer, 2004, p. 421) and so be particularly high in ethnocentrism, prejudice, and right-wing political orientation. And, second, Altemeyer (1998) suggested that the combination of high-SDO leaders and high-RWA followers would form a "lethal union" that would be particularly conducive to groups making and engaging in seriously unethical decisions and actions.

In apparent support of the double-high hypothesis, Altemeyer (2004) found that people with double highs had markedly higher levels of prejudice than persons who were high on just SDO or just RWA. However, it was subsequently pointed out that Altemeyer had not tested for interactions between RWA and SDO and that his findings might be due to the additive effects of each on prejudice. This was confirmed by a meta-analysis of findings from 16 separate samples, which showed strong additive effects for RWA and SDO on prejudice but no significant interactive effects (Sibley, Robertson, & Wilson, 2006).

A study of the "lethal union" that investigated the combination of followers with high RWA and leaders with high SDO found more unethical decisions than for either on their own, but the research design was not able to test for interactions, so the findings could simply have reflected the well-documented additive effects of RWA and SDO (Son Hing, Bobocel, Zanna, & McBride, 2007). Overall, therefore, although independent, additive effects of RWA and SDO on prejudice and a range of social, political, and intergroup phenomena have been extensively documented, no evidence has yet supported the hypotheses of interaction between them, and the idea of a lethal union still needs to be adequately tested.

Conclusions: Authoritarianism in Its Third Stage

Altemeyer's (1981) development of the RWA Scale demonstrated that authoritarianism was a viable individual-difference construct and revitalized interest and research on authoritarianism. The RWA Scale integrated a wide range of social, political, and intergroup attitudes and beliefs along a single tightly organized individual-difference di-

mension that was measured reliably and was relatively stable over long periods of time. Not surprisingly, therefore, Altemeyer (1988, 1996) followed earlier authoritarianism theorists in viewing this as a personality dimension, and this assumption powerfully influenced his and others' research and thinking about the construct.

When the SDO Scale was shown to be as powerful a predictor of sociopolitical and intergroup phenomena as RWA but distinct from it, Altemeyer (1998) extended this conceptual framework by seeing SDO and RWA as two independent but complementary authoritarian personalities—the dominant and the submissive authoritarians, respectively. However, during the 1990s this assumption was questioned, and a new view of RWA and SDO as social-attitude dimensions expressing motivationally based values emerged, opening up questions that had been neglected and leading to the development of new theories.

Fourth Stage: New Perspectives on Authoritarianism

Reassessing the View of Authoritarianism as Personality

There are a number of reasons why the view of authoritarianism as a personality dimension has began to be questioned. First, the items on authoritarianism measures—whether the F, D, C, RWA, or SDO scales—are statements of beliefs and attitudes of a broadly ideological nature and do not describe behavioral dispositions or traits, as the items of personality inventories typically do (Duckitt, 1989, 2001; Feldman & Stenner, 1997; Rosier & Willig, 2002; Saucier, 2000; Stone, Lederer, & Christie, 1993, p. 232). Indeed, Pratto and colleagues (1994; see also Pratto et al., 2006) have generally described their SDO Scale as a measure of enduring beliefs rather than of personality. The assumption that these social-attitude and belief items measure personality rather than social attitudes or values has never been empirically tested or verified. For example, as noted already, the research reviewed by Altemeyer (1996) to show that the RWA Scale measured three covarying personality traits actually investigated social attitudes and beliefs broadly covered in the item content of the RWA Scale. And although the strong genetic influence demonstrated on RWA would be consistent with RWA being a personality dimension, it would be equally compatible with one or more personality dimensions influencing RWA but not being isomorphic with it.

Strong empirical evidence also suggests that authoritarianism measures, and the RWA Scale in particular, seem better viewed as measuring a dimension of social attitudes and values that might be influenced by personality but is not itself a dimension of personality. First, the research on twin studies already reviewed indicated that RWA was not influenced by early childhood familial environments that would be shared by twin siblings. Instead, as Altemeyer (1996) concluded, it seems to form mainly in late adolescence and early adulthood. These environmental influences seem more compatible with RWA as a social attitude or value dimension than as personality. Second, RWA, SDO, and similar measures have also been shown to be highly reactive to priming, situational manipulations, or sociopolitical changes (Duckitt & Fisher, 2003; Guimond, Dambrun, Michinov, & Duarte, 2003; Huang & Liu, 2005; Sales, 1973; Sales & Friend, 1973; Schmitt, Branscombe, & Kappen, 2003).

And third, investigations of the structure of sociopolitical attitudes and sociocultural values have typically revealed two roughly orthogonal dimensions, with one corresponding closely to RWA and the other to SDO (Duckitt, 2001, Table 3). Investigators have usually labeled the RWA-like dimension as social conservatism, traditionalism, or collectivism versus personal freedom, openness, or individualism and the SDO-like dimension as economic conservatism and belief in inequality, or power distance versus social welfare, egalitarianism, or humanitarianism. Moreover, the social conservatism dimension of social attitudes, when reliably measured, has correlated powerfully with the RWA Scale and scaled with it as a single general factor or dimension (Forsyth, 1980; Raden, 1999; Saucier, 2000). For example, Saucier (2000), in a large-scale study of social attitudes, obtained a correlation of .77 between the RWA Scale and attitudinal measures of social conservatism. Central to

these two social-attitude dimensions seem to be two distinct sets of motivationally based higher order sociocultural values, with RWA correlated with conservation or conservatism values (such as tradition, social conformity, cohesion, social harmony) and SDO correlated with valuing power, dominance, hierarchy, and inequality in society. Stangor and Leary (2006) have also interpreted these dimensions as expressing the two core values of conservatism (versus liberalism, freedom, or openness) and egalitarianism (versus power and hierarchy).

New Theories and New Research Issues

These considerations have increasingly led researchers to adopt a new view of authoritarianism, with RWA and SDO seen not as personality but as social-attitude dimensions expressing basic social values (Duckitt, 1989, 2001; Duriez & Van Hiel, 2002; Feldman, 2003; Kreindler, 2005). This view has opened up new issues that had been obscured and neglected because of the personality assumption. One that had been completely neglected in the case of RWA (though less so for SDO) was that of identifying the central, core values that integrate and give the diverse attitudinal content of the dimension its coherence. Second was the issue of understanding the psychological and social bases of these dimensions; what personality or social environmental influences shape them and how? And third was that of why and how dimensions such as RWA and SDO affect prejudice, political preferences, and other outcomes.

An important feature of these new theories that contrasts with the earlier personality approaches has involved giving greater emphasis to social or group factors, both as underlying the motivational values thought to be expressed in authoritarian attitudes and in shaping their effects, such as prejudice. Four of these new theories—that is, the group-cohesion model (Duckitt, 1989), Feldman and Stenner's (1997) interactionist model, Jost and colleagues' (2003) motivated-cognition model, and Kreindler's (2005) dual-group-process model—tend to be partial theories focusing only on either RWA or SDO or only on either their causes or effects. A fifth approach, the dual-process motivational model (Duckitt, 2001), integrates most of the factors specified by these four theories to provide a more comprehensive approach to explaining how both situational and dispositional factors underlie the motivational values expressed in both RWA and SDO and how these generate their effects on prejudice and politics. Each of these theories is briefly described.

The group-cohesion model (Duckitt, 1989) was the first clearly systematized social or group approach to authoritarianism and focused only on RWA. This model suggested that the core idea being expressed by the items of the RWA Scale was that of attitudes to the subordination of individual autonomy to group authority. These authoritarian attitudes were seen as direct expressions of the need for and the value of group cohesion. This implied that authoritarianism was a group phenomenon and could be characteristic of any social group, though as typically studied using measures such as the F Scale or the RWA Scale, the salient social group would be the societal or national group. This need for societal group cohesion was seen as being a joint product of the degree to which people identified with their societal groups and the degree to which people perceived threats to the cohesion of that group. Outgroup dislike or prejudice would therefore be caused by perceiving outgroups as threatening ingroup cohesion or security in some way. Evidence supporting this model has been reported by Stellmacher and Petzel (2005), but in general it has not yet been subject to systematic empirical testing.

Kreindler's (2005) dual-group-processes model (DGPM) also sees authoritarianism as a group phenomenon and makes similar predictions about the causes of RWA. Like the group-cohesion model, the DGPM sees the primary causal determinants of RWA as a joint product of group identification and the perception of threat to the group, though it suggests that the threats that really matter are threats to the norms of the group rather than threats to the group's cohesion. Outgroup prejudice therefore arises when persons high in RWA are hostile to persons seen as threatening group norms.

The DGPM sees SDO resulting from identification with high-status groups, which is thereby expressed in valuing inequality and hierarchy and causes dislike and derogation of lower-status groups. This model has also not been subject to much empirical testing, but several studies have shown that experimental manipulations and real-world events that make peoples' membership in high-status groups salient increase SDO (e.g., Huang & Liu, 2005; Schmitt et al., 2003). There is also research indicating that making particular group identities salient can influence the relationship between RWA and outgroup attitudes in a manner broadly consistent with the model (e.g., Verkuyten & Hagendoorn, 1998).

Both the preceding models explain the causes and effects (at least in terms of prejudice) of authoritarianism largely or entirely in terms of social situational factors. A third approach, Jost and colleagues' (2003) motivated-cognition theory of political conservatism, focuses only on causes, which it sees as both dispositional and situational. This theory sees RWA (and closely related constructs or measures such as the F, C, or D scales) expressing attitudinal resistance to change and SDO expressing attitudinal support for inequality as two components of political conservatism. Conservatism, and therefore both RWA and SDO, expresses motives to manage and reduce threat and uncertainty, which arise from social situational factors likely to activate threat and uncertainty and dispositional factors that index the strength of personal needs to avoid uncertainty and threat. A meta-analysis showed that indicators of these factors did correlate as expected with RWA, SDO, and other indices of political conservatism (Jost et al., 2003). However, it has been pointed out that these findings were less convincing for SDO than for RWA. RWA and related constructs supplied the bulk of the indices used, and their correlations were typically much stronger than those obtained for SDO. Thus the effects obtained for SDO might have been spurious and due to the positive correlation between RWA and SDO (Duckitt & Sibley, 2009).

A fourth theory, Feldman and Stenner's (1997; Feldman, 2003; Stenner, 2005) interactionist model, focuses on RWA and its effects. It sees RWA as expressing the value of social conformity. Social-situational factors that threaten social conformity will activate this value or disposition for persons high in RWA and generate authoritarian reactions. This interactive hypothesis has been empirically supported in research on authoritarian reactions such as outgroup prejudice and support for hard-line right-wing social and political policies (Feldman, 2003; Feldman & Stenner, 1997; Rikert, 1998; Stenner, 2005). Evidence also suggests that the kind of behavioral rigidity and biased judgments or decision making that Altemeyer (1996) tried to demonstrate in persons high in RWA seems to occur only under conditions of threat (Lavine, Lodge, & Freitas, 2005; Schultz & Searleman, 2002). This approach and these findings suggest that social-environmental threat might not only cause RWA but also elicit authoritarian reactions in interaction with authoritarian attitudes and values.

Finally, a dual-process motivational (DPM) model provides a broad approach to explaining both RWA and SDO and their effects, incorporating most of the mechanisms proposed by these new theories. Like the Jost and colleagues (2003) model, it sees RWA and SDO caused by both personality–dispositional factors and by social-environmental factors, but with different factors causing RWA and SDO. The DPM model proposes that RWA and SDO represent two basic dimensions of social or ideological attitudes, with each expressing motivational goals or values made chronically salient for individuals by their world-views and personalities (Duckitt, 2001). High RWA expresses the motivational goal and value of establishing or maintaining collective security, that is, social order, cohesion, and stability. This motivational goal or value is made chronically salient for the individual by the belief that the social world is inherently dangerous and threatening, a belief that is influenced by exposure to and socialization in social environments that are threatening and dangerous. The predisposing personality dimension is social conformity (which, in terms of the Big Five, comprises low openness and high conscientiousness), which leads individuals to value order, stability, and security, as well as influencing their beliefs about how dangerous or threatening their social world may be.

In contrast, SDO stems from the underlying personality dimension of tough- versus tender-mindedness (i.e., low agreeableness in terms of the Big Five). Tough-minded personalities view the world as a ruthlessly competitive jungle in which the strong win and the weak lose. This worldview is also influenced by exposure to and socialization in social environments characterized by inequality, group dominance, and competition over power, status, and resources. Being tough-minded and holding this competitive-jungle worldview makes chronically salient the motivational goals and values of power, dominance, and superiority over others, which are expressed in the social attitudes of SDO. This account of the origins of RWA and SDO has been supported by correlational findings using structural equation modeling, by longitudinal research showing the expected causal effects for these personality and social worldview variables on RWA and SDO, and by experimental research manipulating or making salient particular social or group environments and showing the expected effects on worldview beliefs, RWA, and SDO (see Duckitt & Sibley, 2009, for a review; see also Sibley & Duckitt, 2008).

Like Feldman (2003) and Stenner's (2005) interactionist model for RWA and Kreindler's dual-group-process model for both RWA and SDO, the DPM model sees the effects of RWA and SDO as activated and directed by social-environmental influences. For example, persons high in RWA value collective security. Therefore, outgroup prejudice will be activated in persons high in RWA by the perception of threats to collective security from particular outgroups or minorities. Persons high in SDO value power, dominance, and superiority over others. Consequently, such persons derogate outgroups low in power or status (in order to justify their relatively superiority) or outgroups competing with their own groups over relative power, status, and resources. Studies have supported these hypotheses by showing that RWA and SDO correlate with the different kinds of outgroup prejudice expected from the model (RWA with prejudice against dangerous outgroups, SDO with prejudice against low-status outgroups) and that the effect of RWA on outgroup dislike is mediated by perceived outgroup threat, whereas the effect of SDO on outgroup dislike is mediated by competitiveness over relative group status and superiority (Duckitt, 2006; Duckitt & Sibley, 2007).

Conclusions:
Authoritarianism in Its Fourth Stage

The fourth stage of authoritarianism research has involved an important shift away from seeing authoritarianism as personality to viewing RWA and SDO as attitudinal expressions of motivationally based social values. This shift has generated new theories that have focused on the kind of values and motives that might underlie RWA and SDO, how social-environmental and dispositional factors have shaped these values, and how these values might interact with social-situational factors to trigger authoritarian actions and reactions.

General Conclusions:
Authoritarianism and Its Vicissitudes

The idea of an authoritarian personality that can explain patterns of relatively stable individual differences in a broad range of social, political, and intergroup attitudes and reactions emerged early in the 20th century. Since then, the construct has had a checkered history, during which there have been marked changes in how it has been measured and conceptualized.

One set of changes moved away from trying to measure the entire range of attitudes and beliefs originally deemed to comprise the authoritarian syndrome on a single psychometric dimension. These early measures invariably failed and led to a loss of confidence in the validity and utility of the construct. These changes culminated with the discovery that this broad social attitudinal domain comprised two distinct dimensions, which are today best measured by the RWA and SDO scales and seem to comprehensively organize individuals' social, political, and intergroup attitudes and their many manifestations and expressions.

Another set of changes has come more recently. This has involved challenging the conception of authoritarianism as personality, be it one dimension or two. The new approaches see the two dimensions of authoritarianism, RWA and SDO, not as personality dimensions but rather as two distinct social-attitudinal dimensions expressing two sets of motivationally based social values. These newer theories focus on trying to clarify the

values that lie at the core of RWA, the ways social-environmental factors influence RWA and SDO on their own or in conjunction with personality, and how and why RWA and SDO influence and have their effects on social, political, and intergroup attitudes and reactions.

References

Adorno, T., Frenkel-Brunswik, E., Levinson, D., & Sanford, N. (1950). *The authoritarian personality.* New York: Harper.
Allport, G. (1954). *The nature of prejudice.* Reading, MA: Addison-Wesley.
Altemeyer, B. (1981). *Right-wing authoritarianism.* Winnipeg, Manitoba, Canada: University of Manitoba Press.
Altemeyer, B. (1988). *Enemies of freedom: Understanding right-wing authoritarianism.* San Francisco: Jossey-Bass.
Altemeyer, B. (1996). *The authoritarian specter.* Cambridge, MA: Harvard University Press.
Altemeyer, B. (1998). The other "authoritarian personality." In M. Zanna (Ed.), *Advances in experimental social psychology* (Vol. 30, pp. 47–92). San Diego, CA: Academic Press.
Altemeyer, B. (2002). Dogmatic behavior among students: Testing a new measure of dogmatism. *Journal of Social Psychology, 142,* 713–721.
Altemeyer, B. (2004). Highly dominating, highly authoritarian personalities. *Journal of Social Psychology, 144,* 421–447.
Brown, R. (1965). *Social psychology.* New York: Free Press.
Christie, R., & Jahoda, M. (Eds.). (1954). *Studies in the scope and method of "the authoritarian personality."* Glencoe, IL: Free Press.
Doty, R., Peterson, B., & Winter, D. (1991). Threat and authoritarianism in the United States, 1978–1987. *Journal of Personality and Social Psychology, 61,* 629–640.
Duckitt, J. (1989). Authoritarianism and group identification: A new view of an old construct. *Political Psychology, 10,* 63–84.
Duckitt, J. (1992). *The social psychology of prejudice.* New York: Praeger.
Duckitt, J. (2001). A dual-process cognitive-motivational theory of ideology and prejudice. In M. P. Zanna (Ed.), *Advances in experimental social psychology* (Vol. 33, pp. 41–113). San Diego, CA: Academic Press.
Duckitt, J. (2006). Differential effects of right wing authoritarianism and social dominance orientation on outgroup attitudes and their mediation by threat from competitiveness to outgroups. *Personality and Social Psychology Bulletin, 32,* 684–696.
Duckitt, J., & Fisher, K. (2003). The impact of social threat on worldview and ideological attitudes. *Political Psychology, 24,* 199–222.
Duckitt, J., & Sibley, C. G. (2007). Right wing authoritarianism, social dominance orientation, and the dimensions of generalized prejudice. *European Journal of Personality, 21,* 113–130.

Duckitt, J., & Sibley, C. G. (2009). In J. Jost, A. Kay, & H. Thorisdottir (Eds.), *Social and psychological bases of ideology and system justification* (pp. 242–313). Oxford, UK: Oxford University Press.

Duriez, B., Soenens, B., & Vansteenkiste, M. (2007). In search of the antecedents of adolescent authoritarianism: The relative contribution of parental goal promotion and parenting style dimensions. *European Journal of Personality, 21,* 507–527.

Duriez, B., & Van Hiel, A. (2002). The march of modern fascism: A comparison of social dominance orientation and authoritarianism. *Personality and Individual Differences, 32,* 1199–1213.

Ekehammar, B., & Akrami, N. (2003). The relation between personality and prejudice: A variable and person-centered approach. *European Journal of Personality, 17,* 449–464.

Farnen, R., & Meloen, J. (2000). *Democracy, authoritarianism, and education: A cross-national empirical survey.* New York: St. Martin's.

Feldman, S. (2003). Enforcing social conformity: A theory of authoritarianism. *Political Psychology, 24,* 41–74.

Feldman, S., & Stenner, K. (1997). Perceived threat and authoritarianism. *Political Psychology, 18,* 741–770.

Forsyth, D. (1980). A taxonomy of ethical ideologies. *Journal of Personality and Social Psychology, 39,* 175–184.

Fromm, E. (1941). *Escape from freedom.* New York: Rinehart.

Guimond, S., Dambrun, M., Michinov, N., & Duarte, S. (2003). Does social dominance generate prejudice?: Integrating individual and contextual determinants of intergroup cognitions. *Journal of Personality and Social Psychology, 84,* 697–721.

Huang, L., & Liu, J. (2005). Personality and social structural implications of the situational priming of social dominance orientation. *Personality and Individual Differences, 38,* 267–276.

Jost, J., Glaser, J., Kruglanski, A., & Sulloway, F. (2003). Political conservatism as motivated social cognition. *Psychological Bulletin, 129,* 339–375.

Krauss, S. (2002). Romanian authoritarianism 10 years after communism. *Personality and Social Psychology Bulletin, 28,* 1255–1264.

Kreindler, S. (2005). A dual group processes model of individual differences in prejudice. *Personality and Social Psychology Review, 9,* 90–107.

Lavine, H., Lodge, M., & Freitas, K. (2005). Threat, authoritarianism, and selective exposure to information. *Political Psychology, 26,* 219–244.

Leak, G., & Randall, B. (1995). Clarification of the link between right-wing authoritarianism and religiousness: The role of religious maturity. *Journal of the Scientific Study of Religion, 34,* 245–252.

Martin, J. (2001).The authoritarian personality, 50 years later: What lessons are there for political psychology? *Political Psychology, 22,* 1–26.

Maslow, A. (1943). The authoritarian character structure. *Journal of Social Psychology, 18,* 401–411.

McCann, S. (1999). Threatening times and fluctuations in American church memberships. *Personality and Social Psychology Bulletin, 25,* 325–336.

McCourt, K., Bouchard, T. J., Lykken, D., Tellegen, A., & Keyes, M. (1999). Authoritarianism revisited: Genetic and environmental influences examined in twins reared apart and together. *Personality and Individual Differences, 27,* 985–1014.

McFarland, S. (1998, July). *Toward a typology of prejudiced persons.* Paper presented at the annual meeting of the International Society of Political Psychology, Montreal, Quebec, Canada.

McFarland, S. (2006). *Prejudiced people: Individual differences in explicit prejudice.* Unpublished manuscript.

McFarland, S., & Adelson, S. (1996, July). *An omnibus study of personality, values, and prejudice.* Paper presented at the annual meeting of the International Society of Political Psychology, Vancouver, British Columbia, Canada.

McFarland, S., Ageyev, V., & Abalakina, M. (1990). Authoritarianism in the former Soviet Union. *Journal of Personality and Social Psychology, 63,* 1004–1010.

Meloen, J. (1983). *De autoritaire reaktie in tijden van welvaart en krisis [The authoritarian response in times of prosperity and crisis].* Unpublished doctoral dissertation, University of Amsterdam.

Moghaddam, F., & Vuksanovic, V. (1990). Attitudes and behavior towards human rights across different contexts: The role of right-wing authoritarianism, political ideology, and religiosity. *International Journal of Psychology, 25,* 455–474.

Newcomb, T., Koenig, K., Flacks, R., & Warwick, D. (1967). *Persistence and change: Bennington College and its students after 25 years.* New York: Wiley.

Peterson, B., Doty, R., & Winter, D. (1993). Authoritarianism and attitudes to contemporary social issues. *Personality and Social Psychology Bulletin, 19,* 174–184.

Pratto, F., Sidanius, J., & Levin, S. (2006). Social dominance theory and the dynamics of intergroup relations: Taking stock and looking forward. *European Review of Social Psychology, 17,* 271–320.

Pratto, F., Sidanius, J., Stallworth, L., & Malle, B. (1994). Social dominance orientation: A personality variable predicting social and political attitudes. *Journal of Personality and Social Psychology, 67,* 741–763.

Raden, D. (1999). Is anti-Semitism currently part of an authoritarian attitude syndrome? *Political Psychology, 20,* 323–244.

Reich, W. (1975). *The mass psychology of fascism.* Harmondsworth, UK: Penguin.

Rikert, E. (1998). Authoritarianism and economic threat: Implications for political behavior. *Political Psychology, 19,* 707–720.

Roccato, M., & Ricolfi, L. (2005). On the correlation between right-wing authoritarianism and social dominance orientation. *Basic and Applied Social Psychology, 27,* 187–200.

Rokeach, M. (1954). The nature and meaning of dogmatism. *Psychological Review, 61,* 194–204.

Rokeach, M. (1960). *The open and the closed mind.* New York: Basic Books.

Rosier, M., & Willig, C. (2002). The strange death of the authoritarian personality: 50 years of psychological and political debate. *History of the Human Sciences, 15,* 71–96.

Sales, S. (1973). Threat as a factor in authoritarianism: An analysis of archival data. *Journal of Personality and Social Psychology, 28,* 44–57.

Sales, S., & Friend, K. E. (1973). Success and failure

as determinants of level of authoritarianism. *Behavioral Science, 18,* 163–172.

Saucier, G. (2000). Isms and the structure of social attitudes. *Journal of Personality and Social Psychology, 78,* 366–385.

Schmitt, M., Branscombe, N., & Kappen, D. (2003). Attitudes toward group-based inequality: Social dominance or social identity. *British Journal of Social Psychology, 42,* 161–186.

Schultz, P., & Searleman, A. (2002). Rigidity of thought and behavior: 100 years of research. *Genetic, Social, and General Psychology Monographs, 128,* 165–207.

Schultz, P., & Stone, W. (1994). Authoritarianism and attitudes toward the environment. *Environment and Behavior, 26,* 25–37.

Sibley, C. G., & Duckitt, J. (2008). Personality and prejudice: A meta-analysis and theoretical review. *Personality and Social Psychology Review, 12,* 248–279.

Sibley, C. G., Robertson, A., & Wilson, M. S. (2006). Social dominance orientation and right-wing authoritarianism: Additive and interactive effects. *Political Psychology, 27,* 755–768.

Sibley, C. G., Wilson, M., & Duckitt, J. (2007). Effects of dangerous and competitive worldviews on right-wing authoritarianism and social dominance orientation over a five-month period. *Political Psychology, 28,* 357–371.

Sidanius, J., & Pratto, F. (1999). *Social dominance: An intergroup theory of social hierarchy and oppression.* Cambridge, UK: Cambridge University Press.

Skitka, L., Mullen, E., Griffin, T., Hutchinson, S., & Chamberlin, B. (2002). Dispositions, scripts, or motivated correction: Understanding ideological differences in explanations for social problems. *Journal of Personality and Social Psychology, 92,* 67–81.

Son Hing, L., Bobocel, D., Zanna, M., & McBride, M. (2007). Authoritarian dynamics and unethical decision making: High social dominance orientation leaders and high right-wing authoritarianism followers. *Journal of Personality and Social Psychology, 92,* 67–81.

Stangor, C., & Leary, M. (2006). Intergroup beliefs: Investigations from the social side. In M. Zanna (Ed.), *Advances in experimental social psychology* (Vol. 38, pp. 243–281). New York: Academic Press.

Stellmacher, J., & Petzel, T. (2005). Authoritarianism as a group phenomenon. *Political Psychology, 26,* 245–274.

Stenner, K. (2005). *The authoritarian dynamic.* Cambridge, UK: Cambridge University Press.

Stone, W., Lederer, G., & Christie, R. (1993). The status of authoritarianism. In W. Stone, G. Lederer, & R. Christie (Eds.), *Strength and weakness: The authoritarian personality today* (pp. 229–245). New York: Springer.

Stößell, K., Kämpfe, N., & Riemann, R. (2006). The Jena twin registry and the Jena twin study of social attitudes. *Twin Research and Human Genetics, 9,* 783–786.

Tarr, H., & Lorr, M. (1991). A comparison of right-wing authoritarianism, conformity, and conservatism. *Personality and Individual Differences, 12,* 307–311.

Van Hiel, A., Duriez, B., & Kossowska, M. (2006). The presence of left-wing authoritarianism in Western Europe and its relationship with conservative ideology. *Political Psychology, 27,* 769–793.

Van Hiel, A., & Mervielde, I. (2002). Explaining conservative beliefs and political preference: A comparison of social dominance orientation and authoritarianism. *Journal of Applied Social Psychology, 32,* 965–976.

Verkuyten, M., & Hagendoorn, L. (1998). Prejudice and self-categorization: The variable role of authoritarianism and in-group stereotypes. *Personality and Social Psychology Bulletin, 24,* 99–110.

Walker, W., Rowe, R., & Quinsey, V. (1993). Authoritarianism and sexual aggression. *Journal of Personality and Social Psychology, 65,* 1036–1045.

Whitley, B., & Lee, S. (2000). The relationship of authoritarianism and related constructs to attitudes toward homosexuality. *Journal of Applied Social Psychology, 30,* 144–170.

Wilson, G. (Ed.). (1973). *The psychology of conservatism.* London: Academic Press.

Wylie, L., & Forest, J. (1992). Religious fundamentalism, right-wing authoritarianism, and prejudice. *Psychological Reports, 71,* 1291–1298.

CHAPTER 21

■ ● ▲ ◆ ■ ● ▲ ◆

The Need for Cognition

RICHARD E. PETTY
PABLO BRIÑOL
CHRIS LOERSCH
MICHAEL J. MCCASLIN

As conceptualized by Cacioppo and Petty (1982), the need for cognition (NC) refers to the tendency for people to vary in the extent to which they engage in and enjoy effortful cognitive activities. Some individuals have relatively little motivation for cognitively effortful tasks, whereas other individuals consistently engage in and enjoy cognitively challenging activities. Of course, people can fall at any point in the distribution. For people high in NC, thinking satisfies a desire and is enjoyable. For people low in NC, thinking can be a chore that is engaged in mostly when some incentive or reason is present.

Background and Measurement

Since its introduction, NC has been examined in a large number of studies. In a comprehensive review over a decade ago (Cacioppo, Petty, Feinstein, & Jarvis, 1996), well over 100 studies examining NC were described. Since then, over 100 additional publications have appeared. To date, over 1,000 publications have either cited the original article on NC (Cacioppo & Petty, 1982) or the short version of the scale (Cacioppo, Petty, & Kao, 1984). Given the small amount of space allocated here, we can only begin to outline some of the major

themes in NC work, and we are not able to cover all of the interesting studies that have been conducted. Nevertheless, we aim to illustrate the major conceptual findings. Most important, the available evidence indicates that as NC increases, people are more likely to think about a wide variety of things, including their own thoughts. This enhanced thinking often produces more consequential (e.g., enduring) judgments and can sometimes provide protection from common judgmental biases. At other times, however, enhanced thinking can exacerbate a bias or even reverse it. We begin our review with a brief history of the NC concept and its measurement. Then we turn to the role of NC in current dual-process and system theories of judgment. We conclude with a summary of some of the key research areas in which the NC construct has proven useful.

The NC construct was originally conceptualized by Cohen, Stotland, and Wolfe (1955) as reflecting a need to make sense of the world. Therefore, greater NC was associated with preference for structure and clarity in one's surroundings, making it appear closer to contemporary scales that measure need for structure (see Webster & Kruglanski, 1994) than to the current definition. Because Cohen's original NC measurement device was no longer available, Cacioppo and Petty (1982) developed a new scale to reflect their new conceptualization but retained the term *need for cognition* in acknowledgement of the pioneering efforts of Cohen and colleagues.

Cacioppo and Petty (1982) proposed that NC is a stable individual difference in the tendency to engage in and enjoy cognitively effortful activities across a wide range of domains. NC was conceptualized as reflecting a stable intrinsic motivation that developed over time rather than a need in the traditional sense (i.e., a source of energy that motivates behavior). In this conceptualization, the emphasis is on cognitive processing rather than particular cognitive outcomes. The idea that NC taps into differences in motivation rather than ability is supported by research showing that NC is only moderately related to measures of cognitive ability (e.g., verbal intelligence) and continues to predict relevant outcomes after cognitive ability is controlled (see Cacioppo et al., 1996).

Although the NC scale was originally developed as a 34-item inventory (Cacioppo & Petty, 1982), the most commonly used version contains 18 statements that people rate on 5-point scales to reflect how characteristic the statement is of themselves (Cacioppo et al., 1984). Some examples of scale items are "I prefer complex to simple tasks" and "Thinking is not my idea of fun" (reverse scored). The scale has high internal consistency (reflecting one factor) and test–retest reliability. The scale also demonstrates good convergent and discriminant validity. For instance, the scale correlates highly with a recent scale designed to assess elaborated forms of thinking and judgment (Eigenberger, Critchely, & Sealander, 2006) but is uncorrelated with social desirability (Fletcher, Danilovics, Fernandez, Peterson, & Reeder, 1986; for correlations with many other variables, see Cacioppo et al., 1996; Petty & Jarvis, 1996). Sometimes fewer than 18 items have been used to assess NC with success (e.g., Verplanken, 1991), and a two-item version of the scale was developed for and used in the 2000 National Election Study (Bizer et al., 2002).

NC and Theories of Judgment

Cacioppo and Petty (1982) developed the NC construct at a time when dual-process theories of judgment were beginning to become popular in social psychology. In particular, the elaboration likelihood model (Petty & Cacioppo, 1981, 1986), the heuristic systematic model (Chaiken, 1987), and still other dual-process theories (see Chaiken & Trope, 1999) proposed that some judgments were thoughtfully based on a careful consideration of the information presented, whereas other judgments were based on a more cursory analysis. Within the context of the dual-process theories, NC was used as a way to determine the mechanism by which individuals' judgments would be formed or changed. Considerable research has suggested that individuals low in NC are, absent some incentive to the contrary, more likely to rely on simple cues in a persuasion situation (Haugtvedt, Petty, & Cacioppo, 1992) and on stereotypes alone in judging other people (Carter, Hall, Carney, & Rosip, 2006) than are those high in NC. Those high in NC are more likely to consider all of the pertinent information. Thus, as explained further later, if cues and stereotypes have any impact on individuals high in NC, it is more likely to be an indirect effect and to occur by a mechanism that requires some cognitive effort (e.g., Wegener, Clark, & Petty, 2006).

Although the 1980s and 1990s were dominated by *dual-process* models of judgment, the most recent decade has brought forth various *dual-system* theories. One system has been referred to as emotional, impulsive, intuitive, implicit, or slow learning and is contrasted with the other system, which is labeled as cognitive, reflective, rational, explicit, or fast learning (Petty & Briñol, 2006). The dual-system theories share with the dual-process models the idea that judgments are sometimes deliberative and sometimes are not but also propose that high- and low-thought judgments depend on different mental systems that act independently and rely on distinct brain structures (e.g., Lieberman, 2000). As was the case with some dual-process models, some dual-system approaches have explicitly incorporated the NC construct. In particular, in his cognitive–experiential self-theory, Epstein (2003) uses a slightly modified NC scale to tap into the rational system, whereas the *Faith in Intuition* Scale (e.g., "I am a very intuitive person") is used to tap the experiential system (Epstein, Pacini, Denes-Raj, & Heier, 1996).

The rational system is assumed to be logical, verbal, and relatively affect free, whereas the experiential system is assumed to be intuitive, based on images, and highly dependent on affect. Because the NC scale is used to tap the rational system, one might expect that those high in NC would *not* rely on intuition, images, or affect. However, empirically, the NC and Faith in Intuition scales are uncorrelated, suggesting that individuals both high and low in NC make use of their intuitions, images, and emotions in forming their judgments. Indeed, the evidence suggests that individuals high and low in NC use their intuitions, images, and emotions in different ways.

Specifically, research indicates that affect, intuitions, and images, like any other mental content, can affect judgments in a variety of relatively thoughtful or nonthoughtful ways. When a person is not thinking much, the input (whether emotion, intuition, or image) is used in a rather direct way, having implications for judgment consistent with its valence (e.g., positive images lead to positive judgments). However, when thinking is higher, the impact on judgment is indirect because the input serves in some other capacity (e.g., biasing the thoughts that are generated). Thus it may be confusing to think of NC as assessing "rationality" (Epstein & Pacini, 1999) because one might expect purely rational outcomes from a rational system. However, individuals high in NC can be highly influenced by their intuitions, emotions, and images, but in thoughtful ways. This point is not always appreciated, as it is sometimes assumed that only people low in NC are influenced by these factors. For example, McMath and Prentice-Dunn (2005) suggested that individuals low in NC invariably respond more to images than to text. Rather, images can have an impact under both high and low thinking conditions, but by different mechanisms (e.g., see Miniard, Bhatla, Lord, Dickson, & Unnava, 1991). Thus it is preferable to refer to NC as tapping into the tendency to engage in extensive thinking. To the extent that this thinking is influenced (biased) by irrational intuitions, emotions, or images, the outcome of the thinking need not be rational.

In one study investigating the impact of intuitions on those who vary in NC, Jordan, Whitfield, and Zeigler-Hill (2007) examined the relationship between individuals' deliberative (explicit) versus intuitive (implicit) self-esteem. The key result was that individuals who were high in their faith in intuition showed a larger correlation between their implicit and explicit self-esteem scores than those low in this trait. However, faith in intuition moderated the correlation mostly for people high rather than low in NC.[1] This finding is consistent with other work on metacognition showing that confidence in mental content is more important for individuals high rather than low in NC. That is, just as individuals high in NC rely on their subjective experiences only to the extent that they have confidence in them, so too do they rely on any salient mental contents primarily when perceived validity is high (see Petty, Briñol, Tormala, & Wegener, 2007).

Over the past 25 years, NC has been examined in a wide variety of areas. For example, in the domain of survey research, it has been shown that individuals high in NC provide more thoughtful survey responses and are less likely to satisfice in their answers (Krosnick, 1991). People high in NC not only engage in more thinking, but they are also more aware of their thinking. Thus research shows that people high in NC are more likely to experience lucid dreaming (Blagrove & Hartnell, 2000; Patrick & Durndell, 2004), which is the awareness that one is dreaming. Although there are numerous studies relating NC to many phenomena, we have selected four broad domains to illustrate the utility of the NC construct: attitudes and persuasion, social cognition and decision making, interpersonal relations, and various more applied domains.

Attitudes and Persuasion

Reliance on Effortful Evaluation versus Low-Effort Processes

The psychology of persuasion focuses on which variables produce changes in individuals' beliefs and attitudes and the mechanisms by which they do so. Consistent with the idea that NC is associated with effortful thinking, people high in NC tend to form attitudes on the basis of an effortful analysis of the quality of the relevant information in a persuasive message (e.g., discriminating between strong and weak arguments—

Cacioppo, Petty, & Morris, 1983; discriminating between diagnostic and nondiagnostic information—Chang, 2007). In contrast, absent any incentive to the contrary, individuals low in NC tend to treat variables as simple cues. These include factors such as the attractiveness (e.g., Haugtvedt, Petty, & Cacioppo, 1992) or credibility (Priester & Petty, 1995) of the message source (see also Briñol, Petty, & Tormala, 2004; Kaufman, Stasson, & Hart, 1999), the appearance and frame (e.g., positive vs. negative, gains vs. losses) of the message (e.g., Chatterjee, Heath, Milberg, & France, 2000; Smith & Levin, 1996; Zhang & Buda, 1999), and their own emotional states (Briñol, Petty, & Barden, 2007; Petty, Schumann, Richman, & Strathman, 1993).

However, individuals low in NC can be motivated to scrutinize the available information carefully and eschew reliance on cues if situational circumstances are motivating—such as when the message is of high personal relevance (Axsom, Yates, & Chaiken, 1987), when there is some uncertainty regarding the communication (Priester & Petty, 1995; Priester, Dholakia, & Fleming, 2004; Smith & Petty, 1996; Ziegler, Diehl, & Ruther, 2002), when the medium through which they receive the information is entertaining or engaging (e.g., when it uses comic strips) (Bakker, 1999; Stephan & Brockner, 2007), when the message matches some aspect of the recipient's self-concept (e.g., Brannon & McCabe, 2002; Evans & Petty, 2003), and when the message includes emotional contents (Vidrine, Simmons, & Brandon, 2007; see also Haddock, Maio, Arnold, & Huskinson, 2008). When strong arguments are presented, increasing thinking enhances persuasion, but when weak arguments are presented, increasing thinking diminishes persuasion. It is important to note that the normally extensive thinking of individuals high in NC can be undermined when a message is framed as being for people who do not like to think (Wheeler, Petty, & Bizer, 2005) or when the thinking is demanded rather than spontaneous (Lassiter, Apple, & Slaw, 1996; Leone & Ensley, 1986).

Because individuals high (vs. low) in NC typically engage in more thinking, they also tend to have stronger attitudes (e.g., more accessible in memory, resistant to change, and having more impact on subsequent behavior) (e.g., Haugtvedt & Petty, 1992; Ruiter, Verplanken, De Cremer, & Kok, 2004; see Petty, Haugtvedt, & Smith, 1995). If individuals high in NC are told that they based their attitudes on simple cues rather than on a careful assessment of the message arguments, they feel ambivalent about their attitudes, which can undermine attitude strength (Tormala & DeSensi, 2008). Also, because individuals high (vs. low) in NC engage in more thinking, they tend to form stronger automatic associations among attitude objects (Briñol, Petty, & McCaslin, 2009), and to generalize their changes to other, related beliefs (e.g., Murphy, Holleran, Long, & Zeruth, 2005).

Metacognition

Individuals high in NC not only tend to generate more thoughts than those low in NC, but they are also more likely to think about their thoughts (i.e., engage in metacognition; Petty et al., 2007). For example, following thought generation, individuals high in NC are more likely to evaluate their thoughts for validity, a process called *self-validation* (Petty, Briñol, & Tormala, 2002). The more valid thoughts are seen to be, the more likely they are to be used in forming judgments. Many variables have been shown to affect thought confidence and subsequent thought reliance for individuals high but not low in NC, including whether people were nodding rather than shaking their heads during thought generation (Briñol & Petty, 2003) or experiencing ease rather than difficulty in thought generation (Tormala, Falces, Briñol, & Petty, 2007; Tormala, Petty, & Briñol, 2002). Thought confidence has also been increased for individuals high (vs. low) in NC if following thought generation they learned that the message source was of high versus low credibility (Briñol, Petty, & Tormala, 2004), were made to feel powerful rather than powerless (Briñol, Petty, Valle, Rucker, & Becerra, 2007), or were led to believe that their thoughts were shared by similar others (Petty et al., 2002). Enhanced thought confidence can increase persuasion when thoughts are favorable toward the proposal but decrease it when thoughts are mostly unfavorable.

Not only do individuals high in NC think about the thoughts that they have generated to a message, but they also think about the process by which they either changed their attitudes or resisted change. First, people high in NC are typically aware of the greater thought they put into their judgments and as a result tend to have more confidence in their opinions than individuals low in NC (Barden & Petty, 2008). Furthermore, when people high in NC change their attitudes, they become more confident of their new opinions if they believe that they have considered both sides of the issue rather than just one side (Rucker & Petty, 2004; Rucker, Petty, & Briñol, 2008). On the other hand, if people have resisted persuasion, they can become more confident in their original attitude if they are impressed with their resistance (Petty, Tormala, & Rucker, 2004), such as when they think they have resisted strong arguments rather than weak ones (Tormala & Petty, 2004).

Finally, as a result of their enhanced thinking and concern about validity, individuals high (vs. low) in NC are more likely to correct their judgments for any perceived judgmental biases that might be operating (e.g., DeSteno, Petty, Rucker, Wegener, & Braverman, 2004; for a review, see Wegener & Petty, 1997). For example, DeSteno, Petty, Wegener, and Rucker (2000) found that when an irrelevant source of emotion was made salient, people high in NC adjusted their judgments in a direction opposite to the perceived biasing impact of the emotion (see also Briñol, Rucker, Tormala, & Petty, 2004).

Multiple Roles for Variables Depending on NC

We have noted that the same variables can have an impact on the judgments of individuals high and low in NC, but the mechanism of impact is often different. For example, variables that operate as simple cues for individuals low in NC can influence attitudes for those with high NC, but by different mechanisms, such as biasing thoughts or validating thoughts. To illustrate, in one study (Petty et al., 1993), participants viewed a commercial for a pen embedded in a television program that invoked either a happy or a neutral affective state. Participants both high and low in NC developed more favorable attitudes

toward the pen when they were happy. However, emotion worked differently for those high and low in NC. For individuals high in NC, emotion biased the thoughts that were generated (i.e., a happy state led to more favorable thoughts being produced that mediated attitude change). For individuals low in NC, a happy state produced more favorable attitudes without affecting thoughts (i.e., happiness served as a simple cue). In a similar vein, Priluck and Till (2004) found that a deliberative aspect of conditioning—contingency awareness—mediated the classical conditioning effect for individuals high (but not low) in NC.

Other Attitudinal Effects

In other research, NC has been related to a number of well-established attitudinal phenomena, such as the *mere thought effect* (Smith, Haugtvedt, & Petty, 1994) and *primacy* and *recency* effects (e.g., Petty, Tormala, Hawkins, & Wegener, 2001; see Briñol & Petty, 2005, for a review). Recent research has shown that individuals high (vs. low) in NC are more susceptible to the *sleeper effect*. In this paradigm, individuals both high and low in NC initially discount a strong persuasive message due to its association with a negative cue (e.g., low credibility source), but persons high in NC become more influenced over time. The reason is thought to be that individuals high but not low in NC had engaged in more processing of the strong message arguments, so the attitudes from this emerged once the negative cue was forgotten (Priester, Wegener, Petty, & Fabrigar, 1999).

Social Cognition and Decision Making

At the most basic level, NC affects the amount of thought that goes into a decision. Thus, those high in NC tend to think more about available options prior to making a decision (Levin, Huneke, & Jasper, 2000) and are more likely to search for additional information before coming to a judgmental conclusion (Yang & Lee, 1998). Perhaps surprisingly, both high and low levels of NC have been related to various biases in judgment. Across a variety of studies, those low in NC tend to show greater amounts of bias when this bias is created by a reliance on mental shortcuts. Alternatively, when the bias is created through effortful thought, individuals high in NC tend to be more strongly affected. When a bias can come about through either route, individuals both low and high in NC can show the effect, but it will be produced by different mechanisms. We highlight various research findings that illustrate NC's role in producing judgmental bias.

False Memories

One domain in which high thought leads to more bias is in the creation of false memories. In a common paradigm, participants are first asked to memorize lists of related words (e.g., *table, sit, legs*). After this task, recognition memory is tested by having participants go through a larger list that contains both studied and nonstudied items. The critical items in this task are nonstudied words that are semantically related to those contained in the studied list (e.g., *chair*). Individuals high in NC are more likely to show false memory for these lures (Graham, 2007). Because individuals high in NC elaborate each list item and have stronger interconnections in memory, they are more likely to think about and access the semantically related (but nonpresented) items and therefore show greater false memory for them.

Halo Effects

One bias presumed to be on the opposite end of the thinking continuum from false memories is the halo effect, a phenomenon in which people rate attractive or likeable others as superior on a variety of other trait dimensions (e.g., intelligence; Feingold, 1992). Perlini and Hansen (2001) argued that because this effect can occur when people rely on their stereotypes of attractive others alone to judge a novel target (rather than individuating this person), those low in NC would be more susceptible to this bias. However, individuals high in NC also showed a smaller halo effect. Although not explicitly studied, it is possible that instead of their relying on target attractiveness as a

simple cue, the thoughts of participants high in NC were biased in a favorable direction by the target's attractiveness (as was the case for happiness; see Petty et al., 1993).

Anchoring

One well-studied judgmental bias is the anchoring effect—the tendency for an activated irrelevant number to influence numeric estimates (Tversky & Kahneman, 1974). In one study, Epley and Gilovich (2006) asked students questions that elicited self-generated anchors, such as "When was George Washington elected president?" (eliciting an anchor of 1776). The responses to these questions provided by individuals low in NC were more influenced by the starting anchors. Because individuals high in NC engage in greater levels of thought, they tend to entertain a greater range of possible values and subsequently provided estimates further from the initial anchor value. Importantly, although this specific process renders individuals low in NC more susceptible to a starting anchor, other anchoring mechanisms tend to emerge more strongly when one thinks extensively about the judgment and when one's thoughts are biased by the anchor (e.g., see Mussweiler & Strack, 2001, on selective accessibility). When this is the case, those high in NC can show equal or greater judgmental bias from the anchor (Blankenship, Wegener, Petty, Detweiler-Bedell, & Macy, 2008).

Priming

Another area in which bias can be exacerbated by extensive thinking is priming. In a series of studies (Petty, DeMarree, Briñol, Horcajo, & Strathman, 2008), NC affected the degree to which participants subtly primed with openness (or resistance) judged an ambiguous individual in a prime-consistent manner. Because primes often affect judgments by biasing one's interpretation of a target (Higgins, Rholes, & Jones, 1977), those who think more about the target have more opportunities for the prime to have an effect. Furthermore, because those high in NC are also more likely to think about the validity of their thoughts, these individuals are less likely to show priming effects when a construct is primed in a blatant manner because they are more likely to correct for any perceived biasing impact of the prime. If individuals high in NC overcorrect for a perceived assimilative bias, they can show a reverse effect of the prime (i.e., contrast; see also Martin, Seta, & Crelia, 1990).

Stereotyping

As a final example of how the same variable can create bias in those high or low in NC via different mechanisms, consider a study on stereotyping (Crawford & Skowronski, 1998) in which participants were presented with a hypothetical criminal assault case in which the defendant was described as either Hispanic or Caucasian. In addition to the crime details, participants also read about three kinds of behaviors that this individual had performed prior to the crime—behaviors consistent with the criminal stereotype (negative and incriminating), inconsistent (positive and exculpating), and neutral.

Although individuals both low and high in NC were biased by the defendant's ethnicity, the nature of this bias was quite different. Those low in NC simply relied on the Hispanic stereotype to form their guilt judgments. In contrast, those high in NC elaborated carefully on the crime details they received and were able to avoid an overall guilt bias. However, individuals high in NC showed a bias in memory for the behaviors performed by the defendant such that they recalled a greater percentage of the guilt-implying behaviors when the defendant was Hispanic. Although this was not examined, this memory bias could lead to a guilt bias on a delayed assessment (see also Wegener et al., 2006).

Interpersonal Relations

Although most work on NC has examined its operation with respect to intrapersonal cognition, some studies have shown that people who vary in NC also behave differently in interpersonal contexts. For example, research suggests that those high in NC typically take a more involved role in dyads and other small-group settings, such as entering into discussions earlier (Henningsen & Henningsen, 2004) and speaking longer than those low in NC (Shestowsky & Horowitz, 2004).

In some cases, interacting with an individual high in NC can be beneficial for all those involved. For instance, Schei, Rognes, and Mykland (2006) found that better joint outcomes were obtained for buyer–seller dyads in which the seller was high in NC, and Smith, Kerr, Markus, and Stasson (2001) showed that in collective settings, those high (versus low) in NC were less likely to engage in social loafing. In other cases, though, individuals high in NC can have a negative impact on interpersonal interactions. For example, Henningsen and Henningsen (2004) showed that in a group setting, those high in NC are more likely to promote the discussion of information that is already known by other group members, thereby limiting the productivity of group discussions. Shestowsky and Horowitz (2004) provided evidence that, despite the fact that individuals high in NC were seen as more active and persuasive, they were *less* responsive to differences in the quality of arguments presented by a confederate than those low in NC, perhaps because they were distracted by focusing on presenting their own ideas. In addition, Briñol and colleagues (2005) showed that although people high in NC were able to generate more convincing arguments in a group setting than those low in NC (see also Shestowsky, Wegener, & Fabrigar, 1998), they were also less efficient in reaching group consensus as the size of the group increased. Briñol and colleagues reasoned that group discussions can become deadlocked due to fierce counterarguing among individuals high in NC who hold different opinions. However, when individuals high in NC receive training in interpersonal skills, they can adapt their behavior in a way that enhances group performance (Briñol et al., 2007).

Applied Areas: Law and Health

NC has been of interest to researchers in a number of applied areas. Some, such as survey research, advertising, and the media, were mentioned in earlier sections of this chapter. Two other domains in which NC has had an impact are in law and health. These are noted next.

Research in psychology and law has shown that differences in the amount and depth of thinking between individuals high and low in NC can influence legal judgments. For example, one study (Sargent, 2004) showed that the greater attributional complexity of individuals high (vs. low) in NC led them to endorse less punitive judgments. Another study (Leippe, Eisenstadt, Rauch, & Seib, 2004) provided evidence for a curvilinear relationship between NC and jurors' likelihood of convicting a defendant in a particular case, such that those either very low or high in NC were least likely to convict. The authors speculated that individuals low in NC failed to appreciate the merits of the case and that individuals very high in NC saw even minor flaws as weaknesses. A third study suggested that individuals high in NC are more likely to correct for perceived biasing agents in a trial (Sommers & Kassin, 2001; see Wegener, Kerr, Fleming, & Petty, 2000, for a review).

Recent studies have also shown that NC can lead to a greater understanding of health-related phenomena. For instance, just as beliefs are better predictors of attitudes for individuals high rather than low in NC, Hittner (2004) found that participants' cognitive expectations about the positive and negative outcomes of drinking alcohol were more strongly associated with actual drinking behavior as NC increased. Similarly, Ruiter and colleagues (2004) showed that although participants both high and low in NC reported more fear arousal after reading a high- (vs. low-) threat message about breast cancer, the high-threat appeal favorably influenced relevant attitudes and behaviors only for those high in NC. In contrast, threat was associated with negative attitudes toward breast self-examination and was unrelated to behavior for those low in NC. Importantly, NC is also relevant to crafting persuasive health appeals. In one study (Williams-Piehota, Scheider, Pizarro, Mowad, & Salovey, 2003), women high in NC were significantly more likely to obtain a mammography within 6 months when given a complex versus a simple message, and in another study (Bakker, 1999), presenting information about AIDS in a simple cartoon format rather than a text format proved more effective for individuals low in NC, whereas the reverse was true for those high in NC.

Summary and Conclusions

Based on the reviewed findings, it is clear that need for cognition (NC), the tendency to engage in and enjoy thinking, is an individual difference that is relevant across many different areas of inquiry, ranging from attitudes and persuasion, judgment and decision making, interpersonal and group interactions, and important applied settings. A number of general conclusions emerge from this chapter. First, and most important, individuals high in NC tend to think more than those low in NC about all kinds of information, including their own thoughts (metacognition). Second, however, it is noteworthy that individuals low in NC are capable of and can be motivated to exert extensive thinking, and individuals high in NC can decide not to think under certain circumstances, such as when the message does not seem challenging. Third, these differences in the extent of thinking between individuals high and low in NC can result in different outcomes in response to the same treatment. For example, if people experience happiness (versus sadness) after receiving a weak persuasive message, the happiness would induce more persuasion for individuals low in NC by serving as a simple positive cue but would lead to less persuasion for individuals high in NC by instilling more confidence in their negative thoughts. Fourth, even when individuals high and low in NC show the same outcome, the underlying processes (e.g., cue effect vs. biased processing) and further consequences can differ (e.g., weaker attitudes for individuals low than high in NC). Fifth, although the mechanisms usually differ, individuals high and low in NC can both be susceptible to various biases, regardless of the nature and the source of the biasing factor (e.g., an anchor, a stereotype, or an emotional state). Sixth, individual differences in NC are relevant to understanding not only how people process information (e.g., as targets of influence) but also how they behave (e.g., as persuasive agents). Seventh, different levels of NC can be associated with both positive or negative, accurate or inaccurate, and rational or irrational outcomes, depending on the circumstances involved. For example, high levels of NC can be beneficial in some domains (e.g., buyer–seller dyads) but can also yield negative outcomes in other situations (e.g., reaching consensus in large-group discussions). Finally, we have seen how NC relates not only to some classic topics in psychology (e.g., the sleeper effect, halo effects, priming, group influence) but also to more recent phenomena (e.g., dual-system models, metacognition). Although our review of the literature has been illustrative rather than exhaustive, it provides a reasonably coherent picture of the proclivities of those who vary in NC and the utility of this construct in a wide variety of basic and applied domains.

Note

1. The moderational impact of NC was not shown in a second study that used a substantially smaller sample and a truncated NC scale.

References

Ahlering, R. F., & Parker, L. D. (1989). Need for cognition as a moderator of the primacy effect. *Journal of Research in Personality, 23,* 313–317.

Axsom, D., Yates, S. M., & Chaiken, S. (1987). Audience response as a heuristic cue in persuasion. *Journal of Personality and Social Psychology, 53,* 30–40.

Bakker, A. B. (1999). Persuasive communication about AIDS prevention: Need for cognition determinates the impact of message format. *AIDS Education and Prevention, 11,* 150–162.

Barden, J., & Petty, R. E. (2008). The mere perception of elaboration creates attitude certainty: Exploring the thoughtfulness heuristic. *Journal of Personality and Social Psychology, 95,* 489–509.

Bizer, G. Y., Krosnick, J. A., Holbrook, A. L., Petty, R. E., Rucker, D. D., & Wheeler, S. C. (2002, September). *The impact of personality on political beliefs and behavior: Need for cognition and need to evaluate.* Paper presented at the annual meeting of the American Political Science Association, Boston.

Blagrove, M., & Hartnell, S. J. (2000). Lucid dreaming: Associations with internal locus of control, need for cognition and creativity. *Personality and Individual Differences, 28,* 41–47.

Blankenship, K. L., Wegener, D. T., Petty, R. E., Detweiler-Bedell, B., & Macy, C. L. (2008). Elaboration and consequences of anchored estimates: An attitudinal perspective on numerical anchoring. *Journal of Experimental Social Psychology, 44,* 1465–1476.

Brannon, L. A., & McCabe, A. E. (2002). Schema-derived persuasion and perception of AIDS risk. *Health Marketing Quarterly, 20,* 31–48.

Briñol, P., Becerra, A., Díaz, D., Horcajo, J., Valle, C., & Gallardo, I. (2005). El efecto de la necesidad de cognición sobre la influencia interpersonal [The impact of need for cognition on interpersonal influence]. *Psicothema, 17,* 666–671.

Briñol, P., Horcajo, J., Díaz, D., Valle, C., Becerra, A., & De Miguel, J. (2007). El efecto de la formación sobre la influencia interpersonal [The effect of training on interpersonal influence]. *Psicothema, 19,* 401–405.

Briñol, P., & Petty, R. E (2003). Overt head movements and persuasion: A self-validation analysis. *Journal of Personality and Social Psychology, 84,* 1123–1139.

Briñol, P., & Petty, R. E. (2005). Individual differences in persuasion. In D. Albarracín, B. T. Johnson, & M. P. Zanna (Eds.), *The handbook of attitudes and attitude change* (pp. 575–616). Hillsdale, NJ: Erlbaum.

Briñol, P., Petty, R. E., & Barden, J. (2007). Happiness versus sadness as determinants of thought confidence in persuasion: A self-validation analysis. *Journal of Personality and Social Psychology, 93,* 711–727.

Briñol, P., Petty, R. E., & McCaslin, M. J. (2009). Changing attitudes on implicit versus explicit measures: What is the difference? In R. E. Petty, R. H. Fazio, & P. Briñol (Eds.), *Attitudes: Insights from the new implicit measures* (pp. 285–326). New York: Psychology Press.

Briñol, P., Petty, R. E., & Tormala, Z. L. (2004). The self-validation of cognitive responses to advertisements. *Journal of Consumer Research, 30,* 559–573.

Briñol, P., Petty, R. E., Valle, C., Rucker, D. D., & Becerra, A. (2007). The effects of message recipients' power before and after persuasion: A self-validation analysis. *Journal of Personality and Social Psychology, 93,* 1040–1053.

Briñol, P., Rucker, D., Tormala, Z. L., & Petty, R. E. (2004). Individual differences in resistance to persuasion: The role of beliefs and meta-beliefs. In E. S. Knowles & J. A. Linn (Eds.), *Resistance and persuasion* (pp. 83–104). Mahwah, NJ: Erlbaum.

Cacioppo, J. T., & Petty, R. E. (1982). The need for cognition. *Journal of Personality and Social Psychology, 42,* 116–131.

Cacioppo, J. T., Petty, R. E., Feinstein, J. A., & Jarvis, W. B. G. (1996). Dispositional differences in cognitive motivation: The life and times of individuals varying in need for cognition. *Psychological Bulletin, 119,* 197–253.

Cacioppo, J. T., Petty, R. E., & Kao, C. F. (1984). The efficient assessment of "need for cognition." *Journal of Personality Assessment, 48,* 306–307.

Cacioppo, J. T., Petty, R. E., & Morris, K. (1983). Effects of need for cognition on message evaluation, argument recall, and persuasion. *Journal of Personality and Social Psychology, 45,* 805–818.

Carter, J. D., Hall, J. A., Carney, D. R., & Rosip, J. C. (2006). Individual differences in the acceptance of stereotyping. *Journal of Research in Personality, 40,* 1103–1118.

Chaiken, S. (1987). The heuristic model of persuasion. In M. P. Zanna, J. M. Olson, & C. P. Herman (Eds.), *Social influence: The Ontario Symposium* (Vol. 5, pp. 3–39). Hillsdale, NJ: Erlbaum.

Chaiken, S., & Trope, Y. (Eds.). (1999). *Dual-process theories in social psychology.* New York: Guilford Press.

Chang, C. (2007). Diagnostic advertising content and individual differences. *Journal of Advertising, 36,* 75–84.

Chatterjee, S., Heath, T. B., Milberg, S. J., & France, K. R. (2000). The differential processing of price in gains and losses: The effects of frame and need for cognition. *Journal of Behavioral Decision Making, 13,* 61–75.

Cohen, A. R., Stotland, E., & Wolfe, D. M. (1955). An experimental investigation of need for cognition. *Journal of Abnormal and Social Psychology, 51,* 291–294.

Crawford, M. T., & Skowronski, J. (1998). When motivated thought leads to heightened bias: High need for cognition can enhance the impact of stereotypes on memory. *Personality and Social Psychology Bulletin, 24,* 1075–1088.

DeSteno, D., Petty, R. E., Rucker, D. D., Wegener, D. T., & Braverman, J. (2004). Discrete emotions and persuasion: The role of emotion-induced expectancies. *Journal of Personality and Social Psychology, 86,* 43–56.

DeSteno, D., Petty, R. E., Wegener, D. T., & Rucker, D. D. (2000). Beyond valence in the perception of likelihood: The role of emotion specificity. *Journal of Personality and Social Psychology, 78*(3), 397–416.

Eigenberger, M. E., Critchely, C., & Sealander, K. A. (2006). Individual differences in epistemic style: A dual-process perspective. *Journal of Research in Personality, 41,* 3–24.

Epley, N., & Gilovich, T. (2006). The anchoring-and-adjustment heuristic: Why the adjustments are insufficient. *Psychological Science, 17*(4), 311–318.

Epstein, S. (2003). Cognitive–experiential self-theory of personality. In T. Millon & M. J. Lerner (Eds.), *Handbook of psychology: Vol. 5. Personality and social psychology* (pp. 159–184). Hoboken, NJ: Wiley.

Epstein, S., & Pacini, R. (1999). Some basic issues regarding the dual-process theories from the perspective of cognitive–experiential self-theory. In S. Chaiken & Y. Trope (Eds.), *Dual-process theories in social psychology* (pp. 462–482). New York: Guilford Press.

Epstein, S., Pacini, R., Denes-Raj, V., & Heier, H. (1996). Individual differences in intuitive-experiential and analytical–rational thinking styles. *Journal of Personality and Social Psychology, 71,* 390–405.

Evans, L., & Petty, R. E. (2003). Self-guide framing and persuasion: Responsibly increasing message processing to ideal levels. *Personality and Social Psychology Bulletin, 29,* 313–324.

Feingold, A. (1992). Good-looking people are not what we think. *Psychological Bulletin, 111*(2), 304–341.

Fletcher, G. J. O., Danilovics, P., Fernandez, G., Peterson, D., & Reeder, G. D. (1986). Attributional complexity: An individual difference measure. *Journal of Personality and Social Psychology, 51,* 875–884.

Graham, L. M. (2007). Need for cognition and false memory in the Deese–Roediger–McDermott paradigm. *Personality and Individual Differences, 42*(3), 409–418.

Haddock, G., Maio, G., Arnold, K., & Huskinson, T. (2008). Should persuasion be affective or cognitive: The moderating effects of need for affect and need for cognition. *Personality and Social Psychology Bulletin, 34,* 769–778.

Haugtvedt, C. P., & Petty, R. E. (1992). Personality and persuasion: Need for cognition moderates the persistence and resistance of attitude changes. *Journal of Personality and Social Psychology, 63,* 308–319.

Haugtvedt, C. P., Petty, R. E., & Cacioppo, J. T. (1992). Need for cognition and advertising: Understanding the role of personality variables in consumer behavior. *Journal of Consumer Psychology, 1,* 239–260.

Henningsen, D. D., & Henningsen, M. L. M. (2004). The effect of individual difference variables on information sharing in decision-making groups. *Human Communication Research, 30,* 540–555.

Higgins, E. T., Rholes, W. S., & Jones, C. R. (1977). Category accessibility and impression formation. *Journal of Experimental Social Psychology, 13*(2), 141–154.

Hittner, J. B. (2004). Alcohol use among American college students in relation to need for cognition and expectations of alcohol's effects on cognition. *Current Psychology: Developmental, Learning, Personality, Social, 23,* 173–187.

Jordan, C. H., Whitfield, M., & Zeigler-Hill, V. (2007). Intuition and the correspondence between implicit and explicit self-esteem. *Journal of Personality and Social Psychology, 93,* 1067–1079.

Kaufman, D. Q., Stasson, M. F., & Hart, J. W. (1999). Are the tabloids always wrong or is that just what we think?: Need for cognition and perceptions of articles in print media. *Journal of Applied Social Psychology, 29,* 1984–1997.

Krosnick, J. A. (1991). Response strategies for coping with the cognitive demands of attitude measures in surveys. *Applied Cognitive Psychology, 5,* 213–236.

Lassiter, G. D., Apple, K. J., & Slaw, R. D. (1996). Need for cognition and thought-induced attitude polarization: Another look. *Journal of Social Behavior and Personality, 11,* 647–665.

Leippe, M. R., Eisenstadt, D., Rauch, S. M., & Seib, H. M. (2004). Timing of eyewitness expert testimony, jurors' need for cognition, and case strength as determinants of trial verdicts. *Journal of Applied Psychology, 89,* 524–541.

Leone, C., & Ensley, E. (1986). Self-generated attitude change: A person by situation analysis of attitude polarization and attenuation. *Journal of Research in Personality, 20,* 434–446.

Levin, I. P., Huneke, M. E., & Jasper, J. D. (2000). Information processing at successive stages of decision making: Need for cognition and inclusion–exclusion effects. *Organizational Behavior and Human Decision Processes, 82,* 171–193.

Lieberman, M. D. (2000). Intuition: A social cognitive neuroscience approach. *Psychological Bulletin, 126,* 109–137.

Martin, L. L., Seta, J. J., & Crelia, R. A. (1990). Assimilation and contrast as a function of people's willingness and ability to expend effort in forming an impression. *Journal of Personality and Social Psychology, 59*(1), 27–37.

McMath, B. F., & Prentice-Dunn, S. (2005). Protection motivation theory and skin cancer risk: The role of individual differences in responses to persuasive appeals. *Journal of Applied Social Psychology, 35,* 621–643.

Miniard, P., Bhatla, S., Lord, K. R., Dickson, P. R.,

& Unnava, H. R. (1991). Picture-based persuasion processes and the moderating role of involvement. *Journal of Consumer Research, 18,* 92–107.

Murphy, P. K., Holleran, T. A., Long, J. F., & Zeruth, J. A. (2005). Examining the complex roles of motivation and text medium in the persuasion process. *Contemporary Educational Psychology, 30,* 418–438.

Mussweiler, T., & Strack, F. (2001). The semantics of anchoring. *Organizational Behavior and Human Decision Processes, 86*(2), 234–255.

Patrick, A., & Durndell, A. (2004). Lucid dreaming and personality: A replication. *Dreaming, 14,* 234–239.

Perlini, A. H., & Hansen, S. D. (2001). Moderating effects of need for cognition on attractiveness stereotyping. *Social Behavior and Personality, 29,* 313–321.

Petty, R. E., & Briñol, P. (2006). Understanding social judgment: Multiple systems and processes. *Psychological Inquiry, 17,* 217–223.

Petty, R. E., Briñol, P., & Tormala, Z. L. (2002). Thought confidence as a determinant of persuasion: The self-validation hypothesis. *Journal of Personality and Social Psychology, 82,* 722–741.

Petty, R. E., Briñol, P., Tormala, Z. L., & Wegener, D. T. (2007). The role of metacognition in social judgment. In A. W. Kruglanski & E. T. Higgins (Eds.), *Social psychology: Handbook of basic principles* (2nd ed., pp. 254–284). New York: Guilford Press.

Petty, R. E., & Cacioppo, J. T. (1981). *Attitudes and persuasion: Classic and contemporary approaches.* Dubuque, IA: Brown.

Petty, R. E., & Cacioppo, J. T. (1986). *Communication and persuasion: Central and peripheral routes to attitude change.* New York: Springer-Verlag.

Petty, R. E., DeMarree, K. G., Briñol, P., Horcajo, J., & Strathman, A. J. (2008). Need for cognition can magnify or attenuate priming effects in social judgment. *Personality and Social Psychology Bulletin, 34,* 900–912.

Petty, R. E., Haugtvedt, C., & Smith, S. M. (1995). Elaboration as a determinant of attitude strength: Creating attitudes that are persistent, resistant, and predictive of behavior. In R. E. Petty & J. A. Krosnick (Eds.), *Attitude strength: Antecedents and consequences* (pp. 93–130). Mahwah, NJ: Erlbaum.

Petty, R. E., & Jarvis, B. G. (1996). An individual differences perspective on assessing cognitive processes. In N. Schwarz & S. Sudman (Eds.), *Answering questions: Methodology for determining cognitive and communicative processes in survey research* (pp. 221–257). San Francisco: Jossey-Bass.

Petty, R. E., Schumann, D. W., Richman, S. A., & Strathman, A. J. (1993). Positive mood and persuasion: Different roles for affect under high- and low-elaboration conditions. *Journal of Personality and Social Psychology, 64*(1), 5–20.

Petty, R. E., Tormala, Z., Hawkins, C., & Wegener, D. T. (2001). Motivation to think and order effects in persuasion: The moderating role of chunking. *Personality and Social Psychology Bulletin, 27,* 332–344.

Petty, R. E., Tormala, Z. L., & Rucker, D. D. (2004). Resisting persuasion by counterarguing: An attitude strength perspective. In J. T. Jost, M. R. Banaji, &

D. A. Prentice (Eds.), *Perspectivism in social psychology: The yin and yang of scientific progress* (pp. 37–51). Washington, DC: American Psychological Association.

Priester, J., Wegener, D., Petty, R. E., & Fabrigar, L. (1999). Examining the psychological processes underlying the sleeper effect: The elaboration likelihood model explanation. *Media Psychology, 1,* 27–48.

Priester, J. R., Dholakia, U. M., & Fleming, M. A. (2004). When and why the background contrast effect emerges: Thought engenders meaning by influencing the perception of applicability. *Journal of Consumer Research, 31,* 491–501.

Priester, J. R., & Petty, R. E. (1995). Source attributions and persuasion: Perceived honesty as a determinant of message scrutiny. *Personality and Social Psychology Bulletin, 21,* 637–654.

Priluck, R., & Till, B. D. (2004). The role of contingency awareness, involvement, and need for cognition in attitude formation. *Journal of the Academy of Marketing Science, 32,* 329–344.

Rucker, D. D., & Petty, R. E. (2004). When resistance is futile: Consequences of failed counterarguing for attitude certainty. *Journal of Personality and Social Psychology, 86,* 219–235.

Rucker, D. D., Petty, R. E., & Briñol, P. (2008). What's in a frame anyway?: A meta-cognitive analysis of one- versus two-sided message framing. *Journal of Consumer Psychology, 18,* 137–149.

Ruiter, R. A. C., Verplanken, B., De Cremer, D., & Kok, G. (2004). Danger and fear control in response to fear appeals: The role of need for cognition. *Basic and Applied Social Psychology, 26,* 13–24.

Sargent, M. (2004). Less thought, more punishment: Need for cognition predicts support for punitive responses to crime. *Personality and Social Psychology Bulletin, 30,* 1485–1493.

Schei, V., Rognes, J. K., & Mykland, S. (2006). Thinking deeply may sometimes help: Cognitive motivation and role effects in negotiation. *Applied Psychology: An International Review, 55,* 73–90.

Shestowsky, D., & Horowitz, L. M. (2004). How the Need for Cognition Scale predicts behavior in mock jury deliberations. *Law and Human Behavior, 28,* 305–337.

Shestowsky, D., Wegener, D. T., & Fabrigar, L. R. (1998). Need for cognition and interpersonal influence: Individual differences in impact on dyadic decisions. *Journal of Personality and Social Psychology, 74,* 1317–1328.

Smith, B. N., Kerr, N. A., Markus, M. J., & Stasson, M. F. (2001). Individual differences in social loafing: Need for cognition as a motivator in collective performance. *Group Dynamics: Theory, Research, and Practice, 5,* 150–158.

Smith, S. M., Haugtvedt, C. P., & Petty, R. E. (1994). Need for cognition and the effects of repeated expression on attitude accessibility and extremity. *Advances in Consumer Research, 21,* 234–237.

Smith, S. M., & Levin, I. P. (1996). Need for cognition and choice framing effects. *Journal of Behavioral Decision Making, 9,* 283–290.

Smith, S. M., & Petty, R. E. (1996). Message framing and persuasion: A message processing analysis. *Personality and Social Psychology Bulletin, 22,* 257–268.

Sommers, S. R., & Kassin, S. M. (2001). On the many impacts of inadmissible testimony: Selective compliance, need for cognition, and the overcorrection bias. *Personality and Social Psychology Bulletin, 27*, 1368–1377.

Stephan, J., & Brockner, J. (2007). Spaced out in cyberspace?: Evaluations of computer-based information. *Journal of Applied Social Psychology, 37*, 210–226.

Tormala, Z. L., & DeSensi, V. L. (2008). The perceived informational basis of attitudes: Implications for subjective ambivalence. *Personality and Social Psychology Bulletin, 34*, 275–287.

Tormala, Z. L., Falces, C., Briñol, P., & Petty, R. E. (2007). Ease of retrieval effects in social judgment: The role of unrequested cognitions. *Journal of Personality and Social Psychology, 93*, 143–157.

Tormala, Z. L., & Petty, R. E. (2004). Resistance to persuasion and attitude certainty: The moderating role of elaboration. *Personality and Social Psychology Bulletin, 30*, 1446–1457.

Tormala, Z. L., Petty, R. E., & Briñol, P. (2002). Ease of retrieval effects in persuasion: A self-validation analysis. *Personality and Social Psychology Bulletin, 28*, 1700–1712.

Tversky, A., & Kahneman, D. (1974). Judgment under uncertainty: Heuristics and biases. *Science, 185*(4157), 1124–1131.

Verplanken, B. (1991). Persuasive communication of risk information: A test of cue versus message processing effects in a field experiment. *Personality and Social Psychology Bulletin, 17*, 188–193.

Vidrine, J. I., Simmons, V. N., & Brandon, T. H. (2007). Construction of smoking-relevant risk perceptions among college students: The influence of need for cognition and message content. *Journal of Applied Social Psychology, 37*, 91–114.

Webster, D. M., & Kruglanski, A. W. (1994). Individual differences in need for cognitive closure. *Journal of Personality and Social Psychology, 67*, 1049–1062.

Wegener, D. T., Clark, J. K., & Petty, R. E. (2006). Not all stereotyping is created equal: Differential consequences of thoughtful versus non-thoughtful stereotyping. *Journal of Personality and Social Psychology, 90*, 42–59.

Wegener, D. T., Kerr, N. L., Fleming, M. A., & Petty, R. E. (2000). Flexible corrections of juror judgments: Implications for jury instructions. *Psychology, Public Policy, and Law, 6*, 629–654.

Wegener, D. T., & Petty, E. (1995). Flexible correction processes in social judgment: The role of naive theories in corrections for perceived bias. *Journal of Personality and Social Psychology, 68*(1), 36–51.

Wegener, D. T., & Petty, R. E. (1997). The flexible correction model: The role of naive theories in bias correction. In M. P. Zanna (Ed.), *Advances in experimental social psychology* (Vol. 29, pp. 141–208). San Diego, CA: Academic Press.

Wheeler, S. C., Petty, R. E., & Bizer, G. Y. (2005). Self-schema matching and attitude change: Situational and dispositional determinants of message elaboration. *Journal of Consumer Research, 31*, 787–797.

Williams-Piehota, P., Schneider, T. R., Pizarro, J., Mowad, L., & Salovey, P. (2003). Matching health messages to information-processing styles: Need for cognition and mammography utilization. *Health Communication, 15*, 375–392.

Yang, Y., & Lee, H. J. (1998). The effect of response mode, prior knowledge, and need for cognition on consumers' information acquisition process. *Korean Journal of Industrial and Organizational Psychology, 11*, 85–103.

Zhang, Y., & Buda, R. (1999). Moderating effects of need for cognition on responses to positively versus negatively framed advertising messages. *Journal of Advertising, 28*, 1–15.

Ziegler, R., Diehl, M., & Ruther, A. (2002). Multiple source characteristics and persuasion: Source inconsistency as a determinant of message scrutiny. *Personality and Social Psychology Bulletin, 28*, 496–508.

CHAPTER 22

■ ● ▲ ◆ ■ ● ▲ ◆

Optimism

CHARLES S. CARVER
MICHAEL F. SCHEIER

Optimists are people who expect good things to happen to them; pessimists are people who expect bad things to happen to them. This is a dimension of individual differences that has a long history in folk psychology. And folk wisdom has long held that it is important in human affairs. Research over the past two decades suggests that this particular aspect of folk wisdom is right. This simple difference among people—anticipating good versus anticipating bad—relates to a number of processes underlying behavior. The ways in which optimists and pessimists differ have a big impact on their lives. These people differ in how they approach problems; they differ in how, and how well, they cope with adversity; and they differ in their social relationships. This chapter describes some of those reflections of this individual-difference variable.

Scientific definitions of optimism and pessimism focus on expectations for the future, thereby linking these ideas to a long line of expectancy-value models of motivation. Expectancy-value theories assume that behavior reflects the pursuit of goals: desired states or actions. People try to fit their behaviors to what they see as desirable. The more important a goal is to the person, the greater its *value* (for more detail, see Austin & Vancouver, 1996; Carver & Scheier, 1998; Higgins, 2006). The second element is *expectancy*—confidence that the goal can

be attained. If people doubt that a goal can be reached, effort toward it may sag even before the action starts. People confident about an eventual outcome will persevere even in the face of great adversity.

Confidence and doubt can pertain to narrow and limited contexts (the ability to make a putt longer than 20 feet), to moderately broad contexts (the ability to make positive impressions in social situations), and to even broader contexts. Put differently, expectancies can be situated (Armor & Taylor, 1998) or generalized (Scheier & Carver, 1992). Optimism and pessimism represent generalized versions of confidence and doubt, pertaining to most situations in life rather than just one or two. Thus optimists should tend to be confident and persistent in the face of challenges (even if progress is difficult or slow). Pessimists should be doubtful and hesitant in these situations. Such differences in how people confront adversity have implications for the manner in which people cope with stress.

There are at least two ways to think about generalized expectancies and how to measure them. One is to measure them directly, asking people (in one fashion or another) whether they think their outcomes will be good or bad (Scheier & Carver, 1992). This approach, which we have taken in our own work on this topic, adds no conceptual complexity to what we have said so far. Our preferred measure is the Life Orientation Test—Revised, or LOT-R (Scheier, Carver, & Bridges, 1994). It consists of a series of statements (e.g., "I'm always optimistic about my future," "I rarely count on good things happening to me" [reversed]) to which people indicate the extent of their agreement or disagreement on a multipoint scale. Other measures have also been created that similarly consist of statements about good and bad outcomes, with respondents indicating their agreement or disagreement with the statement (e.g., Dember, Martin, Hummer, Howe, & Melton, 1989). Such generalized expectancies, which pertain to the person's entire life space, are what we mean by *optimism* and *pessimism*.

Another approach to measuring optimism relies on the idea that people's expectancies for the future stem from their interpretations of the past (Peterson & Seligman, 1984). If past failures are seen as reflecting stable causes, expectancies will be pessimistic, because the cause (which is relatively permanent) is likely to remain in force. If past failures are seen as reflecting unstable causes, the outlook for the future may be brighter, because the cause may no longer be there. Some define optimism and pessimism in terms of patterns of attributions made about the causes of events (e.g., Peterson & Seligman, 1984; see also Furnham, Chapter 18, this volume) and make the inference that the attributions result in expectancies. This view differs from ours in important ways, but both share the theme that expectations for the future affect people's actions and experiences.

Each of these measures gives a continuous distribution of scores. Writers often refer to optimists and pessimists as though they were distinct categories of people, but this is a verbal convenience. People actually range from very optimistic to very pessimistic, with most falling somewhere between. Another issue that should be mentioned is that although trait optimism is thought of as a stable trait, moment-to-moment confidence is subject to situational influences as well. For example, as people prepare themselves to encounter threats or undesired outcomes, their momentary states of confidence may shift downward, whether they are basically optimists or pessimists (Sweeny, Carroll, & Shepperd, 2006).

One final issue that also bears mention is that there has been some controversy about whether the optimism construct should be viewed as one bipolar dimension or whether there are two separable dimensions, one pertaining to the affirmation of optimism and the other pertaining to affirmation of pessimism. There have been cases in which separating those qualities has led to better prediction of outcomes (Marshall, Wortman, Kusulas, Hervig, & Vickers, 1992; Robinson-Whelen, Kim, MacCallum, & Kiecolt-Glaser, 1997), but this does not always happen. A number of studies aimed at settling the issue have arrived at different answers, with some concluding that a unidimensional view is accurate (Rauch, Schweizer, & Moosbrugger, 2007) and others concluding that there are two dimensions (Herzberg, Glaesmer, & Hoyer, 2006). For the sake of simplicity in presentation, in this chapter we treat optimism–pessimism as one dimension. Keep in mind, however, that in some situations what matters may be the extent to which people endorse versus reject a pessimistic outlook rather than endorse versus reject an optimistic outlook, and vice versa.

In this chapter we describe some ways in which individual differences in optimism versus pessimism, measured as expectations for one's future, relate to variations in other important aspects of life (see also Segerstrom, 2006a). Manifestations of optimism are grouped here into four sets: subjective well-being, coping responses, physical well-being, and social relationships.

Optimism and Subjective Well-Being

One straightforward influence of optimism and pessimism is on how people feel when facing problems. When people confront difficulty, the emotions they experience range from excitement and eagerness to anger, anxiety, and depression. The balance among such feelings relates to differences in optimism. Optimists expect good outcomes, even when things are hard. This expectation yields a relatively positive mix of feelings. Pessimists expect bad outcomes. This expectation yields more negative feelings—anxiety, anger, sadness, or even despair (Carver & Scheier, 1998; Scheier & Carver, 1992).

Relations between optimism and distress have been examined in people facing a wide range of difficulties, including students entering college (Aspinwall & Taylor, 1992; Brissette, Scheier, & Carver, 2002); survivors of missile attacks (Zeidner & Hammer, 1992); people caring for cancer patients (Given et al., 1993) or Alzheimer's patients (Hooker, Monahan, Shifren, & Hutchinson, 1992; Shifren & Hooker, 1995); and people dealing with childbirth (Carver & Gaines, 1987), coronary artery bypass surgery (Fitzgerald, Tennen, Affleck, & Pransky, 1993; Scheier et al., 1989), aging (Giltay, Zitman, & Kromhout, 2006), failed attempts at *in vitro* fertilization (Litt, Tennen, Affleck, & Klock, 1992), bone marrow transplantation (Curbow, Somerfield, Baker, Wingard, & Legro, 1993), cancer (Carver et al., 1993; Friedman et al., 1992), and the progression of AIDS (Taylor et al., 1992).

The studies vary in complexity and thus in what they can show. Researchers sometimes examine responses to an adverse event at one time point. Such studies consistently show that greater pessimism relates to reports of experiencing more distress. What those studies *cannot* show is whether pessimists had more distress even before this particular adverse event. Other studies assess people at multiple times. This gives a better picture of how distress shifts over time and changing circumstances. It also allows researchers to control for initial levels of distress. We focus here on this sort of research.

A very early study of optimism and emotional well-being (Carver & Gaines, 1987) examined the development of depressed feelings after childbirth. Women completed the original LOT and a depression scale in the last third of their pregnancies. They completed the depression measure again 3 weeks after delivery. Optimism was related to lower depression symptoms at initial assessment, and optimism predicted lower depression postpartum, controlling for the initial levels. Thus optimism conferred resistance to postpartum depressive symptoms.

Several projects have studied people dealing with coronary artery bypass. One assessed people a month before surgery and 8 months afterward (Fitzgerald et al., 1993). Optimists had less presurgical distress and (controlling for presurgical life satisfaction) more postsurgical life satisfaction. Opti-

mism about life appeared to lead to a specific optimism about the surgery, and from there to satisfaction with life. A similar study by Scheier and colleagues (1989) found that optimists retained higher quality of life even up to 5 years after the surgery.

Optimism has also been studied in the context of other health crises. An example is treatment for breast cancer (Carver et al., 1993). Women were interviewed at diagnosis, the day before surgery, a few days after surgery, and 3, 6, and 12 months later. Optimism (at initial assessment) predicted less distress over time, controlling for effects of medical variables and earlier distress. Thus optimism predicted not just lower initial distress but also resilience against distress during the following year. A study of head and neck cancer patients yielded similar results (Allison, Guichard, & Gilain, 2000). Patients were assessed before treatment and 3 months afterward. Optimists reported higher quality of life before treatment and also posttreatment, controlling for initial ratings.

Another medical context in which optimism has been studied is *in vitro* fertilization, a procedure that lets people overcome fertility problems. This study focused on people whose attempts at *in vitro* fertilization were unsuccessful (Litt et al., 1992). Eight weeks beforehand, the researchers measured optimism, expectancies for fertilization success, distress, and the impact of infertility on participants' lives. Two weeks after notification of a negative pregnancy test, distress was measured again. None of the initial variables predicted follow-up distress (controlling for Time 1 distress) except optimism.

Yet another context in which effects of optimism have been examined is treatment for ischemic heart disease. In this study (Shnek, Irvine, Stewart, & Abbey, 2001), pessimism related to more symptoms of depression shortly after hospitalization for this disease. Furthermore, pessimism related to more symptoms of depression at a 1-year follow-up, even when controlling for earlier depression and a variety of other variables.

Not only does optimism have a positive effect on the psychological well-being of people dealing with medical conditions, but it also influences well-being among caregivers. One project studied a group of cancer patients and their caregivers (Given et al., 1993). Caregivers' optimism predicted less depression and less impact of caregiving on their physical health. Similar results were found in research on caregiver spouses of Alzheimer's patients (Hooker et al., 1992; Shifren & Hooker, 1995): Optimism related to lower depression and greater well-being.

Other studies have looked at events that are challenging, but less extreme. For example, the start of college is a stressful time, and studies have examined students adjusting to their first semester of college (Aspinwall & Taylor, 1992; Brissette et al., 2002). Optimism and other variables were assessed when the students first arrived on campus. Measures of well-being were obtained at the end of the semester. Higher initial optimism predicted less distress at the end of the semester, along with greater development of friendship networks.

Indeed, the simple process of aging confronts people with a variety of circumstances that are difficult to adjust to. A Dutch study of older men examined the role of personality at the initial assessment as a predictor of depression across a 15-year follow-up (Giltay et al., 2006). Optimism proved to predict significantly lower cumulative incidence of depression symptoms.

Optimism, Pessimism, and Coping

If optimists experience less distress than pessimists when dealing with difficulties, is it just because they are cheerful? Apparently not, because the differences often remain even when statistical controls are included for prior distress. There have to be other explanations. This section addresses one of them: coping strategies. In many ways, this is just a more detailed depiction of the broad behavioral tendencies discussed at the outset. That is, people who are confident about the future continue trying, even when it's hard. People who are doubtful try to escape the adversity by wishful thinking, they employ temporary distractions that do not help to solve the problem, and they sometimes even stop trying.

Differences in coping that correspond to this divergence in behavior have been observed in several studies. Early projects found that optimistic students reported both situational coping responses and general coping styles that differed from those of pessimists (Scheier, Carver, & Bridges, 2001). Optimism related to problem-focused coping, especially in controllable situations. Optimism also related to positive reframing and a tendency to accept the situation's reality. Optimism related to less denial and less of an attempt to distance oneself from the problem. Thus optimists appear generally to be approach copers, and pessimists appear to be avoidant copers.

Other projects have studied coping strategies in specific contexts. Indeed, several studies described earlier also looked at coping. In their study of coronary artery bypass surgery, Scheier and colleagues (1989) assessed attentional-cognitive strategies as ways of dealing with the experience. Before surgery, optimists more than pessimists reported making plans for their future and setting goals for recovery. Optimists also focused less on negative aspects of the experience— distress and symptoms. Once surgery was past, optimists were more likely than pessimists to report seeking out information about what the physician would require of them in the months ahead. Optimists also were less likely to say that they were suppressing thoughts about their symptoms. There was also evidence that the positive impact of optimism on quality of life 6 months later occurred through the indirect effect of these differences in coping.

The study of failed *in vitro* fertilization described earlier (Litt et al., 1992) also examined coping. Pessimism related to escape as a coping response. Escape, in turn, led to more distress after the fertilization failure. Optimists were also more likely than pessimists to report feeling they had benefited from the experience, for example, by becoming closer to their spouses.

Information on coping also comes from the study of AIDS patients described earlier (Taylor et al., 1992). Optimism predicted positive attitudes and tendencies to plan for recovery, seek information, and reframe bad situations more positively. Optimists used less fatalism, self-blame, and escapism, and they didn't focus on negative aspects of the situation or try to suppress thoughts about their symptoms. Optimists also appeared to accept unchangeable situations rather than trying to escape them.

Relations between optimism and coping also have been studied among cancer patients. Stanton and Snider (1993) found that pessimistic women used more cognitive avoidance in coping with an upcoming biopsy than optimists. The avoidance appeared to mediate the relation of pessimism to prebiopsy distress. Cognitive avoidance prebiopsy also predicted postbiopsy distress among women with positive diagnoses.

Another study of cancer patients, mentioned earlier, examined how women coped with treatment for breast cancer during the first year (Carver et al., 1993). Both before and after surgery, optimism was related to coping that involved accepting the reality of the situation, placing as positive a light on it as possible, and trying to relieve the situation with humor. Pessimism was related to denial and tendencies to give up at each time point. The coping responses related to optimism and pessimism were also related to distress. Further analyses revealed that the effect of optimism on distress was largely indirect through coping, particularly postsurgery.

Another study also examined the role of coping in women treated for breast cancer (Schou, Ekeberg, & Ruland, 2005). Two coping strategies mediated the relationship between optimism and pessimism and quality of life 1 year after diagnosis. The greater fighting spirit of optimists (assessed before diagnosis) predicted better quality of life at the 1-year follow-up. Hopelessness/helplessness (reported by pessimists) predicted poorer quality of life.

In sum, it appears that optimists differ from pessimists both in stable coping tendencies and in the coping responses generated when confronting stressful situations (for a detailed review, see Solberg Nes & Segerstrom, 2006). In general, optimists use more problem-focused coping strategies than pessimists. When problem-focused coping is not a possibility, optimists turn to strategies such as acceptance, use of humor, and positive reframing. Pessimists tend to cope through overt denial and by mentally and behaviorally disengaging from the goals with which the stressor is interfering.

Particularly noteworthy is the contrast between acceptance and active denial. Denial (refusing to accept the reality of the situation) means trying to maintain a worldview that is no longer valid. Acceptance implies restructuring one's perceptions to come to grips with the situation. This does not mean giving up. That response does not help. In fact, reacting to illness with resignation may actually hasten death (Greer, Morris, Pettingale, & Haybittle, 1990; Reed, Kemeny, Taylor, Wang, & Visscher, 1994). Acceptance of the diagnosis has very different consequences. By accepting that life is compromised (but not over), people develop adaptive parameters within which to live the time that is left. Acceptance may actually serve the purpose of keeping the person goal-engaged and, indeed, "life-engaged" (Scheier & Carver, 2001).

Promoting Well-Being

Another aspect of coping is proactive or preventive coping, processes that promote good health and well-being rather than just reacting to adversity. Perhaps optimists take active steps to ensure positive outcomes in their future. This would resemble problem-focused coping, except that it is intended to prevent a stressor from arising.

There are many ways in which this might occur. An example is seeking knowledge pertaining to areas of potential risk. One study investigated heart attack–related knowledge in a group of middle-aged adults. It might be assumed that adults who are optimistic about their health would not make much effort to learn about risks related to heart attacks. Those high in dispositional optimism, however, actually knew more about the risk factors than those who were less optimistic (Radcliffe & Klein, 2002).

Proactive efforts in health promotion have also been examined among patients in a cardiac rehabilitation program (Shepperd, Maroto, & Pbert, 1996). Optimism was related to success in lowering levels of saturated fat, body fat, and an index of overall coronary risk. Optimism was also related to increases in exercise. Another study of the lifestyles of coronary artery bypass patients 5 years after surgery found optimists more likely than pessimists to be taking vitamins and eating low-fat foods and to be enrolled in a cardiac rehabilitation program (Scheier & Carver, 1992).

Another proactive health-related behavior concerns HIV risk. By avoiding certain sexual practices (e.g., sex with unknown partners), people reduce risk of infection. One study of HIV-negative gay men found that optimists reported fewer anonymous sexual partners than pessimists (Taylor et al., 1992). This suggests that optimists were making efforts to reduce their risk, thus safeguarding their health.

Optimists appear to take action to minimize health risks. They do not simply stick their heads in the sand and ignore threats to well-being. They attend to risks, but selectively. They focus on risks that are applicable to them and that relate to potentially serious health problems (Aspinwall & Brunhart, 1996). If the potential health problem is minor, or if it is unlikely to bear on them, they are not especially vigilant. Optimists appear to scan their surroundings for threats to well-being but save their behavioral responses for threats that are truly meaningful.

Is it paradoxical that people who expect good things to happen take active steps to make sure good things *do* happen? Maybe. But years of experience presumably teach people that their own efforts play an important part in many kinds of outcomes in life. Optimists may be more confident than pessimists that their efforts will be successful. For that reason, they are quicker to engage in those efforts when there is a need for them.

Pessimism and Health-Defeating Behaviors

We have characterized optimists throughout this chapter as being persistent in trying to reach goals. Theory suggests that pessimists are less persistent and more likely to give up. There is, in fact, evidence of giving-up tendencies among pessimists, with bad consequences. For example, giving up may underlie various forms of substance abuse, such as excessive alcohol use, which is often seen as an escape from problems. This suggests that pessimists should be more vulnerable than optimists to such maladaptive behavior. Evidence supports this reasoning.

One study of women with family histories of alcoholism found that pessimists in that group were more likely than optimists to report drinking problems (Ohannessian, Hesselbrock, Tennen, & Affleck, 1994). In another study, people who had been treated for

alcohol abuse were followed as they entered an aftercare program. Pessimists were more likely to drop out of that program and to return to drinking than were optimists (Strack, Carver, & Blaney, 1987). Yet another study (Park, Moore, Turner, & Adler, 1997) found that optimistic pregnant women were less likely to engage in substance abuse during the course of their pregnancies.

A more recent study examined a different indicator of giving up: the disruption of normal social activities. Breast cancer patients reported illness-related disruption of social activities after treatment (Carver, Lehman, & Antoni, 2003). At each assessment, pessimism predicted more disruption, along with emotional distress and fatigue. When confronted with a health threat, pessimism led to a withdrawal from the very social activities that are important to a normal life.

Giving up can be reflected in many ways. Alcohol dulls awareness of failures and problems. People can ignore problems by distracting themselves with other activities. Sometimes, though, giving up is more complete. Sometimes people give up not just on specific goals, but on their lives, by suicide. Some are more vulnerable to suicide than others. It is commonly assumed that depression is the best indicator of suicide risk. But at least one study found that pessimism was actually a stronger predictor of this act, the ultimate disengagement from life (Beck, Steer, Kovacs, & Garrison, 1985).

In sum, a sizeable body of evidence indicates that pessimism can lead people into self-defeating patterns. The result can be less persistence, more avoidance coping, health-damaging behavior, and potentially even an impulse to escape from life altogether. Without confidence about the future, there may be nothing to sustain life.

Does Optimism Have a Down Side in Coping and Goal Pursuit?

Although most evidence on coping and confronting difficulty links optimism to adaptive, engaged coping, some have asked whether the optimistic stance on life may also have a down side. Confidence and persistence are good, but they can potentially lead to problems. Consider gambling, a form of entertainment that can create major problems for people who engage in it too much.

Problem gambling can result in loss of large amounts of money, and it often leads to additional problems in work and relationships. Gibson and Sanbonmatsu (2004) reasoned that gambling is a context in which positive expectancies and the resulting persistence might be counterproductive. They found a variety of worrisome tendencies among optimists. They had more positive expectations for gambling than did pessimists, and they were also less likely to reduce their betting after poor outcomes. The people studied in that research were not people with gambling problems. But this pattern suggests the possibility that optimists may be more likely to develop such problems than pessimists.

Another set of studies deals with the question of whether the persistence of optimists results in problems because they are unable to recognize what they cannot accomplish. More simply, perhaps they don't know when it is best to quit. Certainly there are circumstances in which people must recognize that goals have been lost and that the adaptive course is to turn away from their pursuit (Wrosch, Scheier, Carver, & Schulz, 2003). Does the persistence that follows from optimism prevent that from occurring?

One project relevant to this question was based on the reasoning that greater persistence should lead to the development of greater goal conflict, partly because commitment to many goals causes people to spread their resources thinner (Segerstrom & Solberg Nes, 2006). Two studies (one of them prospective) found evidence that optimism did relate to such an elevation in goal conflict. However, this conflict did not have adverse psychological consequences. Evidence from the second study suggested that optimistic people balanced expectancy, value, and cost of goal pursuit more effectively than did pessimistic people. They were committed to more incompatible goals, but they were more efficient at managing the conflict.

Another project (Aspinwall & Richter, 1999) examined participants' willingness to disengage from tasks on which they were unable to succeed (the task actually was impossible). In one condition, there was no alternative task to turn to; in other conditions, there was an alternative. Optimism related to faster disengagement from the impossible task when there was an alternative task to

switch to. In effect, they gave up on a task they could not master in order to turn to a similar task that they *could* master. Indeed, if they had been led to think that the other task measured a somewhat different skill, they even outperformed the less optimistic people.

Yet another set of studies deals with the question of whether optimism causes people to see only what they want to see and ignore threats. The initial evidence suggested the opposite: that optimists pay closer attention to information about health threats than pessimists, provided the threat is serious and relevant to them (Aspinwall & Brunhart, 1996). More recently, Luo and Isaacowitz (2007) found the opposite pattern. Several other studies have found that optimism is associated with an attentional bias toward positive rather than negative stimuli (Isaacowitz, 2005; Segerstrom, 2001). For example, optimism has been linked to shorter times looking at pictures of skin cancers (Isaacowitz, 2005). Exactly how to interpret the aggregated information is not clear. It may be, for example, that optimists prefer to attend to positively valenced stimuli but are quick to encode threat-related information when that information is perceived as useful to them.

In sum, there are cases in which optimism has a down side. The question of when there are costs as well as benefits to optimism is certain to receive additional scrutiny in future work.

Optimism and Physical Well-Being

The previous sections included frequent mention of stress and coping with medical problems. As implied by that, much of the work on optimism has been conducted in the domain of health psychology. Some of that research has gone on to examine optimism and physical well-being. The general line of thinking underlying such research is that optimists may be less reactive than pessimists to the general stresses of life; that the lower physiological stress responses may (over many years) result in less physical wear and tear on the body; and that the end result may be better physical health and potentially greater longevity.

In one study of physical well-being, middle-aged women were tested for carotid intima thickness—an index of atherosclerosis in the carotid artery—at a baseline and a 3-year follow-up (Matthews, Raikkonen, Sutton-Tyrrell, & Kuller, 2004). Pessimism at the initial assessment predicted increases in intima thickness at follow-up. Optimists experienced almost no increase over the 3-year period.

In another project, Scheier and colleagues (1999) examined patterns of rehospitalization after coronary artery bypass surgery. The need for rehospitalization is very common in this population, but optimism significantly predicted lower likelihood of that occurring and a longer time before it occurred. Ironson and colleagues (2005) tested prospective links between optimism, coping, and disease progression among persons with HIV. Optimists displayed more proactive coping, less avoidant coping, and less disease progression.

Individual differences in healing and immunity have also been examined. In one study, men receiving biopsies were followed throughout the healing process (Ebrecht et al., 2004). The sample was split into "slow healing" and "fast healing" groups. Slow healers had significantly lower optimism than the fast healers. In another study, older adults received an influenza vaccine, and optimism predicted a significantly better immune response 2 weeks later (Kohut, Cooper, Nickolaus, Russell, & Cunnick, 2002; for a broader review of optimism and immunity, see Szondy, 2004). Other research has found, however, that optimism was related to lower immune response under very high challenge (Segerstrom, 2005, 2006b). Segerstrom (2005, 2006b) suggests that the reduction under high challenge may reflect the greater engagement of optimists in dealing behaviorally with the challenge.

Research to date suggests that optimism is a psychological construct that is relevant to biological outcomes. One study even found that optimism predicts longer life—among 900 older Dutch persons, those reporting a high level of optimism at baseline were less likely to die over the next 10 years (Giltay, Geleijnse, Zitman, Hoekstra, & Schouten, 2004). The evidence on biological outcomes is less consistent than for self-reports of health (Rasmussen, Scheier, & Greenhouse, 2009), but relations between optimism and physical well-being surely deserve further study.

Optimism and Interpersonal Relations

Although health psychology has been the main arena for studying effects of optimism and pessimism, not all research on this individual difference has been health focused. Indeed, some of the work on stress and coping also had other facets. For example, a study by Brissette and colleagues (2002) that was described earlier examined how new students coped with the challenge of starting college. However, this study also made the point that optimists experienced greater increases in their social networks across the first semester of school than did pessimists.

Associations between social networks and expecting positive outcomes in the future have also been found in other research (MacLeod & Conway, 2005). Yet other work has found that optimistic women under treatment for breast cancer were less likely to withdraw from their social activities due to their treatment than were less optimistic women (Carver, Lehman, & Antoni, 2003). In fact, there is some evidence that social networks and optimism have mutually reinforcing effects: Segerstrom (2007) found that the development of social networks over a 10-year period was related to increases in optimism over that same period.

A number of people have by now characterized optimism as representing a positive resource for relationships, both general social networks and close relationships. Why do optimists have better social connections than pessimists? One contributing factor is that optimists are easier to like than pessimists. Several studies have confirmed that people are more accepting of someone who expressed positive expectations for the future and more rejecting of a person who expressed negative expectations (Carver, Kus, & Scheier, 1994; Helweg-Larsen, Sadeghian, & Webb, 2002). Another study found that actual social interactions with optimistic people are more positive than those with less optimistic people (Räikkönen, Matthews, Flory, Owens, & Gump, 1999). In yet another study, pessimism among men who were about to undergo coronary artery bypass surgery was related to higher reports of caregiver burden from their wives 18 months later (Ruiz, Matthews, Scheier, & Schulz, 2006).

Another contributor may be that optimists tend to see most things in the best light, including things pertaining to their relationships. This might make the optimist more satisfied in the relationship even if things are not perfect. Indeed, a recent study of close relationships found that optimists had higher relationship satisfaction than pessimists and that this difference was mediated by perceptions of the supportiveness of their partners (Srivastava, McGonigal, Richards, Butler, & Gross, 2006). Of course, it might be possible that their partners really *are* more ready to be supportive than the partners of pessimists, because optimists are easier to like (and thus support) than pessimists. This study controlled for that possibility, however. Even with that control, optimists perceived more supportiveness than pessimists. Evidence that optimists perceive greater social support than pessimists also comes from several other sources (e.g., Abend & Williamson, 2002; Trunzo & Pinto, 2003).

Yet another reason why optimism may represent a resource for relationships is that optimists work harder at their relationships (or work more effectively), consistent with their greater engagement with other tasks. Fitting this view, the relationship partners of optimists also express more satisfaction with their relationships than the partners of pessimists (Srivastava et al., 2006). In another part of that study, Srivastava and colleagues (2006) asked the couples to engage in a conversation in the laboratory about the area of their current greatest disagreement. After the conversation, the couples made ratings about their own behavior and their partners' behavior during the interaction. From this was created an index of positive engagement (being a good listener, not criticizing, trying to understand the other's point of view). A week later, the couples were asked how well the conflict had been resolved at that point.

Results indicated the following flow of associations: Optimism (as noted previously) predicted perceptions of supportiveness, which predicted more positive engagement in the conflict discussion. More positive engagement predicted better conflict resolution a week later. These effects occurred in the individual's own reports and in the reports of the partners, as well. Finally, mediational analysis suggested that the beneficial effect of optimism on conflict resolution was par-

tially mediated by perceptions of supportiveness and by positive engagement.

This project had one more step. One year later the couples were contacted and were asked about the status of the relationship. About a third of the couples had broken up by that time. Men's optimism (but not women's optimism) was a significant predictor of relationship survival, and again there was evidence of partial mediation by perceptions of partner supportiveness. This was the only part of the study in which a gender difference emerged. Srivastava and colleagues (2006) noted that men's social support tends to be more bound up in their partners, whereas women tend to have support from multiple sources. Perhaps this rendered the difference in partner supportiveness more salient and more important for the men.

Another recent project examined the possibility that optimism would be associated with an orientation to relationships that fosters effective problem solving, just as optimism is related to task-focused coping when confronting stress. This project (Assad, Donnellan, & Conger, 2007) studied married couples across a 2-year period. Participants completed measures of cooperative problem-solving behaviors, both for themselves and for their spouses, and they were videotaped while discussing diverse aspects of their relationship. Raters coded the tapes for relationship quality and negative interactions. Optimism was associated positively with relationship quality and inversely with negative interactions. Optimism was also associated with reports of higher levels of cooperative problem solving.

This study also examined prediction of relationship status 2 years later. In this case, women's optimism (but not men's) was a significant predictor of relationship survival. Among those who were still married, optimism at Time 1 predicted relationship quality, even when controlling for earlier relationship quality.

In sum, although there are relatively few studies of the role of optimism in relationships, what evidence does exist is consistent in indicating that pessimists have a rockier road than do optimists. Given how important close relationships are to life (Uchino, 2004), this represents yet one more area in which the optimist appears to have the advantage.

Can Pessimists Become Optimists?

Given the many ways in which optimists' lives seem to be better than those of pessimists, many ask if optimism can be acquired. Yes, change is possible, but there remain questions about how large a change can be reasonably expected and how permanent it will be. There also remain questions about whether an induced optimistic view acts in the same way—has the same beneficial effects—as a naturally occurring optimistic view.

The most straightforward way to turn a pessimist into an optimist is probably the set of techniques known collectively as cognitive-behavioral therapies. The logic behind them is that people with problems make negative distortions in their minds. The negative thoughts cause negative affect and induce people to stop trying to reach their goals. We would imagine that the interior monologue of the pessimist is filled with such distortions. The therapies aim to make the cognitions more positive, thereby reducing distress and fostering renewed effort. The key, then, may be to train oneself to think and act in the ways optimists think and act (Segerstrom, 2006a).

It is important to recognize, though, that it can be unwise to substitute an unquestioning optimism for an existing doubt. Sometimes people are pessimistic because they have overly high aspirations. They demand perfection from themselves, hardly ever see it, and accordingly develop doubts about their adequacy. What someone with this pattern needs is realistic goals and practice setting alternative goals to replace those that cannot be attained (Carver & Scheier, 2003; Wrosch, Scheier, Carver, & Schulz, 2003).

Concluding Comments and Future Directions

A large and growing literature indicates that people who dispositionally hold positive expectations for the future respond to difficulty or adversity in more adaptive ways than people who hold negative expectations. Expectancies influence how people approach these situations, and they influence the success with which people deal with them. There are some ways in which the focused efforts and persistence of the optimist can go awry, but they are few in number compared with the benefits that optimism seems to confer. Optimism has been linked to better emotional well-being, more effective coping strategies, and even to better outcomes in several areas of physical health. The advantages of optimism also seem to translate into the domains of interpersonal relationships: Optimists are better liked than pessimists, they benefit from their natural tendency to see things in the best light, and they appear to engage more productive effort in the sorts of problem solving that keep relationships alive.

Given the accumulation of evidence, it is clear that optimism is an individual-difference variable that plays a central role in human experience. Several questions remain, however. First, little is known about developmental antecedents of optimism. We know that socioeconomic status during childhood plays a role (Heinonen et al., 2006), but other factors must surely be involved, and they have not yet been identified systematically.

Second, more needs to be known about the structure of optimism and pessimism. As our discussion of measurement issues made clear, one model construes optimism and pessimism as a single, bipolar dimension. A second model construes optimism and pessimism as two dimensions that are only moderately correlated. Research needs to address the validity of these two models. This means routinely analyzing studies in both ways, with optimism and pessimism treated as a bipolar dimension and also as two distinct dimensions, and comparing the utility of these models.

Finally, very little systematic work has explored interventions to assist pessimistic persons to deal more effectively with adversity in their lives. We know that this is a relatively stable characteristic over time and that there is a genetic component to the variations among people. Still, even if this quality is resistant to change, change has been documented in certain contexts. Attention needs to be devoted to the components that might be included in intervention efforts and to study the effectiveness of these interventions in concrete settings.

Acknowledgments

Preparation of this chapter was facilitated by support from the National Cancer Institute (Grant No. CA64710), the National Science Foundation (Grant No. BCS0544617), and the National Heart, Lung, and Blood Institute (Grant Nos. HL65111, HL65112, HL076852, and HL076858).

References

Abend, T. A., & Williamson, G. M. (2002). Feeling attractive in the wake of breast cancer: Optimism matters, and so do interpersonal relationships. *Personality and Social Psychology Bulletin, 28,* 427–436.

Allison, P. J., Guichard, C., & Gilain, L. (2000). A prospective investigation of dispositional optimism as a predictor of health-related quality of life in head and neck cancer patients. *Quality of Life Research, 9,* 951–960.

Armor, D. A., & Taylor, S. E. (1998). Situated optimism: Specific outcome expectancies and self-regulation. In M. Zanna (Ed.), *Advances in experimental social psychology* (Vol. 30, pp. 309–379). San Diego, CA: Academic Press.

Aspinwall, L. G., & Brunhart, S. N. (1996). Distinguishing optimism from denial: Optimistic beliefs predict attention to health threats. *Personality and Social Psychology Bulletin, 22,* 993–1003.

Aspinwall, L. G., & Richter, L. (1999). Optimism and self-mastery predict more rapid disengagement from unsolvable tasks in the presence of alternatives. *Motivation and Emotion, 23,* 221–245.

Aspinwall, L. G., & Taylor, S. E. (1992). Modeling cognitive adaptation: A longitudinal investigation of the impact of individual differences and coping on college adjustment and performance. *Journal of Personality and Social Psychology, 61,* 755–765.

Assad, K. K., Donnellan, M. B., & Conger, R. D. (2007). Optimism: An enduring resource for romantic relationships. *Journal of Personality and Social Psychology, 93,* 285–297.

Austin, J. T., & Vancouver, J. B. (1996). Goal constructs in psychology: Structure, process, and content. *Psychological Bulletin, 120,* 338–375.

Beck, A. T., Steer, R. A., Kovacs, M., & Garrison, B. (1985). Hopelessness and eventual suicide: A 10-year prospective study of patients hospitalized with suicidal ideation. *American Journal of Psychiatry, 142,* 559–563.

Brissette, I., Scheier, M. F., & Carver, C. S. (2002). The role of optimism in social network development, coping, and psychological adjustment during a life transition. *Journal of Personality and Social Psychology, 82,* 102–111.

Carver, C. S., & Gaines, J. G. (1987). Optimism, pessimism, and postpartum depression. *Cognitive Therapy and Research, 11,* 449–462.

Carver, C. S., Kus, L. A., & Scheier, M. F. (1994). Effects of good versus bad mood and optimistic versus pessimistic outlook on social acceptance versus rejection. *Journal of Social and Clinical Psychology, 13,* 138–151.

Carver, C. S., Lehman, J. M., & Antoni, M. H. (2003). Dispositional pessimism predicts illness-related disruption of social and recreational activities among breast cancer patients. *Journal of Personality and Social Psychology, 84,* 813–821.

Carver, C. S., Pozo, C., Harris, S. D., Noriega, V., Scheier, M. F., Robinson, D. S., et al. (1993). How coping mediates the effect of optimism on distress: A study of women with early stage breast cancer. *Journal of Personality and Social Psychology, 65,* 375–390.

Carver, C. S., & Scheier, M. F. (1998). *On the self-regulation of behavior.* New York: Cambridge University Press.

Carver, C. S., & Scheier, M. F. (2003). Three human strengths. In L. G. Aspinwall & U. M. Staudinger (Eds.), *A psychology of human strengths: Fundamental questions and future directions for a positive psychology* (pp. 87–102). Washington, DC: American Psychological Association.

Curbow, B., Somerfield, M. R., Baker, F., Wingard, J. R., & Legro, M. W. (1993). Personal changes, dispositional optimism, and psychological adjustment to bone marrow transplantation. *Journal of Behavioral Medicine, 16,* 423–443.

Dember, W. M., Martin, S. H., Hummer, M. K., Howe, S. R., & Melton, R. S. (1989). The measurement of optimism and pessimism. *Current Psychology: Research and Reviews, 8,* 102–119.

Ebrecht, M., Hextall, J., Kirtley, L.-G., Taylor, A. M., Dyson, M., & Weinman, J. (2004). Perceived stress and cortisol levels predict speed of wound healing in healthy male adults. *Psychoneuroendocrinology, 29,* 798–809.

Fitzgerald, T. E., Tennen, H., Affleck, G., & Pransky, G. S. (1993). The relative importance of dispositional optimism and control appraisals in quality of life after coronary artery bypass surgery. *Journal of Behavioral Medicine, 16,* 25–43.

Friedman, L. C., Nelson, D. V., Baer, P. E., Lane, M., Smith, F. E., & Dworkin, R. J. (1992). The relationship of dispositional optimism, daily life stress, and domestic environment to coping methods used by cancer patients. *Journal of Behavioral Medicine, 15,* 127–141.

Gibson, B., & Sanbonmatsu, D. M. (2004). Optimism, pessimism, and gambling: The downside of optimism. *Personality and Social Psychology Bulletin, 30,* 149–160.

Giltay, E. J., Geleijnse, J. M., Zitman, F. G., Hoekstra, T., & Schouten, E. G. (2004). Dispositional optimism and all-cause and cardiovascular mortality in a prospective cohort of elderly Dutch men and women. *Archives of General Psychiatry, 61,* 1126–1135.

Giltay, E. J., Zitman, F. G., & Kromhout, D. (2006). Dispositional optimism and the risk of depressive symptoms during 15 years of follow-up: The Zutphen Elderly Study. *Journal of Affective Disorders, 91,* 45–52.

Given, C. W., Stommel, M., Given, B., Osuch, J., Kurtz, M. E., & Kurtz, J. C. (1993). The influence of cancer patients' symptoms and functional states on patients' depression and family caregivers' reaction and depression. *Health Psychology, 12,* 277–285.

Greer, S., Morris, T., Pettingale, K. W., & Haybittle, J. L. (1990, January 6). Psychological response to breast cancer and 15-year outcome. *Lancet, 335,* 49–50.

Heinonen, K., Räikkönen, K., Matthews, K. A., Scheier, M. F., Raitakari, O. T., Pulkki, L., et al. (2006). Socioeconomic status in childhood and adulthood: Associations with dispositional optimism and pessimism over a 21-year follow-up. *Journal of Personality, 74,* 1111–1126.

Helweg-Larsen, M., Sadeghian, P., & Webb, M. S. (2002). The stigma of being pessimistically biased. *Journal of Social and Clinical Psychology, 21,* 92–107.

Herzberg, P. Y., Glaesmer, H., & Hoyer, J. (2006). Separating optimism and pessimism: A robust psychometric analysis of the revised Life Orientation Test (LOT-R). *Psychological Assessment, 18,* 433–438.

Higgins, E. T. (2006). Value from hedonic experience and engagement. *Psychological Review, 113,* 439–460.

Hooker, K., Monahan, D., Shifren, K., & Hutchinson, C. (1992). Mental and physical health of spouse caregivers: The role of personality. *Psychology and Aging, 7,* 367–375.

Ironson, G., Balbin, E., Stuetzle, R., Fletcher, M. A., O'Cleirigh, C., Laurenceau, J.-P., et al. (2005). Dispositional optimism and the mechanisms by which it predicts slower disease progression in HIV: Proactive behavior, avoidant coping, and depression. *International Journal of Behavioral Medicine, 12,* 86–97.

Isaacowitz, D. M. (2005). The gaze of the optimist. *Personality and Social Psychology Bulletin, 31,* 407–415.

Kohut, M. L., Cooper, M. M., Nickolaus, M. S., Russell, D. R., & Cunnick, J. E. (2002). Exercise and psychosocial factors modulate immunity to influenza vaccine in elderly individuals. *Journals of Gerontology: Series A. Biological Sciences and Medical Sciences, 57A,* 557–562.

Litt, M. D., Tennen, H., Affleck, G., & Klock, S. (1992). Coping and cognitive factors in adaptation to *in vitro* fertilization failure. *Journal of Behavioral Medicine, 15,* 171–187.

Luo, J., & Isaacowitz, D. M. (2007). How optimists face skin cancer information: Risk assessment, attention, memory, and behavior. *Psychology and Health, 22,* 963–984.

MacLeod, A. K., & Conway, C. (2005). Well-being and the anticipation of future positive experiences: The role of income, social networks, and planning ability. *Cognition and Emotion, 19,* 357–374.

Marshall, G. N., Wortman, C. B., Kusulas, J. W., Hervig, L. K., & Vickers, R. R., Jr. (1992). Distinguishing optimism from pessimism: Relations to fundamental dimensions of mood and personality. *Journal of Personality and Social Psychology, 62,* 1067–1074.

Matthews, K. A., Raikkonen, K., Sutton-Tyrrell, K., & Kuller, L. H. (2004). Optimistic attitudes protect against progression of carotid atherosclerosis in healthy middle-aged women. *Psychosomatic Medicine, 66,* 640–644.

Ohannessian, C. M., Hesselbrock, V. M., Tennen, H., & Affleck, G. (1994). Hassles and uplifts and generalized outcome expectancies as moderators on the relation between a family history of alcoholism and drinking behaviors. *Journal of Studies on Alcohol, 55,* 754–763.

Park, C. L., Moore, P. J., Turner, R. A., & Adler, N. E. (1997). The roles of constructive thinking and optimism in psychological and behavioral adjustment during pregnancy. *Journal of Personality and Social Psychology, 73,* 584–592.

Peterson, C., & Seligman, M. E. P. (1984). Causal explanations as a risk factor for depression: Theory and evidence. *Psychological Review, 91,* 347–374.

Radcliffe, N. M., & Klein, W. M. P. (2002). Dispositional, unrealistic, and comparative optimism: Differential relations with the knowledge and processing of risk information and beliefs about personal risk. *Personality and Social Psychology Bulletin, 28,* 836–846.

Räikkönen, K., Matthews, K. A., Flory, J. D., Owens, J. F., & Gump, B. B. (1999). Effects of optimism, pessimism, and trait anxiety on ambulatory blood pressure and mood during everyday life. *Journal of Personality and Social Psychology, 76,* 104–113.

Rasmussen, H. N., Scheier, M. F., & Greenhouse, J. B. (2009). *Optimism and physical health: A meta-analytic review.* Manuscript submitted for publication.

Rauch, W. A., Schweizer, K., & Moosbrugger, H. (2007). Method effects due to social desirability as a parsimonious explanation of the deviation from unidimensionality in LOT-R scores. *Personality and Individual Differences, 42,* 1597–1607.

Reed, G. M., Kemeny, M. E., Taylor, S. E., Wang, H.-Y., & Visscher, B. R. (1994). "Realistic acceptance" as a predictor of decreased survival time in gay men with AIDS. *Health Psychology, 13,* 299–307.

Robinson-Whelen, S., Kim, C., MacCallum, R. C., & Kiecolt-Glaser, J. K. (1997). Distinguishing optimism from pessimism in older adults: Is it more important to be optimistic or not to be pessimistic? *Journal of Personality and Social Psychology, 73,* 1345–1353.

Ruiz, J. M., Matthews, K. A., Scheier, M. F., & Schulz, R. (2006). Does who you marry matter for your health?: Influence of patients' and spouses' personality on their partners' psychological well-being following coronary artery bypass surgery. *Journal of Personality and Social Psychology, 91,* 255–267.

Scheier, M. F., & Carver, C. S. (1992). Effects of optimism on psychological and physical well-being: Theoretical overview and empirical update. *Cognitive Therapy and Research, 16,* 201–228.

Scheier, M. F., & Carver, C. S. (2001). Adapting to cancer: The importance of hope and purpose. In A. Baum & B. L. Andersen (Eds.), *Psychosocial interventions for cancer* (pp. 15–36). Washington, DC: American Psychological Association.

Scheier, M. F., Carver, C. S., & Bridges, M. W. (1994). Distinguishing optimism from neuroticism (and trait anxiety, self-mastery, and self-esteem): A reevaluation of the Life Orientation Test. *Journal of Personality and Social Psychology, 67,* 1063–1078.

Scheier, M. F., Carver, C. S., & Bridges, M. W. (2001). Optimism, pessimism, and psychological well-being. In E. C. Chang (Ed.), *Optimism and pessimism: Implications for theory, research, and practice* (pp. 189–216). Washington, DC: American Psychological Association.

Scheier, M. F., Matthews, K. A., Owens, J. F., Magovern, G. J., Lefebvre, R. C., Abbott, R. A., et al. (1989). Dispositional optimism and recovery from coronary artery bypass surgery: The beneficial effects on physical and psychological well-being. *Journal of Personality and Social Psychology, 57,* 1024–1040.

Scheier, M. F., Matthews, K. A., Owens, J. F., Schulz, R., Bridges, M. W., Magovern, G. J., Sr., et al. (1999). Optimism and rehospitalization following coronary artery bypass graft surgery. *Archives of Internal Medicine, 159,* 829–835.

Schou, I., Ekeberg, O., & Ruland, C. M. (2005). The mediating role of appraisal and coping in the relationship between optimism–pessimism and quality of life. *Psycho-Oncology, 14,* 718–727.

Segerstrom, S C. (2001). Optimism and attentional bias for negative and positive stimuli. *Personality and Social Psychology Bulletin, 27,* 1334–1343.

Segerstrom, S. C. (2005). Optimism and immunity: Do positive thoughts always lead to positive effects? *Brain, Behavior, and Immunity, 19,* 195–200.

Segerstrom, S. C. (2006a). *Breaking Murphy's law: How optimists get what they want from life—and pessimists too.* New York: Guilford Press.

Segerstrom, S. C. (2006b). How does optimism suppress immunity?: Evaluation of three affective pathways. *Health Psychology, 25,* 653–657.

Segerstrom, S. C. (2007). Optimism and resources: Effects on each other and on health over 10 years. *Journal of Research in Personality, 41,* 772–786.

Segerstrom, S. C., & Solberg Nes, L. (2006). When goals conflict but people prosper: The case of dispositional optimism. *Journal of Research in Personality, 40,* 675–693.

Shepperd, J. A., Maroto, J. J., & Pbert, L. A. (1996). Dispositional optimism as a predictor of health changes among cardiac patients. *Journal of Research in Personality, 30,* 517–534.

Shifren, K., & Hooker, K. (1995). Stability and change in optimism: A study among spouse caregivers. *Experimental Aging Research, 21,* 59–76.

Shnek, Z. M., Irvine, J., Stewart, D., & Abbey, S. (2001). Psychological factors and depressive symptoms in ischemic heart disease. *Health Psychology, 20,* 141–145.

Solberg Nes, L., & Segerstrom, S. C. (2006). Dispositional optimism and coping: A meta-analytic review. *Personality and Social Psychology Review, 10,* 235–251.

Srivastava, S., McGonigal, K. M., Richards, J. M., Butler, E. A., & Gross, J. J. (2006). Optimism in close relationships: How seeing things in a positive light makes them so. *Journal of Personality and Social Psychology, 91,* 143–153.

Stanton, A. L., & Snider, P. R. (1993). Coping with breast cancer diagnosis: A prospective study. *Health Psychology, 12,* 16–23.

Strack, S., Carver, C. S., & Blaney, P. H. (1987). Predicting successful completion of an aftercare program following treatment for alcoholism: The role of dispositional optimism. *Journal of Personality and Social Psychology, 53,* 579–584.

Sweeny, K., Carroll, P. J., & Shepperd, J. A. (2006). Is optimism always best? *Current Directions in Psychological Science, 15,* 302–306.

Szondy, M. (2004). Optimism and immune functions. *Mentalhigiene es Pszichoszomatika, 5,* 301–320.

Taylor, S. E., Kemeny, M. E., Aspinwall, L. G., Schneider, S. G., Rodriguez, R., & Herbert, M. (1992). Optimism, coping, psychological distress, and high-risk sexual behavior among men at risk for acquired immunodeficiency syndrome (AIDS). *Journal of Personality and Social Psychology, 63,* 460–473.

Trunzo, J. J., & Pinto, B. M. (2003). Social support as a mediator of optimism and distress in breast cancer survivors. *Journal of Consulting and Clinical Psychology, 4,* 805–811.

Uchino, B. N. (2004). *Social support and physical health: Understanding the health consequences of relationships.* New Haven, CT: Yale University Press.

Wrosch, C., Scheier, M. F., Carver, C. S., & Schulz, R. (2003). The importance of goal disengagement in adaptive self-regulation: When giving up is beneficial. *Self and Identity, 2,* 1–20.

Zeidner, M., & Hammer, A. L. (1992). Coping with missile attack: Resources, strategies, and outcomes. *Journal of Personality, 60,* 709–746.

CHAPTER 23

■ ● ▲ ◆ ■ ● ▲ ◆

The Need for Cognitive Closure

ARIE W. KRUGLANSKI
SHIRA FISHMAN

As people acquire knowledge about the world, they generate and test hypotheses using relevant information. Such cognitive activities do not have a distinct point of termination, and the process of generating hypotheses could go on indefinitely, as could the examination of more and more information intended to validate these hypotheses. The need for cognitive closure has been conceptualized as a motivational "stopping mechanism" that applies "brakes" to the epistemic process and allows crystallized judgments to form (Kruglanski, 1989). The need for closure is closely related to phenomena such as closed- and open-mindedness that have been addressed by prior psychological theories, including those of Piaget and Freud (for a review, see Kruglanski, 2004, Chapter 4). Particularly well-known in this regard are notions of authoritarianism (Adorno, Frenkel-Brunswik, Levinson, & Sanford, 1950; Altemeyer, 1981), dogmatism (Rokeach, 1960), and uncertainty orientation (Sorrentino & Short, 1986). These formulations have often adopted a psychodynamic perspective, highlighted the socialization antecedents of closed- and open-mindedness, and viewed closed-mindedness as largely an indicator of problematic psychosexual development. As a consequence, closed- and open-mindedness in those frameworks were conceptualized and opera-tionalized as dimensions of individual differences. By contrast, need-for-closure research has emphasized the epistemic functions of closed- and open-mindedness. Hence, in addition to measuring individual differences in the need for closure, the research has considered situational circumstances whereby an individual may evaluate the epistemic costs and benefits of closure (or openness) at a given point in time.

Because knowledge-formation processes underlie large portions of human interaction, the need for closure appears to have important implications for social behavior, including (1) intrapersonal processes such as impression formation and social judgment, (2) interpersonal processes including persuasion, communication, and empathy, (3) intragroup processes such as pressures to uniformity (Festinger, 1950), and (4) intergroup processes including ingroup favoritism, outgroup derogation, and assimilation and acculturation of immigrants. In this chapter, we review the theory of the need for closure and its varied implications. We also identify gaps in current knowledge on closed- and open-mindedness and suggest directions for further research.

The need for closure (NFC) has been defined as a desire for a definite answer to a question, as opposed to uncertainty, confusion, or ambiguity (Kruglanski, 1989). It is assumed that the motivation toward closure varies along a continuum anchored at one end with a strong NFC and at the other end with a strong need to avoid closure. The NFC is elevated when the perceived benefits of possessing closure and/or the perceived costs of lacking closure are high (Kruglanski & Webster, 1996; Webster & Kruglanski, 1994). Likewise, the need to avoid closure is elevated when the perceived benefits of lacking closure and the perceived costs of possessing closure are high. These benefits and costs vary according to situational factors and individual differences.

Situational Determinants

A wide variety of situational factors affect the need for closure. The NFC may be heightened in situations in which a decision is required immediately, as, for example, under time pressure (see Chiu, Morris, Hong, & Menon, 2000; Kruglanski & Freund, 1983), or in situations in which a judgment is required, as opposed to those in which the individual is at liberty to abstain from forming a definite opinion. Additionally, a variety of conditions that render information processing difficult, laborious, or otherwise unpleasant may increase the NFC because closure renders further processing unnecessary. Such conditions include environmental noise (see Kruglanski, Webster, & Klem, 1993), tedium and dullness of the cognitive task (see Webster, 1993b), fatigue or low energy, the arduousness of information processing (see Webster, Richter, & Kruglanski, 1996), and alcoholic intoxication, which limits the capacity for systematic thought (see Webster, 1993a). The NFC is also higher when closure is known to be valued by others, because closure may earn their esteem and appreciation (see Mayseless & Kruglanski, 1987).

Conversely, the NFC may be diminished in situations that highlight the costs of closure and the benefits of openness. In some circumstances, the costs of closure may be rendered salient by the fear of invalidity (Kruglanski & Freund, 1983), which stems from concerns about committing a costly judgmental error. Validity and closure are not necessarily at odds, but they may pull information processing in opposite directions. For example, when the need for closure is elevated, an individual may consider limited information and rely on preconceived notions or stereotypes. When the need for closure is lower, however, one may be willing to consider ample evidence before making up one's mind. Such epistemic dynamics prompted by the NFC are not assumed to be consciously accessible to the knower but, rather, exert their effects implicitly and typically outside of awareness.

Individual Differences

People exhibit stable personal differences in the degree to which they value closure. Some people may form definitive, and perhaps extreme, opinions regardless of the situation, whereas others may resist making decisions even in the safest environments. To measure such individual differences, Webster and Kruglanski (1994) developed the Need for Closure Scale (NFCS), consisting of a series of statements to which participants respond along a continuum from "strongly agree" to "strongly disagree." Structural analysis on the scale reveals that the best fit is a single-factor model with interitem correlations in five domains (Webster & Kruglanski, 1994). The factors are (1) the desire for order and structure, (2) discomfort with ambiguity, (3) decisiveness, (4) desire for predictability about the future, and (5) closed-mindedness. Studies have shown that the factors are unidimensional and consistent across a variety of national and international samples (Cratylus, 1995; Pierro et al., 1995; Webster & Kruglanski, 1994). The NFCS has been translated into several languages (e.g., Arabic, Cantonese, Croatian, Dutch, French, German, Hebrew, Italian, Japanese, Korean, Mandarin, and Spanish), affording a cross-cultural investigation of closed- and open-mindedness. The results of numerous studies (e.g., Cratylus, 1995; De Grada, Kruglanski, Mannetti, Pierro, & Webster, 1996; Kossowska, Van Hiel, Chun, & Kruglanski, 2002; Pierro et al., 1995) indicate that the NFCS has the same basic meaning and structure cross-nationally and that the ratings can be meaningfully compared across different countries and cultures.

The Urgency
and Permanence Tendencies

Research suggests that the NFC may instill two general tendencies in an individual: the *urgency* tendency and the *permanence* tendency. The urgency tendency refers to the inclination to "seize" on closure quickly. People under a heightened NFC desire closure immediately and experience postponement of closure as bothersome. The permanence tendency refers to the desire to perpetuate closure, giving rise to the dual inclination to preserve, or "freeze" on, past knowledge and to avoid having to consider other incoming information. Individuals under a heightened NFC may thus desire an enduring closure and, in extreme cases, abhor letting go of closure. The urgency and permanence notions both rest on the assumption that people under a heightened NFC experience the absence of closure as aversive. They may wish to terminate this unpleasant state quickly (the urgency tendency) and keep it from recurring (the permanence tendency). The processes of seizing and freezing have implications for human social behavior across a wide variety of domains.

Intrapersonal Processes

As noted, the NFC represents a stopping mechanism that allows for a formation of firm conclusions. Importantly, then, individual differences in NFC should be associated with the types of information sought in social judgments, as well as the speed and confidence with which those judgments are formed.

Hypothesis Generation
and Subjective Confidence

In reaching a firm conclusion, individuals often generate multiple hypotheses to account for known facts and choose among those hypotheses on the basis of additional evidence. The processes of seizing and freezing, evoked by the NFC, may restrict the tendency to continue generating alternative hypotheses. To examine this possibility, participants were shown photos of parts of common objects (e.g., a comb or a tooth-brush) taken from unusual angles to disguise their identity. Results showed that individuals high in NFC generated fewer hypotheses about the identity of the objects compared with those low in NFC (Mayseless & Kruglanski, 1987). Thus it seems that people who are high in NFC will restrict the number of hypotheses that they will entertain before reaching a given judgment.

One may expect that generating fewer hypotheses would lead to lower confidence in one's decision. Ironically, however, a reduction in hypothesis generation may lead to the opposite effect. Individuals who are high in NFC may be less aware of competing judgmental possibilities and, therefore, may be more confident that their selection is correct. Indeed, elevated judgmental confidence under heightened NFC has been manifested in numerous studies (Kruglanski & Webster, 1991; Kruglanski et al., 1993; Mayseless & Kruglanski, 1987; Webster, 1993b). These findings suggest that in the absence of extensive information processing and the awareness of multiple competing possibilities, individuals may be more confident in their decisions; therefore, people with a heightened need for closure, by virtue of their assurance in their decisions, show an inverse relationship between judgmental confidence and the extent of information processing.

Impression Formation

In forming impressions of other people, NFC should similarly increase the need to "seize" and "freeze" on information, thus limiting the search for new information. In other words, individuals high in NFC should seek less information about another person before making a decision. In a study in which students were asked to play the role of a manager faced with a hiring decision, those who experienced high (vs. low) NFC requested significantly fewer pages of relevant information prior to forming their impression of the job candidate (Webster et al., 1996). In contrast, individuals low (vs. high) in NFC sought more information on the candidate prior to their decision. In another study, individuals high in NFC spent less time searching for information presented on a screen as compared with individuals low in NFC (Mayseless & Kruglanski, 1987). Thus, individuals high in NFC may seek less information about another person before reaching a conclusion or forming a definite impression about this person.

Cue Utilization

NFC also appears to heighten people's reliance on initial information. The urgency tendency predisposes an individual to quickly "seize" on early cues and utilize them toward the formation of initial judgments, whereas the permanence tendency predisposes an individual to "freeze" or fixate on those particular judgments. Research on a variety of seemingly diverse social-psychological topics has lent support to these ideas.

Primacy Effects in Impression Formation

A primacy effect refers to the tendency to base one's social impressions on early information about that person, to the relative neglect of subsequent, potentially relevant information. From the present perspective, primacy effects exemplify the seizing-and-freezing tendencies that are assumed to be stronger for individuals who are high in NFC. Indeed, when individuals are high in NFC, primacy effects are augmented (Webster & Kruglanski, 1994). In addition, the higher the individual's NFC, the stronger the magnitude of the primacy effect.

The Correspondence Bias

The correspondence bias (Jones, 1979), or the fundamental attribution error (Ross, 1977), refers to the attributor's tendency to overascribe an actor's behavior to her or his unique attitudes or personality and to underestimate the power of the situation. Just as with primacy and anchoring effects, the correspondence bias reflects the seizing-and-freezing tendencies of individuals who are high in NFC. Webster (1993b) asked participants to complete a typical attitude-attribution task in which they estimated a target's attitude after hearing her deliver a speech criticizing student exchange programs with foreign universities. The speech was allegedly prepared under either high- or low-choice conditions. As in previous re-

search, despite the other student not having had any choice in writing the essay, participants reported that the student's actual attitude was similar to the perspective taken in the essay. However, this effect was magnified when individuals were high rather than low in NFC.

Stereotype Application

Increased application of prevalent social stereotypes and prejudices to various social judgments may represent a particularly striking case of seizing and freezing under a heightened NFC. Because culturally prevalent stereotypes constitute knowledge structures that may readily come to mind, they may be particularly likely to serve as bases for judging stereotyped targets when the perceiver is high (vs. low) in NFC. This possibility was supported in several studies and with several different stereotypic contents, such as the stereotypes of Ashkenazi and Sephardic Israelis (Kruglanski & Freund, 1983), of women in management (Jamieson & Zanna, 1989), and of soccer hooligans and nurses (Dijksterhuis, van Knippenberg, Kruglanski, & Schaper, 1996).

Construct Accessibility

Stereotypes are more accessible to individuals who are high in the need for closure, coming to mind more easily when they are confronted with a judgmental target. Indeed, Ford and Kruglanski (1995) found that, compared with individuals low in NFC, those high in NFC relied to a greater extent on a previously primed concept when judging an ambiguous target.

Recency Effects

In some circumstances, NFC may lead to recency effects rather than primacy effects, depending on construct accessibility. Specifically, timing of the impression-formation goal should moderate the use of primacy versus recency heuristics. When the impression-formation goal exists from the start, high NFC should predict an enhanced primacy effect due to a seizing and freezing on the initial information. However, when the impression-formation goal is introduced following exposure to the stimulus materials, participants should rely on their memories of the information, and high (vs. low) NFC should predict a stronger recency effect. Data from experimental studies confirm these predictions (Richter & Kruglanski, 1999).

Taken together, the research on intrapersonal processes demonstrates that people who are high in NFC seek less information, generate fewer hypotheses, and rely on early, initial information when making judgments. Paradoxically, despite the reliance on less, and perhaps incomplete, information, individuals high in NFC display greater confidence in their decisions.

Interpersonal Phenomena

The processing of information about one's interaction partners and the formation of online judgments about their feelings, cognitions, and probable actions is fundamental to social relations and should be consequential for interpersonal relationships. The seizing-and-freezing tendencies fostered by a heightened NFC should, therefore, exert important effects at the interpersonal level of analysis.

Perspective Taking and Empathy

Taking another's perspective often requires substantial cognitive effort, as one needs to overlook one's own perspective and focus on the perspective of another. In this vein, if the need for cognitive closure reduces individuals' readiness to put effort into mental processing and predisposes them to seize and freeze on early information, it may reduce perspective taking and empathic concerns when individuals high in the need for closure interact with dissimilar others. To examine this possibility, Webster-Nelson, Klein, and Irvin (2003) had participants read descriptions of a person who was either similar or dissimilar to themselves. Under a heightened NFC (experienced through mental fatigue), the ability to take a different perspective was reduced when the target was dissimilar to the participant. Similarly, the ability to show empathy was lower when the target was dissimilar. As expected, no differences

in perspective taking and empathy emerged when the target and participant were similar to each other.

Interpersonal Communication

When conveying messages to others, speakers often take the audience's perspective into account and make reference to the realities that both parties share. However, under time pressure, speakers are less likely to reference common ground. As time pressure has been one of the major ways in which NFC has been operationalized (Kruglanski & Freund, 1983; Shah, Kruglanski, & Thompson, 1998), a high-level NFC may reduce the amount of effort communicators invest in their search for common ground. As a consequence, communications by individuals high in NFC may be excessively biased in the direction of the communicator's own perspective, which might reduce their comprehensibility to listeners. Richter and Kruglanski (1999) investigated this hypothesis by asking participants to write descriptions of figures and then, on a subsequent visit, to match the descriptions to the pictures. Participants high (vs. low) in NFC used significantly fewer words in their descriptions, and their descriptions were less likely to be matched with the figure, as compared with descriptions written by individuals low in NFC.

The way that individuals converse with each other should also be affected by NFC. If NFC induces the tendency to seek permanent knowledge and reduce ambiguity, then individuals high in NFC should prefer abstract descriptions and category labels to concrete, situational descriptions. Indeed, evidence supports this idea (Boudreau, Baron, & Oliver, 1992; Mikulincer, Yinon, & Kabili, 1991). In another study, individuals with high (vs. low) NFC preferred to ask more abstract interview questions (Rubini & Kruglanski, 1997). A subsequent study found that abstract questions from individuals high in NFC elicited more abstract answers from respondents. The level of abstraction was, in turn, related to liking, with more abstract questions eliciting less liking from respondents. The latter decrease in liking occurred because the subject of abstract questions is usually an object (e.g., because dogs are ...) rather than the self (e.g., because I like dogs ...).

Individuals high in NFC prefer abstract labels because they can be applied across a variety of situations, implying epistemic permanence. In different terms, abstract expressions are "multifinal" (Kruglanski, Shah, Fishbach, et al., 2002) in that they satisfy multiple goals (provide multiple closures) with a single means and thus should be preferred. A set of studies by Chun and Kruglanski (2005) demonstrated that individuals high in NFC preferred proverbs that espoused the multifinality idea (e.g., "killing two birds with one stone") as compared with proverbs that argued the opposite (e.g., "if you run after two hares, you will catch neither"). Furthermore, people who are high in NFC pursue multifinality even at the expense of quality or cost. Finally, when the number of goals was held constant, individuals high in NFC chose fewer means to achieve the goal.

Transference

Andersen and colleagues' work (e.g., Andersen & Berk, 1998; Andersen & Chen, 2002; Andersen & Cole, 1990) on the transference effect in social judgment demonstrates how a significant other's schema stored in memory can be applied to a new individual who resembles the significant other in some way. Information about a new individual who is similar to a significant other may activate the significant-other schema, which is then used to make (often inaccurate) inferences about the newly encountered individual. Such transference effects have been explained in terms of the high accessibility of the significant other's representation in memory. Given that NFC implies seizing and freezing on accessible constructs, the transference effect should be more pronounced under high NFC. Indeed, research by Pierro and Kruglanski (2008) found that the transference effect is more pronounced for individuals high rather than low in NFC.

In summary, individual differences in NFC, as well as situational differences in NFC, have important implications for social interaction. Individuals high in NFC (vs. low in NFC) have greater difficulty taking other people's perspectives and empathizing with them. While communicating with others, individuals high in NFC are focused on their own perspective, making it more difficult for others to understand their views and communications. Individuals high in NFC prefer to use abstract labels, which can be applied across various situations. Lastly, individuals high in NFC are quick to apply significant-other schemas to individuals who resemble them superficially, potentially producing substantial errors of person perception.

Group Processes

As a result of the tendency to seize and freeze on accessible information, individuals high in NFC exhibit a number of intriguing behavioral tendencies within group settings.

Task versus Socioemotional Orientation

When assigned a group task, group members may choose to focus on either task or socioemotional goals. Because the task represents the most accessible construct for defining the situation (because it is the obvious reason for individuals finding themselves in that situation), people who are high in NFC may be more task oriented than socioemotionally oriented. De Grada, Kruglanski, Mannetti, and Pierro (1999) asked groups of four students to role-play the managers of four corporate departments while negotiating a monetary reward for a meritorious worker. Participants high in NFC produced a higher proportion of task-oriented responses and a lower proportion of positive social-emotional acts than participants low in NFC.

Consensus Striving

Within a group, individuals strive toward homogeneity of opinions (Festinger, 1950). From an NFC perspective, such homogeneity is essential for epistemic certainty; if so, individuals high in NFC should show a higher desire for consensus. Consistent with that prediction, De Grada and colleagues (1999) found that during a negotiation session within a group, members of groups composed of individuals high in NFC felt greater pressure toward uniformity as compared with members of groups low in NFC. Blind coders, unaware of differences in group composition, confirmed this finding by rating social pressures higher in groups with high (vs. low) NFC. In a different research paradigm, Kruglanski and colleagues (1993) found that when individuals high in NFC entered the situation with considerable certainty in their views, they refused to change their views, even when others disagreed with them; whereas when individuals high in NFC entered the situation with little confidence in their views, they showed a greater inclination to change their own views toward their partner's opinion.

Individuals can also seek consensus by rejecting members who deviate from the majority opinion (Festinger, 1950). In a situation in which groups were required to reach consensus on an issue, individuals high (vs. low) in NFC showed greater tendency to reject an opinion deviate (Kruglanski & Webster, 1991). Importantly, when the groups were able to use a majority rule to reach a conclusion, high NFC did not predict rejection of a deviate. Therefore, only when collective closure is required (via consensus agreement) is there a tendency to derogate the deviate.

Consensus can also be built around shared information, and groups tend to focus their discussions around such shared information (Stasser & Stewart, 1992; Stasser & Titus, 1985, 1987). Webster (1993b) found that during group discussion, NFC was inversely correlated with the tendency to bring up unique information (information that was possessed solely by some and not by other group members). Thus individuals high in NFC seem to focus on shared information, presumably in order to create consensus more quickly, which allows them to achieve closure. In the absence of generating new ideas, a group may actually become less creative, especially to the extent that it focuses on shared information. Indeed, Chirumbolo, Mannetti, Pierro, Areni, and Kruglanski (2005) found that groups composed of individuals high (vs. low) in NFC tend to produce fewer ideas, to elaborate on those ideas less fully, and to be less creative in a mock advertising task.

Given the desire for consensus within the high-NFC group, such groups should support leaders who make quick and decisive decisions. Thus groups high in NFC may prefer an autocratic leadership style, which

allows fewer opinions to be voiced during the course of the discussion. Indeed, a number of studies have found that groups composed of individuals high in NFC foster the emergence of autocratic leadership to a greater extent than groups that are composed of individuals low in NFC (De Grada et al., 1999; Pierro, Mannetti, De Grada, Livi, & Kruglanski, 2003).

Further exploring autocratic leadership, Pierro and Kruglanski (2008) studied the influence styles preferred by leaders high in NFC and their subordinates. "Soft" power bases allow greater autonomy and are less controlling than "hard" power bases (Raven, Schwarzwald, & Koslowsky, 1998). Results showed that subordinates high in NFC prefer "hard" social influence tactics, whereas subordinates low in NFC prefer "soft" tactics. Similarly, supervisors who are high in NFC tend to employ "hard" tactics, whereas those low in NFC tend to employ "soft" tactics. Finally, evidence suggests that organizations are more effective to the extent that the types of tactics used by the supervisor fit the preferences of the subordinates (Pierro & Kruglanski, 2008).

The desire to have consensus might imply an unwillingness to embrace change. A study by Livi (2002) found that, over time and with turnover, the norms established at initial stages of group formation persisted more in groups whose members were high in NFC than in groups whose members were low in NFC. Similarly, research conducted in organizational settings has shown that individuals high in NFC have trouble coping with organizational change (Kruglanski, Pierro, Higgins, & Capozza, 2007). However, in a culture that is very supportive of such change, individuals high in NFC had an easier time coping with change. In other words, although individuals high in NFC are generally averse to change, they are also generally supportive of the "social reality" of their particular organization. Thus, when the existing social reality supports change, individuals high in NFC adjust better to changes in the workplace.

Taken together, the research on group processes and NFC indicates that individuals with high NFC desire consensus and homogeneity among group members. As such, they are willing to engage in activities perceived as likely to achieve and maintain stability, including focusing on the task at hand, pressuring others to change their opinions, rejecting those who hold different opinions, sharing less information with others, and supporting an autocratic leadership style.

Intergroup Processes

To the individual, the ingroup represents an important provider of social knowledge concerning norms for acting and thinking. Because of this, the ingroup can provide closure to the individual. If the ingroup is valued partly because it constitutes a closure provider, it should be valued more by individuals high versus low in NFC. Shah, Kruglanski, and Thompson (1998) investigated this hypothesis in a study in which participants believed they would be competing in a group of two members against another similar group. After reading alleged self-descriptions of their partners and competitors, individuals high in NFC reported more liking for their own teammates and less liking toward the members of the other teams than individuals low in NFC.

If the ingroup represents a stable social reality, individuals high in NFC should prefer groups that are homogeneous in their composition over heterogeneous groups. Homogeneous (vs. heterogeneous) groups are likely to agree on their basic worldviews and may thus come to consensus faster. If individuals high in NFC attach particular value to consensus, they should prefer homogeneous groups, but this should be true only to the extent that the views of a given homogeneous group agree with the individual's own views. Consistent with this analysis, Kruglanski, Shah, Pierro, and Mannetti (2002) found that individuals high (vs. low) on NFC had a greater preference for homogeneous (vs. heterogeneous) groups, but only when the group's opinions were similar (vs. dissimilar) to their own opinions.

Related experiments by Dechesne, Schultz, Kruglanski, Fishman, and Orehek (2007) found that individuals high (vs. low) in NFC preferred groups with impermeable (vs. permeable) boundaries, but only when the groups were perceived as homogeneous, suggesting a greater likelihood of consensus. Thus, if a group represents a source of stable social reality, as is likely to be the case with homogenous groups, individuals high

in NFC are likely to want to maintain that reality; this may be achieved by keeping (potentially dissimilar) others out of the group.

The Linguistic Intergroup Bias

The linguistic intergroup bias (LIB) is the tendency for group members to describe the positive characteristics of the ingroup and the negative characteristics of the outgroup in abstract terms, thereby implying stable traits. In contrast, individuals describe the negative characteristics of the ingroup and the positive characteristics of the outgroup in concrete terms, implying that the characteristics are situationally specific rather than fundamental (Maass & Arcuri, 1992). A study by Webster, Kruglanski, and Pattison (1997) found that individuals high (vs. low) in NFC used significantly more abstract terms when describing positive ingroup and negative outgroup behaviors, thereby exhibiting the LIB.

In summary, research on the dynamics of NFC in intergroup contexts suggests that individuals high in NFC seek to protect and maintain their ingroups. Indeed, individuals high in NFC are biased toward their own ingroups. They exhibit greater liking for ingroup members and greater LIB. Furthermore, individuals high in NFC prefer ingroups that are homogeneous as well as similar to themselves; once those groups are established, they support attempts to maintain the group and exclude others from the group.

Conclusions and Future Directions

NFC has been conceptualized as the desire for a definite answer, as opposed to uncertainty or ambiguity. Because NFC allows individuals to reach a decision in the process of knowledge formation, NFC has important implications for social interaction. Individual differences in NFC predict behavior at the intrapersonal, interpersonal, group, and intergroup levels of analysis. Individuals high in NFC generate fewer hypotheses and seek less information before making a decision. Similarly, they are focused on their own perspectives and have difficulty taking the perspectives of others. They seek closure within groups, pressuring others or changing their own opinions in order to reach group consensus. Finally, they prefer solid boundaries to their own homogenous groups. In all, individuals high in NFC desire quick closure, seizing and freezing on information that is quickly and efficiently able to provide such closure.

Though considerable knowledge exists concerning the situational antecedents of the need for closure and its varied consequences, a substantial gap exists in understanding the conditions and circumstances that prompt the development of individual differences in the need for closure. Intriguing recent work by Kossowska and her colleagues (Kossowska, Orehek, & Kruglanski, in press; Legierski & Kossowska, 2008) suggests that individuals with low working memory capacity may develop a high need for closure. In this vein, Kossowska and colleagues (in press) found that individual differences in working memory capacity are correlated with individual differences in the need for closure. In addition, individual differences in working memory capacity were found to mediate the relation between individual differences in the need for closure, the type of information sought in a judgmental task (i.e., simple vs. complex information), and the extent of information search exhibited by participants. These results are promising, yet their correlational nature prevents firm conclusions as to the causal relations between working memory capacity and need for closure. Further probing, perhaps exploring the brain mechanisms involved in closed-mindedness, is needed to fully understand the nature of these relations.

In addition, possible developmental antecedents of individual differences in need for closure merit further explorations. Though prior work on individual differences in closed- and open-mindedness (e.g., Adorno et al., 1950; Rokeach, 1960; Sorrentino & Short, 1986) emphasized psychosexual development as a fundamental antecedent of these differences, little empirical evidence to date exists concerning these claims. Additional aspects of the socialization context might also foster individual differences in closed- and open-mindedness. For instance, disagreements between one's parents during early childhood might give rise to an aversive uncertainty, inducing a stable need for closure. Growing up in unstable physi-

cal (e.g., during war times) and economic circumstances (e.g., during an economic depression) might also induce a sense of profound and aversive uncertainty contributing to one's craving for assurance and predictability. In short, despite the considerable work thus far on the need for cognitive closure, substantial further work is needed to fully understand this fundamental aspect of human behavior.

References

Adorno, T. W., Frenkel-Brunswik, E., Levinson, D. J., & Sanford, R. N. (1950). *The authoritarian personality.* New York: Harper.
Altemeyer, B. (1981). *Right-wing authoritarianism.* Winnipeg, Manitoba, Canada: University of Manitoba Press.
Andersen, S. M., & Berk, M. S. (1998). The social-cognitive model of transference: Experiencing past relationships in the present. *Current Directions in Psychological Science, 7,* 1–7.
Andersen, S. M., & Chen, S. (2002). The rational self: An interpersonal social-cognitive theory. *Psychological Review, 109,* 619–645.
Andersen, S. M., & Cole, S. W. (1990). "Do I know you?": The role of significant others in general social perception. *Journal of Personality and Social Psychology, 59,* 384–399.
Boudreau, L. A., Baron, R., & Oliver, P. V. (1992). Effects of expected communication target expertise and timing of set on trait use in person description. *Personality and Social Psychology Bulletin, 18,* 447–452.
Chirumbolo, A., Mannetti, L., Pierro, A., Areni, A., & Kruglanski, A. W. (2005). Motivated closed-mindedness and creativity in small groups. *Small Group Research, 36,* 59–82.
Chiu, C., Morris, M. W., Hong, Y., & Menon, T. (2000). Motivated cultural cognition: The impact of implicit cultural theories on dispositional attribution varies as a function of need for closure. *Journal of Personality and Social Psychology, 78,* 247–259.
Chun, W. Y., & Kruglanski, A. W. (2005). Consumption as a multiple goal pursuit without awareness. In F. R. Kardes, P. M. Herr, & J. Nantel (Eds.), *Applying social cognition to consumer-focused strategy* (pp. 25–43). Mahwah, NJ: Erlbaum.
Cratylus. (1995). De Nederlandse Need for Closure Schaal (The Netherlands Need for Closure Scale). *Nederlandse Tijdschrift Voor de Psychologie, 50,* 231–232.
Dechesne, M., Schultz, J., Kruglanski, A. W., Fishman, S., & Orehek, E. (2007). *Psychology of boundary conditions: Need for closure and the allure of group impermeability.* Manuscript submitted for publication.
De Grada, E., Kruglanski, A. W., Mannetti, L., & Pierro, A. (1999). Motivated cognition and group interaction: Need for closure affects the contents and processes of collective negotiations. *Journal of Experimental Social Psychology, 35,* 346–365.

De Grada, E., Kruglanski, A. W., Mannetti, L., Pierro, A., & Webster, D. M. (1996). Un'analisi stutturale comparative delle versioni USA e italiana della scala di "Bisogno di chiusura cognitive" di Webster and Kruglanski [A comparative structural analysis of the U.S. and Italian versions of the "Need for Cognitive Closure" Scale of Webster and Kruglanski]. *Testing, Psicometria, Metodologia, 3*, 5–18.

Dijksterhuis, A., van Knippenberg, A., Kruglanski, A. W., & Schaper, C. (1996). Motivated social cognition: Need for closure effects on memory and judgment. *Journal of Experimental Social Psychology, 32*, 254–270.

Festinger, L. (1950). Informal social communication. *Psychological Review, 57*, 271–282.

Ford, T. E., & Kruglanski, A. W. (1995). Effects of epistemic motivations on the use of accessible constructs in social judgment. *Personality and Social Psychology Bulletin, 21*, 950–962.

Jamieson, D. W., & Zanna, M. P. (1989). Need for structure in attitude formation and expression. In A. R. Pratkanis, S. J. Breckler, & A. G. Greenwald (Eds.), *Attitude structure and function* (pp. 383–406). Hillsdale, NJ: Erlbaum.

Jones, E. E. (1979). The rocky road from act to disposition. *American Psychologist, 34*, 107–117.

Kossowska, M., Orehek, E., & Kruglanski, A. W. (in press). Motivation towards closure and cognitive resources: An individual differences approach. In A. Gruszka, G. Mathews, & B. Szymura (Eds.), *Handbook of individual differences in cognition: Attention, memory and executive control*. New York: Springer.

Kossowska, M., Van Hiel, A., Chun, W. Y., & Kruglanski, A. W. (2002). The Need for Closure scale: Structure, cross-cultural invariance, and comparison of mean ratings between European-American and East Asian samples. *Psychologica Belgica, 42*, 267–286.

Kruglanski, A. W. (1989). *Lay epistemics and human knowledge: Cognitive and motivational bases*. New York: Plenum Press.

Kruglanski, A. W. (2004). *The psychology of closed-mindedness*. New York: Psychology Press.

Kruglanski, A. W., & Freund, T. (1983). The freezing and unfreezing of lay-inferences: Effects on impressional primacy, ethnic stereotyping, and numerical anchoring. *Journal of Experimental Social Psychology, 19*, 448–468.

Kruglanski, A. W., Pierro, A., Higgins, E. T., & Capozza, D. (2007). "On the move" or "staying put": Locomotion, need for closure and reactions to organizational change. *Journal of Applied Social Psychology, 37*, 1305–1340.

Kruglanski, A. W., Shah, J. Y., Fishbach, A., Friedman, R., Chun, W., & Sleeth-Keppler, D. (2002). A theory of goals systems. In M. P. Zanna (Ed.), *Advances in experimental social psychology* (Vol. 34, pp. 331–378). New York: Academic Press.

Kruglanski, A. W., Shah, J. Y., Pierro, A., & Mannetti, L. (2002). When similarity brings content: Need for closure and the allure of homogeneous and self-resembling groups. *Journal of Personality and Social Psychology, 83*, 648–662.

Kruglanski, A. W., & Webster, D. M. (1991). Group members' reactions to opinion deviates and conformists at varying degrees of proximity to decision deadline and of environmental noise. *Journal of Personality and Social Psychology, 61*, 212–225.

Kruglanski, A. W., & Webster, D. M. (1996). Motivated closing of the mind: "Seizing" and "freezing." *Psychological Review, 103*, 263–283.

Kruglanski, A. W., Webster, D. M., & Klem, A. (1993). Motivated resistance and openness to persuasion in the presence or absence of prior information. *Journal of Personality and Social Psychology, 65*, 861–876.

Legierski, J., & Kossowska, M. (2008). *Epistemic motivation, working memory and diagnostic information search*. Unpublished manuscript, Jagielonski Uniwersytet, Krakow, Poland.

Livi, S. (2002). *Il bisogna di chiuscora cognitiva e la transmissione delle norme nei piccoli gruppi [The need for cognitive closure and norm-transmission in small groups]*. Unpublished doctoral dissertation, University of Rome La Sapienza.

Maass, A., & Arcuri, L. (1992). The role of language in the persistence of stereotypes. In G. Semin & K. Fiedler (Eds.), *Language, interaction and social cognition* (pp. 129–143). Newbury Park, CA: Sage.

Mayseless, O., & Kruglanski, A. W. (1987). What makes you so sure?: Effects of epistemic motivations on judgmental confidence. *Organizational Behavior and Human Decision Processes, 39*, 162–183.

Mikulincer, M., Yinon, A., & Kabili, D. (1991). Epistemic needs and learned helplessness. *European Journal of Personality, 5*, 249–258.

Pierro, A., & Kruglanski, A. W. (2008). "Seizing and freezing" on a significant-person schema: Need for closure and the transference effect in social judgment. *Personality and Social Psychology Bulletin, 34*, 1492–1503.

Pierro, A., Mannetti, L., Converso, D., Garsia, V., Miglietta, A., Ravenna, M., et al. (1995). Caratteristiche strutturali della versione italiana della scale di bisogno di chiusura cognitiva (di Webster and Kruglanski) [Structural characteristics of the Italian version of the Need for Cognitive Closure Scale (of Webster and Kruglanski)]. *Testing, Psicometria, Metodologia, 2*, 125–141.

Pierro, A., Mannetti, L., De Grada, E., Livi, S., & Kruglanski, A. W. (2003). Autocracy bias in informal groups under need for closure. *Personality and Social Psychology Bulletin, 29*, 405–417.

Raven, B. H., Schwarzwald, J., & Koslowsky, M. (1998). Conceptualizing and measuring a power/interaction model of interpersonal influence. *Journal of Applied Social Psychology, 28*, 307–332.

Richter, L., & Kruglanski, A. W. (1999). Motivated search for common ground: Need for closure effects on audience design in interpersonal communication. *Personality and Social Psychology Bulletin, 25*(9), 1101–1114.

Rokeach, M. (1960). *The open and closed mind*. New York: Basic Books.

Ross, L. (1977). The intuitive psychologist and his shortcomings: Distortions in the attribution process. In L. Berkowitz (Ed.), *Advances in experimental social psychology* (Vol. 10, pp. 173–220). New York: Academic Press.

Rubini, M., & Kruglanski, A. W. (1997). Brief encounters ending in estrangement: Motivated language use and interpersonal rapport in the question–answer paradigm. *Journal of Personality and Social Psychology, 72,* 1047–1060.

Shah, J. Y., Kruglanski, A. W., & Thompson, E. P. (1998). Membership has its (epistemic) rewards: Need for closure effects on ingroup bias. *Journal of Personality and Social Psychology, 75,* 383–393.

Sorrentino, R. M., & Short, J. C. (1986). Uncertainty orientation, motivation and cognition. In R. M. Sorrentino & E. T. Higgins (Eds.), *Handbook of motivation and cognition: Vol. 1. Foundations of social behavior* (pp. 189–206). New York: Guilford Press.

Stasser, G., & Stewart, D. (1992). Discovery of hidden profiles by decision-making groups: Solving a problem versus making a judgment. *Journal of Personality and Social Psychology, 63*(2), 426–434.

Stasser, G., & Titus, W. (1985). Pooling of unshared information in group decision making: Biased information sampling during discussion. *Journal of Personality and Social Psychology, 48*(6), 1467–1478.

Stasser, G., & Titus, W. (1987). Effects of information load and percentage of shared information on the dissemination of unshared information during group discussion. *Journal of Personality and Social Psychology, 53*(1), 83–93.

Webster, D. M. (1993a). *Groups under the influence: Need for closure effects on information sharing in decision making groups.* Unpublished doctoral dissertation, University of Maryland.

Webster, D. M. (1993b). Motivated augmentation and reduction of the overattribution bias. *Journal of Personality and Social Psychology, 65*(2), 261–271.

Webster, D. M., & Kruglanski, A. W. (1994). Individual differences in need for cognitive closure. *Journal of Personality and Social Psychology, 67,* 1049–1062.

Webster, D. M., Kruglanski, A. W., & Pattison, D. A. (1997). Motivated language use in intergroup contexts: Need for closure effects on the linguistic intergroup bias. *Journal of Personality and Social Psychology, 72,* 1122–1131.

Webster, D. M., Richter, L., & Kruglanski, A. W. (1996). On leaping to conclusions when feeling tired: Mental fatigue effects on impressional primacy. *Journal of Experimental Social Psychology, 32,* 181–195.

Webster-Nelson, D., Klein, C. F., & Irvin, J. E. (2003). Motivational antecedents of empathy: Inhibiting effects of fatigue. *Basic and Applied Social Psychology, 25,* 37–50.

CHAPTER 24

■ ● ▲ ◆ ■ ● ▲ ◆

Integrative Complexity

PETER SUEDFELD

The idea that stable individual differences exist in the ways that people process information, evaluate data, and make decisions—in other words, in their cognitive processes—became salient in psychological theorizing in the 1960s. Of course, this idea had precursors: intelligence, obviously a cognitive processing characteristic, had for decades been studied as an unchanging attribute; and authoritarianism, although usually considered to be a personality factor, has cognitive components such as intolerance of ambiguity, rigidity of beliefs, stereotyping, and preference for simple rules to guide decisions and behavior.

But with the cognitive revolution that transformed psychology, thinking as a topic in itself, as well as its personality-related aspects, attracted increasing interest (e.g., Schroder & Suedfeld, 1971; Scott, Osgood, & Peterson, 1979). As the limitations of drive theories became increasingly clear, psychologists proposed intrinsic motives such as sensation-seeking, exploration, novelty, agency, play, and others whose relation to biological needs or physiological homeostasis were not obvious (e.g., Berlyne, 1960; Zuckerman, 1979).[1] Two characteristics of such motives also emerged: They comprised both cognitive and emotional components, and people differed in the degree to which they experienced and were driven by them.

This chapter traces the development of one line of theory and research within the tradition that has become known as cognitive complexity (Bieri, 1955). "Cognitive complexity" subsumes a variety of specific approaches, but the general foundation is the idea that a nonhomeostatic variable can be identified that involves how people deal with the flow of information that impinges on them throughout their lives. It was hypothesized that stable differences exist in the way that individuals react when that information flow becomes too meager or too lavish. In the first case, people may either magnify (sharpen) aspects of available information or generate their own, whereas in the other case, they select what information to attend to while ignoring the rest, clump bits of information into categories so that the distinct pieces are reduced in number, ignore differences among different inputs (leveling), and so on.

Three of the cognitive complexity approaches have continued to generate considerable amounts of research—need for closure (Kruglanski & Webster, 1996), need for cognition (Cacioppo & Petty, 1982), and conceptual complexity (Harvey, Hunt, & Schroder, 1961; Schroder, Driver, & Streufert, 1967). The first two of these, which are discussed in other chapters (Kruglanski & Fishman, Chapter 23, this volume; Petty, Briñol, Loersch, & McCaslin, Chapter 21, this volume) are closely related to each other; and other constructs, such as the theories of uncertainty orientation (Sorrentino, Roney, & Hanna, 1992) and telic dominance (Apter, 1989), also have components that are very similar to both need for closure and need for cognition. The third construct—conceptual complexity and its major offshoots—is the focus of this chapter.

The various conceptual and empirical relationships among formulations of cognitive complexity raise the question of how many such traits really exist, what they are, and the extent to which these theories are overlapping or redundant. It is certainly the case that their psychometric measures are correlated, but no overarching correlation matrix incorporating all of these variables has been published. For the sake of clarity, and to reduce clutter in the field (or at least to make sense of the clutter), such an analysis would be very valuable.

Another issue, which lies at the heart of this chapter, is the degree to which these theories actually describe individual differences, including cognitive processes, that underlie behavior, imparting a relatively high level of stability that characterizes the individual's responses across time, environmental conditions, specific problems or issues, and other dynamic variables. The approach with which this chapter is primarily concerned, conceptual/integrative complexity theory, recognized from the beginning that "concepts are jointly determined by the totality of external (situational) and internal (dispositional) factors at the given time operating in mutual interdependence" (Harvey et al., 1961, p. 15). Note that the existence of a trait-like ("dispositional") characteristic is assumed, and this assumption underlies most of the early research. Later emphasis shifted to the consideration of how dynamic variables affected current (i.e., state) cognition, the individual's underlying trait predisposition being only inferred.

However, both early and late in the history of this research tradition, researchers recognized that although the relative importance of trait and state factors varies depending on a host of factors, the final cognitive process is always the result of an interaction between these two large categories of influences. This chapter traces chronologically the major versions of this approach—conceptual systems theory and the theories of conceptual complexity (subsuming interactive complexity) and integrative complexity—and summarizes a sampling of the research inspired by each.

Conceptual Systems Theory

Basic Concepts

Conceptual complexity theory was formulated as a systems theory of personality development related to childrearing strategies (Harvey et al., 1961). The model was inspired by George Kelly's (1955) psychology of personal constructs to posit cognitive differentiation as one of the basic components of trait-like differences in thinking. Differentiation was defined as the perception of clearly articulated parts within a situation, whereas integration involves relating these parts to each other and to previously established constructs. In broad outline, differentiation and integration have remained the hallmark variables of this school of thought throughout the subsequent years and give every indication of remaining so. The inclusion of integration also separates this theory and its successors from most other cognitive personality models (e.g., Bieri, 1955; Hermann, 1980).

According to systems theory, differentiation and integration develop or fail to develop differently in a series of personality types through four stages of conceptual development. Progress from one stage to the next is dependent on how family rules were generated and applied. Briefly, the predisposition (or ability; the distinction is not totally clear in the theory) for either concrete or abstract thinking is based on how family rules are established and the reliability or unreliability of reward and punishment.

If rules are laid down by the parents and consistently lead to reward for compliance and punishment for transgression (reliable unilateral training), the child learns to trust and obey authority (System I conceptual structure). If the outcomes of rule observance or violation are not consistent (unilateral unreliable training), counterdependence and rebelliousness (System II) follow. Systems I and II are characterized as concrete modes of thought. If rules are developed through interaction between the parents and the child, the result is abstract thinking. If, when the child breaks a rule, the parent steps in to shield the child from adverse consequences (interdependent protective training), the individual comes to expect help and support from others (System III). However, if the parents allow natural consequences to occur—except when these would be dangerous or seriously damaging—the child learns to search for and process relevant information before making decisions (System IV). "Arrestation" at a particular stage can occur if childrearing methods prevent differentiations that would lead to more abstract integration.

Measurement and Research

Harvey and colleagues (1961) emphasized multiple measurement methods to identify the conceptual systems level that particular individuals attained. These included what would normally be considered experimental manipulations (such as criticizing participants and interpreting their reactions to negative comments, including them in a conformity experiment, and so on), which seems a circular method. Conceptual level is inferred from the participant's behavior, which is attributed to the characteristics of thinking at that particular level. Theoretical constructs that were thought to overlap with conceptual systems could also provide the basis of what we might call measurement by analogue. That is, measures of authoritarianism, dogmatism, and rigidity tap some of the characteristics of System I; a Machiavellianism scale and some responses on a measure of field independence indicate System II; and so on. There were also paper-and-pencil tests designed to measure systems-level functioning, including a Sentence Completion Test that was the forerunner of the later Paragraph Completion Test, described later.

Much of the research mustered in the Harvey and colleagues (1961) book to support systems theory had been conducted in different theoretical contexts. For example, Harvey and colleagues cited research on field independence, cognitive rigidity,

avoidance of ambiguity, and the authoritarian personality, all of which have factors in common with the various systems (and with cognitive personality theories in general). Research specifically aimed at the systems model showed that: (1) people functioning at a System I level made more extreme judgments about others than those at Systems II, III, and IV; (2) System II is associated with heightened sensitivity to control by others and with disengagement from feedback, commitment, and responsibility; (3) System III individuals are especially open to other people and their reactions to oneself; and (4) System IV functioning emphasizes the person's own standards and autonomy, as well as a high level of sensitization to information.

In a stock-market simulation, concrete-level groups minimized diversity, both from the environment and within the team; sought less information; and were less active, as well as less cohesive (Tuckman, 1964). Other studies looked at social perception, attitude change in response to persuasive messages, and behavioral rigidity (e.g., response modification after critical feedback and generalization–extinction curves) as a function of system level. Applied researchers have used measures of system-level functioning in studies of trainer–trainee and teacher–student relationships (e.g., Hunt, 1966; Hunt & Joyce, 1967), and Tuckman's (1965) theory of group development proposed four stages that are essentially the same as Harvey et al.'s four systems.

In one experiment, Harvey (1963) found that System IV participants were able to construct and present counterattitudinal speeches better than the other three groups, regardless of whether or not they expected the speeches to be heard by a committee that had the power to make decisions concerning the position espoused in the speech. This finding was interpreted as reflecting higher tolerance for cognitive dissonance and greater cognitive flexibility at this level of structure. System II participants performed the worst when they expected to speak publicly but not otherwise, presumably because of their distrust of authority and unwillingness to expose their products to the committee. System III participants performed the worst in the private condition, but better than Systems I and II in the public condition, perhaps because they trusted authority and had experienced positive reinforcement in the past in their dealings with people in authority.

Conceptual Complexity Theory[2]

Basic Concepts

Although the systems theory generated a respectable volume of research, some of the scientists who developed the theory and the studies soon moved in a different direction. In conceptual complexity theory (Schroder et al., 1967), the developmental aspect of the original theory was dropped, as were the stages. More important, the modified theory primarily concerned the structure of thought rather than its content.

Because this version of the theory viewed complexity as a fully structural rather than a content variable, the complexity score was defined by levels of differentiation and integration rather than by the attitude or opinion expressed. For example, the beliefs that rules should always be followed and that rules are made to be broken are opposite in content but equivalent in structure: Neither belief shows any sign that the speaker recognizes nuances, contingencies, or different arguments (no differentiation), and in the absence of differentiation, integration is not possible. Both statements would be scored at the lowest level of conceptual complexity, in contrast with conceptual systems scoring (Harvey et al., 1961), in which the first statement would be scored as reflecting System I thinking and the second, System II. Although they thought of complexity as a dimension, Schroder and colleagues (1967) still referred to four levels of conceptual complexity. However, they acknowledged that these levels are actually nodal points along a continuum of any number of possible levels. The lowest ("concrete") level is characterized by compartmentalized, rigid, and absolutistic cognitive rules. At a moderately low level, the individual generates alternative ways of looking at concepts and recognizes some areas of autonomous choice. At the moderately high, more "abstract," level, more dimensions are perceived, and combinatorial rules for organizing (matching, comparing)

them are developed. At the highest level, one finds alternative combinations, general laws, more diversity, self-generated rules, and flexibility.

Measurement

Although several methods for assessing conceptual complexity were described by Schroder et al. and other researchers (see Streufert & Streufert, 1978, for a comprehensive review), the most frequently used instrument was, and remains, the Paragraph Completion Test (PCT). The PCT is a semiprojective measure in which the individual is presented with a series of sentence stems consisting of one or a few words and is asked to complete a sentence starting with the stem and then to continue writing on the same topic until time is up (usually 1–2 minutes), when they go to the next stem.

Two stems are used to represent each of three major areas about which people commonly need to make decisions—uncertainty, relations to authority, and social rejection. The specific word or phrase that begins each item can vary depending on the nature of the participant sample. For example, with undergraduate research volunteers, one of the authority stems is "Parents. ... " With older participants, this would not be appropriate, and the researcher would select a stem that would better represent authority to that group. The completed paragraphs are scored on a 1–7 scale in ascending order of complexity, and the final score for the individual is the mean of the six paragraph scores. As the scoring system developed, scores of 1 and 3 came to represent the concrete levels of undifferentiated and differentiated but not integrated conceptual structures, whereas 5 and 7 marked abstract, integrated thinking. Scores of 2, 4, and 6 were used to mark the implicit or implied, but not clearly stated, emergence of the next higher level. A highly detailed scoring manual has been developed that is appropriate for scoring both conceptual (trait) and integrative (state) complexity (Baker-Brown et al., 1992). In the latter version, the terms *concrete* and *abstract* are dropped, as are verbal labels attached to specific levels of complexity. Scorers can be trained and qualified either in face-to-face workshops or online.

Research

Despite the emphasis on structure, conceptual complexity scores are correlated with a number of ostensibly content-based variables, possibly because the latter have some structural components. Complexity is negatively correlated with authoritarianism and dogmatism and positively correlated with both convergent thinking (crystallized intelligence) and divergent thinking. The correlations are low, however, usually accounting for less than 10% of the variance, so that conceptual complexity is clearly not just an aspect of traditional attitudinal or cognitive factors (Schroder et al., 1967; Suedfeld & Coren, 1992).

Personality traits that are positively related to conceptual complexity include sociability, warmth, nurturance, nonconformity, and sensation seeking. Highly complex individuals also tend to be more ambitious and dominant (Coren & Suedfeld, 1995), although a study of MBA students in a multiday workshop showed that they are also low in social compliance and conscientiousness and are perceived by others as self-centered, easily bored, and—despite low scores on a narcissism scale—narcissistic (Tetlock, Peterson, & Berry, 1993). Conceptually complex leaders in a negotiation experiment were rated as higher on tolerance for uncertainty, assumption of leader role, consideration for others, and predictive accuracy; less complex leaders were perceived as higher on initiating structure, emphasizing production, and demanding reconciliation (Streufert, Streufert, & Castore, 1968).

Besides such explorations of the relationship between conceptual complexity and other traits, the theory impelled a considerable amount of experimental research. A much-favored tool has been the use of simulations, perhaps because complex situations were thought to be necessary to evoke differences between people who differed in conceptual complexity. Before the days of widespread computer use, the simulations were role-playing situations in which participants (usually university students) took the part of national leaders, military commanders, business executives, and the like. Groups were composed to be homogeneous in their level of trait complexity, and the researchers analyzed their decision-making processes, strategies, and outcomes under conditions that differed in information load, ambiguity and uncertainty, success and failure, and so on.

From the beginning, conceptual complexity research emphasized how trait complexity predicted the reactions of experimental participants to variations in the informational environment. Findings cited in Schroder and colleagues (1967) showed that more cognitively complex participants used more dimensions to judge other players in an internation simulation, were better at tracking information that was not immediately available in a stock market simulation, showed a higher level of information search and processing in a tactical war game, expressed greater doubt and uncertainty as stimuli became more ambiguous, and made decisions that were more connected to each other and to changes in the environment than less complex participants. Complex groups used more, and more complex, descriptions and integrated past feedback better, regardless of information load. In both the simulations and other experimental situations (e.g., restricted environmental stimulation), suboptimal and superoptimal levels of information input resulted in performance becoming less complex. At extremely high and extremely low information load, the information-processing differences between abstract and concrete participants diminished. The same occurred under conditions of high levels of either failure or success feedback.

Not all of the relevant experiments used the simulation paradigm. For example, one interesting study (Harris & Highlen, 1982) found that the successful solving of anagrams was positively related to complexity, presumably because of greater cognitive flexibility. Not only that, but in an inescapable-aversive-noise (learned helplessness) paradigm, conceptually simpler participants showed a significant performance decrement, whereas complex participants actually improved.

In field experiments with Peace Corps trainees who responded to statements related to racial prejudice and to reasons for joining the Peace Corps, less conceptually complex participants rated more statements as categorically accepted *or* rejected than did complex participants matched for intelligence, dogmatism, authoritarianism, cognitive differentiation, and verbal fluency. The complex group also generated less racially prejudiced statements than did the simple group (Coffman, 1967). The finding of greater extremity of opinions associated with low complexity was confirmed by an impression-formation experiment that showed that low-complexity students made more extreme judgments of the target person across positive, negative, and neutral sets than more complex individuals (Frauenfelder, 1974).

The interaction between environmental and trait complexity variables led to another version of this model, the interactive complexity theory (Streufert & Streufert, 1978). In this approach, complexity is conceptualized as "dimensionality," with a major distinction between unidimensional and multidimensional thinking as the counterparts of the earlier concrete–abstract categories. The theory acknowledges domain specificity, the idea that people may function at different levels of dimensionality in different cognitive areas. It also recaptures some of the earlier attention to developmental influences; in this formulation, authoritarian but multidimensional parents may inculcate hierarchical multidimensionality in their children (i.e., the ability to perceive and use several dimensions, but only in fixed order and rigid interrelationships). By contrast, flexible multidimensionality is achieved by children whose parents are multidimensional thinkers and foster this trait in their children by letting them experience the world through play and trial and error.

A novel aspect of the interactive theory was that it went far beyond the traditional focus of cognitive psychology. The research looked at the effects of the curvilinear functions of information load interacting with trait complexity on outcomes such as affect, interpersonal attraction, social influence, person perception, attitude formation and change, and motivation (Streufert & Streufert, 1978). In his later work, Streufert switched his attention to how environmental and conceptual complexity function in organizations (e.g., Streufert & Swezey, 1986). Using more sophisticated simulations and groups made up of actual managers rather than university students, the research looked again at some old topics (e.g., the effects of information load) and some new ones,

such as leadership, organizational complexity, managerial and organizational performance, and the relationship among conceptual complexity, problem content, arousal, and health.

Integrative Complexity Theory

Basic Concepts

Integrative complexity theory is an offshoot of conceptual complexity theory and is closely related to interactive complexity theory. However, its focus is not on the trait complexity that sets the boundaries within which the person operates. Rather, the topic of interest is complexity as a dependent variable—that is, the level of complexity revealed in the individual's oral or written utterances, conceived to be a product of an interaction between the complexity trait and a host of other situational and internal variables. The situational factors include characteristics such as information load, time pressure, potential rewards and punishments, the number and relative importance of problems facing the person at a given period of time, and the level of noise (both literal and figurative) in the environment. Internal factors studied include fatigue, emotional arousal, motivation, and perceived likelihood of success.

The foundational assumption is that the level of expressed complexity fluctuates on the basis of these and other influences. For example, the cognitive manager model (Suedfeld, 1992) postulates that complex information processing uses up more resources (such as time, effort, thought, and energy) than simple processing and that good cognitive managers will therefore deal with problems at a level of complexity that conserves needed resources—that is, at the lowest level commensurate with a high probability of success, tempered by the perceived importance of the problem within the array of problems needing to be solved within the same time frame.

Furthermore, under high levels of stress—stemming from imbalance between the number and importance of problems and the resources available to solve them—a phenomenon known as disruptive stress is observed, leading to a reduced level of complexity, even though the problem solver may know that this will be inadequate to solve the problem. Thus, many European diplomats knew in the summer of 1914 that their world was spiraling toward chaos but could think of no way to avert disaster, even though only a few years earlier, they had been able to generate a clever peaceful solution to an impending showdown between France and Germany over spheres of influence in North Africa.

As the example illustrates, another major departure from previous aspects of complexity theory is in the sources of data used. Integrative complexity research focuses on archival materials from biography and autobiography, history, the media, and other published or recorded documentation. Studies have concentrated on how trait (conceptual) complexity interacts with endogenous and environmental factors to determine the complexity of thinking in the specific situation, as well as on identifying factors that lead to generally predictable changes in state complexity across levels of trait complexity.

Integrative complexity researchers usually make no special effort to assess trait complexity. (Indeed, this would be impossible in most cases, given their usual sources of data.) Instead, their interest is in the level at which the person is operating at some, usually important, time, such as national leaders during a political campaign or international confrontation, generals before and during battle, or ordinary people facing life crises.

Measurement

The measurement of integrative complexity uses the same 1–7 scale and the same scoring manual as the Paragraph Completion Test. However, the material to be scored, although it includes the PCT, is mostly drawn from archival collections. Data may be taken from books, letters, diaries, media interviews, speeches to legislatures or the public, memoranda, military orders, audio or videotapes, and other sources that reflect a person's level of thinking. To avoid biased scoring, the material is collected by a member of the research staff who is unaware of the hypotheses, who selects paragraphs (the unit of analysis) at random if sampling from a larger population of paragraphs is necessary, and who, as far as possible, removes all identifying information from the materials before passing them to the scorers. As a

rule, more than one qualified scorer works with the dataset, and reliability between the scorers is always calculated.

Research

The first study in this aspect of complexity (Suedfeld & Rank, 1976) looked at the reasons that some leaders of victorious revolutions maintain their eminent positions in the postrevolution government, whereas others lose their positions, as well as their freedom or their lives in many cases. As can be seen, this is an individual difference with very serious real-life (as opposed to laboratory) consequences for the person. It turned out that a low level of complexity predicted long-term success during the armed struggle, with a rise to a significantly higher level of complexity when the revolutionary movement became the governing party. Leaders who failed to show this rise fell by the wayside after victory (e.g., Trotsky, Guevara), as did those whose initially high level of complexity made them mistrusted by their comrades as being insufficiently committed to the cause (e.g., Alexander Hamilton), a common reaction to people who are high in trait complexity.

Later research showed that this pattern is not unique to revolutionaries. In democratic elections in several countries, campaign speeches have been found to be generally lower in complexity than postvictory speeches. Furthermore, individual differences are important. Presidents of the United States who failed to show a substantial increase in complexity from before to after their election were among the least highly regarded by professional political scientists and historians (Suedfeld, 1994; Tetlock, 1981).

Integrative complexity while in high office may be related to continued success. Andrei Gromyko, for example, managed to retain eminent positions in Soviet foreign policy from the start of his career under Stalin in the 1930s through all the vicissitudes of history through the reign of Gorbachev in the 1980s. He was also the only one among his contemporary statesmen in the United States and the U.S.S.R. whose complexity did not diminish—and, in fact, increased—during the domestic and international crises of that half-century. A similar resistance to disruptive stress was shown by several other long-serving leaders, including the Duke of Wellington and Canadian Prime Minister Lester Pearson (Wallace & Suedfeld, 1988). Whether resistance to disruptive stress is the same as high trait complexity, correlated with it, or orthogonal to it remains to be investigated.

High trait complexity, while perhaps enhancing the person's likelihood of success under some difficult conditions, is no panacea under constant and worsening stress. General Robert E. Lee's pre–Civil War writings showed consistently high complexity, from which high trait complexity may be inferred. In the first years of the war, commanding against Union generals whose state complexity was lower than his, he repeatedly gained victory or at least managed to avoid severe defeat by superior numbers. However, toward the end of the war, after years of attrition in manpower and resources, and for the first time facing an enemy commander of equivalent or higher complexity (U. S. Grant), Lee's series of unlikely successes came to an end. Interestingly, from his surrender at Appomattox to the end of his life, he regained his earlier high complexity level (Suedfeld, Corteen, & McCormick, 1986). Lee is one of the best examples of the interplay between conceptual complexity and environmental conditions, an interplay that determines the level of integrative complexity.

As implied earlier, high complexity is not necessarily a key to success. Under some conditions, it is in fact counterproductive. This is probably the case when the situation requires rapid, clear-cut decisions, such as when the country is under attack or when one is up against an implacable opponent. During the 1938 Munich conference, for example, Prime Minister Chamberlain's complexity was almost half again as high as Adolf Hitler's (Suedfeld, 1988), but the latter's intransigence prevailed because of Chamberlain's willingness to accept successive compromises that redounded to Germany's benefit. Similar patterns may characterize some negotiations in today's international system. For example, Tibon (2000) reported that strong Israeli supporters of peace negotiations between Israel and Palestinians were higher in complexity than those who were less supportive. It does seem that with parties who are willing to accept some compromise, more complex negotiations are associated with more progress (Liht, Suedfeld, & Krawczyk, 2005). However, extensive research on negotiations, as opposed to confrontations, remains to be done.

In contrast to Chamberlain, Winston Churchill dogmatically maintained that Hitler and the Nazis must be dealt with by arms buildups and stern displays of force. Churchill claimed that appeasement through flexible negotiation encouraged further aggression. Most historians today agree, with the 20/20 vision that hindsight affords, that Churchill was right. Throughout the 1930s, Churchill maintained a simple stance toward Hitler's Germany, whereas Chamberlain continued to discuss the problem at a complex level until shortly prior to the outbreak of war in 1939 (Tetlock & Tyler, 1996).

A drop in complexity just before war breaks out characterizes national leaders and their subordinates across many international confrontations. International crises that end in war are consistently preceded by such a drop, whereas negotiated solutions come at the end of exchanges that show maintained or increased complexity. In addition, surprise strategic attacks are forecast by a drop in the complexity of communications from the eventual attacker, but not from the target. However, the target's complexity becomes as low as the attacker's immediately after the attack occurs. This general pattern has been reliable from the Russo-Japanese War through the Iraqi invasion of Kuwait, during regional wars, world wars, and persistent rivalries (Suedfeld & Bluck, 1988). But within the pattern, some leaders seem to have chronically higher (or lower) levels of complexity than others; thus the complexity of a nation's policies may shift when the leadership of that nation changes. For example, Mikhail Gorbachev displayed decidedly higher complexity scores than his Soviet predecessors (Tetlock & Boettger, 1989). There may also be individual differences in maintaining complexity under stress and in the ability to recognize and act on the need to shift complexity levels, as mentioned earlier. Such individual differences within leadership groups and their influence on group decision making need further research.

In general, aggressive or otherwise uncompromising strategies, even if they do not result in war, are accompanied by low complexity among leaders (e.g., Conway, Suedfeld, & Tetlock, 2001). There are also spread-of-effect phenomena in which policymakers of nations that are politically or geographically remote from the conflict show less disruption of complexity than those directly involved or close to the line of fire. Similarly, although the head of state shows more pronounced effects than subordinates within the leadership group, war or imminent war produces reduced complexity in a wide variety of elites, even those who have no role in national policy or wartime strategy, such as novelists, scientists, editorial writers, eminent psychologists, and the like (see Suedfeld, 2003).

Complexity is also involved in political ideology. The old debate about whether authoritarianism in its cognitive incarnation (rigidity, closed-mindedness, rule-based decisions, avoidance of uncertainty and ambiguity, all-or-nothing thinking, etc.) exists on both the left and the right of the political spectrum has been inconclusive, despite attempts to resolve it by fiat or redefinition (e.g., Altemeyer, 1988; Duckitt, Chapter 20, this volume). However, studies of conceptual complexity have found lower levels of complexity among members of ideologically based parties, left or right, than among more pragmatic ones (Suedfeld, Bluck, Loewen, & Elkins, 1994).

Tetlock (1986) hypothesized that, in Western democracies, liberalism has a special need to reconcile two basic, important, but often mutually contradictory values—freedom and equality. This need to accommodate value conflict leads to higher levels of complexity among center-left parties than among those further from the center in either direction, which hold one or the other value as central and are therefore willing to compromise on the other. The model is not restricted to the political arena but, rather, is relevant to any situation in which value conflict is a component of ideology. Supporting evidence has been found among political groups in the U.S.S.R., the United States, Britain, and Canada; in the United States before the Civil War; in groups involved in a Canadian controversy about sustainable forest management; and in students writing value-related essays. Van Hiel and Mervielde (2003), however, reported significant positive correlations between integrative

complexity on the one hand and both political extremism and political interest on the other. They attribute the discrepancy from previous findings to differences in the participant samples used, but the issue clearly calls for further research.

Although much of integrative complexity research has focused on political topics, there have been other issues of interest. For example, Woike (1994) used the concepts of differentiation and integration to test the theory that these were linked to agency and communion as general orientations, with men tending to emphasize the former and women the latter. Using a revised version of the integrative complexity measurement technique, she reported that in descriptions of a positive or negative life experience, the predicted gender difference in the percentages of differentiation versus integration was found regardless of whether the event described was pleasant or unpleasant, but that no such difference was found in a neutral condition. A second experiment found congruent results when participants high in either intimacy or power motivation were primed to watch for either leadership or friendly cooperation in a tape of a job interview. Participants high in power motivation used differentiation more, and those high in intimacy motivation used integration, regardless of their gender, and the motivation–priming combination predicted differentiation and integration more strongly than gender did.

Gruenfeld, Thomas-Hunt, and Kim (1998) tested the finding that members of a majority generally show higher integrative complexity than a competing minority. Because there has been some controversy as to whether this difference reflects the structure of thought or only impression management, Gruenfeld and colleagues used an experimental paradigm that manipulated a private versus public communication condition. Their results showed that the majority–minority difference exists under both conditions, confirming inferences from archival research that the complexity score is a measure of thought and not merely of self-presentation to an audience.

de Vries and Walker (1987) had student participants take the PCT and write an essay defending their own attitude concerning capital punishment. They found that the essays were higher in complexity than the PCT responses, possibly because the participants were more interested in the former. This would have been predicted by the cognitive-manager model (Suedfeld, 1992). The authors also reported an interesting curvilinear function, supporting the value conflict model, with those who rated themselves as neutral on the subject writing more complex essays than did both strong opponents and strong proponents of capital punishment.

In another study, de Vries, Blando, and Walker (1995) found that more pleasant than unpleasant events were mentioned in life-review interviews. However, complexity was higher when the individual was recalling unpleasant, undesirable, intense events or events that had been unexpected, for which the interviewee was not responsible and to which the interviewee had not adjusted.

Studies of scientists have been few, but interesting. Presidents of the American Psychological Association give less complex presidential addresses during times of national crisis; the presidents who were rated as more eminent by other psychologists show higher complexity than their less eminent counterparts; and the speeches of presidents whose areas and scientific approaches are more in the area of social rather than biological science are more complex (Suedfeld, 1985). Feist (1994) expanded this approach to study characteristics of professors of physics, chemistry, and biology, who agreed to be interviewed about their research and teaching. Both Suedfeld (1985) and Feist (1994) showed that their participants were substantially higher in complexity overall (means above 3.5) than most research samples. Feist did find differences across the three disciplines, but only the overall results are mentioned here. Scientists who thought in complex ways about their research were cited more frequently, were rated by peers as more eminent, and were rated by observers as exploitative, fastidious, deceitful, manipulative, and not socially poised, giving, or sensitive to others. They rated themselves as having high standards, rapid tempo, and a narcissistic working style (cf. the findings concerning graduate students in business, cited previously; Tetlock et al., 1993). Feist also found that scientists who thought in complex ways about education and teaching were perceived by others as warm, charming, gregarious, and not condescending.

Their self-ratings showed broad interests, not playing hunches, enjoying difficult problems (need for cognition?), and not being motivated by money. Perhaps surprisingly, complexity scores in the two domains of research and teaching had a zero correlation; although domain specificity has been reported before, the frequently assumed close relationship between research and teaching would imply otherwise.

One unusual study (Suedfeld, de Vries, Bluck, Wallbaum, & Schmidt, 1996) tested whether there exists an intuitive common-sense understanding of complexity that parallels the everyday, generally accepted understanding of the concept of intelligence. Undergraduates (who had not taken a course that covered cognitive complexity theory) completed the PCT. They then compared their own responses with two sets of described solutions. One of these sets consisted of four "prototype paragraphs" written by expert scorers to represent general information processing at complexity levels of 1, 3, 5, and 7 (see the earlier section on the measurement of complexity); the second set comprised actual PCT responses to the same stems, taken from previous studies and scored 1, 3, 5, or 7. Last, the participants were asked how a list of 17 factors would have affected their responses. The factors included both endogenous and environmental influences that previous research had shown to have reliable effects on integrative complexity, such as accountability, value conflict, and distraction.

The results were reassuring if one believes that ecological validity includes some congruity with what people other than social scientists sense to be "real" qualities of human personality and behavior. Although the participants were not good at estimating the complexity of their own PCT responses (i.e., the general prototypes they chose as most similar to their own were generally not at the same level of complexity), they were quite accurate in matching the prototype paragraphs with actual PCT completions from previous studies. In fact, some of them scored at $r = .85$ or higher with the experts' scoring, which is the threshold for qualification as an independent scorer! Their pick of the "most comfortable" response was reliably more complex than their own paragraphs; and they were very accurate in estimating how situational variables would affect complexity, reaching statistical significance in the correct direction on 16 of the 17 variables listed.

Conclusions and Future Directions

Studies of integrative complexity, which have tended to focus on archival materials, are high in ecological validity. By the same token, their internal validity is compromised because it is difficult to eliminate all possible confounds or extraneous variables and to identify causal relationships between complexity and the decision process by manipulating independent variables. For example, we cannot tell whether reduced complexity (perhaps in response to disruptive stress) leads to situation-simplifying decisions such as ceasing to negotiate and going to war or whether, once such a decision is made, reduced complexity of communications follows.

The range of relevant factors, the course of resource mustering, use, and exhaustion, and the impact of these variables on decisions in fields other than politics are open questions. So is the possibility that training or life experience (such as exposure to several cultures; Tadmore & Tetlock, 2006) can enable people to reach higher levels of complexity or develop a better understanding of the appropriate level for a particular problem-solving effort. From an applied point of view, there is a need for more predictive studies in a variety of settings in which formal or informal negotiations can have drastically different outcomes (e.g., compromise, aggression, postponement, breaking off relations, referral to a third party), including politics, business, interpersonal relations, and so on.

There are enough unknowns to leave room for a great deal of innovative and important research, and what we already know about conceptual and integrative complexity justifies the effort of doing that research. People differ in trait complexity and in their ability to address decisions and problems at the appropriate level of state complexity. These differences interact with other personality and cognitive factors to play important roles in personal and societal life.

The emphasis on political applications of integrative complexity theory has been beneficial (what is there in psychology that is more dramatic and more important than issues of war or peace?). These decisions, and the personalities of the people who make them, are relevant and interesting. Because much of what we know about integrative complexity was developed in this context, psychologists are not the only people who are interested in the topic. Furthermore, because there is no reason to believe that how complexity operates and what affects it applies only to politics, testing it in other settings is an attractive possibility.

Notes

1. Zuckerman (1979) was an early exponent of neurophysiological bases underlying such differences.
2. In some publications based on conceptual complexity theory, the term *integrative complexity* is used. For the sake of clarity, in this chapter that term is reserved for its most current usage, which emphasizes (1) the nature of complex thinking as a variable resource and (2) its application to unobtrusive, frequently archival datasets.

References

Altemeyer, B. (1988). *Enemies of freedom: Understanding right-wing authoritarianism.* San Francisco: Jossey-Bass.

Apter, M. J. (1989). *Reversal theory: Motivation, emotion, and personality.* London: Routledge.

Baker-Brown, G., Ballard, E. J., Bluck, S., de Vries, B., Suedfeld, P., & Tetlock, P. E. (1992). The conceptual/integrative complexity scoring manual. In C. P. Smith (Ed.), *Motivation and personality: Handbook of thematic content analysis* (pp. 401–418). New York: Cambridge University Press.

Berlyne, D. B. (1960). *Conflict, arousal, and curiosity.* New York: McGraw-Hill.

Bieri, J. (1955). Cognitive complexity–simplicity and predictive behavior. *Journal of Abnormal and Social Psychology, 51,* 263–268.

Cacioppo, J. T., & Petty, R. E. (1982). The need for cognition. *Journal of Personality and Social Psychology, 42,* 116–131.

Coffman, T. L. (1967, April). *The integrative complexity of attitudes as a dependent and independent variable in social judgment.* Paper presented at the meeting of the Eastern Psychological Association, Boston.

Conway, L. G., III, Suedfeld, P., & Tetlock, P. E. (2001). Integrative complexity and political decisions that lead to war or peace. In D. J. Christie,

R. V. Wagner, & D. Winter (Eds.), *Peace, conflict, and violence: Peace psychology for the 21st century* (pp. 66–75). Englewood Cliffs, NJ: Prentice-Hall.

Coren, S., & Suedfeld, P. (1995). Personality correlates of conceptual complexity. *Journal of Social Behavior and Personality, 10*, 229–242.

de Vries, B., Blando, J., & Walker, L. J. (1995). The review of life's events: Analyses of content and structure. In B. Haight & J. Webster (Eds.), *The art and science of reminiscing: Theory, research, methods, and applications* (pp. 123–137). Washington, DC: Taylor & Francis.

de Vries, B., & Walker, L. J. (1987). Conceptual/integrative complexity and attitudes toward capital punishment. *Personality and Social Psychology Bulletin, 13*, 448–457.

Feist, G. J. (1994). Personality and working style predictors of integrative complexity: A study of scientists' thinking about research and teaching. *Journal of Personality and Social Psychology, 67*, 474–484.

Frauenfelder, K. J. (1974). Integrative complexity and extreme responses. *Psychological Reports, 34*, 770.

Gruenfeld, D. H., Thomas-Hunt, M. C., & Kim, P. H. (1998). Cognitive flexibility, communication strategy, and integrative complexity in groups: Public versus private reactions to majority and minority status. *Journal of Experimental Social Psychology, 34*, 202–226.

Harris, R. M., & Highlen, P. S. (1982). Cognitive complexity and susceptibility to learned helplessness. *Social Behavior and Personality, 10*(2), 183–188.

Harvey, O. J. (1963). *Cognitive determinants of role playing* (Technical Report No. 3, Contract No. 1147(07)). Alexandria, VA: Department of Defense.

Harvey, O. J., Hunt, D., & Schroder, H. M. (1961). *Conceptual systems and personality organization.* New York: Wiley.

Hermann, M. G. (1980). Explaining foreign policy behavior using the personal characteristics of leaders. *International Studies Quarterly, 24*, 7–46.

Hunt, D. E. (1966). A model for analyzing the training of training agents. *Merrill–Palmer Quarterly of Behavior and Development, 12*, 137–156.

Hunt, D. E., & Joyce, B. R. (1967). Teacher trainee personality and initial teaching style. *American Educational Research Journal, 4*, 253–259.

Kelly, G. A. (1955). *The psychology of personal constructs: Vol. 1. A theory of personality.* New York: Norton.

Kruglanski, A. W., & Webster, D. M. (1996). Motivated closing of the mind: "Seizing" and "freezing." *Psychological Review, 103*, 263–268.

Liht, J., Suedfeld, P., & Krawczyk, A. (2005). Integrative complexity in face-to-face negotiations between the Chiapas guerrillas and the Mexican government. *Political Psychology, 26*(4), 543–552.

Schroder, H. M., Driver, M. J., & Streufert, S. (1967). *Human information processing.* New York: Holt, Rinehart & Winston.

Schroder, H. M., & Suedfeld, P. (Eds.). (1971). *Personality theory and information processing.* New York: Ronald Press.

Scott, W. A., Osgood, D. W., & Peterson, C. (1979). *Cognitive structure: Theory and measurement of individual differences.* New York: Wiley.

Sorrentino, R. M., Roney, C. J. R., & Hanna, S. E. (1992). Uncertainty orientation. In C. P. Smith (Ed.), *Motivation and personality: Handbook of thematic content analysis* (pp. 419–427). New York: Cambridge University Press.

Streufert, S., & Streufert, S. C. (1978). *Behavior in the complex environment.* Washington, DC: Winston.

Streufert, S., Streufert, S. C., & Castore, C. H. (1968). Leadership in negotiations and the complexity of conceptual structure. *Journal of Applied Psychology, 52*, 218–223.

Streufert, S., & Swezey, R. W. (1986). *Complexity, managers, and organizations.* New York: Academic Press.

Suedfeld, P. (1985). American Psychological Association Presidential addresses: The relation of integrative complexity to historical, professional, and personal factors. *Journal of Personality and Social Psychology, 49*, 1643–1651.

Suedfeld, P. (1988). Are simple decisions always worse? *Society, 25*, 25–27.

Suedfeld, P. (1992). Cognitive managers and their critics. *Political Psychology, 13*, 435–453.

Suedfeld, P. (1994). President Clinton's policy dilemmas: A cognitive analysis. *Political Psychology, 15*, 337–349.

Suedfeld, P. (2003). Integrative complexity in political contexts. In J. Kawata & Y. Araki (Eds.), *Handbook of political psychology* (pp. 52–62). Tokyo: Hokuju Shuppan.

Suedfeld, P., & Bluck, S. (1988). Changes in integrative complexity prior to surprise attacks. *Journal of Conflict Resolution, 32*, 626–635.

Suedfeld, P., Bluck, S., Loewen, L., & Elkins, D. J. (1994). Sociopolitical values and integrative complexity of members of student political groups. *Canadian Journal of Behavioural Science, 26*, 121–141.

Suedfeld, P., & Coren, S. (1992). Cognitive correlates of conceptual complexity. *Personality and Individual Differences, 13*, 1193–1199.

Suedfeld, P., Corteen, R. S., & McCormick, C. (1986). The role of integrative complexity in military leadership: Robert E. Lee and his opponents. *Journal of Applied Social Psychology, 16*, 498–507.

Suedfeld, P., de Vries, B., Bluck, S., Wallbaum, A. B. C., & Schmidt, P. W. (1996). Intuitive perceptions of decision-making strategy: Naive assessors' concepts of integrative complexity. *International Journal of Psychology, 31*, 177–190.

Suedfeld, P., & Rank, D. A. (1976). Revolutionary leaders: Long-term success as a function of conceptual complexity. *Journal of Personality and Social Psychology, 34*, 169–178.

Tadmore, C. T., & Tetlock, P. E. (2006). Biculturalism: A model of the effects of second-culture exposure on acculturation and integrative complexity. *Journal of Cross-Cultural Psychology, 37*(2), 173–190.

Tetlock, P. E. (1981). Pre- to post-election shifts in presidential rhetoric: Impression management or cognitive adjustment? *Journal of Personality and Social Psychology, 41*, 207–212.

Tetlock, P. E. (1986). A value pluralism model of ideological reasoning. *Journal of Personality and Social Psychology, 50,* 819–827.

Tetlock, P. E., & Boettger, R. (1989). Cognitive and rhetorical styles of traditionalist and reformist Soviet politicians: A content analysis study. *Political Psychology, 10,* 209–232.

Tetlock, P. E., Peterson, R., & Berry, J. M. (1993). Flattering and unflattering personality portraits of integratively simple and complex managers. *Journal of Personality and Social Psychology, 64*(3), 500–511.

Tetlock, P. E., & Tyler, A. (1996). Churchill's cognitive and rhetorical style: The debates over Nazi intentions and self-government for India. *Political Psychology, 17,* 149–170.

Tibon, S. (2000). Personality traits and peace negotiations: Integrative complexity and attitudes toward the Middle East peace process. *Group Decision and Negotiation, 9*(1), 1–15.

Tuckman, B. W. (1964). Personality structure, group composition, and group functioning. *Sociometry, 27,* 469–487.

Tuckman, B. W. (1965). Developmental sequence in small groups. *Psychological Bulletin, 63,* 384–399.

Van Hiel, A., & Mervielde, I. (2003). The measurement of cognitive complexity and its relationship with political extremism. *Political Psychology, 24*(4), 781–801.

Wallace, M. D., & Suedfeld, P. (1988). Leadership performance in crisis: The longevity–complexity link. *International Studies Quarterly, 32,* 439–451.

Woike, B. A. (1994). The use of differentiation and integration processes: Empirical studies of "separate" and "connected" ways of thinking. *Journal of Personality and Social Psychology, 67*(1), 142–150.

Zuckerman, M. (1979). *Sensation seeking: Beyond the optimal level of arousal.* Hillsdale, NJ: Erlbaum.

PART V

■ ● ▲ ◆

MOTIVATIONAL DISPOSITIONS

CHAPTER 25

■ ● ▲ ◆ ■ ● ▲ ◆

Conscientiousness

BRENT W. ROBERTS
JOSHUA J. JACKSON
JENNIFER V. FAYARD
GRANT EDMONDS
JENNA MEINTS

Conscientiousness is defined as individual differences in the propensity to follow socially prescribed norms for impulse control, to be goal directed, to plan, and to be able to delay gratification and to follow norms and rules (John & Srivastava, 1999). Most researchers are familiar with the term *conscientiousness* because of its inclusion in the Big Five taxonomy of personality traits: Extraversion, Agreeableness, Conscientiousness, Emotional Stability, and Openness/Intellect (Goldberg, 1993). There are a few things to note about the origin of the term *conscientiousness* in the context of the Big Five. First, conscientiousness is a personality trait, which is defined as a "tendency to respond in certain ways under certain circumstances" (Tellegen, 1988, p. 622), or, more generally speaking, the tendency to think, feel, and behave in a relatively enduring and consistent fashion across time in trait-affording situations. Clearly, given its definition, conscientiousness should be an important correlate of a wide swath of social behavior.

Speaking in historical terms, traits associated with the domain of conscientiousness have some of the longest histories in psychology. Beginning with Freud's idea of the superego and the subsidiary concepts of the ego ideal and conscience, dispositions related to conscientiousness, such as achievement and control, have been studied for over 100 years. In the interim between Freud and the Big Five, related constructs were studied under terms such as *impulsivity* (Eysenck), *norm-favoring* (Gough), *social conformity* (Comrey), and even *Judging versus Perceiving* (i.e., the Myers–Briggs Type Indicator).

A third thing to note about the term *conscientiousness* is that it is something of a historical artifact. Many terms have been used to describe this family of traits. The term *conscientiousness* was somewhat arbitrarily assigned because of fealty to the individual who first identified the Big Five (e.g., Norman, 1963). Many have complained that the terms used to describe the Big Five, like all scale, measure, or factor labels, are less than ideal because they are (1) unwieldy, (2) inaccurate, or (3) vague. In the case of conscientiousness, the term turns out to be a fairly good compromise. The alternative descriptors, such as *constraint* (Tellegen), *work* (Jackson), and *superego strength* (Cattell), overemphasize specific aspects of conscientiousness. The term *conscientiousness*, being somewhat broad and ambiguous in its meaning, is better suited to represent the family of traits that define this domain, which are described in this chapter.

Finally, Goldberg (1993) used the term *Big Five* for a reason. The Big Five are big. Not big in the sense that they are important, but big in the sense that each of the Big Five is best considered a broad domain of traits, not a unitary construct. This point seems to be increasingly lost on the current generation of personality inventory consumers, as the preference appears to be to use short measures under the assumption that measuring a single dimension of conscientiousness, or any of the remaining Big Five, is a sufficient representation of the domain. This is like arguing that oranges, apples, and bananas are interchangeable because they are all fruit. Conscientiousness is clearly not unidimensional and consists of several relatively distinct facets that, like different fruit, are not identical.

What, then, is the composition of the family of traits within the conscientiousness domain? Several studies have focused on identifying the lower order structure of conscientiousness using two approaches. One route to identifying the structure of conscientiousness is to examine lexically derived trait adjectives, as was done to develop the Big Five (e.g., Goldberg, 1993). A second route to identifying the underlying domain of conscientiousness is an examination of the factor structure of personality inventories that measure conscientiousness-related traits. Across both approaches research has arrived at some semblance of consensus on the replicable facets of conscientiousness. In a lexical study (Roberts, Bogg, Walton, Chernyshenko, & Stark, 2004), five components found in previous lexical research on the lower order structure of conscientiousness were identified: industriousness (tenaciousness vs. laziness), reliability (dependability vs. unreliability), orderliness (organization vs. sloppiness), impulse control (cautiousness vs. carelessness), and decisiveness (decisiveness vs. indecisiveness). Unlike previous research, two additional, interpretable facets were found: formalness and conventionality. Both of these dimensions appeared to represent blends of conscientiousness, with high and low openness to experience, respectively.

In a second study of scales drawn from personality inventories, the factor structure of 36 different scales assessing aspects of conscientiousness was examined (Roberts, Chernyshenko, Stark, & Goldberg, 2005).

The 36 measures of conscientiousness were best subsumed by six factors: Impulse Control, Conventionality, Reliability, Industriousness, Order, and Virtue. Interestingly, there is striking convergence across the lexical and questionnaire studies: Industriousness, Reliability, Order, Impulse Control, and Conventionality replicated across these disparate samples and assessment techniques, suggesting that, at a minimum, these five factors make up the underlying structure of conscientiousness. Two aspects of this five-facet interpretation of conscientiousness are worth noting. First, no existing personality inventory includes all five, which renders any existing system of assessing conscientiousness inadequate. Most inventories fail to incorporate the conventionality facet, which is often mistakenly identified as an aspect of low openness. Despite this preconception, across these two studies conventionality was more strongly related to conscientiousness than to openness. Furthermore, in both studies the remaining facets of conscientiousness showed good levels of convergent and discriminant validity with the remaining Big Five, with the exception of the reliability facet. The latter is almost equivalently correlated with conscientiousness and agreeableness.

This more differentiated model of conscientiousness provides the starting point for documenting the relation of conscientiousness to social behaviors. As is seen in the following section, it allows us to organize previous research literature in order to discover which aspect of conscientiousness is most important for a variety of phenomena. In this chapter we review the association between conscientiousness and four domains: behavior (social and otherwise), emotion, motivation, and social cognition. Given the fact that conscientiousness is a personality trait that reflects relatively consistent patterns of thoughts, feelings, and behaviors, it should come as no surprise that it is associated with behaviors (health behavior), feelings (guilt and shame), and thoughts (motivations and social cognition). It is the association between conscientiousness and these outcomes that may help to explain why conscientiousness, in turn, predicts so many significant life outcomes, such as health, longevity, occupational success, and marital stability (Roberts, Kuncel, Shiner, Caspi, & Goldberg, 2007).

Conscientiousness and Behavior

How does a conscientious person behave? Based on the definition, a conscientious individual will be likely to show up to appointments early, follow society's rules, keep a clean and tidy room, work hard, and cut him- or herself off before he or she has one too many cocktails. Conscientiousness is thought to shape how people experience, interpret, and hence respond and behave in the social world. Conceptual definitions aside, what do the empirical data say about the link between conscientiousness and behavior?

To organize the behaviors associated with conscientiousness, we examine the relationship between conscientiousness and behaviors associated with significant life outcomes. Conscientiousness is associated with a number of outcomes that span the gamut from disease and health (Goodwin & Friedman, 2006) to education and occupations (Judge, Higgins, Thoreson, & Barrick, 1999; Noftle & Robins, 2007) to relationships (Roberts & Bogg, 2004; Tucker, Kressin, Spiro, & Ruscio, 1998) and even to criminal history (Krueger et al., 1994). Many different behaviors are thought to play a part in shaping the development of these outcomes. By using these life outcomes as an organizing scheme, we hope to identify a wide range of behaviors that are associated with conscientiousness and to explain its potential significance for multiple domains.

Previous research has shown that relative to other factors conscientiousness is a strong predictor of longevity (Friedman et al., 1993; Roberts, Kuncel, et al., 2007; Weiss & Costa, 2005). Specific behaviors associated with conscientiousness have been identified as a possible reason for this association. A comprehensive meta-analysis of the relationship between conscientiousness and the nine different health-related behaviors that are among the leading causes of mortality—alcohol use, disordered eating (including obesity), drug use, lack of physical activity, risky sexual practices, risky driving practices, tobacco use, suicide, and violence—demonstrated that conscientiousness predicted every category of health-related behavior relevant to longevity (Bogg & Roberts, 2004). Interestingly, the facet with the highest correlation with health behaviors was not impulse control, as expected, but conventionality. Apparently, adherence to social norms has more pervasive effects on health behaviors than other components of conscientiousness. Although some social norms are related to risky health behaviors, such as excessive drinking in college, these behaviors are usually short lived. In contrast, norms for health-facilitating behaviors, such as exercising, eating well, not smoking, and drinking in moderation, are much more pervasive (Linnan, LaMontagne, Stoddard, Emmons, & Sorensen, 2005). Clearly, conventional people are not only picking up on these norms but also adhering more strongly to them.

In turn, conscientiousness is positively related to health behaviors that could prevent mortality, such as seeing a doctor regularly and checking smoke alarms (Chuah, Drasgow, & Roberts, 2006). Additionally, the conventionality and reliability facets of conscientiousness predict whether patients adhere to medical regimens, which play a significant role in subsequent health and longevity (Insel, Reminger, & Hsiao, 2006). These findings suggest that conscientious individuals perform a number of behaviors that both lead to better health and safeguard against disease.

In the realm of education and work, a number of studies have linked high levels of conscientiousness, especially the industriousness facet, with higher grades in a variety of educational settings (Abe, 2005; Duckworth & Seligman, 2005; Noftle & Robins, 2007). The positive relation between conscientiousness and achievement continues into the workforce, with conscientiousness predicting long-term occupational attainment and income above and beyond cognitive ability (Judge et al., 1999). These associations with educational and occupational attainment can again be partially explained by behaviors associated with conscientiousness. For example, conscientiousness predicts behaviors that are associated with success in educational and occupational domains, such as study habits, time management, procrastination, and absenteeism (Conte & Jacobs, 2003; Duckworth, Peterson, Matthews, & Kelly, 2007; Graziano & Ward, 1992; Scher & Osterman, 2002). Evidence also suggests that conscientious individuals tend to persist when faced with difficult challenges and problems, such as schoolwork, rather than neglecting and avoiding these situations (O'Brien & DeLongis, 1996).

Similarly, success in the labor force is related to behaviors that are associated with conscientiousness. For example, conscientiousness is one of the best predictors of job performance (Barrick & Mount, 1991). Conscientiousness also predicts a number of behaviors related to job performance, such as absenteeism (Ones, Viswesvaran, & Schmidt, 2003), decision making and treatment of subordinates (LePine, Hollenbeck, Ilgen, & Hedlund, 1997), leadership skills (Judge, Bono, Ilies, & Gerhardt, 2002), and counterproductive work behaviors such as stealing and fighting with coworkers (Roberts, Harms, Caspi, & Moffitt, 2007). Conscientiousness also influences how individuals search for jobs and to what types of jobs people apply for, thus shaping the possibilities for advancement, success, and satisfaction (Mount, Barrick, Scullen, & Rounds, 2005).

In terms of relationships, conscientious individuals are less likely to get divorced (Roberts & Bogg, 2004; Roberts, Kuncel, et al., 2007; Tucker et al., 1998). This makes sense given the fact that relationship satisfaction is predicted by partners' levels of conscientiousness (Robins, Caspi, & Moffitt, 2000; Watson, Hubbard, & Wiese, 2000). Also, a number of key behaviors associated with conscientiousness are thought to contribute to relationship quality. For example, conscientiousness is related to a number of specific behaviors that alone are directly related to divorce, such as extramarital affairs, spousal abuse, and alcohol abuse (Buss, 1991; Buss & Shackelford, 1997). Based on these patterns, conscientiousness plays a critical role in developing and maintaining successful relationships.

More generally, conscientious behaviors are likely to shape the quality of long-term relationships. For example, individuals low in conscientiousness are not as responsible, tend to disclose personal information inappropriately, are less responsive to their partners, have poorer social support, act more condescendingly, and are not as proficient at holding back comments that might cause turmoil in a relationship (Buss, 1991; Finkel & Campbell, 2001; Vohs & Ciarocco, 2004). Over time these behaviors could con-

tribute to partners' feeling dissatisfied with their relationship. In contrast, individuals higher in conscientiousness tend to be better at managing conflicts that inevitably arise in relationships (Buss, 1992; Finkel & Campbell, 2001; Jensen-Campbell & Graziano, 2001). Moreover, conscientious individuals might actually provoke fewer disagreements and have fewer conflicts because their behaviors evoke less criticism, as they are generally controlled, organized, responsible, and hardworking. These behaviors can result in stronger bonds in relationships, which should contribute to greater marital and relationship stability (Baumeister & Leary, 1995; Lodi-Smith & Roberts, 2007).

In addition to the significant domains of work and love, conscientiousness is inversely related to a number of maladaptive life outcomes, such as unemployment, homelessness, and being incarcerated (Caspi, Wright, Moffitt, & Silva, 1998; De Fruyt & Mervielde, 1999; Kokko & Pulkkinen, 2000; Patrick, Hicks, Krueger, & Lang, 2005). Criminal acts have long been associated with the impulsivity facet of conscientiousness (Eysenck & Gudjonsson, 1989; Krueger, Caspi, Moffitt, White, & Stouthamer-Loeber, 1996), which can lead to a host of problems above and beyond jail time, such as difficulties gaining future employment. In addition to criminal activity, people low in conscientiousness have trouble saving money and have different borrowing practices than conscientious individuals do (Brandstatter & Guth, 2000; Nyhus & Webley, 2001). Behaviors associated with money extend into purchasing behavior, in which conscientiousness is associated with planning upcoming shopping purchases and not spontaneously buying unneeded items (Verplanken & Herabadi, 2001). Additionally, low levels of conscientiousness are associated with watching television more often (Persegani et al., 2002), which may reflect a lack of responsibility that can lead to maladaptive outcomes. Interestingly, this lack of responsibility manifests itself in an increase in accidental injuries (Vollrath, Landolt, & Ribi, 2003). Furthermore, parents who are low in conscientiousness are more likely to have children who injure themselves (van Aken, Junger, Verhoeven, van Aken, & Dekovic, 2007).

These findings illustrate the broad influence of conscientiousness on a variety of behaviors. These behaviors in turn have profound effects on one's health, educational and occupational attainment, relationships, and even social standing. Interestingly, most of these behaviors go above and beyond the definition and content of conscientiousness measures, suggesting that conscientiousness is an underlying cause of these behaviors (Tellegen, 1991).

Conscientiousness and Emotion

At first glance, conscientiousness seems to be primarily a behaviorally oriented construct, emphasizing actions related to impulse control, reliability, conventionality, industriousness, and orderliness (Roberts, Bogg, et al., 2004). However, conscientiousness does, despite appearances, have a connection to emotions. Two meta-analyses have shown that conscientiousness is correlated with positive affect, negative affect, happiness, and life satisfaction, with effects that are quite close in magnitude to those of extraversion and neuroticism (DeNeve & Cooper, 1998; Heller, Watson, & Ilies, 2004). Clearly conscientiousness is not devoid of emotional consequences and possibly even encompasses some emotional content.

Why would conscientiousness be linked to both positive and negative affect and especially to life satisfaction? Interestingly, the connection between conscientiousness and emotions can be found in Freud's (1961) discussion of the superego. The conscience, which inhibits or controls behavior, is driven by guilt. When people violate internal standards of decorum, they respond with the emotion of guilt—if they are properly socialized. Conversely, attaining or exceeding the implicit standards of the ego ideal (e.g., achieving what the parent values) will result in pride and positive affect. If conscientiousness captures the same processes identified by Freud in his description of the superego, then we would expect that the strongest link to emotion would be found for emotions in the family of guilt and pride, which fall into the special subcategory of "self-conscious emotions" (Tracy & Robins, 2004), and that these specific emotions would account for the relation of conscientiousness to positive and negative affect.

Within the domain of self-conscious emotions, a distinction is made between the capacity to experience guilt (and shame) and the actual experience of guilt (Tangney, 1996), which is critical for understanding the resulting pattern of associations with conscientiousness. For example, in one study, conscientiousness was moderately related to three measures of guilt (Einstein & Lanning, 1998). However, the results differed dramatically, depending on whether the outcome was the experience of guilt (termed *anxious guilt*) or the capacity for guilt (termed *empathic guilt*). Conscientiousness was negatively related to the experience of guilt and positively related to the capacity for guilt—conscientious people tended to experience guilt less frequently, but highly conscientious people felt guilt more intensely when it was experienced. Similarly, in a second study, guilt proneness, or the capacity for guilt, was (moderately positively) related to conscientiousness, whereas the experience of guilt and shame was more (strongly negatively) correlated with conscientiousness (Abe, 2003). A third study replicated the negative relations between conscientiousness and the experience of shame (Rolland & De Fruyt, 2003).

These relationships become even stronger when analyzed in terms of "shame-free" guilt and "guilt-free" shame. A study on the relation between procrastination and guilt and shame proneness found low correlations with conscientiousness (Fee & Tangney, 2000). However, since guilt and shame proneness were substantially correlated, these researchers used partial correlations to compute measures of shame-free guilt and guilt-free shame. Correlations between these "pure" measures and conscientiousness were more pronounced. Thus the true magnitude of these relationships may be obscured in previous studies that did not adequately separate guilt from shame.

Research has demonstrated that guilt often arises from interpersonal situations—either by directly wronging another or by not living up to others' standards, even when someone has done nothing wrong per se (Baumeister, Stillwell, & Heatherton, 1994). It could be that conscientious individuals' increased capacity for guilt, together with guilt's interpersonal nature, is one of the primary forces behind the above-average interpersonal functioning associated with conscientious-ness (Jensen-Campbell & Malcolm, 2007). Thus experiencing guilt may drive conscientious people to continue to behave conscientiously through promoting reparative actions aimed at either correcting wrongdoing or striving for adherence to one's own and others' standards, helping to maintain and strengthen interpersonal relationships.

Considering these findings, conscientiousness could be an important influencing factor on the experience of positive and negative affect through its relation to guilt and shame. People who are more conscientious may avoid situations that engender guilt and shame and by doing so experience elevated levels of positive affect and lower levels of negative affect. Moreover, when confronted with their own actions that may have caused another person some emotional or physical harm, conscientious individuals will be more likely to try to make amends or repair the damaged relationship, thus making their life experiences more positive going forward. Finally, guilt may be a factor in promoting conscientious behaviors that in turn lead to better interpersonal relationships. From this, we can see that conscientiousness does play a significant role in emotion and life satisfaction, mostly through avoiding negative actions and through creating life experiences that will be more intrinsically satisfying.

Conscientiousness and Motivation

Conscientiousness has often been described as a "motivational trait," which raises the question of how motivations differ from traits. Motivation has to do with both the desire to achieve an end and marshalling the resources at some point in time to serve that end (Roberts & Wood, 2006). Given the content of conscientiousness scales and the clear relationship between conscientiousness and achievement outcomes, some may be tempted to simply construe conscientiousness and motivation as identical concepts. The available data suggest that conscientiousness and motivation are better seen as relatively independent but related constructs that have a complex and as yet not fully elaborated relationship.

For example, in a study examining the interface between personality traits and multiple approaches to motivation, the industriousness facet of conscientiousness was a key factor in predicting personal strivings (Emmons & McAdams, 1991). Specifically, individuals higher on measures of industriousness generated lists of personal goals that exhibit more achievement-oriented themes (Emmons & McAdams, 1991), yet the magnitude of the association was modest at best. This supports the assertion that the content of individuals' goals is meaningfully related to conscientiousness but that the two constructs are not interchangeable.

Conscientiousness is similarly related to major life goals. Major life goals are defined as a person's aspirations to shape his or her life context and establish general life structures such as having a career, a family, and a certain kind of lifestyle (Roberts & Robins, 2000). Across two studies, conscientiousness was found to be positively associated with economic goals, such as wanting a prestigious occupation with a high standard of living (Roberts & Robins, 2000), and with social and relationship goals, which focus on making an impact on others in need and establishing a strong family structure (Roberts, O'Donnell, & Robins, 2004).

Within the domain of work, conscientiousness has been associated with key motivational constructs related to job performance. For example, conscientiousness is related to autonomous goal setting and commitment to goals (Barrick, Mount, & Strauss, 1993; Gerhardt, Rode, & Peterson, 2007; Klein & Lee, 2006), which in turn are related to job performance. More conscientious individuals also expect to perform better and select more difficult goals, both of which operate as mediators between conscientiousness and task performance (Gellatly, 1996).

Conscientiousness also relates to the way goals are strategically employed (Bajor & Baltes, 2003). Specifically, conscientious people will more efficiently select goals, optimize existing goals, and compensate across goals. Selection, optimization, and compensation (SOC) represent three broad strategies for successfully coping with discrepancies between resources and demands across the life course. Individuals employing a selection strategy in response to circumstances in which resources are limited may reduce the number of goals they are committed to or may organize their goals in a coherent hierarchy. Optimization refers to steps taken to enhance or maintain strategies relevant to selected goals. Compensation involves the application of alternate goal-relevant strategies when previously used strategies or resources are no longer available.

Conscientiousness shows moderate correlations with selection, optimization, and compensation strategies (Wiese, Freund, & Baltes, 2000). Bajor and Baltes (2003) further demonstrated that SOC variables are correlated with autonomous goal setting, goal expectancies, and goal commitment. More important, they found that SOC strategies mediated the relationship between conscientiousness and job performance. This effect was stronger for managerial jobs. Overall, these results suggest not only that highly conscientious individuals show greater propensities to select and commit to challenging goals but also that, in situations in which they have the opportunity to exercise autonomy, they are more likely to employ successful strategies for maximizing performance.

There are many ways that the connection between conscientiousness and motivation can be conceptualized and studied. We have described how conscientiousness is related to goal content, appraisals of those goals, and expected goal-related outcomes. Additionally, all of these goal-relevant variables are related to important outcomes. Having and committing to goals are demonstrative of one level of motivation-relevant behavior. These can be thought of as aspects relating to the desire component of motivation. Managing and selecting goals and resources represents a higher order perspective on motivation and its connection to conscientiousness. Further developing an explicit taxonomy of motivational constructs related to conscientiousness will likely allow us to better understand how this important personality variable leads to so many beneficial long-term outcomes.

Conscientiousness and Social Cognition

Social-cognitive models have historically theorized that social cognition influences and predicts human behavior and that social-cognitive units of analysis supersede or replace personality traits in the prediction of behavior (Bandura, 1982). For example, one's attitude toward a behavior influences that person's actual behavior. If the individual's attitude toward the behavior is positive, then one is more likely to perform the behavior. Recently, researchers have considered the possibility that personality traits are linked to social-cognitive units of analysis in a hierarchical structure (e.g., Roberts & Pomerantz, 2004). In this type of hierarchy, social-cognitive variables would mediate the relationship of personality traits, such as conscientiousness, and relevant outcomes, such as health behaviors. The implication in this conceptualization is that personality traits and social-cognitive units of analysis should be linked.

Several studies have reported linkages between conscientiousness and various social-cognitive units of analysis. Highly conscientious individuals have reported higher levels of perceived behavioral control over intended actions (e.g., Courneya, Bobick, & Schinke, 1999), less influence from perceived situational constraints (Gerhardt et al., 2007), and less effect from perceived stress (Besser & Shackelford, 2007) than individuals low in conscientiousness. Highly conscientious individuals also report fewer externalizing and attention problems (Jensen-Campbell & Malcolm, 2007), higher trait emotional intelligence (e.g., Petrides & Furnham, 2001), and stronger locus of control and coping skills (Saklofske, Austin, Galloway, & Davidson, 2007). Additionally, highly conscientious individuals possess higher levels of self-management (Gerhardt et al., 2007), of promotion and prevention foci at work (Wallace & Chen, 2006), and of self-regulatory learning strategies (Bidjerano & Yun Dai, 2007). Conscientiousness has also been associated with numerous attitudes, such as having a positive attitude toward exercise behaviors (Courneya et al., 1999) and toward health-protective behaviors (Conner & Abraham, 2001), as well as a negative attitude toward arriving late to work (Foust, Elicker, & Levy, 2006).

Of all the social-cognitive variables, self-efficacy is by far the most commonly studied and influential (Gist & Mitchell, 1992). According to Bandura, "perceived self-efficacy is concerned with judgments of how well one can execute courses of action required to deal with prospective situations" (1982, p. 122). Conscientiousness has been associated with self-efficacy in the study of health outcomes through its incorporation into the theory of planned behavior (Ajzen, 1985). For example, conscientiousness was significantly correlated with attitudes toward health-protective behaviors and health-protective self-efficacy in one sample of British university students, whereas it was significantly correlated only with attitude toward health-protective behaviors and exercise in a second sample (Conner & Abraham, 2001). Similarly, conscientiousness was positively correlated with instrumental attitude toward exercise, as well as affective attitude toward exercise, but not exercise self-efficacy, in a study of American students (Rhodes, Courneya, & Hayduk, 2002).

Additionally, conscientiousness has been consistently associated with various types of vocational self-efficacy modeled with social-cognitive career theory (Lent, Brown, & Hackett, 1994). In most of these studies, conscientiousness has shown significant correlations with investigative, social, enterprising, and conventional self-efficacies (Hartman & Betz, 2007; Larson, Wei, Wu, Borgen, & Bailey, 2007; Nauta, 2004; Rottinghaus, Lindley, Green, & Borgen, 2002). These findings indicate that highly conscientious individuals report higher levels of ability than individuals low in conscientiousness to succeed at jobs that focus on examining, analyzing, and solving complex problems (investigative); helping, training, and enlightening others (social); influencing, persuading, and leading others (enterprising); and working with data, details, and instructions (conventional) (Holland, 1997).

Furthermore, highly conscientious individuals report higher levels of self-efficacy than individuals low in conscientiousness for succeeding at tasks that involve science, mathematics, writing, helping, teaching, teamwork, public speaking, leadership, office services, organizational management, data management, and project management (Hartman & Betz, 2007). Conscientiousness also has been significantly correlated with job-search self-efficacy in American samples (Brown, Cober, Kane, Levy, & Shalhoop, 2006; Côté, Saks, & Zikic, 2006), and with preinterview and postinterview self-efficacies

in a Singaporean sample (Tay, Ang, & Van Dyne, 2006).

Beyond self-efficacy for health outcomes and vocational activities, conscientiousness has been significantly associated with generalized self-efficacy in work settings (Burke, Matthiesen, & Pallesen, 2006; Judge & Ilies, 2002). These studies indicate that highly conscientious individuals report higher levels of self-efficacy for succeeding at all tasks encountered in a work setting without regard to the tasks' nature or requirements. Moreover, there is some evidence that highly conscientious individuals report even higher levels of self-efficacy for succeeding at high-complexity tasks than at low-complexity tasks (Chen, Casper, & Cortina, 2001). In a meta-analysis of the effect of training on task performance, conscientiousness was a significant predictor of pretraining self-efficacy and posttraining self-efficacy (Colquitt, LePine, & Noe, 2000). Subsequent research has shown similar associations between conscientiousness and pretest learning self-efficacy in a classroom environment (Lee & Klein, 2002).

Bogg (2006) conducted a series of studies that included an examination of correlations between the various facets of conscientiousness and exercise self-efficacy. The construct of exercise self-efficacy was delineated into six subscales that each represented a participant's self-efficacy to overcome a specific barrier to exercise, including negative affect, excuse making, exercising alone, exercise inconvenience, resistance of others, and bad weather. The most important facet of conscientiousness for exercise self-efficacy was industriousness, which was correlated with all six self-efficacy scales. Reliability was significantly correlated with four exercise self-efficacies: negative affect, excuse making, exercise inconvenience, and resistance of others, whereas impulse control was significantly correlated with three self-efficacies: exercising alone, exercise inconvenience, and resistance of others. Orderliness was significantly correlated with only one self-efficacy, exercise inconvenience, and conventionality yielded no significant correlations at all. If these results generalize, one would expect the industriousness facet of conscientiousness to be the most consistent predictor of exercise self-efficacy.

The results from studies that have incorporated conscientiousness into models including self-efficacy are quite consistent with hierarchical models of personality that assume traits, such as conscientiousness, to be broad predictors of multiple outcomes, including self-efficacy. Conscientiousness predicts self-efficacies associated with health behaviors, with some evidence for the specific facet of industriousness being the core predictor of self-efficacy. Moreover, conscientiousness is a significant predictor of vocational self-efficacy, job-search self-efficacy, and generalized work self-efficacy. As a whole, these significant associations between conscientiousness and self-efficacy suggest that conscientiousness should be hierarchically incorporated into social-cognitive models that predict various behaviors.

Conclusion

As we have shown in this chapter, conscientiousness has pervasive correlates with multiple important life outcomes, including success at work, marital satisfaction and stability, health, and longevity. The link to important life outcomes is predicated on and partially explained by the particular behaviors, feelings, and thoughts that conscientiousness predicts. Conscientious people behave in ways that facilitate achievement, social interaction, and health. They tend to be more prosocial and hardworking in achievement settings, more reliable in interpersonal relationships, and more careful with health-related behaviors. In turn, these behaviors are the proximal mechanisms that explain better achievement, stable relationships, and a longer life. Similarly, conscientious people tend to experience more adaptive emotions, motivations, and cognitions.

The pervasive correlates of conscientiousness makes sense when traits are considered to be hierarchical systems in which the lower order manifestations of traits are the state-like features of the disposition (Roberts & Jackson, 2008; Roberts & Pomerantz, 2004). Yet this poses an interesting dilemma for categorizing conscientiousness. One needs to go no further than the scheme used to organize this book, which is an excellent representation of the field of in-

dividual differences, to see the issue. In the current tome, conscientiousness is categorized as a motivational disposition, which is not unreasonable. Nonetheless, as seen in our review, conscientiousness, like most personality traits, has links to interpersonal functioning, emotions, cognitions, and self-related constructs. Thus conscientiousness could have been categorized into any one or all of the categories that divide this book.

A second issue related to the organizational scheme of this book (and our field of social/personality psychology) is the fact that we take the organizational scheme seriously. That is, by labeling our constructs "self," "motivational," or "emotion," researchers can avoid confronting the fact that they are all studying highly related constructs. The distinction, for example, between the constructs of self-control, self-regulation, and conscientiousness is difficult to describe. Clearly, self-control and self-regulation (especially behavioral self-regulation) are lower order facets of conscientiousness. By overlooking these links, the field both needlessly proliferates new constructs and ignores opportunities to leverage complementary strengths. As noted earlier, understanding the proximal, state-like aspects of a trait domain is critical for understanding the causal pathways from trait to outcome (see Roberts, Kuncel, et al., 2007). It also provides a pathway to understanding how personality traits develop (Roberts & Caspi, 2003). The proximal interpersonal, emotional, cognitive, and motivational mechanisms underlying conscientiousness explains why conscientiousness exhibits both continuity and change over time—issues that are poorly dealt with in classic personality trait psychology (Roberts & Wood, 2006).

In sum, conscientiousness is the trait domain that sits on the fulcrum between indulging one's impulses and controlling oneself in order to meet higher order ambitions. The trait domain of conscientiousness is multifaceted, containing components such as self-control, industriousness, and conventionality. Consistent with a hierarchical model of dispositions, conscientiousness-related traits predict a whole host of behaviors, emotions, and thoughts that, in turn, appear to have functional significance for the well-being, success, and survival of individuals.

References

Abe, J. A. (2003). Shame, guilt, and personality judgment. *Journal of Research in Personality, 38,* 85–104.

Abe, J. A. A. (2005). The predictive value of the five-factor model of personality with preschool-age children: A nine-year follow-up study. *Journal of Research in Personality 39,* 423–442.

Ajzen, I. (1985). From intentions to actions: A theory of planned behavior. In J. Kuhl & J. Beckmann (Eds.), *Action control: From cognition to behavior* (pp. 11–39). Heidelberg, Germany: Springer-Verlag.

Bajor, J. K., & Baltes, B. B. (2003) The relationship between selection optimization with compensation, conscientiousness, motivation, and performance. *Journal of Vocational Behavior, 63,* 347–367.

Bandura, A. (1982). Self-efficacy mechanism in human agency. *American Psychologist, 37*(2), 122–147.

Barrick, M. R., & Mount, M. K. (1991). The Big Five personality dimensions and job performance: A meta-analysis. *Personnel Psychology, 44,* 1–26.

Barrick, M. R., Mount, M. K., & Strauss, J. P. (1993). Conscientiousness and performance of sales representatives: Test of the mediating effects of goal setting. *Journal of Applied Psychology, 78,* 715–722.

Baumeister, R. F., & Leary, M. R. (1995). The need to belong: Desire for interpersonal attachments as a fundamental human motivation. *Psychological Bulletin, 117,* 497–529.

Baumeister, R. F., Stillwell, A. M., & Heatherton, T. F. (1994). Guilt: An interpersonal approach. *Psychological Bulletin, 115,* 243–267.

Besser, A., & Shackelford, T. (2007). Mediation of the effects of the Big Five personality dimensions on negative mood and confirmed affective expectations by perceived situational stress: A quasi-field study of vacationers. *Personality and Individual Differences, 42*(7), 1333–1346.

Bidjerano, T., & Yun Dai, D. (2007). The relationship between the Big Five model of personality and self-regulated learning strategies. *Learning and Individual Differences, 17*(1), 69–81.

Bogg, T., & Roberts, B. W. (2004). Conscientiousness and health behaviors: A meta-analysis of the leading behavioral contributors to mortality. *Psychological Bulletin, 130,* 887–919.

Bogg, T. D. (2006). *Conscientiousness and the transtheoretical model of change in exercise: Integrating trait and social cognitive frameworks in the prediction of behavior.* Unpublished doctoral dissertation, University of Illinois, Urbana–Champaign.

Brandstatter, H., & Guth, W. (2000). A psychological approach to individual differences in intertemporal consumption patterns. *Journal of Economic Psychology, 21,* 465–479.

Brown, D., Cober, R., Kane, K., Levy, P., & Shalhoop, J. (2006). Proactive personality and the successful job search: A field investigation with college graduates. *Journal of Applied Psychology, 91*(3), 717–726.

Burke, R., Matthiesen, S. B., & Pallesen, S. (2006). Personality correlates of workaholism. *Personality and Individual Differences, 40*(6), 1223–1233.

Buss, D. M. (1991). Conflict in married couples: Personality predictors of anger and upset. *Journal of Personality, 59*(4), 663–703.

Buss, D. M. (1992). Manipulation in close relationships: The five factor model of personality in interactional context. *Journal of Personality, 60,* 477–499.

Buss, D. M., & Shackelford, T. K. (1997). From vigilance to violence: Mate retention tactics in married couples. *Journal of Personality and Social Psychology, 72,* 346–361.

Caspi, A., Wright, B. R., Moffitt, T. E., & Silva, P. A. (1998). Early failure in the labor market: Childhood and adolescent predictors of unemployment in the transition to adulthood. *American Sociological Review, 63,* 424–451.

Chen, G., Casper, W. J., & Cortina, J. M. (2001). The roles of self-efficacy and task complexity in the relationships among cognitive ability, conscientiousness, and work-related performance: A meta-analytic examination. *Human Performance, 14*(3), 209–230.

Chuah, S. C., Drasgow, F., & Roberts, B. W. (2006). Personality assessment: Does the medium matter? No. *Journal of Research in Personality, 40,* 359–376.

Colquitt, J. A., LePine, J. A., & Noe, R. A. (2000). Toward an integrative theory of training motivation: A meta-analytic path analysis of 20 years of research. *Journal of Applied Psychology, 85*(5), 678–707.

Conner, M., & Abraham, C. (2001). Conscientiousness and the theory of planned behavior: Toward a more complete model of the antecedents of intention and behavior. *Personality and Social Psychology Bulletin, 27*(11), 1547–1561.

Conte, J. M., & Jacobs, R. R. (2003). Validity evidence linking polychronicity and Big 5 personality dimensions to absence, lateness, and supervisory ratings of performance. *Human Performance, 16,* 107–129.

Côté, S., Saks, A., & Zikic, J. (2006). Trait affect and job search outcomes. *Journal of Vocational Behavior, 68*(2), 233–252.

Courneya, K. S., Bobick, T. M., & Schinke, R. J. (1999). Does the theory of planned behavior mediate the relation between personality and exercise behavior? *Basic and Applied Social Psychology, 21,* 317–324.

De Fruyt, F., & Mervielde, I. (1999). RIASEC types and Big Five traits as predictors of employment status and nature of employment. *Personnel Psychology, 52,* 701–727.

DeNeve, K. M., & Cooper, H. (1998). The happy personality: A meta-analysis of 137 personality traits and subjective well-being. *Psychological Bulletin, 124,* 197–229.

Duckworth, A. L., Peterson, C., Matthews, M. D., & Kelly, D. R. (2007). Grit: Perseverance and passion for long-term goals. *Journal of Personality and Social Psychology, 92*(6), 1087–1101.

Duckworth, A. L., & Seligman, M. E. P. (2005). Self-discipline outdoes IQ predicting academic performance in adolescents. *Psychological Science, 16,* 939–944.

Einstein, D., & Lanning, K. (1998). Shame, guilt, ego development, and the five-factor model of personality. *Journal of Personality, 66,* 555–582.

Emmons, R. A., & McAdams, D. P. (1991). Personal strivings and motive dispositions: Exploring the links. *Personality and Social Psychology Bulletin*, 17, 648–654.

Eysenck, H. J., & Gudjonsson, G. (1989). *The causes and cures of criminality*. New York: Plenum Press.

Fee, R. L., & Tangney, J. P. (2000). Procrastination: A means of avoiding shame or guilt? *Journal of Social Behavior and Personality*, 15, 167–184.

Finkel, E. J., & Campbell, W. K. (2001). Self-control and accommodation in relationships: An interdependence analysis. *Journal of Personality and Social Psychology*, 81, 263–277.

Freud, S. (1961). *Civilization and its discontents*. New York: Norton.

Foust, M. S., Elicker, J. D., & Levy, P. E. (2006). Development and validation of a measure of an individual's lateness attitude. *Journal of Vocational Behavior*, 69(1), 119–133.

Friedman, H. S., Tucker, J. S., Tomlinson-Keasey, C., Schwartz, J. E., Wingard, D. L., & Criqui, M. H. (1993). Does childhood personality predict longevity? *Journal of Personality and Social Psychology*, 65, 176–185.

Gellatly, I. R. (1996). Conscientiousness and task performance: Test of cognitive process model. *Journal of Applied Psychology*, 81(5), 474–482.

Gerhardt, M. W., Rode, J. C., & Peterson, S. J. (2007). Exploring mechanisms in the personality–performance relationship: Mediating roles of self-management and situational constraints. *Personality and Individual Differences*, 43, 1344–1355.

Gist, M. E., & Mitchell, T. R. (1992). Self-efficacy: A theoretical analysis of its determinants and malleability. *Academy of Management Review*, 17, 183–211.

Goldberg, L. R. (1993). The structure of phenotypic personality traits. *American Psychologist*, 48, 26–34.

Goodwin, R. D., & Friedman, H. S. (2006). Health status and the five-factor personality traits in a nationally representative sample. *Journal of Health Psychology*, 11, 643–654.

Graziano, W. G., & Ward, D. (1992). Probing the Big Five in adolescence: Personality and adjustment during a developmental transition. *Journal of Personality*, 60, 425–440.

Hartman, R., & Betz, N. (2007). The five-factor model and career self-efficacy: General and domain-specific relationships. *Journal of Career Assessment*, 15(2), 145–161.

Heller, D., Watson, D., & Ilies, R. (2004). The role of person versus situation in life satisfaction: A critical examination. *Psychological Bulletin*, 130, 574–600.

Holland, J. L. (1997). *Making vocational choices: A theory of vocational personalities and work environments* (3rd ed.). Odessa, FL: Psychological Assessment Resources.

Insel, K. S., Reminger, S. L., & Hsiao, C.-P. (2006). The negative association of independent personality and medication adherence. *Journal of Aging and Health*, 18, 407–418.

Jensen-Campbell, L. A., & Graziano, W. G. (2001). Agreeableness as a moderator of interpersonal conflict. *Journal of Personality*, 69, 323–361.

Jensen-Campbell, L. A., & Malcolm, K. T. (2007). The importance of conscientiousness in adolescent interpersonal relationships. *Personality and Social Psychology Bulletin*, 33(3), 368–383.

John, O. P., & Srivastava, S. (1999). The Big Five trait taxonomy; History, measurement, and theoretical perspectives. In L. A. Pervin & O. P. John (Eds.), *Handbook of personality: Theory and research* (Vol. 2, pp. 102–138). New York: Guilford Press.

Judge, T. A., Bono, J. E., Ilies, R., & Gerhardt, M. W. (2002). Personality and leadership: A qualitative and quantitative review. *Journal of Applied Psychology*, 87, 765–780.

Judge, T. A., Higgins, C. A., Thoresen, C. J., & Barrick, M. R. (1999). The Big Five personality traits, general mental ability, and career success across the life span. *Personnel Psychology*, 52, 621–652.

Judge, T. A., & Ilies, R. (2002). Relationship of personality to performance motivation: A meta-analytic review. *Journal of Applied Psychology*, 87, 797–807.

Klein, H. J., & Lee, S. (2006). The effects of personality on learning: The role of goal setting. *Human Performance*, 19(1), 43–66.

Kokko, K., & Pulkkinen, L. (2000). Aggression in childhood and long-term unemployment in adulthood: A cycle of maladaptation and some protective factors. *Developmental Psychology*, 36, 463–472.

Krueger, R. F., Caspi, A., Moffitt, T. E., White, J. L., & Stouthamer-Loeber, M. (1996). Delay of gratification, psychopathology, and personality: Is low self-control specific to externalizing problems? *Journal of Personality*, 64, 107–129.

Krueger, R. F., Schmutte, P. S., Caspi, A., Moffitt, T. E., Campbell, K., & Silva, P. A. (1994). Personality traits are linked to crime among men and women: Evidence from a birth cohort. *Journal of Abnormal Psychology*, 103, 328–338.

Larson, L. M., Wei, M., Wu, T., Borgen, F. H., & Bailey, D. C. (2007). Discriminating among educational majors and career aspirations in Taiwanese undergraduates: The contribution of personality and self-efficacy. *Journal of Counseling Psychology*, 54(4), 395–408.

Lee, S., & Klein, H. J. (2002). Relationships between conscientiousness, self-efficacy, self-deception, and learning over time. *Journal of Applied Psychology*, 87(6), 1175–1182.

Lent, R. W., Brown, S. D., & Hackett, G. (1994). Toward a unifying social cognitive theory of career and academic interest, choice, and performance. *Journal of Vocational Behavior*, 45, 79–122.

LePine, J. A., Hollenbeck, J. R., Ilgen, D. R., & Hedlund, J. (1997). Effects of individual differences on the performance of hierarchical decision-making teams: Much more than g. *Journal of Applied Psychology*, 82, 803–811.

Linnan, L., LaMontagne, A. D., Stoddard, A., Emmons, K. M., & Sorensen, G. (2005). Norms and their relationship to behavior in worksite settings: An application of the Jackson return potential model. *American Journal of Health Behavior*, 29, 258–268.

Lodi-Smith, J. L., & Roberts, B. W. (2007). Social investment and personality: A meta-analytic analysis of the relationship of personality traits to investment in work, family, religion, and volunteerism. *Personality and Social Psychology Review*, 11, 68–86.

Mount, M. K., Barrick, M. R., Scullen, S. M., & Rounds, J. (2005). Higher order dimensions of the Big Five personality traits and the Big Six vocational interest types. *Personnel Psychology, 58*, 447–478.

Nauta, M. (2004). Self-efficacy as a mediator of the relationships between personality factors and career interests. *Journal of Career Assessment, 12*(4), 381–394.

Noftle, E. E., & Robins, R. (2007). Personality predictors of academic outcomes: Big Five correlates of GPA and SAT scores. *Journal of Personality and Social Psychology, 93*, 116–130.

Norman, W. T. (1963). Toward an adequate taxonomy of personality attributes: Replicated factor structure in peer nomination personality ratings. *Journal of Abnormal and Social Psychology, 66*, 574–583.

Nyhus, E. K., & Webley, P. (2001). The role of personality in household saving and borrowing behaviour. *European Journal of Personality, 15*, 85–103.

O'Brien, T. B., & DeLongis, A. (1996). The interactional context of problem-, emotion-, and relationship-focused coping: The role of the Big Five personality factors. *Journal of Personality, 64*, 775–811.

Ones, D. S., Viswesvaran, C., & Schmidt, F. L. (2003). Personality and absenteeism: A meta-analysis of integrity tests. *European Journal of Personality, 17*, 19–38.

Patrick, C. J., Hicks, B. M., Krueger, R. F., & Lang, A. R. (2005). Relations between psychopathy facets and externalizing in a criminal offender sample. *Journal of Personality Disorders, 19*, 339–356.

Persegani, C., Russo, P., Carucci, C., Nicolini, M., Papeschi, L. L., & Trimarchi, M. T. (2002). Television viewing and personality structure in children. *Personality and Individual Differences, 32*, 977–990.

Petrides, K. V., & Furnham, A. (2001). Trait emotional intelligence: Psychometric investigation with reference to established trait taxonomies. *European Journal of Personality, 15*, 425–448.

Rhodes, R. E., Courneya, K. S., & Hayduk, L. A. (2002). Does personality moderate the theory of planned behavior in the exercise domain? *Journal of Sport and Exercise Psychology, 24*(2), 120–132.

Roberts, B. W., & Bogg, T. (2004). A 30-year longitudinal study of the relationships between conscientiousness-related traits and the family structure and health-behavior factors that affect health. *Journal of Personality, 72*, 325–354.

Roberts, B. W., Bogg, T., Walton, K. E., Chernyshenko, O. S., & Stark, S. E. (2004). A lexical investigation of the lower-order structure of conscientiousness. *Journal of Research in Personality, 38*, 164–178.

Roberts, B. W., & Caspi, A. (2003). The cumulative continuity model of personality development: Striking a balance between continuity and change in personality traits across the life course. In R. M. Staudinger & U. Lindenberger (Eds.), *Understanding human development: Lifespan psychology in exchange with other disciplines* (pp. 183–214). Dordrecht, The Netherlands: Kluwer Academic.

Roberts, B. W., Chernyshenko, O., Stark, S., & Goldberg, L. (2005). The structure of conscientiousness: An empirical investigation based on seven major personality questionnaires. *Personnel Psychology, 58*, 103–139.

Roberts, B. W., Harms, P. D., Caspi, A., & Moffitt, T. E. (2007). Predicting the counterproductive employee in a child-to-adult prospective study: Evidence from a 23-year longitudinal study. *Journal of Applied Psychology, 92*, 1427–1436.

Roberts, B. W., & Jackson, J. J. (2008). Sociogenomic personality psychology. *Journal of Personality, 76*, 1523–1544.

Roberts, B. W., Kuncel, N., Shiner, R. N., Caspi, A., & Goldberg, L. (2007). The power of personality: A comparative analysis of the predictive validity of personality traits, SES, and IQ. *Perspectives in Psychological Science, 2*, 313–345.

Roberts, B. W., O'Donnell, M., & Robins, R. W. (2004). Goal and personality trait development in emerging adulthood. *Journal of Personality and Social Psychology, 87*, 541–550.

Roberts, B. W., & Pomerantz, E. M. (2004). On traits, situations, and their integration: A developmental perspective. *Personality and Social Psychology Review, 8*(4), 402–416.

Roberts, B. W., & Robins, R. W. (2000). Broad dispositions, broad aspirations: The intersection of the Big Five dimensions and major life goals. *Personality and Social Psychology Bulletin, 26*, 1284–1296.

Roberts, B. W., & Wood, D. (2006). Personality development in the context of the neo-socioanalytic model of personality. In D. Mroczek & T. Little (Eds.), *Handbook of personality development* (pp. 11–39). Mahwah, NJ: Erlbaum.

Robins, R. W., Caspi, A., & Moffitt, T. E. (2000). Two personalities, one relationship: Both partners' personality traits shape the quality of a relationship. *Journal of Personality and Social Psychology, 79*, 251–259.

Rolland, J. P., & De Fruyt, F. (2003). The validity of FFM personality dimensions and maladaptive traits to predict negative affects at work: A six month prospective study in a military sample. *European Journal of Personality, 17*, 101–121.

Rottinghaus, P. J., Lindley, L. D., Green, M. A., & Borgen, F. H. (2002). Educational aspirations: The contribution of personality, self-efficacy, and interests. *Journal of Vocational Behavior, 61*, 1–19.

Saklofske, D. H., Austin, E. J., Galloway, J., & Davidson, K. (2007). Individual difference correlates of health-related behaviours: Preliminary evidence for links between emotional intelligence and coping. *Personality and Individual Differences, 42*(3), 491–502.

Scher, S. J., & Osterman, N. M. (2002). Procrastination, conscientiousness, anxiety, and goals: Exploring the measurement and correlates of procrastination among school-aged children. *Psychology in the Schools, 39*, 385–398

Tangney, J. P. (1996). Conceptual and methodological issues in the assessment of shame and guilt. *Behaviour Research and Therapy, 34*, 741–754.

Tay, C., Ang, S., & Van Dyne, L. (2006). Personality, biographical characteristics, and job interview success: A longitudinal study of the mediating effects of interviewing self-efficacy and the moderating effects of internal locus of causality. *Journal of Applied Psychology, 91*(2), 446–454.

Tellegen, A. (1988). The analysis of consistency in personality assessment. *Journal of Personality, 56*, 621–663.

Tellegen, A. (1991). Personality traits: Issues of definition, evidence, and assessment. In D. Cicchetti & W. Grove (Eds.), *Thinking clearly about psychology: Essays in honor of Paul Everett Meehl* (Vol. 2, pp. 10–35). Minneapolis: University of Minnesota Press.

Tracy, J. L., & Robins, R. W. (2004). Putting the self in the self-conscious emotions: A theoretical model. *Psychological Inquiry, 1*(5), 103–125.

Tucker, J. S., Kressin, N. R., Spiro, A., & Ruscio, J. (1998). Intrapersonal characteristics and the timing of divorce: A prospective investigation. *Journal of Social and Personal Relationships, 15*, 211–225.

van Aken, C., Junger, M., Verhoeven, M., van Aken, A. G., & Dekovic, M. (2007). Externalizing behaviors and minor unintentional injuries in toddlers: Common risk factors? *Journal of Pediatric Psychology, 32*, 230–244.

Verplanken, B., & Herabadi, A. (2001). Individual differences in impulse buying tendency: Feeling and no thinking. *European Journal of Personality, 15*, 71–83.

Vohs, K. D., & Ciarocco, N. J. (2004). Interpersonal functioning requires self-regulation. In R. F. Baumeister & K. D. Vohs (Eds.), *Handbook of self-regulation: Research, theory, and applications* (pp. 392–410). New York: Guilford Press.

Vollrath, M., Landolt, M. A., & Ribi, K. (2003). Personality of children with accident-related injuries. *European Journal of Personality, 17*, 299–307.

Wallace, C., & Chen, G. (2006). A multilevel integration of personality, climate, self-regulation, and performance. *Personnel Psychology, 59*(3), 529–557.

Watson, D., Hubbard, B., & Wiese, D. (2000). General traits of personality and affectivity as predictors of satisfaction in intimate relationships: Evidence from self- and partner ratings. *Journal of Personality, 68*, 413–449.

Weiss, A., & Costa, P. T. (2005). Domain and facet personality predictors of all-cause mortality among Medicare patients aged 65 to 100. *Psychosomatic Medicine, 67*, 1–10.

Wiese, B. S., Freund, A. M., & Baltes, P. B. (2000). Selection, optimization, and compensation: An action-related approach to work and partnership. *Journal of Vocational Behavior, 57*(3), 273–300.

CHAPTER 26

■ ● ▲ ◆ ■ ● ▲ ◆

Achievement Motivation

David E. Conroy
Andrew J. Elliot
Todd M. Thrash

The pursuit of competence is ubiquitous in our daily experiences at work, school, and play. Achievement motivation theories seek to explain the processes that energize, direct, and sustain efforts to be competent (A. J. Elliot & Dweck, 2005). Although research has often emphasized outcomes such as performance and related processes (e.g., level of aspiration, persistence, enjoyment), competence pursuits typically occur in social contexts—either before an evaluative audience (real or imagined) or as a part of a team or group with a shared goal. Thus social behavior is another significant outcome that may be explained, at least in part, by achievement motivation.

Some of the most well-established approaches to understanding achievement motivation have focused on constructs such as levels of aspiration (Lewin, Dembo, Festinger, & Sears, 1944), achievement motives (McClelland, Atkinson, Clark, & Lowell, 1953), test anxiety (Mandler & Sarason, 1952), risk taking (Atkinson, 1957), attributions (Weiner & Kukla, 1970), perceived competence (Harter, 1983), achievement goals (Maehr & Nicholls, 1980), self-efficacy (Bandura, 1997), and implicit theories (Dweck, 1999; for a review, see Thrash & Hurst, 2008). This chapter focuses specifically on the motive- and goal-based approaches to achievement motivation that have been integrated in the hierarchical model of achievement

motivation (Elliot, 1999; Elliot & Church, 1997). We begin by describing key theoretical concepts and tenets in the motive and goal-based approaches, with particular attention to how these concepts are measured and their implications for social behavior. Following this introduction, we review extant research linking both motives and goals to social behavior. The chapter concludes with our perspective on an agenda for future research in this area.

Motive-Based Approaches to Achievement Motivation

In a seminal study of individual differences in college-age men, Murray (1938) posited the existence of a variety of *needs* that underlie human behavior. Needs may represent either "a temporary happening ... [or] a more or less consistent trait of personality" (p. 61). They were conceptualized as hypothetical entities that represent "potentiality or readiness to respond in a certain way under given conditions" (p. 61) and as "a force which organizes perception, apperception, intellection, conation and action in such a way as to transform in a certain direction an existing, unsatisfying situation" (p. 63).

Several of the desired effects on perception, cognition, affect, and behavior noted by Murray (1938) were specifically linked to the pursuit of competence. For example, the *need for achievement* was conceived as "the desire or tendency to do things as rapidly and/or as well as possible" (p. 164). Likewise, the *need for infavoidance* represents a desire "to avoid humiliation, to quit embarrassing situations or to avoid conditions which may lead to belittlement: the scorn, derision or indifference of others, to refrain from action because of fear of failure" (p. 192). These two needs parallel the appetitive and aversive achievement motives that later emerged in the motive-based approach to achievement motivation.

Achievement Motives

The seminal theorizing and research on achievement motives per se was conducted by David McClelland, John Atkinson, and their colleagues (e.g., Atkinson, 1957; McClelland, Atkinson, Clark, & Lowell, 1953). They conceived of motives as the learned association between "a cue [and] a change in an affective situation" (McClelland et al., 1953, p. 28). In other words, motives link cognitive representations of environmental cues with learned affective responses to those cues in such a fashion that the cue is sufficient to arouse an anticipatory affective response and to energize corresponding achievement behavior in a particular direction.

This definition raises an important question: Which emotions energize achievement behavior? At the broadest level of analysis, any pleasant emotion linked to success or unpleasant emotion linked to failure could provide the foundation for an achievement motive. Such a broad-based approach has merits, but it also limits us to relatively straightforward approach–avoid behavioral predictions for achievement motives based on the hedonic principle. A more common approach has focused on emotions that are most central to competence pursuits.

From this perspective, it is important to recognize that competence has close relations to the self. Self-perceptions emerge from perceptions of competence (Harter, 1983), and, from a very early age, competence and incompetence appear to generate self-evaluative emotional responses (Heckhausen, 1984; Lewis, Alessandri, & Sullivan, 1992; Lewis, Sullivan, Stanger, & Weiss,

1989; Stipek, Recchia, & McClintic, 1992). One class of emotions can be distinguished for their unique role in self-evaluative processing: the self-conscious or social emotions (Tracy, Robins, & Tangney, 2007). These emotions include pride and shame, which are the two exemplars most frequently posited to be associated with achievement motives. Anticipatory pride in succeeding was proposed as the basis for the need for achievement (nAch), and anticipatory shame in failing was proposed as the basis for fear of failure (FF) (Atkinson, 1957; McClelland et al., 1953).

Assessing Achievement Motives

Murray (1938) held that humans were unlikely to be aware of the motivations underlying their behavior. As such, he developed a projective ("apperceptive") method using the Thematic Apperception Test (TAT; Murray, 1943) for assessing individual differences. McClelland and colleagues (1953) later adapted this fantasy-based method and developed a scoring protocol for assessing the need for achievement using this approach (for a summary of differences between these methods, see Winter, 1999). Other scoring systems also have been developed for both nAch and FF (Birney, Burdick, & Teevan, 1969; Heckhausen, 1963; Schultheiss, 2001; Winter, 1994). Tables 26.1 and 26.2 summarize the thematic content that these different systems code for nAch and FF, respectively.

As seen in Table 26.1, the McClelland and colleagues (1953) system for nAch has the most extensive set of coding categories. Because it was empirically derived, the relevance of some categories is not intuitive and may even be theoretically questionable. For example, it is not clear why nAch scores should increase when achievement imagery depicts negative affective states, negative anticipatory goal states, or unsuccessful instrumental activities. The Heckhausen (1963) coding system was developed in part to address these limitations and to provide a more theoretically congruent measure of the nAch motive. It is a simpler system, with only six major coding categories, but it was not available for English-language researchers until translated by Schultheiss (2001). Winter (1994) developed a system for coding running text that may be the most flexible of

TABLE 26.1. Summary of Thematic Categories in Implicit Need for Achievement Coding Systems

McClelland, Atkinson, Clark, & Lowell (1953)	Heckhausen (1963) (English translation by Schultheiss, 2001)	Winter (1994)
Achievement imagery[a]	Need for achievement and success	Adjectives that positively evaluate performances
Stated need for achievement	Instrumental activity to achieve success	Goals or performances that are described in ways that suggest positive evaluation
Instrumental activity (successful, doubtful, or unsuccessful)	Expectation of success	Mention of winning or competing with others
Anticipatory goal states (positive or negative)	Praise	Failure, doing badly, or other lack of excellence
Obstacles or blocks (personal or environmental)	Positive affect	Unique accomplishments
Nurturant press	Success theme	
Affective states (positive or negative)		
Achievement theme		

[a]Stories in which achievement imagery is altogether absent receive a negative achievement motivation score. Those in which achievement imagery is doubtful receive a zero score.

the available coding systems because it can be applied to any data that are at least partly imaginative (e.g., speeches, conversations, fictional writing). This system is similar to the Heckhausen system in that the number of coding categories is limited compared with the McClelland and colleagues system; however, the content of the categories is somewhat unique compared with the other systems. This coding system also focuses exclusively on approach-based motives and does not differentiate them from avoidance-based motives—a nuance that may help to explain why text concerning "failure, doing badly, or other lack of excellence" (Winter, 1994, p. 10) is coded positively for the achievement motive.

The categories in the two major coding systems for FF are summarized in Table 26.2. The Heckhausen (1963) system has

seven major coding categories and is theoretically consistent with prevailing concepts of FF. Working independently of Heckhausen, Birney and colleagues (1969) used an approach similar to that of McClelland and colleagues (1953) to develop a system for coding Hostile Press in stories. This Hostile Press score was based on imagery depicting a threat presented by the situation to the participant and interpreted as an indicator of FF. Not surprisingly, this coding system is also vulnerable to concerns about content relevance. For example, it is not clear from a theoretical standpoint why one would infer high FF from stories that depict successful instrumental activity, anticipation of successful goal attainment, or pleasant affective reactions. Overall, we concur with the conclusions of McClelland (1987) and Schultheiss (2001)—the Heckhausen coding

TABLE 26.2. Summary of Thematic Categories in Implicit Fear of Failure Coding Systems

Heckhausen (1963) (English translation by Schultheiss, 2001)	Birney, Burdick, & Teevan (1969)
Need to avoid failure	Hostile Press imagery
Instrumental activity to avoid failure	Need press relief
Expectation of failure	Successful/unsuccessful instrumental activity
Criticism	Goal anticipation
Negative affect	Affective reactions to press
Failure	Blocks
Failure theme	Press thema

system provides the best fantasy-based approach for assessing nAch and FF motives.

The more recently developed fantasy-based methods for assessing achievement motives are quite refined and are less vulnerable to methodological criticisms that were frequently leveled in the 20th century (for details on these improved methods, see Schultheiss & Pang, 2007; Smith, 1992). The Picture Story Exercise described by Schultheiss and Pang (2007) is one example of a methodologically rigorous protocol for administering and scoring fantasy-based measures that yields psychometrically sound scores for motives. In addition to the projective measures described previously, the nAch and FF were also commonly assessed using self-report measures (e.g., Atkinson & Litwin, 1960; Conroy, Metzler, & Willow, 2002; Feather, 1965; Hagtvet & Benson, 1997; Herman, 1990; Jackson, 1974; Spence & Helmreich, 1983). Examples of items used to assess nAch include "I like to work hard" and "Once I undertake a task, I persist" (Spence & Helmreich, 1983, p. 42). Examples of items used to assess FF include "When I am failing, it is embarrassing if others are there to see it" and "When I am failing, I believe that my doubters feel that they were right about me" (Conroy et al., 2002, p. 90). In our view, the self-report measures that presently provide the most valid scores for nAch and FF are the Work–Family Orientation Questionnaire (particularly the work-mastery score; Spence & Helmreich, 1983) and the Performance Failure Appraisal Inventory (Conroy et al., 2002), respectively. Semiprojective tests have even been proposed to try to capitalize on the strengths of both projective and self-report assessments (e.g., Schmalt, 1999), although these measures have been used less frequently than either projective or self-report measures.

One source of great controversy and, ultimately, insight in the achievement motivation literature is the fact that scores from projective and self-report measures tend to correlate less strongly than would be expected if they were assessing a common motive (Spangler, 1992). Critics from either side often took this as evidence that the other approach did not yield valid scores of the relevant motive. In early writings, what we now call self-attributed or explicit (i.e., questionnaire-based) scores were intentionally distinguished and even distanced from motives by denying them status as a motive and calling them instead *values* (e.g., deCharms, Morrison, Reitman, & McClelland, 1955). McClelland later backed off this position and recognized the existence of explicit motives as a separate motivational system (McClelland, Koestner, & Weinberger, 1989). This theoretical reconciliation was based on the conclusion that different motivational systems exist: a primitive implicit motive system that is grounded in affective arousal and a cognitively elaborated system that is based on an "elaborate system of explicit goals, desires, and commitments" (McClelland et al., 1955, p. 700). The former system is expressed in fantasy-based measures such as the Picture Story Exercise, whereas the latter is consciously accessible and may be assessed using self-report methods.

Schultheiss (2007) linked these motivational systems and their corresponding assessment methods to different memory systems—implicit motives and fantasy-based measures tap into nondeclarative memory systems of which the individual is not consciously aware, whereas explicit motives and self-report questionnaires tap into declarative memory systems of which the individual is consciously aware. The differences in these underlying memory systems may help to explain differences in the outcomes predicted by implicit and explicit motives. The nondeclarative memories tapped by implicit motives may be linked to procedural learning and Pavlovian conditioning that likely underlie the acquisition of skills, habits, and emotional associations. In contrast, the declarative memory system tapped by explicit motives may be linked most directly to outcomes based in semantic and episodic memories, such as conscious attitudes, retrospective judgments, and future intentions. Much remains to be learned about why implicit and explicit motives differ, but the ideas articulated by Schultheiss (2007; Schultheiss & Pang, 2007) provide fruitful ground for theory development and testing.

A significant emerging line of work in this area examines the factors that influence the relationship between implicit and explicit achievement motives. As Thrash, Elliot, and Schultheiss (2007) noted, the conclusion that implicit and explicit nAch are largely uncorrelated is reminiscent of early reports of poor consistency between traits and behavior and between attitudes and behavior (Mischel, 1968; Wicker, 1969). In both of these prior consistency literatures, researchers subsequently uncovered two types of evidence that traits or attitudes are more systematically related to behavior than had been apparent in early research. First, methodological refinements resulted in stronger consistency coefficients. Second, consistency itself was found to vary systematically as a function of moderator variables. In parallel to the developments in these literatures, motive researchers have documented two classes of factors—methodological factors and moderator variables—that predict the degree of association between implicit and explicit nAch.

Regarding a methodological factor, Thrash and colleagues (2007) argued that the correlation between implicit and explicit nAch may have been underestimated in past research due to poor correspondence of content between implicit and explicit measures. Many popular measures of explicit nAch are based on Murray's (1938) conceptualization of nAch (e.g., Jackson, 1974), whereas McClelland and colleagues' (1953) widely used coding system for implicit nAch was derived empirically by examining how achievement imagery changes when the motive is and is not aroused. One unintended consequence of this approach was that the coding system deviates from Murray's conceptualization of the nAch (Koestner & McClelland, 1990). For example, the scoring system used by McClelland and colleagues counts negative anticipatory goal-state imagery toward the nAch score (e.g., "The boy thinks he just can't make it through college"; p. 129)—this content is exclusive of the achievement need described by Murray (1938). Thrash and colleagues reported that implicit nAch, assessed using Schultheiss's (2001) translation of Heckhausen's coding system, was uncorrelated with three existing measures of explicit nAch (rs = .00, .00, and .02); in contrast, it was significantly correlated with a new measure of explicit nAch (r = .17) that was designed to closely match the implicit nAch coding system in content. This finding indicates that implicit and explicit nAch are systematically related, albeit weakly, when assessed with measures that are properly matched for content.

Several studies have sought a fuller characterization of the relationship between implicit and explicit nAch by identifying dispositional variables that function as moderators. Thrash and Elliot (2002) examined the moderating role of *self-determination*, which refers to autonomy or authenticity (Deci & Ryan, 1985). Thrash and Elliot argued that feelings of self-determination reflect the development of explicit values that are well aligned with deeply grounded implicit motivational tendencies. As expected, self-determination was found to moderate the relation between implicit and explicit nAch. Implicit nAch was a robust predictor of explicit nAch among individuals high in self-determination (r = .40) but was unrelated to explicit nAch among individuals low in self-determination (r = –.07).

More recently, Thrash and colleagues (2007) examined three additional dispositional moderators: private body consciousness, self-monitoring, and preference for consistency. *Private body consciousness* refers to a sensitivity to internal bodily processes (Miller, Murphy, & Buss, 1981). Thrash and colleagues proposed that private body consciousness may promote congruence between implicit and explicit nAch, because the effects of implicit motive arousal are embodied and may be perceptible as diffuse gut feelings or surges of energy. *Self-monitoring* is the tendency to monitor the social environment and to adjust one's behavior or attitudes accordingly (Snyder & Gangestad, 1986). Self-monitoring was posited to impede congruence, because the achievement values internalized from the social environment are less likely to correspond to one's implicit motives than are internally generated values. *Preference for consistency* refers to a tendency to seek consistency among cognitions (Cialdini, Trost, & Newsom, 1995). Preference for consistency was expected to predict greater congruence, because individuals high in this trait would be more motivated to reconcile discrepancies between explicit motives and any rudimentary knowledge of one's implicit motives. Results showed that all three traits moderated the association between implicit and explicit nAch. Moreover, all three traits functioned as independent moderators, suggesting that multiple, distinct processes are responsible for motive congruence.

In related research on the congruence between implicit motives and explicit goals, Brunstein (2001) reported that state-oriented individuals, who have a tendency toward indecisiveness and hesitation (as opposed to action-oriented individuals, who have a tendency toward decisiveness and initiative), are more likely to adopt goals that are incongruent with implicit motives. More recently, Baumann, Kaschel, and Kuhl (2005) reported that state orientation predicted incongruence between implicit and explicit nAch only when individuals were under stress. In addition, motive incongruence led to lower well-being and partially mediated the effect of the state orientation × stress interaction on well-being.

Summary of Motive-Based Approaches

The motive-based approaches to achievement motivation are based on relatively stable individual differences in affective associations with success and failure. Motives exist at two levels of analysis—implicit motives that are grounded in deeply rooted affective structures and are not readily accessible to awareness and explicit motives that are grounded in consciously held values, beliefs, or attitudes. These motive systems do not necessarily converge for all individuals, and the available evidence indicates that they predict quite different outcomes. Recent research has shown that implicit and explicit nAch are not strictly independent and that methodological and dispositional factors influence the association between them. Poor alignment between implicit and explicit nAch is associated with low levels of well-being.

Strengths of this motive-based approach to achievement motivation include the focus on how behavior is energized (via learned anticipatory affect, particularly involving pride and shame) and the general distinction between approach and avoidance orientations for achievement behavior (Elliot, 1997). Two major limitations of this approach have also been identified: (1) It does not differentiate beyond omnibus approach or avoidance strivings and (2) as decontextualized constructs, motives are not well suited for predicting context-specific processes and outcomes (Elliot, 1997). This latter point is important because motives are decontextualized with respect to both the specific achievement context and time. In theory, motives may be "canalized," or channeled into specific achievement contexts (e.g., sports or classroom achievement) in different individuals (Thrash & Elliot, 2001), but researchers have generally not exploited this fact to maximize the predictive validity of their instruments (Thrash & Hurst, 2008).

From a methodological perspective, it should also be noted that it can be difficult to interpret many findings in the achievement-motives literature. Researchers often focused their analyses on "resultant motivation" scores that represented the difference between standardized scores for nAch and FF in a sample. Large positive and large negative resultant scores have clear interpretations (i.e., high scores for one motive and low scores for the other), but it is less clear what resultant scores of zero indicate about the level of individual motives. Participants may have scored high for both motives, average for both motives, or low for both motives. In contemporary research, it is preferable to examine main and interactive effects of the achievement motives instead of losing valuable information by calculating a resultant motivation score.

Goal-Based Approaches to Achievement Motivation

An alternative approach to studying achievement motivation emerged in the form of achievement goal theory. Achievement goal theory grew from the observation of two very different patterns of responses to failure among young children: a *mastery response*, characterized by low-effort attributions, persistence, increased competence expectancies, selection of challenging tasks, and improved performance; and a *helpless response*, characterized by low-ability attributions, unpleasant affect, decreased competence expectancies, selection of easy tasks, and reduced performance (Diener & Dweck, 1978, 1980; Dweck, 1975). Dweck (1986; Dweck & Elliott, 1983; E. S. Elliott & Dweck, 1988) proposed that these responses reflected different goals that children adopt in achievement pursuits. Some view achievement pursuits as opportunities to learn and to increase their competence (learning goals);

others view achievement pursuits as opportunities to establish their standing with respect to intelligence or ability in comparison with their peers (performance goals). Learning goals were presumed to facilitate mastery responses because they orient the person to the process of learning and improving. In contrast, performance goals were thought to engender helpless responses because they orient the person to factors outside of his or her control and create a threatening environment for achievement pursuits.

A similar approach grew from the work of Nicholls (1976, 1978, 1984) on developmental changes in children's conceptions of ability. In early childhood, children possess an undifferentiated concept of ability that equates competence with learning and effort. By trying hard, they are able to improve and therefore feel competent. Around age 12, children begin to differentiate between two primary internal sources of achievement outcomes: effort and ability. This differentiated concept of ability leads to changes in how children construe competence. Ability is now inferred from the amount of effort required to produce a successful performance—outperforming a peer while exerting minimal effort would lead to perceptions of greater ability than if one had to work very hard to outperform a peer. Nicholls (1984) extended these ideas about different conceptions of ability by proposing that they are the basis for two major achievement goals. People who pursued competence in an undifferentiated sense—meaning that they focused on effort and learning—were said to be in a state of *task involvement*. People who pursued competence in a differentiated sense—meaning that they focused on demonstrating ability by outperforming others with an economy of effort—were said to be in a state of *ego involvement*. These task and ego states of involvement represented the purpose of achievement behavior and overlap considerably with the aims or foci of behavior associated with learning and performance goals, respectively.

These converging lines of work provided the foundation for what has come to be known as the dichotomous model of achievement goals. The dichotomous model of achievement goals inspired a large volume of research that consistently demonstrated adaptive qualities of task involvement and

learning goals and mixed consequences for ego involvement and performance goals. For example, whereas task involvement and learning goals exhibit consistent positive relations with intrinsic motivation for a task, ego involvement and performance goals typically exhibit a mixed profile of null and negative relations. To resolve ambiguities about the consequences of this goal, Elliot (1997; Elliot & Harackiewicz, 1996) proposed that it was necessary to consider the valence of goals in addition to how competence is defined in the goal.

The valence of an achievement goal refers to whether the individual is focused on succeeding (an approach goal) or on not failing (an avoidance goal). Early goal theorists intimated that avoiding incompetence may be a relevant achievement goal (e.g., Nicholls, Patashnick, Cheung, Thorkildsen, & Lauer, 1989); however, research in the dichotomous-goals tradition focused explicitly on approach-valenced achievement goals that differed only in how competence was defined. Crossing the *definition of competence* (task- or self-referenced competence vs. normatively referenced competence) with the *valence of the competence-based possibility represented in the goal* (e.g., being competent vs. avoiding incompetence) yields the 2 × 2 achievement-goal framework proposed by Elliot (1999; see also Elliot & McGregor, 2001) and depicted in Figure 26.1.

Mastery-approach (MAp) goals focus the person on performing a task as well as possible (task-referenced competence) or surpassing his or her previous level of performance on that task (self-referenced competence). For example, a student with an MAp goal could strive to ace an exam or to exceed his or her score on previous exams in that course. *Mastery-avoidance (MAv) goals* focus the person on not making mistakes (avoiding task-referenced incompetence) or on maintaining a previously established level of performance (avoiding self-referenced incompetence). A politician with an MAv goal might be focused on not making a mistake in a speech or on not doing worse than she or he did while practicing the speech. *Performance-approach (PAp) goals* focus the person on outperforming others (normatively referenced competence), such as the salesperson who is focused on producing the best sales figures in her or his division. Fi-

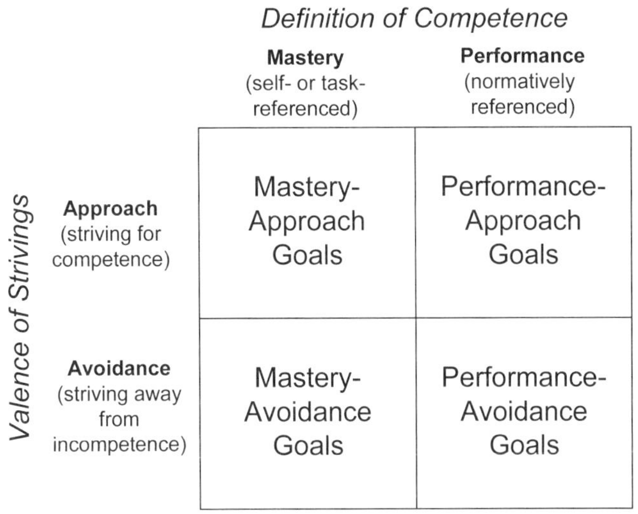

Definition of Competence

	Mastery (self- or task-referenced)	Performance (normatively referenced)
Approach (striving for competence)	Mastery-Approach Goals	Performance-Approach Goals
Avoidance (striving away from incompetence)	Mastery-Avoidance Goals	Performance-Avoidance Goals

Valence of Strivings

FIGURE 26.1. The 2 × 2 achievement goal framework. From Elliot and McGregor (2001, p. 502). Copyright 2001 by the American Psychological Association. Adapted by permission.

nally, *performance-avoidance (PAv) goals* focus the person on not being outperformed by others (avoiding normatively referenced incompetence), such as the swimmer whose primary objective is to avoid finishing last in his or her qualifying heat during a meet. An emerging body of evidence from social-personality, educational, sports, and industrial/organizational psychology has made it increasingly apparent that considering both dimensions of achievement goals (i.e., definition of competence and goal valence) enhances the predictive power of the goal construct (for a review, see Moller & Elliot, 2006).

Summary of Goal-Based Approaches

Goal-based approaches to achievement motivation are based on the different competence-based aims or purposes of achievement strivings. Early research focused on a dichotomous model of goals that emphasized the distinction between mastery- and performance-based definitions of competence. Recent work has convincingly demonstrated the conceptual and predictive value of attending to the approach–avoidance valence of goals. The corresponding 2 × 2 achievement-goal framework has received substantial attention, and results consistently demonstrate

that these four goals have unique profiles of antecedents and consequences.

The strengths and weaknesses of the goal-based approach to achievement motivation generally complement those of the motive-based approach reviewed earlier (Elliot, 1997). Recall that the motive-based approach emphasizes the energization of achievement behavior but offers only general insight into how such behavior is directed (e.g., toward competence, away from incompetence). The goal-based approach offers little with respect to the energization of achievement behavior, but it specifically accounts for the different ways that individuals can orient their achievement behavior to feel competent (e.g., definitions of competence). The dynamic nature of the goal construct itself also makes it possible to account for intraindividual variability in the quality of achievement strivings that is more difficult within the motive-based tradition.

The Hierarchical Model of Achievement Motivation

The hierarchical model of achievement motivation was proposed to integrate these complementary approaches and to increase the conceptual clarity of the achievement motivation literature (Elliot, 1997, 1999, 2005; Elliot & Church, 1997; Elliot & McGregor, 1999). In a nutshell, the hierarchical model of achievement motivation posits achievement goals as proximal regulators of achievement-related processes and outcomes. In the Lewinian tradition, a host of individual differences, situational factors, and their interactions can serve as antecedents of these goals (Elliot, 1999). These factors include neurophysiological predispositions, motives, self-based variables, relational variables, and the motivational climate surrounding the activity, to name but a few examples.

Of all these variables, achievement motives are perhaps the most robust and well-established antecedents of achievement goals. The nAch orients people to the possibility of success and increases the likelihood of MAp, PAp, and MAv goal adoption; the FF orients people to the possibility of failure and increases the likelihood of MAv, PAp, and PAv goal adoption (Conroy & Elliot, 2004; Elliot & McGregor, 2001; Elliot & Murayama, 2008). Although the hierarchical model of achievement motivation posits a sequential path from stable individual differences (motives) to dynamic self-regulatory strategies (goals) to achievement-related processes and outcomes, it does not preclude the possibility of direct effects from individual differences to achievement-related processes and outcomes. The remainder of this chapter reviews what is known about links between achievement motivation and social behavior and frames an agenda for future research in this area.

Achievement Motives and Social Behavior

Research on achievement motives has largely focused on predicting and explaining outcomes such as academic achievement, entrepreneurial activity, challenge seeking, and persistence (Koestner & McClelland, 1990; McClelland et al., 1953). It is somewhat surprising that social behaviors have received so little attention given their important role in determining achievement outcomes. Most of the research involving social behaviors has focused on identifying factors that contribute to the socialization of achievement motives.

We exclude this developmentally oriented research from our review and focus instead on social behaviors that are plausible *consequences* of implicit and explicit achievement motives.

Implicit Motives

Two studies have linked children's implicit nAch with peer perceptions. In the first study, children high in nAch in a kibbutz were perceived by their peers as having greater learning and leadership abilities (Lifshitz, 1974). Children high in nAch also have higher sociometric status than children low in nAch, as indicated by their peers' expressing a greater preference to work and play with them (Teevan, Diffenderfer, & Greenfield, 1986). Thus it appears that implicit nAch in childhood is valuable for establishing status.

When implicit nAch is aroused, people exhibit decreased interpersonal sensitivity—they are less accurate in rating the characteristics of people with whom they work (Berlew & Williams, 1964). Decreased accuracy of social perception may be a cost of devoting limited attentional resources to the achievement task. On the other hand, implicit nAch has been linked with more cooperative behavior during a prisoner's dilemma task, especially when one's partner initially exhibits cooperative behavior (Terhune, 1968). Cooperating on this task represents the best strategy for ensuring mutual productivity with minimal risk and therefore satisfies the need to excel, as well as the need to be efficient in one's achievement pursuits. As a whole, these findings suggest that implicit nAch facilitates task-relevant behavior to the exclusion of broader social perceptions.

Less is known about the social consequences of implicit FF. One study documented that Reserve Officer Training Corps (ROTC) cadets who scored high in implicit FF were less active in structuring roles for themselves or group members during training exercises (Dapra, Zarrillo, Carlson, & Teevan, 1985). These cadets also demonstrated less initiative during training exercises compared with cadets low in FF. Dapra and colleagues (1985) suggested that cadets high in FF may come across as less assertive because they are concerned about earning the approval of others. This interpretation is consistent with the finding that implicit FF was associated with greater impression management during a purported creativity test (Cohen & Teevan, 1974). Birney and colleagues (1969) also reported a series of studies demonstrating that FF was linked with greater conformity to others' judgments and opinions, but that this association exists only when the person is in a social context. Collectively, these results suggest that relational concerns and insecurities are intertwined with implicit FF. Young adults appear to regulate these concerns with appeasing behaviors. In contrast, maternal reports indicate that children high in FF engage in more attention-seeking behavior than children low in FF (Singh, 1992).

Overall, these results present a picture of two implicit motives with quite different social consequences. Implicit nAch appears to facilitate successful social interactions, although the achievement pursuit may draw the individual's attention to the task, may reduce the accuracy of person perception, and may enhance social status. On the other hand, implicit FF may inhibit social behavior in different ways at different points in life. Children high in FF may act out and engage in problem behaviors to solicit parental attention, whereas young adults may inhibit agentic behavior because their concerns over social approval and acceptance take precedence over genuine competence.

Explicit Motives

Compared with the implicit-motives literature, considerably less evidence is available regarding links between explicit achievement motives and social behaviors. The following review is limited to studies that focused on nAch or FF; related constructs such as test anxiety are beyond the scope of this coverage. Studies that focused on resultant motivation (i.e., standardized nAch minus standardized FF) also were excluded, because it is impossible to interpret which motive is responsible for any observed effects. Unfortunately, this delimitation leads us to exclude some very interesting studies concerning achievement motivation and leadership (e.g., Sorrentino, 1973; Sorrentino & Field, 1986; Sorrentino & Sheppard, 1978).

In one study that specifically examined explicit motives and social behavior, the nAch was linked with prosocial and noncompliant behaviors in the workplace (Puffer, 1987). Supervisors in a chain of retail stores rated employees who were high in nAch as demonstrating more prosocial behaviors, such as assisting coworkers and pursuing solutions to customer service problems. They also rated these employees as demonstrating fewer noncompliant behaviors, such as complaining about work conditions, lying to customers, and taking excessive breaks. In another study, high nAch participants allocated rewards to a partner based on the partner's performance instead of the partner's reward-allocation strategy (O'Malley & Schubarth, 1984). These findings are consistent with proposals that the nAch orients people toward efficient and just behaviors in their competence pursuits; however, the study neither evaluated nor controlled for the influence of FF.

Explicit FF has been linked to self-protective behavior. Children high in FF engage in cheating more frequently than peers low in FF, presumably to enhance their probability of avoiding failure (Monte & Fish, 1987; Shelton & Hill, 1969). In college students, FF has been shown to negatively predict students' likelihood of telling their parents about their performance on a task they just completed if they failed at the task and to positively predict their likelihood of telling their parents if they succeeded at the task (McGregor & Elliot, 2005).

Emerging results from our research also suggest that achievement motives have distinct relations with different forms of interpersonal problems. Anticipatory pride (i.e., explicit nAch) has a very limited association with interpersonal problems; if anything, low levels of the nAch may be associated with submissive interpersonal problems (Conroy, Elliot, & Pincus, 2009). On the other hand, anticipatory shame (i.e., explicit FF) is associated with significant interpersonal distress. This distress is reported by individuals high in FF themselves, as well as being reported by knowledgeable peers. Although self-reported FF was not associated with specific interpersonal problems, peers described friends high in FF as being more exploitable, overly nurturant, and intrusive than friends low in FF.

In another study that focused on college students with high FF, two clusters of self-reported interpersonal-problem profiles emerged (Wright, Pincus, Conroy & Elliot, in press). The first cluster of people with high FF, labeled Appeasers, had problem profiles characterized by submissive behavior. The second cluster of people with high FF, labeled Aggressors, had problem profiles characterized by dominant to hostile–dominant behavior. These problem profiles converged with distinctive styles for coping with shame: appeasement/withdrawal and rage (Gilbert & McGuire, 1998; Lewis, 1971). The extent to which these individual differences in shame regulation influence broader aspects of social behavior, productivity, and well-being will need to be established in future research.

Summary

Looking at the literature reviewed so far, it is clear that achievement-motive research has sampled only a very limited scope of social behaviors. Methodological difficulties have plagued this literature, as implicit and explicit motives have not always been distinguished clearly. Despite these limitations, two working conclusions can be drawn: (1) Explicit nAch is associated with high-quality task engagement and social behaviors in support of productivity and status, and (2) explicit FF is associated with self-protective behavior that creates interpersonal difficulties. As this literature grows, we anticipate that constructs will be operationalized more consistently, studies will control complementary motives, and designs will shift to focus on patterns of behavioral variability *within* people who vary in motive strength to strengthen conclusions that can be drawn regarding the influence of achievement motives on social behavior.

Achievement Goals and Social Behavior

In contrast to the achievement-motive literature, a broad range of social behaviors have been linked to achievement goals, and it is apparent that many of these social behaviors have strong interpersonal components. That is, they reflect elements of agency and communion—the primary dimensions of interpersonal behavior (Bakan, 1966; Kiesler,

1996; Leary, 1957; Wiggins, 1991). Agentic behaviors involve variability along an axis ranging from dominance to submission. Communal behaviors involve variability along an axis from friendly to hostile, although the hostile end represents cold/distant behaviors rather than open hostility. These dimensions are independent and form the interpersonal circumplex (Kiesler, 1996; Leary, 1957) shown in Figure 26.2. This circumplex encapsulates behavioral phenotypes that vary in terms of their agentic and communal properties. These behaviors are often identified within octants of the interpersonal circumplex and include pure forms of dominant, submissive, friendly, and hostile behaviors, as well as agentic–communal hybrids such as friendly–dominant, friendly–submissive, hostile–submissive, and hostile–dominant behaviors. The interpersonal circumplex model provides a useful organizing framework for reviewing and interpreting the literature on achievement goals and interpersonally based social behavior. Other important social behaviors have less pronounced interpersonal components. These outcomes typically involve group processes and are reviewed in a later section.

Interpersonal Social Behaviors

Submissive to Friendly–Submissive Behavior: Help Seeking

Help seeking is among the most well-investigated social consequences of achievement goals and has received substantial attention in research on academic achievement. Help seeking refers to a class of strategies used by self-regulated learners when they need assistance with a task. These strategies may be adaptive when students seek instrumental help that supports their autonomy in the achievement pursuit (e.g., requesting a hint on how to proceed) or maladaptive when they simply request executive or expedient help to complete the task (e.g., requesting a solution; Nelson-LeGall, 1985). Adaptive help seeking appears to be greater for people who adopt MAp goals (Butler & Neuman, 1995; Karabenick, 2003; Linnenbrink, 2005; Ryan & Pintrich, 1997). Expedient help seeking is negatively associated with MAp goals in some studies (Linnenbrink, 2005) and unassociated with MAp

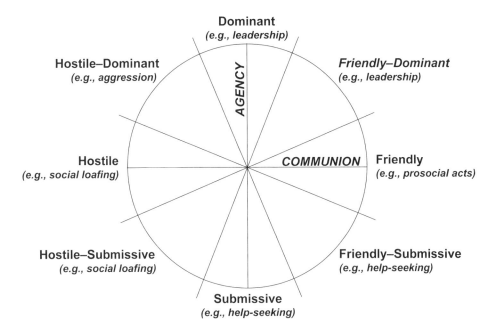

FIGURE 26.2. The interpersonal circle with illustrative examples of social behaviors that have been linked to achievement goals.

goals in other studies (Karabenick, 2003). Avoidance of help seeking has been linked with low levels of MAp goals (Linnenbrink, 2005), as well as high levels of MAv and PAv goals (Karabenick, 2003; Middleton & Midgley, 1997). Such avoidance has been positively associated with PAp goals in college students, but not in elementary school students (Karabenick, 2003; Linnenbrink, 2005).

Ryan and Pintrich (1997) provided additional evidence that linked achievement goals with attitudes toward help seeking. Not surprisingly, a focus on learning and improving (i.e., MAp goals) has been associated with more positive attitudes toward help seeking. Students with MAp goals are also less likely to endorse a belief that their teachers will have negative reactions to help seeking. In contrast, PAp goals have been linked to perceptions that help seeking leads to negative reactions from both teachers and peers. Ryan and Pintrich concluded that attitudes toward help seeking may provide an indirect pathway for achievement goals to influence help-seeking behavior (or the avoidance thereof).

Friendly Behavior: Prosocial Behaviors

This category involves prototypically communal behaviors in which the focus is on connecting and forming a positive bond with another social being. Cheung, Ma, and Shek (1998) focused on self-reported tendencies to engage in helping behavior, to cooperate and share, to maintain empathic and friendly relations with others, and to go along with social norms. In their sample of Chinese adolescents, MAp goals were consistently associated with high levels of these prosocial behaviors, whereas PAp goals were not associated with any of these prosocial behaviors. In a related study, students with dominant MAp goals expressed a greater willingness to cooperate with their peers, regardless of the peers' social status, whereas students with dominant PAp and PAv goals expressed a preference for cooperating with ingroup and high-status peers (Levy, Kaplan, & Patrick, 2004). These findings suggest that status concerns may moderate relations between performance-based achievement goals and communal behavior during competence pursuits. LePine (2005) found that MAp goals were associated with judges' ratings of respectful and supportive communication from members of a triad whose achievement pursuit was disrupted. When the triad was given a difficult goal, PAp goals were negatively associated with judges' ratings of respectful and supportive communication; PAp goals were unassociated with judges' ratings when triads were given an easy goal. In the sport domain, MAp goals have been positively associated with athletes' respect for their opponents, rules, and officials, whereas PAp goals have been negatively associated with these important indicators of sportspersonship (Stornes & Ommundsen, 2004). The PAp goal effects were somewhat moderated by athletes' perceptions of the motivational climate; a strong mastery-motivational climate weakens relations between PAp goals and poor sportspersonship.

Dominant Behavior (Hostile to Friendly): Leadership

One of the central challenges of leadership involves influencing others. Although there are many ways of exerting influence (see House & Singh, 1987), leadership in its varied styles remains a prototypically agentic interpersonal behavior. Yamaguchi (2001) used a qualitative analysis to compare the leadership styles that emerged in 10 groups of children working on a task. Groups that were given MAp goals at the beginning of the task exhibited a shared leadership style between the members, whereas groups that were given PAp goals exhibited a dominant leadership style in which one member "overtook and overpowered the [task] and group processes" (p. 683). This effect is consistent with other findings that children who adopt performance-based goals are exceedingly focused on social status (e.g., Levy et al., 2004).

Hostile–Dominant Behavior: Aggression

Aggressive behavior involves an immediate intent to injure another individual (Anderson & Bushman, 2002). Limited research exists on links between achievement goals and aggressive behavior. An early study in the sport domain found that aggressive behavior was perceived as more legitimate by athletes who had low MAp goals and moderately high PAp goals (Duda, Olson, & Templin, 1986). Self-reported use of aggression to gain a competitive advantage has also been linked with high PAp goals in athletes (Stornes & Ommundsen, 2004). Based on these limited results, it appears that normative definitions of competence (performance-based goals) are associated with the potential for increased aggressive behavior—perhaps because individuals with performance-based goals are so preoccupied with social status that, in their basest moments, they resort to primitive means of attaining it.

Hostile to Hostile–Submissive Behavior: Social Loafing

Social loafing refers to the phenomenon of a "decrease in individual effort due to the social presence of other persons" (Latané, Williams, & Harkins, 1979, p. 823). This behavior is submissive because the individual is reducing her or his efforts to influence the group or the group's performance. The fact that such behavior may harm the group suggests that it may be a hostile interpersonal process, although that need not always be the case. Social loafing in academic work has been positively associated with students' PAp goals, but not their MAp goals (Linnenbrink, 2003). From a different perspective, athletes with high PAp goals are more likely to report that their teammates are withholding effort during performances; however, goals were not associated with athletes' reports that they themselves would withhold effort if they perceived teammates to be loafing (Hoigaard & Ommundsen, 2007). Performance-based achievement goals may lead to effort reductions because ability is inferred in part from the amount of effort an individual must expend to be successful at a task (Nicholls, 1984). In other words, the hostile–submissive act of withholding effort may actually be a strategy for demonstrating competence in group work. One would assume that this effect would be more pronounced for individuals focused on avoiding incompetence than for those focused on being competent.

Group Processes

There are many possible examples of social behaviors that do not map directly onto the interpersonal circle. Three relevant examples that have been linked to achievement goals involve information exchange, conflict regulation, and role structure adaptation within groups.

Information Exchange

Dyadic and group achievement processes frequently require people to share information about task requirements or the situation in which the task is being performed. As a bidirectional process, information exchange can be characterized both by people's openness to sharing information with others and by the degree to which they implement information that they receive from others. Achievement goals can influence these exchange processes by orienting individuals either toward reciprocity (when they are interested in developing competence) or exploitation (when they seek to enhance their status relative to others) in their information exchanges (Poortvliet, Janssen, Van Yperen, & Van de Vliert, 2007). One experiment demonstrated that performance-based goals resulted in less openness in sharing information and greater utilization of high- but not low-quality information compared with both mastery-based goals and a condition in which participants were not assigned a particular achievement goal (Poortvliet et al., 2007). Goal valence manipulations had no effect on information exchanges in this study. The effects of performance-based relative to mastery-based goals in the experiment were at least partially mediated by hypothesized reciprocity and exploitation orientations. These findings suggest that mastery-based goals engender more cooperative behavior than performance-based goals.

Conflict Regulation

When people work together, disagreements are inevitable. Cognitively and socially focused strategies for dealing with such disagreements have been identified (Doise & Mugny, 1984). Epistemic conflict-regulation strategies involve evaluating the factual accuracy of each proposition in the disagreement, whereas relational conflict-regulation strategies focus on self-protection by asserting the superiority of one's own position. As expected, MAp goals have been associated with the use of epistemic conflict-regulation strategies, whereas PAp goals have been associated with the use of relational conflict-regulation strategies (Darnon, Muller, Schrager, Pannuzzo, & Butera, 2006).

Role Structure Adaptation

When a group's performance on a task is disrupted and roles need to change, the group members' success in adapting to their new roles will influence their groups' performance. In a computer-based decision-making task for triads, LePine (2005) created an equipment failure that disrupted normal communication channels between members, thereby forcing them to adapt their communications. Neither MAp nor PAp goals had direct links with participants' success in adapting to their new roles in the communication process; however, both goals interacted with the difficulty of a group's goals to predict their likelihood of adapting. MAp goals positively predicted role structure adaptation when groups had difficult goals, and PAp goals negatively predicted role structure adaptation when groups had difficult goals. Neither achievement goal was associated with role structure adaptation when groups had easy goals. Thus it appears that, under challenging situations, mastery-based goals may promote more flexible social behavior than performance-based goals.

Summary

Achievement goals have been linked to a variety of social behaviors that vary in their levels of agency and communion. Based on the evidence reviewed here, it is clear that performance-based goals are more strongly and consistently associated with social behavior than are mastery-based goals. This difference reflects the heightened sensitivity to social comparisons that performance-based goals engender. Moreover, these performance-based goals seem to orient individuals to their status and lead to more agentic variation in interpersonal behavior (e.g., dominance, social loafing). In contrast, mastery-based goals appear to facilitate communal behaviors (e.g., help seeking, prosocial acts).

We offer a few caveats to these conclusions. First, social behavior is a very complex phenomenon, and a relatively narrow range of behavior has been studied. Some of the seemingly simple behaviors that were reviewed may have multiple components (e.g., help seeking) (Nelson-LeGall, 1985), and it may be simplistic to cast all of these behaviors into a single interpersonal circumplex octant. Second, few studies have examined the social impact of avoidance goals. It will be important to determine how this characteristic of achievement goals influences social behaviors. Finally, most research in this area has focused on individual differences in goals and has not considered how the motivational climate might influence social behavior (either as a main effect or in an interaction with states of goal involvement).

Future Directions

This chapter opened with the proposal that competence strivings frequently involve social behavior and that achievement motivation theories should speak to these processes as well as proximal achievement processes and outcomes. The evidence reviewed herein clearly indicates that individual differences in achievement motivation are associated with different patterns of social behavior.

Looking forward, we see great potential for using achievement motivation theories to explain social behavior during competence pursuits. As noted at the beginning of this chapter, many approaches have been employed in achievement motivation research, and this chapter focused on two specific approaches that have been integrated in the hierarchical model of achievement motivation (Elliot, 1999). Other approaches, such as those that focus on attributions for achievement outcomes or implicit theories of intelligence and ability, also seem to hold great promise for explaining social behavior during competence pursuits.

One of the challenges in moving this literature forward will be the sheer scope of possible social behaviors that can be investigated. The interpersonal circumplex may provide a valuable framework for generating hypotheses and organizing findings in this complex domain. Not every social behavior is neatly captured by this model, and we do not advocate limiting investigations to interpersonal behaviors alone. Nevertheless, we encourage researchers to consider ways in which they can anchor their measures of social behavior in broad nomological networks to facilitate future theorizing.

Finally, it seems appropriate to conclude by returning to a fundamental point in individual-differences research. Both the person and situation are important factors to consider when predicting social behavior. Our best chance for understanding how achievement motivation influences social behavior will require us to engage in more process-focused research that highlights consistencies in behavioral variability as a function of situational characteristics (e.g., Mischel & Shoda, 1995).

References

Anderson, C. A., & Bushman, B. J. (2002). Human aggression. *Annual Review of Psychology, 53*, 27–51.

Atkinson, J. W. (1957). Motivational determinants of risk-taking behavior. *Psychological Review, 64*, 359–372.

Atkinson, J. W., & Litwin, G. (1960). Achievement motive and test anxiety conceived as motive to approach success and motive to avoid failure. *Journal of Abnormal and Social Psychology, 60*, 52–64.

Bakan, D. (1966). *The duality of human existence: Isolation and communion in Western man.* Boston: Beacon Press.

Bandura, A. (1997). *Self-efficacy: The exercise of control.* New York: Freeman.

Baumann, N., Kaschel, R., & Kuhl, J. (2005). Striving for unwanted goals: Stress-dependent discrepancies between explicit and implicit achievement motives reduce subjective well-being and increase psychosomatic symptoms. *Journal of Personality and Social Psychology, 89*, 781–799.

Berlew, D. E., & Williams, A. F. (1964). Interpersonal sensitivity under motive arousing conditions. *Journal of Abnormal and Social Psychology, 68*, 150–159.

Birney, R. C., Burdick, H., & Teevan, R. C. (1969). *Fear of failure.* New York: Van Nostrand Reinhold.

Brunstein, J. C. (2001). Persönliche Ziele und Handlungs- versus Lageorientierung: Wer bindet sich an realistische und bedürfniskongruente Ziele? [Personal goals and action versus state orientation: Who builds a commitment to realistic and need-congruent goals?]. *Zeitschrift für Differentielle und Diagnostische Psychologie, 22*, 1–12.

Butler, R., & Neuman, O. (1995). Effects of task and ego achievement goals on help-seeking behaviors and attitudes. *Journal of Educational Psychology, 87*, 261–271.

Cheung, P. C., Ma, H. K., & Shek, D. T. L. (1998). Conceptions of success: Their correlates with prosocial orientation and behaviour in Chinese adolescents. *Journal of Adolescence, 21*, 31–42.

Cialdini, R. B., Trost, M. R., & Newsom, J. T. (1995). Preference for consistency: The development of a valid measure and the discovery of surprising behavioral implications. *Journal of Personality and Social Psychology, 69*, 318–328.

Cohen, R. J., & Teevan, R. C. (1974). Fear of failure and impression management: An exploratory study. *Psychological Reports, 35*, 1332.

Conroy, D. E., & Elliot, A. J. (2004). Fear of failure and achievement goals in sport: Addressing the issue of the chicken and the egg. *Anxiety, Stress, and Coping, 17*, 271–285.

Conroy, D. E., Elliot, A. J., & Pincus, A. L. (2009). The expression of achievement motives in interpersonal problems. *Journal of Personality, 77*, 445–526.

Conroy, D. E., Metzler, J. N., & Willow, J. P. (2002). Multidimensional fear of failure measurement: The Performance Failure Appraisal Inventory. *Journal of Applied Sport Psychology, 14*, 76–90.

Dapra, R. A., Zarrillo, D. L., Carlson, T. K., & Teevan, R. C. (1985). Fear of failure and indices of leadership utilized in the training of ROTC cadets. *Psychological Reports, 56*, 27–30.

Darnon, C., Muller, D., Schrager, S. M., Pannuzzo, N., & Butera, F. (2006). Mastery and performance goals predict epistemic and relational conflict regulation. *Journal of Educational Psychology, 98*, 766–776.

deCharms, R., Morrison, H. W., Reitman, W., & McClelland, D. C. (1955). Behavioral correlates of directly and indirectly measured achievement motivation. In D. C. McClelland (Ed.), *Studies in motivation* (pp. 414–423). New York: Appleton-Century-Crofts.

Deci, E. L., & Ryan, R. M. (1985). *Intrinsic motivation and self-determination in human behavior.* New York: Plenum Press.

Diener, C. I., & Dweck, C. S. (1978). An analysis of learned helplessness: Continuous changes in performance, strategy, and achievement cognitions following failure. *Journal of Personality and Social Psychology, 36*, 451–462.

Diener, C. I., & Dweck, C. S. (1980). An analysis of learned helplessness: II. The processing of success. *Journal of Personality and Social Psychology, 39*, 940–952.

Doise, W., & Mugny, G. (1984). *The social development of the intellect.* Oxford, UK: Pergamon Press.

Duda, J. L., Olson, L. K., & Templin, T. J. (1986). The relationship of task and ego orientation to sportsmanship attitudes and the perceived legitimacy of injurious acts. *Research Quarterly for Exercise and Sport, 62*, 79–87.

Dweck, C. S. (1975). The role of expectations and attributions in the alleviation of learned helplessness. *Journal of Personality and Social Psychology, 31*, 674–685.

Dweck, C. S. (1986). Motivational processes affecting learning. *American Psychologist, 41*, 1040–1048.

Dweck, C. S. (1999). *Self-theories: Their role in motivation, personality, and development.* Philadelphia: Psychology Press.

Dweck, C. S., & Elliott, E. S. (1983). Achievement motivation. In P. H. Mussen (Series Ed.) & E. M. Hetherington (Vol. Ed.), *Handbook of child psychology: Vol. 4. Socialization, personality, and social development* (4th ed., pp. 643–691). New York: Wiley.

Elliot, A. J. (1997). Integrating the "classic" and "contemporary" approaches to achievement motivation: A hierarchical model of approach and avoidance achievement motivation. In M. Maehr & P. Pintrich (Eds.), *Advances in motivation and achievement* (Vol. 10, pp. 143–179). Greenwich, CT: JAI Press.

Elliot, A. J. (1999). Approach and avoidance motivation and achievement goals. *Educational Psychologist, 34*, 169–189.

Elliot, A. J. (2005). A conceptual history of the achievement goal construct. In A. J. Elliot & C. S. Dweck (Eds.), *Handbook of competence and motivation* (pp. 52–72). New York: Guilford Press.

Elliot, A. J., & Church, M. A. (1997). A hierarchical model of approach and avoidance achievement motivation. *Journal of Personality and Social Psychology, 72*, 218–232.

Elliot, A. J., & Dweck, C. S. (2005). Competence and motivation: Competence as the core of achievement motivation. In A. J. Elliot & C. S. Dweck (Eds.), *Handbook of competence and motivation* (pp. 2–12). New York: Guilford Press.

Elliot, A. J., & Harackiewicz, J. M. (1996). Approach and avoidance achievement goals and intrinsic motivation: A meditational analysis. *Journal of Personality and Social Psychology, 70*, 968–980.

Elliot, A. J., & McGregor, H. A. (1999). Test anxiety and the hierarchical model of approach and avoidance achievement motivation. *Journal of Personality and Social Psychology, 76*, 628–644.

Elliot, A. J., & McGregor, H. A. (2001). A 2 × 2 achievement goal framework. *Journal of Personality and Social Psychology, 80*, 501–519.

Elliot, A. J., & Murayama, K. (2008). On the measurement of achievement goals: Critique, illustration, and application. *Journal of Educational Psychology, 100*, 613–628.

Elliott, E. S., & Dweck, C. S. (1988). Goals: An approach to motivation and achievement. *Journal of Personality and Social Psychology, 54*, 5–12.

Feather, N. (1965). The relationship of expectation of success to achievement and test anxiety. *Journal of Personality and Social Psychology, 1*, 118–126.

Gilbert, P., & McGuire, M. T. (1998). Shame, status, and social roles: Psychobiology and evolution. In P. Gilbert & B. Andrews (Eds.), *Shame: Interpersonal behavior, psychopathology, and culture* (pp. 99–125). New York: Oxford University Press.

Hagtvet, K., & Benson, J. (1997). The motive to avoid failure and test anxiety responses: Empirical support for integration of two research traditions. *Anxiety, Stress, and Coping, 10*, 35–57.

Harter, S. (1983). Developmental perspectives on the self-system. In P. H. Mussen (Series Ed.) & E. M. Hetherington (Vol. Ed.), *Handbook of child psychology: Vol. 4. Socialization, personality and social development* (4th ed., pp. 275–386). New York: Wiley.

Heckhausen, H. (1963). *Hoffnung und Furcht in der Leistungsmotivation [Hope and fear components of achievement motivation].* Meisenheim am Glan, Germany: Anton Hain.

Heckhausen, H. (1984). Emergent achievement behavior: Some early developments. In J. Nicholls (Ed.), *Advances in motivation and achievement: The development of achievement motivation* (Vol. 3, pp. 1–32). Greenwich, CT: JAI Press.

Herman, W. (1990). Fear of failure as a distinctive personality trait measure of test anxiety. *Journal of Research and Development in Education, 23*, 180–185.

Hoigaard, R., & Ommundsen, Y. (2007). Perceived social loafing and anticipated effort reduction among young football (soccer) players: An achievement goal perspective. *Psychological Reports, 100*, 857–875.

House, R. J., & Singh, J. V. (1987). Organizational behavior: Some new directions for I/O psychology. *Annual Review of Psychology, 38,* 669–718.

Jackson, D. N. (1974). *Manual for the Personality Research Form.* Goshen, NY: Research Psychology Press.

Karabenick, S. A. (2003). Seeking help in large college classes: A person-centered approach. *Contemporary Educational Psychology, 28,* 37–58.

Kiesler, D. J. (1996). *Contemporary interpersonal theory and research: Personality, psychopathology, and psychotherapy.* New York: Wiley.

Koestner, R., & McClelland, D. C. (1990). Perspectives on competence motivation. In L. A. Pervin (Ed.), *Handbook of personality: Theory and research* (pp. 527–548). New York: Guilford Press.

Latané, B., Williams, K., & Harkins, S. (1979). Many hands make light the work: The causes and consequences of social loafing. *Journal of Personality and Social Psychology, 37,* 822–832.

Leary, T. (1957). *Interpersonal diagnosis of personality.* New York: Oxford University Press.

LePine, J. A. (2005). Adaptation of teams in response to unforeseen change: Effects of goal difficulty and team composition in terms of cognitive ability and goal orientation. *Journal of Applied Psychology, 90,* 1153–1167.

Levy, I., Kaplan, A., & Patrick, H. (2004). Early adolescents' achievement goals, social status, and attitudes towards cooperation with peers. *Social Psychology of Education, 7,* 127–159.

Lewin, K., Dembo, T., Festinger, L., & Sears, P. S. (1944). Level of aspiration. In J. M. Hunt (Ed.), *Personality and the behavior disorders: A handbook based on experimental and clinical research* (pp. 333–378). New York: Ronald Press.

Lewis, H. B. (1971). *Shame and guilt in neurosis.* New York: International Universities Press.

Lewis, M., Alessandri, S. M., & Sullivan, M. W. (1992). Differences in shame and pride as a function of children's gender and task difficulty. *Child Development, 63,* 630–638.

Lewis, M., Sullivan, M. W., Stanger, C., & Weiss, M. (1989). Self-development and self-conscious emotions. *Child Development, 60,* 146–156.

Lifshitz, M. (1974). Achievement motivation and coping behavior of normal and problematic preadolescent kibbutz children. *Journal of Personality Assessment, 38,* 138–143.

Linnenbrink, E. A. (2003). *The dilemma of performance goals: Promoting students' motivation and learning in cooperative groups.* Unpublished doctoral dissertation, University of Michigan, Ann Arbor.

Linnenbrink, E. A. (2005). The dilemma of performance-approach goals: The use of multiple goal contexts to promote students' motivation and learning. *Journal of Educational Psychology, 97,* 197–213.

Maehr, M. L., & Nicholls, J. G. (1980). Culture and achievement motivation: A second look. In N. Warren (Ed.), *Studies in cross-cultural psychology* (Vol. 3, pp. 221–267). New York: Academic Press.

Mandler, G., & Sarason, S. B. (1952). A study of anxiety and learning. *Journal of Abnormal and Social Psychology, 47,* 166–173.

McClelland, D. C. (1987). *Human motivation.* New York: Cambridge University Press.

McClelland, D. C., Atkinson, J. W., Clark, R. A., & Lowell, E. L. (1953). *The achievement motive.* East Norwalk, CT: Appleton-Century-Crofts.

McClelland, D. C., Koestner, R., & Weinberger, J. (1989). How do self-attributed and implicit motives differ? *Psychological Review, 96,* 690–702.

McGregor, H. A., & Elliot, A. J. (2005). The shame of failure: Examining the link between fear of failure and shame. *Personality and Social Psychology Bulletin, 31,* 218–231.

Middleton, M. J., & Midgley, C. (1997). Avoiding the demonstration of lack of ability: An underexplored aspect of goal theory. *Journal of Educational Psychology, 89,* 710–718.

Miller, L. C., Murphy, R., & Buss, A. H. (1981). Consciousness of body: Private and public. *Journal of Personality and Social Psychology, 41,* 397–406.

Mischel, W. (1968). *Personality and assessment.* New York: Wiley.

Mischel, W., & Shoda, Y. (1995). A cognitive-affective system theory of personality: Reconceptualizing situations, dispositions, dynamics, and invariance in personality structure. *Psychological Review, 102,* 246–268.

Moller, A. C., & Elliot, A. J. (2006). The 2 × 2 achievement goal framework: An overview of empirical research. In A. V. Mitel (Ed.), *Focus on educational psychology* (pp. 307–326). Hauppauge, NY: Nova Science.

Monte, C. F., & Fish, J. M. (1987). The fear-of-failure personality and academic cheating. In R. Schwarzer, H. M. van der Ploeg, & C. D. Spielberger (Eds.), *Advances in test anxiety research* (Vol. 6, pp. 87–103). Amsterdam: Swets & Zeitlinger.

Murray, H. A. (1938). *Explorations in personality.* New York: Oxford University Press.

Murray, H. A. (1943). *Thematic Apperception Test.* Cambridge, MA: Harvard University Press.

Nelson-Le Gall, S. (1985). Help-seeking behavior in learning. In E. W. Gordon (Ed.), *Review of research in education* (Vol. 12, pp. 55–90). Washington, DC: American Educational Research Association.

Nicholls, J., Patashnick, M., Cheung, P., Thorkildsen, T., & Lauer, J. (1989). Can achievement motivation succeed with only one conception of success? In F. Halisch & J. Van der Bercken (Eds.), *International perspectives on achievement motivation* (pp. 187–208). Amsterdam: Swets & Zeitlinger.

Nicholls, J. G. (1976). Effort is virtuous, but it's better to have ability: Evaluative responses to perceptions of effort and ability. *Journal of Personality and Social Psychology, 31,* 306–315.

Nicholls, J. G. (1978). The development of concepts of effort and ability, perception of own attainment, and the understanding that difficult tasks require more ability. *Child Development, 49,* 800–814.

Nicholls, J. G. (1984). Achievement motivation: Conceptions of ability, subjective experience, task choice, and performance. *Psychological Review, 91,* 328–346.

O'Malley, M. N., & Schubarth, G. (1984). Fairness and appeasement: Achievement and affiliation motives in interpersonal relations. *Social Psychology Quarterly, 47,* 364–371.

Poortvliet, P. M., Janssen, O., Van Yperen, N. W., & Van de Vliert, E. (2007). Achievement goals and interpersonal behavior: How mastery and performance goals shape information exchange. *Personality and Social Psychology Bulletin, 33*, 1435–1447.

Puffer, S. M. (1987). Prosocial behavior, noncompliant behavior, and work performance among commission salespeople. *Journal of Applied Psychology, 72*, 615–621.

Ryan, A. M., & Pintrich, P. R. (1997). "Should I ask for help?": The role of motivation and attitudes in adolescents' help seeking in math class. *Journal of Educational Psychology, 89*, 329–341.

Schmalt, H.-D. (1999). Assessing the achievement motive using the grid technique. *Journal of Research in Personality, 33*, 109–130.

Schultheiss, O. C. (2001). *Manual for the assessment of hope of success and fear of failure.* Unpublished manuscript, University of Michigan.

Schultheiss, O. C. (2007). A memory-systems approach to the classification of personality tests: Comment on Meyer and Kurtz (2006). *Journal of Personality Assessment, 89*, 197–201.

Schultheiss, O. C., & Pang, J. S. (2007). Measuring implicit motives. In R. W. Robins, R. F. Fraley, & R. Krueger (Eds.), *Handbook of research methods in personality psychology* (pp. 322–344). New York: Guilford Press.

Shelton, J., & Hill, J. P. (1969). Effects of cheating on achievement anxiety and knowledge of peer performance. *Developmental Psychology, 1*, 449–455.

Singh, S. (1992). Hostile Press measure of fear of failure and its relation to child-rearing attitudes and behavior problems. *Journal of Social Psychology, 132*, 397–399.

Smith, C. P. (1992). *Motivation and personality: Handbook of thematic content analysis.* Cambridge, UK: Cambridge University Press.

Snyder, M., & Gangestad, S. (1986). On the nature of self-monitoring: Matters of assessment, matters of validity. *Journal of Personality and Social Psychology, 51*, 125–139.

Sorrentino, R. M. (1973). An extension of theory of achievement motivation to the study of emergent leadership. *Journal of Personality and Social Psychology, 26*, 356–368.

Sorrentino, R. M., & Field, N. (1986). Emergent leadership over time: The functional value of positive motivation. *Journal of Personality and Social Psychology, 50*, 1091–1099.

Sorrentino, R. M., & Sheppard, B. H. (1978). Effects of affiliation-related motives on swimmers in individual versus group competition: A field experiment. *Journal of Personality and Social Psychology, 36*, 704–714.

Spangler, W. D. (1992). Validity of questionnaire and TAT measures of need for achievement: Two meta-analyses. *Psychological Bulletin, 112*, 140–154.

Spence, J. T., & Helmreich, R. L. (1983). Achievement-related motives and behaviors. In J. T. Spence (Ed.), *Achievement and achievement motives: Psychological and sociological approaches* (pp. 10–74). San Francisco: Freeman.

Stipek, D., Recchia, S., & McClintic, S. (1992). Self-evaluation in young children. *Monographs of the Society for Research in Child Development, 57* (Serial No. 226).

Stornes, T., & Ommundsen, Y. (2004). Achievement goals, motivational climate and sportspersonship: A study of young handball players. *Scandinavian Journal of Educational Research, 48*, 205–221.

Teevan, R. C., Diffenderfer, D., & Greenfield, N. (1986). Need for achievement and sociometric status. *Psychological Reports, 58*, 446.

Terhune, K. W. (1968). Motives, situation and interpersonal conflict within prisoners' dilemma. *Journal of Personality and Social Psychology, 8*, 1–24.

Thrash, T. M., & Elliot, A. J. (2001). Delimiting and integrating achievement motive and goal constructs. In A. Efklides, J. Kuhl, & R. M. Sorrentino (Eds.), *Trends and prospects in motivation research* (pp. 3–21). Boston: Kluwer.

Thrash, T. M., & Elliot, A. J. (2002). Implicit and self-attributed achievement motives: Concordance and predictive validity. *Journal of Personality, 70*, 729–755.

Thrash, T. M., Elliot, A. J., & Schultheiss, O. C. (2007). Methodological and dispositional predictors of congruence between implicit and explicit need for achievement. *Personality and Social Psychology Bulletin, 33*, 961–974.

Thrash, T. M., & Hurst, A. (2008). Approach and avoidance motivation in the achievement domain: Integrating the achievement motive and achievement goal traditions. In A. J. Elliot (Ed.), *Handbook of approach and avoidance motivation* (pp. 215–231). New York: Psychology Press.

Tracy, J. T., Robins, R. W., & Tangney, J. P. (2007). *The self-conscious emotions: Theory and research.* New York: Guilford Press.

Weiner, B., & Kukla, A. (1970). An attributional analysis of achievement motivation. *Journal of Personality and Social Psychology, 15*, 1–20.

Wicker, A. W. (1969). Attitudes versus actions: The relationship of verbal and overt behavioral responses to attitude objects. *Journal of Social Issues, 25*, 41–78.

Wiggins, J. S. (1991). Agency and communion as conceptual coordinates for the understanding and measurement of interpersonal behavior. In D. Cicchetti & W. M. Grove (Eds.), *Thinking clearly about psychology: Essays in honor of Paul E. Meehl* (pp. 89–113). Minneapolis: University of Minnesota Press.

Winter, D. G. (1994). *Manual for scoring motive imagery in running text* (4th ed.). Unpublished manuscript, University of Michigan, Ann Arbor.

Winter, D. G. (1999). Linking personality and "scientific" psychology: The development of empirically derived Thematic Apperception Test measures. In L. Gieser & M. I. Stein (Eds.), *Evocative images: The Thematic Apperception Test and the art of projection* (pp. 107–124). Washington, DC: American Psychological Association.

Wright, A. G. C., Pincus, A. L., Conroy, D. E., & Elliot, A. J. (in press). The pathoplastic relationship between interpersonal problems and fear of failure. *Journal of Personality.*

Yamaguchi, R. (2001). Children's learning groups: A study of emergent leadership, dominance, and group effectiveness. *Small Group Research, 32*, 671–697.

CHAPTER 27

■ ● ▲ ◆ ■ ● ▲ ◆

Belonging Motivation

MARK R. LEARY
KRISTINE M. KELLY

Human beings are an unusually social species. Although many other animals live in herds, flocks, schools, troupes, and other social groupings, none are as chronically immersed in such a wide array of relationships as human beings. People not only live in groups and establish a variety of relationships with other individuals, but they are also pervasively concerned with the degree to which they are accepted by those with whom they interact. In fact, evidence suggests that people possess a "need to belong" that motivates them to seek and maintain some minimum number of strong and abiding relationships with both individuals and groups (Baumeister & Leary, 1995). This motive has been referred to by a number of terms—such as the need to belong, motivation for acceptance, and belonging motivation—and we use the latter term to acknowledge the fact that the degree to which people are motivated to be accepted and to belong springs from a variety of sources, only one of which is the innate "need" to belong described by Baumeister and Leary (1995).

All normal human beings desire some degree of social acceptance and belonging, and people who show absolutely no interest in interpersonal relationships invariably display signs of psychological dysfunction. Yet,

like virtually all motives, belonging motivation varies across individuals. Some people are strongly motivated to foster and maintain belonging and acceptance across a wide variety of people, groups, and situations, whereas others manifest a weaker desire to establish and maintain social connections. Our goal in this chapter is to describe and explain these individual differences in belonging motivation.

Research on belonging motivation is quite new. Although researchers have been interested for many years in personality variables—such as extraversion and need for affiliation—that involve the degree to which people are motivated to interact with others, as well as the ways in which people seek approval and affirmation, these variables do not involve the desire for acceptance and belonging that is central to the construct of belonging motivation. Given that concerted research on belonging motivation can be traced back only to 1995, many of the findings described in this chapter are unpublished (and much of it is from our own work). Yet, the existing data show that belonging motivation is an important attribute that relates to social behavior and emotion in ways that differ from more widely studied constructs such as extraversion and affiliation motivation.

Measurement

The only well-validated measure that was explicitly designed to assess the degree to which people desire acceptance and belonging is the 10-item Need to Belong Scale (Leary, Kelly, Cottrell, & Schreindorfer, 2008). Sample items on the scale include "I want other people to accept me," "I try hard not to do things that will make other people avoid or reject me," and "I have a strong need to belong." The scale possesses high internal and test–retest reliability (coefficient alpha = .81; 10-week test–retest coefficient = .87), and across nine studies, Leary and colleagues (2008) provided strong converging evidence that the scale is a valid measure of individual differences in belonging motivation.

However, other ways of measuring belonging motivation have also been proposed. For example, Panicia (2000) asked people to rate the degree to which they want 24 other people to like and accept them. Target individuals included family members, friends, acquaintances, authority figures, strangers, and people in a variety of professional roles (e.g., hair cutter, professor, store clerk, pizza delivery person). Scores on this measure correlate very highly ($r = .61$) with those on the Need to Belong Scale, as one would expect. Along the same lines, Olthof and Goossens (2008) had children rate the importance of being accepted by each of their classmates as an indication of their belonging motivation.

Some researchers have used a single-item measure consisting of only ratings of the statement, "I have a strong need to belong," the item on the Need to Belong Scale with the highest item–total correlation of the 10 scale items (Knowles & Gardner, 2006). Not surprisingly, this item shows the same pattern of relationships with other measures as the Need to Belong Scale does, although the magnitudes of the relationships are slightly weaker.

Seeking Acceptance

Affiliation

As noted, behavioral researchers have been interested for many years in individual differences in sociality, focusing on traits such as extraversion, sociability, and affiliation motivation that involve, in one way or another, the degree to which people interact with others. Conceptually, belonging motivation is distinct from these constructs in emphasizing the motive to obtain social acceptance and belonging. In contrast, extraversion is a broad, multifaceted trait that involves warmth, gregariousness, assertiveness, activity, excitement seeking, and positive emotion (see Wilt & Revelle, Chapter 3, this volume) but does not necessarily entail efforts to obtain acceptance or group belonging. Similarly, the traits of sociability and affiliation motivation (or need for affiliation) reflect a preference for interacting with other people rather than being alone and a tendency to seek out and interact with other people (Cheek & Buss, 1981; Hill, 1987). But neither of these constructs necessarily entails a desire for acceptance and belonging.

Although the desire for acceptance is distinct from the frequency with which people interact with others, social acceptance is necessarily facilitated by interpersonal contact. Thus one would expect that people who more highly desire to be accepted by other people might tend to seek more opportunities for social interaction than those who have a weaker desire for acceptance. Consistent with this expectation, studies show that people who more greatly desire acceptance and belonging are more likely to be extraverted than introverted and tend to score higher on measures of sociability than people who desire acceptance and belonging less strongly (Leary et al., 2008). Similarly, studies that have examined the relationship between the Need to Belong Scale and measures of need for affiliation, such as those developed by Edwards (1954) and by Jackson (1967), have found low to moderate correlations between belonging motivation and affiliation motivation (Kelly, 1999).

Importantly, Hill (1987) showed that people who score high in affiliation motivation may be motivated to affiliate with others for at least four distinct reasons that involve efforts to obtain emotional support, social attention, the positive stimulation that other people often provide, and social comparison information (see Hill, Chapter 28, this volume). Scores on the Need to Belong Scale correlate similarly with each of Hill's subscales that measure these four bases of affiliation motivation (Leary et al., 2008). This finding may indicate that people seek belonging for the same kinds of reasons that motivate them to affiliate with others—that is, to obtain support, attention, stimulation, or social comparison information. We suspect, however, that although people do affiliate for the four reasons that Hill identified, the primary reason may be to obtain acceptance and belonging.

Clearly, people who score high in belonging motivation tend to be more sociable and affiliation motivated than those who score low. But do people high in belonging motivation actually spend less time alone? The answer appears to be "no," for Need to Belong scores did not predict the frequency with which participants in one study reported engaging in solitary behaviors during the past week. However, although participants with higher scores reported being alone just as often as those with lower scores, they expressed a stronger dislike for doing things by themselves.

Taken together, these patterns show that, although belonging motivation correlates with extraversion, sociability, and affiliation motivation, it is a distinct construct. Because people cannot easily achieve acceptance and belonging without affiliating with other people, one would expect a small to moderate correlation between belonging motivation and motives to affiliate and socialize, which is what is found.

Establishing Social Connections

At its most basic level, belonging motivation stimulates people to establish and maintain relationships with other individuals and groups. Accordingly, one would expect strong belonging needs to be linked with larger social networks. Our own unpublished data support this hypothesis. Individuals who score high on the Need to Belong Scale reported having more close friends and a larger social support network and were more likely to use Facebook (the online community) as a social networking tool (Carton, Young, & Kelly, 2008; Kelly, 2008). Overall, these data demonstrate that people's actual social connections and feelings of belonging and acceptance coincide with their belonging motivation.

Belonging motivation explicitly involves values and goals that entail establishing social connections with other people. For example, a study of the basic life values that are associated with belonging motivation showed that people who score high in belonging motivation place a greater value on friendship, love, and social recognition than those who score low, outcomes that clearly reflect a focus on one's social connections. Similarly, we have unpublished data showing that belonging motivation is strongly associated with the goal of "pleasing others." In contrast, belonging motivation is not associated with the degree to which people endorse values that are irrelevant to being accepted by other people, such as the value that they place on inner harmony, freedom, wisdom, and pleasure (Leary et al., 2008).

Although little research has examined how the values of people who are high in belonging motivation relate to specific interpersonal behaviors, the available evidence shows that people who are high in belonging motivation are more attuned to cues that involve evaluation and rejection, as well as to opportunities to connect socially with other people, than people who are low in belonging motivation. For example, Morrison, Wheeler, and Smeesters (2007) reported small correlations between the need to belong and self-monitoring—the tendency to monitor and control one's behavior in order to behave appropriately to the social context and to make desired impressions on others.

Similarly, people who scored higher on the Need to Belong Scale were more accurate in identifying emotional expressions depicted in pictures of angry, happy, fearful, and sad faces than participants who scored lower (Knowles, Gardner, Pickett, & Turner, 2004). They were also better at interpreting paralanguage by accurately recognizing positive and negative vocal tones, even when the tone of voice was incongruent with the valence of the word spoken. Finally, Need to Belong scores were related to greater empathic accuracy in that people scoring high in need to belong were more often correct in their construal of what another person was thinking or feeling than those who scored lower.

In another set of studies, Kelly and her colleagues examined the relationship between belonging motivation and interpersonal perception (Kelly & Tee, 2005, 2006; Kelly, Tee, & Ferry, 2005). Participants first completed the Need to Belong Scale and then engaged in various interpersonal perception tasks. Analyses revealed that belonging motivation was positively correlated with accuracy in identifying intimate relationships between other people, as measured by the Interpersonal Perception Task. However, no differences were found between people who scored low versus high in belonging motivation in identifying other types of relationships, such as those based on kinship, status, or competition. In subsequent studies (Kelly & Tee, 2006), college students engaged in a 1-minute social interaction with a stranger and then completed personality measures for both their interaction partners and themselves. Results indicated that participants high in belonging motivation were more accurate at judging conscientiousness in others, an interesting finding given that people are typically better at judging more visible traits, such as extraversion, that are easily observed during social interactions (Funder & Dobroth, 1987). In another study of interpersonal perception, Kelly, Tee, and Ferry (2005) found that participants who were high in belonging motivation more accurately identified people who told lies versus truths (on videotape) than those who were low in belonging motivation. Overall, the results of studies of interpersonal perception reveal that belonging motivation is associated with patterns of social sensitivity that may be particularly relevant to one's acceptance by others. People high in belonging motivation were more accurate in identifying close relationships (but not those based on kin, status, or competition), as well as more proficient at detecting deception and judging other people's conscientiousness, characteristics that are especially important in close relationships.

Paradoxically, although people high in belonging motivation are generally more accurate in decoding others' expressions and paralanguage, they may nonetheless underestimate rejection cues in certain situations. Consistent with other research showing that people's motives, goals, and anxieties sometimes bias their interpretations of social cues (Hilton & Darley, 1991; Stevens & Fiske, 1995), Carvallo and Pelham (2006) found that participants who scored high in the

need to belong reported experiencing less personal discrimination due to their gender than participants who scored low in need to belong, while at the same time reporting that, as a group, members of their gender experienced greater discrimination. This difference in judgments of personal versus group discrimination held even after controlling for individual differences in stigma consciousness, gender identity, and public collective self-esteem. According to Carvallo and Pelham, these patterns suggest that "the drive for social acceptance colors people's judgments of others in ways consistent with the belief that one will not be subject to interpersonal rejection" (p. 103). People high in the need to belong do not like to think of themselves as being personally discriminated against and thus may downplay or ignore indications that they have been devalued or mistreated.

Given that people often cooperate with others as a way to gain approval and acceptance and that noncooperators are often disliked and rejected (Danheiser & Graziano, 1982), one might expect that people who are high in belonging motivation cooperate more than those who are low. In a study that tested this hypothesis, De Cremer and Leonardelli (2003) found that participants who scored high on the Need to Belong Scale cooperated more than those low in the need to belong in a public-goods dilemma that involved splitting money between themselves and a group, but only when they believed that they were participating in a large, eight-person group. When they thought they were in a smaller, four-person group, belonging motivation was not related to participants' contributions. The authors explained this pattern by suggesting that because larger groups afford fewer opportunities for the kinds of interactions that promote acceptance and belonging, participants relied more heavily on cooperation to increase their acceptance in larger groups. Interestingly, Need to Belong scores were also related to the decisional frustration that participants experienced when trying to decide how much money to contribute to the group versus keep for themselves, possibly because they were more conflicted by the tradeoff between personal gain and social belonging.

Individual differences in belonging motivation also have implications for the degree to which people are responsive to the goals that other people have for them. Morrison and colleagues (2007, Study 3) found that among participants who had low achievement aspirations but whose mothers had achievement goals for them, those who were high in belonging motivation performed better on an achievement-relevant task after being primed to think about their mothers. Those who scored low in the need to belong, in contrast, did not perform better after being primed. To say it differently, scores on the Need to Belong Scale correlated positively with performance in the mother-prime condition but not in the control-prime condition. Thus people high in belonging motivation may be especially willing to strive to meet the goals that significant others have for them.

Another indication that belonging motivation leads people to seek acceptance is the finding that belonging motivation is associated with the degree to which people value having wealth and material possessions, presumably because they believe that money and possessions increase their chances of social acceptance. Indeed, scores on both an ad hoc measure of belonging motivation and the Need to Belong Scale correlated with materialist values and with the belief that buying material goods facilitates acceptance. Furthermore, the belief that materialism promotes acceptance fully mediated the relationship between belonging motivation and materialism (Rose & DeJesus, 2007).

Along these same lines, people who are high in belonging motivation seem to be more likely to engage in risky behaviors that might facilitate social inclusion, approval, and acceptance. For example, college students who scored higher in belonging motivation reported drinking alcohol significantly more than those who scored lower (Mathes, Kelly, & Carton, 2008). Results further indicated that this effect may occur because students who use alcohol heavily are rewarded by being invited to go out and have a good time, whereas those who abstain from drinking are less well liked and sometimes excluded from social gatherings (Carton, Kelly, Serra, & Mathes, 2008). Whether people who are high in belonging motivation also engage in other risky behaviors that promote acceptance is an important topic for future research.

Indirect Means of Feeling Accepted

People cannot always obtain the degree of acceptance and belonging that they desire, either because opportunities for acceptance are not currently available or because they have been explicitly rejected. In such instances, people may use tactics that make them feel accepted even when actual acceptance is unavailable. Research suggests that people who are high in belonging motivation use such tactics more commonly than those who are low in it.

Some people seem to derive emotional benefits from the parasocial relationships that they have with actors, newscasters, and celebrities that they see on television. Research on parasocial relationships shows that TV viewers regard favorite television performers as emotionally closer to them than an acquaintance but not as close as a friend (Koenig & Lessan, 1985), reflecting a notable degree of interpersonal connection. Theorists have assumed that people form parasocial relationships with public figures to fill unmet social needs and reduce loneliness (Koenig & Lessan, 1985; Rubin, Perse, & Powell, 1985), but little is known regarding when people use parasocial relationships to bolster feelings of acceptance. A series of studies by Knowles and Gardner (2003, 2008) showed that people who scored high in belonging motivation have closer and more intense attachments to their favorite television characters, even seeking "social support" from television characters, who keep them company when they are alone. Oddly, people high in belonging motivation were even more likely to seek the company and support of cartoon characters. They are also more likely to endorse God as a source of social support (Carton et al., 2008), which suggests that they capitalize on the interpersonal elements of a variety of contexts.

Similarly, people sometimes satisfy their desire for acceptance indirectly in ways that do not actually increase their acceptance by other people. Gardner, Pickett, Jefferies, and Knowles (2005) suggested that, in the same way that people may snack in order to tide them over to the next full meal, people who feel inadequately connected may "snack" on symbolic reminders of their social connections until they can engage in actual supportive interactions. Social snacking may take the form of rereading letters or e-mail messages from friends and loved ones, reminiscing about previous times when one was accepted or loved, daydreaming about significant others, or looking at photographs of family, friends, or romantic partners. Importantly, social snacking is more common among people who score high in belonging motivation (Gardner, Knowles, & Jefferies, in press).

As we have seen, people fulfill their desire for acceptance and belonging by seeking acceptance in face-to-face interactions, as well as via surrogate communications (e.g., photographs, e-mails) and real and imagined relationships (e.g., with beloved celebrities and God). We have additional data showing that people remember (or misremember) the nature of their social connections differently, depending on their belonging motivation. In a study of belonging motivation, social exclusion, and social networking websites, Kelly (2008) found that people who are high in belonging motivation who were primed with a social task (using Facebook) estimated that they had significantly more friends than those with lower belonging motivation and those who were primed with a nonsocial task (using Wikipedia, the online encyclopedia). Furthermore, after experiencing social exclusion, people who were high in belonging motivation indicated that they spend three times more hours per week browsing Facebook than those with lower belonging motivation. Overall, it appears that having a strong motive to be accepted and belong evokes construals of personal social memories in ways that help to satisfy that motive.

Social Deprivation

Most motives tend to become stronger, or at least more salient, when they remain unsatisfied. Along these lines, Baumeister and Leary (1995) suggested that the degree to which people desire acceptance and belonging increases when their need for belonging is unmet, as does their experience of negative emotions. Although Baumeister and Leary were discussing state-like changes in belonging motivation, their analysis raises the question of whether stable individual differences in belonging motivation are tied to feeling disconnected, rejected, lonely, or left out and to the tendency to experience negative emotions.

Perceived Rejection and Lack of Connections

Leary and colleagues (2008) presented considerable evidence that belonging motivation is not related to the degree to which people believe that they are accepted and belong. Specifically, no relationships were found between scores on the Need to Belong Scale and seven distinct measures of perceived acceptance, received social support, perceived belonging, loneliness, alienation, and related constructs (all $rs < |.10|$). Perhaps most notably, no relationship between Need to Belong scores and loneliness was found in three different samples (Leary et al., 2008; Walker, Green, Richardson, & Hubertz, 1996).

Null results are always equivocal, but to the extent that these particular findings can be trusted, they suggest that people who typically perceive that they lack acceptance, belonging, social support, or adequate social networks do not necessarily score higher in the disposition to desire acceptance and belonging. Thus, although state-like desires for acceptance may increase when people feel inadequately accepted at a particular moment in time (e.g., Baumeister & Leary, 1995), individual differences in belonging motivation do not appear to arise from a perceived lack of social connections.

Fear of Rejection and Other Negative Emotions

People who are highly motivated to obtain a particular outcome typically worry more that the motive will not be fulfilled than people who are less motivated to obtain it. Thus we might expect that people high in belonging motivation are more sensitive to and worried about possible rejection and more likely to experience negative emotions that are linked to interpersonal concerns, such as social anxiety and hurt feelings. However, the evidence for such a link is mixed.

First, belonging motivation has been found to be unrelated to rejection sensitivity (Downey & Feldman, 1996). Thus being motivated by acceptance and belonging does not relate to the tendency to anxiously expect rejection in interpersonal situations.

However, this conclusion is clouded by the fact that scores on the Rejection Sensitivity Questionnaire are a function of both the expectation that one will be rejected and the degree to which one is concerned or anxious about being rejected. As a result, we do not know whether fears of rejection, unconfounded with people's interpersonal expectations, are related to belonging motivation.

On the face of it, these findings involving rejection sensitivity appear to be contradicted by data showing that belonging motivation correlates moderately with scores on the Fear of Criticism and Rejection factor of the Sociotropy–Autonomy Scale (Beck, Epstein, Harrison, & Emery, 1983). However, this finding, too, must be interpreted with caution because of uncertainly regarding what the Fear of Criticism and Rejection subscale actually measures. Inspection of the items from this subscale suggests that they do not predominantly measure "fear" of rejection and criticism. Rather, they deal with the desire to be liked, attentiveness to signs of social approval, feelings of unease and distress when one is uncertain of obtaining approval, and behaviors that people enact in order to be liked and accepted (such as being nice, trying not to hurt other people's feelings, and doing things to please other people). Thus this subscale appears to assess thoughts, feelings, and behaviors that are broadly associated with desiring approval and acceptance, coupled with concerns regarding disapproval and rejection. Thus this subscale appears to measure roughly the same general construct as the Need to Belong Scale, with which it correlates (Leary et al., 2008).

Although people who are high in belonging motivation do not perceive that they are generally less accepted than those who are low, they nonetheless show emotional indications that they are concerned about acceptance. High belonging motivation is associated with emotions that reflect concerns with other people's impressions, evaluations, and approval. For example, scores on the Need to Belong Scale correlate with the tendency to experience social anxiety when speaking or performing in front of an audience, with feelings of shyness in social encounters, and with embarrassability (Leary et al., 2008). They are also associated with concern over

making mistakes and the failure to live up to one's own expectations (Findley & Kelly, 2008b). In each case, these emotions reflect concerns that one may make an undesired impression on others, an impression that might lead to rejection (Leary & Buckley, 2000).

Belonging motivation correlates particularly highly with the propensity to experience hurt feelings. One theory of hurt feelings suggests that people's feelings are hurt when they do not believe that others value having relationships with them as much as they wish (Leary, Springer, Negel, Ansell, & Evans, 1998). Thus people who greatly desire acceptance feel more hurt when they perceive that others do not adequately value their relationships.

Excessively High and Low Belonging Motivation

The desire for social acceptance and belonging is presumably a highly adaptive characteristic that facilitated survival and reproduction throughout human evolution (Baumeister & Leary, 1995). Even so, as is the case with most motives, excessively low and high levels of belonging motivation appear to be associated with emotional and behavioral difficulties.

High Belonging Motivation

As noted, people who are very highly motivated to be accepted are more likely to experience negative emotions when they are not certain that others will perceive and accept them as they would like. Research shows that people who are high in belonging motivation score higher on measures of audience anxiousness, shyness, and embarrassability than those who score low, and they are also more likely to have their feelings hurt by other people. More generally, belonging motivation is associated with the tendency to experience negative affect, as reflected in measures of negative affectivity and neuroticism. Although unpleasant, these feelings are not necessarily dysfunctional unless they become strong enough to interfere with effective behavior or to lead people to avoid interactions and relationships in which they fear rejection.

Although direct evidence on this point does not exist, we suspect that very high belonging motivation is associated with social anxiety disorder (or social phobia). Social anxiety disorder is characterized by overwhelming anxiety, often accompanied by excessive self-consciousness, in social situations (American Psychiatric Association, 1994). Social anxiety disorder can be limited to only one particular type of situation (such as speaking in public or interacting with members of the other sex) or so broad that a person experiences anxiety in most of their dealings with other people. At the core, people with social anxiety disorder are concerned about the degree to which others will accept or reject them (Leary & Buckley, 2000), and to that extent very high belonging motivation can sometimes be debilitating.

Additionally, exceedingly high need to belong is associated with decisional procrastination (Findley & Kelly, 2008a, 2008b), possibly because people fear making "wrong" decisions that might lead others to devalue or reject them. Given that difficulty in making decisions has been linked not only to failure to complete important tasks but also to provoking anger and rejection from others (Ferrari, 1994), procrastination seems to be self-defeating, especially for people who are highly motivated to affiliate with and be accepted by others.

Low Belonging Motivation

The question of whether low need to belong is associated with negative outcomes is somewhat difficult to answer because, in an absolute sense, very few people have an objectively low need to belong. For example, if we examine the semantic meaning of people's responses on the Need to Belong Scale, the percentage of people who report a genuinely low level of belonging motivation (i.e., 2 or below on a 5-point scale) is only about 20% (Leary et al., 2008). Put differently, scores on the Need to Belong Scale are normally distributed around a "moderately high" level of belonging motivation. Such a distribution of scores makes conceptual sense if one assumes that people need to be moderately motivated to maintain acceptance and belonging in order to fare well in their everyday lives. From a functional

perspective, healthy people should have at least a moderate desire for acceptance and belonging, particularly given that evolutionary pressures would have favored those who made every effort to be integrated into their social groups. Even in the modern world, a person who has no desire for acceptance or belonging would fare poorly in most social, occupational, and romantic pursuits.

Evidence that excessively low belonging motivation may include a dysfunctional side is provided by the finding that low need to belong correlates with tendencies toward schizoid personality disorder, which is characterized by a chronic pattern of social detachment (Leary et al., 2008). People diagnosed with schizoid tendencies find little value in close relationships, do not enjoy their relationships, and lack close friends and confidants other than first-degree relatives (American Psychiatric Association, 1994). They also appear indifferent to praise or criticism from other people, which might reflect a lack of concern about being valued and accepted. To be sure, people with schizoid personality disorder typically show a broad array of problems (for example, they often appear emotionally cold or show flattened affect), but low belonging motivation appears to be among them.

Conclusions

The history of the measurement of individual differences suggests that, after a construct has been investigated for a while, questions often arise regarding whether the construct should be assessed in a more nuanced fashion that acknowledges more refined variations in the attribute. For example, global measures of locus of control gave way to multidimensional measures (see Furnham, Chapter 18, this volume), and domain-specific measures of trait self-esteem were developed to assess self-esteem in academic, athletic, social, and other settings (Bosson & Swann, Chapter 36, this volume). Along these lines, the question may be raised whether belonging motivation is a single motivation or a cluster of motives associated with being accepted into various kinds of groups and relationships. In our view, both broad and domain-specific approaches to belonging motivation are needed. As this chapter shows, individual differences in the broad tendency to seek acceptance and belonging predict people's goals, thoughts, emotions, and behaviors in important ways. Even so, we do not doubt that an individual may be notably more motivated to be accepted in some relationships and contexts than in others.

Most of the content of social psychology is predicated on the fact that human beings desire to develop social connections of various kinds with one another. Indeed, little else in the field makes sense without the recognition that people have a desire for acceptance and belonging. Likewise, individual differences in a broad array of cognitive, emotional, and behavioral phenomena appear to reflect differences among people in the strength of their belonging motivation and in the idiosyncratic ways that they attempt to foster social acceptance and belonging.

References

American Psychiatric Association. (1994). *Diagnostic and statistical manual of mental disorders* (4th ed.). Washington, DC: Author.

Baumeister, R. F., & Leary, M. R. (1995). The need to belong: Desire for interpersonal attachments as a fundamental human motivation. *Psychological Bulletin, 117,* 497–529.

Beck, A. T., Epstein, N., Harrison, R. P., & Emery, G. (1983). *Development of the Sociotropy–Autonomy Scale: A measure of personality factors in psychopathology.* Unpublished manuscript, University of Pennsylvania, Philadelphia.

Carton, A. D., Kelly, K. M., Serra, R. N., & Mathes, E. W. (2008, May). *Lascivious and inebriated: College student enforcement of sex and alcohol norms.* Paper presented at the annual meeting of the Midwestern Psychological Association, Chicago.

Carton, A. D., Young, M. S., & Kelly, K. M. (2008). *Changes in perceived social support and quality of relationships among formerly homeless persons receiving assertive community treatment services.* Manuscript submitted for publication.

Carvallo, M., & Pelham, B. W. (2006). When fiends become friends: The need to belong and perceptions of personal and group discrimination. *Journal of Personality and Social Psychology, 90,* 94–108.

Cheek, J. M., & Buss, A. H. (1981). Shyness and sociability. *Journal of Personality and Social Psychology, 41,* 330–339.

Danheiser, P. R., & Graziano, W. G. (1982). Self-monitoring and cooperation as a self-presentational strategy. *Journal of Personality and Social Psychology, 42,* 497–505.

De Cremer, D., & Leonardelli, G. J. (2003). Cooperation in social dilemmas and the need to belong: The moderating effect of group size. *Group Dynamics: Theory, Research, and Practice, 7,* 168–174.

Downey, G., & Feldman, S. (1996). Implication of rejection sensitivity for intimate relationships. *Journal of Personality and Social Psychology, 70,* 1327–1343.

Edwards, A. L. (1954). *Manual—Edwards Personal Preference Schedule.* New York: Psychological Corporation.

Ferrari, J. R. (1994). Dysfunctional procrastination and its relationship with self-esteem, interpersonal dependency, and self defeating behaviors. *Personality and Individual Differences, 17,* 673–679.

Findley, M. B., & Kelly, K. M. (2008a, March). Procrastination as an indicator of inclusionary status: Delaying work inhibits social connections. In J. Ferrari (Chair), *Revealing the procrastinator's self: Social, personality, cognitive, and perceptual perspectives.* Symposium presented at the annual meeting of the Eastern Psychological Association, Boston.

Findley, M. B., & Kelly, K. M. (2008b, May). *The role of perfectionism in fulfilling the need to belong.* Paper presented at the annual meeting of the Midwestern Psychological Association, Chicago.

Funder, D. C., & Dobroth, K. M. (1987). Differences between traits: Properties associated with interjudge agreement. *Journal of Personality and Social Psychology, 52,* 409–418.

Gardner, W., Jefferies, V. E., & Knowles, M. L. (in press). Never alone: The interdependent self as a buffer from rejection. *Journal of Personality and Social Psychology.*

Gardner, W. L., Pickett, C. L., Jefferies, V., & Knowles, M. (2005). On the outside looking in: Loneliness and social monitoring. *Personality and Social Psychology Bulletin, 31,* 1549–1560.

Gifford, R. (1982). Afilliativeness: A trait measure in relation to single-act and multiple-act behavioral criteria. *Journal of Research in Personality, 16,* 128–134.

Hill, C. A. (1987). Affiliation motivation: People who need people … but in different ways. *Journal of Personality and Social Psychology, 52,* 1008–1018.

Hilton, J. L., & Darley, J. M. (1991). The effects of interaction goals on person perception. In M. P. Zanna (Ed.), *Advances in experimental social psychology* (Vol. 24, pp. 235–267). San Diego, CA: Academic Press.

Jackson, D. N. (1967). *Personality Research Form manual.* Goshen, NY: Research Psychologists Press.

Kelly, K. M. (1999). *Measurement and manifestation of the need to belong.* Unpublished doctoral dissertation, University of Tennessee, Knoxville, TN.

Kelly, K. M. (2008). [Fulfilling belonging needs with Facebook]. Unpublished raw data.

Kelly, K. M., & Tee, A. J. (2005). [Need to belong and interpersonal perception]. Unpublished raw data.

Kelly, K. M., & Tee, A. J. (2006). [Need to belong and personality judgments.] Unpublished raw data.

Kelly, K. M., Tee, A. J., & Ferry, S. (2005, January). *Belongingness and the detection of lies.* Paper presented at the meeting of the Society for Personality and Social Psychology, New Orleans.

Knowles, M. L., & Gardner, W. L. (2003, May). *When the Friends are your friends: Parasocial relationships among individuals with a high need to belong.* Paper presented at the meeting of the Midwestern Psychological Association, Chicago.

Knowles, M. L., & Gardner, W. L. (2006, May). *Parasocial "friendships" among individuals with high belonging needs*. Paper presented at the meeting of the Midwestern Psychological Association, Chicago.

Knowles, M. L., & Gardner, W. L. (2008, February). *"I'll be there for you ... :" Favorite television characters as social surrogates*. Paper presented at the meeting of the Society for Personality and Social Psychology, Albuquerque, NM.

Knowles, M. L., Gardner, W. L., Pickett, C., & Turner, E. (2004, May). *Tuning in: Belonging needs and sensitivity to facial displays*. Paper presented at the meeting of the Midwestern Psychological Association, Chicago.

Koenig, F., & Lessan, G. (1985). Viewers' relationships to television personalities. *Psychological Reports, 57,* 263–266.

Leary, M. R., & Buckley, K. (2000). Social anxiety as an early warning system: A refinement and extension of the self-presentational theory of social anxiety. In S. G. Hofman & P. M. DiBartolo (Eds.), *Social phobia and social anxiety: An integration* (pp. 321–334). New York: Allyn & Bacon.

Leary, M. R., Kelly, K. M., Cottrell, C. A., & Schreindorfer, L. S. (2008). *Individual differences in the need to belong: Mapping the nomological net.* Manuscript submitted for publication.

Leary, M. R., Springer, C., Negel, L., Ansell, E., & Evans, K. (1998). The causes, phenomenology, and consequences of hurt feelings. *Journal of Personality and Social Psychology, 74,* 1225–1237.

Mathes, E. W., Kelly, K. M., & Carton, A. D. (2008). *Are college students punished with social rejection for not drinking heavily and engaging in casual sex?* Manuscript in preparation.

Morrison, K. R., Wheeler, S. C., & Smeesters, D. (2007). Significant other primes and behavior: Motivation to respond to social cues moderates pursuit of prime-induced goals. *Personality and Social Psychology Bulletin, 33,* 24–46.

Murray, H. A. (1938). *Explorations in personality.* New York: Oxford University Press.

Olthof, T., & Goossens, F. A. (2008). Bullying and the need to belong: Early adolescent bullying-related behavior and the acceptance they desire and receive from particular classmates. *Social Development, 17,* 24–46.

Panicia, N. (2000). [A measure of sociotropic breadth]. Unpublished raw data, Wake Forest University, Winston-Salem, NC.

Rose, P., & DeJesus, S. P. (2007). A model of motivated cognition to account for the link between self-monitoring and materialism. *Psychology and Marketing, 24,* 93–115.

Rubin, A. M., Perse, E. M., & Powell, R. A. (1985). Loneliness, parasocial interaction, and local television news viewing. *Human Communication Research, 12,* 155–180.

Stevens, L. E., & Fiske, S. T. (1995). Motivation and cognition in social life: A social survival perspective. *Social Cognition, 13,* 189–214.

Walker, S., Green, L. R., Richardson, D. R., & Hubertz, M. J. (1996, November). *Correlates of the need to belong*. Paper presented at the meeting of the Society of Southeastern Social Psychologists, Virginia Beach, VA.

CHAPTER 28

■ ● ▲ ◆ ■ ● ▲ ◆

Affiliation Motivation

CRAIG A. HILL

The desire to experience and maintain close relations with other people is generally viewed as a core attribute of human beings (Baumeister & Leary, 1995; Leary & Kelly, Chapter 27, this volume). Within social and personality psychology, the desire for warm relations with others is called *affiliation motivation*. Affiliation motivation has been operationalized in slightly different ways by different theorists but is typically conceptualized as the desire to associate and interact with other people, particularly in warm, harmonious ways. Various measures of affiliation motivation differ in the degree to which they focus on the desire for being with other people, for harmonious and warm relationships, or for closeness and intimacy, and some writers have used the term *intimacy motivation* (McAdams, 1980, 1982, 1992) to distinguish a newer measure that emphasizes the desire for closeness from other measures of affiliation motivation that focus on the desire for social interaction. In this chapter, the term *affiliation motivation* is used except when discussing work that explicitly involves intimacy motivation.

One of the most prominent conceptualizations of affiliation motivation was advanced by Murray (1938) within his theory of manifest needs or motives. The theory proposes that twenty fundamental motives underlie all human behavior. A motive is conceived as a psychological force within the individual that directs mental processes and behavior to eliminate unsatisfying conditions and produce a more satisfying state of affairs. One of the 20 core needs within Murray's system is the affiliation motive—the desire to experience "a mutually enjoyed, enduring, harmoniously co-operating and reciprocating relation with another person" (p. 175). In fact, within the body of research based on Murray's theory, the affiliation motive is one of three motives considered to be among the most important, along with the achievement motive (see Conroy, Elliot, & Thrash, Chapter 26, this volume) and the power motive (see Fodor, Chapter 29, this volume; Stewart & Chester, 1982). This is evidenced by the fact that the preponderance of research within this tradition has been devoted to these three motives.

These motive dimensions likewise are identified as core aspects of human personality in the theoretical perspective advanced by Bakan (1966) in the form of two essential trait domains, *agency* and *communion*. Agency is the tendency to strive for or behave in a way that advances an individual's individuality and well-being by asserting and protecting oneself and mastering or controlling one's environment. Both achievement motivation and power motivation may be viewed as aspects of agency. Within this perspective, these types of motivation are referred to as *assertive motivations* (Veroff, 1982).

The trait domain of communion is characterized by a desire and striving for relatedness and connection with others, that is, feeling a sense of union, belonging, and empathy with fellow human beings. Communion also involves mutually felt, reciprocated enjoyment of contact among individuals, as well as compassion, concern, and desire for cooperation. The motivation for affiliation (and intimacy) is therefore clearly a component of the core personality dimension of communion. Sufficient levels of agency are seen as essential to an individual's ability to take care of his or her needs in order to survive and flourish. Yet an extreme degree of agency without an accompanying concern for others and their well-being is thought to be harmful and unhealthy. Extreme agency in the absence of substantial communion is referred to as *unmitigated agency* (Bakan, 1966). Communion, therefore, is considered to be as necessary for health and well-being as agency, with one serving as a balancing and stabilizing force to the other.

Historically, the conceptual linkage between affiliation motivation and achievement motivation as central aspects of human personality has been intensified by their association with issues related to gender. Based on early research on achievement motivation, males were thought to be motivated to achieve success by the prospect of experiencing satisfaction on attaining their own internalized standards of excellence. In contrast, females were thought to be motivated by the prospect of receiving social rewards, such as praise and recognition (Hoffman, 1972; Stein & Bailey, 1973). By extension, males were believed to be motivated primarily by achievement needs, and females were thought to be motivated primarily by affiliation needs (Hoffman, 1972; Kelemen, 1980). Contrary to this early theoretical view, research has demonstrated that the nature of achievement motivation is similar for women and men, although small gender differences in the strength of achievement motives have been documented for self-report measures (Spence & Helmreich, 1983). This issue of gender differences in affiliation motivation is addressed later in this chapter.

Four major conceptualizations of affiliation motivation have spurred a substantial amount of research on the topic. Each perspective is presented individually, along with the measurement instruments developed to investigate the perspective and the evidence that has accumulated to support it.

The Implicit–Motive Perspective

Virtually all conceptualizations of affiliation motivation derive from the Murray theory of manifest needs. The version of this theory that has produced the most prolific program of research is that advanced by McClelland, Atkinson, and their colleagues (McClelland, Atkinson, Clark, & Lowell, 1953). This version incorporated concepts from the learning theory tradition to elaborate on the process by which a motive instigates behavior. Atkinson (1966) described a motive as a tendency to approach a certain class of incentives in order to obtain satisfaction associated with those incentives. Incentives are aspects of behavior, interpersonal interaction, or the environment that provide a pleasurable or rewarding experience. Motives are conceived as being aroused in response to incentives that are available in particular situations; once aroused, motives then influence behavior. The strength of motive arousal is a direct function of the dispositional strength of an individual's motive, that is, the stable, characteristic strength of his or her motive relative to other individuals. Motives are therefore considered to be a type of trait intrinsic to the individual that produce typical patterns of behavior across different situations and over time. Furthermore, individual differences exist in the strength of the various motives.

Implicit versus Self-Attributed Motives

Motives measured through the thematic apperception, or thought-sampling, process have been viewed by advocates of the method as assessing the tendency to obtain pleasure out of engaging in a behavior or activity itself (McClelland, Koestner, & Weinberger, 1992), such as social interaction or expressing intimate feelings for another person (i.e., affiliation). Motives measured in this way have therefore been called *implicit motives*. In contrast, motives measured by self-report methods, such as questionnaires and interviews, are thought to represent conscious, explicitly constructed self-perceptions. Advocates of this perspective, therefore, have called self-reported motivations *self-attributed motives*. Self-attributed motives are thought to be activated and to influence behavior when explicit demand is strong in a social situation, that is, when a social incentive is salient. Drawing on concepts generated within the learning theory tradition, McClelland and his colleagues (1992) proposed that implicit motives reflect operant tendencies (self-generated behavior focused on attaining rewards), whereas self-attributed motives reflect respondent tendencies (reacting to stimuli in the environment).

The basis for the distinction between implicit and self-attributed motives is twofold. First, McClelland and his colleagues (1992) have concluded that scores derived from the Thematic Apperception Test (TAT) assessing a specific motive (such as affiliation motivation, achievement motivation, power motivation) do not correlate to a great extent with scores on self-report questionnaires that assess the same motive. However, Emmons and McAdams (1991) disputed this conclusion. The second basis for the distinction between implicit and self-attributed motives is that measures of the two types of motivation tend to correlate with different kinds of behavior. According to McClelland and colleagues, "implicit motives predict spontaneous behavioral trends over time, whereas self-attributed motives predict immediate specific responses to specific situations or choice behavior" (p. 52). The conclusions reached by McClelland and his colleagues, however, are at odds with those of theorists and researchers who have found stable correlations between self-reported dispositional motivations, including affiliation motivation, with emotions over a 3-year period (Izard, Libero, Putnam, & Haynes, 1993; Wong & Csikszentmihalyi, 1991b).

Perhaps the most useful perspective for understanding the distinction between motivations assessed by the two methods is to consider them to be analogous to implicit and explicit attitudes (Fazio & Olson, 2003; Wilson, Lindsey, & Schooler, 2000). Implicit and explicit attitudes have been conceived as separate and independent systems within the model of dual attitudes (Wilson et al., 2000). Conceiving of implicit and explicit motivation as distinct, relatively independent

systems would account for the differences in patterns of correlations that have been found for the TAT and self-report questionnaires.

The TAT Measure of Affiliation Motivation

The administration of the TAT, sometimes called the Picture Story Exercise (PSE), involves having people write stories concerning situations portrayed in four to six pictures. Scores are assigned to the content of the stories by individuals trained in the coding scheme, which was developed by comparing responses of individuals who were assumed to be in a state of aroused affiliation motivation with the responses of individuals who were thought to be in a state in which affiliation motivation was not aroused (Atkinson, Heyns, & Veroff, 1954; Rosenfeld & Franklin, 1966; Shipley & Veroff, 1952). For example, in the initial studies (Atkinson et al., 1954; Shipley & Veroff, 1952), researchers hypothesized that affiliation motivation was aroused for a group of college men who had just undergone an evaluation by their peers; this was thought to activate thoughts and feelings concerning others, as well as to create desires related to positive relations with others. The coding system involves detecting themes in the stories related to concern about initiating, establishing, and maintaining positive social interactions and relationships. The underlying type of relationship in the themes of the story may be characterized as a concern about having friendly interactions (Heyns, Veroff, & Atkinson, 1992).

Scores on the TAT affiliation motivation scale are generally sufficiently stable, as indicated by test–retest correlations, for relatively short periods of time. Coefficients for scores measured approximately a year apart in two studies were .56 (Lundy, 1985) and .66 (Koestner & Franz, 1989). However, the correlation for scores compared over a 10-year period was only .30 (Koestner & Franz, 1989). Similarly, internal consistency coefficients are frequently not very high for the scoring systems of many of the motive dimensions, including affiliation motivation. Although not specific to affiliation motivation, a review by Entwisle (1972) of evidence regarding the reliability of the achievement motivation scoring system indicates that coefficients are generally in the range of .30 to .40.

Advocates of the TAT method argue that critics have exaggerated the low reliability of the system by including studies in their reviews that were not methodologically sound and by excluding studies with higher reliability (Smith, 1992). Studies that have been based on higher interscorer agreement, that include stimulus pictures that are conceptually relevant to the motivation dimension under consideration, and that have included six or more pictures in the measurement process have obtained internal consistency and stability coefficients in the .50 to .60 range (Smith, 1992).

The stipulations required to elevate internal reliability to acceptable levels indicate that responses on the TAT are sensitive to factors unrelated to the stimulus items (pictures) themselves. In fact, Atkinson and Birch (Atkinson, 1982; Atkinson & Birch, 1970, 1978) explained the low internal consistency by proposing a theory of the dynamics of action. According to this view, rather than a given motive exerting a constant influence, the effects of dispositional motives on behavior vary over time. The reason is that experiencing gratification by engaging in motive-relevant behavior decreases the tendency to engage in the behavior over the interval of time in which the behavior is performed; this is essentially the process of satiation. Writing stories to the TAT stimulus pictures is a behavior that provides gratification relevant to the motive expressed in a given story. Consequently, the influence of the motive on behavior declines as a story is created, allowing other motives to move to the forefront in influencing behavior. The tendency to write themes relevant to the first motive diminishes in subsequent pictures. In other words, the very process of measuring a motive causes the influence of the motive to decline, resulting in variability of motive scores across TAT pictures. Proponents of the TAT thought-sampling method therefore argue that classic test theory, which presumes a stable influence of traits across time, does not pertain to the method. Furthermore, they cite studies demonstrating relationships between TAT motive scores and theoretically predicted behavioral outcomes as evidence for the validity of the thought-sampling method.

Correlates of TAT Affiliation Motivation Scores

As noted, affiliation motivation is conceptualized as a desire for warm, close relations with others. Yet research based on the coding scheme developed in early studies indicated that scores also correlate with negative social tendencies and outcomes (Koestner & McClelland, 1992). Specifically, people who have high affiliation motivation scores are more likely to be unpopular with their peers than those with low scores (Atkinson et al., 1954; Crowne & Marlowe, 1964; Shipley & Veroff, 1952; Skolnick, 1966), and they experience greater social anxiety as well (Byrne, 1962; Mussen & Jones, 1957). In a study of adolescent girls, those with high affiliation motivation scores were quieter, more submissive, and less assertive, qualities that seem inconsistent with the conceptualization of affiliation motivation. Furthermore, women who scored high in affiliation motivation and who were characterized by low self-control and greater life stress had a stronger tendency to physically or psychologically abuse their romantic partners (Skolnick, 1966). People who are high in affiliation motivation are also more likely to have had mothers who did not comfort them as children when they cried at night (McClelland, 1989), suggesting early experience with social rejection. In fact, some writers have suggested that high scores on the TAT affiliation motive dimension may be more accurately conceived as measuring social anxiety, dependency, or fear of rejection (Boyatzis, 1973; Koestner & McClelland, 1992; Shipley & Veroff, 1952).

Nonetheless, people with strong affiliation motivation engage to a greater extent in a wide range of social behaviors, including visiting friends, making phone calls, and writing letters to peers (Boyatzis, 1973; Constantian, 1981; Lansing & Heyns, 1959). People with strong affiliation motivation as measured by the TAT also engage in more interactions throughout the day (McClelland, 1985), including at work (Noujaim, 1968). They are also more likely to desire interaction with other people when they are by themselves (McClelland, 1985), and women with high affiliation motivation scores are more interested in becoming involved in long-term romantic relationships (Bickman, 1975).

People with greater affiliation motivation are more sensitive to social demands and the reactions of others. They are more likely to comply with requests (Walker & Heyns, 1962) and to avoid competitive situations (McClelland, 1975; Terhune, 1968), and they perform more poorly when in competition (Karabenick, 1977). In general, they prefer to avoid conflict with others (Exline, 1962). Such behaviors are consistent with the interpretation of the TAT affiliation motivation dimension as reflecting a concern about negative evaluation by others and a fear of not being liked. Furthermore, the dimension may be characterized as general insecurity and dependency. People with high scores are sensitive to evaluative feedback related to their performance on tasks and desire relationship-relevant feedback rather than competence-related feedback in group activity settings. They also prefer to work with friends rather than with experts (French, 1956). Again, this pattern indicates a concern about receiving information about their competence; friends are more likely to be considerate of, and concerned about, their feelings and to avoid conveying unfavorable information about their performance. Along these lines, people high in affiliation motivation tend to perform better if the focus is on an affiliative outcome. They even obtain better grades in classes led by supportive, caring instructors (McKeachie, 1961).

Intimacy Motivation as an Alternate to Affiliation Motivation

Because the TAT affiliation motivation scoring system assesses the desire to avoid rejection by others, a type of social anxiety, McAdams (1980) developed a scoring system intended to focus more directly on a positive desire for contact with others, as originally conceived by Murray (1938). Intimacy motivation is the desire for "a mutually enjoyed, reciprocal, egalitarian union" (McAdams, 1980, p. 135). According to McAdams (1982, 1992), the theoretical basis for the intimacy scoring system was the conceptualization of Being-Love (B-Love) compared with Deficiency-Love (D-Love) proposed by Maslow (1954, 1968). Being-Love is the desire to share emotional communion with another person who is not concerned with attaining or receiving benefits from the person and who is undemanding and nonintrusive. Being-Love involves joy and satisfaction in the mere experience of the relationship with the other person rather than having an endpoint at which the desire for involvement with the other person is fulfilled and begins to subside. In contrast, Deficiency-Love is concerned with filling a deficit or void in a person's life, and involvement with another person is sought to obtain the resource that is absent. The intimacy motivation that McAdams (1980, 1982, 1992) has conceptualized and assessed through the TAT scoring system is focused on the desire to experience Being-Love.

The procedure employed in measuring intimacy motivation within McAdams's perspective involves creating stories in response to pictures used within the TAT tradition. As with affiliation motivation, the coding scheme was created by comparing responses of individuals who were assumed to be in a state of aroused motivation with those of individuals who were in a state in which intimacy motivation was not aroused. Four samples were initially employed to develop the coding scheme. In one, the individuals thought to be in a state of aroused intimacy motivation were those who had just been inducted into a fraternity or sorority "during friendly, joyful celebrations" (McAdams, 1992, p. 225). The other samples involved individuals at a large dance party, dating couples who had obtained high scores on a self-report measure of being in love, and those who participated in a series of games and discussions that were designed to promote intimacy (McAdams, 1992).

Test–retest reliability of TAT intimacy motivation scores was reported to be .48 for high school students assessed over a 1-year period (Lundy, 1985), a moderate level of stability at best. As is the case for all TAT motive scoring systems, proponents of the TAT method maintain that traditional techniques for assessing reliability are not relevant to evaluating TAT scoring systems (Atkinson, 1992).

Correlates of TAT Intimacy Motivation Scores

In contrast to people who score high in TAT affiliation motivation, those with high intimacy motivation scores are not less popular with their peers. Rather, they are perceived as friendly, sincere, loving, affectionate, and cooperative (McAdams, 1980; McAdams & Losoff, 1984; McAdams & Powers, 1981). People with high intimacy motivation scores display more nonverbal behaviors that promote intimacy and positive feelings, such as eye contact, smiling, and laughter. They are also more likely to include other people in the way they talk (using more words such as *we* and *us* rather than *I* and *me*), as well as more likely to engage all members of a group in discussions. Furthermore, individuals with high intimacy motivation tend to be less controlling and directive in group projects (McAdams & Powers, 1981).

Intimacy motivation as measured by the TAT also relates to positive feelings about relationships and higher quality interactions. In an experience-sampling study in which participants reported their feelings and behaviors throughout the day, greater intimacy motivation was associated with a greater percentage of thoughts about other people and relationships, involvement in a greater number of conversations, and more positive feelings when around others (McAdams & Constantian, 1983). Within friendships, individuals with high intimacy motivation report engaging in more one-on-one interactions, as well as self-disclosing and listening more in conversations with others (McAdams, Healy, & Krause, 1984).

Furthermore, intimacy motivation is associated with psychological well-being and adjustment, as well as psychological health over long periods of time. In one study, intimacy motivation scores obtained for Harvard men in the early 1950s were strongly related to their job satisfaction and happiness with marriage 17 years later (McAdams & Vaillant, 1982). Intimacy motivation has been found in a large study to correlate with self-reported satisfaction with women's roles in life and general happiness (McAdams & Bryant, 1987). Men high in intimacy motivation were less likely to report anxiety, substance abuse, and psychosomatic symptoms. High levels of intimacy motivation may benefit women and men psychologically in different ways, according to McAdams (1989, 1992). Women with a strong desire for intimacy may have a greater sense of identity and self-value, whereas men high in intimacy

motivation may feel more secure and able to explore what they are like as individuals.

The Jackson Perspective

Jackson (1984, 1989) developed a self-report questionnaire, the Personality Research Form (PRF), to measure 20 of the fundamental motivations or needs proposed by Murray (1938). Jackson characterized the fundamental motivations as traits, specifically motivational dispositions, that influence the behaviors in which individuals engage to attain their goals. A number of researchers have employed the PRF to measure individual differences in affiliation motivation to examine issues relevant to the desire for closeness with others, but a systematic program of research has not been conducted within this perspective to document the theoretical framework of dispositional affiliation motivation.

The Measurement of Dispositional Affiliation Motivation

The PRF is a theory-based measure of 20 of the needs proposed by Murray, comprising 352 items in the version called PRF-E (that is, form E). After the creation of an initial pool of items, the instrument was developed based on psychometric principles to hone its empirical properties and construct validity. The items consist of statements to which respondents indicate *true* or *false* with respect to whether a given statement describes their typical proclivity or behavior. Examples of statements measuring affiliation motivation are "I try to be in the company of friends as much as possible," "Sometimes I have to make a real effort to be social" (reverse scored), and "I spend lots of time visiting friends."

The PRF-E scales were constructed by narrowing an initial pool of 100 items per scale down to 20 items each (Helmes & Jackson, 1977). Statements were eliminated based on empirical criteria to reduce social desirability and redundancy, maximize the internal consistency of each scale, and minimize the similarity of items on one scale to those of other scales (enhancing discriminant validity). Factor analysis of the PRF has demonstrated extremely high factorial integrity of the instrument in that all but two of the items loaded on the theoretically expected factor and did not load substantially on the other factors. The mean factor loading of affiliation motivation items on the affiliation motivation scale was .39, whereas the mean factor loading of these items on other scales was .09.

Correlates of the PRF Affiliation Motivation Scale

A number of studies employing the PRF in general (as opposed to focusing on the affiliation motivation scale) are concerned with psychometric issues involving the comparison of personality measures with one another and establishing the construct validity of measures. A bibliography available from the Research Psychologists Press, which publishes the PRF, attests to the largely psychometric focus of much research (SIGMA Assessment Systems, 2008). Only a few studies have examined affiliation motivation in particular.

The PRF affiliation motivation scale has been shown to correlate with the expressivity scale of the Personal Attributes Questionnaire (Spence, Helmreich, & Stapp, 1975), a measure of expressiveness or communion (Moneta & Csikszentmihalyi, 2003). Communion was discussed previously as one of two core aspects of personality, the one with which affiliation motivation is strongly aligned conceptually and theoretically. Characteristics constituting the measure of expressiveness are *understanding of others, aware of the feelings of others, kind, able to devote self completely to others, helpful to others, gentle, warm in relations to others,* and *emotional.* As would be expected, high school students with stronger dispositional affiliation motivation as measured by the PRF more often wished to be with friends and less often wanted to be alone (Wong & Csikszentmihalyi, 1991a).

On the other hand, the affiliation motivation scale is negatively related to measures of narcissism, which involves being dominant, feeling a sense of entitlement, possessing inflated self-worth, and yet being dependent on social approval and sensitive to being slighted or rejected (Sturman, 2000). Scores on the PRF affiliation motivation scale were negatively correlated with the Superior-ity/Arrogance and Exploitive/Entitlement subscales of the Narcissistic Personality Inventory (Raskin & Hall, 1979). The affiliation motivation scale was additionally negatively associated with the Narcissism–Hypersensitivity Scale (Serkownek, 1975) and the Ego Sensitivity Scale, both measures of covert narcissism (Pepper & Strong, 1958).

Although people generally prefer coworkers who are highly affiliative, people with strong affiliation motivation have even greater preference for working with affiliative colleagues (Tett & Murphy, 2002). Furthermore, affiliation motivation affects a range of issues related to working with others on tasks. Klein and Pridemore (1992) examined the effects of cooperating with another person on a learning project among a sample of education majors in college. Participants who scored high in affiliation motivation performed more poorly on a test of knowledge following the learning project when they worked on the project by themselves compared with working with a partner. The authors suggested that the involvement of other people influences the task-related motivation of learners with high affiliation motivation. Social interaction may make the task more interesting for those who desire close interaction with others. As an aside, individuals with low affiliation motivation spent more time working on the project overall and performed better on the test of knowledge, regardless of whether they worked alone or with a partner, possibly as a result of more time investment.

In a follow-up study (Klein & Schnackenberg, 2000), participants with low affiliation motivation expressed a greater desire to work alone on projects in the future, whereas those with high affiliation motivation indicated more interest in working with a partner on future projects. Dyads high in affiliation motivation also engaged in more task-related group behaviors than dyads low in affiliation motivation, although they also engaged in more behaviors that were irrelevant to task progress. In this study, no effect was found for affiliation motivation on knowledge attained or on a task involving application of knowledge.

Affiliation motivation is also related to people's expectations about a task, even before beginning it. Stronger affiliation motivation was associated with a tendency to emphasize the affiliative aspects of an upcoming project in which individuals were to teach others about incorporating software packages in workplace and school settings (Griner & Smith, 2000). This occurred despite the fact that the project was designed to involve both achievement-related features and affiliation-related features. However, people with stronger affiliation motivation additionally appraised the task-related (achievement) aspects as especially important and anticipated experiencing greater interest and less boredom during the project than participants who were low in affiliation motivation.

Affiliation motivation as measured by the PRF predicted improvement in psychological symptoms of 33 inpatients over the course of a 3-week group psychotherapy program (Ratto & Hurley, 1995). Psychological symptoms—as indicated by two measures—declined over the course of psychotherapy. Dispositional affiliation motivation was negatively associated with both measures of posttest symptoms at a substantial level. Ratto and Hurley (1995) speculated that inpatients who were high in affiliation motivation may have felt less threatened in the group therapy setting, contributing to a heightened sense of security, compared with patients low in affiliation motivation. Individuals low in affiliation motivation may need special assistance in developing trust in such interpersonal situations.

Reprising the issue of implicit and explicit motivation, Hofer and colleagues (Hofer, Busch, Chasiotis, & Kiessling, 2006) demonstrated that congruence between implicit affiliation motivation and explicit affiliation motivation was related to individuals' level of identity achievement. Implicit motivation was assessed with the TAT method, and explicit motivation was measured with the PRF. Specifically, people with high levels of both implicit and explicit motivation were more likely to be classified in the identity achievement status, as opposed to moratorium, foreclosure, and diffusion statuses (Marcia, 1994). Identity achievement involves having a meaningful commitment to one's own values and goals after a period of exploration. The other statuses involve lower commitment or less personal exploration to achieve the commitment, or lower

levels of both commitment and exploration. Those with low implicit affiliation motivation did not tend to differ in terms of identity status, regardless of their standing in terms of explicit affiliation motivation. Explicit affiliation motivation was positively associated with identity achievement, although this was not the case for implicit motivation. Congruence of implicit and explicit motives may permit people to develop a self-concept and identity that straightforwardly and accurately reflects the characteristics that they possess.

Congruence of motivations between people are likewise important with respect to interpersonal relationships. Meyer and Pepper (1977) found that married couples characterized by greater adjustment were those in which the individuals were more similar to one another with respect to motives for affiliation, aggression, autonomy, and nurturance. No evidence was found to support the notion of complementarity, that individuals who have opposite types of needs are better suited for one another in relationships.

The Mehrabian Two-Motive Perspective

Mehrabian (1970) developed two measures that are potentially relevant to understanding affiliation motivation—one designed to assess affiliative tendency (MAFF) and the other to assess sensitivity to rejection (MSR). Affiliative tendency is the disposition to have generalized positive expectations about social relationships, to anticipate that social interactions will be pleasant and rewarding, and to engage in behavior based on these positive expectations. In contrast, sensitivity to rejection is the disposition to have generalized negative expectations about social relationships, to be fearful and apprehensive that social interactions will produce rejection and pain, and to engage in behavior based on these negative expectations. The two dimensions are conceptualized as independent rather than as opposing tendencies (Mehrabian, 1994).

However, empirical evidence indicates that sensitivity to rejection is not an element of, nor relevant to, affiliation motivation at all. Instead, it is virtually equivalent to dispositional dominance, or possibly power motivation, in the reverse direction. Consequently, it is not considered further in this section.

The MAFF is a self-report questionnaire that was developed from an initial pool of items drawn from other measures and new items written specifically for the scale. The final items were selected based on several rounds of analysis and modification of items. It consists of 26 items that may be grouped into a number of correlated factors. The MAFF possesses adequate internal consistency and substantial test–retest reliability and is only slightly correlated with measures of social desirability (Mehrabian, 1994).

Correlates of the MAFF

The MAFF correlates with other measures of affiliation motivation, as well as other measures that are conceptually related to affiliation motivation. These include scales that measure liking for other people in general, belief in the goodness of people, concern for the welfare of others, and willingness to self-disclose. The scale is also highly correlated with the Jackson PRF affiliation motivation scale. Scales inversely related to the MAFF assess the inability to experience pleasure in social relationships, loneliness or the absence of social contacts, social alienation, avoidance of social contacts related to discomfort around others, and general anxiety. The MAFF is also somewhat correlated with psychological well-being (Mehrabian, 1994).

People with higher scores on the MAFF tend to assume that others will have similar attitudes to theirs (Mehrabian & Ksionzky, 1971) and to perceive that individuals with whom they have interacted have similar attitudes (Mehrabian & Ksionzky, 1985). They likewise assume that they are compatible with a variety of different types of individuals (Mehrabian & Ksionzky, 1971), possibly as a result of the tendency to perceive others as similar to them. In the same vein, people who are high in affiliative tendency perceive another person who has been portrayed in an ambiguous way with respect to affiliative tendencies as more affiliative (Solar & Mehrabian, 1973).

As would be expected of those with stronger affiliation motivation, people who have higher scores on the MAFF engage in more affiliative behaviors during spontaneous social interaction (Ksionzky & Mehrabian, 1980; Mehrabian, 1971; Mehrabian & Diamond, 1971; Mehrabian & Ksionzky, 1972). This is true under conditions of anxiety-provoking social situations, as well, such as when pairs of men and women believed that they would evaluate each other regarding their social attractiveness. In a study that evaluated social behavior in such a setting, people who scored high in affiliative tendency engaged in more positive affiliative behaviors. In the process, they made their partners more relaxed, were liked more, and elicited more affiliative behaviors from their partners (Mehrabian & Ksionzky, 1985).

A Multidimensional Model of Affiliation Motivation

The approaches discussed thus far view affiliation motivation as a monolithic trait, but evidence suggests that people may be motivated to affiliate with others for a number of distinct reasons that have implications for understanding their behavior. To address this possibility, Hill (1987) proposed the multidimensional model of affiliation motivation, which maintains that motivation for interpersonal closeness and intimacy consists of four different, but related, desires, specifically the desires for (1) positive stimulation, (2) emotional support, (3) social comparison, and (4) attention. The rationale for this more detailed view of affiliation motivation is that understanding of motivation is enhanced by distinguishing among factors that motivate a general class of behavior (Buss, 1986; Foa & Foa, 1974; Spence & Helmreich, 1983; Veroff, 1986). As Atkinson (1966) observed, "The names of given motives—such as achievement—are really classes of incentives which produce essentially the same kind of experience of satisfaction. ... The general aim of one class of motives ... is to maximize satisfaction of some kind" (p. 13). Veroff (1986) noted additional advantages of proposing a more nuanced view of subtypes of motives, such as documenting developmental trends in which one aspect of a motive increases or decreases while other aspects change in different ways or remain the same. Additionally, differentiation among various motive subtypes is likely to permit more accurate prediction of the influence of social situations on behavior.

Murray (1938) and a variety of social psychologists, as well as related empirical research, provide a basis for identifying desire for positive stimulation, emotional support, social comparison, and attention as specific aspects of affiliation motivation (see Hill, 1987, for a discussion of the theoretical issues justifying the four proposed motive subtypes).

The *positive stimulation* aspect of affiliation motivation is the desire to obtain pleasant affective and cognitive stimulation from contact and interaction with others. This is the desire to receive gratification from harmonious relationships and a sense of communion. It involves a desire for affection, love, intimacy, and belongingness. The *emotional support* aspect of affiliation motivation is the desire to obtain relief from stressful or fearful situations by receiving sympathy, compassion, and nurturance from others. The *social comparison* aspect of affiliation motivation is the desire to reduce uncertainty, ambiguity, and confusion through obtaining information about others' behavior, attitudes, opinions, and expectations. The *attention* aspect of affiliation motivation is the desire to be held in high regard and to receive praise and adulation from other people (Hill, 1987).

A Measure of the Four Aspects of Affiliation Motivation

The Interpersonal Orientation Scale (IOS), a self-report questionnaire, was designed to measure each of the four subtypes of affiliation motivation (Hill, 1987). The development process involved writing statements that reflected the four proposed motive subtypes. The response format was a 5-point Likert scale with response anchors ranging from "Not at all true" to "Completely True" in reference to the extent to which each statement describes a respondent's typical feelings. Through a series of analyses of the items, subsequent revision of the wording of a few statements, and elimination of others, a final set of 26 items was obtained. The proposed model of four affiliation motive subtypes was supported by factor analyses of responses from two large samples. Factor solutions were extremely similar for women

and men. (Additionally, a fifth set of items was constructed to represent a dimension of interpersonal skills to establish that motivation is different from social ability. Factor analyses supported this proposal in that the interpersonal skill items loaded distinctly on a separate factor in all analyses.) The four scales are moderately correlated with one another, ranging from .27 to .58. Internal consistency coefficients (alphas) in the initial study (Hill, 1987) ranged from .70 for the Social Comparison scale for men to .86 for the Emotional Support scale for men; most were .78 or above.

Correlates of the Four IOS Scales

All four scales were correlated with sociability, the tendency to self-disclose during interactions with others, emotional vulnerability (being needful of others' approval), and self-monitoring (the tendency to attend to social cues and to modify behavior to conform with social expectations). The Positive Stimulation scale and the Emotional Support scale were especially strongly associated with sociability, as well as measures of expressivity (or communion; Bakan, 1966) and empathic concern (the tendency to experience the same emotions others are believed to be experiencing); the Social Comparison scale and Attention scale were not correlated with expressivity or empathic concern. On the other hand, the Social Comparison and Attention scales were associated with public self-consciousness, the tendency to focus on oneself when in the presence of others; the other two affiliation motivation scales were not correlated with this dimension (Hill, 1987). All four scales were moderately positively correlated with sociotropy (Clark, Steer, Beck, & Ross, 1995), the tendency to be extremely committed to the importance of positive social interactions (Beck, 1987).

The discriminant validity of the IOS scales was established by the absence of correlations with measures that were theoretically and conceptually unrelated to affiliation motivation. These included a measure of instrumentality or agency (the counterpart to communion; Bakan, 1966), achievement motivation, self-esteem, shyness, and social desirability (need for approval).

The discriminant validity of each scale was also established in the initial study by

Hill (1987) through a procedure in which individuals imagined how they would behave in four situations described in vignettes. Each vignette portrayed a situation that is specifically relevant to one of the affiliation motivation subtypes but less relevant to the other affiliation motivation subtypes. As predicted, the vignette about a party situation was most highly associated with the Positive Stimulation scale, whereas the vignette about a stressful, frightening situation was most strongly correlated with the Emotional Support scale. The vignette about a job interview emphasizing one's capabilities relative to others was most highly correlated with the Social Comparison scale. Finally, the vignette about concern over receiving recognition for one's contribution on a project at work was most strongly associated with the Attention scale.

All four aspects of affiliation motivation are correlated with affect intensity (Blankstein, Flett, Koledin, & Bortolotto, 1989). Those with stronger affiliative needs have a tendency to experience more intense emotions. This finding supports the position that interaction with others provides a source of stimulation that some people desire more strongly.

One line of research has focused on the affiliation motivation component of desire for emotional support because of its direct relevance to coping with stress and enhancing well-being. Individuals with stronger desire for emotional support were shown to express greater desire to discuss personal problems with another person only when that person was warm and compassionate. When the other person was viewed as not at all warm and compassionate, those with strong emotional support need were extremely averse to talking about their problems (Hill, 1991). In contrast, those who were low in the desire for emotional support did not distinguish between the two types of confidants, being only moderately interested in talking with either person. A similar effect was obtained for the Positive Stimulation scale. The results of the study are consistent with the incentive view of motivation in that individuals with high motivation are interested primarily in interactions that provide desired incentives (such as warmth and support).

A follow-up study (Hill, 1996) examined the influence of both the desire for emotional support and interpersonal skill on the nature of interaction between pairs of unacquainted individuals. The interactions focused on personal problems that each individual was currently experiencing or that were still of concern to them. The emotional support aspect of affiliation motivation was associated with a greater tendency to express understanding, offer encouragement, and compliment their partners, three responses that reflect emotional support (Cohen & Wills, 1985). Analyses indicated that individuals with a strong need for emotional support provided greater levels of emotional support to their partners, regardless of whether the partners reciprocated or not.

Highly interpersonally skilled participants were more likely to discuss ways for the partners to deal effectively with emotions related to their problems as well as to offer more suggestions, a type of informational support. Interpersonally skilled individuals engaged in both types of behaviors (discussing ways to deal with negative emotions and making suggestions) to a greater extent regardless of whether the partners reciprocated with similar types of behavior that focused on the interpersonally skilled individuals' problems.

This set of findings indicates that people who desire emotional support are not self-centered or self-indulgent, focusing only on their own problems. In fact, this type of individual provided greater emotional support to his or her partner despite the fact that some partners did not offer emotional support to them. People with strong interpersonal skills focused primarily on strategies for helping the partners deal effectively with their negative emotions. This finding indicates that interpersonally skilled individuals possess the sensitivity, confidence, and expertise necessary to carry out helping behaviors effectively.

Dispositional affiliation motivation has also been shown to relate to cancer patients' interest in receiving emotional support from their spouses, specifically, having their spouses show concern and provide comfort (Manne, Alfieri, Taylor, & Dougherty, 1999). Affiliation motivation was not associated with an interest in receiving instrumental support (providing assistance with treatment, doing chores), however. This study examined the joint effects of the Emotional

Support scale, the Positive Stimulation scale, and the Attention scale in a path analysis model.

The dispositional motivation to affiliate for emotional support is additionally associated with perceptions of the quality of emotional support that people receive from family members and friends (Hill, 1997). Specifically, people with stronger emotional support needs were more satisfied with their support providers, but only if the providers were perceived as possessing greater expressiveness (communion), such as being warm, sensitive, and compassionate. If providers were not emotionally expressive, participants expressed less satisfaction than those who had lower motivation to affiliate to obtain emotional support. This pattern is consistent with the findings of the Hill (1991) study, in that people with a high desire for emotional support are sensitive to and selective about the quality of the experiences they have with others.

Affiliation motivation in the pursuit of positive social stimulation also contributes to the organizational identification of virtual employees, employees in a company who work outside of traditional centralized offices, such as in their homes. Employees with a stronger desire for positive social stimulation report higher levels of organizational identification. However, even those with a lower desire for social stimulation express strong identification when they feel that they receive support from colleagues and supervisors (Wiesenfeld, Raghuram, & Garud, 2001). Other research has demonstrated that perceived organizational support—the sense that one's employer values one's contributions and cares about one's well-being—affects work-related performance primarily for those with stronger dispositional affiliation motivation (Armeli, Eisenberger, Fasolo, & Lynch, 1998). The explanation proposed by the authors for this qualified relationship is that workers who feel valued, and especially those who are concerned about social relationships, feel an obligation to repay the organization. In this study, state police patrol officers with stronger desires for emotional support, attention, and positive stimulation who felt supported by their employers made more arrests for driving under the influence of alcohol and gave more citations for speeding. No such effect for perceived organiza-

tional support was found for officers with lower affiliation motivation.

Gender Differences

Evidence regarding gender differences in dispositional affiliation motivation as assessed by projective measures is generally inconclusive (Wong & Csikszentmihalyi, 1991a). Some studies based on projective measures have found no differences (Chusmir, 1985; Hyland & Mancini, 1985), whereas others have found that women have higher affiliation motivation than men (Agrawal & Upadhyay, 1983; McAdams & Constantian, 1983; McAdams, Lester, Brand, McNamara, & Lensky, 1988; Schroth, 1985). Thus a major review of research concerning the TAT measure of affiliation motivation led Stewart and Chester (1982) to conclude that the evidence is inconsistent regarding gender differences. Nonetheless, in another review, Minton and Schneider (1980) concluded that women obtain higher scores on projective measures. One factor that may contribute to inconsistent findings is the fact that projective measures typically possess relatively low internal consistency and test–retest reliability (Entwisle, 1972; Koestner & Franz, 1989).

In contrast, studies based on self-report questionnaires of affiliation motivation generally find gender differences, with women scoring higher than men (Minton & Schneider, 1980; Moffitt, Spence, & Goldney, 1986; Schroth, 1985; Wong & Csikszentmihalyi, 1991a). An important caveat to this conclusion is that gender differences actually occur as a function of the particular aspect of affiliation motivation. Within the multidimensional model of affiliation motivation (Hill, 1987), women usually have higher scores than men on the Positive Stimulation scale and the Emotional Support scale, although men are typically no different from women with respect to scores on the Social Comparison scale and the Attention scale.

The positive social stimulation and emotional support aspects are highly similar to the broader personality dimension of communion or expressivity. The positive social stimulation aspect is most likely the component of affiliation motivation that other, more general measures tap. The social comparison and attention aspects of affiliation motivation appear to represent other components of the interpersonal domain that overlap with communion but are more self-focused. That is, they involve concerns more directed at ensuring one's own well-being than do the positive stimulation and emotional support dimensions. Recall that the emotional support aspect of affiliation motivation involves a strong reciprocal concern for the emotional well-being of others (Hill, 1996).

Conclusion

Substantial evidence supports the construct of affiliation motivation as conceived originally by Murray (1938) in its various incarnations. These include (1) the implicit-motive perspective within the McClelland–Atkinson–McAdams tradition, (2) the Jackson perspective, (3) the Mehrabian perspective (at least with respect to the construct of affiliative tendency), and (4) the Hill multidimensional model of affiliation motivation. The two exceptions that have not received support as versions of the Murray conception of affiliation motivation are (1) the initial construct assessed by the TAT scoring system for affiliation motivation devised by Shipley and Veroff (1952) and (2) the construct of sensitivity to rejection proposed by Mehrabian (1970).

The personality dimension assessed by the original TAT scoring system is characterized by negative social proclivities, such as unpopularity, social anxiety, reticence, submissiveness, unassertiveness, and compliance. This type of anxiety involves insecurity about one's qualities and a concern about rejection and being harmed; people with high scores on this dimension want to avoid conflict and competition. When under stress, they may be more likely to abuse individuals who are close to them.

These attributes are similar to those associated with sensitivity to rejection as proposed by Mehrabian (1970). Although he identified the dimension as the opposite pole of dominance (that is, submissiveness), sensitivity to rejection also encompasses insecurity, social anxiety, brittleness, and emotional vulnerability. These characteristics are not consistent with the construct of

affiliation motivation as conceptualized by other theorists, including McAdams, Jackson, Mehrabian, and Hill. In fact, sensitivity to rejection scores are unrelated to affiliative tendency scores. Moreover, TAT research has indicated that lower intimacy motivation is not characteristically associated with a "fear of intimacy," which was proposed by early theorists as the reason that men obtain lower dispositional intimacy scores on average than women (McAdams, 1992). Sensitivity to rejection and fear of intimacy are clearly different constructs from affiliation motivation.

Finally, the multidimensional model of affiliation motivation provides a more detailed and nuanced view of dispositional interests and desires that motivate people to seek positive interaction with others. All four motivation dimensions correlate with measures of sociability, self-disclosure, and the tendency to be sensitive to social cues from others. Yet each dimension displays a different pattern of relationships with factors and situations specific to a given dimension, which has been established by research demonstrating their discriminant validity.

The motivation for positive social stimulation is associated more strongly than the other motivational dimensions with interest in entertaining and fun social settings, such as parties, despite the fact that it is also related to a desire for intimacy and communion. The motivation for emotional support is associated at a higher level with interest in receiving comfort and solace in stressful or frightening situations while also being related to a desire for intimacy and to provide comfort to others. The dispositional motivation for social comparison is more strongly correlated with the desire to obtain self-relevant information in an ambiguous setting than the other motivational dimensions, while also being associated with a desire to socialize with others in general. Finally, the motivation to receive attention from others is related at a higher level with the desire to seek recognition and praise, although it, too, is linked to a desire to be sociable in general. Targeting specific aspects of the motivation to affiliate permits greater precision in understanding and predicting social behavior while also recognizing the complexity and richness of social motivation and behavior.

References

Agrawal, T. D., & Upadhyay, S. N. (1983). Sex and age differences in affiliation behavior. *Psychological Studies, 28*, 25–29.

Armeli, S., Eisenberger, R., Fasolo, P., & Lynch, P. (1998). Perceived organizational support and police performance: The moderating influence of socioemotional needs. *Journal of Applied Psychology, 83*, 288–297.

Atkinson, J. W. (1966). Motivational determinants of risk-taking behavior. In J. W. Atkinson & N. T. Feather (Eds.), *A theory of achievement motivation* (pp. 11–29). New York: Wiley.

Atkinson, J. W. (1982). Motivational determinants of thematic apperception. In A. J. Stewart (Ed.), *Motivation and society: A volume in honor of David C. McClelland* (pp. 3–40). San Francisco: Jossey-Bass.

Atkinson, J. W. (1992). Motivational determinants of thematic apperception. In C. P. Smith (Ed.), *Motivation and personality: Handbook of thematic content analysis* (pp. 21–48). New York: Cambridge University Press.

Atkinson, J. W., & Birch, D. (1970). *The dynamics of action.* New York: Wiley.

Atkinson, J. W., & Birch, D. (1978). *An introduction to motivation* (2nd ed.). New York: Van Nostrand.

Atkinson, J. W., Heyns, R. W., & Veroff, J. (1954). The effect of experimental arousal of the affiliation motive on thematic apperception. *Journal of Abnormal and Social Psychology, 49*, 277–288.

Bakan, D. (1966). *The duality of human existence.* Boston: Beacon Press.

Baumeister, R. F., & Leary, M. R. (1995). The need to belong: Desire for interpersonal attachments as a fundamental human motivation. *Psychological Bulletin, 117*, 497–529.

Beck, A. T. (1987). Cognitive model of depression. *Journal of Cognitive Psychotherapy, 1*, 2–27.

Bickman, L. D. (1975). *Personality constructs of senior women planning to marry or to live independently soon after college.* Unpublished doctoral dissertation, University of Pennsylvania.

Blankstein, K. R., Flett, G. L., Koledin, S., & Bortolotto, R. (1989). Affect intensity and dimensions of affiliation motivation. *Personality and Individual Differences, 10*, 1201–1203.

Boyatzis, R. E. (1973). Affiliation motivation. In D. C. McClelland & R. S. Steele (Eds.), *Human motivation: A book of readings* (pp. 252–276). Morristown, NJ: General Learning Press.

Buss, A. H. (1986). *Social behavior and personality.* Hillsdale, NJ: Erlbaum.

Byrne, D. (1961). Anxiety and the experimental arousal of affiliation need. *Journal of Abnormal and Social Psychology, 63*, 660–662.

Chusmir, L. H. (1985). Motivation of managers: Is gender a factor? *Psychology of Women Quarterly, 9*, 153–159.

Clark, D. A., Steer, R. A., Beck, A. T., & Ross, L. (1995). Psychometric characteristics of revised sociotropy and autonomy scales in college students. *Behaviour Research and Therapy, 33*, 325–334.

Cohen, S., & Wills, T. A. (1985). Stress, social support, and the buffering hypothesis. *Psychological Bulletin, 98*, 310–357.

Constantian, C. A. (1981). *Attitudes, beliefs, and behavior in regard to spending time alone.* Unpublished doctoral dissertation, Harvard University.

Crowne, D. P., & Marlowe, D. (1964). *The approval motive.* New York: Wiley.

Depue, R. A. (2006). Interpersonal behavior and the structure of personality: Neurobehavioral foundation of agentic extraversion and affiliation. In T. Canli (Ed.), *Biology of personality and individual differences* (pp. 60–92). New York: Guilford Press.

Emmons, R. A., & McAdams, D. P. (1991). Personal strivings and motive dispositions: Exploring the links. *Personality and Social Psychology Bulletin, 17*, 648–654.

Entwisle, D. R. (1972). To dispel fantasies about fantasy-based measures of achievement motivation. *Psychological Bulletin, 77*, 377–391.

Exline, R. V. (1962). Need affiliation and initial communication behavior in problem solving groups characterized by low interpersonal visibility. *Psychological Reports, 10*, 79–89.

Fazio, R. H., & Olson, M. A. (2003). Implicit measures in social cognition research: Their meaning and uses. *Annual Review of Psychology, 54*, 297–327.

Foa, U. G., & Foa, E. B. (1974). *Social structures of the mind.* Springfield, IL: Thomas.

French, E. G. (1956). Motivation as a variable in work-partner selection. *Journal of Abnormal and Social Psychology, 53*, 96–99.

Griner, L. A., & Smith, C. A. (2000). Contributions of motivational orientation to appraisal and emotion. *Personality and Social Psychology Bulletin, 26*, 727–740.

Helmes, E., & Jackson, D. N. (1977). The item factor structure of the Personality Research Form. *Applied Psychological Measurement, 1*, 185–194.

Heyns, R. W., Veroff, J., & Atkinson, J. W. (1992). A scoring manual for the affiliation motive. In C. P. Smith (Ed.), *Motivation and personality: Handbook of thematic content analysis* (pp. 211–223). New York: Cambridge University Press.

Hill, C. A. (1987). Affiliation motivation: People who need people .. but in different ways. *Journal of Personality and Social Psychology, 52*, 1008–1018.

Hill, C. A. (1991). Seeking emotional support: The influence of affiliative need and partner warmth. *Journal of Personality and Social Psychology, 60*, 112–121.

Hill, C. A. (1996). Interpersonal and dispositional influences on problem-related interactions. *Journal of Research in Personality, 30*, 1–22.

Hill, C. A. (1997). Relationship of expressive and affiliative personality dispositions to perceptions of social support. *Basic and Applied Social Psychology, 19*, 133–161.

Hofer, J., Busch, H., Chasiotis, A., & Kiessling, F. (2006). Motive congruence and interpersonal identity status. *Journal of Personality, 74*, 511–541.

Hoffman, L. W. (1972). Early childhood experiences and women's achievement motives. *Journal of Social Issues, 28*, 129–155.

Hyland, M. E., & Mancini, A. V. (1985). Fear of success and affiliation. *Psychological Reports, 57*, 714.

Izard, C. E., Libero, D. Z., Putnam, P., & Haynes, O. M. (1993). Stability of emotion experiences and their relations to traits of personality. *Journal of Personality and Social Psychology, 64,* 847–860.

Jackson, D. N. (1984). *Personality Research Form manual.* Port Huron, MI: Research Psychologists Press.

Jackson, D. N. (1989). *Personality Research Form manual* (4th ed.). Goshen, NY: Research Psychologists Press.

Karabenick, S. A. (1977). Fear of success, achievement and affiliative dispositions, and the performance of men and women under individual and competitive situations. *Journal of Personality, 45,* 117–149.

Kelemen, V. P., Jr. (1980). Achievement and affiliation: A motivational perspective of sex differences. *Social Behavior and Personality, 8,* 1–11.

Klein, J. D., & Pridemore, D. R. (1992). Effects of co-operative learning and need for affiliation on performance, time on task, and satisfaction. *Education Technology Research and Development, 40*(4), 39–47.

Klein, J. D., & Schnackenberg, H. L. (2000). Effects of informal cooperative learning and the affiliation motive on achievement, attitude, and student interactions. *Contemporary Educational Psychology, 25,* 332–341.

Koestner, R., & Franz, C. (1989, March). *Life changes and the reliability of TAT motive assessment.* Paper presented at the meeting of the Eastern Psychological Association, Boston.

Koestner, R., & McClelland, D. C. (1992). The affiliation motive. In C. P. Smith (Ed.), *Motivation and personality: Handbook of thematic content analysis* (pp. 205–210). New York: Cambridge University Press.

Ksionzky, S., & Mehrabian, A. (1980). Personality correlates of self-disclosure. *Social Behavior and Personality, 8,* 145–152.

Lansing, J. B., & Heyns, R. W. (1959). Need affiliation and frequency of four types of communication. *Journal of Abnormal and Social Psychology, 58,* 365–372.

Lundy, A. (1985). The reliability of the Thematic Apperception Test. *Journal of Personality Assessment, 49*(2), 141–145.

Manne, S., Alfieri, T., Taylor, K., & Dougherty, J. (1999). Preferences for spousal support among individuals with cancer. *Journal of Applied Social Psychology, 29,* 722–749.

Marcia, J. E. (1994). The empirical study of ego identity. In H. A. Bosma, T. L. G. Graafsma, H. D. Grotevant, & D. J. De Levita (Eds.), *Identity and development: An interdisciplinary approach* (pp. 67–79). Thousand Oaks, CA: Sage.

Maslow, A. H. (1954). *Motivation and personality.* New York: Harper & Row.

Maslow, A. H. (1968). *Toward a psychology of being.* New York: Van Nostrand.

McAdams, D. P. (1980). A thematic coding system for the intimacy motive. *Journal of Research in Personality, 14,* 413–432.

McAdams, D. P. (1982). Intimacy motivation. In A. J. Stewart (Ed.), *Motivation and society: A volume in honor of David C. McClelland* (pp. 133–171). San Francisco: Jossey-Bass.

McAdams, D. P. (1989). *Intimacy: The need to be close.* New York: Doubleday.

McAdams, D. P. (1992). The intimacy motive. In C.

P. Smith (Ed.), *Motivation and personality: Handbook of thematic content analysis* (pp. 224–253). New York: Cambridge University Press.

McAdams, D. P., & Bryant, F. (1987). Intimacy motivation and subjective mental health in a nationwide sample. *Journal of Personality, 55,* 395–413.

McAdams, D. P., & Constantian, C. A. (1983). Intimacy and affiliation motives in daily living: An experience sampling analysis. *Journal of Personality and Social Psychology, 45,* 851–861.

McAdams, D. P., Healy, S., & Krause, S. (1984). Social motives and patterns of friendship. *Journal of Personality and Social Psychology, 41,* 828–838.

McAdams, D. P., Lester, R. M., Brand, P. A., McNamara, W. J., & Lensky, D. B. (1988). Sex and the TAT: Are women more intimate than men? Do men fear intimacy? *Journal of Personality Assessment, 52,* 397–409.

McAdams, D. P., & Losoff, M. (1984). Friendship motivation in fourth- and sixth-graders: A thematic analysis. *Journal of Social and Personal Relationships, 1,* 11–27.

McAdams, D. P., & Powers, J. (1981). Themes of intimacy in behavior and thought. *Journal of Personality and Social Psychology, 40,* 573–587.

McAdams, D. P., & Vaillant, G. E. (1982). Intimacy motivation and psychosocial adjustment: A longitudinal study. *Journal of Personality Assessment, 46,* 586–593.

McClelland, D. C. (1975). *Power: The inner experience.* New York: Irvington (Halsted Press/Wiley).

McClelland, D. C. (1985). *Human motivation.* Glenview, IL: Scott, Foresman.

McClelland, D. C. (1989). Motivational factors in health and disease. *American Psychologist, 44,* 675–683.

McClelland, D. C., Atkinson, J. W., Clark, R. A., & Lowell, E. L. (1953). *The achievement motive.* New York: Appleton-Century-Crofts.

McClelland, D. C., Koestner, R., & Weinberger, J. (1992). How do self-attributed and implicit motives differ? In C. P. Smith (Ed.), *Motivation and personality: Handbook of thematic content analysis* (pp. 49–72). New York: Cambridge University Press.

McKeachie, W. J. (1961). Motivation, teaching methods, and college learning. In M. R. Jones (Ed.), *Nebraska Symposium on Motivation: 1961* (Vol. 9, pp. 111–142). Lincoln: University of Nebraska Press.

Mehrabian, A. (1970). The development and validation of measures of affiliative tendency and sensitivity to rejection. *Educational and Psychological Measurement, 30,* 417–428.

Mehrabian, A. (1971). Verbal and nonverbal interaction of strangers in a waiting situation. *Journal of Experimental Research in Personality, 5,* 127–138.

Mehrabian, A. (1994). Evidence bearing on the Affiliative Tendency (MAFF) and Sensitivity to Rejection (MSR) Scales. *Current Psychology: Developmental, Learning, Personality Social, 13*(2), 97–117.

Mehrabian, A., & Diamond, S. G. (1971). The effects of furniture arrangement, props, and personality on social interaction. *Journal of Personality and Social Psychology, 20,* 18–30.

Mehrabian, A., & Ksionzky, S. (1970). Models for

affiliative and conformity behavior. *Psychological Bulletin, 74,* 110–126.

Mehrabian, A., & Ksionzky, S. (1971). Anticipated compatibility as a function of attitude or status similarity. *Journal of Personality, 39,* 225–241.

Mehrabian, A., & Ksionzky, S. (1972). Some determiners of social interaction. *Sociometry, 35,* 588–609.

Mehrabian, A., & Ksionzky, S. (1985). Social behavior under interpersonal stress. *International Journal of Small Group Research, 1,* 51–68.

Meyer, J. P., & Pepper, S. (1977). Need compatibility and marital adjustment in young married couples. *Journal of Personality and Social Psychology, 35,* 331–342.

Minton, H. L., & Schneider, F. W. (1980). *Differential psychology.* Belmont, CA: Brooks & Cole.

Moffitt, P. F., Spence, N. D., & Goldney, R. D. (1986). Mental health in marriage: The role of need for affiliation, sensitivity to rejection and other factors. *Journal of Clinical Psychology, 42,* 68–76.

Moneta, G. B., & Csikszentmihalyi, M. (2003). Internalized gender role attributes and motivational dispositions in talented teenagers. *Psychology, 10*(2 & 3), 181–191.

Murray, H. A. (1938). *Explorations in personality.* New York: Oxford University Press.

Mussen, P. H., & Jones, M. C. (1957). Self-conceptions, motivations and interpersonal attitudes of late- and early-maturing boys. *Child Development, 28,* 243–256.

Noujaim, K. (1968). *Some motivational determinants of effort allocation and performance.* Unpublished doctoral dissertation, Massachusetts Institute of Technology.

Pepper, L. J., & Strong, P. N. (1958). *Judgmental scales for the MF scale of the MMPI.* Unpublished manuscript.

Raskin, R. N., & Hall, C. S. (1979). A narcissistic personality inventory. *Psychological Reports, 45,* 590.

Ratto, R., & Hurley, J. R. (1995). Outcomes of inpatient group psychotherapy associated with dispositional and situational affiliativeness. *Group, 19*(3), 163–172.

Rosenfeld, H. M., & Franklin, S. S. (1966). Arousal of need for affiliation in women. *Journal of Personality and Social Psychology, 3,* 245–248.

Rosenheim, E., & Neumann, M. (1981). Personality characteristics of sexually dysfunctioning males and their wives. *Journal of Sex Research, 17,* 124–138.

Schroth, M. L. (1985). The effect of differing measuring methods on the relationship of motives. *Journal of Psychology, 119,* 213–218.

Serkownek, K. (1975). *Subscales for scale 5 and 0 of the MMPI.* Unpublished manuscript.

Shipley, T. E., & Veroff, J. (1952). A projective measure of need for affiliation. *Journal of Experimental Psychology, 43,* 349–356.

SIGMA Assessment Systems. (2008). *Personality Research Form (PRF) research bibliography.* Retrieved January 4, 2008, from *www.rpp.on.ca/bibliographies/prfbibliography.pdf.*

Skolnick, A. (1966). Motivational imagery and behavior over twenty years. *Journal of Consulting Psychology, 30*(6), 463–478.

Smith, C. P. (1992). Reliability issues. In C. P. Smith (Ed.), *Motivation and personality: Handbook of thematic content analysis* (pp. 126–139). New York: Cambridge University Press.

Solar, D., & Mehrabian, A. (1973). Impressions based on contradictory information as a function of affiliative tendency and cognitive style. *Journal of Experimental Research on Personality, 6,* 339–346.

Spence, J. T., & Helmreich, R. L. (1983). Achievement-related motives and behaviors. In J. T. Spence (Ed.), *Achievement and achievement motives: Psychological and sociological approaches* (pp. 10–74). San Francisco: Freeman.

Spence, J. T., Helmreich, R. L., & Stapp, J. (1975). Ratings of self and peers on sex role attributes and their relation to self-esteem and conceptions of masculinity and femininity. *Journal of Personality and Social Psychology, 32,* 29–39.

Stein, A. H., & Bailey, M. M. (1973). The socialization of achievement orientation in females. *Psychological Bulletin, 80,* 345–366.

Stewart, A. J., & Chester, N. L. (1982). Sex differences in human social motives: Achievement, affiliation, and power. In A. J. Stewart (Ed.), *Motivation and society: A volume in honor of David C. McClelland.* San Francisco: Jossey-Bass.

Sturman, T. S. (2000). The motivational foundations and behavioral expressions of three narcissistic styles. *Social Behavior and Personality, 28,* 393–408.

Terhune, K. W. (1968). Motives, situation and interpersonal conflict within prisoners' dilemma. *Journal of Personality and Social Psychology, 8*(Pt. 2, Monograph Suppl.), 1–24.

Tett, R. P., & Murphy, P. J. (2002). Personality and situations in co-worker preference: Similarity and complementarity in worker compatibility. *Journal of Business and Psychology, 17,* 223–243.

Veroff, J. (1982). Assertive motivations: Achievement versus power. In A. J. Stewart (Ed.), *Motivation and society: A volume in honor of David C. McClelland* (pp. 99–132). San Francisco: Jossey-Bass.

Veroff, J. (1986). Contextualism and human motives. In D. R. Brown & J. Veroff (Eds.), *Frontiers of motivational psychology: Essays in honor of John W. Atkinson* (pp. 132–145). Berlin: Springer-Verlag.

Walker, E. L., & Heyns, R. N. (1962). *An anatomy for conformity.* Englewood Cliffs, NJ: Prentice-Hall.

Wiesenfeld, B. M., Raghuram, S., & Garud, R. (2001). Organizational identification among virtual workers: The role of need for affiliation and perceived work-based social support. *Journal of Management, 27,* 213–229.

Wilson, T. D., Lindsey, S., & Schooler, T. Y. (2000). A model of dual attitudes. *Psychological Review, 107,* 101–126.

Wong, M. M., & Csikszentmihalyi, M. (1991a). Affiliation motivation and daily experience: Some issues on gender differences. *Journal of Personality and Social Psychology, 60,* 154–164.

Wong, M. M., & Csikszentmihalyi, M. (1991b). Motivation and academic achievement: The effects of personality traits and the quality of experience. *Journal of Personality, 59,* 539–574.

CHAPTER 29

■ ● ▲ ◆ ■ ● ▲ ◆

Power Motivation

EUGENE M. FODOR

The power motive (often referred to as *n* Power) involves a need to influence, control, or impress other people and, as a corollary, to achieve recognition or acclaim for one's power-oriented actions. Impact can occur through a variety of means, notably, forceful action toward or against others, vigorous efforts at controlling their behavior, and ostentatious display of valued personal characteristics. Reactions from other people can take the form of admiration, astonishment, even fear. Guided in part by the seminal studies of Veroff (1957) and Ullman (1972), David Winter (1967, 1973, 1992) developed the measure that forms the basis for most research on the power motive. This measure is the Picture Story Exercise (PSE), first developed by Winter's mentor, David McClelland (1958), but later fashioned by Winter into an instrument to assess power motivation. Instructions to the research participant are to write *vivid, imaginative* stories about a series of pictures (usually six) that were selected as moderately elicitative of the power motive. The participant understands that these stories that he or she writes should answer certain questions:

1. What is happening? Who are the people?
2. What has led up to the situation? That is, what has happened in the past?

3. What is being thought? What is wanted? By whom?
4. What will happen? What will be done?

Trained scorers later code these individual stories according to the coding system that Winter devised.

Here is a story that in a recent experiment received the highest *n* Power score for a single picture from among 259 male and female college students. The picture shows a sea captain (as signified by the uniform) speaking to a person aboard ship whose back is turned toward the viewer. *Italicized phrases* represent scoring categories. Each category commands a score of 1 for its first appearance, but not when or if it recurs later in the story.

There is a new ship. It has just been built and it is traveling to America from Ireland. The man with the hat is *the head of the mob* in Ireland and he *wants the ship to carry some illegal drugs and weapons* and he asks the captain kindly at first. Then *the captain refuses and says this is his ship and there is no way he is going to do that* and get arrested and never see his grandchildren again. *The mob guy tries to bribe him* with a lot of money *but that doesn't work. Captain takes the money and throws it into the sea. Mob guy gets mad and grabs him and leads him over to the edge and strangles him and says, "I have your grandchildren and

426

your daughter" and then shows him some pictures of them tied up. The captain is shivering scared and starts sweating and crying and begs for their lives. The mob guy smiles and lights up a cigar and takes a puff and says let my men get on board with the stuff and when you get to America, and my stuff is safe, you can have your precious family back! Captain does what he tells him.

The rater first determines whether power imagery (designated as Pow Im) is present. If it is, the rater determines whether there is evidence for additional scoring categories, of which there is a possible total of 11. If no Pow Im is present, the story receives a score of zero. The head of the mob, we read at the beginning of the story, wants the captain to approve the transport of illegal contraband. This desired activity concerns a wish to exert control over the captain, as does the entire story. Pow Im is clearly present, for a score of 1. *Head of the mob* signifies negative prestige of actor (Pa–) and suggests status of a kind likely to attract attention. The phrase *wants the ship to carry some illegal drugs and weapons* directly connotes a need or wish to exert power (N). The captain's refusal to comply with the mob leader's request constitutes a block to the power need (Bw), a thwarting of the mob leader's power attempt. Trying to bribe the captain is an instrumental activity oriented toward the exercise of power (I). The captain takes the money the mob head offers as a bribe and throws it into the sea. Again we see a block to the expression of power, that is, block in the world (Bw) *or* instrumental activity (I), now emanating from the captain. Regardless of which coding category the rater chooses, the category has already appeared in the story, and no additional point enters into the score. The mob head gets mad—a clear sign that he is experiencing negative affect on failure to achieve the power goal (G–). The mob head grabs the captain by the neck and shows him pictures of the daughter and grandchildren tied up, again an "I," but a repeat. The captain shivers, thereby showing his fear, and begs for their lives. This entire scenario shows that through his power-motivated actions the mob leader has produced a strong effect (Eff) on the captain. The mob leader smiles, lights up a cigar, and takes a puff, thereby evincing positive affect associated

with attainment of the power goal (G+). The rest of the sentence, beginning with "says," once more points toward instrumental activity (I). The captain's compliance, as stated in the last sentence, illustrates another Eff. The story receives a score of 8. There are only three additional coding categories: Pa+, positive prestige of actor; Ga+, anticipation of successful attainment of the power goal; and Ga–, anticipation of goal failure. As with G– (negative affect associated with goal failure), Ga– suggests a preoccupation with thoughts of power, albeit possible failure in its pursuit.

As the reader reflects on the story of the mob leader and the captain, the impression may be that power motivation invariably produces harmful consequences. Although some stories high in power imagery so suggest, power motivation may energize the pursuit of noble causes that enormously benefit the human condition (McClelland & Burnham, 1976). As Winter (1973) observed, "power is like *fire*: it can do useful things; it can be fun to play with and to watch; but it must be constantly guarded and trimmed back, lest it burn and destroy" (p. xviii). President Franklin Roosevelt, for example, implemented the Social Security system as a measure to ameliorate poverty among the aged, clearly an act of humanitarian value. Winter (1987) ranked Roosevelt's inaugural address a full standard derivation above the mean in power motivation by comparison with all U.S. presidents. (The procedure for scoring inaugural addresses closely approximates the PSE scoring system.)

People sometimes intuitively presume that there is a fundamental incompatibility between *n* Power and need for affiliation (*n* Affiliation), the desire to establish, maintain, or restore positive affect in relations with others (see Hill, Chapter 28, this volume). Actually, this is not necessarily true. The college student who wrote the foregoing story scored distinctly high in *n* Affiliation, as well as *n* Power. Also, Winter's analysis of presidential inaugural addresses found the highest scores among presidents for President John F. Kennedy in both power motivation (essentially tied with Harry Truman) and affiliation motivation (roughly tied with both Bushes). Any combination of the basic needs measured by the PSE is possible. The third basic need arising from the McClelland tradition, and the one researchers have studied the most, is need for achievement (*n* Achievement), which translates as a need to perform well according to a standard of excellence.

An important distinction exists between PSE and self-report measures of motivation (Winter, 1999). PSE measures are inferred, that is, *implicit*. They are projective tests thought to reflect motives that are largely nonconscious. The research participant does not directly describe the thoughts residing within but rather tells a story about a picture, from which the rater infers inner motivational dynamics. Self-report inventories, by contrast, describe what the participant believes are the motives that shape his or her intents and actions. They are *explicit*, residing squarely within the conscious mind. Later I show that these two kinds of measures reflect different aspects of motivation.

The McClelland Model

The model that best explains implicit motives comes from the thinking of McClelland (1958, 1976, 1985; McClelland, Koestner, & Weinberger, 1989). Motives, by his reasoning, shape how we configure and react to the social stimuli we encounter in various walks of life. For example, a power-motivated manager encounters a mild-mannered, compliant, but largely friendless subordinate. The manager cannot tell us why, but, consistent with the evidence that Winter (1973) and Fodor, Wick, and Hartsen (2006) present, the manager likes that person, promotes him to a supervisory position, and places him within his "inner circle" of close advisers. By possessing the personal characteristics that he does, the subordinate constitutes an *activity incentive* for the power-motivated person, a high-probability opportunity to exercise influence and control. Activity incentives can apply to any of the three fundamental implicit motives—need for achievement, need for affiliation/intimacy, or need for power. What activity incentives do is signal the possibility for emotionally reinforcing activity that is specific to a given motive. When the activity incentive closely coincides with a motive and successfully results in an emotionally reinforcing activity, the individual experiences

what Woike (1994) characterizes as an emotional "kick," a surge in pleasurable affect. For the power-motivated person, feelings of strength, vigor, and energy derive from activities prompted by the appropriate activity incentive. In partial support of this idea, McClelland and colleagues (1989) obtained evidence that the act of registering impact on others results in the hormonal release of norepinephrine, which is known to be associated with pleasure. Sometimes an activity incentive presents itself, but the successful exercise of power that the power-motivated individual anticipates does not occur. The result, according to McClelland (1976), is what he termed *power stress*. Indeed, the mere *anticipation* of failure to exercise power (a Ga– in the Winter coding system) may be sufficient to cause power stress.

Implicit versus Explicit Motives

The PSE is conceived as a projective test that measures nonconscious motivation. For this reason, researchers regard the PSE as measuring *implicit* motives (Winter, 1999). The motives it assesses are implicit in the sense that the rater must infer them from what the research participant writes; they are not *explicitly* stated.

The question that immediately presents itself is, Why the distinction between implicit and explicit motives? That is, why not study human motivation by simply administering self-report measures? The answer is that the two kinds of measures (the PSE vs. self-report measures) do not correlate with one another, even though at face they appear to measure the same motives. Moreover, to the extent that they both measure important psychological processes, those processes appear to be different for the two kinds of measures.

Schultheiss and Brunstein (2001) compared the PSE measures for the achievement, affiliation, and power motives against the German NEO Five-Factor Inventory (NEO-FFI; Borkenau & Ostendorf, 1993). They found no significant correlations between the PSE measures and Extraversion, Neuroticism, Openness to experience, Conscientiousness, or Agreeableness. The PSE, therefore, measures something conceptually different from what psychologists believe to be the fundamental dimensions of personality. More to the point, Schultheiss and Brunstein also correlated the same three PSE measures against their supposed counterparts in the German Personality Research Form (PRF; Stumpf, Angleitner, Wieck, Jackson, & Beloch-Till, 1985), specifically, the scales designated as Achievement, Affiliation, and Dominance. Again, there were no significant correlations between the PSE and the self-report measures. Similar findings appear in earlier work by deCharms, Morrison, Reitman, and McClelland (1955). The pattern of empirical findings here documented clearly suggests that PSE measures yield evidence for psychological variables that are separate and distinct from those that one can deduce from self-reports.

Winter, John, Stewart, Klohnen, and Duncan (1998) proposed that *motive* (as reflected in PSE scores) and *trait* (as determined by self-report measures) constitute conceptually different aspects of motivation. They hypothesized that motives and traits can combine in various ways to channel behavior over the life course. The nonconscious wishes and goals that are the stuff of which motives are made, Winter and colleagues reason, do not in themselves steer the individual toward fulfillment. This is where traits come in. Traits serve a channeling function, guiding the individual hither and thither in ways that optimize motive expression, drawing the person toward certain activities and away from others.

To make their point, Winter and colleagues (1998) reported a longitudinal analysis of Radcliffe and Mills college women over a span of years. They examined the interactive effect of the affiliation and power motives on the one hand (PSE measures) in combination with introversion–extraversion on the other (self-report measures). Their principal findings matched prediction. High *n* Affiliation in combination with high extraversion resulted in heavy commitment to volunteer work at midlife. High *n* Affiliation combined with low extraversion (introversion) did not eventuate in significant volunteer activity; neither did *n* Affiliation or extraversion in and by itself. Extraverts experience less electrical activity within the ascending reticular activating system than do introverts, evidence suggests, so they seek out social reinforcement, turning up

the volume, so to speak; whereas introverts already experience high levels of electrical activity, perhaps higher than they want, so they turn away from social stimulation (Bullock & Gilliland, 1993; Stewart, 1996). Introverts high in affiliation motivation see volunteer work as bringing on too much arousal. Extraverts high in *n* Affiliation, by contrast, hunger for the social reinforcement that volunteer activity delivers. Work and family roles, by the same logic, blend well for those women who are extraverts high in *n* Affiliation, but not for introverts high in *n* Affiliation. The combination (work and family) occurred more frequently among extraverts high in *n* Affiliation than it did for introverts high in *n* Affiliation. Introverts high in *n* Affiliation may have found the process of balancing work against family too arousing, whereas affiliation-motivated extraverts probably welcomed the hustle and bustle the balancing act required. Intimate relationships likewise may well have proven excessively overarousing, conflictual, and perhaps even threatening to the affiliation-motivated introverts. Winter and colleagues indeed found that it was they who experienced higher rates of separation and divorce and also stress in their close relationships.

Turning to the power motive, Winter and colleagues (1998) found that high *n* Power in combination with extraversion often produced entry into *impact* careers such as teaching and management. These same women also valued more highly the work relationships in their chosen careers than did power-motivated women who were introverts. The central thesis behind this research on both affiliation and power motives is that the PSE measures something very different from self-report inventories, something more in the nature of wishes and fantasies, real in their own right but not perfect predictors of *long-term* trends in behavior.

Power Stress

McClelland (1976) saw power stress as a social situation, actual or anticipated, that arouses the power motive and either blocks the power motive or has the potential for doing so. For example, one might attempt to persuade a colleague to share participation in a proposed research venture for which the colleague has valued technical skills, only to meet with a reaction of no interest. Persons known to be prone to cardiovascular disease, McClelland noted, look in many ways like persons high in *n* Power. Most notably, they are aggressive and competitively striving, seeming to derive satisfaction from outdoing others. Steele (1973) found that a power-arousal manipulation did increase epinephrine output as a correlate of sympathetic arousal in research participants whose measured *n* Power increased in response to the power-arousal manipulation. No such effect resulted from an achievement-arousal manipulation. The general adaptation syndrome (Selye, 1973) is believed to cause cardiovascular illness when it is aroused often and to a high degree. Epinephrine production is integrally associated with the general adaptation syndrome, as are increased heart rate, increased blood pressure, and glycogen conversion from the liver into blood glucose.

The McClelland (1979, 1982) hypothesis proposes two separate mechanisms by which power stress can occur among persons who are high in *n* Power. The first is *activity inhibition*—an internal control mechanism that restricts the outward expression of anger and assertiveness. The second is the occurrence of social circumstances that by their very nature prevent the power motive from expressing itself. An example would be a person presenting a strong counterargument to a position on which the power-motivated person has taken a firm stand. Either method—one internal, the other external to the self—can thwart the power motive and, according to McClelland, produce cardiovascular distress if repeated many times.

McClelland's (1979) inquiries into the nature of power stress led him to what he termed the *blocked power motive syndrome*, namely, high *n* Power, low *n* Affiliation, and high activity inhibition. The role of *n* Affiliation is that it prompts people to seek out the comfort of friends in times of duress, sharing their discontent and essentially soliciting the solace and alleviation from anxiety that friends can provide (McClelland, 1985). In an important study of this topic, largely because it was prospective rather than concurrent in its design, McClelland (1979) examined PSE protocols that college men had written 20 years previously, sought out these

same men, and obtained blood pressure readings. Men who had shown PSE evidence for the blocked power motive syndrome now showed elevated blood pressure readings compared with men who had then exhibited alternative motive patterns. The readings, on average, were only slightly below the level ordinarily regarded as having medical significance. McClelland, Davidson, Floor, and Saron (1980) subsequently investigated the possible role of epinephrine in the blocked power motive syndrome, using male prison inmates as participants. Those inmates who reported high levels of power stress during recent months and who exhibited the blocked power motive syndrome in their PSE protocols showed high epinephrine concentration in the urine as compared with inmates with other motive patterns.

Friedman and Rosenman (1974) conducted extensive studies on what they termed *Type A* versus *Type B* personalities. More than normal individuals, Type A's were irritable, always in a hurry, hard driving, and tense. Also, they gave evidence of repressed anger. Type B's, by contrast, were much more relaxed and easygoing, willing to go with the flow. Friedman and Rosenman found that Type A's were more likely to experience heart attacks than were Type B's. The "driven" quality of Type A behavior, they reasoned, produced a more chronically active sympathetic nervous system that was likely to put a strain on the cardiovascular system. Chronic sympathetic activation increases heart rate and releases epinephrine. Both effects can damage the cardiovascular system. Suppressed assertiveness and the implication of catecholamine release through the sympathetic nervous system both constitute attributes of Type A behavior and thereby connect with aspects of the blocked power motive syndrome (McClelland, 1976, 1985). Power motivation per se, however, does not correlate with Type A behavior, nor does *n* Achievement or *n* Affiliation (Matthews & Saal, 1978). The power motive must incur blockage to its expression for the deleterious effect on the cardiovascular system to occur (McClelland, 1976, 1985).

It will be recalled that McClelland (1979) hypothesized that power stress could occur in either of two ways: (1) in the blocked power motive syndrome, as discussed in the previous paragraphs, and (2) through social events that thwart expression of the power motive. What is needed to explore the second possibility, he wrote, are experiments that present "strong situational challenges" (p. 189) to the power motive. I conducted some experiments to pursue McClelland's suggestion. The difference from the McClelland research was that I regarded n Power as high if it was in the top third of the overall PSE distribution. For assignment to the blocked power motive syndrome, McClelland regarded a T-score of 45 as qualifying if it was higher than the T-score for n Affiliation (a T-score of 50 is the average for a distribution). The higher cutoff for designating persons as high in n Power implies a hypothesis that if high enough, power motivation by itself is sufficient to produce power stress given appropriately instigating circumstances.

Heeding McClelland's call for experiments that present "strong situational challenges" to the power need, I designed a pair of industrial simulation experiments using male college students as research participants. The first experiment (Fodor, 1984) simulated for the college student "supervisor" a hard-to-manage work crew of high school students in the next room. The task, ostensibly, was construction of Tinkertoy models from pictured diagrams. Actually, there were no workers. Their production and voiced comments to the supervisor were preprogrammed, the voiced comments coming through the intercom system at the end of each of the six trials. Worker comments in the group-stress condition connoted tension within the group: concern about not meeting the standard or beating out the competition, fear that they would not earn much money (the supervisor was authorized to grant pay increases or decreases), and concern that they would not be invited back for another experiment. Instructions to the supervisor stated that it was his task to use any and all means at his disposal to improve worker performance. His efforts, however, were to no avail. Productivity held at roughly the 40th percentile according to the stated norms. The nonstress condition remained at approximately the 80th percentile throughout, and worker comments were strictly neutral. Student supervisors high in n Power scored distinctly high on the General Activation subscale of Thayer's (1978) Activation–

Deactivation Adjective Check List at the end of the power-stress session, higher than supervisors low in n Power, and higher than all supervisors in the nonstress sessions. The General Activation subscale consists of the following adjectives: *activated, active, energetic, full of pep, lively, peppy, vigorous, wakeful*, and *wide awake*. In validating the General Activation subscale, Thayer exposed people to an experimental procedure that was designed to stimulate physiological arousal. General Activation scores showed a substantial correlation with a composite physiological index that combined heart rate and skin conductance.

In the second industrial simulation experiment, students high or low in power motivation acted as "president" of Modern World Electronics (Fodor, 1985). Presiding over two "managers"—one in marketing and the other in production engineering—the president's responsibility was to reconcile any conflict that might arise between the two managers and guide the group toward an amicable solution. He further understood that his ability to mediate and resolve conflict signified managerial capability. The issue concerned whether the company should or should not manufacture and market a portable sunlamp. The two managers in the power-stress condition had opposing role scripts, urging one manager to argue for, the other against the proposal. Each had in his script four arguing points for his position. Instructions were that he introduce these arguments forcibly but not let on that he was being prompted by the script. Managers assigned to the control condition both had role scripts exhorting them to favor the project. Electromyographic (EMG) recordings from the forearm extensor muscle served as the stress measure. Presidents high in n Power evinced higher EMG readings in the conflict condition than did presidents low in n Power and higher than all presidents placed in the control condition.

The hypothalamic–pituitary–adrenal (HPA) axis offers clues as to how researchers may effectively examine the physiological consequences of power stress. McClelland (1989) saw cortisol as playing a mediating role in organizing the general adaptation syndrome. Noting that the HPA axis releases cortisol in response to psychological stressors, Wirth, Welsh, and Schultheiss (2006) experimentally induced defeat in a competitive contest. They hypothesized that high-power individuals are more stressed by a defeat than low-power individuals and that this should manifest itself in increased cortisol release. Specifically, student participants worked on varying forms of the Number Track Ring Task, a reaction-based cognitive task. Half of the participants were led to experience social defeat, the other half social victory. Among the various forms that power stress may assume, losing out against another in competition surely ranks high in its impact value for the power-oriented person. And so the evidence demonstrated. Salivary cortisol proved to be high for participants high in n Power who experienced social defeat but not for those low in the power motive.

Winter (1973) found that students high in n Power chose as close friends students who were not well known by other students— students who posed minimal threat to the power-motivated students' assertiveness and desire for control. He also found that power-motivated men had a preference for unassertive, compliant wives. What about the prospect of hiring an assertive, strong-willed subordinate? Would such a person not constitute a power stress to the power-motivated person, posing a threat to the successful exercise of power? We obtained evidence that this appears to be the case (Fodor et al., 2006). College men imagined themselves interviewing for employment a candidate who came across on video either as strongly assertive (but not unpleasant) or as nonassertive and compliant. They further were to imagine themselves as that person's superior should he be hired. Viewing the assertive candidate, high-power participants showed stronger EMG readings from the corrugator brow (frown) muscle than did participants scoring low in the power motive and stronger readings than all participants viewing the compliant candidate. A scale measuring negative affect toward the candidate displayed the same pattern and correlated highly with the corrugator EMG readings.

Leadership and the Power Motive

Extrapolating from previous research and then thinking that the essence of leadership capability resided with the achievement mo-

tive rather than n Power or n Affiliation, McClelland and Winter (1969) described a groundbreaking program for fostering entrepreneurial success among businessmen in India. They conducted the initial and most extensive program in two different provinces in India, focusing their efforts toward inculcating the achievement motive. They based their design on the extensive research literature documenting what is known about the precursors and correlates of n Achievement. The businesses of which participants were a part typically involved only a small number of employees. Two years after the training program ended, men trained in the achievement motive attained higher scores than a control group on a business activity index. That is, they gave evidence of greater effort to improve the functioning of their respective business operations, such as broadening the product line (e.g., selling women's saris in addition to bicycles), adding a new salesperson to expand the sales territory, or hiring an accountant to improve bookkeeping efficiency. In addition, men trained in n Achievement, more frequently than controls, created a second business, hired more people to work for them, and increased business revenue more. A follow-up program on a more limited scale further strengthened the emerging impression that n Achievement was the core ingredient of managerial success. Looking at initial managerial hires at a major U.S. firm, researchers in the McClelland group (McClelland & Winter, 1969) now conducted a version of the program that controlled for the "Hawthorne effect," the possibility that all the individual attention may have contributed to the success of the India program. Managers in the control group received instruction in the basic functions of management (accounting, production, marketing, etc.), thereby matching the group trained in n Achievement for amount of attention shown to participants. Managers in both groups were tracked over a period of several years to see who advanced most through the managerial hierarchy. The cadre trained in the achievement motive won out over the people who learned principles of management.

To explore this question further, McClelland and Burnham (1976) examined sales division managers at a major corporation. Sales management is a good managerial category to study because there are relatively unambiguous quantitative measures that one can apply across different divisions to determine performance level. McClelland and Burnham wanted to know whether PSE profiles for managers of the best-performing divisions differed from those of the worst-performing divisions. Surprisingly, the best-performing sales managers were high in *n* Power, not *n* Achievement! Indeed, *n* Achievement was no higher for the best-performing than for the worst-performing managers. Moreover, the best-performing managers scored low on *n* Affiliation and high on activity inhibition. (Activity inhibition is indexed by the number of times the word *not* appears throughout a protocol, a seemingly simple measure that has proven to have predictive value.) McClelland and Burnham named this constellation of traits the *leadership motive profile*, or LMP (high *n* Power, low *n* Affiliation, and high activity inhibition). The reader will note that this is the same motive pattern that McClelland and his associates (McClelland, 1979, 1982; McClelland et al., 1980) later found to be implicated in power stress. The finding may have surprised them, because power motivation conjures up ugly images in the popular mind of a tyrannical type of person who is insensitive to the needs of subordinates.

McClelland and Burnham (1976) administered an organizational climate questionnaire to all of the salespersons in each division and discovered two climate dimensions that appeared to be associated with high sales performance for a division (i.e., sales divisions for which LMP characterized the division managers). These dimensions were *organizational clarity* and *team spirit*. Organizational clarity means that individual employees have a clear definition of what the organization's performance expectations are. Team spirit refers to a proclivity to identify with the organization, working toward common goals. The motto of the Three Musketeers—all for one, one for all—captures the essential meaning of team spirit.

Because there was no easy way to compare production divisions against one another (they manufacture entirely different products), McClelland and Burnham (1976) administered the organizational climate questionnaire to all employees within the various production divisions. Sure enough, leaders of those divisions high in organizational clarity and team spirit generally exhibited LMP; leaders of divisions low in those climate dimensions rarely did so.

As a corollary step, McClelland and Boyatzis (1982) examined managers who participated in a managerial assessment experience when they first came to work for AT&T. The PSE was among the many exercises and tests that were part of the program. McClelland and Boyatzis tracked these managers over a 16-year period and found that LMP correlated with their level of managerial placement at the end of that period, whereas those high in *n* Achievement usually settled at a lower managerial level. LMP has a number of features in its favor. People who are high in power motivation *orchestrate* the performance of others. They are charismatic (House, Woycke, & Fodor, 1988). Think of Jack Welch, the legendary CEO of General Electric (Stater, 1999), Winston Churchill, or Franklin Roosevelt. These were people endowed with a capacity to inspire others. Power-motivated managers tend to use others as a means toward achievement of organizational goals.

As McClelland and Burnham (1976) observed, leadership is an influence game. It requires manipulative intent, the power of persuasion. Persons high in *n* Achievement, the evidence shows, tend to do tasks themselves rather than make optimal use of others (McClelland, 1985). Affiliation motivation detracts from leader effectiveness because it places a premium on soliciting the good will and liking of others at the expense of organizational goals. McClelland and Burnham emphasized that managers must be *universalistic* in how they make and invoke policy decisions. If managers make exceptions in order to cultivate the good will of individual employees, overall morale may suffer, eroding the all-important organizational climate dimensions of organizational clarity and team spirit.

The significance of high activity inhibition as an aspect of LMP requires some explanation. High activity inhibition means controlling one's emotions ("don't let them see you sweat") but also more than that. Persons low in activity inhibition too often "say what's on their minds" and let fly feelings that cause psychological distress to others and thereby diminish subordinates' willingness to commit wholeheartedly to organizational goals. On assuming leadership of Continental Airlines, Gordon Bethune garnered much acclaim from the business community and the press for the finesse with which he converted the troubled airline into an industry leader. When asked by a TV journalist what lesson he had learned from his former boss at Northwest Airlines, Bethune said the man taught him to check his tongue and temper. Also, one of Bethune's strategies was to award generous bonuses to employees when the airline was performing well. The evidence suggests that leaders characterized by LMP can be a source of guidance and inspiration.

The question naturally arises, Is it possible to have incompetent leaders who nevertheless fit the leadership motive profile? What about a leader who fits the profile but leads the group toward nonhumanitarian or self-aggrandizing ends? Does this occur frequently enough to cause concern? Common observation suggests that perhaps it does. Thus it may make sense to distinguish between leadership (an ability to guide others toward stated or privately conceived goals) and the values that guide the leader's actions. Both considerations figure prominently into our deliberations on whom we want as leaders.

Another chapter in the leadership literature as it pertains to power motivation is Winter's (1987) study of presidential inaugural addresses and their correlation with presidential performance. Winter developed a scoring system that he applied to the first inaugural address of all elected presidents throughout U.S. history. His method was closely predicated on the PSE procedure and assessed n Achievement, n Affiliation/ Intimacy, and n Power. Scholars often ask whether speechwriters can accurately infer the motive pattern of the president for whom they compose these addresses. What has been written on this topic suggests that these speechwriters are highly perceptive in their appraisals, similar to persons who evaluate potential jurors for defense attorneys (Ritter & Medhurst, 2003).

Power motivation significantly correlated with two measures of presidential greatness: rankings by recognized presidential historians and the occurrence of great decisions, again as cited by presidential historians.

The Social Security system as it arose during the administration of Franklin Roosevelt illustrates a great decision, as does Abraham Lincoln's issuance of the Emancipation Proclamation that freed the slaves. Both initiatives altered the fabric of American life. Unfortunately, power motivation in presidents also correlates highly with war entry, consistent perhaps with the known relationship between n Power and aggression. Pursuing the same line of thinking, we can imagine that the bold, assertive demeanor that characterizes a power-motivated president might arouse a degree of hostility in others. Winter (1987) did indeed find a correlation between n Power and assassination attempts. John Kennedy and Harry Truman received the highest n Power scores among all U.S. presidents. Both experienced assassination attempts, one successful. Ronald Reagan, also the recipient of such an attempt, likewise scored distinctly high in power motivation. These various findings neatly integrate with what we know about power motivation, in both its positive and negative aspects.

In a recent and highly ambitious study, Winter (2007) examined eight pairs of crises, one crisis in the pair leading to war and the other to peaceful negotiation. He applied content analysis to government statements, speeches, press conferences, and diplomatic documents drawn from each crisis to determine various motivational states implicit in the wording of communications attributable to key decision makers. The assumption by Winter and others is that when emotions run high, when accurate information is scarce, and when there exists a time urgency, psychological factors can tip the balance between peace and war. Winter took great care to pair match crises such that a single pair occurred at a similar time in history, in the same (or a similar) country, and centered on the same (or similar) political issues. Trained raters were blind as to the research hypotheses and, where possible, to the side of the conflict that authored a given communication. Documents within each pair were randomly mixed before coding. Also, it was absolutely critical to select documents within each pair that were formally similar to one another with respect to the kind of document. For many paired crises, archival collections existed of government-to-government communications.

Illustrative of crises that Winter (2007) examined were two that are familiar to students of American history. One concerned United States territorial expansion in the years 1845–1846, specifically the Mexican War as it related to U.S. annexation of Texas and the Oregon boundary dispute with Canada. The Mexican War eventuated in military confrontation, the Oregon boundary dispute in peaceful compromise. The second crisis was the escalating economic, political, and social conflict between North and South: the Compromise of 1850 versus the Civil War, the latter a truly tragic episode. Another pair focused on Iraq in Kuwait: noninvasion in 1961, invasion in 1991. In cases of this sort, ratings were applied only to parties to the conflict, not to peripheral parties or to those who become involved afterward.

Consistent with prior evidence, power motivation emerged as the principal predictor of war entry. Surprising at first glance is the finding that ratings of responsibility likewise correlated with war entry. Winter's (2007) scoring system for responsibility involves reference to an abstract moral standard, including legality, and fittingness of manners or behavior as appropriate or inappropriate. Obligation to rules and regulations and sympathetic concern for others or groups also figure into the scoring system. By Winter's reasoning, responsibility can take an ugly turn in times of crisis when people perceive that the *other* party lacks responsibility and when responsibility demands protection of oneself and one's own group. These cognitions can prompt a sense of time urgency, coupled with an expressed need to secure the survival of one's core values. Power motivation in combination with high responsibility appears to constitute a potent force that leads to conflict escalation and war entry but couched in the language of altruistic concern for one's own nation.

Government communications obviously constitute a collaborative effort by multiple individuals, including speechwriters. Winter (2007) suggested that they reasonably represent the climate of thinking and value orientation that prevail within an interacting group at a given time. These communications can be viewed as proxies that average out prevailing motivational sentiments that exist among closely interacting persons.

The practical applications of these findings are obvious. It would be possible to monitor government-to-government communications in times of crisis, anticipating escalation or even possible movement toward war. Alternatively, analysis might reveal a deescalating temper of mind among conflicting parties, thereby opening the opportunity for compromise and peaceful resolution of differences. Communications from key political figures also might contain important clues on what their constituencies can expect from them by way of aggressive or conciliatory initiatives in dealing with adversarial nations.

The available evidence for small groups implies a negative influence from power-motivated leaders. Recall that *n* Power as an aspect of the LMP produces a positive influence on productivity only in relation to large aggregates of subordinates, situations in which one-on-one interaction with subordinates is minimal. The leader in those instances inspires and motivates from a distance, essentially orchestrating the actions of others. We did an experiment that explored some implications of Janis's (1982) concept of *groupthink*, which he defined as faulty group decision making prompted by various social forces that arise within the group (Fodor & Smith, 1982). Janis examined foreign relations fiascos that U.S. government and military officials perpetrated in their advisory group roles at various points in history, such as the failure to anticipate the attack on Pearl Harbor, escalation of the Korean War, the Bay of Pigs invasion of Cuba, and escalation of the Vietnam War. A reading of history (along with Winter's [1987] inaugural-address analyses of the presidents) suggests that the leaders who officiated over the deliberations leading to each of these fiascoes were distinctly high in power motivation.

We arranged five-person discussion groups of college students for the imagined purpose of determining whether they as managers should recommend the manufacture and marketing of a new microwave oven (Fodor & Smith, 1982). Each "manager" had a role script with six items of information, some items favoring and some opposing the decision. For example, the following items of information were among those available to the group member designated as manager of production engineering:

1. At present, concern exists over the 10 mW per square centimeter radiation allowance on all of the new ovens. Microwave repairmen working in fields of radiation as low as 10–22 mW per square centimeter developed inflammation of the blood vessels, which was attributed to their frequent exposure to microwaves.
2. While the company has not done any production of this type, the actual production process will fit in well with the current production of magnetron tubes (the largest component part of the microwave ovens). (Fodor & Smith, 1982, p. 181)

The role scripts instructed group members to introduce information from their scripts in a natural manner as they saw fit, not making it obvious that they were receiving prompts from the script. The assigned group leader (president) had scored either in the top or bottom third on the PSE for *n* Power among the many students who took the test. The president understood that he (all presidents were male) had major responsibility for guiding the group to its final decision. Observing through a one-way mirror, we recorded two outcome measures: number of informational items from the role scripts coming forth into the actual discussion and number of distinctly different proposals made. Flowers (1977) had previously argued that these two outcome measures satisfactorily determine the occurrence of groupthink. By both measures, groupthink was more in evidence when the leader was high in *n* Power than when he was low. Completing a 7-point scale afterward, group members reported having received greater influence from their leader if he was high in *n* Power than if he was low.

Creativity

Looking back to McClelland's (1989) conceptualization of activity incentives, one may ponder the many ways that power-motivated people may envisage impact of a kind that brings recognition. Some we have already encountered in this chapter, but the list is endless. Some harm the human condition, some enhance it. What about opportunities to perform creatively in science, the arts, and engineering design? Such opportunities meet McClelland's definition of activity incentives for the power motive.

A series of experiments do suggest that arousal of the power motive can lead to heightened creativity (Fodor, 1990; Fodor & Carver, 2000; Fodor & Greenier, 1995). The design of these three experiments followed a similar pattern. College students at a predominantly technological university first rendered a written solution to an engineering-design problem. The experimenter examined the solution and provided written feedback, accompanied by a rating. The feedback signified the degree of recognition that the experimenter felt the proposed solution was likely to command from the engineering and scientific community. This feedback was simulated as part of the experimental procedure. The nature of the problem was such that the student could generate a solution with ease but without any certainty about how creative it was. The feedback, be it positive or negative, was couched in the language of power imagery, that is, having or not having potential impact. The student then attempted solution to a second and more demanding problem or completed the Remote Associates Test of creativity (Mednick & Mednick, 1967). The Remote Associates Test is the creativity test for which the greatest evidence of validity exists (Dacey, 1989). Evidence shows it to be a *state* as well as a *trait* measure of creativity (Isen, Daubman, & Nowicki, 1987), so that various experimental manipulations can alter people's scores. When the dependent measure was a proposed solution to a second engineering problem, qualified judges trained in the use of Amabile's (1983) creativity scales completed sets of ratings.

Positive feedback on the first solution, suggestive of impact and recognition, enhanced subsequent creative performance in power-motivated persons; negative feedback, using imagery that implied absence of impact, diminished creative performance in power-motivated persons. These findings did not occur with persons low in power motivation. That a striving for recognition and acclaim can promote creative thought is well documented by Watson's (1968) autobiographical account of the driving force behind his and Francis Crick's discovery of the molecular makeup of DNA. They shocked the scientific community by unabashedly stating that a prime motive was their quest for the Nobel Prize. In a similar vein, sociologist Robert

Merton (1973) wrote of the "race for prior-ity" as a key element in the pursuit of scien-tific discovery.

An important point is that *n* Achievement also fosters creativity, but the underlying mechanism may be different. When they have recently experienced negative feedback on a prior effort at creative performance, achievement-motivated persons improve their creative performance on a subsequent task, whereas power-motivated persons show diminished creativity during the sec-ond task (Fodor & Carver, 2000). This find-ing is consistent with research indicating that negative feedback results in improved task performance in persons who are high in *n* Achievement (McClelland, 1985). As Win-ter (1973) observed, achievement-motivated persons may not like news of failure, but it goads them on to greater effort. In essence, it serves as a basis for new information that can modify future performance. Persons who are high in power motivation, by con-trast, may perceive failure as an inability to impress another person or an aggregate of persons, thereby thwarting their need to register impact and receive acclaim. In other words, failure to impress may represent a power stress. Winter suggested that in this sense the goals of persons high in *n* Power may be short rather than long term.

Power Motivation and Emotion

Closely integrated with McClelland's con-cept of power stress is research evidence linking power motivation with emotion. McClelland and colleagues (1989) theorized that individuals engage in behaviors that im-pact the social environment in ways that link to their dominant motives. Individuals high in *n* Power, by this reasoning, should enact behaviors that create and maintain a feel-ing of energy and personal excitement. Ac-cordingly, Woike (1994) attempted to induce specific affective states by asking power- and intimacy-motivated individuals to vividly recall an event that had made them very happy or an event that occurred yesterday and was ordinary. Immediately thereafter, research participants completed a question-naire on their current affective state. Using McAdams's (1982) scoring system for auto-biographical memories, Woike found that

individuals high in *n* Power generally used more power imagery in their recollections of the happy event (personal strength, control, vigor, prestige, and recognition) and indi-viduals high in *n* Intimacy wrote memories more associated with intimacy imagery (in-volving loving, caring, empathy, and close-ness to people) when recalling a happy event. In their questionnaire responses, power-motivated individuals in the pleasant-recall condition reported more excitement and anger than did individuals high in *n* Inti-macy in the same condition. Anger energizes one's efforts to create impact and therefore elicits positive emotions, such as excitement, in power-motivated persons (Woike & Mc-Adams, 2005).

Taking account of McClelland's moti-vational theory (McClelland, 1985; Wein-berger & McClelland, 1990), Zurbriggen and Sturman (2002) hypothesized that mo-tives are linked to specific primary emo-tions. They asked people to vividly imagine successful experiences at satisfying each of three motives—power, achievement, and affiliation/intimacy—and then report the degree to which they experienced various emotional states during the visualizations. Instructions for the power visualization were to "think about a time when you were able to persuade someone to do something, or to convince someone of something (to bring them around to your point of view)." Consistent with McClelland's prediction, high levels of anger were experienced during the power visualization but not during the achievement or affiliation/intimacy visual-izations. Contrary to McClelland's reason-ing, however, excitement was not associated with the power visualization but rather with the achievement visualization.

Building upon McClelland's (1989) theo-retical analysis of how incentives activate im-plicit motives, Schultheiss and Hale (2007) considered the way that faces expressing various emotions might affect allocation of attention in power- and affiliation-motivated individuals. They used as incentives faces known to express joy, anger, and surprise, paired side by side with faces with a neutral expression. Previous studies have shown that facial expressions consistently elicit certain attributions as to the motives they express (Knutson, 1996). Joyful faces elicit high ratings for both dominance and affiliation, whereas angry faces rate high on dominance but low on affiliation. A dominant expression from another person, Schultheiss and Hale hypothesized, signals lack of control by the power-motivated person. Anger and joy, therefore, should figure as *disincentives* for these persons, constituting cues that should divert their attention. Surprise, on the other hand, implies that the power-motivated person has had impact and therefore should rivet the power-motivated person's attention.

Schultheiss and Hale (2007) employed the dot-probe task (Mogg & Bradley, 1999), which presents an emotional face and a neutral face side by side. The computer screen then masks the faces. A dot next appears in the position of either the emotional or the neutral face just previously seen. The participant's response latency in attending to the dot reflects the degree of attention the participant directed toward the emotional face. A previous focus on the emotional face should produce a short latency if the dot replaces that face; a previous focus on the neutral face (and away from the emotional face) should result in a long latency, again if the dot replaces the emotional face. Power-motivated individuals attended to the low-dominance surprised faces, facial expressions that had likely provided reward value for them in the past. They oriented away from anger faces, as these would pose a threat. Affiliation-motivated persons proved to be highly vigilant toward anger faces, consistent with evidence that persons high in *n* Affiliation are rejection-sensitive.

Some Concluding Thoughts

As in so much of the research on the relation of personality to social behavior, we look back historically with some surprise as we note the directions that research traditions have taken. With power motivation, two recent trends are especially noticeable, and possibly a third. One, as the preceding section suggests, concerns the interconnection between *n* Power and emotion. Indications are that this trend will continue into the near future.

Another growing trend, to which some of the foregoing discussion alludes, is an interest in physiological substrates of the power motive and the other implicit motives as well. In presenting his seminal work on the power motive, Winter (1973) commented, "A general explanation of the physiological mechanisms of all motivated behavior ... would be valuable if it were complete and accurate" (p. 24). Advances in the technology for studying physiological mechanisms that underlie psychological processes are opening new research vistas. Illustrative of future possibilities is a pilot study by Welsh (2003) that made use of positron emission tomography. Welsh presented aversive images of mutilated bodies to persons high in need for intimacy and also persons high in need for power. These images activated the right fusiform gyrus, a portion of the brain that evaluates the socioempathic implications of images, as when people process faces. Her hypothesis was that intimacy motivation would accentuate this process, as the neuroimaging data suggested it had. With power-motivated persons, on the other hand, these same aversive images activated brain regions implicated in defending the self against threat, namely the right pons, an area involved in the startle reflex, and the superior frontal gyrus, an area involved in deception and angry face processing. These findings, although tentative, make sense in terms of what we know about the intimacy and power motives.

Another interesting development is a means for determining testosterone level through analysis of a person's saliva. Schultheiss and colleagues (2005) found evidence for a connection between *n* Power and testosterone level. Pairs of men competed on several rounds of a contest that the experimenters had programmed to result predominantly in success or in failure. For men high in power motivation, more than for those scoring low, success resulted in an increase in gonadal steroid testosterone within the saliva, whereas failure produced a decrease, again more for men scoring high than for those scoring low in *n* Power. The association between testosterone level in men and predilections toward aggression and dominance is well established (Mazur & Booth, 1998). High or rising levels of testosterone, Schultheiss and colleagues theorized, motivates dominance, thus priming assertive behavior. Defeat-induced decreases in testosterone, on the other hand, constitute impact failure and diminish attempts to dominate others. Women's testosterone levels did not react in the same way.

On a totally different note, Winter's (2007) recent analysis of power motivation as it relates to escalation or deescalation of conflict offers a possible avenue for exploring labor–management negotiations. Should organizational psychologists obtain evidence that parallels what Winter found, they might possibly develop diagnostic criteria and intervention techniques that could forestall the injurious personal and economic consequences that accompany the breakdown of negotiations.

Advances in methodology have been the catalyst for many of the recent findings in our quest to better understand power motivation. Theories by themselves merely whet the appetite for further understanding, but advances in methodology bring theories to fruition.

References

Amabile, T. M. (1983). *The social psychology of creativity*. New York: Springer-Verlag.

Borkenau, P., & Ostendorf, F. (1993). *NEO-Fünf-Faktoren Inventar (NEO-FFI) nach Costa and McCrae: Handaniveisung [NEO-Five-Factor Inventory (NEO-FFI) according to Costa and McCrae: Manual]*. Göttingen, Germany: Hogrefe.

Bullock, W. A., & Gilliland, K. (1993). Eysenck's arousal theory of introversion–extraversion: A converging measures investigation. *Journal of Personality and Social Psychology, 64*, 113–123.

Dacey, J. S. (1989). *Fundamentals of creative thinking*. New York: Lexington Books.

deCharms, R., Morrison, H. W., Reitman, W. R., & McClelland, D. C. (1955). Behavioral correlates of directly and indirectly measured achievement motivation. In D. C. McClelland (Ed.), *Studies in motivation* (pp. 414–423). New York: Appleton-Century-Crofts.

Flowers, M. L. (1977). A laboratory test of some implications of Janis's groupthink hypothesis. *Journal of Personality and Social Psychology, 35*, 888–896.

Fodor, E. M. (1984). The power motive and reactivity to power stresses. *Journal of Personality and Social Psychology, 47*, 853–859.

Fodor, E. M. (1985). The power motive, group conflict, and physiological arousal. *Journal of Personality and Social Psychology, 49*, 1408–1415.

Fodor, E. M. (1990). The power motive and creativity of solutions to an engineering problem. *Journal of Research in Personality, 24*, 338–354.

Fodor, E. M., & Carver, R. A. (2000). Achievement and power motives, performance feedback, and creativity. *Journal of Research in Personality, 34*, 380–396.

Fodor, E. M., & Greenier, K. D. (1995). The power motive, self-affect, and creativity, *Journal of Research in Personality, 29*, 242–252.

Fodor, E. M., & Smith, T. (1982). The power motive as an influence on group decision making. *Journal of Personality and Social Psychology, 42*, 178–185.

Fodor, E. M., Wick, D. P., & Hartsen, K. M. (2006). The power motive and affective response to assertiveness. *Journal of Research in Personality, 40*, 598–610.

Friedman, M., & Rosenman, R. H. (1974). *Type A behavior and your heart*. New York: Fawcett.

House, R. J., Woycke, J., & Fodor, E. M. (1988). Charismatic and noncharismatic leaders: Differences in behavior and effectiveness. In J. S. Conger & R. N. Kanungo (Eds.), *Charismatic leadership: The elusive factor in organizational effectiveness* (pp. 98–121). San Francisco: Jossey-Bass.

Isen, A. M., Daubman, K. A., & Nowicki, G. P. (1987). Positive affect facilitates creative problem solving. *Journal of Personality and Social Psychology, 52*, 1122–1131.

Janis, I. L. (1982). *Groupthink: Psychological studies of policy decisions and fiascoes* (2nd ed.). Boston: Houghton Mifflin.

Knutson, B. (1996). Facial expressions of emotion influence interpersonal trait inferences. *Journal of Nonverbal Behavior, 20*, 165–182.

Matthews, K. A., & Saal, F. E. (1978). Relationship of the Type A coronary-prone behavior pattern to achievement, power, and affiliation motives. *Psychosomatic Medicine, 40*, 631–636.

Mazur, A., & Booth, A. (1998). Testosterone and dominance in men. *Behavioral and Brain Sciences, 21*, 353–397.

McAdams, D. P. (1982). Experiences of intimacy and power: Relationships between personal motives and autobiographical memory. *Journal of Personality and Social Psychology, 42*, 292–302.

McClelland, D. C. (1958). Methods of measuring human motivation. In J. W. Atkinson (Ed.), *Motives in fantasy, action, and society* (pp. 7–42). Princeton, NJ: Van Nostrand.

McClelland, D. C. (1976). Sources of stress in the drive for power. In G. Serban (Ed.), *Psychopathology and human adaptation* (pp. 247–270). New York: Plenum Press.

McClelland, D. C. (1979). Inhibited power motivation and high blood pressure in men. *Journal of Abnormal Psychology, 88*, 182–190.

McClelland, D. C. (1982). The need for power, sympathetic activation, and illness. *Motivation and Emotion, 6*, 31–41.

McClelland, D. C. (1985). *Human motivation*. Glenview, IL: Scott, Foresman.

McClelland, D. C. (1989). Motivational factors in health and disease. *American Psychologist, 41*, 675–683.

McClelland, D. C., & Boyatzis, R. E. (1982). The leadership motive pattern and long-term success in management. *Journal of Applied Psychology, 67*, 737–743.

McClelland, D. C., & Burnham, D. H. (1976, March–April). Power is the great motivator. *Harvard Business Review, 54*, 100–110.

McClelland, D. C., Davidson, R. J., Floor, E., & Saron, C. (1980). Power motivation, catecholamine secretion, immune function and illness reports. *Journal of Human Stress, 6,* 11–19.

McClelland, D. C., Koestner, R., & Weinberger, J. (1989). How do self-attributed and implicit motives differ? *Psychological Review, 96,* 690–702.

McClelland, D. C., & Winter, D. G. (1969). *Motivating economic achievement.* New York: Free Press.

Mednick, S. A., & Mednick, M. T. (1967). *Remote Associates Test: Experimenter's manual.* Boston: Houghton Mifflin.

Merton, R. K. (1973). *The sociology of science.* Chicago: University of Chicago Press.

Mogg, K., & Bradley, B. P. (1999). Some methodological issues in assessing attentional biases for threatening faces in anxiety: A replication study using a modified version of the probe detection task. *Behavior Research and Therapy, 37,* 595–604.

Ritter, K., & Medhurst, M. J. (2003). *Presidential speechwriting: From the new deal to the Reagan revolution and beyond.* College Station: Texas A & M University Press.

Schultheiss, O. C., & Brunstein, J. C. (2001). Assessment of implicit motives with a research version of the TAT: Picture profiles, gender differences, and relations to other personality measures. *Journal of Personality Assessment, 77,* 71–86.

Schultheiss, O. C., & Hale, J. A. (2007). Implicit motives modulate attentional orienting to facial expression of emotion. *Motivation and Emotion, 31,* 13–24.

Schultheiss, O. C., Wirth, M. M., Torges, C. M., Pang, J. S., Villacorta, M. A., & Welsh, K. M. (2005). Effects of implicit power motivation on men's and women's implicit learning and testosterone changes after social victory or defeat. *Journal of Personality and Social Psychology, 88,* 174–188.

Selye, H. (1973). The evolution of the stress concept. *American Scientist, 61,* 672–699.

Slater, R. (1999). *Jack Welch and the GE way: Management insights and leadership secrets of the legendary CEO.* New York: McGraw-Hill.

Steele, R. S. (1973). *The physiological concomitants of psychogenic motive arousal in college males.* Unpublished doctoral dissertation, Harvard University.

Stewart, G. L. (1996). Reward structure as a moderator of the relationship between extraversion and sales performance. *Journal of Applied Psychology, 81,* 619–627.

Stumpf, H., Angleitner, A., Wieck, T., Jackson, D. N., & Beloch-Till, H. (1985). *Deutsche Personality Research Form (PRF).* Göttingen, Germany: Hogrefe.

Thayer, R. E. (1978). Factor analytic and reliability studies on the Activation–Deactivation Adjective Check List. *Psychological Reports, 42,* 747–756.

Ullman, J. S. (1972). The need for influence: Development and validation of a measure, and comparison with the need for power. *Genetic Psychology Monographs, 85,* 157–214.

Veroff, J. (1957). Development and validation of a projective measure of power motivation. *Journal of Abnormal Psychology, 54,* 1–8.

Watson, J. D. (1968). *The double helix.* New York: Atheneum.

Weinberger, J., & McClelland, D. C. (1990). Cognitive versus traditional motivational models: Irreconcilable or complementary? In E. T. Higgins & R. M. Sorrentino (Eds.), *Handbook of motivation and cognition: Vol. 2. Foundations of social behavior* (pp. 562–597). New York: Guilford Press.

Welsh, K. M. (2003, August). *Implicit motives and brain activation in emotion.* Paper presented at the convention of the American Psychological Association, Toronto, Ontario, Canada.

Winter, D. G. (1967). *Power motivation in thought and action.* Unpublished doctoral dissertation, Harvard University.

Winter, D. G. (1973). *The power motive.* New York: Free Press.

Winter, D. G. (1987). Leader appeal, leader performance, and the motive profiles of leaders and followers. *Journal of Personality and Social Psychology, 52,* 196–202.

Winter, D. G. (1992). Power motivation revisited. In C. P. Smith (Ed.), *Motivation and personality: Handbook of thematic content analysis* (pp. 301–310). Cambridge, UK: Cambridge University Press.

Winter, D. G. (1999). Linking personality and "scientific" psychology: The development of empirically derived Thematic Apperception Test measures. In L. Geiser & M. I. Stein (Eds.), *Evocative images: The Thematic Apperception Test and the art of projection* (pp. 107–124). Washington, DC: American Psychological Association.

Winter, D. G. (2007). The role of motivation, responsibility, and integrative complexity in crisis escalation: Comparative studies of war and peace crises. *Journal of Personality and Social Psychology, 92,* 920–937.

Winter, D. G., John, O. P., Stewart, A. J., Klohnen, E. C., & Duncan, L. E. (1998). Traits and motives: Toward an integration of two traditions in personality research. *Psychological Review, 105,* 230–250.

Wirth, M. M., Welsh, K. M., & Schultheiss, O. C. (2006). Salivary cortisol changes in humans after winning or losing a dominance contest depend on implicit power motivation. *Hormones and Behavior, 49,* 346–352.

Woike, B. A. (1994). Vivid recollection as a technique to arouse implicit motive-related affect. *Motivation and Emotion, 18,* 335–349.

Woike, B. A., & McAdams, D. P. (2005). Motives. In V. J. Derlaga, B. A. Winstead, & W. H. Jones (Eds.), *Personality: Contemporary theory and research* (pp. 156–189). Belmont, CA: Thomson Wadsworth.

Zurbriggen, E. L., & Sturman, T. S. (2002). Linking motives and emotions: A test of McClelland's hypothesis. *Personality and Social Psychology Bulletin, 28,* 521–535.

CHAPTER 30

■ ● ▲ ◆ ■ ● ▲ ◆

Social Desirability

RONALD R. HOLDEN
JENNIFER PASSEY

Social desirability is the tendency for people to present themselves in a generally favorable fashion (Holden, 2001). Particularly within the field of self-report assessment of personality and attitudes, the topic of social desirability has been and remains the source of long-standing and sometimes acrimonious argument. Like a forest fire, disagreements regarding the topic have ranged from the incendiary blazes of the 1960s to controlled flames in the 1970s and 1980s. During the 1990s, some believed the fire had been extinguished, but the first decade of the 2000s has seen that the debate still smolders.

Various definitions of social desirability have been offered. Edwards (1957) defined the concept as the tendency of individuals to endorse personality self-statements with socially desirable scale values and to reject self-statements with socially undesirable scale values. Crowne and Marlowe (1960) indicated that social desirability reflects people's need to gain approval by appearing in a culturally appropriate and acceptable manner. Jackson (1984) defined the term as the description of the self in terms judged as desirable or as favorable self-presentation. More recently, Paulhus (1991) has viewed social desirability as the tendency to give responses that make the individual look good.

Self-report measurement of noncognitive attributes is ubiquitous. Consider the many instances in which inventories, questionnaires, and surveys are used. For example, children, adolescents, and adults routinely complete personality and vocational interest inventories as part of assessments associated with career choices. Job applicants commonly answer personality and integrity questionnaires during employment selection procedures. Psychiatric and counseling clients typically undergo personality testing as a component of clinical evaluation or intervention assessment procedures. Incarcerated individuals often undergo personality testing prior to court proceedings, as part of a correctional facility admissions procedure, or in advance of custody release. Furthermore, people participating in research commonly respond to surveys as part of investigations that may span a wide diversity of psychological and nonpsychological areas. Thus few adults have not completed a self-report vocational interest, personality, personnel, clinical evaluation, or research instrument at some time during their lives. Yet what evidence is there that an individual's responses are valid and do not merely index self-presentation styles (i.e., socially desirable responding)? Consider, therefore, that the stylistic responding associated with social desirability could be a major impediment for accurate measurement in what constitutes a significant enterprise in society.

441

History of the Issue

The potential impact of social desirability on psychological testing has a long history. Projective approaches to assessment are based on the assumption that the private world of the individual is covert and jealously guarded and that, because of a variety of defenses, one must evaluate signs rather than samples of behavior (Frank, 1948; Goodenough, 1946). Furthermore, within structured (i.e., nonprojective) assessment, Steinmetz (1932) referred to research in the 1920s in which E. K. Strong, Jr., manipulated self-presentation instructions to Stanford students so that they would complete the Strong Vocational Interest Blank so as to qualify as engineers. Subsequently, concerns about socially desirable responding have been noted by Meehl (1945), who, at the time, advocated an empirical structured approach to test construction, and by Ellis (1946), who described the limitations associated with rational approaches to structured test construction.

In the 1950s and 1960s, the issue of social desirability became more contentious. Jackson and Messick (1961, 1962a, 1962b) published a series of articles indicating that the variance in the scales of the Minnesota Multiphasic Personality Inventory (MMPI), one of the most widely used self-report personality inventories, could be explained largely in terms of response styles. They estimated that over 30% of the common variance in MMPI scale scores was attributable to a social desirability dimension. Not to be outdone, Edwards and Walker (1961) suggested that because the MMPI was so saturated with social desirability variance, the entire 566-item instrument could be replaced by a 39-item social desirability scale. According to these critics, one of the most professionally popular and technologically sophisticated personality measures of its time could be interpreted as reflecting response styles rather than dimensions of personality. Of course, heated responses to this position arose, but, nonetheless, there emerged the recognition that social desirability was an important force to be reckoned with when constructing self-report measures of noncognitive constructs. In the 1970s, this recognition was codified in notable publications by Jackson (1970, 1973), who indicated that "to construct psychological measures in disregard

for sources of method variance is to court disaster" (Jackson, 1971, p. 240).

Perhaps measures of social desirability can reflect both relevant content and stylistic responding. Consider a controversial debate in the 1980s regarding the overlap between measures of socially desirable responding and the concept of hopelessness (Holden & Mendonca, 1984; Holden, Mendonca, & Mazmanian, 1985; Linehan & Nielsen, 1981, 1983; Nevid, 1983; Strosahl, Linehan, & Chiles, 1984). The Beck Hopelessness Scale (Beck, Weissman, Lester, & Trexler, 1974), a self-report measure that represents the preeminent psychological predictor of suicide in prospective studies (Beck, Brown, Berchick, Stewart, & Steer, 1990; Beck, Steer, Kovacs, & Garrison, 1985; Brown, Beck, Steer, & Grisham, 2000), apparently is contaminated overwhelmingly with social desirability bias. Despite this saturation of supposedly irrelevant response variance, the scale statistically predicts subsequent suicidal behavior and postdicts previous suicide attempts. Thus actual behavior is predictable from something that seems to be highly infected with the threat to construct validity of social desirability.

As a more detailed example of this issue, consider items from the Beck Hopelessness Scale, which measures a psychological construct that is highly relevant for predicting suicide risk. For the responses of 78 psychiatric patients in crisis (including 10 suicide attempters and 41 suicide ideators), Mendonca, Holden, Mazmanian, and Dolan (1983) reported item–Hopelessness scale and item–Desirability scale correlations (based on Jackson's [1984] Desirability Scale). The researchers also calculated a differential reliability index (DRI; Jackson, 1984, p. 31) that represented the portion of item variance associated with the Hopelessness scale after removing the item's shared variance with social desirability.

The item–Hopelessness scale correlations indicated that all of the scale's items were strongly related to total Hopelessness scale scores. This is not surprising and replicates findings associated with the scale's development (Beck et al., 1974). However, values for item–Desirability scale correlations indicated that Hopelessness scale items are heavily laden with variance attributable to stylistic responding. Furthermore, the DRI values suggested that most items on the Hopelessness scale would fail to meet standards (e.g., Jackson, 1984, 1989) for being adequately distinct from response-style variance. In general, therefore, the scale and its items appear not to measure anything other than a supposedly irrelevant response style. It could even be suggested that the scale developers should go back the drawing board. Or should they? Again, empirical studies indicate that the Hopelessness scale predicts actual behavior—behavior that is of substantial and societal significance (e.g., death by suicide).

Although concerns about social desirability appeared to subside for a while, as personality assessment regained prominence with the ascendance of the Big Five model of personality within industrial/organizational and personnel contexts, social desirability reemerged as a potential issue. Given that job applicants' self-report for Big Five constructs (i.e., Neuroticism, Extraversion, Openness, Agreeableness, Conscientiousness) could predict job performance, a concern about socially desirable responding, in particular impression management, seemed logical. However, prominent validity studies by Hough, Eaton, Dunnette, Kamp, and McCloy (1990), Barrick and Mount (1996), and Piedmont, McCrae, Riemann, and Angleitner (2000) seemed to indicate that, at a group level, social desirability does not attenuate self-report personality scale validity, leading some to suggest that the issue is a "red herring" (Ones, Viswesvaran, & Reiss, 1996). More recently, however, findings suggest that this putative red herring may be important after all (Holden, 2007, 2008). Holden (2007) indicated that, averaged over personality scales, socially desirable responding can account for 10–15% of the variability of the prediction in peer criterion ratings. Furthermore, under high-stakes testing associated with the military, White, Young, and Rumsey (2001) reported that the validity of personality measures that predict duty performance and attrition is severely compromised as a function of social desirability.

Where does this leave us? It appears that social desirability can contaminate self-report scales and, consequently, threaten scales' construct validity. In such instances, scale score interpretations are ambiguous.

For example, does a normatively elevated score on a self-report measure of orderliness represent a respondent's true level of being orderly or the individual's tendency to answer in terms of social desirability?

In other circumstances, however, social desirability may not be a contaminant but, rather, a legitimate aspect of the construct being measured. As an example, it could be theorized that appearing socially desirable is an inherent component of the individual-difference variable of affiliation motivation (i.e., people who have a greater desire to affiliate may tend to describe themselves positively to others). Although, for a specific construct, such an interpretation could be appropriate, applying this reasoning to a set of individual differences does raise an important consideration (Holden, 2001). If social desirability is a legitimate facet of many different individual-difference constructs (e.g., achievement, affiliation, agreeableness, nurturance) and if negative social desirability (i.e., social undesirability) is also a true component of certain person variables (e.g., depression, hopelessness, impulsivity, psychopathy), then these constructs are not conceptually distinct and should not be theorized, measured, or interpreted as such. Presently, discerning whether social desirability is part of the construct being measured or an interfering response style is not an easy task and is not well established either theoretically or empirically.

How does social desirability relate to other personality variables? This seemingly straightforward question is not answered readily. Difficulties arise because social desirability is not well defined theoretically, because measures of social desirability are quite varied, and because the structure of social desirability is not completely articulated. Historically, social desirability scales have been associated with personality variables of honesty, need for approval, and ego resiliency. However, subscales of social desirability have also been shown to correlate, with at least a medium effect size (i.e., $r >$ .30), with every domain scale of the Big Five personality traits (Paulhus, 2002).

More recently, in a novel statistical residualization approach to characterizing social desirability bias as a departure from reality, Paulhus (2002) identified egoistic and moralistic biases as the chief facets of social desirability bias. The egoistic bias of social desirability focuses on a narcissistic exaggeration of agency-related traits such as dominance, courage, emotional stability, intelligence, and creativity. Also associated with this bias are personality characteristics of ego resilience, achievement via independence, social potency, perceived capability, lack of distress, and personal growth (Paulhus & John, 1998). Social desirability's moralistic bias exaggerates communion-related traits such as duty, agreeableness, and impulse control (Paulhus, 2002). Related personality traits are ego control, achievement via conformity, nurturance, social closeness, interpersonal sensitivity, restraint, and socialization (Paulhus & John, 1998). These innovative characterizations of social desirability await further empirical confirmation.

Because researchers are far from reaching a consensus on the contamination-versus-legitimate content issue, test developers and users should be alert to the potential deleterious effects of social desirability. Two suggestions may be particularly relevant. First, although many personality dimensions (e.g., hopelessness) could have content aspects of socially desirable responding as part of their constructs, if a goal is to construct multiscale inventories with relatively distinct and independent scales, then item selection procedures that minimize social desirability will serve to foster greater scale independence. Conversely, item selection techniques that enhance scale orthogonality should attenuate the socially desirable responding associated with the resultant personality scales. Second, in situations in which the motivation to distort self-report exists, the use of a separate scale of socially desirable responding is recommended. Even if the content scale has been developed to reduce the impact of socially desirable responding, an independent index of test-respondent motivation can alert test users to particular individuals whose scores may reflect stylistic rather than content responding.

Measurement

Although a plethora of scales are available to measure social desirability, five of the more noted ones are mentioned here. These scales have been and are more prominent because of their popularity, their psychometric properties, and the reputations of their developers.

The Edwards Social Desirability Scale (Edwards, 1957) comprises items from the MMPI. The scale includes 39 true–false items that were selected by judges who unanimously agreed on the direction of keying when asked to respond in a socially desirable fashion. In assessing scale internal-consistency reliability, a coefficient alpha of .79 has been reported with a sample of university students (Holden & Fekken, 1989). Sample items include "My hands and feet are usually warm enough" (true-keyed), "I am very seldom troubled by constipation" (true-keyed), and "I find it hard to keep my mind on a task or job" (false-keyed).

The Marlowe–Crowne Social Desirability Scale (Crowne & Marlowe, 1960) focuses on culturally sanctioned and approved but unlikely behavior. In this way this scale's items avoid psychopathology content. Items were devised and selected based on consideration of various personality inventories, judged social desirability ratings, and item–total associations. Holden and Fekken (1989) reported a coefficient-alpha scale reliability of .78 for an undergraduate sample. Sample items include "Before voting, I thoroughly investigate the qualifications of all the candidates" (true-keyed), "There have been occasions when I felt like smashing things" (false-keyed), and "I have never deliberately said something that hurt someone's feelings" (true-keyed).

The Personality Research Form (Form E) Desirability Scale (Jackson, 1984) consists of 16 true–false items. Items represent heterogeneous content and have relatively extreme values of scaled desirability. Jackson reported a Spearman–Brown corrected split-half reliability of .68 for college students. Sample items include "I am quite able to make correct decisions on difficult questions" (true-keyed), "I am never able to do things as well as I should" (false-keyed), and "My life is full of interesting activities" (true-keyed).

The Balanced Inventory of Desirable Responding (Version 7) Self-Deceptive Enhancement Scale (Paulhus, 1998) focuses on an unconscious favorability bias. This scale comprises 20 items answered on 5-point rating scales ranging from 1 (*not true*) to 5 (*very true*). With items scored dichotomously, this scale assesses a pervasive lack of insight associated with narcissistic overconfidence. Paulhus reported scale coefficient-alpha reliability coefficients ranging from .70 for college students to .75 for the general population. Sample items include "My first impressions of people usually turn out to be right" (positively keyed), "It would be hard for me to break any of my bad habits" (negatively keyed), and "I don't care what other people really think of me" (positively keyed).

The Balanced Inventory of Desirable Responding (Version 7) Impression Management Scale (Paulhus, 1998) consists of 20 items responded to on 5-point rating scales. Items are scored dichotomously, and the scale assesses faking, lying, and dissimulation. Coefficient-alpha reliability for the scale is reported by Paulhus as .81 for college students and .84 for prison entrants. Sample items include "I sometimes tell lies if I have to" (negatively keyed), "I never cover up my mistakes" (positively keyed), and "There have been occasions when I have taken advantage of someone" (negatively keyed).

Structure

Although social desirability is commonly regarded as a single response style, evidence suggests that the structure may be more complex. In a factor analysis of 30 scales of stylistic responding (including more than just social desirability scales), Wiggins (1964) reported three factors associated with social desirability: Alpha (unfavorable vs. favorable self-evaluation); Gamma (a lying factor); and Cautious, Controlled Good Impression. In also analyzing at the scale level, Paulhus's (1984) analysis of various response-style measures identified self-deception and impression management as two distinct components of socially desirable responding. More recently, Paulhus (2002) suggested a revision of the structure, now indicating four socially desirable responding aspects (self-deceptive enhancement, agency management, self-deceptive denial, and communion management).

Complementing the scale-level results, lower level analyses also indicate the multidimensional nature of social desirability. O'Grady (1988), in analyzing six miniscales

of the Edwards and Marlowe–Crowne social desirability scale items, concluded that the two scales measure distinct factors. Holden and Fekken (1989) factor analyzed responses to 92 items from three social desirability scales and uncovered eight first-order and two higher order factors. In interpreting their solution, they did not rule out the possibility that factors could represent both style and substance and indicated that the two higher order social desirability factors represented a Sense of Own General Capability and Interpersonal Sensitivity. Contained within the Sense of Own General Capability factor were facets of focused and realistic thinking (e.g., no difficulty concentrating), social integration (e.g., a sense of being cared for), self-confidence (e.g., not being self-conscious), hardiness (e.g., seldom being ill), and acceptance of responsibility (e.g., actions following words). For Interpersonal Sensitivity, subcomponents of considerateness (e.g., never deliberately hurting someone), social sensitivity (e.g., always being courteous), and tolerance (e.g., not resenting doing favors) were uncovered.

Regardless of whether scales, miniscales, or items are analyzed, a consensus emerges that at least two correlated but distinct higher order factors of social desirability exist, one emphasizing the self and one focusing on others. These factors may include both content and style and, consequently, may or may not indicate distortions from accuracy. That is, although departures from veridicality will be indicated by extreme scores on these factors, extreme scores do not necessarily imply invalid responding.

Recent Investigations into Social Desirability

Given the potential detrimental effects of social desirability, the extent of its possible impact should be considered. The following is a nonexhaustive review of recent social desirability investigations conducted in prominent research areas. Though many of these explorations may be preliminary, and although in some areas only a handful of studies have been conducted, future studies will likely build on these examinations. Thus we refrain from drawing general conclusions in anticipation both of future work and of the evolution of theories and measurements of social desirability.

Psychological Well-Being

Studies examining anxiety, mental health, and life satisfaction tend to involve self-report measures that may be influenced by individual differences in social desirability. Within anxiety research, measures of competitive state anxiety and social desirability correlated between .38 and .70 for high-level soccer players assessed just prior to competition (Smith, Driver, Lafferty, Burrell, & Devonport, 2001). Likewise, Riketta (2004) indicated that social desirability could inflate the relationship between self-esteem and anxiety by approximately 9% of the variance.

Other studies have demonstrated differential effects of social desirability on anxiety by gender. For example, math anxiety has been negatively associated with measures of social desirability for men but not for women (Zettle & Houghton, 1998). In another study, Grossbard, Cumming, Standage, Smith, and Smoll (2007) found that social desirability was negatively associated with performance anxiety for women. Furthermore, the observed relationship between goal orientations and performance anxiety was reduced when controlling for social desirability.

In one investigation of children (Dadds, Perrin, & Yule, 1998), self-reported anxiety and social desirability did not correlate for either boys or girls at any age. However, social desirability partially explained discrepancies between child and teacher reports of anxiety. For girls, social desirability was positively associated with teacher ratings of child anxiety. Furthermore, consideration of social desirability improved agreement between teacher and child anxiety ratings and between these ratings and clinician ratings. Among boys rated as anxious by their teachers, those boys self-reporting high anxiety had significantly lower social desirability scores than did those boys self-reporting low anxiety. Thus social desirability appears to be an important construct to consider when examining several forms of anxiety.

Social desirability may be important for other aspects of mental health and well-being as well. For self-reported mental health, the proportion of "true" responses on positively worded items and the proportion of "false" responses on negatively worded items were positively and negatively associated, respectively, with the social desirability scale values of items (Huang, Liao, & Chang, 1998). These findings indicated that the relationship between the social desirability scale value of an item and the proportion of social desirability responses can be described as V-shaped, not linear. For dispositional optimism, Rauch, Schweizer, and Moosbrugger (2007) reported that deviation from unidimensionality of observed optimism scores could be accounted for by including a method effect factor of positively worded items and that this factor was differentially associated with dimensions of social desirability. Whereas the impression-management dimension correlated significantly with the Method factor, the self-deceptive dimension correlated significantly with the General Optimism factor.

Social desirability has also been examined with respect to coping. Gravdal and Sandal (2006) examined whether impression-management and self-deception facets of social desirability were differentially related to measures of coping strategies, defense mechanisms, and self-efficacy in students. In factor analyses, self-deception grouped with self-efficacy, active problem solving, depressive reactions, and comforting cognitions on an Active Coping factor, whereas impression management and social desirability clustered together on a separate factor labeled Other-Deception. Athletic coping skills in undergraduates have been demonstrated to be unrelated to an impression-management component of social desirability but strongly affected by self-deception (Bourgeois, Loss, Meyers, & LeUnes, 2003). In a study of employed adult students that examined coping with work stress, high social desirability predicted direct action coping, whereas low social desirability predicted alcohol use as a coping mechanism (Gianakos, 2002). Other researchers, however, in investigating whether different types of social desirability influence the identification of individuals with repressive coping styles in adults, have found no relationship between facets of social desirability and a repressive coping style (Furnham, Petrides, & Spencer-Bowdage, 2002).

Recent research examining the relationship between social desirability and emotion has indicated that social desirability is positively associated with emotional intelligence (Mesmer-Magnus, Viswesvaran, Deshpande, & Joseph, 2006). Furthermore, emotional intelligence was a significant predictor of social desirability over and above self-esteem and overclaiming alone. In studies examining responses to emotional advertising, men reported a less pleasant viewing experience and a less favorable attitude toward the advertisement when a stereotype-incongruent advertisement was viewed with another man, whereas their responses were not affected by the presence of another man when they were exposed to a stereotype-congruent advertisement (Fisher & Dubé, 2005). Therefore, research has emerged in several areas showing a significant influence of social desirability on well-being.

Other research, however, indicates that scales in the domain of adjustment function independently of social desirability. For example, some measures of life satisfaction appear to be untainted by social desirability in adolescents (Gilman & Barry, 2003) and younger and older adults (Laicardi, Baldassarri, & Artistico, 2001). Furthermore, Rogers, Reinecke, and Setzer (2004) revealed a strong association, independent of social desirability, between childhood attachment experience and cognitive vulnerability in a sample of clinically depressed adults. Likewise, Cramer (2000) found that, although social desirability was positively associated with satisfaction, social support, and mental health, the association between these latter two constructs remained relatively unchanged when social desirability was controlled for. Future research will be needed to examine the full extent and boundaries of the effects of social desirability on self-reported well-being.

Rather than having a construct definition, social desirability, as measured by self-report scales, is traditionally viewed as a response style that threatens the construct validity of other self-report scales. Nevertheless, social desirability scale scores, in and of themselves, show interesting relationships with behavioral and non-self-report measures. In particular, the relationship of social desirability and suicide appears to be stable and generalizable. Linehan and Neilsen (1981)

reported that social desirability scale scores correlated negatively ($r = -.25$) with the presence of a previous suicide attempt for a sample drawn from the general community. Among psychiatric patients, social desirability correlated negatively with clinicians' ratings of patients' suicidal desire ($r = -.34$), suicide preparation ($r = -.22$), and suicide ideation ($r = -.30$) (Holden, Mendonca, & Serin, 1989). Holden and colleagues (1989) also found that, for male federal inmates, social desirability correlated negatively ($r = -.29$) with a history of a previous suicide attempt. Similarly, Ivanoff and Jang (1991) found that, for male state inmates, social desirability scale scores correlated negatively with clinician-rated suicide ideation ($r = -.44$) and a previous history of suicidal behavior ($r = -.32$). Thus it appears that there is substantive as well as stylistic variance in measures of social desirability. Perhaps this is the reason that social desirability may be evolving into a concept for which some now indicate that, in measuring this response-style concept, there is a "necessity of demonstrating departure-from-reality" (Paulhus, 2002, p. 49). Thus many current self-report scales of social desirability may lack a necessary exaggeration-from-veridicality aspect or at least confound it with true content associated with other constructs.

Self-Knowledge and Goals

Just as social desirability may influence self-reported measures of psychological well-being, it may also affect measures of self-knowledge. Social desirability is positively associated with the evaluative component of self-knowledge: self-esteem (Mesmer-Magnus et al., 2006). Social desirability also moderates the relationship between implicit and explicit self-esteem such that the relationship is stronger under conditions of high or low self-deception depending on the type of implicit measure used (Riketta, 2005). Self-knowledge has been found to be significantly influenced by social desirability, but the amount of influence differs as a function of the self-knowledge domain (Meleddu & Guicciardi, 1998). Specifically, social desirability effects are weaker for the anxiety domain than for the extraversion domain in that the ideal self is a better predictor of the actual self for extraversion than for anxiety.

These investigations indicate a consistent impact of social desirability on the measurement of self-knowledge.

Social psychology has seen increased interest in studies examining aspects of motivation. Accordingly, recent research has investigated whether social desirability influences goal orientation related to work and academics (Tan & Hall, 2005). Social desirability was negatively associated with learning goals and positively related to performance-avoidance goals, whereas performance-approach goals were uncontaminated by social desirability. Grossbard and colleagues (2007) reported that social desirability was negatively associated with ego orientation in adolescent men and women and positively associated with task orientation in women and that it reduced the relationship between goal orientations and performance anxiety in women. Though the reasons for these complex relationships require further investigation, social desirability appears to be related to people's goals and motivations.

Culture

Research suggests that cultural orientation may be associated with socially desirable responding. Middleton and Jones (2000) explored differences in overall social desirability across Eastern and Western cultures. Significant differences existed such that students from Asian countries reported higher social desirability than students from the United States and Canada. Across several studies, European Americans, compared with Asian Americans, scored higher on self-deception and lower on impression-management facets of social desirability, and individualism was positively associated with self-deception, whereas collectivism was positively associated with impression management (Lalwani, Shavitt, & Johnson, 2006). Keillor, Owens, and Pettijohn (2001) investigated differences in social desirability in 15- to 65-year-olds across cultures and observed higher social desirability in Malaysian compared with U.S. and French samples.

Contrary to the research that demonstrates significant relations between cultural orientation and social desirability, some studies demonstrate a lack of cultural differences in self-enhancement. For example,

Cuixia, Jian, and Zhongfang (2003) reported that Chinese college students' ratings of item social desirability and estimates of the percentage of others who would behave in the manner described by these items indicated self-enhancement and honesty similar to that for American college students. Chinese college students perceived that they did more desirable and fewer undesirable activities than others and chose to give more honest responses to undesirable items that were perceived to be more neutral than desirable items. Future research will need to determine whether different samples and methodologies account for these discrepancies or, alternatively, whether self-enhancement is an exception to the influence of culture on social desirability.

Relationships, Attraction, and Gender Roles

In exploring love styles, Davies (2001) found that social desirability was associated with traditional gender-role socialization such that social desirability negatively correlated with possessive, dependent love styles (*mania*) in men and women. Furthermore, for men, social desirability was positively related to romantic, passionate (*eros*) and game-playing (*ludus*) love and negatively associated with all-giving, selfless love (*agape*). For women, social desirability was positively related to agape and negatively related to ludus.

The susceptibility of attachment-style measures to impression-management and self-deception aspects of social desirability has been examined in college students (Leak & Parsons, 2001). All attachment measures examined were influenced by impression-management tendencies, and two of three were influenced by self-deception. Maltby and Day (2000) examined whether the importance of romantic acts was associated with social desirability and found that endorsement of romantic acts was positively related to social desirability in both men and women. Loving and Agnew (2001) developed a measure of social desirability (including impression-management and self-deception components) for use in relationship research with dating and married couples. Impression-management scores were higher in public versus private conditions, and self-deception was associated with several relationship-quality measures. Therefore, impression-management and self-deception dimensions of social desirability appear to be relevant to measures that are used in relationship research.

On the other hand, the relationship between ratings of attractiveness and social desirability is inconsistent. An investigation of whether age and attractiveness of targets was associated with ratings of social desirability revealed that young and older adults rated younger, unattractive targets as possessing fewer socially desirable traits (Perlini, Bertolissi, & Lind, 1999). Overall, younger judges rated attractive targets as high in socially desirable traits, and older male judges rated older attractive targets as less socially desirable than younger attractive targets. Conversely, in another study, young and elderly women's ratings of men indicated that neither age nor attractiveness influenced ratings of socially desirable traits (Perlini, Marcello, Hansen, & Pudney, 2001). Thus it seems that, whereas measures of love and attachment are more consistently affected by social desirability concerns, the results for attraction alone are mixed.

Physical Health

A large number of investigations have examined the influence of social desirability on aspects of self-reported physical health, such as weight loss and dieting. For example, Carels, Cacciapaglia, Rydin, Douglass, and Harper (2006) examined the association between social desirability and percentage of body weight loss in obese participants. Higher social desirability was associated with self-reports of greater weight control competence and weight loss self-efficacy, fewer calories and dietary lapses, and more positive attitudes toward dieting. Higher social desirability was also associated with less weight loss over a 6-month intervention. In addition, Klesges and colleagues (2004) reported that social desirability was associated with overestimates of physical activity, underestimates of sweetened beverage preferences, and lower ratings of weight concerns and dieting behaviors in African American girls. Socially desirable responding also distorted the relationship of body mass index with self-reports of physical activity and energy intake.

For children, Baxter and colleagues (2004) investigated the association between general social desirability and social desirability vis-à-vis ratings of food. Whereas one food factor (including items about drinking milk, eating vegetables, and finishing all of one's food) was associated with social desirability, another food factor (with questions about eating fast food, drinking soda, and eating too much) was not related to social desirability. The predictive validity of a theory of planned behavior for healthy food choices in adults revealed that social desirability had minimal influence on the relationships between model components (Armitage & Conner, 1999).

Research has also explored the relationship between social desirability and eating disorders in adolescents (Miotto, De Coppi, Frezza, Rossi, & Preti, 2002). For male and female adolescents, a negative association was found between social desirability and scores on eating-disorder measures. In a study of eating-disorder prevention in seventh- and eighth-grade girls, Tilgner, Wertheim, and Paxton (2004) found that social desirability had a low correlation with body dissatisfaction, drive for thinness, bulimic tendencies, intention to diet, and size discrepancy.

In research by Watson and colleagues (2006), controlling for social desirability appeared to have little influence on the correlations between self-efficacy (for either physical activity or fruit and vegetable consumption) and actual behaviors. However, when using multidimensional item-response theory, the relationships between efficacy and behavior were substantially reduced when controlling for social desirability. Motl, McAuley, and DiStefano (2005) found little evidence of an influence of social desirability on self-report measures of physical activity in young adults, with only a small relationship between social desirability and physical activity for one of the two social desirability measures used.

Effects of social desirability have also been explored with respect to other important aspects of physical health, including sexual health. In studying the accuracy of self-reported sexual behavior among Botswana women, respondents have pointed to shame and the fear of public talk about them as key factors contributing to inaccurate self-reports (Chillag et al., 2006). Meston, Heiman, Trapnell, and Paulhus (1998) assessed the impact of self-deception and impression-management facets of social desirability on undergraduate students' sexuality self-reports. Sexual adjustment was associated with self-deception variables for both sexes, whereas a number of intrapersonal and interpersonal sexual behaviors for women and unrestricted sexual attitudes and fantasies for men were negatively associated with impression management. Furthermore, the associations between impression management and sexuality measures were significant even after controlling for general personality and conservatism.

The influence of self-deceptive social desirability on the accuracy of self-reported HIV serostatus was studied in active injection-drug users (Latkin & Vlahov, 1998). For respondents who scored low on self-deception, the sensitivity of self-reported HIV serostatus was 81% as compared with 63% for those individuals who scored high on self-deception. However, for a study examining the relationship between social desirability and self-reported condom use behavior in sex workers in the Philippines, no relationship was found (Morisky, Ang, & Sneed, 2002). Furthermore, Keffala and Stone (1999) found that social desirability was not related to psychologists' decisions to maintain or break confidentiality of HIV-positive patients across 16 scenarios of varying risk, danger, and situation.

Willebrand, Wikehult, and Ekselius (2005) found that among former burn patients, high social desirability was associated with poorer perceived health on the burn-specific health subscales of heat sensitivity, work, and body image. However, another study examining reported somatic and emotional health in adults found no influence for social desirability (Sheridan, Mulhern, & Martin, 1999).

Other aspects of physical health have also been explored. A study of the relationship between social desirability and self-reported heroin cravings revealed that high social desirability was related to lower self-reported cravings but was not related to physiological craving measures and did not moderate the relation between self-reported and physiological craving indices (Marissen, Franken, Blanken, van den Brink, & Hendriks, 2005). Sloan, Bodapati, and Tucker (2004) examined whether social desirability influ-

enced reporting of marijuana and cocaine drug use by arrestees in the United States. In comparing self-reports with the results of urinalysis tests of drug use, social desirability was related to reporting such that arrestees who tested positive for cocaine were 15 times more likely to misreport their drug use than those who tested positive for marijuana.

Thus a large body of work has demonstrated that social desirability appears to exert at least some influence on self-reported measures of physical health and could have impact on several areas that are significant to society. In addition to the research mentioned here on psychological well-being, self-knowledge, motivation, relationships, and culture, social desirability continues to be of interest among social and personality psychologists.

Summary

As research on social desirability continues to evolve, additional promising avenues and techniques emerge. Holden and his colleagues (Holden & Kroner, 1992; Holden, Kroner, Fekken, & Popham, 1992) have identified the use of response latencies as a behaviorally based method for assessing socially desirable responding in general and faking in particular. In their model, responses that are incongruent with a faking schema take longer to produce than schema-congruent answers. From the perspective of item-response theory, Zickar and his associates (Zickar, Gibby, & Robie, 2004; Zickar & Robie, 1999) have applied this item-response approach toward the modeling of induced socially desirable responding. Their work indicates that patterns of induced faking are heterogeneous rather than homogeneous in nature. This, again, suggests that socially desirable responding is a multidimensional phenomenon. Employing signal-detection methods, Paulhus and his collaborators (Paulhus, Harms, Bruce, & Lysy, 2003; Williams, Paulhus, & Harms, 2001) have developed an operationalized implementation of social desirability. In this technique, the overclaiming of knowledge involves a self-serving distortion that relates to other self-report measures of socially desirable self-deceptive enhancement. Furthermore, this approach represents a relatively subtle and unobtrusive measure of socially desirable responding.

Social desirability is a multidimensional response style that has the potential to compromise the accurate measurement of noncognitive individual differences assessed by self-report. The extent of this disruption may be substantial depending on the domain and context of the assessment. Scales of social desirability can reflect both content and stylistic responding, and, in some domains, the content component of a social desirability scale can be relevant for the domain being measured. Distinguishing relevant content responding from irrelevant stylistic responding is challenging, both theoretically and operationally. Although new directions in social desirability research may assist in separating substance from style, in the interim, prudent scale users should remain alert to social desirability response styles as potential threats to the construct validity of self-reports.

Acknowledgment

Preparation of this chapter was supported, in part, by a grant from the Social Sciences and Humanities Research Council of Canada.

References

Armitage, C. J., & Conner, M. (1999). Predictive validity of the theory of planned behaviour: The role of questionnaire format and social desirability. *Journal of Community and Applied Social Psychology, 9*, 261–272.

Barrick, M. R., & Mount, M. K. (1996). Effects of impression management and self-deception on the predictive validity of personality constructs. *Journal of Applied Psychology, 81*, 261–272.

Baxter, S. D., Smith, A. F., Litaker, M. S., Baglio, M. L., Guinn, C. H., & Shaffer, N. M. (2004). Children's social desirability and dietary reports. *Journal of Nutrition Education and Behavior, 36*, 84–89.

Beck, A. T., Brown, G., Berchick, R. J., Stewart, B. L., & Steer, R. A. (1990). Relationship between hopelessness and ultimate suicide: A replication with psychiatric outpatients. *American Journal of Psychiatry, 147*, 190–195.

Beck, A. T., Steer, R. A., Kovacs, M., & Garrison, B. (1985). Hopelessness and eventual suicide: A 10-year prospective study of patients hospitalized with suicidal ideation. *American Journal of Psychiatry, 142*, 559–563.

Beck, A. T., Weissman, A., Lester, D., & Trexler, L. (1974). The measurement of pessimism: The Hope-

lessness scale. *Journal of Consulting and Clinical Psychology, 42*, 861–865.

Bourgeois, A. E., Loss, R., Meyers, M. C., & LeUnes, A. D. (2003). The Athletic Coping Skills Inventory: Relationship with impression management and self-deception aspects of socially desirable responding. *Psychology of Sport and Exercise, 4*, 71–79.

Brown, G. K., Beck, A. T., Steer, R. A., & Grisham, J. R. (2000). Risk factors for suicide in psychiatric outpatients: A 20-year prospective study. *Journal of Consulting and Clinical Psychology, 68*, 371–377.

Carels, R. A., Cacciapaglia, H. M., Rydin, S., Douglass, O. M., & Harper, J. (2006). Can social desirability interfere with success in a behavioral weight loss program? *Psychology and Health, 21*, 65–78.

Chillag, K., Guest, G., Bunce, A., Johnson, L., Kilmarx, P. H., & Smith, D. K. (2006). Talking about sex in Botswana: Social desirability bias and possible implications for HIV-prevention research. *African Journal of AIDS Research, 5*, 123–131.

Cramer, D. (2000). Social desirability, adequacy of social support and mental health. *Journal of Community and Applied Social Psychology, 10*, 465–474.

Crowne, D. P., & Marlowe, D. (1960). A new scale of social desirability independent of psychopathology. *Journal of Consulting Psychology, 24*, 349–354.

Cuixia, L., Jian, X., & Zhongfang, Y. (2003). A compromise between self-enhancement and honesty: Chinese self-evaluations on social desirability scales. *Psychological Reports, 92*, 291–298.

Dadds, M. R., Perrin, S., & Yule, W. (1998). Social desirability and self-reported anxiety in children: An analysis of the RCMAS Lie Scale. *Journal of Abnormal Child Psychology, 26*, 311–317.

Davies, M. F. (2001). Socially desirable responding and impression management in the endorsement of love styles. *Journal of Psychology: Interdisciplinary and Applied, 135*, 562–570.

Edwards, A. E. (1957). *The social desirability variable in personality assessment and research.* New York: Dryden.

Edwards, A. L., & Walker, J. N. (1961). A short form of the MMPI: The SD Scale. *Psychological Reports, 8*, 485–486.

Ellis, A. (1946). The validity of personality questionnaires. *Psychological Bulletin, 43*, 385–440.

Fisher, R. J., & Dubé, L. (2005). Gender differences in responses to emotional advertising: A social desirability perspective. *Journal of Consumer Research, 31*, 850–858.

Frank, L. F. (1948). *Projective methods.* Springfield, IL: Thomas.

Furnham, A., Petrides, K. V., & Spencer-Bowdage, S. (2002). The effects of different types of social desirability on the identification of repressors. *Personality and Individual Differences, 33*, 119–130.

Gianakos, I. (2002). Predictors of coping with work stress: The influences of sex, gender role, social desirability, and locus of control. *Sex Roles, 46*, 149–158.

Gilman, R., & Barry, J. (2003). Life satisfaction and social desirability among adolescents in a residential treatment setting: Changes across time. *Residential Treatment for Children and Youth, 21*, 19–42.

Goodenough, F. L. (1946). Semantic choice and personality structure. *Science, 104*, 451–456.

Gravdal, L., & Sandal, G. M. (2006). The two-factor

model of social desirability: Relation to coping and defense, and implications for health. *Personality and Individual Differences, 40,* 1051–1061.

Grossbard, J. R., Cumming, S. P., Standage, M., Smith, R. E., & Smoll, F. L. (2007). Social desirability and relations between goal orientations and competitive trait anxiety in young athletes. *Psychology of Sport and Exercise, 8,* 491–505.

Holden, R. R. (2001). Social desirability. In W. E. Craighead & C. B. Nemeroff (Eds.), *The Corsini encyclopaedia of psychology and behavioral science* (3rd ed., Vol. 4, pp. 1557–1558). New York: Wiley.

Holden, R. R. (2007). Socially desirable responding does moderate scale validity both in experimental and in nonexperimental contexts. *Canadian Journal of Behavioural Science, 39,* 184–201.

Holden, R. R. (2008). Underestimating the effects of faking on the validity of self-report personality scales. *Personality and Individual Differences, 44,* 311–321.

Holden, R. R., & Fekken, G. C. (1989). Three common social desirability scales: Friends, acquaintances, or strangers? *Journal of Research in Personality, 23,* 180–191.

Holden, R. R., & Kroner, D. G. (1992). Relative efficacy of differential response latencies for detecting faking on a self-report measure of psychopathology. *Psychological Assessment, 4,* 170–173.

Holden, R. R., Kroner, D. G., Fekken, G. C., & Popham, S. M. (1992). A model of personality test item response dissimulation. *Journal of Personality and Social Psychology, 63,* 272–279.

Holden, R. R., & Mendonca, J. D. (1984). Hopelessness, social desirability, and suicidal behavior: A need for conceptual and empirical disentanglement. *Journal of Clinical Psychology, 40,* 1342–1345.

Holden, R. R., Mendonca, J. D., & Mazmanian, D. (1985). Relation of response set to observed suicide intent. *Canadian Journal of Behavioural Science, 17,* 359–368.

Holden, R. R., Mendonca, J. D., & Serin, R. C. (1989). Suicide, hopelessness, and social desirability: A test of an interactive model. *Journal of Consulting and Clinical Psychology, 57,* 500–504.

Hough, L. M., Eaton, N. K., Dunnette, M. D., Kamp, J. D., & McCloy, R. A. (1990). Criterion-related validities of personality constructs and the effect of response distortion on those validities. *Journal of Applied Psychology, 75,* 581–595.

Huang, C. Y., Liao, H. Y., & Chang, S. H. (1998). Social desirability and the clinical self-report inventory: Methodological reconsideration. *Journal of Clinical Psychology, 54,* 517–528.

Ivanoff, A., & Jang, S. J. (1991). The role of hopelessness and social desirability in predicting suicidal behavior: A study of prison inmates. *Journal of Consulting and Clinical Psychology, 59,* 394–399.

Jackson, D. N. (1970). A sequential system for personality scale development. In C. D. Spielberger (Ed.), *Current topics in clinical and community psychology* (Vol. 2, pp. 61–96). New York: Academic Press.

Jackson, D. N. (1971). The dynamics of structured personality tests: 1971. *Psychological Review, 78,* 229–248.

Jackson, D. N. (1973). Structured personality assessment. In B. B. Wolman (Ed.), *Handbook of general*

psychology (pp. 775–792). Englewood Cliffs, NJ: Prentice-Hall.

Jackson, D. N. (1984). *Personality Research Form manual* (3rd ed.). Port Huron, MI: Research Psychologists Press.

Jackson, D. N. (1989). *Basic Personality Inventory manual.* Port Huron, MI: Sigma Assessment Systems.

Jackson, D. N., & Messick, S. (1961). Acquiescence and desirability as response determinants on the MMPI. *Educational and Psychological Measurement, 21,* 771–790.

Jackson, D. N., & Messick, S. (1962a). Response styles and the assessment of psychopathology. In S. Messick & J. Ross (Eds.), *Measurement in personality and cognition* (pp. 129–155). New York: Wiley.

Jackson, D. N., & Messick, S. (1962b). Response styles on the MMPI: Comparison of clinical and normal samples. *Journal of Abnormal and Social Psychology, 65,* 285–299.

Keffala, V. J., & Stone, G. L. (1999). Role of HIV serostatus, relationship status of the patient, homophobia, and social desirability of the psychologist on decisions regarding confidentiality. *Psychology and Health, 14,* 567–584.

Keillor, B., Owens, D., & Pettijohn, C. (2001). A cross-cultural/cross-national study of influencing factors and socially desirable response biases. *International Journal of Market Research, 43,* 63–84.

Klesges, L. M., Baranowski, T., Beech, B., Cullen, K., Murray, D. M., Rochon, J., et al. (2004). Social desirability bias in self-reported dietary, physical activity and weight concerns measures in 8- to 10-year-old African-American girls: Results from the Girls Health Enrichment Multisite Studies (GEMS). *Preventive Medicine: An International Journal Devoted to Practice and Theory, 38,* S78–S87.

Laicardi, C., Baldassarri, F., & Artistico, D. (2001). Unidimensionality of life satisfaction and its relation to social desirability: A confirmatory study of a short form of the Life Satisfaction Scale. *Psychological Reports, 88,* 253–261.

Lalwani, A. K., Shavitt, S., & Johnson, T. (2006). What is the relation between cultural orientation and socially desirable responding? *Journal of Personality and Social Psychology, 90,* 165–178.

Latkin, C. A., & Vlahov, D. (1998). Socially desirable response tendency as a correlate of accuracy of self-reported HIV serostatus for HIV seropositive injection drug users. *Addiction, 93,* 1191–1197.

Leak, G. K., & Parsons, C. J. (2001). The susceptibility of three attachment style measures to socially desirable responding. *Social Behavior and Personality, 29,* 21–30.

Linehan, M. M., & Nielsen, S. L. (1981). Assessment of suicide ideation and parasuicide: Hopelessness and social desirability. *Journal of Consulting and Clinical Psychology, 49,* 773–775.

Linehan, M. M., & Nielsen, S. L. (1983). Social desirability: Its relevance to the measurement of hopelessness and suicidal behavior. *Journal of Consulting and Clinical Psychology, 51,* 141–143.

Loving, T. J., & Agnew, C. R. (2001). Socially desirable responding in close relationships: A dual-component approach and measure. *Journal of Social and Personal Relationships, 18,* 551–573.

Maltby, J., & Day, L. (2000). Romantic acts as a correlate of social desirability, neuroticism, and extraversion. *Journal of Psychology: Interdisciplinary and Applied, 134,* 462–464.

Marissen, M. A. E., Franken, I. H. A., Blanken, P., van den Brink, W., & Hendriks, V. M. (2005). The relation between social desirability and different measures of heroin craving. *Journal of Addictive Diseases, 24,* 91–103.

Meehl, P. E. (1945). The dynamics of "structured" personality assessment. *Journal of Clinical Psychology, 1,* 296–303.

Meleddu, M., & Guicciardi, M. (1998). Self-knowledge and social desirability of personality traits. *European Journal of Personality, 12,* 151–168.

Mendonca, J. D., Holden, R. R., Mazmanian, D., & Dolan, P. J. (1983). The influence of response style on the Beck Hopelessness Scale. *Canadian Journal of Behavioural Science, 15,* 237–247.

Mesmer-Magnus, J., Viswesvaran, C., Deshpande, S., & Joseph, J. (2006). Social desirability: The role of over-claiming, self-esteem, and emotional intelligence. *Psychology Science, 48,* 336–356.

Meston, C. M., Heiman, J. R., Trapnell, P. D., & Paulhus, D. L. (1998). Socially desirable responding and sexuality self-reports. *Journal of Sex Research, 35,* 148–157.

Middleton, K. L., & Jones, J. L. (2000). Socially desirable response sets: The impact of country culture. *Psychology and Marketing, 17,* 149–163.

Miotto, P., De Coppi, M., Frezza, M., Rossi, M., & Preti, A. (2002). Social desirability and eating disorders: A community study of an Italian school-aged sample. *Acta Psychiatrica Scandinavica, 105,* 372–377.

Morisky, D. E., Ang, A., & Sneed, C. D. (2002). Validating the effects of social desirability on self-reported condom use behavior among commercial sex workers. *AIDS Education and Prevention, 14,* 351–360.

Motl, R. W., McAuley, E., & DiStefano, C. (2005). Is social desirability associated with self-reported physical activity? *Preventive Medicine: An International Journal Devoted to Practice and Theory, 40,* 735–739.

Nevid, J. S. (1983). Hopelessness, social desirability, and construct validity. *Journal of Consulting and Clinical Psychology, 51,* 139–140.

O'Grady, K. E. (1988). The Marlowe–Crowne and Edwards social desirability scales: A psychometric perspective. *Multivariate Behavioral Research, 23,* 87–101.

Ones, D. S., Viswesvaran, C., & Reiss, A. D. (1996). Role of socially desirable responding in personality testing for personnel selection: The red herring. *Journal of Applied Psychology, 81,* 660–679.

Paulhus, D. L. (1984). Two-component models of socially desirable responding. *Journal of Personality and Social Psychology, 46,* 598–609.

Paulhus, D. L. (1991). Measurement and control of response bias. In J. P. Robinson, P. R. Shaver, & L. S. Wrightsman (Eds.), *Measure of personality and social psychological attitudes* (Vol. 1, pp. 17–59). San Diego, CA: Academic Press.

Paulhus, D. L. (1998). *Paulhus Deception Scales (PDS): The Balanced Inventory of Desirable Responding—7 user's manual.* North Tonawanda, NY: Multi-Health Systems.

Paulhus, D. L. (2002). Socially desirable responding: The evolution of a construct. In H. I. Braun, D. N. Jackson, & D. E. Wiley (Eds.), *The role of constructs in psychological and educational measurement* (pp. 49–69). Mahwah, NJ: Erlbaum.

Paulhus, D. L., Harms, P. D., Bruce, N., & Lysy, D. C. (2003). The over-claiming technique: Measuring self-enhancement independent of ability. *Journal of Personality and Social Psychology, 84,* 890–904.

Paulhus, D. L., & John, O. P. (1998). Egoistic and moralistic biases in self-perception: The interplay of self-deceptive styles with basic traits and motives. *Journal of Personality, 66,* 1025–1060.

Perlini, A. H., Bertolissi, S., & Lind, D. L. (1999). The effects of women's age and physical appearance on evaluations of attractiveness and social desirability. *Journal of Social Psychology, 139,* 343–354.

Perlini, A. H., Marcello, A., Hansen, S. D., & Pudney, W. (2001). The effects of male age and physical appearance on evaluations of attractiveness, social desirability and resourcefulness. *Social Behavior and Personality, 29,* 277–287.

Piedmont, R. L., McCrae, R. R., Riemann, R., & Angleitner, A. (2000). On the invalidity of validity scales: Evidence from self-reports and observer ratings in volunteer samples. *Journal of Personality and Social Psychology, 78,* 582–593.

Rauch, W. A., Schweizer, K., & Moosbrugger, H. (2007). Method effects due to social desirability as a parsimonious explanation of the deviation from unidimensionality in LOT-R scores. *Personality and Individual Differences, 42,* 1597–1607.

Riketta, M. (2004). Does social desirability inflate the correlation between self-esteem and anxiety? *Psychological Reports, 94,* 1232–1234.

Riketta, M. (2005). Gender and socially desirable responding as moderators of the correlation between implicit and explicit self-esteem. *Current Research in Social Psychology, 11,* 14–28.

Rogers, G. M., Reinecke, M. A., & Setzer, N. J. (2004). Childhood attachment experience and adulthood cognitive vulnerability: Testing state dependence and social desirability hypotheses. *Journal of Cognitive Psychotherapy, 18,* 79–96.

Sheridan, C. L., Mulhern, M. A., & Martin, D. (1999). The role of social desirability, negative affectivity, and female reproductive system symptoms in differences in reporting symptoms by men and women. *Psychological Reports, 85,* 54–62.

Sloan, J. J., III, Bodapati, M. R., & Tucker, T. A. (2004). Respondent misreporting of drug use in self-reports: Social desirability and other correlates. *Journal of Drug Issues, 34,* 269–292.

Smith, D., Driver, S., Lafferty, M., Burrell, C., & Devonport, T. (2001). Social desirability bias and direction modified Competitive State Anxiety Inventory—2. *Perceptual and Motor Skills, 95,* 945–952.

Steinmetz, H. L. (1932). Measuring ability to fake occupational interest. *Journal of Applied Psychology, 16,* 123–130.

Strosahl, K. D., Linehan, M. M., & Chiles, J. A. (1984). Will the real social desirability scale please stand up? Hopelessness, depression, social desirability, and the prediction of suicidal behavior. *Journal of Consulting and Clinical Psychology, 52,* 449–457.

Tan, J. A., & Hall, R. J. (2005). The effects of social desirability bias on applied measures of goal orientation. *Personality and Individual Differences, 38*, 1891–1902.

Tilgner, L., Wertheim, E. H., & Paxton, S. J. (2004). Effect of social desirability on adolescent girls' responses to an eating disorders prevention program. *International Journal of Eating Disorders, 35*, 211–216.

Watson, K., Baranowski, T., Thompson, D., Jago, R., Baranowski, J., & Klesges, L. M. (2006). Innovative application of a multidimensional item response model in assessing the influence of social desirability on the pseudo-relationship between self-efficacy and behavior. *Health Education Research, 21*, 85–97.

White, L. A., Young, M. C., & Rumsey, M. G. (2001). ABLE implementation issue and related research. In J. P. Campbell & D. J. Knapp (Eds.), *Exploring the limits of personnel selection and classification* (pp. 525–558). Mahwah, NJ: Erlbaum.

Wiggins, J. S. (1964). Convergences among stylistic response measures from objective personality tests. *Educational and Psychological Measurement, 24*, 551–562.

Willebrand, M., Wikehult, B. R., & Ekselius, L. (2005). Social desirability, psychological symptoms, and perceived health in burn injured patients. *Journal of Nervous and Mental Disease, 193*, 820–824.

Williams, K., Paulhus, D. L., & Harms, P. (2001, June). *The over-claiming questionnaire: Invulnerable to faking and warning about foils.* Paper presented at the annual convention of the American Psychological Society, Toronto, Ontario, Canada.

Zettle, R. D., & Houghton, L. L. (1998). The relationship between mathematics anxiety and social desirability as a function of gender. *College Student Journal, 32*, 81–86.

Zickar, M. J., Gibby, R. E., & Robie, C. (2004). Uncovering faking samples in applicant, incumbent, and experimental data sets: An application of mixed-model item response theory. *Organizational Research Methods, 7*, 168–190.

Zickar, M. J., & Robie, C. (1999). Modeling faking good on personality items: An item-level analysis. *Journal of Applied Psychology, 84*, 551–563.

CHAPTER 31

■ ● ▲ ◆ ■ ● ▲ ◆

Sensation Seeking

MARVIN ZUCKERMAN

The sensation-seeking construct was developed as part of a theory of individual differences in response to the experimental situation of sensory deprivation (Zuckerman, 1969; Zuckerman, Kolin, Price, & Zoob, 1964). The first Sensation Seeking Scale (SSS) was developed to measure the postulated trait of "optimal level of stimulation/optimal level of arousal" (Zuckerman, 1969, Postulate III, p. 429). We soon realized that the SSS had a broader construct validity beyond predicting and explaining responses to sensory deprivation. The conceptual basis for sensation seeking also changed as research accumulated. It was apparent that sensation seeking was a motive for many kinds of behaviors that reflected a preference for novelty, as well as intensity and variety of stimulation.

The theory and research on sensation seeking is described in three books (Zuckerman, 1979, 1994b, 2007) and many book chapters and articles focusing on particular areas of research. These are cited and the general results described to avoid the need for citation to numerous articles on a particular subject. Some research articles or those with specific salience are also included.

The most recent definition of sensation seeking is: "Sensation seeking is a trait defined by the seeking of varied, novel, complex, and intense sensations and experiences, and the willingness to take physical, social,

legal, and financial risks for the sake of such experience" (Zuckerman, 1994b, p. 27). Note that risk is not an essential part of the trait. It is not accurate to equate sensation seeking solely with risky behavior. Many things that sensation seekers do are not risky. If there is risk it is often ignored, minimized, or tolerated and may even increase positive arousal to the activities that are risky.

Eysenck and Costa and McCrae conceived of sensation seeking as a facet of extraversion, but our factor-analytic studies have shown that it is a relatively independent and major dimension of personality. Within Eysenck's "Big Three," it is most strongly related to psychoticism, and within the Costa and McCrae "Big Five," it is primarily correlated (inversely) with conscientiousness (Zuckerman, Kuhlman, Joireman, Teta, & Kraft, 1993).

Measures of Sensation Seeking

The first form of the SSS (Form II; Zuckerman et al., 1964) was a general scale describing a need for varied and intense stimulation and arousal in human activities and preferences. Items were selected in terms of their correlation with the first unrotated factor. It was soon apparent that there might be more than a general factor, so items were written for an experimental Form III. The first unrotated factor was similar, but rotation identified four other factors: Thrill and Adventure Seeking (TAS), Experience Seeking (ES), Disinhibition (Dis), and Boredom Susceptibility (BS). The general scale and new scales for the subfactors were included in the SSS Form IV (Zuckerman, 1971). The subscales are briefly described:

TAS describes the seeking of arousal through extreme sports involving unusual sensations and risks, such as skydiving, scuba diving, or flying. Most of the items are expressed as intentions rather than actual experiences, for example, "I would like to. ... "

ES is the seeking of novel experiences through the mind and senses, travel, music, art, and people. It also represents social nonconformity and a desire to associate with unconventional people.

Dis is the seeking of intense experiences in parties, social drinking, and sex. Although some items describe behavioral preferences, others are general attitudes, for example, "I like to have new and exciting experiences even if they are a little unconventional or illegal."

BS items involve an intolerance for repetitive experience and boring people and restlessness when exposed to such conditions. An example of a forced-choice item is: "A. The worst social sin is to be a bore; B. The worst social sin is to be rude."

Form V contained subscales of 10 items, each selected to enhance increased convergent validity within scales and discriminant validity between scales. The substitution of a Total score, sum of the four subscales, replaced the general scale in Forms II and IV (Zuckerman, Eysenck, & Eysenck, 1978). The four subfactors of sensation seeking have been generally replicated in studies of translated scales in many different countries (Zuckerman, 1994b).

Forms II, IV, and V of the SSS were developed in isolation from other personality factors. Beginning in the late 1980s we began a series of factor analyses with the goal of providing a trait classification for *Psychobiology of Personality* (Zuckerman, 1991). All of the subscales of SSS-V, as well as other scales for sensation seeking, impulsivity, sociability, socialization, activity, neuroticism, and anxiety, were included in the factor analyses. One of the factors that consistently emerged in a five-factor analysis was described as Impulsive Unsocialized Sensation Seeking (Zuckerman, 1994a).

Analyses of items within all of the scales was done to develop a five-factor test of personality, the Zuckerman–Kuhlman Personality Questionnaire (ZKPQ; Zuckerman, 1994a, 2002b, 2008; Zuckerman et al., 1993). One of the replicable factors was called Impulsive Sensation Seeking (ImpSS), because it included both impulsivity, in the form of spontaneous reactions without planning, and general sensation-seeking items reflecting the need for excitement and novelty without the specification of particular activities. The 19-item scale may be scored for the two subfactors, impulsivity and sensation seeking, as well as the total.

Aluja and colleagues (2006) developed a shortened (50-item) cross-cultural form of the ZKPQ with English, Spanish, French, and German versions. The ImpSS, like the other four subscales, contains only 10 items, but alpha reliability coefficients range from .72 to .74.

Arnett (1994) developed a short form of the SSS with items selected to represent two qualities of stimuli attractive to sensation seekers: novelty and intensity. There are 10 items for each. Although the internal reliabilities are relatively low, the scale has been correlated with a variety of risky behaviors.

Hoyle, Stephenson, Palmgreen, Lorch, and Donohew (2002) devised a Brief Sensation-Seeking Scale appropriate for young and older adolescents using two items from each of the four subscales of the SSS-V, avoiding mention of alcohol or drugs. Only a total score is used. This scale has been used in drug prevention campaigns, as described in a subsequent section.

Cloninger (1987b) is the only other personality theorist to include sensation seeking as one of the major dimensions of personality. He devised a scale called Novelty Seeking (NS). In its most recent form it includes subscales for exploratory excitability, impulsiveness, extravagance, and disorderliness (Cloninger, Svrakic, & Przybeck, 1993). The shorter form of the NS scale correlates very highly with the ImpSS scale (Zuckerman & Cloninger, 1996) and highly with the SSS-V Total score.

Russo and colleagues (1993) constructed an SSS form appropriate for children ages 9–14. Three subscales were developed from an item factor analysis: Thrill and Adventure Seeking, Social Disinhibition, and Drug and Alcohol Attitudes. The latter scale is a measure of a specific attitude rather than a personality factor.

Risky Behavior

Volunteering and Risk Appraisal

In the 1960s we were doing experiments in sensory deprivation and hypnosis. We noticed that our paid volunteers for both types of experiments looked like high sensation seekers. We confirmed this impression, asking for volunteers from students at three universities. The volunteers for both experiments scored higher on the SSS-II general scale than nonvolunteers. Subsequent studies by others showed that volunteering by high sensation seekers depended on the type of experiment. Any study offering a chance at an unusual or novel type of experience (e.g., sensory deprivation, hypnosis, drugs, gambling, sensitivity training, brain wave control, training in transcendental meditation, and encounter groups) attracted high sensation seekers. However, sensation seeking was unrelated to volunteering for more mundane experiments in learning or social psychology. Subsequent research showed that risk appraisal and expectations of experiencing anxiety versus expectations of experiencing positive arousal influenced the approach or avoidance behavior related to volunteering.

Risk appraisal across a variety of activities, even those never experienced, is negatively related to sensation seeking (Zuckerman, 1979, 1994b, 2007). High sensation seekers tend to rate riskiness lower than low sensation seekers. But even in experiments in which risk appraisal is the same in high and low sensation seekers, the anxiety gradient rises more steeply and the anticipation of positive affect (elation) decreases with appraised riskiness of the experiment in low sensation seekers, whereas in high sensation seekers the slope of the anxiety gradient is less steep, and the anticipated positive emotion does not decline with in-

creased riskiness. The result is a cross of the approach–avoidance gradient, with avoidance predominating earlier along the risk continuum in low sensation seekers.

Volunteering for dangerous military or civilian assignments is also more characteristic of high sensation seekers. Israeli soldiers who volunteered for combat units were higher in sensation seeking than other recruits. Many of them engaged in scuba diving in their free time (Hobfoll, Rom, & Segal, 1989). Trait anxiety was unrelated to these voluntary choices. Among those who actually engaged in combat, those who received medals for bravery were higher sensation seekers than other soldiers (Neria, Solomon, Ginzburg, & Dekel, 2000).

Sociability, Relationships, and Sex

In the "alternative five" model, Impulsive Sensation Seeking (ImpSS) and Sociability are independent factors (Zuckerman, 2002b). At the trait level, sensation seeking (SSS-V) is only weakly correlated with Eysenck's E scale and ImpSS with the NEO Extraversion scale (Zuckerman, et al., 1993). However, in a situation of close confinement with a stranger, low sensation seekers showed much more stress and distress than high sensation seekers (Zuckerman, Persky, Link, & Basu, 1968). High sensation seekers engage in self-disclosure with both casual and close friends (Franken, Gibson, & Mohan, 1990). In an interview, high sensation seekers show more spontaneous interactive behavior: fast reactions, eye gaze, posture, vocalization, smiles, and laughter (Cappella & Green, 1984).

Comparing the SSS with Hendrick and Hendrick's (1986) scales for love styles, the Total SSS was positively related to the Ludus style (playful, less committed love) and negatively related to the Pragma style (rational appraisal of mate's potential for a long-term relationship). The SSS Dis and BS subscales had the highest correlations with Ludus.

Thornquist, Zuckerman, and Exline (1991) studied the relations between the SSS and relationships among unmarried heterosexual partners in current relationships. They found moderate positive correlations between SSS scores of partners, a finding similar to those found for married couples, indicating a role for the sensation-seeking trait in assortative mating. In both partners Total SSS was negatively related to relationship satisfaction, liking, and loving and positively related to consideration of alternatives outside of the relationship. The most satisfactory relationships were between two low sensation seekers, and the least satisfactory were between two high sensation seekers. When one partner is low and the other is high on sensation seeking, there is usually conflict, not only about sex but in general preferences for life activities and choice of friends.

Nonverbal interactions between members of a pair were also studied. Women high in sensation seeking looked more at their partners and spoke more to them. Mutual gaze correlated with the woman's SSS when she was speaking but did not when the male was speaking. Women high in sensation seeking tend to command attention from their mates when they are speaking but do not necessarily give it when their mates are speaking.

The negative relation between sensation seeking and relationship satisfaction is also found for married or cohabiting couples (Schroth, 1991). Divorced men have higher scores on the SSS than both married and single men, and divorced women have higher scores than married women (Zuckerman & Neeb, 1980).

In the general population there are high correlations between SSS scores of spouses, indicating a high degree of assortative mating not typically found for other personality traits. However, the correlations between couples entering couple therapy are lower than those of happily married couples (Ficher, Zuckerman, & Neeb, 1981; Ficher, Zuckerman, & Steinberg, 1988). Low sensation-seeking scores in the male partners relative to the female's scores were related to sexual dissatisfaction in both partners. The reverse was not necessarily true. Donaldson (1989) reported similar findings among married and intimate college students.

Studies relating the SSS to sexual attitudes and behavior in college students conducted during the 1970s showed that sensation seeking was related to sexually permissive attitudes and variety of sexual experience and partners (Zuckerman, 1994b, 2007). There seemed to be less risk related to impulsive and promiscuous sex in the 1970s because of birth control pills

and effective treatments for the prevalent sexually transmitted diseases. This complacency changed in the 1980s with the AIDs epidemic.

Hoyle, Fejfar, and Miller (2000) reviewed all studies relating personality traits to sexual risk taking through 1999. Of all tests used in these studies, the SSS had the highest correlations with risky sex, including number of partners, unprotected sex (not using condoms), and high-risk sex with strangers. Zuckerman (2007) reviewed subsequent studies from 2000 to 2004 and found that the SSS and other versions of the scale predicted risky sexual behavior in large-scale studies of young adolescent, college, and community populations. In adolescents, sensation seeking and impulsivity were related to the use of alcohol or drugs before having sex.

Zuckerman (2007) also reviewed studies of risky sexual behavior among gay men. Many of these studies were conducted by Kalichman and his colleagues (Kalichman, Heckman, & Kelly, 1996), who developed scales for sexual sensation seeking and nonsexual sensation seeking. Most studies show that both the specific and general types of sensation seeking are related to number of sexual partners, to anal sex without using condoms, and to using alcohol and drugs before and during sex. The direct effect of sensation seeking accounts for 80% of the association with unprotected anal sex among gay men, whereas alcohol and drug use account for only 20% (Kalichman et al., 1996). Sensation seeking accounted for the relationship between substance use and high-risk sexual behavior in gay men.

Smoking (Tobacco), Drinking, and Drugs

Several studies we conducted in a college population during the 1970s and 1980s showed that smokers were higher in sensation seeking than nonsmokers. Although the prevalence of smoking had diminished in males (but not in females) during the 1980s, the relationship between sensation seeking and smoking was still a significant one. Another study conducted at a nearby university in 1993 showed the same differences between smoking prevalence in participants high and low in sensation seeking (Kuman, Pekala, & Cummings, 1993).

Between 1995 and 2003 six large-sample studies of middle and high school students showed relationships between various sensation-seeking scales, including ImpSS, and smoking prevalence and prediction (see Zuckerman, 2007, Table 4.1). Zuckerman and Kuhlman (2000) found that smoking, drinking, drugs, and risky sex were all intercorrelated and correlated with the ZKPQ ImpSS.

Early studies of drinking in college students found relationships between heavy drinking and sensation seeking. These findings have been supported in more recent studies of high school and college students and the general population in several countries.

Most heavy drinking by college students occurs in social situations in which social disinhibition is a primary motive for both sexes. Sexual disinhibition is another motive for men (Beck, Thombs, Mahoney, & Fingar, 1995). Katz, Fromme, and D'Amico (2000) found that positive social and sexual expectancies were positively related and that risk expectancy was negatively related to sensation seeking. However, the relationship between sensation seeking and heavy drinking was *not* mediated by expectancies. Sensation or novelty seeking is high in alcoholics, particularly Cloninger's (1987a) Type 2 alcoholic, characterized by early age of onset, antisocial personality, and low harm avoidance.

Marijuana and other drug use is even more highly related to sensation seeking than is drinking in high school and college populations. These findings, beginning in the 1970s, have persisted into this century (e.g., Wagner, 2001). Jaffe and Archer (1987) compared the SSS and other personality scales in prediction power for the use of drugs in a college population. The SSS was the most powerful predictor of the use of 7 of the 10 classes of drug and polydrug use. Substance abusers were *low* in anxiety sensitivity. Within the drug-using community, polydrug use is more highly related to sensation seeking than the use of any one specific type of drug, although there is some preference for stimulants and psychedelic drugs among polydrug abusers. The qualities of intensity and novelty are provided by these drugs, in addition to the disinhibition also produced by alcohol and depressant drugs. Many polydrug users alternate or mix stimulant and depressant drugs, including alcohol, to suit their moods and situational needs. The SSS-Total and ImpSS are predictors of negative outcome in the treatment of cocaine abuse (Ball, 1995; Patkar et al., 2004).

A series of laboratory and community studies showed the effectiveness of sensation-seeking theory in designing communications for the prevention and reduction of marijuana use in adolescent populations (Donohew, Bardo, & Zimmerman, 2004). The laboratory studies showed that messages with high-stimulation characteristics (novel, complex, intense, exciting, fast paced) were more effective than low-stimulation messages in increasing intent to call a drug hotline, particularly in high sensation seekers using drugs. A campaign using television ads with high-stimulation values reduced overall marijuana usage in two counties following 4-month campaigns (Palmgreen, Donohew, Lorch, Hoyle, & Stephenson, 2001).

Effect of Social Predictors of Sensation Seeking on the Trait

Does sensation seeking increase the likelihood of drug use, or does drug use increase sensation seeking? The causal relationships between social-psychological variables and sensation seeking are best investigated in longitudinal studies. Stacy, Newcomb, and Bentler (1991) studied such predictors in a 9-year longitudinal study of sensation seeking from adolescence to adulthood. In addition to adolescent sensation seeking itself as a predictor of adult levels of the trait, other predictors involved social conformity, emotional distress, drug use, social support, and peer deviance. Only the sensation-seeking factor in adolescence directly predicted the same factor in adulthood using structural equation modeling. However, some social predictors, particularly social support, predicted specific subscales of sensation seeking. Lower social support during adolescence predicted high ES and BS in adulthood beyond the prediction from the adolescent levels of these subtraits. Of course, social support may represent the familial reactions to earlier manifestations of the nonconforming behavior involved in ES. Family support may moderate the effects of adolescent sensation seeking and its persistence or nonpersistence into adulthood.

Risky Driving, Sports, and Vocations

These activities are related to the specific part of the broader sensation-seeking trait called thrill and adventure seeking (TAS). However, studies that use the forms of the SSS with subscales usually find that risky behaviors related to TAS are also related to at least one of the other subscales (Zuckerman, 1994b, 2007).

Risky driving behavior includes speeding far above the posted limits, following other cars too closely at high speeds, frequent and abrupt lane changes, driving while intoxicated, and generally aggressive driving. Jonah (1997) reviewed 40 studies of sensation seeking and risky driving and found that the "vast majority" of these studies showed positive relationships between them. Correlations were generally in the .30–.40 range depending on gender (men do more risky driving), the form of the SSS used, and the particular measure(s) of risky driving. Sensation seekers find a kind of positive arousal in speed (Whissel & Bigelow, 2003).

Some of these studies used behavioral tests, actually observing participants driving during runs along preselected routes (Burns & Wilde, 1995; Heino, 1996). In the Heino (1996) study drivers made risk estimates for each section of road, and heart rate was measured. High sensation seekers drove faster than low sensation seekers, depending on the type of road, but there was no difference in perceptions of risk and heart rate. They also tended to follow the car in front of them more closely. It is interesting that risk appraisal and arousal heart rate could not explain the faster driving of high sensation seekers. Perhaps the heightened risk and arousal is subjectively positive for high and negative for low sensation seekers. Sensation seekers are less inclined to use their seat belts, suggesting an indifference to risk.

Not surprisingly, high sensation seekers have more citations for traffic violations and driving while intoxicated. Surprisingly, accident records are not consistently related to sensation seeking, perhaps because such records include the blameless as well as those responsible. Another possibility is that high sensation seekers are more skilled drivers, compensating for their risky driving habits.

Zuckerman (1983), in a review of studies of participants in various sports, concluded that high sensation seekers were particularly attracted to high-risk sports such as parachuting and skydiving, scuba diving, mountain climbing, and downhill skiing, whereas participants in low-risk sports were just average in sensation seeking. Research since that date has generally confirmed this hypothesis (Goma-i-Freixanet, 2004; Jack & Ronan, 1998). Skydivers, mountain climbers, rock climbers, white-water canoeists, hang gliders, cave explorers, scuba divers, and downhill skiers all tend to be higher on sensation seeking. As we might expect, they score higher on the TAS subscale, but they usually score higher on the ES subscale, as well. The latter difference shows that novel sensations are part of the reward for these activities. Participants in medium-risk or team sports, including swimmers and baseball, soccer, and football players, tend to be average in sensation seeking. Participants in some sports, such as golf, volleyball, and marathon running, are actually lower on sensation seeking.

Goma-i-Freixanet (1995, 2001) compared those engaging in high-risk sports with other groups of risk takers, including criminals incarcerated for armed robbery and those with risky prosocial jobs such as firefighters, police officers, prison wardens, ambulance drivers, forest firefighters, and lifeguards. Among males, the sportsmen scored higher on the SSS Total and a modified Total score, excluding TAS, than prosocial risk takers and controls. But they did not score as high as the criminal risk takers on these scales. Among females, the sportswomen scored higher than the prosocial risk takers and the controls but did not differ from the criminals on these two scales. They scored lower than the criminals on a separate scale for impulsivity. The groups who worked in risky vocations scored higher on Total SSS than controls, but this was due only to their higher scores on TAS.

Other studies on specific vocations have shown some attracting high sensation seekers (Zuckerman, 1994b, 2007). Norwegian paratroopers, Swedish Air Force pilots, Israeli applicants for risky security-related jobs, Spanish firefighters, American air traffic controllers, physicians and nurses working in emergency rooms, and rape crisis counselors had higher SSS scores than control groups in less risky or stressful jobs. Other vocational groups, such as naval fliers and naval divers, scored higher on TAS but actually lower than controls on ES and Dis, perhaps as a function of the lower social desirability of the latter.

Within some groups some members have higher scores related to their risky behavior. For instance, Israeli soldiers who were decorated for bravery in the 1973 war scored higher on a short form of the SSS than others who fought in the war (Neria et al., 2000). Within a group of police patrolmen scoring average on the SSS and a general risk scale, those engaging in high-speed chases scored higher on both of these scales (Homant, Kennedy, & Howton, 1994).

Antisocial, Criminal, and Delinquent Behavior

In the study by Goma-i-Freixanet (1995), violent criminals scored significantly higher on the Total and all of the SSS subscales than participants in risky sports, risky vocational, and control groups. In the female groups the criminals scored higher than the risky vocational and control groups on the SSS Total, ES, and Dis scales, but not the female risky sports group (Goma-i-Freixanet, 2001). Imprisoned male delinquents scored higher than controls on ES and BS but not TAS or Dis scales (Romero, Luengo, & Sobral, 2001). However, other studies have shown that Dis in early adolescence predicts delinquent behavior in later adolescence (Newcomb & McGee, 1991; White, Labouvie, & Bates, 1985).

Horvath and Zuckerman (1993) found that SSS Total was highly correlated with self-reports (made anonymously) of delinquent and criminal behavior in college students. Sensation seeking and criminal behavior also correlated with risk appraisals for criminal behavior, but risk appraisal did *not* mediate the relationship between sensation seeking and criminal behavior. Instead sensation seeking mediated the relationship between risk appraisal and criminal behavior. It is probable that engaging in some kind of criminal behavior without getting caught lowers the perceived riskiness of the behavior.

Summary: Risk Taking

Sensation seeking was defined as the willingness to take risks for the sake of the reward of arousing stimulation. The acceptance of physical risk by high sensation seekers is shown in their driving behavior and their engagement in risky sports and in risky vocations and activities within vocations. Such behavior in prosocial vocations is often admirable, but the pursuit of sensation in criminal antisocial activities is the darker side of the trait.

Risky sensation seeking is the outcome of a conflict between the anticipation of pleasure from a risky activity and the anticipation of anxiety related to the perceived risk. High sensation seekers have a stronger anticipation of reward and a weaker anticipation of anxiety or punishment and therefore are more likely to engage in these activities, whereas low sensation seekers are more likely to avoid them.

Preferences in Art, Media, and Music

Sensation seeking is not related only to risky behavior. Entertainment preferences reflect the qualities of stimulation in the definition of the trait: novelty, intensity, complexity, and variety (Zuckerman, 1994b, 2006). High sensation seekers show a stronger orienting reflex, a physiological (skin conductance, heart rate) response to novel stimuli on their first presentations but not on repetition. They are particularly responsive to stimuli that are interesting to them and intense. Their cortical evoked response is augmented by high-intensity stimulation, whereas evoked responses of low sensation seekers tend to be reduced by intense stimuli.

High sensation seekers like novel and complex designs, whereas lows like simple and symmetrical ones. High sensation seekers like paintings with high tension and semiabstract or abstract styles and Pop art. They also like erotic and violent themes in art or photographs. Low sensation seekers like paintings with low tension and realistic styles and dislike violent or morbid themes in art.

Similarly, high sensation seekers enjoy and go to movies with horror and explicit

sexual themes. In television the high sensation seekers like violent action-adventure
programs, whereas the lows like game shows
and news programs. Given a chance to select
programs, high sensation seekers tend to do
more channel switching, showing a need for
variety and a boredom susceptibility.

Sensation seeking correlates positively
with a liking for rock music, particularly
hard rock, and negatively with a liking for
religious and bland soundtrack music. However, those who score high on the ES subscale like a broader variety of music, including folk and classical, in addition to hard
and soft rock. Intensity of sound, particularly the drums and loud bass of the amplified guitars, dissonance, and "edginess" of
lyrics, are qualities of music appreciated by
high sensation seekers.

Psychobiology of Sensation Seeking

The explanation for differences in impulsive sensation seeking is a psychobiological
one involving genetics, psychophysiology,
psychopharmacology, and neuropsychology
(Zuckerman, 1994b, 1995, 2005). According to this model, the attraction to novel
and intense sensations and activities is a
function of genetic predispositions toward
impulsive approach based on dopaminergic
activity in the reward pathways in the limbic brain, dysregulated by low levels of the
enzyme monoamine oxidase type B. The
hormone testosterone also potentiates the
approach mechanism. A weak behavioral
inhibitory mechanism is a function of in-
sensitivity of serotonergic inhibitory systems. Weak arousal or fearlessness in the
face of risk is a function of attenuated no-
radrenergic reactivity. Sensation seeking is
affected by the balance between the three
behavioral mechanisms (approach, inhibition, and arousal) and the biological systems underlying them. This might be called
the "three-monoamine theory," as contrasted with theories only involving one monoamine for impulsivity and sensation seeking
(e.g., Cloninger, 1987b).

As we have seen, cognitive phenomena
such as expectations and risk appraisal are
involved in the relationships of the trait with
some of the behavioral phenomena, but not
always as mediators. My explanations have

been largely at the psychobiological level
and involve comparative models (Zuckerman, 1984, 1991, 1994b, 1995, 1996, 2003,
2005, 2007). A full account of this theory
and research can be found in these references.

Genetic twin studies of sensation seeking including separated twins have shown a
high degree of heritability for the SSS and
most of its subscales (Zuckerman, 2002a).
A specific gene for the dopamine 4 receptor (DRD4) was found to be associated
with novelty seeking, a scale highly correlated with ImpSS (Ebstein et al., 1996).
Replications have been inconsistent, but a
meta-analysis shows a small but significant
effect comparing the long allele form with
the shorter form (Schinka, Letsch, & Crawford, 2002). What is interesting is that this
form of the gene is also associated with the
strength of the orienting reflex response to
novel stimuli in infants, with heroin and
alcohol abuse and gambling in adults and
with attention-deficit hyperactivity disorder
in children. Other genes are also involved,
additively and interactively, in the personality trait and forms of psychopathology. This
may explain why associations are weak and
sometimes difficult to replicate.

Insights into the neurochemical basis of
sensation seeking have been derived from
comparisons of selectively bred strains of
exploratory and novelty-reactive rats and
those who are more neophobic (Dellu, Piazza, Mayo, LeMoal, & Simon, 1996; Siegel
& Driscoll, 1996). The exploratory strains
have more dopamine in the nucleus accumbens and are more dopaminergic reactive to
stimulant drugs or stress. The nucleus accumbens is a reward nucleus in the medial
forebrain bundle hypothesized to be more
reactive in human sensation seekers. More
inhibited rats respond to novelty and stress
with increases in serotonin, an inhibitory
neurotransmitter acting antagonistically to
dopamine.

Studies of brain neurochemistry in humans rely largely on metabolites of the neu-
rotransmitters in cerebrospinal fluid (CSF)
or on blood or hormonal indices of reactivity
of the neurotransmitter to stimulants. Basal
levels of metabolites have shown little relationship to sensation and novelty seeking.
However, responses to neurochemical ago-
nists show a greater serotonergic reactivity

in low sensation seekers and blunted reactivity in high sensation seekers (see Table 1.4 in Zuckerman, 2007). The findings on relationships with dopaminergic reactivity have been mixed. Recent brain imaging studies, however, have shown greater reactivity of the dopaminergic system in the ventral striatum or nucleus accumbens and greater dopaminergic reactivity and sensitization to amphetamine in high novelty seekers (Boileau et al., 2006; Leyton et al., 2002). These tentative results support the three-monoamine model of sensation seeking (Zuckerman, 1995) and explain the attraction of stimulant drugs for high sensation seekers.

Conclusions

Sensation seeking was a construct designed to predict a narrow range of phenomena in an experimental situation (sensory deprivation). Unexpectedly, it was found to be applicable to a wide variety of behavioral preferences, and the scales used to measure it showed a broad construct validity. The construct involves a tendency to approach and engage in novel and arousing activities and weak inhibition or avoidance associated with the perceived riskiness of these activities. The balance between approach and avoidance in these areas of voluntary risk taking is based on genetic and biological determinants and their interactions with environmental opportunities and influences. The trait of sensation seeking in humans has been connected with explorativeness and novelty seeking in other species through shared biological markers suggesting evolutionary origins. Sensation seeking at some optimal level ensured gene survival: Too little and you starved or failed to mate; too much and you met a premature death.

References

Aluja, A., Rossier, J., Garcia, L. F., Angleitner, A., Kuhlman, M., & Zuckerman, M. (2006). A cross-cultural shortened form of the ZKPQ (ZKPQ-50-cc) adapted to English, French, German, and Spanish languages. *Personality and Individual Differences*, 41, 619–628.

Arnett, J. (1994). Sensation seeking: A new conceptualization and a new scale. *Personality and Individual Differences*, 16, 289–296.

Ball, S. A. (1995). The validity of the alternative five-factor measure of personality in cocaine abusers. *Psychological Assessment*, 7, 148–154.

Beck, K. H., Thombs, D. L., Mahoney, C. A., & Fingar, K. M. (1995). Social context and sensation seeking: Gender differences in college student drinking motivations. *International Journal of the Addictions*, 30, 1101–1115.

Boileau, I., Dagher, A., Leyton, M., Gunn, R. N., Baker, G. B., Diksic, M., et al. (2006). Modeling sensitization to stimulants in humans. *Archives of General Psychiatry*, 63, 1386–1395.

Burns, P. C., & Wilde, G. S. (1995). Risk taking in male taxi drivers: Relationships among personality, observational data and driver records. *Personality and Individual Differences*, 18, 267–278.

Cappella, J. N., & Green, J. O. (1984). The effects of distance and individual differences in arousability on nonverbal involvement: A test of discrepancy arousal theory. *Journal of Nonverbal Behavior, 8*, 259–286.

Cloninger, C. R. (1987a). Neurogenic adaptive mechanisms in alcoholism. *Science, 236*, 410–416.

Cloninger, C. R. (1987b). A systematic method for clinical description and classification of personality variants. *Archives of General Psychiatry, 44*, 573–588.

Cloninger, C. R., Svrakic, D. M.,& Przybeck, T. R. (1993). A psychobiological model of temperament and character. *Archives of General Psychiatry, 50*, 975–990.

Dellu, F., Piazza, P. V., Mayo, W., LeMoal, M., & Simon, H. (1996). Novelty-seeking in rats: Biobehavioural characteristics and possible relationship with the sensation seeking trait in man. *Neuropsychobiology, 34*, 136–145.

Donaldson, S. (1989). Similarity in sensation seeking, sexual satisfaction, and contentment in relationship in heterosexual couples. *Psychological Reports, 64*, 405–406.

Donohew, L., Bardo, M. T., & Zimmerman, R. S. (2004). Personality and risky behavior: Communication and prevention. In R. M. Stelmack (Ed.), *On the psychobiology of personality: Essays in honor of Marvin Zuckerman* (pp. 223–235). Oxford, UK: Elsevier.

Ebstein, R. P., Novick, O., Umansky, R., Priel, B., Osher, Y., Blaine, D., et al. (1996). Dopamine D4 receptor (D4DR) exon III polymorphism associated with the human personality trait of novelty seeking. *Nature Genetics, 12*, 78–80.

Ficher, I. V., Zuckerman, M., & Neeb, M. (1981). Marital compatibility in sensation seeking trait as a factor in marital adjustment. *Journal of Sex and Marital Therapy, 7*, 60–69.

Ficher, I. V., Zuckerman, M., & Steinberg, M. (1988). Sensation seeking congruence in couples as a determinant of marital adjustment: A partial replication and extension. *Journal of Clinical Psychology, 44*, 803–809.

Franken, R. E., Gibson, K. J., & Mohan, P. (1990). Sensation seeking and disclosure to close and casual friends. *Personality and Individual Differences, 11*, 829–832.

Goma-i-Freixanet, M. (1995). Prosocial and antisocial aspects of personality. *Personality and Individual Differences, 19*, 125–134.

Goma-i-Freixanet, M. (2001). Prosocial and antisocial aspects of personality in women: A replication study. *Personality and Individual Differences, 30,* 1401–1411.

Goma-i-Freixanet, M. (2004). Sensation seeking and participation in physical risk sports. In R. M. Stelmack (Ed.), *On the psychobiology of personality: Essays in honor of Marvin Zuckerman* (pp. 185–201). Oxford, UK: Elsevier.

Heino, A. (1996). *Risk taking in car driving: Perceptions, individual differences and effects of safety incentives.* Unpublished doctoral dissertation, University of Groningen.

Hendrick, C., & Hendrick, S. S. (1986). A theory and method of love. *Journal of Personality and Social Psychology, 50,* 392–402.

Hobfoll, S. E., Rom, T., & Segal, B. (1989). Sensation seeking, anxiety, and risk-taking in the Israeli context. In S. Ebstein (Ed.), *Drugs and alcohol use: Issues and facts* (pp. 53–59). New York: Plenum Press.

Homant, R. J., Kennedy, D. B., & Howton, J. D. (1994). Risk taking and police pursuit. *Journal of Social Psychology, 134,* 213–221.

Horvath, P., & Zuckerman, M. (1993). Sensation seeking, risk appraisal, and risky behavior. *Personality and Individual Differences, 14,* 41–51.

Hoyle, R., Fejfar, M. C., & Miller, J. D. (2000). Personality and sexual risk taking: A quantitative review. *Journal of Personality, 68,* 1203–1231.

Hoyle, R., Stephenson, M. T., Palmgreen, P., Lorch, E. P., & Donohew, R. L. (2002). Reliability and validity of a brief measure of sensation seeking. *Personality and Individual Differences, 32,* 401–414.

Jack, S. J., & Ronan, K. R. (1998). Sensation seeking among high- and low-risk sports participants. *Personality and Individual Differences, 25,* 1063–1083.

Jaffe, L. T., & Archer, R. P. (1987). The prediction of drug use among college students from MMPI, MCMI, and sensation-seeking scales. *Journal of Personality, 51,* 243–253.

Jonah, B. A. (1997). Sensation seeking and risky driving: A review and synthesis of the literature. *Accident Analysis and Prevention, 29,* 651–665.

Kalichman, S. C., Heckman, T., & Kelly, J. A. (1996). Sensation seeking as an explanation for the association between substance use and HIV-related risky sexual behavior. *Archives of Sexual Behavior, 25,* 141–154.

Katz, E. C., Fromme, K., & D'Amico, E. J. (2000). Effects of outcome expectancies and personality on young adults' illicit drug use, heavy drinking and risky sexual behavior. *Cognitive Therapy and Research, 24,* 1–22.

Kuman, V. K., Pekala, R. J., & Cummings, J. (1993). Sensation seeking, drug use, and reported paranormal beliefs and experiences. *Personality and Individual Differences, 14,* 685–691.

Leyton, M., Boileau, I., Benkelfat, C., Diksic, M., Baker, G., & Dagher, A. (2002). Amphetamine induced increases in extracellular dopamine, drug wanting, and novelty seeking. *Neuropsychopharmacology, 27,* 1027–1035.

Neria, Y., Solomon, Z., Ginzburg, K., & Dekel, R. (2000). Sensation seeking, wartime performance, and long-term adjustment among Israeli war vet-

erans. *Personality and Individual Differences, 29,* 921–932.

Newcomb, M. D., & McGee, L. (1991). Influence of sensation seeking on general deviance and specific problem behaviors from adolescence to young adulthood. *Journal of Personality and Social Psychology, 61,* 614–628.

Palmgreen, P., Donohew, L., Lorch, E. P., Hoyle, R. H., & Stephenson, M. T. (2001). Television campaigns and adolescent marijuana use: Tests of sensation-seeking targeting. *American Journal of Public Health, 91,* 292–296.

Patkar, A. A., Murray, H. W., Mannelli, P., Gottheil, E., Weinstein, S. P., & Vergare, M. J. (2004). Pretreatment measures of impulsivity, aggression, and sensation seeking are associated with treatment outcome for African-American cocaine dependent patients. *Journal of Addictive Diseases, 23,* 109–122.

Romero, E., Luengo, A., & Sobral, J. (2001). Personality and antisocial behavior: Study of temperamental dimensions. *Personality and Individual Differences, 31,* 329–348.

Russo, M. F., Stokes, G. S., Lahey, B. B., Christ, M. A. G., McBurnett, K., Loeber, R., et al. (1993). A sensation-seeking scale in children: Further refinement and psychometric development. *Journal of Psychopathology and Behavioral Assessment, 15,* 69–86.

Schinka, J. A., Letsch, E. A., & Crawford, F. C. (2002). *DRD4* and novelty seeking: Results of meta-analyses. *American Journal of Medical Genetics, 114,* 643–648.

Schroth, M. L. (1991). Dyadic adjustment and sensation-seeking compatibility. *Personality and Individual Differences, 12,* 467–471.

Siegel, J., & Driscoll, P. (1996). Recent developments in an animal model of visual evoked potential augmenting/reducing and sensation-seeking behavior. *Neuropsychobiology, 34,* 130–135.

Stacy, A. W., Newcomb, M. D., & Bentler, P. M. (1991). Social psychological influences on sensation seeking from adolescence to adulthood. *Personality and Social Psychology Bulletin, 17,* 701–708.

Thornquist, M. H., Zuckerman, M., & Exline, R. V. (1991). Loving, liking, looking and sensation seeking in unmarried college couples. *Personality and Individual Differences, 12,* 1283–1292.

Wagner, M. K. (2001). Behavioral characteristics related to substance abuse and risk-taking, sensation seeking, and self-reinforcement. *Addictive Behaviors, 26,* 115–120.

Whissel, R. W., & Bigelow, B. J. (2003). The speeding attitude scale and the role of sensation seeking in profiling young drivers at risk. *Risk Analysis, 23,* 811–820.

White, W. R., Labouvie, E. W., & Bates, M. E. (1985). The relationship between sensation seeking and delinquency: A longitudinal analysis. *Journal of Research in Crime and Delinquency, 22,* 197–211.

Zuckerman, M. (1969). Theoretical formulations: I. In J. P. Zubek (Ed.) *Sensory deprivation: Fifteen years of research* (pp. 407–432). New York: Appleton-Century-Crofts.

Zuckerman, M. (1971). Dimensions of sensation seeking. *Journal of Consulting and Clinical Psychology, 36,* 45–52.

Zuckerman, M. (1979). *Sensation seeking: Beyond the optimal level of arousal.* Hillsdale, NJ: Erlbaum.

Zuckerman, M. (1983). Sensation seeking and sports. *Personality and Individual Differences, 4,* 285–292.

Zuckerman, M. (1984). Sensation seeking: A comparative approach to a human trait. *Behavioural and Brain Sciences, 7,* 453–471.

Zuckerman, M. (1991). *Psychobiology of personality.* Cambridge, UK: Cambridge University Press.

Zuckerman, M. (1994a). An alternative five-factor model for personality. In C. F. Halverson, Jr., G. A. Kohnstrom, & R. P. Martin (Eds.), *The developing structure of temperament and personality from infancy to adulthood* (pp. 53–68). Hillsdale, NJ: Erlbaum.

Zuckerman, M. (1994b). *Behavioral expressions and biosocial bases of sensation seeking.* New York: Cambridge University Press.

Zuckerman, M. (1995). Good and bad humors: Biochemical bases of personality and its disorders. *Psychological Science, 6,* 325–332.

Zuckerman, M. (1996). The psychobiological model for impulsive unsocialized sensation seeking: A comparative approach. *Neuropsychobiology, 34,* 125–129.

Zuckerman, M. (2002a). Genetics of sensation seeking. In J. Benjamin, R. P. Ebstein, & R. H. Belmaker (Eds.), *Molecular genetics and the human personality* (pp. 193–210). Washington, DC: American Psychiatric Press.

Zuckerman, M. (2002b). Zuckerman–Kuhlman Personality Questionnaire (ZKPQ): An alternative five-factorial model. In B. DeRaad & M. Perugini (Eds.), *Big Five assessment* (pp. 377–396). Seattle, WA: Hogrefe & Huber.

Zuckerman, M. (2003). Biological bases of personality. In T. Millon & M. J. Lerner (Eds.), *Handbook of psychology: Vol. 5. Personality and social psychology* (pp. 85–116). Hoboken, NJ: Wiley.

Zuckerman, M. (2005). *Psychobiology of personality* (2nd ed., rev. and updated). New York: Cambridge University Press.

Zuckerman, M. (2006). Sensation seeking in entertainment. In J. Bryant & P. Vorderer (Eds.), *Psychology of entertainment* (pp. 367–387). Mahwah, NJ: Erlbaum.

Zuckerman, M. (2007). *Sensation seeking and risky behavior.* Washington, DC: American Psychological Association.

Zuckerman, M. (2008). Zuckerman–Kuhlman Personality Questionnaire: An operational definition of the alternative five factorial model of personality. In G. J. Boyle, G. Matthews, & D. H. Saklofske (Eds.), *The Sage handbook of personality theory and assessment* (Vol. 2, pp. 219–238). Los Angeles: Sage.

Zuckerman, M., & Cloninger, B. (1996). Relationships between Cloninger's, Zuckerman's, and Eysenck's dimensions of personality. *Personality and Individual Differences, 21,* 283–285.

Zuckerman, M., Eysenck, S. B. G., & Eysenck, H. J. (1978). Sensation seeking in England and America: Cross-cultural, age, and sex comparisons. *Journal of Consulting and Clinical Psychology, 46,* 139–149.

Zuckerman, M., Kolin, I., Price, L., & Zoob, I. (1964). Development of a sensation-seeking scale. *Journal of Consulting Psychology, 28,* 477–482.

Zuckerman, M., & Kuhlman, M. (2000). Personality and risk-taking: Common biosocial factors. *Journal of Personality, 68,* 999–1029.

Zuckerman, M., Kuhlman, M., Joireman, J., Teta, P., & Kraft, M. (1993). A comparison of three structural models for personality: The Big Three, the Big Five, and the Alternative Five. *Journal of Personality and Social Psychology, 65,* 757–768.

Zuckerman, M., & Neeb, M. (1980). Demographic influences in sensation seeking and expressions of sensation seeking in religion, smoking, and driving habits. *Personality and Individual Differences, 1,* 197–206.

Zuckerman, M., Persky, H., Link, K. E., & Basu, G. K. (1968). Experimental and subject factors determining responses to sensory deprivation, social isolation and confinement. *Journal of Abnormal Psychology, 73,* 183–194.

CHAPTER 32

■ ● ▲ ◆ ■ ● ▲ ◆

Rejection Sensitivity

RAINER ROMERO-CANYAS
VANESSA T. ANDERSON
KAVITA S. REDDY
GERALDINE DOWNEY

Human beings are social animals who have come to rely on conspecifics for cooperation, protection, nourishment, and survival (Axelrod & Hamilton, 1981; Barash, 1977; Baumeister & Leary, 1995). Because people thrive only by forming supportive relationships with others, being liked and accepted by other people has become an important motivation for human beings. This motivation to seek acceptance and avoid rejection from others has been recognized as one of the core human motives since the early days of the discipline (Horney, 1937; Maslow, 1987; McClelland, 1987). More recently, psychologists have shown that the experience of social exclusion and rejection affects people's psychological functioning and behavior, triggering hostility, disrupting self-regulation and effortful cognitive control, decreasing the probability of prosocial behavior, and orienting individuals to seek information about potential sources of acceptance (Baumeister, DeWall, Ciarocco, & Twenge, 2005; Baumeister, Twenge, & Nuss, 2002; Bourgeois & Leary, 2001; Leary, Kowalski, Smith, & Phillips, 2003; Twenge, Baumeister, Tice, & Stucke, 2001; Williams, 2001).

Although most people are concerned with avoiding rejection from important others—such as relatives, friends, and romantic partners—people vary in the intensity of their reactions to rejection or the threat of rejection. The characterization of people who respond intensely to rejection as "rejection sensitive" has a long history in psychiatry. Horney (1937) devoted a chapter to this phenomenon in her work, *The Neurotic Personality of Our Time*. She described a vicious cycle wherein rejection anxiety leads people to respond with rage to "what is felt to be a rejection, but also to the anticipation of a rejection. The hostility provided ... is an important factor in establishing a *vicious cycle* which is difficult to escape from" (pp. 136–137).

These two processes, the concern with rejection and the intense reaction to rejection, are embodied in the concept of rejection sensitivity, an anxious expectation of rejection that is linked to affective and behavioral overreactions to the behavior of significant others. Defining rejection sensitivity as a cognitive–affective processing disposition whereby people anxiously expect, readily perceive, and intensely react to cues of rejection in the behavior of others, Downey and her colleagues explored the rejection sensitivity cycle described by Horney from a perspective that draws on social cognition (and, more recently, social-cognitive neuroscience), perspectives on individual differences, and work on interpersonal relationships (Downey & Feldman, 1996; Downey, Freitas, Michaelis, & Khouri, 1998; Feldman & Downey, 1994). This program of research has produced a testable model that identifies the social and cognitive–affective processes underlying the formation and maintenance of rejection sensitivity.

Downey's model is based on two assumptions. The first is that acceptance–rejection is a privileged dimension of information processing that reflects the fact that human beings need each other for survival. Avoiding rejection is challenging because the pursuit of acceptance entails subjecting oneself to the threat of rejection, particularly from those to whom people feel most connected and who, ironically, have the power to inflict the most painful rejection. Thus those to whom attaining acceptance and avoiding rejection is most important and most challenging may be particularly likely to show extremes of attentiveness and accommodation on the one hand and extremes of hostility and negativity on the other. The second assumption is that rejection sensitivity is a product of people's biological makeup and social history. People learn through experience, in conjunction with inherent biological reactivity to threat, to expect acceptance or rejection, and what they learn can change through new experiences. Thus rejection anxiety can be situation specific. Moreover, people may learn to expect rejection from certain individuals (e.g., a parent) and certain groups (e.g., peers at school but not in the neighborhood). Furthermore, people learn to expect rejection because they possess certain attributes in some contexts but not in others (e.g., women in stereotypically male domains such as the physical sciences and math; young African American men in relation to the police). Hence, to conceptualize rejection sensitivity, it is necessary to rely on an approach to personality that emphasizes individual differences in cognitive–affective processes, that accounts for apparent inconsistencies in behavior across situations, and that provides for personality change.

Rejection sensitivity is conceptualized in Mischel and Shoda's (1995) cognitive–affective processing system (CAPS) framework, which is concerned with understanding how personality processes emerge in specific person-by-situation interactions. Within this CAPS approach, an individual's behavior varies in a systematic manner within situations. Behavior is mediated by a dynamic network of cognitive–affective units shaped by biopsychosocial history—a network that includes expectations, encoding biases, affects, self-regulatory goals, and competencies—that guide responses to triggering cues in specific situations. In this interactionist perspective, behavioral expressions are reflected in stable, contextualized "if ... then" contingencies or personality signatures. This conceptualization allows researchers to ask (1) What are the specific situational features (both internal and external) that trigger this personality signature? and (2) What cognitive–affective units mediate the characteristic "if ... then" signature?

In Downey's model, highly rejection-sensitive people approach social situations in which rejection is possible with anxious expectations of rejection that make them hypervigilant for signs of potential rejection. These expectations are associated with perceptual biases that lead rejection-sensitive people to avoid negative interpersonal situations whenever possible. However, when avoiding these cues of rejection is not possible, the highly rejection-sensitive person feels rejected and reacts intensely with hostile behavior, social avoidance, depression, or socially inappropriate efforts to prevent or obviate the rejection (Ayduk et al., 2000; Downey & Feldman, 1996; Downey, Freitas, et al., 1998). Paradoxically, these reactions often elicit rejection from the target of the behavior, and so the feared outcome becomes a reality for the highly rejection-sensitive person. Because additional experiences of rejection serve to perpetuate the expectations of rejection, the rejection-sensitivity dynamic is strengthened.

Because rejection sensitivity operates within this vicious cycle, it appears to be a dysfunctional system that perpetuates personal and interpersonal difficulties. Alternatively, the rejection-sensitivity dynamic may be functional in helping to defend the person against rejection by significant others. To the extent that an individual has been exposed to the pain of rejection, protecting oneself from rejection while maintaining close relationships will be an important goal, and a protective system such as rejection sensitivity may develop to serve it. We view rejection sensitivity as a defensively motivated system that develops through rejection experiences to defend people against rejection while maintaining connection with the source of the threat. The adaptive value of rejection sensitivity is its ability to trigger quick defensive responses under threat conditions. However, the system becomes maladaptive if activated in situations that require reflective, tactical behavior, when the threat is minimal, or when efforts to prevent rejection undermine other personal goals.

Several strands of evidence suggest that the rejection-sensitivity dynamic operates as a defensive, affectively based system that evolved to guide rapid and intense responses to threats of danger (Davis, 1992; LeDoux, 1996). When rejection is the danger, activation of the rejection-sensitivity system orients and prepares the individual to detect signs of social danger and to be ready to act to avert the danger, escape, or strike out in self-defense. This helps to explain why the behavior of highly rejection-sensitive people can include a mixture of accommodation, withdrawal, and intense hostility and draws attention to the need to account for the specific contexts in which each type of behavior will emerge.

We devote this chapter to an overview of the impact of rejection sensitivity on people's behavior, an overview that also presents evidence for the view that the rejection-sensitivity dynamic operates as a defensive motivational system. We summarize work on sensitivity to interpersonal rejection generally, as well as work on sensitivity to rejection that is based on specific characteristics or social identities. We begin with a description of how the dynamic is measured in research on rejection sensitivity.

Measurement

Given the dynamic conceptualization of rejection sensitivity, individual differences in rejection sensitivity should be most evident in situations in which rejection by important others is a possibility. Anxious expectations of rejection are at the core of rejection sensitivity and are particularly likely to be activated when the person is dependent on a significant other. This assumption is reflected in the operationalization of rejection sensitivity in the Rejection Sensitivity Questionnaire (RSQ; Downey & Feldman, 1996). The RSQ presents a series of interpersonal situations, identified through extensive qualitative pilot work, in which people make a request of someone who is important to them. In addition, researchers have developed and validated measures of rejection sensitivity tailored for particular populations, resulting in measures that reflect specific types of situations in which rejection concerns are likely to be activated. These include measures of sensitivity to rejection for personal reasons tailored to college students, community adults, middle-school children, and incarcerated women and measures of sensitivity to rejection because of status characteristics including race (Chan & Mendoza-Denton, 2008; Mendoza-Denton, Downey, Purdie, Davis, & Pietrzak, 2002), gender (London, Downey, Rattan, & Tyson, 2006), physical appearance (Park, 2007a), and sexual orientation (Pachankis, Goldfried, & Ramrattan, 2008).

A sample situation from the personal RSQ states: "You approach a close friend to talk after doing something that seriously upset him/her." Respondents indicate their expectations of rejection (e.g., by rating the degree to which "I would expect that he/she would want to talk with me to try to work things out") and their concern or anxiety about the outcome (e.g., "How concerned or anxious would you be over whether or not your friend would want to talk with you?"). The level of anxious expectations in each situation is calculated by multiplying the degree of concern by the level of expectation of rejection (which, incidentally, did not covary in a large validation sample; Downey & Feldman, 1996). This operationalization captures the view that rejection sensitivity is a "hot cognition" (Metcalfe & Mischel, 1999) that is activated in situations of threat. Highly rejection-sensitive individuals do not merely expect rejection (as, e.g., telephone solicitors do) but also feel threatened by the possibility of rejection (as telephone solicitors apparently do not). In contrast, people low in rejection sensitivity may tend to expect acceptance and/or to be less concerned about the possibility of rejection. RSQ scores are calculated by averaging the computed RS levels across the situations that constitute the measure. RSQ scores are approximately normally distributed and show a stable one-factor structure, good internal and test–retest reliability (Downey & Feldman, 1996), and discriminant validity in samples of college students (see Downey & Feldman, 1996), adolescents (Downey, Lebolt, Rincon, & Freitas, 1998), and adults (Downey, Berenson, & Kang, 2006).

The RSQ does not tap into a general sensitivity to negative events but, rather, measures specifically fears and expectations of personal rejection by significant others. For example, the RSQ is distinct in terms of its predictive validity from measures of sensitivity to race- or gender-based rejection (Chan & Mendoza-Denton, 2008; London et al., 2006; Mendoza-Denton et al., 2002). Rejection-sensitivity scores are also not redundant with constructs with which RS might be expected to overlap, such as introversion, neuroticism, self-esteem, general attachment style, depression, social anxiety, and social avoidance (Downey & Feldman, 1996). It is also not significantly associated with self-monitoring or with the perspective-taking or empathic-concern dimensions of Davis's empathy measure (Romero-Canyas & Downey, 2008). Rejection sensitivity is, however, associated with the subscale of Davis's empathy measure that assesses the tendency to find other people's distress upsetting. Finally, the RSQ is weakly negatively associated with narcissism.

The Perception of and Immediate Reaction to Rejection Cues

As noted, the network of cognitive–affective units that are theorized to constitute a personality dynamic such as rejection sensitivity include encoding and perceptual biases that moderate behavior. These biases are activated in situations of social threat (Downey, Irwin, Ramsay, & Ayduk, 2004; Downey, Mougios, Ayduk, London, & Shoda, 2004) and influence the processes of detection, interpretation, and reaction to signals of potential rejection. However, rejection sensitivity is unrelated to biases in people's perception of signs of acceptance or positive affect. In other words, rejection sensitivity functions as a defensive system singularly attuned to signs of threat (Downey, Mougios, et al., 2004).

In social interactions, highly rejection-sensitive people are vigilant for cues of the relevant threat (rejection) in the same way that people with severe phobias are vigilant for cues of their particular fear objects. For example, in the presence of rejection-themed art, highly rejection-sensitive people show increased physiological reactivity associated with a vigilant state, as measured using a startle probe paradigm (Downey, Mougios, et al., 2004). However, rejection-sensitive people do not show this heightened response to art that has other negative themes or to positive- or acceptance-themed art.

Although they are vigilant to cues of rejection, rejection-sensitive people also show a bias to ignore information about potential rejection. When the option to avoid rejection—or situations that are likely to result in rejection—exists, the highly rejection-sensitive person is likely to seize it. This avoidance has emerged in work exploring attentional biases in the perception of threatening faces using a visual probe task (Berenson & Downey, 2008b; Mogg, Mathews, & Eysenck, 1992). Rejection sensitivity predicted disrupted attention away from threat stimuli (angry faces) but was unrelated to reactions to neutral stimuli. This resembles the pattern that abused children with post-traumatic stress disorder (PTSD) show (e.g., Pine et al., 2005) and reflects motivated strategies for regulating threat. When detecting and reducing threat are priorities, attentional vigilance for opportunities to avoid the threat sources should be the preferred responses. This strategy may develop as a result of the competition between the motivation to prevent rejection and the motivation to seek acceptance that characterize highly rejection-sensitive people. When seeking to remain close to the source of the potential threat, turning a blind eye to indications of threat keeps that threat at bay, at least at the perceptual and subjective levels. However, in day-to-day life, people face situations in which indications that they are not liked or accepted cannot be avoided.

Once confronted with cues of rejection and with no option to avoid them, highly rejection-sensitive people see those cues as more threatening and negative compared with other people, showing a bias to see more interpersonal negativity. In a study by Romero-Canyas and Downey (2008), participants in an online dating service viewed videos of people they believed were users of the dating service and estimated how negative or positive those people felt. Participants' rejection sensitivity predicted higher estimates of negativity, regardless of the emotions the person in the video had reported feeling. This effect was stronger when participants thought that the people in the videos were potential dating partners but was much weaker when participants thought they would never interact with those people.

In an experiment by Olsson, Carmona, Downey, and Ochsner (2008), participants viewed photos depicting the same person with different facial expressions. These photographs were blends of a photo of a neutral face and of an angry face, and together they made up a spectrum of different combinations of the two emotions. Relative to people low in rejection sensitivity, highly rejection-sensitive people were more likely to classify a face as angry instead of neutral, given only a small proportion of features from the angry photo relative to the number of features from the neutral photo. A small amount of negativity was enough for highly rejection-sensitive people to infer negativity. These biases are associated with the detection of threat, as well as with the activation of defensive strategies that direct the rejection-sensitive people's behavior in interpersonal interactions and that lead to strong reactions to perceived rejection.

Rejection Sensitivity and Immediate Affective Responses to Cues of Rejection

Rejection sensitivity is associated with a tendency to "absorb" or mirror the negative affect of other people. In the study that documented the bias to overestimate negativity (Romero-Canyas & Downey, 2008), both rejection sensitivity and the mood of the person in the video (collected when the video was filmed) predicted the participants' self-reported moods. The more negatively the target person felt, the more negative observers felt, but this effect was magnified for the highly rejection-sensitive observer.

Highly rejection-sensitive people have trouble regulating their intense emotional reactions. The intensity of their negative

emotions in response to cues of rejection is associated with decreased activation in brain areas believed to be involved in the regulation of emotions. In one study (Burklund, Eisenberger, & Lieberman, 2007) in which participants viewed disapproving faces, rejection-sensitivity scores were negatively correlated with activation in the subgenual anterior cingulate cortex, an area that is linked with extinction of fear responses to human faces and with reinterpretation of negative stimuli. In another brain imaging study (Kross, Egner, Ochsner, Hirsch, & Downey, 2007), participants low and high in rejection sensitivity viewed the rejection-themed paintings from Downey, Mougios, and colleagues' (2004) startle study. Participants low in rejection sensitivity showed significantly greater activation in two clusters of the left lateral prefrontal cortex and one cluster in the right dorsal superior frontal gyrus, areas linked to regulation and cognitive control of emotion. Activation in these regions was negatively correlated with participants' reported distress when viewing the rejection-themed slides. Both studies suggest that, relative to people low in rejection sensitivity, people who are high in rejection sensitivity show decreased cognitive control of emotion in the face of cues of rejection, which may account for the distress experienced by people high in rejection sensitivity.

Rejection Sensitivity and Hostile Responses to Rejection

As noted, people who are low versus high in rejection sensitivity differ in their perceptions of cues of rejection, how they think about them, and how they affectively react to them. Actual rejection reveals further differences between people low and high in rejection sensitivity, differences that may result from highly rejection-sensitive people's difficulty in regulating the intense negative affect they experience after rejection, affect that may fuel and magnify impulsive behavior (Ayduk et al., 2000). The resulting intense behaviors have the ironic effect of eliciting rejection from the people from whom the highly rejection-sensitive person seeks acceptance.

One response to rejection that has been extensively documented is increased hostility and aggression (Leary, Twenge, & Quinlivan, 2006). For highly rejection-sensitive people, this link is particularly strong, noticeable even among children. Rejection-sensitive middle-school children react more strongly than less sensitive children to a staged rejection from a class peer. Furthermore, over the course of the school year, they have more hostility-related behavioral problems in the classroom than less rejection-sensitive children (Downey, Lebolt, et al., 1998).

The link between rejection and hostility thoughts is strong and automatic among people who are rejection sensitive. In sequential priming–pronunciation paradigms, rejection-related words facilitate pronunciation of hostility-related words among people who are high in rejection sensitivity but not among people who are low in rejection sensitivity (Ayduk, Downey, Testa, Yen, & Shoda, 1999; Romero-Canyas, Downey, Berenson, Ayduk, & Kang, in press), suggesting an automatic link between rejection and hostile thoughts. These hostile thoughts translate to more hostile behavior for highly rejection-sensitive people. In one study (Ayduk et al., 1999), women expected to meet with a man after exchanging biographical information with him. When the man then refused to meet the participant, rejection-sensitivity scores predicted a more negative evaluation of him.

In diary studies of couples (Ayduk et al., 1999; Downey, Freitas, et al., 1998), rejection sensitivity predicted a greater probability of conflict following a day when highly rejection-sensitive people felt more rejected, suggesting that highly rejection-sensitive women react to rejection with some hostility toward their partners. Similarly, rejection sensitivity predicts greater relationship violence by male college students who were highly invested in their relationships (Downey, Feldman, & Ayduk, 2000). Highly rejection-sensitive people are also more likely to aggress against strangers who reject them, as captured in a study using the hot-sauce paradigm. In this study, highly rejection-sensitive people fed their rejecters a condiment that they knew the rejecters found particularly aversive: hot sauce (Ayduk, Gyurak, & Luerssen, 2007). Similarly, in a study of singers in auditions, rejection sensitivity predicted aggression and derogation of judges following rejection,

as well as indirect efforts to sabotage other singers in the audition (DiBenigno, Romero-Canyas, & Downey, 2007).

The rejection–hostility link is also evident in highly rejection-sensitive people's reactions to distant, powerful others. Rejection-sensitivity scores predict people's withdrawal of support from politicians who people feel betrayed them (Romero-Canyas & Downey, 2003) and expressed hostility toward and distancing from God among religious people who are facing personal difficulties (Anderson, Romero-Canyas, & Downey, 2008).

Clearly, behaving in a hostile way toward others is likely to elicit rejection. Dating couples that include a highly rejection-sensitive person are almost three times more likely than couples without a highly rejection-sensitive person to have separated within a year of the time their rejection sensitivity was measured (Downey, Freitas, et al., 1998). The processes underlying these outcomes have been explored in laboratory work. In one study (Downey, Freitas, et al., 1998), independent raters coded videotapes of couples engaged in discussing a relationship issue. Women's rejection-sensitivity scores predicted greater partner-reported anger, as well as more behavior coded as angry by independent raters. Women high in rejection sensitivity were more hostile, defensive, and negative than women low in rejection sensitivity. This hostility had an impact on their partners' affect such that the coders' ratings of negative behavior accounted for 54% of the effect of women's rejection sensitivity on their partner's negative affect.

In sum, the negative response that highly rejection-sensitive people show to cues of rejection engenders correspondingly negative responses from others. However, highly rejection-sensitive people are also motivated to avoid rejection and to seek acceptance, even when faced with very clear cues indicating that rejection is probable.

Rejection Sensitivity and Efforts to Secure Acceptance

Rejection-sensitive people are highly motivated to prevent rejection. In the course of social interactions, highly rejection-sensitive people will engage in impression-management strategies to prevent rejection from loved ones or new interaction partners. When faced with strong cues that rejection is impending, as when they are turned away from a social group or rejected by a prospective dating partner, highly rejection-sensitive people will make efforts to win back the person who has rejected them.

Efforts to prevent rejection from significant others are evident in early work on rejection sensitivity. In a study of adolescent girls in romantic relationships (Purdie & Downey, 2000), rejection sensitivity correlated positively with greater willingness on the part of girls to "do anything" to keep their boyfriends, even if that meant doing something they thought was wrong. Among low-income women at risk for contracting HIV, higher rejection sensitivity predicted the likelihood of engaging in risky sexual behavior to prevent their sexual partners from leaving them (Berenson & Downey, 2008a). These self-silencing strategies also emerge in novel relationships in situations in which people are given information that suggests that rejection is possible. In a study of self-presentation strategies, when introducing themselves to a group of highly artistic peers who were described as being unathletic, rejection-sensitive participants presented themselves as less athletic using the same rating scale they had used less than an hour earlier to indicate high levels of athleticism to the experimenter. Similarly, rejection sensitivity predicted changes in self-ratings of political conservatism among college students joining a group of peers in a university campus where politically conservative students feel stigmatized and alienated (Romero-Canyas, Downey, Pelayo, & Bashan, 2004). Highly conservative, highly rejection-sensitive men who were randomly assigned to interact with a very liberal group decreased their self-ratings of conservatism at the time of their public presentation to the group. Highly conservative, highly rejection-sensitive men placed in a conservative group did not change their scores.

People high in rejection sensitivity are also more likely than people low in rejection sensitivity to make efforts to regain acceptance from the people who have expressed no interest in them and have rejected them (Romero-Canyas et al., 2008). In a series of studies, after being rejected or accepted by a novel group of peers or dating partners, par-

ticipants reported their willingness to carry out a series of tedious tasks for the group (e.g., cooking dinner for the group, archiving past messages exchanged by group members) and how much money they would donate to a group meeting. After rejection, but not after acceptance, men's rejection-sensitivity scores predicted larger monetary contributions to the group and a greater willingness to perform the tedious tasks.

The rejection-avoidance behaviors that highly rejection-sensitive people adopt may not always yield the desired result. People who fear rejection and are asked to sacrifice personal interests for their partners are more likely to end their relationships than people who had no such concerns (Impett, Gable, & Peplau, 2005). Highly rejection-sensitive people's apparently ingratiating behavior after rejection may elicit mistrust and suspicion from the social targets whom they pursue, leading to eventual rejection. In addition, a highly rejection-sensitive person's willingness to transform him- or herself into a different person to gain acceptance may have long-term costs leading to unstable relationships and troubled affect.

The Link between Rejection Sensitivity and Health Problems

The findings we have reviewed thus far suggest that people who are rejection sensitive react strongly to rejection and that their overreactions often have negative consequences for them. In combination with other psychological dynamics, rejection sensitivity predicts poor mental health. Rejection-sensitive children tend to be socially avoidant and lonely (London, Downey, Bonica, & Paltin, 2007). The same pattern is evident among college students, for whom rejection sensitivity also predicts a smaller number of close friends, a smaller number of significant dating relationships, and longer periods of time before entering relationships (Berenson, Kang, & Downey, 2008; Downey et al., 2000).

Rejection sensitivity also predicts strong internalization of rejection experiences, predicting depression following interpersonal losses associated with rejection (Ayduk, Downey, & Kim, 2001). Rejection-sensitivity scores obtained 2 weeks before the start of the school year predicted more depressive symptoms at the end of the school year for participants who had experienced a partner-initiated breakup during the 6 months preceding the end of the school year. Rejection sensitivity was unrelated to depressive symptoms among women who had initiated the breakups or who had not experienced any breakups. For male college students who viewed themselves as conservative, rejection sensitivity predicted a higher number of depressive symptoms, as well as a lowered sense of belonging at their liberal university (Romero-Canyas, Downey, & Cavanaugh, 2003). These correlations are not evident among highly rejection-sensitive, liberal men who did not expect peer rejection because of their beliefs.

The Association of Rejection Sensitivity and Personality Disorders

Sensitivity to rejection, conceptualized as a tendency to overreact to rejection, is one of the diagnostic criteria for some forms of psychopathology, such as depression and borderline personality disorder (American Psychiatric Association, 1994). There are clear parallels in the perceptual processes, behaviors, and outcomes between rejection sensitivity and borderline personality disorder (BPD) and avoidant personality disorder (APD). BPD is characterized by impulsivity, instability in mood, and self-directed harm or injury. APD is characterized by social inhibition, feelings of inadequacy, and avoidance of social interaction. At the core of both disorders is a fear of rejection or abandonment that leads to volatile relationships and low self-concept clarity. People with BPD or APD have significantly higher levels of rejection sensitivity than healthy controls, and the relationship between BPD and high rejection sensitivity holds even when controlling for depression (Berenson, 2008). This suggests that rejection sensitivity might play a role in the processing of social information among people who are diagnosed as having BPD or APD.

Consistent with this hypothesis, Berenson (2008) found that people with APD and especially those with BPD selectively attended to, detected, interpreted, and reacted to social threat cues in ways that reflect high rejection sensitivity. Berenson also showed

that people with BPD avoided angry faces and showed less attention to happy faces, whereas people with APD show a bias toward angry faces. Hence, patients with BPD behaved like highly rejection-sensitive people. In the paradigm used in the studies of overestimation of negativity, people with BPD perceived significantly more negativity and slightly less positivity in faces and were more certain about their interpretations than control participants. People with BPD or APD also showed a lower threshold for detecting angry faces in angry–afraid morphed faces. Finally, when asked to imagine that close others might be losing interest in them, people with BPD reported a higher likelihood of losing control of their tempers, gratifying impulsive urges including harm to themselves, and a lower likelihood of talking to close others to improve the relationships. In response to the same scenario, people with APD reported imagining that they would withdraw and feel worthless.

Eating and Body Dysmorphic Disorders

Being sensitive to rejection based on physical appearance or attractiveness has specific physical and mental health implications. Atlas (2004) found that appearance-related sensitivity (measures of feelings of attractiveness and investment in one's appearance) together with rejection sensitivity predicted a drive for thinness and symptoms of bulimia. Park (2007a) and her colleagues developed an appearance-based rejection-sensitivity measure to capture the dynamic of anxiously expecting rejection because of one's appearance or physical attractiveness. High appearance-based rejection sensitivity is strongly associated with body dysmorphic disorder and predicts intent to undergo cosmetic surgery for social rather than personal reasons (Park, DiRaddo, & Harwin, 2007). People high in appearance-based rejection sensitivity experience distress when interacting with others in situations in which they believe appearance is important (Park, 2007b).

As the work on appearance-based rejection sensitivity illustrates, people can be rejection sensitive with regard to particular aspects of themselves. Specific concerns, situations, or aspects of the person can be the basis for concerns about rejection. For example, social identities can be a source of concern about rejection from others, particularly social identities that in the larger sociocultural and sociohistorical sphere have been stigmatized and historically discriminated against. Anxiously expecting rejection because of a social identity has specific implications for behavior, cognition, and emotion. These implications are explored extensively in research looking at status-based rejection sensitivity, which we summarize next.

Sensitivity to Status-Based Rejection

Belonging to a group that has been historically stigmatized or excluded from certain domains can have serious consequences for physical health and psychological well-being. Intergroup differences (black vs. white, women vs. men) have traditionally been the focus of studies on the implications of stigma for health, well-being, belonging, and achievement, but increasing attention has been directed to the intragroup differences in stigma's effect on these outcomes (London et al., 2006; Mendoza-Denton et al., 2002).

Building on Downey's personal rejection-sensitivity model, the status-based rejection sensitivity models posit that past experiences of rejection or discrimination based on one's social identity or status (e.g., race, gender, age, socioeconomic status) can lead people to anxiously expect such rejection in situations in which rejection is possible (London et al., 2006; Mendoza-Denton et al., 2002; Mendoza-Denton, Page-Gould, & Pietrzak, 2006; Pietrzak, 2004). These expectations influence behavioral and affective responses to indications of race-based rejection, driving the individual to avoid environments and organizations in which these cues abound and people who are perceived to represent these organizations. A growing body of research offers compelling evidence of how expecting rejection from others can affect interpersonal relationships, as well as relationships with institutions. This section reviews the effect of status-based rejection sensitivity on physical and psychological well-being, institutional belonging, academic achievement, and decision making for some of the traditionally stigmatized groups for whom rejection sensitivity measures have been developed.

Race-Based Rejection Sensitivity among African Americans

Race-based rejection sensitivity is defined as the anxious expectation of rejection based on one's race or ethnicity (Mendoza-Denton et al., 2002, 2006). Just like personal rejection sensitivity, status-based rejection is context specific and activated in situations in which the threat is likely, such as in majority white environments. Race-based rejection sensitivity is measured using the Race-Based Rejection Sensitivity Questionnaire (RSQ-race), which describes 12 ambiguous scenarios in which racial/ethnic discrimination is possible (Mendoza-Denton et al., 2002). An example of a scale item is: "Imagine that you are in a pharmacy, trying to pick out a few items. While you are looking at the different brands, you notice one of the clerks glancing your way" (Mendoza-Denton et al., 2002). Respondents rate their expectations of rejection and their anxiety in the situation, and these scores are used to compute the anxious expectations of rejection. The original RSQ-race was designed using scenarios that elicit concerns about race-based rejection from African American students, but it has been shown to be effective in measuring race-based rejection sensitivity in Hispanic Americans living in urban environments.

In a sample of African American college students at a predominantly white university, Mendoza-Denton and colleagues (2002) found that students high in race-based rejection sensitivity reported feeling a lower sense of belonging with the university as a whole and with their peers and professors and less trust in the university and its representatives (Mendoza-Denton et al., 2002). Mendoza-Denton, Pietrzak, and Downey (2008) found that this lower sense of belonging and institutional trust was most pronounced among students who were also high in ethnic identity. Evidence that the race-based rejection-sensitivity dynamic is situationally activated comes from a study comparing African American students at a predominantly white university to those at a historically black one. Anderson, London, and Downey (2008) found that race-based rejection sensitivity predicted a lower sense of belonging only at the predominantly white university; there was no effect of race-based rejection sensitivity on sense of belonging at the historically black university, where the threat of race-based rejection was highly unlikely. Anderson and Downey (2005) replicated this finding in a study of race-based rejection sensitivity among high school students. Significantly, positive experiences with people from the threatening group attenuate the effects of race-based rejection sensitivity on African Americans. Hence, having quality friendships with white students increased sense of belonging among highly race-based rejection-sensitive African American students at a predominantly white college (Mendoza-Denton et al., 2006).

The discomfort experienced by students high in race-based rejection sensitivity in predominantly white environments may motivate them to avoid or at least minimize further discomfort by avoiding people who represent the rejecting authorities. Among African American students at predominantly white universities and among African American and Hispanic students at predominantly white and Asian high schools, race-based rejection sensitivity predicted less academic help seeking and use of available resources, such as attending professors' and teaching assistants' office hours and review sessions (Anderson et al., 2008; Mendoza-Denton et al., 2002). In an experimental study, London, Downey, and Dweck (2008) found that after receiving feedback on essays, African American participants high in race-based rejection sensitivity who believed that the evaluating professor was aware of their race were less willing to meet the professor to discuss improving their essays relative to peers low in RS-race. In challenging academic settings in which seeking help is crucial in managing difficult coursework, avoiding uncomfortable but potentially beneficial situations may translate into academic underachievement. Indeed, Mendoza-Denton and colleagues (2002) found that students high in race-based rejection sensitivity exhibited a decline in grade point average over their 4 years at a competitive predominantly white university.

The desire to avoid the discomfort of potential rejection makes the prospect of attending a predominantly white college unattractive to high school students who are high in race-based rejection sensitivity. This is especially true for students high in RS-race who have extensive exposure to predominantly white environments, such as students in predominantly white high schools. In Anderson and colleagues' study (2008), African American and Hispanic students' scores on the RSQ-race predicted a preference for colleges with more students of color, whether these were fictitious colleges or real colleges to which they desired to apply. In focus group discussions, students offered such explanations as, "I just can't repeat this experience. There needs to be enough Black people in my college for me to be comfortable" (Anderson, 2005). Of course, institutional racial composition is not the only factor considered in the college choice of minority students. Although factors such as proximity to home and availability of financial aid all influence the choice of where students decide to attend college, the racial makeup of a given college may be very important in the college transition of students high in RS-race, as evidenced by the adverse outcomes for students high in RS-race seen in Mendoza-Denton and colleagues (2002).

African Americans and Hispanics in majority white settings may be more at risk for compromised health if they score high in race-based rejection sensitivity due to the higher probability of perceiving race-based rejection. Pietrzak (2004) found that students high in race-based rejection sensitivity reported more somatic symptoms, such as stomachache and pounding heart, after reading a vignette about a negative racial incident or after recalling a recent personal negative racial experience. Furthermore, these students are also more likely to respond to such experiences with self-silencing or strong emotional outbursts (e.g., crying, yelling), reactions that are likely to further their isolation (Pietrzak, 2004; Velilla, Mendoza-Denton, London, & Downey, 2001).

Race–Based Rejection Sensitivity among Asian Americans

Because Asian American stereotypes and discrimination experiences differ from those of other ethnic minorities in the United States (Oyserman & Sakamoto, 1997), a scale specific to the stigmatizing and discriminating experiences of Asian Americans was developed (rejection sensitivity—Asian; Chan & Mendoza-Denton, 2008). Asian Americans as a group have lower self-esteem than African Americans and Hispanic Americans and are at higher risk for anxiety, depression, and socioemotional maladjustment (cf. Chan & Mendoza-Denton, 2008). This process of lowered personal esteem as a result of group discrimination is a form of internalized stigma that results from individuals not differentiating between discrimination aimed at one's social groups and negative behavior aimed at one as an individual. Consistent with this approach in which Asian Americans internalize stigma, being high in rejection sensitivity—Asian predicts lower self-esteem. Mediational analysis shows that shame, a self-directed negative emotion particularly relevant in interpersonal contexts of rejection or discrimination, is the mechanism by which high rejection sensitivity leads to lower self-esteem among Asian participants (Chan & Mendoza-Denton, 2008). Being high in race-based rejection sensitivity has no such implication for African Americans. Work on rejection sensitivity—Asian demonstrates that race-based rejection concerns are activated in different contexts and can lead to disparate outcomes depending on the racial group. Consistent with the process-based approach that characterizes research using the rejection-sensitivity model, culturally salient values and experiences are important in understanding how rejection sensitivity affects people's emotions and behaviors.

Gender-Based Rejection Sensitivity

Although they are not a numerical minority, as African Americans and Asian Americans are in North America, women have been historically excluded or underrepresented in several professions, such as law and business, and continue to be underrepresented in math and science. Negative stereotypes about women's abilities and skills in these fields are widespread, and thus women experience stereotype threat in the same way as African Americans. London and colleagues (2006) proposed a model of gender-based rejection sensitivity to account for individual differences in the expectation, perception of, and reaction to gender-based discrimination. The gender-based rejection-sensitivity model posits that past experiences with gender discrimination can lead women to anxiously expect, readily perceive, and react strongly to discrimination in contexts in which gender discrimination is likely.

Rejection sensitivity—gender predicts lower institutional belonging and higher self-silencing among college students (London et al., 2008). In an experimental study in which participants believed that their essays were read and evaluated by a highly esteemed male professor, women who scored high in gender-based rejection sensitivity and who believed their gender was known to the professor expected to receive lower grades on their essays. Upon receiving ambiguous feedback, women high in rejection sensitivity—gender were less likely to want to meet with the professor to work on improving the essay (London et al., 2008). Gender-based rejection sensitivity also has implications for physical and psychological well-being. In a diary study of incoming law school students, rejection sensitivity—gender was associated with more negative affect over the course of the 3-week diary period, as well as with greater somatic responses (i.e., headaches, stomachaches) to stressful events.

Sexual Orientation–Based Rejection Sensitivity

Like members of other minority groups, gay, lesbian, and bisexual individuals experience rejection and discrimination. Unlike members of ethnic minority groups, however, gay, lesbian, and bisexual individuals often do not share their stigmatized minority status with their close others, such as their parents. As such, the possibility of parental rejection based on group membership is substantially higher among gay, lesbian, and bisexual individuals than it is for ethnic minority groups, for example. Pachankis and colleagues (2008) examined the relationship between parental rejection based on sexuality, anxious expectations of rejection based on sexuality, and internalized homophobia—the tendency to see oneself and other gay individuals as inferior and shameful, which leads to the rejection of one's own sexual identity and difficulty in relationships with others. The authors created and validated a gay-related rejection-sensitivity scale and found that the relationship between parental rejection and gay-related rejection sensitivity was mediated by internalized homophobia.

In other words, internalized homophobia is the mechanism by which parental rejection leads to gay-related rejection sensitivity.

Gay-related rejection sensitivity also influences interpersonal behavior such that those who are high in gay-related rejection sensitivity are less likely to assert their needs in relationships (Pachankis et al., 2008); this unassertiveness or acquiescence can lead to a range of risky behaviors, such as unsafe sexual practices.

Summary

Like sensitivity to personal rejection, sensitivity to status-based rejection has important consequences for individuals and their relationships with others. The anxiety felt by those who expect to be rejected due to their social identity may lead them to experience more interpersonal difficulties, in addition to heightened somatic reactions to their status-based stress. In order to manage this anxiety, they may engage in avoidance behaviors, such as self-silencing, disengagement, and failing to use available resources. These behaviors may, in turn, undermine achievement of academic and social goals. Further research should try to identify individual-level and institutional-level interventions that will reduce the threat experienced by people who are highly sensitive to rejection based on status and allow them to achieve and thrive in all environments.

Conclusion

Rejection sensitivity affects interpersonal behavior by biasing people toward perceiving and reacting to threat in ways that may compromise existing relationships and impair the formation of new ones. This pattern can lead to a wide range of difficulties, including discomfort, social awkwardness, psychopathology, and academic troubles. As much of the research suggests (e.g., Ayduk et al., 2008), the ability to control emotions effortfully may curtail some of the negative outcomes associated with being high in rejection sensitivity by preventing impulsive behaviors and preventing the person from experiencing emotions that lead to negative outcomes and that motivate behaviors that could result in rejection from others. Institutional programs, interventions, and positive relationships with outgroup members may help people who are high on status-based rejection sensitivity to cope with threatening environments.

The research summarized here illustrates that the rejection-sensitivity model is useful in explaining people's concerns with rejection and acceptance. It has allowed researchers to study these concerns and their effects on social functioning using a broad array of methods and at multiple levels, from the social to the neural. The dynamic "if ... then" approach and the process-oriented theoretical underpinnings of the work also allow researchers to look at how the individual's response affects his or her social world, eliciting behaviors from others that in turn affect the individual and strengthen or weaken his or her sensitivity to rejection. Current work exploring how to attenuate the effect of rejection sensitivity may yield interventions that can result in greater quality of relationships for people high in rejection sensitivity.

References

American Psychiatric Association. (1994). *Diagnostic and statistical manual of mental disorders* (4th ed.). Washington, DC: Author.

Anderson, V. (2005). [Focus group interviews on students' college decisions]. Unpublished raw data.

Anderson, V. T., & Downey, G. (2005). [Race-based rejection sensitivity among high school students at predominantly black and Hispanic high schools and predominantly White and Asian high schools]. Unpublished raw data.

Anderson, V. T., London, B., & Downey, G. (2008). *Institutional effects of race based rejection sensitivity: Implications for college choice and institutional engagement.* Manuscript submitted for publication.

Anderson, V. T., Romero-Canyas, R., & Downey, G. (2008). *Rejection sensitivity predicts attributing distressing events to powerful others. It's all in God's hands and he doesn't love me.* Unpublished manuscript, Columbia University.

Atlas, J. G. (2004). Interpersonal sensitivity, eating disorder symptoms, and eating/thinness expectancies. *Current Psychology: Developmental, Learning, Personality, Social, 22,* 368–378.

Axelrod, R., & Hamilton, W. D. (1981). The evolution of cooperation. *Science, 211,* 1390–1396.

Ayduk, Ö., Downey, G., & Kim, M. (2001). Rejection sensitivity and depressive symptoms in women. *Personality and Social Psychology Bulletin, 27,* 868–877.

Ayduk, Ö., Downey, G., Testa, A., Yen, Y., & Shoda,

Y. (1999). Does rejection elicit hostility in rejection sensitive women? *Social Cognition, 17*, 245–271.

Ayduk, Ö., Gyurak, A., & Luerssen, A. (2007). Individual differences in the rejection–aggression link in the hot sauce paradigm: The case of rejection sensitivity. *Journal of Experimental Social Psychology, 44*, 775–782.

Ayduk, Ö., Mendoza-Denton, R., Mischel, W., Downey, G., Peake, P. L. K., & Rodriguez, M. (2000). Regulating the interpersonal self: Strategic self-regulation for coping with rejection sensitivity. *Journal of Personality and Social Psychology, 79*, 776–792.

Ayduk, O. N., Zayas, V., Downey, G., Cole, A. B., Shoda, Y., & Mischel, W. (2008). Rejection sensitivity and executive function: Joint predictors of borderline personality features. *Journal of Research in Personality, 42*, 151–168.

Barash, D. P. (1977). *Sociobiology and behavior.* Oxford, UK: Elsevier North-Holland.

Baumeister, R. F., DeWall, C. N., Ciarocco, N. J., & Twenge, J. M. (2005). Social exclusion impairs self-regulation. *Journal of Personality and Social Psychology, 88*, 589–604.

Baumeister, R.F., & Leary, M. R. (1995). The need to belong: Desire for interpersonal attachments as a fundamental human motivation. *Psychological Bulletin, 117*, 497–529.

Baumeister, R. F., Twenge, J. M., & Nuss, C. K. (2002). Effects of social exclusion on cognitive processes: Anticipated aloneness reduces intelligent thought. *Journal of Personality and Social Psychology, 83*, 817–827.

Berenson, K. R. (2008). *Rejection sensitivity as an antecedent of borderline personality disorder.* Manuscript in preparation.

Berenson, K. R., & Downey, G. (2008a). *Rejection sensitivity and increased risky sexual behavior for women at risk for contracting sexually transmitted illnesses.* Unpublished manuscript, Columbia University.

Berenson, K. R., & Downey, G. (2008b). *Rejection sensitivity predicts attention bias away from threatening faces.* Unpublished manuscript, Columbia University.

Berenson, K. R., Kang, J., & Downey, G. (2008). *Rejection sensitivity and intimate relationship in the transition to young adulthood.* Manuscript in preparation.

Bourgeois, K. S., & Leary, M. R. (2001). Coping with rejection: Derogating those who choose us last. *Motivation and Emotion, 25*, 101–111.

Burklund, L. J., Eisenberger, N. I., & Lieberman, M. D. (2007). The face of rejection: Rejection sensitivity moderates dorsal anterior cingulated activity to disapproving facial expressions. *Social Neuroscience, 2*, 238–253.

Chan, W., & Mendoza-Denton, R. (2008). *Status-based rejection sensitivity among Asian Americans: Implications for psychological distress.* Manuscript submitted for publication.

Davis, M. (1992). The role of the amygdala in fear and anxiety. *Annual Review of Neuroscience, 15*, 353–375.

DiBenigno, J., Romero-Canyas, R., & Downey, G. (2007, January). *Do rejection sensitivity and performance predict extreme reactions to rejection for performing artists?* Poster presented at the annual meeting of the Society for Personality and Social Psychology, Memphis, TN.

Downey, G., Berenson, K. R., & Kang, J. (2006). *The Adult Rejection Sensitivity Questionnaire (A-RSQ).* Unpublished questionnaire, Columbia University.

Downey, G., Feldman, S., & Ayduk, O. (2000). Rejection sensitivity and male violence in romantic relationships. *Personal Relationships, 7*, 45–61.

Downey, G., & Feldman, S. I. (1996). Implications of rejection sensitivity for intimate relationships. *Journal of Personality and Social Psychology, 70*, 1327–1343.

Downey, G., Freitas, A. L., Michaelis, B., & Khouri, H. (1998). The self-fulfilling prophecy in close relationships: Rejection sensitivity and rejection by romantic partners. *Journal of Personality and Social Psychology, 75*, 545–560.

Downey, G., Irwin, L., Ramsay, M., & Ayduk, Ö. (2004). Rejection sensitivity and girls' aggression. In M. M. Moretti, C. L. Odgers, & M. A. Jackson (Eds.), *Girls and aggression: Contributing factors and intervention principles* (pp. 7–25). New York: Kluwer Academic/Plenum Press.

Downey, G., Lebolt, A., Rincon, C., & Freitas, A. L. (1998). Rejection sensitivity and children's interpersonal difficulties. *Child Development, 69*, 1074–1091.

Downey, G., Mougios, V., Ayduk, Ö., London, B. E., & Shoda, Y. (2004). Rejection sensitivity and the defensive motivational system: Insights from the startle response to rejection cues. *Psychological Science, 15*, 668–673.

Feldman, S., & Downey, G. (1994). Rejection sensitivity as a mediator of the impact of childhood exposure to family violence on adult attachment behavior. *Development and Psychopathology, 6*, 231–247.

Horney, K. (1937). *The neurotic personality of our time.* New York: Norton.

Impett, E. A., Gable, S. L., & Peplau, L. A. (2005). Giving up and giving in: The costs and benefits of daily sacrifice in intimate relationships. *Journal of Personality and Social Psychology, 89*, 327–344.

Kross, E., Egner, T., Ochsner, K., Hirsch, J., & Downey, G. (2007). Neural dynamics of rejection sensitivity. *Journal of Cognitive Neuroscience, 19*, 945–956.

Leary, M. R., Kowalski, R. M., Smith, L., & Phillips, S. (2003). Teasing, rejection, and violence: Case studies of the school shootings. *Aggressive Behavior, 29*, 202–214.

Leary, M. R., Twenge, J. M., & Quinlivan, E. (2006). Interpersonal rejection as a determinant of anger and aggression. *Personality and Social Psychology Review, 10*, 111–132.

LeDoux, J. E. (1996). *The emotional brain: The mysterious underpinnings of emotional life.* New York: Simon & Schuster.

London, B., Downey, G., Bonica, C., & Paltin, I. (2007). Social causes and consequences of rejection sensitivity. *Journal of Research on Adolescence, 17*, 481–506.

London, B., Downey, G., & Dweck, C. (2008). *The student's dilemma: Coping responses to stereotype threat.* Manuscript in preparation.

London, B., Downey, G., Rattan, A., & Tyson, D. (2006). *Gender rejection sensitivity: Theory, validation, and implications for the psychosocial well-being and achievement outcomes of women.* Unpublished manuscript.

Maslow, A. (1987). *Motivation and personality* (3rd ed.). New York: Harper & Row.

McClelland, D. C. (1987). *Human motivation.* Cambridge, UK: Cambridge University Press.

Mendoza-Denton, R., Downey, G., Purdie, V., Davis, A., & Pietrzak, J. (2002). Sensitivity to status-based rejection: Implications for African American students' college experience. *Journal of Personality and Social Psychology, 83,* 896–918.

Mendoza-Denton, R., Page-Gould, E., & Pietrzak, J. (2006). Mechanisms for coping with status-based rejection expectations. In S. Levin & C. van Laar (Eds.), *Stigma and group inequality: Social psychological perspectives* (pp. 151–169). Mahwah, NJ: Erlbaum.

Mendoza-Denton, R., Pietrzak, J., & Downey, G. (2008). Distinguishing institutional identification from academic goal pursuit: Interactive effects of ethnic identification and race-based rejection sensitivity. *Journal of Personality and Social Psychology, 95,* 1080–1094.

Metcalfe, J., & Mischel, W. (1999). A hot/cool system analysis of delay of gratification: Dynamics of willpower. *Psychological Review, 106,* 3–19.

Mischel, W., & Shoda, Y. (1995). A cognitive–affective system theory of personality: Reconceptualizing situations, dispositions, dynamics, and invariance in personality structure. *Psychological Review, 102,* 246–268.

Mogg, K., Mathews, A., & Eysenck, M. (1992). Attentional bias to threat in clinical anxiety states. *Cognition and Emotion, 6,* 149–159.

Olsson, A., Carmona, S., Downey, G., & Ochsner, K. N. (2008). *Perceiving threat and learning to fear: A processing account of rejection sensitivity.* Manuscript in preparation.

Oyserman, D., & Sakamoto, I. (1997). Being Asian American: Identity, cultural constructs, and stereotype perception. *Journal of Applied Behavioral Science, 33,* 435–453.

Pachankis, J. E., Goldfried, M. R., & Ramrattan, M. E. (2008). Extension of the rejection sensitivity construct to the interpersonal functioning of gay men. *Journal of Consulting and Clinical Psychology, 76,* 306–317.

Park, L. (2007a). Appearance-based rejection sensitivity: Implications for mental and physical health, affect, and motivation. *Personality and Social Psychology Bulletin, 33,* 490–504.

Park, L. (2007b). *Interpersonal dynamics of appearance-based rejection sensitivity.* Manuscript in preparation.

Park, L. E., DiRaddo, A., & Harwin, M. J. (2007). *Appearance-based rejection sensitivity and clinical outcomes: Effects on body dysmorphic disorder and desire for cosmetic surgery.* Manuscript in preparation.

Pietrzak, J. (2004). Race-based rejection sensitivity and ethnic identity: Interactive effects on institutional affiliation and well-being. *Dissertation Abstracts International, 64,* 6379–6453.

Pine, D. S., Mogg, K., Bradley, B. P., Montgomery, L., Monk, C. S., McClure, E., et al. (2005). Attention bias to threat in maltreated children: Implications for vulnerability to stress-related psychopathology. *American Journal of Psychiatry, 162,* 291–296.

Purdie, V., & Downey, G. (2000). Rejection sensitivity and adolescent girls' vulnerability to relationship-centered difficulties. *Child Maltreatment, 5,* 338–349.

Romero-Canyas, R., & Downey, G. (2003, February). *Sensitivity to rejection by groups (rejection sensitivity-G) as a predictor of political behavior.* Poster presented at the conference of the Society of Personality and Social Psychology, Los Angeles.

Romero-Canyas, R., & Downey, G. (2008). *Rejection sensitivity predicts overestimating the negative mood of others and predicts contagion of negative affect.* Manuscript in preparation.

Romero-Canyas, R., Downey, G., Berenson, K., Ayduk, O., & Kang, J. (in press). Rejection sensitivity and the rejection–hostility link in romantic relationships. *Journal of Personality.*

Romero-Canyas, R., Downey, G., & Cavanaugh, T. J. (2003). *Feelings of alienation among college men: The impact of rejection sensitivity and political beliefs.* Unpublished manuscript, Columbia University.

Romero-Canyas, R., Downey, G., Pelayo, R., & Bashan, U. (2004, February). *The threat of rejection triggers social accommodation in rejection sensitive men.* Poster presented at the annual meeting of the Society for Personality and Social Psychology, Austin, Texas.

Romero-Canyas, R., Downey, G., Reedy, K. S., Rodriguez, S., Cavanaugh, T., & Pelayo, R. (2008). *Paying to belong: Who tries. The link between rejection sensitivity and ingratiation after rejection.* Manuscript submitted for publication.

Twenge, J. M., Baumeister, R. F., Tice, D. M., & Stucke, T. S. (2001). If you can't join them, beat them: Effects of social exclusion on aggressive behavior. *Journal of Personality and Social Psychology, 81,* 1058–1069.

Velilla, E., Mendoza-Denton, R., London, B., & Downey, G. (2001, July). *Race based rejection sensitivity in a pre-college sample of students.* Paper presented at the Leadership Alliance Research Symposium, Atlanta, GA.

Williams, K. D. (2001). *Ostracism: The power of silence.* New York: Guilford Press.

CHAPTER 33

■ ● ▲ ◆ ■ ● ▲ ◆

Psychological Defensiveness

Repression, Blunting, and Defensive Pessimism

JULIE K. NOREM

Psychologists from many theoretical perspectives across clinical, personality, social, cognitive, and physiological psychology have been interested in understanding defensive processes. As a result, numerous constructs and operationalizations describe perceptual and information-processing styles and self- and affect-regulation strategies that involve defensive components. Furthermore, individual differences in defensive processes overlap with work on coping, narcissism, self-esteem, self-deception, sensation seeking, introversion and extraversion, the behavioral activation–inhibition system, neuroticism, anxiety, rejection sensitivity, and social desirability, as well as numerous clinical constructs and categories.

Comprehensive review of the ways in which defensiveness potentially plays a role in of all of these phenomena would be beyond the scope of an entire volume, much less a single chapter, so this chapter focuses on constructs that concern how people typically process information in situations in which there is a potential anxiety about specific outcomes. I briefly review three individual-difference dimensions (augmenting–reducing, repression–sensitization, and monitoring–blunting) related to processing sensory, affective, and cognitive stimuli. Then I review research on ways in which the strategies of defensive pessimism and strategic optimism influence cognitive, affective, motivational, social,

and performance consequences for those who use them and how the relative costs and benefits of a strategy vary as a function of specific tasks and contexts.

Individual Differences in Physiological Inhibition and Arousal

Theories concerning individual differences in the relative strength of biologically based aspects of the nervous system have a long history in philosophy, medicine, and psychology. Many of these conceptions focus on physiological phenomena related to inhibition and arousal, responses to environmental stimuli, and reactions to reinforcement contingencies (Traue & Pennebaker, 1993). Pavlov (1927), for example, conceived of "strong" and "weak" nervous systems, and subsequent researchers elaborated his definitions to characterize individual differences in the strength of response to reinforcement contingencies (Hull, 1950; Spence, 1936). Biologically based models typically assert that the goal of the nervous system is to regulate arousal in reaction to stimuli and that efforts to moderate arousal involve inhibiting motoric action, including emotional expression. Arousal differences stem from organic nervous system differences that create differences in perception and physiological experience.

Study of inhibition and arousal, as they relate to repression, emotional expressiveness, and perception, led to several attempts to develop individual-difference models that would capture physiological and psychological patterns of responding. Theorists developed views of individual responses to reward and punishment that are related to the biologically based construct of inhibition, including theories of introversion–extraversion and the behavioral inhibition system and behavioral approach system (Eysenck, 1967; Gray, 1972).

Buck (1976) argued that the biologically based disposition of introversion is associated with higher electrodermal and other physiological reactivity, which, under socialization, leads to the inhibition of expression. Early work found disjunctions between physiological responses (e.g., skin conductance and heart rate) on the one hand and verbal reports and emotional expressiveness/responsiveness on the other hand (Buck, 1976). Research on this disjunction is important to current understanding of defensiveness as exhibited in defensive self-esteem, self-deception, and narcissism. Pennebaker and his colleagues, for example, have done extensive work showing that intentional thought suppression has a number of generally negative physiological consequences (Pennebaker & Chew, 1985; Petrie, Booth, & Pennebaker, 1998).

Nevertheless, this work takes us in a different direction than defensiveness per se in that its focus is on intentional lying or suppression of troublesome emotions and thoughts. Suppression that is initially intentional, of course, may develop into a characteristic or habitual suppression that occurs automatically outside of awareness, which is one way of understanding repression–sensitization, as discussed later. Yet the subdued emotional responses measured by self- and observer reports of introversion do not correspond in any simple way to the verbal–physiological disjunction noted either when people are trying to lie or when they automatically suppress. Indeed, suppression, or lying to oneself that occurs outside of awareness, appears to be more strongly associated with extraverted characteristics than introverted ones (Paulhus & John, 1998). Although use of the term *inhibition* in this early work may suggest to contemporary readers a close asso-

ciation with current usage of *repression* and *defensiveness*, past uses do not correspond to present understandings in a straightforward way.

Augmenters and Reducers

Other models of reaction to stimuli also suggest connections to defensiveness. Petrie posited two perceptual–cognitive styles called augmenting and reducing (A–R). At one extreme she described "augmenters," who magnify or intensify effects of sensory input, and at the other extreme "reducers," who attempt to decrease or attenuate the effect of sensory input (Petrie, 1967). These styles reflect temperamental differences in the modulation of stimulation. She operationalized these styles with the kinesthetic aftereffect measure, in which individuals typically report that a standard block is larger after they have handled a smaller block and smaller after they have handled a larger block. She found individual differences in the size of the kinesthetic aftereffect: Those who are more extreme in their reports of how large the test block is after the smaller block (in the augmenting condition) also tend to be less extreme in their reports of how small the test block is after the larger block (in the reducing condition); they are labeled "augmenters." Others augment less and reduce more and are called "reducers." Petrie (1967) also identified two other groups: moderates, who showed little aftereffect in either condition, and the "stimulus-governed," who exaggerated in both directions. Most research on augmenting–reducing has focused on the former two groups.

Congruent with a focus on a sensory measure, much of the research on these styles has investigated reports of experience with other sensory stimuli; in particular, there has been considerable research on the experience of pain as a function of A–R. In general, augmenters tend to be less tolerant of pain than reducers. Interestingly, they also report greater pain relief from analgesics (Petrie, 1967) and from hypnosis (Morgan, Lezard, Prytulak, & Hilgard, 1970) than reducers do. Petrie's kinesthetic aftereffect method correlates with questionnaire measures of need for sensory stimulation, interest in contact sports, delinquency, and tolerance of cold and pain (Herzog, Williams, & Weintraub, 1985).

Sales (1971) found that reducers seek out and enjoy interesting and intense stimulus situations, whereas augmenters seek out and enjoy quieter and duller stimulus situations; he argued that these styles represent different levels of "need for stimulation." Further results connect A–R to levels of cortical attenuation of incoming stimuli: Research has shown systematic differences between augmenters and reducers in evoked potentials, reaction times, and physiological reactivity (Schwerdtfeger & Baltissen, 2002). These differences are not specific to emotional stimuli (Schwerdtfeger, 2003), which would tend to differentiate A–R from psychodynamic accounts of defensiveness.

Individual differences in physiological sensitivity could include or predispose one to emotional sensitivity that increases subjective need for defensive processing. Psychoanalytic models that focus on defensiveness in response to sexual or aggressive content would have difficulty incorporating such predispositions. Neuroticism as a broad dimension of personality includes aspects of heightened sensitivity and defensiveness, but not in ways that account for disjunctions between physiological and conscious self-reported experience. In contrast, models of defensiveness that focus on threats to self-concept might more easily include this kind of sensitivity. Overall, although descriptions of augmenters and reducers seem on the surface as if they would correspond to certain conceptions of psychological defensiveness, empirical work suggests that they are better understood as part of the constellation of characteristics that make up sensation seeking (see Zuckerman, Chapter 31, this volume) and extraversion (Bruneau, Roux, Perse, & Lelord, 1984; Eysenck, 1973; see Wilt & Revelle, Chapter 3, this volume).

Psychoanalytic and Social-Cognitive Perspectives

Psychoanalytic theory is arguably the most influential source of ideas about defensiveness. Freud (1914) famously argued that human beings are motivated to defend themselves against the intrusion of psychologically painful ideas and affects. An arsenal of de-

fense mechanisms push threatening thoughts and emotions out of conscious awareness and transform them so that they are no longer recognizable (Freud, 1946). Ample research on specific psychoanalytic defensive mechanisms demonstrates that people use distinct cognitive transformations when they face psychological threat (Baumeister, Dale, & Sommer, 1998; Cramer, 1995). There are also defense mechanism inventories derived from psychodynamic assumptions about types of defense mechanisms (for a review, see Davidson & MacGregor, 1998).

There are commonalities between theories that argue that biologically based individual differences in inhibitory and arousal-related neural systems underlie individual differences in physiological and psychological reactions to environmental stimuli, and psychodynamic propositions that individuals are motivated to protect themselves from—that is, keep out of conscious awareness—threatening or anxiety-producing information and thoughts. Both predict individual differences in levels and awareness of anxiety, potential disjunctions between physiological reactivity and verbal behavior, and differences in characteristic modes of responding to threatening or anxiety-producing stimuli.

The "New Look" and Repression–Sensitization

During the post–World War II years, several psychologists developed new theories of perception, cognition, and personality that integrated psychodynamic ideas about defensive processing with a functionalist approach to perception (Bruner & Postman, 1947). The central idea of this "New Look" approach was that motivation influences our perception and processing of stimuli.

From this perspective grew a construct related to individual differences in defensiveness: repression–sensitization (Eriksen, 1966), operationalized by the Repression–Sensitization (R–S) Scale (Byrne, 1961). Repression–Sensitization was initially characterized as a bipolar dimension, the extremes of which represented characteristic and rigid defenses against threatening, aversive, or anxiety-provoking stimuli (Bonanno & Singer, 1995). "Repressors" avoid, deny, or minimize aversive information and anxiety. "Sensitizers," in contrast, seek out as much information as they can about threatening situations and expend considerable effort worrying and ruminating about them.

Byrne's (1961) early scale correlated too highly with anxiety measures, produced conflicting results, and has largely been replaced with new operationalizations. Weinberger, Schwartz, and Davidson (1979) developed the most popular measure of R–S, arguing that the repressor end of the R–S scale confounded repressive individuals with those who were genuinely low in anxiety, whereas the sensitizer end confounded true sensitizers with those who were unsuccessful in their defenses (as opposed to nondefensive) and thus unable to repress their anxiety. Confounding of true person variance with defensive self-reports is an ongoing issue in research on defensiveness.

Weinberger and colleagues (1979) attempted to disentangle these confounds by simultaneously measuring trait anxiety with the Manifest Anxiety Scale (Taylor, 1953) and tendencies to respond in socially desirable ways with the Marlowe–Crowne Social Desirability Scale (Crowne & Marlowe, 1960) to create four groups of individuals. Those low in self-reported trait anxiety and low in social desirability tendencies are nonanxious and nondefensive. Those low in self-reported trait anxiety but high in social desirability are repressors. Those high in self-reported trait anxiety but low in social desirability are sensitizers, whereas those high in both anxiety and social desirability are defensive and highly anxious individuals. Interestingly, until recently, most research using this method has concentrated only on the first three of these groups.

Research on R–S (often described as research on repressive coping) converges somewhat with earlier research on inhibition–expression and augmenting–reducing, in that repressors typically show disjunction between self-reported and autonomic indicators of stress (Weinstein, Averill, Opton, & Lazarus, 1968). Repressors' self-reports suggest less stress than their autonomic responses indicate, whereas sensitizers' self-reports suggest more stress than is reflected in their autonomic responses (Bonanno, Davis, & Singer, 1991; Bonanno & Singer,

1995; Lorig, Singer, Bonanno, & Davis, 1994; Mitchell, 1998; Rohrmann, Netter, Hennig, & Hodapp, 2003).

Repressors tend to encode emotions less complexly (Hansen & Hansen, 1988) and show greater memory failures for both negative and positive emotional events (Davis & Schwartz, 1987). This pattern led Tesser and his colleagues (Mendolia, Moore, & Tesser, 1996) to reason that repressors are hypersensitive to all emotional events but motivated to repress only when they appraise an emotional event as threatening to their self-evaluations; their evidence supports this more specific hypothesis. Subsequent research findings converge with these. For example, repressors show electroencephalographic (EEG) activity associated with anxiety and an absence of cognitive activity when faced with the recall of personally threatening information (Lorig et al., 1994). In addition, sensitizers show stronger emotional reactions to potentially threatening ambiguous stimuli and better memory for such stimuli than repressors (Hock & Krohne, 2004). Furthermore, repressors avoid disturbing self-relevant information when possible, and when they are unable to do so, they rationalize and refute that information (Baumeister & Cairns, 1992).

Monitoring and Blunting

Congruent with the rise of social-cognitive approaches to personality during the 1980s, Miller (1987) used information-processing terms to describe coping strategies that resemble R–S and A–R. Monitoring and Blunting (M–B) refer to sets of strategies, hypothesized to be at least partially independent, for coping with the arousal or anxiety generated by threatening events (Miller, 1987). Miller developed a self-report measure called the Miller Behavioral Style Scale (MBSS) that includes four hypothetical and uncontrollable stressful scenes, followed by eight statements describing characteristically monitoring or blunting reactions. High monitors seek out and attend to information about their performance more than high blunters, whereas high blunters try to distract themselves from, deny, or reinterpret information about stressors. For example, when facing an unpleasant medical procedure, monitors were interested in more in-formation and felt less anxious after receiv-ing it (Miller & Managan, 1983).

As with the original measure of repression–sensitization, one critique of the MBSS is that it may confound nonanxious respon-dents with repressing or blunting respon-dents, and, indeed, the Blunting subscale of the MBSS typically has lower reliability and less predictive validity than the Monitor-ing subscale. The MBSS work has also been criticized for lack of predictive specificity in that some studies show that blunting re-lates to the outcomes measured, some stud-ies show that monitoring predicts outcomes, and some studies use the difference score from the two subscales to predict outcomes. Finally, because the MBSS presents only objectively uncontrollable situations, critics have argued that it may not adequately as-sess systematic variation in response to re-alistic situations in which control is possible (Krohne, 1996).

Which Measure?

Despite different theoretical origins, mea-sures of R–S and M–B both relate to de-fensive tendencies and to some similar out-comes. Each measure also has weaknesses, and there are questions about construct va-lidity, discriminant validity, and general util-ity. In response to some of these questions, Weinberger and Schwartz (1990) developed a measure of repression tendencies as part of the Weinberger Adjustment Inventory (WAI) that includes three factors measured by 10 subscales, two of which are designed to measure repressive tendencies: a Denial of Distress subscale that measures respondents' claims not to be experiencing negative affect and a Repressive Defensiveness subscale that measures suppression of self-serving behav-ior (Weinberger & Schwartz, 1990). These subscales show average correlations of be-tween .4 and .5.

In an analysis comparing several measures of repression-related constructs, including the WAI, the MMBS, the Byrne Repression–Sensitization scale, Weinberger's Repres-sive Coping Scale, Sackeim and Gur's Self-Deception Questionnaire (Sackeim & Gur, 1979), and Paulhus's Self-Deception Ques-tionnaire (Paulhus & Reid, 1991), all except

the MBSS Blunting scale loaded on a single factor, and all correlated significantly with measures of both anxiety and social desir-ability (Turvey & Salovey, 1993). Turvey and Salovey (1993) concluded that, based on psychometric characteristics (high internal consistency and normal distribution of re-sponses) and relative ease of administration (only 22 items), the WAI—Defensiveness scale was the most practically useful. As they noted, however, although their analysis supports the inference that these measures converge on one construct, it does not ad-dress the fundamental question of how this construct is best understood.

All self-report measures of individual differences in defensiveness, when used by themselves, leave open the question of whether systematic variations in response assess repression or denial of threatening negative content or the relative absence of that content. Interpretations of the defensive nature of self-reports rest on assumptions about human experience that are not shared by all theoretical perspectives and that may not apply equally to all individuals. Valid measure of defensive processes may require using two different methodologies (e.g., self-report and physiological measures or self-report and observer reports) because neither alone can demonstrate the specifi-cally defensive nature of processes that can appear identical to nondefensive processes when only one measure is used (Davidson & MacGregor, 1998).

Defensive Pessimism and Strategic Optimism

Research on the cognitive strategies of defen-sive pessimism and strategic optimism devel-oped in the context of the self-enhancement and self-protection research that informed Taylor and Brown's (1988) conclusion that self-enhancement was necessary for posi-tive adaptation and avoidance of depression. Along with other critiques of this conclusion (see Kwan, John, Denny, Bond, & Robins, 2004, for recent arguments), Norem and Cantor (1986a) argued that different indi-viduals will face similar situations with dif-ferent specific goals and that the importance of and approaches used for self-protection will vary across individuals (Norem & Cantor, 1986b). They describe those differences in terms of the strategies individuals use.

Strategies describe coherent patterns of emotions, thoughts, motivations, and behavior as they unfold during the process of pursuing goals (Cantor, Norem, Niedenthal, Langston, & Brower, 1987; Norem, 1989). Although the steps of a particular strategy can be described without reference to the goals or characteristics of the individual using that strategy, strategy coherence follows from an individual's understanding of what he or she is trying to do in a given context. That understanding, in turn, is influenced by prior experiences, self-knowledge, and other aspects of personality.

Defensive pessimism describes a strategy used by anxious individuals who face the challenge of managing their anxiety to prevent it from interfering with achieving success. Defensive pessimism involves expecting negative outcomes prior to a performance, task, or specific situation and reflecting—in concrete and vivid detail—on how those negative outcomes could happen. Expecting bad outcomes is hypothesized to protect one's self-concept if those outcomes occur (hence the pessimism is defensive); therefore, those using defensive pessimism would have little need to make self-serving attributions to protect themselves. Moreover, thinking about how negative outcomes might occur requires a focus away from anxious feelings and toward task-relevant thoughts, which facilitates planning of specific actions to avoid negative outcomes (Showers, 1988).

Most research on defensive pessimism has contrasted it with a strategic optimism. Those who use strategic optimism are typically not aware of being anxious prior to a performance or other self-relevant situation; they feel in control and are optimistic and confident of achieving good outcomes. They set high expectations and actively distract themselves from thinking about possible outcomes. When negative outcomes do occur, they protect their self-concepts by attributing those outcomes to bad luck or other external factors beyond their control. One of the first experimental studies of strategic optimism and defensive pessimism demonstrated that strategic optimists vary their attributions in self-protective or self-enhancing ways according to whether they received, respectively, failure or success feedback, whereas defensive pessimists' attributions did not vary as a function of performance feedback (Norem & Cantor, 1986a).

The initial Optimism–Pessimism Prescreening Questionnaire (OPPQ; Norem & Cantor, 1986a) was a nine-item face-valid self-report measure. This measure has since been revised to create the 17-item Defensive Pessimism Questionnaire (DPQ; Norem, 2001). Questions are worded to reflect the particular domain (e.g., academic, social, recreational) under study, and strategy use shows average cross-situational correlations between .30 and .50. The revised version of the scale correlates at $r = .65$ with the original OPPQ and has both higher reliability (average Cronbach's alpha = .78) and a cleaner factor structure. The DPQ has a 3-year test–retest reliability of $r = .55$ among college women and a 2-month test–retest reliability of $r = .68$ among male and female college students.

Questions on the DPQ load satisfactorily on one major unrotated factor. Oblique rotation produces two correlated factors labeled Reflectivity and Pessimism. Most research using the scales relies on a single score computed by summing the reflectivity and pessimism items (after reverse scoring). Those scoring in the upper third of the distribution are categorized as defensive pessimists, and those in the bottom third are categorized as strategic optimists in prescreening, although one can use continuous scores from the measure.

Research indicates that pessimistic expectations play a crucial role in the defensive pessimism strategy. For example, experimental manipulations that raise defensive pessimists' expectations lead to lower subsequent performance (Norem & Cantor, 1986b). Similarly, manipulations designed to get participants to feel that future successes were subjectively closer than future failures lead to poorer performance for defensive pessimists (Sanna, Chang, Carter, & Small, 2006). Martin and his colleagues, however, have data suggesting that pessimism and reflectivity play different roles over time with respect to other variables (Martin, Marsh, & Debus, 2001a, 2001b; Martin, Marsh, Williamson, & Debus, 2003). Examining how expectations and reflectivity work separately and together will be important in ongoing research.

The DPQ shows small to moderate negative correlations with Extraversion and small to moderate positive correlations with Neuroticism, small positive correlations with Conscientiousness, small negative correlations with Agreeableness, and no consistent correlation with Openness. It correlates negatively and moderately with dispositional optimism, as measured by the Revised Life Orientation Test (Scheier, Carver, & Bridges, 1994). Defensive pessimism does not bear much relationship to attributional or explanatory pessimism. The DPQ has a small positive correlation with the Internal subscale of the Attributional Style Questionnaire (ASQ) and no correlation with the Stable or Global ASQ subscales (Peterson, 1991). Correlations between the DPQ and R–S are typically positive and small to moderate; those between the DPQ and Monitoring are small and positive and those between the DPQ and Blunting are small and negative (Norem, 2001). The DPQ correlates moderately negatively with both the Self-Deception and Impression Management subscales of the Balanced Inventory of Desirable Responding (Paulhus & Reid, 1991).

Defensive Pessimism, Negative Thinking, and Negative Affect

People who use defensive pessimism reliably report higher trait anxiety and lower self-esteem, score higher in negative affect, have more negative expectations for their performances, report more goal conflict, and generate more negative potential outcomes and plans than those who use strategic optimism, despite comparable past performance (Cantor et al., 1987; Norem & Illingworth, 1993, 2004; Sanna, 1998).

There is also evidence that defensive pessimists are simultaneously motivated by the desire to avoid failure and the motivation to achieve success. They focus on specific performance-oriented goals that include both avoiding failure and doing well, and they have a higher ratio of negative to positive self-knowledge than strategic optimists (Elliot & Church, 2003; Yamawaki, Tschanz, & Feick, 2004). Perhaps as a result, they are likely to feel conflicted, particularly in situations in which they value the success that might be obtained.

Research supports the conclusion that defensive pessimists' preparatory negative thinking is importantly different from the negative rumination of depressives. Showers and her colleagues (Showers, 1992; Showers & Reuben, 1990) found that defensive pessimists did not use the avoidant coping methods found among those with depressive disorders and that defensive pessimists did not persist in feeling anxious or in ruminating after stressful events. The focus on the future rather than the past, along with the defensive pessimists' ability to think in concrete terms that readily suggest specific action, explains why defensive pessimists do not seem to be at risk for depression, even though their perspective can be quite negative (Hosogoshi & Kodama, 2006; Norem, 2006; Tomaya, 2005).

Understanding how and why defensive pessimists' negativity is helpful rather than debilitating requires understanding the potential problems created by anxiety. When we are anxious, the dominant response is avoidance of or flight from whatever makes us anxious. Yet often that which makes us anxious (e.g., an attractive potential romantic partner) is also something we are motivated to approach. Anxious individuals thus need a strategy to help them control their urge to flee and allow them instead to act effectively to achieve their goals. One strategy, of course, is to suppress anxiety. Especially in the short term, that can be an effective strategy, though certainly not one without costs and not one available to all individuals. In performance situations, even if the felt emotion of anxiety is repressed, the autonomic correlates of that anxiety may interfere with performance. Suppression requires effort, takes attentional capacity away from the task at hand, and may interfere with performance as a result of ironic processes (Wegner, 1989).

An alternative strategy is self-handicapping, by which individuals preemptively provide themselves with a less incriminating attribution for failure. For example, a socially anxious individual may down a few stiff drinks before approaching a romantic prospect (Jones & Berglas, 1999), thereby both dulling felt anxiety and providing a convenient explanation for rejection. This strategy involves considerable potential costs, however, because most people do not become more socially adept and attractive to others when they are intoxicated. Indeed, repeated reliance on the handicap is likely to lead to deteriorating outcomes over time: "Obnoxious drunk" is hardly a less incriminating social reputation than "socially awkward."

Defensive pessimism, in contrast to self-handicapping, helps anxious individuals focus on thoughts relevant to successful performance of the task at hand. An anxious student using defensive pessimism would think about the possibility of failure on an upcoming test by focusing on the process of preparing for and taking the test. She might first imagine reading the exam and not recognizing important terms or phrases and then rehearse with note cards twice a day for the week before the test. Defensive pessimism involves breaking down large goals into smaller pieces that resemble "implementation intentions," which, according to literature on goal pursuit, provide a clear guide for translating abstract motivations into action (Gollwitzer, 1999); this should ultimately reduce anxiety.

Research supports the hypothesis that defensive pessimism is a self-regulation strategy that helps manage anxiety (Norem, 2008). Defensive pessimists who were distracted prior to a performance task in a laboratory study scored lower on that task and felt less in control and more anxious than when they worked through possible outcomes before the task; anxiety mediated these results (Norem & Illingworth, 1993, Study 1). A conceptual replication of this study using experience-sampling methodology found that defensive pessimists who were prompted to think through what they were doing as they worked on "real life" goals over the course of several weeks reported more progress compared with defensive pessimists whose strategy was not reinforced (1993, Study 2). In both studies, strategic optimists showed the opposite pattern, and there were no main effects of strategy on performance outcomes. In other words, defensive pessimists who used their strategy performed significantly better than defensive pessimists who did not, and both defensive pessimists and strategic optimists performed best (and equivalently well) under conditions that matched their strategies and significantly worse in conditions that interfered with their strategies.

Trying to "think positively" or "just relax" (both frequent admonitions directed toward defensive pessimists) also interferes with performance for defensive pessimists. In an experiment designed to investigate the effect of visualization techniques on performance, defensive pessimists who listened to mastery or relaxation imagery recordings performed significantly more poorly than those who listened to guided imagery recordings of what might go wrong, whereas strategic optimists performed best in the relaxation imagery condition and significantly worse in the other two conditions (Spencer & Norem, 1996).

This pattern occurs across a variety of studies and samples. "Prefactual" and "counterfactual" thinking are mental simulations of possible events prior to their occurrence or after the fact and can involve either upward mental simulation (thinking of outcomes better than those expected or experienced) or downward mental simulation (thinking of outcomes worse than those imagined or experienced). Overall, defensive pessimists prefer to engage in prefactual thinking, whereas strategic optimists prefer to engage in downward counterfactual thinking when performance is disappointing (Sanna, 1996). Each group suffers performance decrements when using the other groups' preferred simulation.

"Cheering up" is ineffective in helping defensive pessimists to control anxiety. Even though defensive pessimists can be put into more positive moods, their performance suffers as a result (Norem & Illingworth, 2004; Sanna, 1998). Sanna (1998) showed that good moods interfere with prefactual mental simulation for defensive pessimists. He argues that they use negative affect as a cue to work harder, which typically leads to better performance. In contrast, strategic optimists rely on "mood repair" through downward counterfactuals (i.e., imagining that things had come out even worse than they did) when experiencing negative outcomes.

Defensive Pessimism and Adaptation

There are few differences in outcome between defensive pessimists and strategic optimists when each group is using its preferred strategy, and each group is vulnerable to performance disruption if prevented from using its strategy. If affect is considered an outcome, however, the balance shifts, because strategic optimists almost always report less negative affect than defensive pessimists. Sanna (1998) suggested, however, that reducing negative affect and increasing positive affect are more important goals for strategic optimists than for defensive pessimists. His data suggest that defensive pessimists are focused on the preparatory functions of their strategy as opposed to the affective functions of the strategic optimists' strategy.

Understanding the implications for adaptation of particular strategies requires paying attention to the ways in which strategies may provide "regulatory fit" between an individual's goals and particular contexts (Higgins, 2005; Norem & Chang, 2001). If we do not assume that minimizing negative affect is always the most important goal, the potential adaptive value of defensive pessimism is easier to see (Kelly et al., 1990; Norem, 2007). Indeed, there are times when being prepared to prevent negative outcomes might be one's primary goal, and the ability to tolerate negative affect might be integral to achieving that goal. For example, defensive pessimists worried more about severe acute respiratory syndrome (SARS) during an outbreak than strategic optimists did, but they also engaged in more recommended preventative efforts (Chang & Sivam, 2004). African American women using defensive pessimism actually performed better on a math test under stereotype threat, whereas African American women who did not use defensive pessimism, demonstrating the typical effects of stereotype threat, performed worse under threat conditions than under no-threat conditions (Perry, 2007).

A large-scale study of African American college retention rates showed that African American students at predominantly white institutions (PWIs) were significantly more likely to use defensive pessimism than those at historically black colleges and universities and that those students who used defensive pessimism had significantly higher retention rates (and rates comparable to those of white students at PWIs) than African American students who did not use defensive pessimism (Brower & Ketterhagen, 2004). Under conditions of perpetual stereotype threat at PWIs, African American students do not have the luxury of short-term failure or a focus on minimizing negative affect, and defensive pessimism may provide their best defensive option.

Chang (1996) has argued that the cultural sensibilities of East Asians and Asian Americans increase the social appropriateness of defensive pessimism, because the cultural context favors self-criticism and modesty over self-enhancement and self-promotion. He has found that pessimism is associated with effective problem solving among Asian Americans.

The potential adaptive benefits of defensive pessimism are also clear when one contrasts it with self-handicapping. Both strategies can be seen as self-protective (Martin, Marsh, & Debus, 2001b), and those using the strategies share anxiety and fear of failure. Yet defensive pessimists are more engaged in self-improvement, work toward more positive goals, and typically perform significantly better than self-handicappers (Eronen, Nurmi, & Salmela Aro, 1998). Among seventh-graders, defensive pessimists were higher than both self-handicappers and control-group students (who were not anxious) in "volitional self-control," and they were better able to manage distractions and competing demands. Defensive pessimist students more strongly endorsed the "good student" self than self-handicappers, indicated that being a good student in the future (as well as avoiding becoming a bad student) was more important to them, and felt more efficacious with respect to those goals than self-handicappers did (Garcia, 1995).

Further research supports the conclusion that anxious individuals who use defensive pessimism do better than other anxious individuals. Socially anxious defensive pessimists are less likely to avoid social interactions and are thus more likely to develop their social skills than are other socially anxious individuals (Schoneman, 2002). Growth-curve analyses of changes in self-esteem during college show that defensive pessimists increased their self-esteem over time, whereas equivalently anxious individuals who did not use defensive pessimism showed decreases in self-esteem (Norem & Andreas Burdzovic, 2007).

Unanswered Questions

Defensive pessimists are often encouraged to be more optimistic by those who view their anxiety as a consequence of their strategy rather than the problem addressed by that strategy. The research reviewed here, in contrast, supports the interpretation that defensive pessimism can be an adaptive coping strategy for managing anxiety. That does not mean, however, that there are no costs to using defensive pessimism, and other people's reactions to the negativity of the strategy may be one of the biggest potential costs. In contrast, strategic optimists, who are typically in better moods and express more self-confidence, may be more immediately likeable and more motivating to be around than defensive pessimists (with the proviso that reactions from others are influenced by cultural and other aspects of contexts). To the extent that their self-confidence is unwarranted, that it prevents attention to relevant feedback, or that it is based on self-aggrandizement at the expense of others, however, strategic optimists may wear out their social welcome over time. Research exploring strategy effectiveness across more situations and longer periods of time, and within different interpersonal relationships and groups, is needed to understand the boundaries of effectiveness for each strategy.

Both defensive pessimists and strategic optimists appear to be vulnerable in situations that do not fit their strategies, and strategy effectiveness may be strongly influenced by flexibility of strategy use (Norem, 1989). At this point, there is little evidence about how flexibly people are able to deploy their strategies. We also know very little about the origins of these strategies or about how difficult it is for people to change strategies. In theory, strategies should be more malleable than many aspects of personality. Yet because defensive pessimism and strategic optimism are both relatively effective, they may tend to be self-perpetuating, particularly given that defensive pessimists tend not to look back and that strategic optimists tend to reframe negative outcomes in positive terms (Norem, 2006). Given the relative effectiveness of defensive pessimism for those who experience manifest anxiety, one of the most intriguing questions is whether anxious people who do not use it can be taught to use it and, if so, whether they experience better outcomes as a result.

Conclusion

The number and variety of results across the augmenting–reducing, repression–sensitization, monitoring–blunting, and defensive pessimism literatures testifies to enduring interest in individual differences in how people experience and react to potentially threatening stimuli and feedback. Two broad observations emerge from examination of these literatures. One is that there are commonalities among the phenomena being studied. Those commonalities center on the phenomenology of anxiety when people are threatened by the prospect of physical or psychological pain, on how intensely and consciously that threat is experienced, and on how individuals direct their attention during that experience. Investigators starting from very different theoretical orientations—ranging from behaviorism to psychodynamic theories through contemporary social-cognitive perspectives—have each developed constructs (and corresponding operationalizations) that capture systematic variance in this experience and predict important aspects of adaptation.

The second observation is that there is little integration across these literatures. This is perhaps not surprising given the different goals and theoretical orientations of the researchers involved. Nevertheless, it seems crucial at this junction to begin systematically to consider ways in which the critiques, limitations, and unanswered questions that arise within each literature might be addressed by empirical work that extends across literatures. The anxiety-management effects of defensive pessimism, for example, would be more fully explained if we knew more about the physiological correlates of the strategy—something better explored in the A–R and R–S literatures—and more about the extent to which those correlates are similar or different across constructs.

The self-concept—its structure, specific content, stability, and associated motivations—is crucial to understanding these constructs, but currently we know relatively little about differential influences of the self across different constructs. We also need more systematic research on the contributions of conscious and nonconscious processing to the development and operation of these individual differences.

The research necessary to pursue integration across constructs will be challenging, because we will need to measure several constructs and to use different kinds of operationalizations within the same study (e.g., physiological and self-report methods, self- and observer reports, independent assessments of adaptation) if we are to make real progress. Nevertheless, we need not be defensive about how far we have come, nor anxious about prospects for future research. The appropriate methods are available, and there is a deep, broad, and fascinating foundation on which to build.

References

Baumeister, R. F., & Cairns, K. B. (1992). Repression and self-presentation: When audiences interfere with self-deceptive strategies. *Journal of Personality and Social Psychology, 62,* 851–862.

Baumeister, R. F., Dale, K., & Sommer, K. L. (1998). Freudian defense mechanisms and empirical findings in modern social psychology: Reaction formation, projection, displacement, undoing, isolation, sublimation, and denial. *Journal of Personality, 66,* 1081–1124.

Bonanno, G. A., Davis, P. J., & Singer, J. L. (1991). The repressor personality and avoidant information processing: A dichotic listening study. *Journal of Research in Personality, 25*(4), 386–401.

Bonanno, G. A., & Singer, J. L. (1995). Repressive personality style: theoretical and methodological implications for health and pathology. In J. L. Singer (Ed.), *Repression and dissociation: Implications for personality theory, psychopathology, and health* (pp. 435–470). Chicago: University of Chicago Press.

Brower, A. M., & Ketterhagen, A. (2004). Is there an inherent mismatch between how black and white students expect to succeed in college and what their college expects from them? *Journal of Social Issues, 60*(1), 95–116.

Bruneau, N., Roux, S., Perse, J., & Lelord, G. (1984). Frontal evoked responses, stimulus intensity control, and the extraversion dimension. *Annals of the New York Academy of Sciences, 425,* 546–550.

Bruner, J. S., & Postman, L. (1947). Emotional selectivity in perception and reaction. *Journal of Personality, 16,* 69–77.

Buck, R. (1976). *Human motivation and emotion.* New York: Wiley.

Byrne, D. (1961). The Repression–Sensitization Scale:
Rationale, reliability, and validity. *Journal of Personality, 29,* 334–349.

Cantor, N., Norem, J. K., Niedenthal, P. M., Langston, C. A., & Brower, A. (1987). Life tasks, self-concept ideals, and cognitive strategies in a life transition. *Journal of Personality and Social Psychology, 53*(6), 1178–1191.

Chang, E. C. (1996). Cultural differences in optimism, pessimism, and coping: Predictors of subsequent adjustment in Asian American and Caucasian American college students. *Journal of Counseling Psychology, 43*(1), 113–123.

Chang, W. C., & Sivam, R.-W. (2004). Constant vigilance: Heritage values and defensive pessimism in coping with severe acute respiratory syndrome in Singapore. *Asian Journal of Social Psychology, 7,* 35–53.

Cramer, P. (1995). Identity, narcissism, and defense mechanisms in late adolescence. *Journal of Research in Personality, 29*(3), 341–361.

Crowne, D. P., & Marlowe, D. (1960). A new scale of social desirability independent of psychopathology. *Journal of Consulting Psychology, 66,* 547–555.

Davidson, K., & MacGregor, M. W. (1998). A critical appraisal of self-report defensive mechanism measures. *Journal of Personality, 66,* 965–992.

Davis, P. J., & Schwartz, G. E. (1987). Repression and the inaccessibility of affective memories. *Journal of Personality and Social Psychology, 52,* 155–162.

Elliot, A. J., & Church, M. A. (2003). A motivational analysis of defensive pessimism and self-handicapping. *Journal of Personality and Social Psychology, 71*(3), 369–396.

Eriksen, C. W. (1966). Defense against ego-threat in memory and perception. *Journal of Abnormal and Social Psychology, 47,* 230–235.

Eronen, S., Nurmi, J. E., & Salmela Aro, K. (1998). Optimistic, defensive–pessimistic, impulsive and self-handicapping strategies in university environments. *Learning and Instruction, 8*(2), 159–177.

Eysenck, H. J. (1967). *The biological basis of personality.* Springfield, IL: Thomas.

Eysenck, H. J. (1973). *On extraversion.* New York: Wiley.

Freud, A. (1946). *The ego and mechanisms of defence.* Oxford, UK: International Universities Press.

Freud, S. (1914). *Psychopathology of everyday life* (A. A. Brill, Trans.). Oxford, UK: Macmillan.

Garcia, T. (1995). The role of motivational strategies in self-regulated learning. In P. R. Pintrich (Ed.), *New directions for teaching and learning* (Vol. 63, pp. 29–42). San Francisco: Jossey-Bass.

Gollwitzer, P. M. (1999). Implementation intentions: Strong effects of simple plans. *American Psychologist, 54,* 493–503.

Gray, J. A. (1972). The psychophysiological nature of introversion–extraversion: A modification of Eysenck's theory. In V. D. Nebylitsyn & J. A. Gray (Eds.), *Biological basis of individual behavior* (pp. 372–399). London: Academic Press.

Hansen, C. H., & Hansen, R. D. (1988). Repression of emotional tagged memories: The architecture of less complex emotions. *Journal of Personality and Social Psychology, 88,* 811–818.

Herzog, T. R., Williams, D. M., & Weintraub, D. J. (1985). Meanwhile, back at personality ranch: The augmenters and reducers ride again. *Journal of Personality and Social Psychology, 48*(5), 1342–1352.

Higgins, E. T. (2005). Value from regulatory fit. *Current Directions in Psychological Science, 14*, 209–213.

Hock, M., & Krohne, H. W. (2004). Coping with threat and memory for ambiguous information: Testing the repressive discontinuity hypothesis. *Emotion, 4*, 65–86.

Hosogoshi, H., & Kodama, M. (2006). Examination of psychological well-being and subjective well-being in defensive pessimists. *Japanese Journal of Psychology, 77*(2), 141–148.

Hull, C. L. (1950). Simple qualitative discrimination learning. *Psychological Review, 57*, 303–313.

Jones, E. F., & Berglas, S. (1999). Control of the attributions about the self through self-handicapping strategies: The appeal of alcohol and the role of underachievement. In R. F. Baumeister (Ed.), *The self in social psychology* (pp. 430–435). Philadelphia: Psychology Press/Taylor & Francis.

Kelly, J. A., St. Lawrence, J. S., Brasfield, T. L., Lemke, A., Amidei, T., Roffman, R. E., et al. (1990). Psychological factors that predict AIDS high-risk versus AIDS precautionary behavior. *Journal of Consulting and Clinical Psychology, 58*(1), 117–120.

Krohne, J. W. (1996). Individual differences in coping. In M. Zeidner & N. S. Endler (Eds.), *Handbook of coping: Theory, research, applications* (pp. 381–409). Oxford, UK: Wiley.

Kwan, V. S. Y., John, O. P., Denny, D. A., Bond, M. H., & Robins, R. W. (2004). Reconceptualizing individual differences in self-enhancement bias: An interpersonal approach. *Psychological Review, 111*(1), 94–110.

Lorig, T. S., Singer, J. L., Bonanno, G. A., & Davis, P. (1994). Repressor personality styles and EEG patterns associated with affective memory and thought suppression. *Cognition and Personality, 14*(3), 203–210.

Martin, A. J., Marsh, H. W., & Debus, R. L. (2001a). A quadripolar need for achievement representation of self-handicapping and defensive pessimism. *American Educational Research Journal, 38*, 583–610.

Martin, A. J., Marsh, H. W., & Debus, R. L. (2001b). Self-handicapping and defensive pessimism: Exploring a model of predictors and outcomes from a self-protection perspective. *Journal of Educational Psychology, 93*(1), 87–102.

Martin, A. J., Marsh, H. W., Williamson, A., & Debus, R. L. (2003). Self-handicapping, defensive pessimism, and goal orientation: A qualitative study of university students. *Journal of Educational Psychology, 95*(3), 617–628.

Mendolia, M., Moore, J., & Tesser, A. (1996). Dispositional and situational determinants of repression. *Journal of Personality and Social Psychology, 70*, 856–867.

Miller, S. M. (1987). Monitoring and blunting: Validation of a questionnaire to assess styles of information seeking under threat. *Journal of Personality and Social Psychology, 52*(2), 345–353.

Miller, S. M., & Managan, C. E. (1983). The interacting effects of information and coping style in adapting to gynecologic stress: Should the doctor tell all? *Journal of Personality and Social Psychology, 45*, 223–236.

Mitchell, D. C. (1998). Repression and relief: Mood and cardiovascular changes following threat, thinking about threat, and threat removal for repressors and nonrepressors. *Dissertation Abstracts International, 58*(9-B), 5180. (University Microfilms No. 1998-95006-081)

Morgan, A. H., Lezard, F., Prytulak, S., & Hilgard, E. R. (1970). Augmenters, reducers, and their reaction to cold pressor pain in waking and suggested hypnotic analgesia. *Journal of Personality and Social Psychology, 16*(1), 5–11.

Norem, J. K. (1989). Cognitive strategies as personality: Effectiveness, specificity, flexibility and change. In D. M. Buss & N. Cantor (Eds.), *Personality psychology: Recent trends and emerging directions* (pp. 45–60). New York: Springer-Verlag.

Norem, J. K. (2001). Defensive pessimism, optimism, and pessimism. In E. C. Chang (Ed.), *Optimism and pessimism: Implications for theory, research and practice* (pp. 77–100). Washington, DC: American Psychological Association.

Norem, J. K. (2006). Defensive pessimism: Positive past, anxious present, and pessimistic future. In L. Sanna & E. C. Chang (Eds.), *Judgments over time: The interplay of thoughts, feelings, and behaviors* (pp. 34–46). Oxford, UK: Oxford University Press.

Norem, J. K. (2007). Defensive pessimism as a positive self-critical tool. In E. C. Chang (Ed.), *Self-criticism and self-enhancement: Theory, research, and clinical implications* (pp. 89–104). Washington, DC: American Psychological Association Press.

Norem, J. K. (2008). Defensive pessimism, anxiety and the complexity of self-regulation. *Social and Personality Compass, 2*, 121–134.

Norem, J. K., & Andreas Burdzovic, J. A. (2007). Understanding journeys: Individual growth analysis as a tool for studying individual differences in change over time. In A. D. Ong & M. v. Dulmen (Eds.), *Handbook of methods in positive psychology* (pp. 477–486). London: Oxford University Press.

Norem, J. K., & Cantor, N. (1986a). Anticipatory and post hoc cushioning strategies: Optimism and defensive pessimism in "risky" situations. *Cognitive Therapy and Research, 10*(3), 347–362.

Norem, J. K., & Cantor, N. (1986b). Defensive pessimism: Harnessing anxiety as motivation. *Journal of Personality and Social Psychology, 51*, 1208–1217.

Norem, J. K., & Chang, E. C. (2001). A very full glass: Adding complexity to our thinking about the implications and applications of optimism and pessimism research. In E. C. Chang (Ed.), *Optimism and pessimism: Implications for theory, research and practice* (pp. 347–367). Washington, DC: American Psychological Association.

Norem, J. K., & Illingworth, K. S. S. (1993). Strategy-dependent effects of reflecting on self and tasks: Some implications of optimism and defensive pessimism. *Journal of Personality and Social Psychology, 65*(4), 822–835.

Norem, J. K., & Illingworth, K. S. S. (2004). Mood and performance among defensive pessimists and strategic optimists. *Journal of Research in Personality, 38*, 351–366.

Paulhus, D. L., & John, O. P. (1998). Egoistic and moralistic biases in self-perception: The interplay of self-deceptive styles with basic traits and motives. *Journal of Personality, 66*(6), 1025–1060.

Paulhus, D. L., & Reid, D. B. (1991). Enhancement and denial in socially desirable responding. *Journal of Personality and Social Psychology, 60,* 307–317.

Pavlov, I. P. (1927). *Conditioned reflexes.* London: Oxford University Press.

Pennebaker, J. W., & Chew, C. H. (1985). Deception, EDA and inhibition of behavior. *Journal of Personality and Social Psychology, 49,* 1427–1433.

Perry, S. (2007, January). *Making lemonade? Defensive coping style moderates the effect of stereotype threat on women's math test performance.* Paper presented at the annual meeting of the Society for Social and Personality Psychology, Memphis, TN.

Peterson, C. (1991). The meaning and measurement of explanatory style. *Psychological Inquiry, 2*(1), 1–10.

Petrie, A. (1967). *Individuality in pain and suffering.* Oxford, UK: University of Chicago Press.

Petrie, K. J., Booth, R. J., & Pennebaker, J. W. (1998). The immunological effects of thought suppression. *Journal of Personality and Social Psychology, 75*(5), 1264–1272.

Rohrmann, S., Netter, P., Hennig, J., & Hodapp, V. (2003). Repression–sensitization, gender, and discrepancies in psychobiological reactions to examination stress. *Anxiety, Stress and Coping: An International Journal, 16*(3), 321–329.

Sackeim, H. A., & Gur, R. C. (1979). Self-deception, other-deception, and self-reported psychopathology. *Journal of Consulting and Clinical Psychology, 47*(1), 213–215.

Sales, S. M. (1971). Need for stimulation as a factor in social behavior. *Journal of Personality and Social Psychology, 19*(1), 124–134.

Sanna, L. J. (1996). Defensive pessimism, optimism, and simulating alternatives: Some ups and downs of prefactual and counterfactual thinking. *Journal of Personality and Social Psychology, 71*(5), 1020–1036.

Sanna, L. J. (1998). Defensive pessimism and optimism: The bitter-sweet influence of mood on performance and prefactual and counterfactual thinking. *Cognition and Emotion, 12*(5), 635–665.

Sanna, L. J., Chang, E. C., Carter, S. E., & Small, E. M. (2006). The future is now: Prospective temporal self-appraisals among defensive pessimists and optimists. *Personality and Social Psychology Bulletin, 32*(6), 727–739.

Scheier, M. F., Carver, C. S., & Bridges, M. W. (1994). Distinguishing optimism from neuroticism (and trait anxiety, self-mastery, and self-esteem): A reevaluation of the Life Orientation Test. *Journal of Personality and Social Psychology, 67*(6), 1063–1078.

Schoneman, S. W. (2002). The role of the cognitive coping strategy of defensive pessimism within the social-evaluative continuum. *Dissertation Abstracts International, 63,* 3024. (University Microfilms No. 2002-95024-319)

Schwerdtfeger, A. (2003). Using affective pictures instead of white noise: Still different response patterns for Petrie-style augmenters and reducers. *Personality and Individual Differences, 34*(2), 253–262.

Schwerdtfeger, A., & Baltissen, R. (2002). Augmenting–reducing paradox lost?: A test of Davis et al.'s (1983) hypothesis. *Personality and Individual Differences, 32,* 257–271.

Showers, C. J. (1988). The effects of how and why thinking on perceptions of future negative events. *Cognitive Therapy and Research, 12,* 225–240.

Showers, C. J. (1992). The motivational and emotional consequences of considering positive or negative possibilities for an upcoming event. *Journal of Personality and Social Psychology, 63*(3), 474–484.

Showers, C. J., & Reuben, C. (1990). Distinguishing defensive pessimism from depression: Negative expectations and positive coping mechanisms. *Cognitive Therapy and Research, 14*(4), 385–399.

Spence, K. W. (1936). The nature of discrimination learning in animals. *Psychological Review, 43,* 427–449.

Spencer, S. M., & Norem, J. K. (1996). Reflection and distraction: Defensive pessimism, strategic optimism, and performance. *Personality and Social Psychology Bulletin, 22*(4), 354–365.

Taylor, J. A. (1953). A personality scale of manifest anxiety. *Journal of Abnormal and Social Psychology, 48,* 285–290.

Taylor, S. E., & Brown, J. D. (1988). Illusion and well-being: A social psychological perspective on mental health. *Psychological Bulletin, 103*(2), 193–210.

Tomaya, M. (2005). Influence of cognitive strategies on test coping strategies and academic achievement: Defensive pessimism and strategic optimism. *Japanese Journal of Educational Psychology, 53*(2), 220–229.

Traue, H. C., & Pennebaker, J. W. (1993). Inhibition and arousal. In H. C. Traue & J. W. Pennebaker (Eds.), *Emotion inhibition and health* (pp. 10–31). Seattle, WA: Hogrefe & Huber.

Turvey, C., & Salovey, P. (1993). Measures of repression: Converging on the same construct? *Imagination, Cognition and Personality, 13*(4), 279–289.

Wegner, D. M. (1989). *White bears and other unwanted thoughts: Suppression, obsession, and the psychology of mental control.* New York: Penguin Books.

Weinberger, D. A., & Schwartz, G. E. (1990). Distress and restraint as superordinate dimensions of self-reported adjustment: A typological perspective. *Journal of Personality, 58,* 381–417.

Weinberger, D. A., Schwartz, G. E., & Davidson, R. J. (1979). Low-anxious, high-anxious, and repressive coping styles: Psychometric patterns and behavioral and physiological responses to stress. *Journal of Abnormal Psychology, 88,* 369–380.

Weinstein, J., Averill, J. R., Opton, E. M. J., & Lazarus, R. S. (1968). Defensive style and discrepancy between self-report and physiological indexes of stress. *Journal of Personality and Social Psychology, 10*(4), 406–413.

Yamawaki, N., Tschanz, B. T., & Feick, D. L. (2004). Defensive pessimism, self-esteem instability, and goal striving. *Cognition and Emotion, 18*(2), 233–249.

PART VI

■ ● ▲ ◆

SELF-RELATED DISPOSITIONS

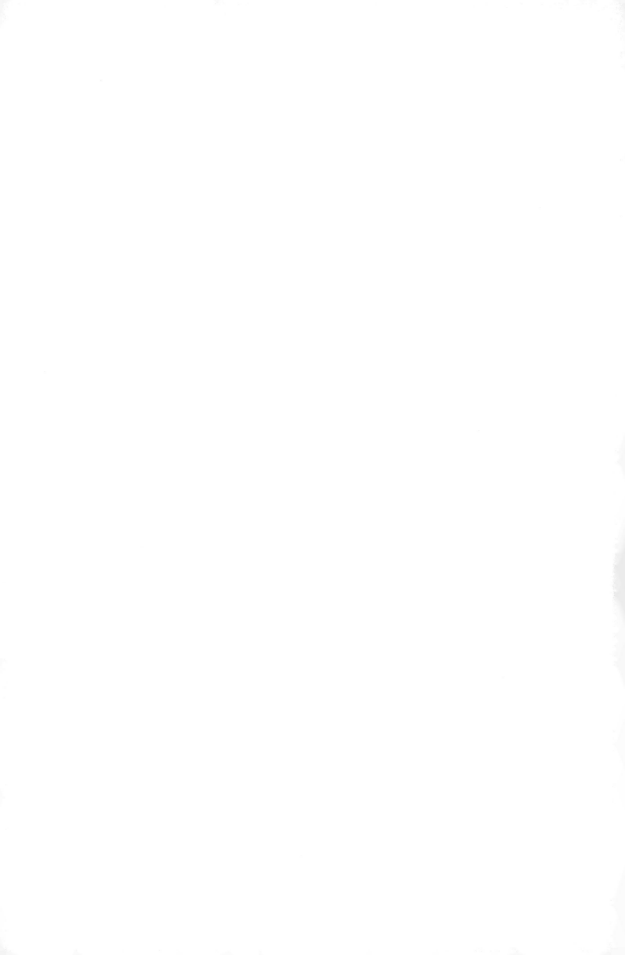

CHAPTER 34

■ ◦ ▲ ◆ ■ ◦ ▲ ◆

Private and Public Self-Consciousness

ALLAN FENIGSTEIN

S elf-consciousness refers to a relatively stable individual difference in the tendency to direct attention and thought toward oneself. As developed by Fenigstein, Scheier, and Buss (1975), the notion of self-focused attention as a personality variable was originally conceived as an extension of Duval and Wicklund's (1972) theory of self-awareness. Self-awareness theory, to a large extent, derived from the recognition of a fundamental distinction between attention directed inward, or back toward the self, versus attention directed outward, away from the self and toward the external environment. Although the self may be regarded as an object of attention, much like any other perceivable object, the theory speculated that the self was, in fact, a unique and significant psychological entity—a speculation borne out by subsequent research showing that the self is an especially elaborate, well-organized, and accessible knowledge structure (e.g., Kihlstrom et al., 1988; Klein & Loftus, 1988; Markus, 1977; Rogers, Kuiper, & Kirker, 1977) that offers an influential interpretive framework for perceiving and making judgments about the world (e.g., Fenigstein & Abrams, 1993; Greenwald, 1980). Self-awareness theory was based on the assumption that attention directed toward the self would also have unique psychological consequences as compared with attention toward anything else.

Self-Consciousness as a Personality Characteristic

The initial research on self-awareness (Duval & Wicklund, 1972) regarded direction of attention, either toward or away from the self, as a variable that is determined by situational stimulus conditions. Specifically, distracting events or engaging activities that require conscious effort were assumed to draw attention toward those occurrences and away from the person. By contrast, stimuli that suggested or reflected an aspect of the person, such as mirrors, the sound of one's own voice, or the presence of an observing audience, were presumed to direct attention back toward the person.

However, researchers soon began to suspect that self-focused attention, in addition to being influenced by transient experimental or situational manipulations, might also be affected by stable dispositional tendencies that differed among individuals. Fenigstein and colleagues (1975) speculated that "some persons constantly think about themselves, scrutinize their behavior or appearance, and mull over their thoughts—to the point of obsessiveness" (p. 22), whereas for others, the "absence of self-consciousness is so complete that they have no understanding of either their own motives or of how they appear to others" (p. 22). These personality differences were identified as a trait variable called *self-consciousness*. *Self-awareness*, in contrast, refers to the psychological *state* of being attentive to the self, whether as a result of transient situational variables, chronic dispositions, or both.

After determining that no psychometric instrument existed to assess individual differences in self-consciousness, Fenigstein and colleagues (1975) constructed the Self-Consciousness Scale (SCS). In designing the scale, several content areas were first identified as relevant to the concept of self-consciousness, and items were then generated, largely on the basis of their face validity, to sample these domains: preoccupation with one's own past, present, or future behavior; awareness of one's own attributes, both positive and negative; sensitivity to inner feelings; introspective behavior; a tendency to visualize oneself; awareness of one's own appearance and style of presentation; and concern over the appraisal of others. Starting with a large pool of questionnaire items, numerous psychometric refinements resulted in a final 23-item scale that has since served as the primary operationalization of self-consciousness.

Private and Public Self-Consciousness

Fenigstein and colleagues' (1975) initial conception of self-consciousness was of a unitary disposition to be more or less attentive to a generalized, homogeneous self. However, repeated factor analyses with different samples consistently demonstrated that there was no such unitary factor. Rather, self-consciousness was composed of two distinct components, one private and one public. The *private self-consciousness* factor identified a tendency to be aware of and attentive to the covert, internal aspects of oneself, such as one's thoughts and feelings. Sample items from this 10-item subscale include "I'm always trying to figure myself out" and "I reflect about myself a lot." *Public self-consciousness* (measured by 7 items) involved an awareness of and interest in the external manifestations of the person, such as appearance, social behavior, and the impression made on others. Sample items include "I'm concerned about the way I present myself to others" and "I'm self-conscious about the way I look." (A third factor in the

SCS, *social anxiety*, may best be regarded as a by-product of public self-consciousness [e.g., Buss, 1980; Leary, 1983], and is addressed later in the chapter.)

The human predilection toward pretense and impression management (e.g., Goffman, 1959; Leary, 1995) suggests that people recognize and understand the difference between the *private*, seemingly more genuine, personal characteristics and intentions that only they are aware of and the *public* aspects of themselves that are seen by, and sometimes disingenuously "presented" to, others (cf. Schlenker, 1980). This distinction between the private and public aspects of the person has been regarded as important in psychology from the earliest days of the discipline (e.g., James, 1890; Jung, 1957). Baumeister (1986) has argued that the need for and realization of a distinction between an "authentic" private and a "presented" public self emerged only within the past few centuries. However, evolutionary theorists, who have emphasized the central role of deceit and its detection in the emergence of the human mind (e.g., Tooby & Cosmides, 1990), would argue that the existence of and ability to recognize differences between private, genuine motives and public, socially presented motives has long been a part of human evolutionary dynamics.

In effect, Fenigstein and colleagues (1975) suggested that the distinction between the private and public aspects of humans may also serve as the basis for two relatively separate individual-difference dimensions: Some persons, when directing attention toward themselves, may be more prone to focus on and think about the private aspects of themselves, such as personal feelings of self-worth, their cognitive faculties, bodily and emotional states, a sense of their inner being, and their future hopes and desires. For others, the public aspects of themselves, such as appearance, dress, and behavioral style, along with thoughts and feelings concerning the recognition or regard received from others, are more salient and of greater interest and thus more likely to draw the individual's self-directed attention.

One may question whether self-consciousness (either private or public) is really a personality variable—that is, a dispositional trait that reflects a relatively chronic state of self-awareness that is independent of external conditions—or whether it is the result of a low threshold for external stimuli that draw attention to the self. The most relevant empirical evidence on this question is research examining the interaction between self-consciousness measures and experimental manipulations of self-awareness; the results, however, are mixed. Consistent with the former possibility, some research has found a *ceiling effect*: Self-awareness manipulations have a stronger effect on persons low in self-consciousness than on those who are already at a high level of self-consciousness (e.g., Carver & Scheier, 1978). However, other research has found that self-awareness manipulations have the greatest impact on persons high, rather than low, in self-consciousness, consistent with the idea that people who are high in self-consciousness are especially sensitive to self-attention-inducing stimuli (e.g., Brockner, 1979). Still other research has found that the combined effects of self-consciousness and self-awareness are additive, suggesting that the disposition and the manipulation are essentially two independent ways of varying the same psychological state (e.g., Scheier, 1976). In sum, the issue of whether self-consciousness is being "pushed" from within the person or being "pulled" from the outside has not yet been resolved.

Relation of Self-Consciousness Factors to Other Personality Variables

Research has suggested that the private and public self-consciousness factors are relatively reliable dimensions (e.g., Fenigstein et al., 1975) that are largely independent of each other. Most studies have found a weak to moderate correlation between them, usually below .30 (see Buss, 1980, and Carver & Scheier, 1981, for reviews; however, see Wicklund & Gollwitzer, 1987, for an alternative view).

Evidence of convergent validity has been found for both factors. Private self-consciousness is correlated with a number of psychological measures to which it is theoretically related, such as Openness to Experience (a Big Five factor), thoughtfulness, reflectiveness, and the use of visual imagery (e.g., Trapnell & Campbell, 1999; Turner, Scheier, Carver, & Ickes, 1978).

Public self-consciousness has been found to relate to variables that suggest an awareness of oneself as an object of attention from others, such as social anxiety (Fenigstein, et al., 1975; Leary, 1983), shyness (Schlenker & Weigold, 1990), sociability (Turner et al., 1978), and self-monitoring, a tendency toward managing one's public impressions (e.g., Briggs, Cheek, & Buss, 1980; Fenigstein, 1979; Turner et al., 1978). That private and public self-consciousness relate to separate sets of variables—one concerned with inner thought and the other dealing with social issues—offers further evidence that they are largely orthogonal dimensions; the presence of one neither precludes nor necessitates the other. Some studies, however, have questioned that independence and suggested a conceptual overlap between the factors. For example, Trapnell and Campbell (1999) found that the dimensions of private and public self-consciousness were both related to the Big Five factor of neuroticism (see later in the chapter for a fuller discussion of the implications of self-consciousness for various forms of psychopathology). It is important to consider, however, that these relationships may be mediated by fundamentally different pathways to disordered behavior, in which case it would still be appropriate to regard the two self-consciousness factors as relatively independent.

Carver and Glass (1976) provided evidence of discriminant validity for the self-consciousness factors. As expected, neither private nor public self-consciousness related to measures of intelligence, need for achievement, test anxiety, or impulsivity. Other studies have shown little relation between self-consciousness and measures of self-esteem (e.g., Brockner et al., 1983) or social desirability (Turner et al., 1978). These findings are consistent with the idea that self-consciousness is a relatively pure attentional tendency; thought or attention may be directed toward aspects of the self that are either positive, neutral, or negative, but by itself, neither public nor private self-consciousness has a reliable relationship with any specific value-laden, self-relevant content.

Since its development, the SCS has become the primary means by which self-consciousness, private or public, is measured. So far, there have been published translations of the SCS into at least 16 other languages

(Arabic, Chinese, Dutch, Estonian, French, German, Greek, Hebrew, Italian, Japanese, Persian, Polish, Portuguese, Spanish, Swedish, and Turkish). The scale has also shown significant heuristic value, having appeared in more than 1,300 published studies and countless dissertations, but it should be said that although SCS-related research is continuing presently, it has slowed down a great deal since the 1980s.

The Self-Attentional Properties of Private and Public Self-Consciousness

A question of fundamental importance to the construct validity of the SCS is whether the two types of self-consciousness both involve self-focused attention. Although the questionnaire items for both subscales sought to identify tendencies or characteristics that were explicitly associated with attention to either private or public aspects of the self, a more definitive response needs to go beyond face validity to independent sources of evidence. Construct validity research concerning the self-attentional properties of private self-consciousness has been clear and consistent. Carver and Scheier (1978) showed that private self-consciousness was associated with self-focused responses on a sentence-completion task. Other studies have demonstrated that private self-consciousness is related to easier access to information about the private self (e.g., Hull & Levy, 1979; Nasby, 1985; Turner, 1980). Finally, many of the findings associated with private self-consciousness effectively parallel those associated with self-attention-inducing stimuli such as mirrors (e.g., Froming, Walker, & Lopyan, 1982; Scheier & Carver, 1977), strongly suggesting that both the experimental and the dispositional findings could be explained most parsimoniously in terms of self-attention. Thus the idea that private self-consciousness measures attention to the self has been generally accepted, even by skeptics of the dispositional approach (e.g., Gibbons, 1990; Wicklund & Gollwitzer, 1987).

Serious questions, however, have been raised regarding the self-attentional properties of public self-consciousness. Gibbons (1990), for example, has argued that directing attention toward the self as a social object involves an *external* rather than a self-orientation in which the person's main focus is on what *others* think of him- or herself. As Fenigstein (1987) pointed out, however, this argument fails to recognize that for a number of influential "self" theorists (e.g., Argyle, 1969; Mead, 1934), attention to or awareness of what others think of the person, rather than detracting or distracting from self-awareness, actually plays a critical role in influencing how one views oneself. In fact, Duval and Wicklund (1972), in their original formulation of self-awareness theory, explicitly defined self-attention in terms of an external perspective, likening it to a process of figuratively coming outside oneself to look back on oneself. In other words, if public self-consciousness involves an "external" perspective on the self, using either the mind's eye to view oneself from the "outside" (cf., Hass, 1984) or taking the presumed viewpoint of another (e.g., Cooley, 1902), that perspective in no way compromises the idea that attention is being directed toward oneself, even if that attention is specifically focused on those aspects of the person that render him or her an object of presumed interest to others.

A number of studies provide direct evidence for the idea that public self-consciousness involves attention toward the self. For example, Franzoi and Brewer (1984), in a naturalistic study of ongoing thought, found that publicly self-conscious persons were especially likely to think about themselves as social objects who were being observed by others. In addition, the trait of public self-consciousness has been associated with either better memory for or memory biased in favor of information specific to the socially observable aspects of the person (e.g., Nasby, 1989a; Turner, Gilliland, & Klein, 1981). Finally, several studies have shown that public self-consciousness is associated with outcomes very similar to those induced by stimuli that heighten attention to the outwardly visible aspects of self, such as an observing audience or a videotape camera (e.g., Fenigstein, 1979, 1984; Froming & Carver, 1981; Hass, 1984). Thus, both theoretically and empirically, strong and consistent evidence supports the self-attentional nature of public self-consciousness.

The Unidimensionality of Private and Public Self-Consciousness

The private and public facets of self-consciousness were originally identified as internally consistent, homogeneous dimensions (Fenigstein et al., 1975). Although a full review of the confirmatory and exploratory factor-analytic studies examining the structure of the SCS are beyond the scope of this chapter, a good deal of that research, using both domestic and foreign samples, has supported the unidimensionality of both the private and public self-consciousness subscales (e.g., Abrams, 1988; Bernstein, Teng, & Garbin, 1986; Britt, 1992; Heinemann, 1979; Nystedt & Smari, 1989; Vleeming & Engels, 1981).

Burnkrant and Page (1984), however, found weak internal consistency for the Private Self-Consciousness subscale and suggested that the Private factor may best be understood as consisting of two dimensions: internal self-awareness (ISA), referring to an awareness of thoughts, feelings, and bodily states; and self-reflectiveness (SR), indicating a tendency toward ruminative thinking about the self. Several subsequent studies have supported that bidimensional structure (e.g., Anderson, Bohon, & Berrigan, 1996; Chang, 1998; Cramer, 2000; Mittal & Balasubramanian, 1987; Piliavin & Charng, 1988).

The distinction between ISA and SR may have implications for different psychological processes associated with self-consciousness. Some research (e.g., Creed & Funder, 1998; Trapnell & Campbell, 1999) has suggested that the distinction may help to explain the apparent paradox of private self-consciousness simultaneously being a source of healthy, adaptive self-knowledge (presumably due to ISA) and also being related to maladaptive and neurotic self-absorption and rumination (as a result of SR). Other research has argued that ISA, by increasing the salience of personal characteristics, makes people *less* susceptible to external influences, whereas SR, by increasing the extent to which incoming information is processed in self-relevant terms, enhances the salience and influence of those external cues (e.g., Wheeler, Morrison, DeMarree, & Petty, 2008).

Consistent with these suggestions, recent studies by Fenigstein (2006) have examined the idea that different aspects of the private self vary in terms of their accessibility, that is, the ease with which these elements come to mind or can be targets of attention (Tversky & Kahneman, 1973). Specifically, the research indicates that when attempting to focus on private self-aspects that involve relatively inaccessible psychological *processes* (see Nisbett & Wilson, 1977), such as the motives for one's behavior, the result is ruminative, self-preoccupying SR. In contrast, when attending to knowable, relatively accessible private psychological *experiences* such as moods, feelings, or beliefs, the result may be a much more adaptive sense of self-knowledge or ISA. Thus far, the findings regarding the differing accessibility of various components of the private self, although suggestive, have not been conclusive. In light of the many studies that have questioned the distinction between ISA and SR as artifactual, rather than real (e.g., Bernstein et al., 1986), and that have challenged the psychometric validity of the distinction (e.g., Britt, 1992), many researchers continue to regard private self-consciousness as a single, unitary dimension, and I follow that practice here.

Research on Private Self-Consciousness

One of the more obvious consequences of attention is that information about the object of attention is made more salient or accessible (Anderson, 1990). Thus, when attention is focused on one's private thoughts or feelings, cognizance of those thoughts or feelings should be increased. Several studies have found a relation between private self-consciousness and more rapid cognitive processing, as well as better memory for information about the private aspects of oneself (e.g., Agatstein & Buchanan, 1984; Hull, Levinson, Young, & Sher, 1983; Mueller, 1982; Turner 1978b, 1980). Private self-consciousness has also been associated with more detailed and articulated personal self-descriptions (e.g., Franzoi, 1983; Nasby, 1985; Turner, 1978a). Finally, persons high compared with those low in self-consciousness tend to offer self-descriptions that are more consistent over time (e.g., Nasby, 1989b) and that correspond more closely with both peer-reported descriptions (e.g., Bernstein & Davis, 1982; Franzoi, 1983) and with participants' subsequent behavior (e.g., Scheier, Buss, & Buss, 1978; Smith & Shaffer, 1986; Underwood & Moore, 1981). Overall, these findings suggest that private self-consciousness is associated with a heightened awareness of the private aspects of oneself and an increased tendency to act in accordance with those aspects.

In addition to its association with increased awareness of self-relevant information, private self-consciousness is associated with heightened awareness, along with intensified experiences, of emotions and other bodily sensations. (The possibility that self-consciousness is related to increased *responsivity* to emotional stimuli, rather than increased *awareness* of internal emotional states, has not been ruled out as an alternative explanation; see, e.g., Hull, Slone, Meteyer, & Matthews, 2002.) Some reviews (e.g., Fejfar & Hoyle, 2000; Gibbons, 1990) have emphasized the relation with negative affect (largely because of the preponderance of research on that relationship), but there is a general acceptance of the view that intensified affect, both positive and negative, is related to private self-consciousness. Private self-consciousness has been shown to correlate positively both with greater laughter in response to humorous stimuli (Porterfield et al., 1988) and with stronger aggression in response to being angered (Scheier, 1976). Similarly, Scheier and Carver (1977) found that in response to both positive and negative emotional stimuli, participants high in private self-consciousness reported more intense affective reactions than those low in private self-consciousness. In the area of sexuality, private self-consciousness is positively associated with responsivity to sexual stimuli (Meston, 2006). Outside the laboratory, research showed that private self-consciousness was related to both stress and associated somatic symptoms among factory workers (Frone & McFarlin, 1989).

A novel application of the relationship between self-consciousness and heightened negative feelings argued that alcohol consumption is a means of reducing self-awareness, which would then minimize existing nega-

tive affect. Hull and Young (1983) found that following failure (and the experience of negative affect), participants high, compared to low, in private self-consciousness engaged in greater alcohol consumption, presumably as a means of reducing their self-critical feelings. Finally, in a test of the relation between private self-consciousness and the clarity of bodily experiences, Scheier, Carver, and Gibbons (1979) found that private self-consciousness correlated with the ability to resist bogus information on a taste test.

Several studies suggest that heightened awareness of private thoughts and feelings is associated not only with increased access to that information but also with an increase in the personal or subjective importance of those self-aspects. Cheek and Briggs (1982), for example, showed that persons high, in comparison with low, in private self-consciousness constructed their identities out of the unique, idiosyncratic, and relatively private elements of their existence, rather than through any social connection with others. Similarly, Fenigstein and Vanable (1993) found that private self-consciousness was more closely associated with a private self-esteem measure, evaluating how highly one valued oneself, than with a measure of public self-esteem, assessing the extent to which persons believed they were valued by others.

Another indication of the relationship between private self-consciousness and the subjective importance of the self is found in studies involving a conflict between situational standards and personal standards. When faced with this conflict, persons high, compared with low, in private self-consciousness tend to emphasize self-standards; they show relatively little concern for social expectations or conformity pressures but instead act in accordance with their own beliefs, values, or characteristics (e.g., Ellis & Holmes, 1982; Froming & Carver, 1981; Greenberg, 1982; Scheier, 1980).

As noted earlier, private self-consciousness increases the extent to which thoughts about the private self are salient and accessible. This increased availability has several interesting cognitive implications, each of which effectively contributes to the subjective importance of the self. One effect of private self-consciousness, as posited in Hull and Levy's (1979) cognitive model of self-awareness, is that conscious (Hull, Van Treuren, Ashford, Propsom, & Andrus, 1988), as well as nonconscious (Hull et al., 2002), information is more likely to be processed or encoded according to its self-relevance. In addition, by activating self-relevant thoughts, self-consciousness may influence subsequent decisions, such as attributional judgments. A number of studies have found a relation between heightened private self-consciousness and the extent to which the self, relative to external stimuli, is perceived as causally responsible for events (e.g., Buss & Scheier, 1976; Fejfar & Hoyle, 2000; Fenigstein & Carver, 1978). In summary, chronic attention to the private self, in the form of dispositional private self-consciousness, is associated with more accessible information regarding private self-aspects, a higher subjective value or importance of those self-aspects relative to external influences, and an increase in the extent to which private self-oriented cognition influences subsequent thoughts or judgments.

Research on Public Self-Consciousness

The psychological consequences of public self-consciousness may be understood as the result of a process of attending to aspects of the self that are public or observable to other people or that constitute one's group identity. Attending to these "outer" aspects of oneself should make one more cognizant of (and, presumably, more knowledgeable about) those self-aspects. Consistent with this argument, research has shown that persons high in public self-consciousness, compared with those who are low in it, had easier access to and better memory for information about the externally displayed aspects of themselves (e.g., Agatstein & Buchanan, 1984; Nasby, 1989a; Turner et al., 1981) and were more aware of their appearance, their gestures, and the public impressions that they were conveying (e.g., Gallaher, 1992; Tobey & Tunnell, 1981).

Evidence also suggests that chronic attention to the public aspects of self increases the extent to which the socially presented, public self is valued as important. Persons high in public self-consciousness were more affected by the esteem they thought others had for them than by a personal sense of self-esteem, compared with people low in public self-consciousness (Fenigstein & Vanable, 1993). In constructing their identities, they also emphasized those self-aspects that related to their public self, such as physical characteristics and group affiliations, over aspects of self that were more private in nature (Cheek & Briggs, 1982). In comparison with privately self-conscious persons, who are not especially concerned with the opinions or desires of others, those who are publicly self-conscious were more responsive to the perceived expectations of others, as evidenced by greater susceptibility to conformity pressures (e.g., Froming & Carver, 1981) and by a willingness to act in ways they thought others would approve, regardless of their own private beliefs (e.g., Greenberg, 1982; Scheier, 1980).

The acute awareness of the socially "presented" self on the part of publicly self-conscious persons is also related to a heightened concern with the impressions they convey to others, particularly with respect to physical appearance (e.g., Cash & LaBarge, 1996; Franzoi, Anderson, & Frommelt, 1990; Solomon & Schopler, 1982), although these concerns may be especially pronounced in women. Miller and Cox (1982) found that among women who were preparing to have their pictures taken, higher public self-consciousness was associated with applying a greater amount of makeup. Furthermore, public self-consciousness is significantly greater among women who are restrained eaters (Blanchard & Frost, 1983) or who have eating disorders (Striegel-Moore, Silberstein, & Rodin, 1993) than among normal controls.

Publicly self-conscious people's concerns with how they are viewed by others extend beyond appearance. Shepherd and Arkin (1989) found that in preparing for a difficult task, persons high in public self-consciousness were more likely than those low in it to engage in self-handicapping, a strategy designed to protect impressions of one's competence in the eyes of others. Another type of impression-management strategy was found in a study of road rage: After being angered by another driver, drivers high, compared with low, in public self-consciousness were less likely to drive aggressively (Millar, 2007). Finally, in a particularly interesting health-related application of the relation between public self-consciousness and social awareness, Raichle and colleagues (2001) found that following treatment for neck or head cancer, patients who were high in public self-consciousness were nearly 13 times more likely than patients low in self-consciousness to discontinue smoking, presumably in an attempt to avoid being perceived as acting in a socially undesirable way.

Public self-consciousness also seems to be related to social judgments, specifically by increasing the extent to which self-conscious people assume that others are aware of or thinking about them. Persons high, compared with low, in public self-consciousness seem to be susceptible to the belief that they are the target of observation by others, perhaps as a result of their own preoccupation with how they are seen by others. Fenigstein and Vanable (1992) found that higher public self-consciousness was associated with feeling that one was being watched, even in the absence of any evidence to that effect. These publicly self-conscious feelings of conspicuousness have also been related to "perceptions of transparency," that is, beliefs that others can accurately "see through" the person and discern his or her personal qualities from observed behavior (e.g., Vorauer & Ross, 1999) and have been proposed as a factor contributing to the sense of "being in the spotlight" (e.g., Gilovich, Medvec, & Savitzky, 2000). As is discussed in more detail later, feelings of being observed may also be associated with the social anxiety that often accompanies public self-consciousness in social situations (e.g., Buss, 1980; Fenigstein et al., 1975; Gibbons, 1990).

Feeling that one is being observed by others also relates to the (not altogether illogical) assumption that other people are very much aware of one's presence and thus are likely to be acting with the person in mind. In one study (Fenigstein, 1979), individuals were ignored by two confederates who were engaged in a conversation between themselves. This situation was intended as an ambiguous social experience in that the others' actions may or may not be relevant to oneself. Persons low in public self-consciousness indicated that they viewed the others' behavior as having little or nothing to do with them and were largely unaffected by the experience. However, persons high in public self-consciousness responded as if they knew that the others were aware of them and could not avoid the inference that they were deliberately being shunned; this personalistic interpretation (cf. Jones & Davis, 1965) resulted in a strong negative reaction to the confederates.

Other studies (e.g., Fenigstein, 1984; Fenigstein & Vanable, 1992) have confirmed the association between high public self-consciousness and the tendency to engage in self-referent interpretations of the behavior of other people. Fenigstein (1984) found that when faced with the possibility that either they or another person had been picked to participate in a classroom demonstration, participants who were high in public self-consciousness overestimated the likelihood that they were the chosen ones, compared with participants who were low on that dimension. In another study, participants were presented with eight hypothetical scenarios, each followed by a neutral or a self-relevant explanation. For example, one scenario presented participants with a situation in which their dates asked to go home early. The possible explanations were either that the date was not feeling well (neutral) or that the date did not want to spend any more time with the person (self-relevant). Public self-consciousness was associated with a tendency to (mis)construe others' actions as being targeted toward the self.

Public self-consciousness has also been associated with egocentrism, the tendency to use one's own thoughts, feelings, or actions as a basis for generating inferences about how others would think or behave. In a series of studies involving a variety of attitudes, behaviors, and causal inferences, Fenigstein and Abrams (1993) had participants answer questions both from their own perspectives and from the perspectives of hypothetical others in the same situation. Higher public self-consciousness was consistently associated with the assumption that other people thought and acted in the same way as oneself.

In sum, these studies suggest that public self-consciousness is associated with greater awareness of oneself as a social object and with the sense of oneself being more prominent in one's thought processes, resulting in a range of self-centered social-cognitive biases.

Specifically, publicly self-conscious persons are prone to exaggerate the extent to which they occupy the attention of others, transform ambiguous or insignificant events into ones that appear to have personal relevance for themselves, overperceive themselves as the cause or target of other's thoughts and actions, and attribute or project their own thoughts and behaviors onto others.

Self-Consciousness and Self-Insight

Although self-consciousness, both private and public, has been associated with greater attention and ready access to certain aspects of the self, it is important to distinguish between heightened awareness of self-related information and the accuracy of that information. That is, self-attention or trait self-consciousness may not always facilitate knowledgeable insight into private or public aspects of the person. For example, although research suggests that private self-consciousness clarifies the experience of internal sensations (e.g., Scheier et al., 1979), other research indicates that, contrary to the notion of mere clarification, the effect of focusing attention on emotional states is to intensify or change them (e.g., Scheier & Carver, 1977). Questions may also be raised about the extent to which self-consciousness facilitates insight into judgments of causality. Much of the relevant research suggests that private self-consciousness, rather than increasing attributional accuracy, instead results in biased judgments of causality involving exaggerated self-attributions (e.g., Buss & Scheier, 1976; Fenigstein, 1979).

Research showing that private self-consciousness heightens the veridicality of self-reports (e.g., Franzoi, 1983; Gibbons, 1990; Scheier et al., 1978), presumably as a function of greater self-insight, is also open to question. Shrauger and Osberg (1981) found that private self-consciousness actually tended to *decrease* the accuracy of self-predictions about one's future behavior. The idea of private self-consciousness leading to a clearer sense of self (e.g., Buss, 1980) is also challenged by the finding that private self-consciousness, rather than enhancing psychological adjustment through self-insight, is associated with higher levels of psychological distress (e.g., Ingram, 1990).

Finally, the so-called veridicality effect is subject to a more parsimonious alternative explanation involving behavioral standards. Self-directed attention is associated with an attempt to match one's behavior to appropriate standards of behavior (e.g., Duval & Wicklund, 1972; Scheier, Fenigstein, & Buss, 1974; Wicklund & Duval, 1971). With regard to self-reports, this suggests that self-consciousness may, in fact, increase the accuracy of these reports, but not necessarily as a result of facilitating self-insight. Rather, it may simply motivate participants to respond in a more appropriate fashion, that is, to be more careful and deliberate in their self-descriptions.

Some of the previously reviewed research on public self-consciousness has already suggested that thinking about how one is viewed by others does not always translate into an accurate understanding of the perspective of others (e.g., Fenigstein, 1984; Fenigstein & Abrams, 1993; Fenigstein & Vanable, 1992). Instead, preoccupation with oneself as a public object of attention often leads to unwarranted or exaggerated assumptions about the extent to which one is the target of others' thoughts. That is, rather than clarifying knowledge about oneself, thinking about oneself as a social object sometimes heightens its accessibility and subjective importance, resulting in a biasing of mental judgments.

The failure of self-consciousness to heighten accurate self-insight is consistent with research on experimental "thoughtfulness" (e.g., Wilson, 1990; Wilson, Dunn, Kraft, & Lisle, 1989). Participants in this research were asked to think about the reasons for their feelings or attitudes, a procedure that may be regarded as a laboratory analogue of the trait of private self-consciousness. These studies consistently found that this manipulated form of private self-focused attention, compared with an absence of self-focused attention, resulted in greater changes in feelings or attitudes but not in greater accuracy regarding the causes or explanations for these thoughts or feelings. That is, directing attention to internal causal processes, either through private self-consciousness or through experimental instructions, does little to provide a clearer, more insightful understanding of them. Thus, although self-consciousness may appear to enhance insight into one's own mental and emotional experiences, the research in support of that claim is inconsistent and equivocal (see Silvia & Gendolla, 2001).

Much of this research suggests a psychological equivalent to the Heisenberg uncertainty principle: Observing a phenomenon changes it. Self-attention or self-consciousness often seem to change the nature of whatever aspect of self is being observed. When attention or thoughtful scrutiny is directed toward self-relevant psychological phenomena such as ongoing affect (e.g., Scheier & Carver, 1977), judgments regarding causality for one's behavior (Buss & Scheier, 1976), the reasons underlying one's attitudes or feelings (e.g., Wilson, 1990), or the self as a social target (e.g., Fenigstein, 1984), the effect of "looking inward," rather than being clarifying or "insightful," instead tends to alter or distort whatever aspect of the self is being thought about. Although it has sometimes been assumed that self-consciousness facilitates self-knowledge, research suggests some skepticism regarding the accuracy of the self-insights gained through self-focused attention.

Self-Consciousness and Psychological Disorders

If self-consciousness undermines self-insight, then to the extent that accurate self-insight is a prerequisite for mental health (as is the prevailing wisdom in clinical psychology), self-consciousness may actually contribute to psychological disorder. That possibility is explored in this section.

Although relatively little research suggests that self-consciousness has positive consequences for mental health, there has been a virtual explosion of research in recent years examining the relation between self-focused attention and clinical disorders (e.g., Ingram, 1990; Nolen-Hoeksema, 2004; Pyszczynski, Greenberg, Hamilton, & Nix, 1991). A number of different pathways by which self-attention or self-scrutiny produces decrements in mood or self-esteem have been examined—by focusing attention on personal shortcomings (e.g., Brockner, 1979; Duval & Wicklund, 1972), by attuning the self to inner contradictions (e.g., Scheier & Carver, 1980), and by preventing people from ignoring or escaping unpleasant or threatening truths about themselves (e.g., Baumeister, 1991; Gibbons, 1990). In addition, it has been argued that self-focused attention is inextricably linked to greater rumination about self-critical thoughts, physical symptoms, or dysphoric emotions, which in turn increases the psychological distress associated with those experiences (e.g., Lyubomirsky & Nolen-Hoeksema, 1993; Wells & Matthews, 1994; Wood, Saltzberg, & Goldsamt, 1990). This section examines three specific forms of psychological dysfunction that have been related to self-consciousness: anxiety, depression, and paranoia.

Anxiety

Researchers have long suspected that heightened attention to the self promotes anxiety, and several studies support this notion (e.g., Izard, 1972; Sarason, 1972; Wine, 1982). Private self-focus has been found to increase awareness of and responsiveness to affective stimuli generally (e.g., Scheier & Carver, 1977) and, more specifically, to the negative affect of anxiety (e.g., Csikszentmihalyi & Figurski, 1982; Gibbons, 1990). To the extent that much of ordinary thought deals with current concerns and unfinished projects (e.g., Singer, 1988), heightened attention to these thoughts, as in the case of self-conscious persons, is likely to provoke discomforting emotions such as anxiety, fear, sadness, and anger. In addition to this "amplification" effect involving the intensification of negative affect, self-consciousness may also contribute to anxiety by directly increasing negative thinking (e.g., Beck & Clark, 1988) or by fostering ruminative, nonproductive coping responses in which people focus on their inadequacies (e.g., Beck & Emery, 1985; Nolen-Hoeksema, 2004) or by contributing to performance deficits (e.g., Carver, Peterson, Follansbee, & Scheier, 1983; Wine, 1971).

An important insight into the relationship between self-attention and anxiety was provided by Izard's (1972) analysis of emotion, which suggests that anxiety in a performance context almost always involves an element of self-evaluation, along with the concern and apprehension that results from self-evaluation. Self-consciousness has also been conceptualized in terms of a real or imaginary evaluative audience composed of the self or others who, in effect, are watching and judging one's performance (Carver & Scheier, 1981; Fenigstein & Vanable, 1992). Thus high self-consciousness may be a significant contributor to the evaluation apprehension that is often associated with anxiety. The relation between self-consciousness and evaluation apprehension may be especially strong in the context of a negative outcome expectancy (e.g., Carver & Scheier, 1981), in which case attention inward may be even more persistent, resulting in excessive, ruminative, and disruptive self-preoccupation, as is presumed to occur in the case of test anxiety (Wine, 1971, 1982) and sexual dysfunction (Barlow, 1986; Bruce & Barlow, 1990).

Social anxiety (or, in the extreme, social phobia) would seem to represent a specifically social form of this evaluation apprehension process. Leary and Kowalski (1995) theorized that social anxiety is a natural, ubiquitous, and even reasonable response to many social situations in which people are motivated to make a favorable impression on others but doubt their ability to do so. Given that public self-consciousness involves a heightened awareness of oneself as an object of attention to others (e.g., Buss, 1980; Fenigstein, 1979), it is reasonable to expect that this form of self-consciousness would be associated with a higher concern regarding the evaluation of others and increased social anxiety. Research has consistently confirmed that public self-consciousness is related to social anxiety and its concomitants (e.g., Cheek & Buss, 1981; Edelmann, 1990; Fenigstein, Scheier, & Buss, 1975; Hope & Heimberg, 1988; Leary & Meadows, 1991; Pilkonis, 1977).

Depression

Several parallels have been noted between the characteristics of depression and those of private self-consciousness, such as self-blaming tendencies and difficulty in engaging in self-deceptive or positive illusions (e.g., Musson & Alloy, 1988). In addition, studies have consistently found positive correlations between measures of private self-focus and depression (e.g., Ingram, Lumry, Cruet, & Sieber, 1987; Smith & Greenberg, 1981). These findings have inspired several theoretical models of depression that accord

a central role to self-focused attention (e.g., Greenberg & Pyszczynski, 1986; Lewinsohn, Hoberman, Teri, & Hautzinger, 1985; Nolen-Hoeksema, 2004; Pyszczynski & Greenberg, 1987).

Many of these models suggest a reciprocal relationship between self-focus and depression, resulting in an ever-increasing, perseverative cycle: Depressed persons engage in greater self-directed attention than nondepressed persons (e.g., Ingram et al., 1987), and self-focus helps to maintain the various affective, cognitive, and behavioral consequences associated with depression. This cycle is often set in motion by the loss of a central source of self-worth, which not only establishes a depressed state but also focuses the person's attention primarily on a sense of oneself that is incapable of restoring self-worth. That self-focus, in the form of self-consciousness, then heightens negative thinking (e.g., Pyszczynski, Hamilton, Herring, & Greenberg, 1989), negative affect (e.g., Wood, Saltzberg, Neale, Stone, & Rachmiel, 1990), low self-esteem (e.g., Pyszczynski, Holt, & Greenberg, 1987), and performance deficits (e.g., Strack, Blaney, Ganellen, & Coyne, 1985), which, in turn, exacerbates the depression. In addition to these reciprocal links between self-consciousness and depressive thought and affect, Wood, Saltzberg, Neale, and colleagues (1990) suggested that depressed persons also tend to use coping responses that resemble the characteristics of self-consciousness: Both involve systematically observing one's behavior and being overly preoccupied with feelings. To the extent that self-consciousness enhances these ruminative tendencies, it may foster emotion-focused coping and interfere with more productive, problem-focused coping, thus heightening and prolonging the depression (Nolen-Hoeksema, 2004).

Paranoia

The idea that paranoia is related to self-consciousness has a long history (e.g., Cameron, 1943; Kraepelin, 1915; Shapiro, 1965), and a program of research by Fenigstein (e.g., Fenigstein, 1984, 1997; Fenigstein & Vanable, 1992) has identified empirical relationships between public self-consciousness and measures of paranoia. The research suggests that as a result of directing one's own attention toward oneself, the self-conscious person may come to believe that others are also directing attention toward him or her. That is, by heightening the salience and subjective importance of the self, self-consciousness may contribute to the distinctly paranoid tendency to perceive oneself as the target of others' thoughts and actions. That misperception, as, for example, when the laughter of others is seen as self-directed, is commonly referred to as an idea (or delusion) of reference and is regarded as one of the hallmark characteristics of paranoid thinking (e.g., Cameron, 1943; Magaro, 1980; Millon, 1981; Swanson, Bohnert, & Smith, 1970).

Paranoia is characterized by self-referential distortions in the way in which others' actions are perceived and interpreted. The relation of paranoia to public self-consciousness, which involves a heightened awareness of those aspects of the person that are potentially observable by others, should, then, not be surprising. As suggested earlier, awareness of one's own observability to others can easily induce a feeling of visibility or conspicuousness (e.g., Fenigstein & Vanable, 1992), resulting in the paranoid-like assumption that others are aware of one's presence and thus are likely to be acting with the person in mind (e.g., Fenigstein, 1979). It is not unreasonable at that point to engage in paranoid interpretations of others' behavior, transforming insignificant and irrelevant events into ones that appear to have personal relevance so that, for example, the appearance of a stranger on the street is taken as an indication that one is being watched or plotted against (e.g., Fenigstein, 1984).

Although the research on self-consciousness and paranoia has been largely concerned with the direct association between self-consciousness and various forms of paranoid behavior, self-focus may also be related to some critical mediating mechanisms that affect paranoia. In particular, to interpret events as if they were intentionally directed toward the self is to engage in personalistic thinking (Heider, 1958; Jones & Davis, 1965). This type of thinking, in which another's behavior is interpreted in terms of their personal intent or dispositions, is both characteristic of paranoia and related to public self-consciousness (Fenigstein, 1984). Paranoid people, for example, rarely accept the idea that bad things just happen (e.g.,

Millon, 1981; Shapiro, 1965) but instead are inclined to regard negative events as evidence for another person's malevolent intentions toward them. Given this dispositional attribution of hostile intent, minor slights become major insults, and, eventually, the accumulation of such occurrences constitutes evidence for a paranoid view of the world as a hostile and threatening place. Recognizing that perspective, other manifestations of paranoia then become comprehensible: suspicion and guardedness, selective attention to signs of trickery or exploitation, misinterpretation of apparently harmless events as malevolent, readiness to take offense and counterattack, and blaming others for one's difficulties. As a result, hostilities become intensified, suspicions are confirmed, and enemies are found everywhere.

Another means by which self-focus may relate to paranoia involves the inability of paranoid people to understand the motivations and perspectives of others (e.g., Millon, 1981) or to examine behavior from any viewpoint other than their own (e.g., Shapiro, 1965). Research has shown that public self-consciousness, perhaps by heightening the salience of one's own perspective, is likewise associated with a diminished capacity to consider others' viewpoints (e.g., Fenigstein & Abrams, 1993). In this way, self-consciousness may contribute to the narrowness and rigidity of paranoid thought—the failure to examine events critically or in a broader context, the extreme selectivity in processing information, and the unwillingness to consider alternative perspectives.

Thus a good deal of evidence suggests that public self-consciousness is associated with a number of thought patterns—in particular, personalistic, self-referential inferences, and rigid egocentrism—that are similar to those observed in paranoid ideation, and these similarities may help explain the relationship between self-consciousness and paranoia.

Conclusion

The purpose of this chapter has been to provide a broad overview of the origins and current understanding of the personality construct of self-consciousness. Growing out of self-awareness theory, one of the most significant discoveries associated with the scale was the reemergence of a long-recognized theoretical distinction between the private and public aspects of the self and the recognition that dispositional self-attention may be directed at either or both of those self-aspects. The scale, which provided both the theoretical structure and the methodology for the study of private and public self-consciousness, has been one of the most heuristic scales in personality research, contributing to an understanding of the content and experience of the self and helping to develop new perspectives and research on alcoholism, depression, eating disorders, shyness and social anxiety, and paranoia.

Previous theoretical accounts of self-focused attention have often emphasized its role as self-evaluative or self-regulatory with respect to personal standards (e.g., Carver & Scheier, 1981; Gibbons, 1990). But in light of the evidence reviewed that questioned the accuracy of self-knowledge gained though self-attention, as well as the myriad relationships between self-consciousness and disordered behavior, the idea that self-consciousness has a strictly regulatory function may be questioned. Instead, this chapter has adopted what may be regarded as an attentional perspective, arguing that a coherent, integrative account of self-directed attention need not assume an automatic self-evaluative or information-seeking orientation but instead may be better served by focusing on the psychological process of attention, which has been shown to have predictable and understandable effects. More specifically, when attention is directed to the private and/or public aspects of the self, the person apparently becomes more aware of those self-characteristics (although that self-knowledge may be subject to bias and distortion). Those self-aspects that are attended to take on greater value or importance in the person's judgments, and an increase occurs in the extent to which the self, as a cognitive organizational system, influences other realms of thought—either by exaggerating the self's role on external events (including other's behavior) or by rendering external information (including other's behavior) as more self-relevant.

Most research on self-consciousness has addressed its implications for a variety of basic cognitive, social, emotional, and psychopathological phenomena, but many larger issues remain: Does self-consciousness have an evolutionary origin, and, if so, what is its functional value? What are its genetic and environmental sources? Is there cross-cultural universality or variation across cultures in self-consciousness? How does self-consciousness develop across time? How can it be modified or treated? Are there any gender differences (e.g., self-consciousness of appearance vs. status)? Some of these issues have been touched on sporadically, but none has received systematic treatment. Perhaps a new generation of researchers will take up the call.

References

Abrams, D. (1988). Self-consciousness scales for adults and children: Reliability, validity, and theoretical significance. *European Journal of Personality, 2,* 11–37.

Agatstein, F. C., & Buchanan, D. B. (1984). Public and private self-consciousness and the recall of self-relevant information. *Personality and Social Psychology Bulletin, 10,* 314–325.

Anderson, E. M., Bohon, L. M., & Berrigan, L. P. (1996). Factor structure of the Private Self-Consciousness scale. *Journal of Personality Assessment, 66,* 144–162.

Anderson, J. R. (1990). *Cognitive psychology.* New York: Freeman.

Argyle, M. (1969). *Social interaction.* New York: Atherton.

Barlow, D. (1986). Causes of sexual dysfunction: The role of anxiety and cognitive interference. *Journal of Consulting and Clinical Psychology, 54,* 14–48.

Baumeister, R. F. (1986). *Identity: Cultural change and the struggle for self.* New York: Oxford University Press.

Baumeister, R. F. (1991). *Escaping the self: Alcoholism, spirituality, masochism, and other flights from the burden of selfhood.* New York: Basic Books.

Beck, A. T., & Clark, D. A. (1988). Anxiety and depression: An information processing perspective. *Anxiety Research, 1,* 23–36.

Beck, A. T., & Emery, G. (1985). *Anxiety disorders and phobias: A cognitive perspective.* New York: Basic Books.

Bernstein, I. H., Teng, G., & Garbin, C. P. (1986). A confirmatory factoring of the self-consciousness scale. *Multivarite Behavioral Research, 21,* 459–475.

Bernstein, W. M., & Davis, M. H. (1982). Perspective-taking, self-consciousness, and accuracy in person perception. *Basic and Applied Social Psychology, 3,* 1–19.

Blanchard, F. A., & Frost, R. O. (1983). Two factors of restraint: Concern for dieting and weight fluctuation. *Behavioral Research and Therapy, 21,* 259–267.

Briggs, S. R., Cheek, J. M., & Buss, A. H. (1980). An

analysis of the Self-Monitoring Scale. *Journal of Personality and Social Psychology, 38,* 679–686.

Britt, T. W. (1992). The Self-Consciousness Scale: On the stability of the three-factor structure. *Personality and Social Psychology Bulletin, 18,* 748–755.

Brockner, J. (1979). Self-esteem, self-consciousness, and task performance: Replications, extensions, and possible explanations. *Journal of Personality and Social Psychology, 37,* 447–461.

Brockner, J., Gardner, M., Bierman, J., Mahan, T., Thomas, B., Weiss, W., et al. (1983). The roles of self-esteem and self-consciousness in the Wortman–Brehm model of reactance and learned helplessness. *Journal of Personality and Social Psychology, 45,* 199–209

Bruce, T. J., & Barlow, D. H. (1990). The nature and role of performance anxiety in sexual dysfunction. In H. Leitenberg (Ed.), *Handbook of social and evaluation anxiety* (pp. 357–384). New York: Plenum Press.

Burnkrant, R. E., & Page, T. J. (1984). A modification of the Fenigstein, Scheier, and Buss Self-Consciousness Scales. *Journal of Personality Assessment, 28,* 629–637.

Buss, A. H. (1980). *Self-consciousness and social anxiety.* San Francisco: Freeman.

Buss, D. M., & Scheier, M. F. (1976). Self-awareness, self-consciousness, and self-attribution. *Journal of Research in Personality, 10,* 463–468.

Cameron, N. (1943). The development of paranoic thinking. *Psychological Review, 50,* 219–233.

Carver, C. S., & Glass, D. C. (1976). The self-consciousness scale: A discriminant validity study. *Journal of Personality Assessment, 40,* 169–172.

Carver, C. S., Peterson, L. M., Follansbee, D. J., & Scheier, M. F. (1983). Effects of self-directed attention on performance and persistence among persons high and low in test anxiety. *Cognitive Theory and Research, 7,* 337–354.

Carver, C. S., & Scheier, M. F. (1978). Self-focusing effects of dispositional self-consciousness, mirror presence, and audience presence. *Journal of Personality and Social Psychology, 36,* 324–332.

Carver, C. S., & Scheier, M. F. (1981). *Attention and self-regulation: A control theory approach to human behavior.* New York: Springer-Verlag.

Cash, T. F., & LaBarge, A. S. (1996). The psychology of cosmetic surgery. *Cognitive Therapy and Research, 20,* 37–50.

Chang, L. (1988). Factor interpretations of the Self-Consciousness Scale. *Personality and Individual Differences, 24,* 635–640.

Cheek, J. M., & Briggs, S. R. (1982). Self-consciousness and aspects of identity. *Journal of Research in Personality, 16,* 401–408.

Cheek, J. M., & Buss, A. H. (1981). Shyness and sociability. *Journal of Personality and Social Psychology, 41,* 330–339.

Cooley, C. H. (1902). *Human nature and the social order.* New York: Scribner's.

Cramer, K. M. (2000). Comparing the relative fit of various factor models of the Self-Consciousness Scale in two independent samples. *Journal of Personality Assessment, 75,* 295–307.

Creed, A. T., & Funder, D. C. (1998). The two faces of private self-consciousness: Self-report, peer report, and behavioral correlates. *European Journal of Personality, 12,* 411–431.

Csikszentmihalyi, M., & Figurski, T. J. (1982). Self-awareness and aversive experiences in everyday life. *Journal of Personality, 50,* 15–28.

Duval, S., & Wicklund, R. A. (1972). *A theory of objective self-awareness.* New York: Academic Press.

Edelmann, R. J. (1990). Chronic blushing, self-consciousness, and social anxiety. *Journal of Psychopathology and Behavioral Assessment, 12,* 119–127.

Ellis, R. J., & Holmes, J. G. (1982). Focus of attention and self-evaluation in social interaction. *Journal of Personality and Social Psychology, 43,* 67–77.

Fejfar, M. C., & Hoyle, R. H. (2000). Effect of private self-awareness on negative affect and self-referent attributions: A quantitative review. *Personality and Social Psychology Review, 4,* 132–142.

Fenigstein, A. (1979). Self-consciousness, self-attention, and social interaction. *Journal of Personality and Social Psychology, 37,* 75–86.

Fenigstein, A. (1984). Self-consciousness and the over-perception of self as a target. *Journal of Personality and Social Psychology, 47,* 860–870.

Fenigstein, A. (1987). On the nature of public and private self-consciousness. *Journal of Personality, 55,* 543–554.

Fenigstein, A. (1997). Paranoid thought and schematic processing. *Journal of Social and Clinical Psychology, 16,* 77–94.

Fenigstein, A. (2006). *Differences in the accessibility of various aspects of the private self.* Unpublished manuscript, Kenyon College.

Fenigstein, A., & Abrams, D. (1993). Self-attention and the egocentric assumption of shared perspectives. *Journal of Experimental Social Psychology, 29,* 287–303.

Fenigstein, A., & Carver, C. S. (1978). Self-focusing effects of heartbeat feedback. *Journal of Personality and Social Psychology, 36,* 1241–1250.

Fenigstein, A., Scheier, M. F., & Buss, A. H. (1975). Public and private self-consciousness: Assessment and theory. *Journal of Clinical and Consulting Psychology, 43,* 522–527.

Fenigstein, A., & Vanable, P. A. (1992). Paranoia and self-consciousness. *Journal of Personality and Social Psychology, 62,* 129–138.

Fenigstein, A., & Vanable, P. A. (1993). *The effects of self-consciousness on private and public self-esteem.* Unpublished manuscript, Kenyon College.

Franzoi, S. L. (1983). Self-concept differences as a function of private self-consciousness and social anxiety. *Journal of Research in Personality, 17,* 275–287.

Franzoi, S. L., Anderson, J., & Frommelt, S. (1990). Individual differences in men's perception of and reactions to thinning hair. *Journal of Social psychology, 130,* 209–218.

Franzoi, S. L., & Brewer, L. C. (1984). The experience of self-awareness and its relation to level of self-consciousness: An experiential sampling study. *Journal of Research in Personality, 18,* 522–540.

Froming, W. J., & Carver, C. S. (1981). Divergent influences of private and public self-consciousness in a compliance paradigm. *Journal of Research in Personality, 15,* 159–171.

Froming, W. J., Walker, G. R., & Lopyan, K. J. (1982).

Public and private self-awareness: When personal attitudes conflict with societal expectations. *Journal of Experimental Social Psychology, 18,* 476–487.

Frone, M. R., & McFarlin, D. B. (1989). Chronic occupational stressors, self-focused attention, and well-being: Testing a cybernetic model. *Journal of Applied Psychology, 74,* 876–883.

Gallaher, P. (1992). Individual differences in nonverbal behavior: Dimensions of style. *Journal of Personality and Social Psychology, 63,* 133–145.

Gibbons, F. X. (1990). Self-attention and behavior: A review and theoretical update. In L. Berkowitz (Ed.), *Advances in experimental social psychology* (Vol. 23, pp. 249–303). New York: Academic Press.

Gilovich, T., Medvec, V. H., & Savitzky, K. (2000). The spotlight effect in social judgment: An egocentric bias in estimates of the salience of one's own actions and appearance. *Journal of Personality and Social Psychology, 79,* 211–222.

Goffman, E. (1959). *The presentation of self in everyday life.* Garden City, NY: Doubleday.

Greenberg, J. (1982). Self-image versus impression management in adherence to distributive justice standards: The influence of self-awareness and self-consciousness. *Journal of Personality and Social Psychology, 44,* 5–19.

Greenberg, J., & Pyszczynski, T. (1986). Persistent high self-focus after failure and low self-focus after success: The depressive self-focusing style. *Journal of Personality and Social Psychology, 50,* 1039–1044.

Greenwald, A. G. (1980). The totalitarian ego: Fabrication and revision of personal history. *American Psychologist, 35,* 603–618.

Hass, R. G. (1984). Perspective taking and self-awareness: Drawing an E on your forehead. *Journal of Personality and Social Psychology, 46,* 788–798.

Heider, F. (1958). *The psychology of interpersonal relations.* New York: Wiley.

Heinemann, W. (1979). The assessment of private and public self-consciousness: A German replication. *European Journal of Personality, 9,* 331–337.

Hope, D. A., & Heimberg, R. G. (1988). Public and private self-consciousness and social phobia. *Journal of Personality Assessment, 52,* 626–639.

Hull, J. G., Levinson, R. W., Young, R. D., & Sher, K. J. (1983). Self-awareness-reducing effects of alcohol consumption. *Journal of Personality and Social Psychology, 44,* 461–473.

Hull, J. G., & Levy, A. S. (1979). The organizational functions of self: An alternative to the Duval and Wicklund model of self-awareness. *Journal of Personality and Social Psychology, 37,* 756–768.

Hull, J. G., Slone, L. B., Meteyer, K. B., & Matthews, A. R. (2002). The nonconsciousness of self-consciousness. *Journal of Personality and Social Psychology, 83,* 406–424.

Hull, J. G., Van Treuren, R. R., Ashford, S. J., Propsom, P., & Andrus, B. W. (1988). Self-consciousness and the processing of self-relevant information. *Journal of Personality and Social Psychology, 54,* 452–465.

Hull, J. G., & Young, R. D. (1983). Self-consciousness, self-esteem, success–failure as determinants of alcohol consumption in male social drinkers. *Journal of Personality and Social Psychology, 44,* 1097–1109.

Ingram, R. E. (1990). Self-focused attention in clinical disorders: Review and a conceptual model. *Psychological Bulletin, 107,* 156–176.

Ingram, R. E., Lumry, A. E., Cruet, D., & Sieber, W. (1987). Attentional processes in depressive disorders. *Cognitive Theory and Research, 11,* 351–360.

Izard, C. (1972). *Patterns of emotion: A new analysis of anxiety and depression.* New York: Academic Press.

James, W. (1890). *The principles of psychology* (Vol. 1). New York: Holt.

Jones, E. E., & Davis, K. E. (1965). From acts to dispositions: The attribution process in person perception. In L. Berkowitz (Ed.), *Advances in experimental social psychology* (Vol. 2). New York: Academic Press.

Jung, C. G. (1957). *The undiscovered self.* New York: New American Library.

Kihlstrom, J. F., Cantor, J., Albright, J., Chew, B., Klein, S., & Niedenthal, P. (1988). Information processing and the study of the self. In L. Berkowitz (Ed.), *Advances in experimental social psychology* (Vol. 21, pp. 145–178). New York: Academic Press.

Klein, S. B., & Loftus, J. (1988). The nature of self-referent encoding: The contributions of elaborative and organizational processes. *Journal of Personality and Social Psychology, 55,* 5–11.

Kraepelin, E. (1915). *Psychiatrie: Ein Lehrbuch [Psychiatry: A textbook]* (7th ed.). Leipzig, Germany: Barth.

Leary, M. R. (1983). Social anxiousness: The construct and its assessment. *Journal of Personality Assessment, 47,* 66–75.

Leary, M. R. (1995). *Self-presentation: Impression management and interpersonal behavior.* Madison, WI: Brown & Benchmark.

Leary, M. R., & Kowalski, R. M. (1995). *Social anxiety.* New York: Guilford Press.

Leary, M. R., & Meadows, S. (1991). Predictors, elicitors, and concomitants of social blushing. *Journal of Personality and Social Psychology, 60,* 254–262.

Lewinsohn, P. M., Hoberman, H., Teri, L., & Hautzinger, M. (1985). An integrative theory of depression. In S. Reiss & R. Bootzin (Eds.), *Theoretical issues in behavior therapy* (pp. 331–359). New York: Academic Press.

Lyubomirsky, S., & Nolen-Hoeksema, S. (1993). Self-perpetuating properties of dysphoric rumination. *Journal of Personality and Social Psychology, 65,* 339–349.

Magaro, P. A. (1980). *Cognition in schizophrenia and paranoia: The interpretation of cognitive processes.* Hillsdale, NJ: Erlbaum.

Markus, H. (1977). Self-schemata and processing information about the self. *Journal of Personality and Social Psychology, 35,* 63–78.

Mead, G. H. (1934). *Mind, self, and society.* Chicago: University of Chicago Press.

Meston, C. M. (2006). The effects of state and trait self-focused attention on sexual arousal in sexually functional and dysfunctional women. *Behavior Research and Therapy, 44,* 515–532.

Millar, M. (2007). The influence of public self-consciousness and anger on aggressive driving. *Personality and Individual Differences, 43,* 2116–2126.

Miller, L. C., & Cox, C. L. (1982). For appearance's sake: Public self-consciousness and makeup use. *Personality and Social Psychology Bulletin, 8*, 748–751.

Millon, T. H. (1981). *Disorders of personality.* New York: Wiley.

Mittal, B., & Balasubramanian, S. K. (1987). Testing the dimensionality of the Self-Consciousness Scales. *Journal of Personality Assessment, 51*, 53–68.

Mueller, J. H. (1982). Self-awareness and access to material rated as self-descriptive or non-descriptive. *Bulletin of the Psychonomic Society, 19*, 323–326.

Musson, R. E., & Alloy, L. B. (1988). Depression and self-directed attention. In L. B. Alloy (Ed.), *Cognitive processes in depression.* New York: Guilford Press.

Nasby, W. (1985). Private self-consciousness, articulation of the self-schema, and recognition memory of trait adjectives. *Journal of Personality and Social Psychology, 49*, 704–709.

Nasby, W. (1989a). Private and public self-consciousness and articulation of the self-schema. *Journal of Personality and Social Psychology, 56*, 117–123.

Nasby, W. (1989b). Private self-consciousness, self-awareness, and the reliability of self-reports. *Journal of Personality and Social Psychology, 56*, 950–957.

Nisbett, R. E., & Wilson, T. D. (1977). Telling more than we can know: Verbal reports on mental processes. *Psychological Review, 84*, 231–259.

Nolen-Hoeksema, S. (2004). Response styles theory. In C. Papageorgiou & A. Wells (Eds.), *Depressive rumination: Nature, theory, and treatment* (pp. 107–124). New York: Wiley.

Nystedt, L., & Smari, J. (1989). Assessment of the Fenigstein, Scheier, and Buss Self-Consciousness Scale: A Swedish translation. *Journal of Personality Assessment, 53*, 342–352.

Piliavin, J. A., & Charng, H. (1988). What is the factorial structure of the private and public self-consciousness scales? *Personality and Social Psychology Bulletin, 14*, 587–595.

Pilkonis, P. A. (1977). Shyness, public and private, and its relationship to other measures of social behavior. *Journal of Personality, 45*, 585–595.

Porterfield, A. L., Mayer, F. S., Dougherty, K. G., Kredich, K. E., Kronberg, M. M., Marsee, K. M., et al. (1988). Private self-consciousness, canned laughter, and responses to humorous stimuli. *Journal of Research in Personality, 22*, 409–423.

Pyszczynski, T., & Greenberg, J. (1987). Self-regulatory perseveration and the depressive self-focusing style: A self-awareness theory of the development and maintenance of depression. *Psychological Bulletin, 102*, 122–138.

Pyszczynski, T., Greenberg, J., Hamilton, J. C., & Nix, J. (1991). On the relationship between self-focused attention and psychological disorder: A critical reappraisal. *Psychological Bulletin, 110*, 538–543.

Pyszczynski, T., Hamilton, J. C., Herring, F. H., & Greenberg, J. (1989). Depression, self-focused attention, and negative memory bias. *Journal of Personality and Social Psychology, 57*, 351–357.

Pyszczynski, T., Holt, K., & Greenberg, J. (1987). Depression, self-focused attention, and expectancies for future positive and negative events for self and others. *Journal of Personality and Social Psychology, 52*, 994–1001.

Raichle, K. A., Christensen, A. J., Ehlers, S., Moran, P. J., Karnell, L., & Funk, G. (2001). Public and private self-consciousness and smoking behavior in head and neck cancer patients. *Annals of Behavioral Medicine, 23*, 120–124.

Rogers, T. B., Kuiper, N. A., & Kirker, W. S. (1977). Self-reference and the encoding of personal information. *Journal of Personality and Social Psychology, 35*, 677–688.

Sarason, I. G. (1972). Experimental approaches to test anxiety: Attention and the uses of information. In C. D. Spielberger (Ed.), *Anxiety: Current trends in theory and research* (Vol. 2, pp. 381–403). Orlando, FL: Academic Press.

Scheier, M. F. (1976). Self-awareness, self-consciousness, and angry aggression. *Journal of Personality, 44*, 627–644.

Scheier, M. F. (1980). Effects of public and private self-consciousness on the public expression of personal beliefs. *Journal of Personality and Social Psychology, 39*, 514–521.

Scheier, M. F., Buss, A. H., & Buss, D. M. (1978). Self-consciousness, self-report of aggressiveness, and aggression. *Journal of Research in Personality, 12*, 133–140.

Scheier, M. F., & Carver, C. S. (1977). Self-focused attention and the experience of emotion: Attraction, repulsion, elation, and depression. *Journal of Personality and Social Psychology, 35*, 625–636.

Scheier, M. F., & Carver, C. S. (1980). Private and public self-attention, resistance to change, and dissonance reduction. *Journal of Personality and Social Psychology, 39*, 390–405.

Scheier, M. F., Carver, C. S., & Gibbons, R. X. (1979). Self-directed attention, awareness of bodily states, and suggestibility. *Journal of Personality and Social Psychology, 37*, 1576–1588.

Scheier, M. F., Fenigstein, A., & Buss, A. H. (1974). Self-awareness and physical aggression. *Journal of Experimental Social Psychology, 10*, 265–273.

Schlenker, B. R. (1980). *Impression management: The self-concept, social identity, and interpersonal relations.* Monterey, CA: Brooks/Cole.

Schlenker, B. R., & Weigold, M. F. (1990). Self-consciousness and self-presentation: Being autonomous versus appearing autonomous. *Journal of Personality and Social Psychology, 59*, 820–828.

Shapiro, D. (1965). *Neurotic styles.* New York: Basic Books.

Shepherd, J. A., & Arkin, R. M. (1989). Determinants of self-handicapping: The moderating role of public self-consciousness and task importance. *Personality and Social Psychology Bulletin, 15*, 252–265.

Shrauger, J. S., & Osberg, T. M. (1981). The relative accuracy of self-predictions and judgments of others in psychological assessment. *Psychological Bulletin, 90*, 322–351.

Silvia, P. J., & Gendolla, G. H. (2001). On introspection and self-perception: Does self-focused attention enable accurate self-knowledge? *Review of General Psychology, 5*, 241–269.

Singer, J. L. (1988). Sampling ongoing consciousness and emotional experience: Implications for health. In M. J. Horowitz (Ed.), *Psychodynamics and cognition* (pp. 297–346). Chicago: University of Chicago Press.

Smith, J. D., & Shaffer, D. R. (1986). Self-consciousness,

self-reported altruism, and helping behavior. *Social Behavior and Personality, 14,* 215–220.

Smith, T. W., & Greenberg, J. (1981). Depression and self-focused attention. *Motivation and Emotion, 5,* 323–331.

Solomon, M. R., & Schopler, J. (1982). Self-consciousness and clothing. *Personality and Social Psychology Bulletin, 8,* 508–514.

Strack, S., Blaney, P. H., Ganellen, R. J., & Coyne, J. C. (1985). Pessimistic self-preoccupation, performance deficits, and depression. *Journal of Personality and Social Psychology, 49,* 1076–1085.

Striegel-Moore, R. H., Silberstein, L. R., & Rodin, J. (1993). The social self in bulimia nervosa: Public self-conscious, social anxiety, and perceived fraudulence. *Journal of Abnormal Psychology, 102,* 297–303.

Swanson, D. W., Bohnert, P. J., & Smith, J. (1970). *The paranoid.* Boston: Little, Brown.

Tobey, E. L., & Tunnell, G. (1981). Predicting our impressions on others: Effects of public self-consciousness and acting, a self-monitoring subscale. *Personality and Social Psychology Bulletin, 7,* 661–669.

Tooby, J., & Cosmides, L. (1990). On the universality of human nature and the uniqueness of the individual: The role of genetics and adaptation. *Journal of Personality, 58,* 17–67.

Trapnell, P. D., & Campbell, J. D. (1999). Private self-consciousness and the five-factor model of personality: Distinguishing rumination from reflection. *Journal of Personality and Social Psychology, 76,* 284–304.

Turner, R. G. (1978a). Effects of differential request procedures and self-consciousness on trait attributions. *Journal of Research in Personality, 12,* 431–438.

Turner, R. G. (1978b). Self-consciousness and speed of processing self-relevant information. *Personality and Social Psychology Bulletin, 4,* 456–460.

Turner, R. G. (1980). Self-consciousness and memory of trait terms. *Personality and Social Psychology Bulletin, 6,* 273–277.

Turner, R. G., Gilliland, L., & Klein, H. M. (1981). Self-consciousness, evaluation of physical characteristics, and physical attractiveness. *Journal of Research in Personality, 15,* 182–190.

Turner, R. G., Scheier, M. F., Carver, C. S., & Ickes, W. (1978). Correlates of self-consciousness. *Journal of Personality Assessment, 42,* 285–289.

Tversky, A., & Kahneman, D. (1973). Availability: A heuristic for judging frequency and probability. *Cognitive Psychology, 5,* 207–232.

Underwood, B., & Moore, B. S. (1981). Sources of behavioral consistency. *Journal of Personality and Social Psychology, 40,* 781–785.

Vleeming, R. G., & Engels, J. A. (1981). Assessment of private and public self-consciousness: A Dutch replication. *Journal of Personality Assessment, 45,* 385–389.

Vorauer, J. D., & Ross, M. (1999). Self-awareness and feeling transparent: Failing to suppress one's self. *Journal of Experimental Social Psychology, 35,* 415–440.

Wells, A., & Matthews, G. (1994). *Attention and emotion: A clinical perspective.* Hillsdale, NJ: Erlbaum.

Wheeler, S. C., Morrison, K. R., DeMarree, K. G., & Petty, R. E. (2008). Does private self-consciousness increase or decrease priming effects?: It depends. *Journal of Experimental Social Psychology, 44,* 882–889.

Wicklund, R. A., & Duval, S. (1971). Opinion change and performance facilitation as a result of objective self-awareness. *Journal of Experimental Social Psychology, 7,* 319–342.

Wicklund, R. A., & Gollwitzer, P. M. (1987). The fallacy of the private-public self-focus distinction. *Journal of Personality, 55,* 492–523.

Wilson, T. D. (1990). Self-persuasion via self-reflection. In J. Olson & M. P. Zanna (Eds.), *Self-inference processes: The Ontario Symposium* (Vol. 6, pp. 43–67). Hillsdale, NJ: Erlbaum.

Wilson, T. D., Dunn, D. S., Kraft, D., & Lisle, D. J. (1989). Introspection, attitude change, and attitude–behavior consistency: The disruptive effects of explaining why we feel the way we do. In L. Berkowitz (Ed.), *Advances in experimental social psychology* (Vol. 19, pp. 123–205). Orlando, FL: Academic Press.

Wine, J. D. (1971). Test anxiety and direction of attention. *Psychological Bulletin, 76,* 92–104.

Wine, J. D. (1982). Evaluation anxiety: A cognitive–attentional construct. In H. W. Krohne & L. C. Laux (Eds.), *Achievement, stress, and anxiety* (pp. 207–222). Washington, DC: Hemisphere.

Wood, J. V., Saltzberg, J. A., & Goldsamt, L. A. (1990). Does affect induce self-focused attention? *Journal of Personality and Social Psychology, 58,* 899–908.

Wood, J. V., Saltzberg, J. A., Neale, J. M., Stone, A. A., & Rachmiel, T. B. (1990). Self-focused attention, coping responses, and distressed mood in everyday life. *Journal of Personality and Social Psychology, 58,* 1027–1036.

CHAPTER 35

■ ● ▲ ◆ ■ ● ▲ ◆

Independent, Relational, and Collective–Interdependent Self-Construals

SUSAN E. CROSS
ERIN E. HARDIN
BERNA GERCEK SWING

Self-construal refers to how individuals define and make meaning of the self in relation to others. In their seminal work, Markus and Kitayama (1991) identified two such self-construals: independent and interdependent. The independent self-construal (IndSC) is characterized by separateness and individuation from others. Demonstrating uniqueness is an important basis of self-esteem. Being "the same person" across situations and communicating assertively are signs of maturity. Social comparison confirms one's uniqueness and internal traits. In contrast, the interdependent self-construal (InterSC) is characterized by the ways in which one is connected to others. Fitting into the group is also an important basis of self-esteem. Changing behavior in response to different situations and regulating emotional expression to maintain group harmony are signs of maturity. The individual strives to subordinate personal goals in order to benefit the group. Social comparison is used to determine whether one is fulfilling obligations within those relationships. Although individuals possess both types of self-construal (Markus & Kitayama, 1991; Singelis, 1994), cultural context typically promotes the development of one or the other more strongly, with IndSC often promoted in Western countries and InterSC promoted in non-Western countries, including parts of Asia, Africa, and Central and South America.

Drawing on Markus and Kitayama's (1991) work, Cross, Bacon, and Morris (2000) described the *relational–interdependent self-construal (RelSC)* as the extent to which people define themselves in terms of close relationships, and they differentiated it from the group-centered collective InterSC. Although much research continues to focus on the two-part distinction between the IndSC and InterSC made by Markus and Kitayama, many others have recognized the value of distinguishing between relational interdependence (based on close, dyadic relationships) and collective interdependence (based on memberships in social groups; see Brewer & Chen, 2007; Sedikides & Brewer, 2001).

In this chapter, we examine the ways that researchers have responded to and elaborated on the original Markus and Kitayama (1991) thesis. Due to space limitations, we focus on research that employs either measures or manipulations of self-construal, excluding research that uses culture as a proxy for self-construal. We begin with a review of the most frequently used means of measuring and manipulating self-construal, followed by a review of the research examining the role of self-construal in cognition, emotion, motivation, and social behavior.

Approaches to Measuring or Manipulating Self-Construal

Measuring Independent and Interdependent Self-Construal

Several measures assess IndSC and InterSC as individual-differences variables as defined by Markus and Kitayama (1991). The most common of these is the Self-Construal Scale (SCS; Singelis, 1994). The SCS provides separate scores for IndSC and InterSC, consistent with theoretical predictions that the two self-construals are orthogonal (Singelis, 1994). Scores on the original 12-item scales demonstrated expected between-groups differences, with Asian Americans being more interdependent and less independent than European Americans. InterSC scores also predicted participants' tendency to make situational attributions for behaviors described in short vignettes. However, the interitem reliabilities of the two scales tend to be adequate at best, with Cronbach's alpha reliabilities hovering around .70 (Singelis, 1994).

Additional items have been added to the SCS, resulting in various versions being used; the 12- and 15-item versions appear to be most common. Although some authors have created a unidimensional self-construal score by reverse-scoring the interdependence items (e.g., Aaker, 2000), such scores are contrary to the intended use of the SCS and to theoretical understanding of self-construal (Singelis, 1994). Although most items have good face validity, several (e.g., "I value being in good health above everything") have been questioned (Hardin, Leong, & Bhagwat, 2004; Levine et al., 2003). The SCS has been used in more than 100 studies and translated into numerous languages.

Another self-report measure of self-construal was developed by Gudykunst and colleagues (1996) based on data from the United States, Japan, Korea, and Australia. The 14-item IndSC scale and 15-item InterSC scale demonstrate adequate to good interitem reliabilities. Although the four national groups did not differ as might be expected in mean scores on the IndSC and InterSC scales, self-construal did predict high- and low-context communication, as expected.

Twenty Statements Test as a Measure of Self-Construal

The Twenty Statements Test (TST; Kuhn & McPartland, 1954) has also been used as a measure of self-construal (e.g., Somech, 2000). Participants are asked to complete 20 sentence stems that begin, "I am. ... " The number of independent (e.g., "I am intelligent"), relational (e.g., "I am John's girlfriend"), and interdependent (e.g., "I am African American") statements generated may then be used as self-construal scores.

Self-Report Measures of Self-Construal: Two or More Factors?

Given that Markus and Kitayama's (1991) self-construal theory posits two dimensions of self-construal, neither Singelis (1994) nor Gudykunst and colleagues (1996) considered more than two factors during development of their scales. However, considerable evidence from a variety of samples suggests that this simple two-factor structure does not provide a good fit to the data from any of the scales (Hardin et al., 2004; Levine et al., 2003). Despite being designed to measure self-construal in terms of independence and interdependence, these measures actually have a multidimensional structure. Content analyses of the TST (Somech, 2000) and factor analyses of Singelis's scale (Hardin, 2006; Hardin et al., 2004; Sato & McCann, 1998) all show that multidimensional structures fit the data better than a simple two-factor structure. For example, Hardin and colleagues (2004) identified a higher order factor structure underlying items on the SCS. The four independence factors (Autonomy/ Assertiveness, Individualism, Behavioral Consistency, and Primacy of Self) and two interdependent factors (Esteem for Group and Relational Interdependence) were replicated in samples of Asian American (Hardin et al., 2004), European American (Hardin, 2006; Hardin et al., 2004), African American and Latino/a (Hardin, 2006) students. Hardin (2006) found that over 50% more variance in social anxiety could be accounted for by specific dimensions of independence and interdependence (e.g., autonomy, behavioral consistency) than by the broader dimensions. Thus there is a clear need for a psychometrically sound measure of multidimensional self-construal.

Measuring Relational Self-Construal

Cross and her colleagues (Cross et al., 2000) created the Relational–Interdependent Self-Construal Scale (RISC) to measure the relational form of interdependent self-construal. Its explicit focus on the individual's self-definition distinguishes it from other measures of communion or expressivity. It has good internal reliability (> .85) and good stability over a 2-month period (test–retest reliability is .76; Cross et al., 2000). Women usually score higher than men (*d*s range from −.17 to −.57). Scores correlate moderately positively with other measures of relatedness but do not correlate with measures of independence. Examination of the incremental utility of the RISC scale showed that it taps self-definition in a unique fashion that is not tapped by other measures of relatedness, expressivity, or communalism (Cross et al., 2000).

Measuring Collective or Group Self-Construal

Whereas the relational–interdependent self is defined in terms of significant dyadic relationships, the collective–interdependent self is defined in terms of significant group memberships. Brewer and Chen (2007) demonstrated that although most existing measures of collectivism and interdependence assess both types of interdependence, relationally oriented items are more than twice as common. Brewer and Chen argued that cross-cultural researchers need to clearly delineate between these two types of interdependence, as they have very different implications and predict different outcomes. For example, whereas men tend to score lower than women on measures of interdependence (see Cross & Madson, 1997), Gabriel and Gardner (1999) demonstrated that distinguishing between relational and collective interdependence yields more nuanced findings: Men score lower than women in terms of relational interdependence but *higher* than women in terms of collective interdependence.

More recently, Harb and Smith (2008) created a Six-Fold Self-Construal Scale that integrates Brewer's work on the personal, relational, and group selves (Brewer & Chen, 2007; Brewer & Gardner, 1996) with Singelis's work on vertical and horizontal individualism and collectivism (IND–COL; Singelis, Triandis, Bhawuk, & Gelfand, 1995). The scale assesses the horizontal and vertical collective self-construal, as well as the horizontal and vertical relational self-construal, the personal self-construal, and a *humanity-bound* self-construal. In samples of college students from the United Kingdom, Lebanon, Syria, and Jordan, reliabilities on all six dimensions were adequate to good, with most reliabilities in the mid-.80s. In light of Brewer and Chen's (2007) call for researchers to distinguish between the relational and collective (or group) interdependence, new measures such as this are likely to be of increasing utility.

Between- and Within-Groups Differences in Self-Construal

These measures have facilitated the explosion in research on self-construal by allowing researchers explicitly to measure self-construals and to test their relations to a range of other cognitive, affective, and behavioral variables (see subsequent sections). The development of these measures has also allowed researchers to explore between- and within-groups differences in self-construal. To the surprise of many, however, the results from such research tend to be inconsistent, often showing that individuals from different countries do not demonstrate the expected differences in self-construal (see Oyserman, Coon, & Kemmelmeier, 2002).

These unexpected or absent between-groups differences led Matsumoto (1999) to conclude that the theory of self-construal is fundamentally flawed, whereas Levine and colleagues (2003) concluded that *measures* of self-construal are flawed. Other authors, however, have argued convincingly that contextual factors may explain the mixed results. Across several studies, Heine, Lehman, Peng, and Greenholtz (2002) obtained expected, unexpected, or absent between-groups differences by manipulating the reference group that participants had in mind when responding to Singelis's (1994) SCS.

They also showed that these *reference-group effects* are attenuated or absent when self-construal scale scores are compared for different ethnic groups within the same country, allowing expected between-groups differences to emerge in such samples (cf. Levine et al., 2003). Thus reference-group effects seem able to account for much of the mixed data on between- and within-groups differences in self-construal, demonstrating that the apparent problems identified by Matsumoto have more to do with measurement issues than with theoretical flaws.

Although demonstrating between- and within-groups differences in levels of self-construal may be important in supporting the theoretical link between culture and self-construal, the purpose of self-construal theory is not solely to explain cultural differences in cognition, emotion, motivation, and behavior. Even if cultures are becoming more similar and do not reliably differ in related constructs such as individualism and collectivism (cf. Matsumoto, 1999), self-construal theory's greatest contribution remains: the identification of independent, relational, and interdependent self-systems as individual-differences variables that predict other psychological phenomena in reliable and theoretically consistent ways.

Manipulations of Self-Construal

The development of priming manipulations allowed researchers to move from reliance on self-report or proxy measures of self-construal to experimental manipulations of these constructs. As a result, researchers can more confidently examine causal hypotheses and within-culture consequences of activation of the three components of self-construal. The premise in this work is that all persons, no matter their cultural background, construct independent, relational, and collective–interdependent self-construals. Cultural practices and affordances, however, result in variability in the elaboration and accessibility of these dimensions.

Two approaches to manipulating self-construal have dominated research. In the first of these, participants read a story about a ruler selecting a general to send to war based on either individualistic concerns (how it would increase the ruler's status; the IndSC prime) or on collective concerns (the general was a member of the ruler's family; the InterSC prime; Trafimow, Triandis, & Goto, 1991). As expected, participants exposed to the IndSC primes described themselves on the TST using more individual, personal terms than did those exposed to the InterSC primes. Participants exposed to the InterSC primes reported more collective and group-oriented responses than did those exposed to the IndSC primes.

Brewer and Gardner (1996) and Gardner, Gabriel, and Lee (1999) introduced a second manipulation of IndSC and InterSC. In this technique, participants read a story about going on a trip, and they circled either singular pronouns (*I, me, mine*; IndSC prime) or plural pronouns (*we, our, us*; InterSC prime). Control conditions included a task in which third-person pronouns (*they, them*) or impersonal pronouns (*it*) were circled. Brewer and Gardner hypothesized that when the InterSC (*we–us*) is primed, others are included in the self, resulting in an increased perception of similarity to others (relative to the *they*-primed control group). Using a reaction-time task, Brewer and Gardner found that *we*-primed participants made judgments of similarity more quickly than those in the *they*-primed condition, but those in the *they*-primed condition made judgments of dissimilarity more quickly than those in the *we*-primed condition. Later, Gardner and colleagues found that InterSC-primed participants endorsed collectivist values and obligations to help more than IndSC-primed participants. These differences were mediated by differences in TST responses: InterSC-primed participants tended to describe themselves in terms of their relationships and group memberships more than did the IndSC-primed participants, and self-descriptions in turn predicted responses to the values and helping measures.

Other priming tasks have also been used successfully in other studies. In their earliest paper, Trafimow and his colleagues (1991) asked participants to write about what made them *similar* to their friends and family (priming the InterSC) or *different* from their friends and family (IndSC). Stapel and Koomen (2001) primed IndSC and InterSC by having participants write a story about themselves, describing either "who I am," using the words *I, me, myself, mine* in each sentence, or "who we are," using the words *we, our, ourselves, ours*." Finally, Kühnen and Hannover (2000) created a scrambled-sentence task in which the four-word sentences either focused on IndSC ("I like being unique") or on InterSC ("I support my team"). Each scrambled sentence also included one word that was related to type of prime—either a word reflecting independence (*assertive*) or a word reflecting interdependence (*help*). The authors varied the salience of the IndSC or InterSC prime by either having participants write down the unscrambled sentence (the "overt" prime) or having the participants write down the unnecessary word (the "subtle" prime). When participants were primed with the overt IndSC prime, they paradoxically viewed themselves as more similar to the target person than when primed with the InterSC prime. But when exposed to the subtle primes, the InterSC primes led to greater perceived similarity than the IndSC prime.

Concerns about Priming Manipulations

Several questions remain about these priming manipulations. First, it is likely that the two most common InterSC manipulations—the story of the ruler sending the general who is a member of his family into battle (Trafimow et al., 1991) and the story of a trip to the city using plural pronouns (Brewer & Gardner, 1996)—make the *relational* self-construal accessible, rather than the collective self. Brewer and Gardner (1996) attempted to tease apart these two dimensions of the InterSC, but they were only partly successful.

Second, researchers have seldom used priming manipulations with non-Western populations. A few studies have included either Asian Americans or Asian students, and their findings are somewhat mixed. Trafimow and colleagues (1991) included a small group of Asian Americans, and the pattern of individual and group cognitions were similar in the two priming conditions to those of the European American participants. Gardner and her colleagues (1999) found that priming the culturally nondominant dimension of self-construal (e.g., InterSC for European Americans and IndSC for East Asians) resulted in greater differences relative to a no-prime condition than priming the culturally dominant self-construal. Finally, an approach developed by Hong, Morris, Chiu, and Benet-Martínez (2000) exposes bicultural Asians to cultural icons from the East (e.g., the Great Wall of China) or from the West (e.g., Mickey Mouse) to prime cultural knowledge systems. This approach likely primes a variety of culture-relevant thoughts, attitudes, beliefs, and goals—some of which will be related to self-construals—but it does not specifically target self-construal.

How Do Self-Construals Shape Behavior?

Self-Construal Influences Cognition and Information Processing

Thinking about the Self

Markus and Kitayama (1991) argued that individuals with InterSC should be especially likely to pay attention to others and the social context of interaction, resulting in self-representations that include social contexts and elaborate cognitive representations of others. Consistent with this hypothesis, people from collectivist cultures (who are presumed to have high InterSC) report more social, collective, or group-oriented responses on the TST than do people from individualistic cultures (e.g., Kanagawa, Cross, & Markus, 2001). Few studies, however, have examined the association between measures of self-construal and TST responses, and their results have not always shown the expected relations (see Bresnahan et al., 2005; Grace & Cramer, 2003). This discrepancy may be due in part to lack of agreement on a standardized coding scheme for TST responses.

Context-Sensitive Self

If persons with high InterSC are sensitive to situational or relational context, then they should tend to describe themselves differently in different situations. This hypothesis has been supported in studies that use culture as a proxy for self-construal (e.g., Suh, 2002), but the results of studies using measures or manipulations are mixed (e.g., Cross, Gore, & Morris, 2003). Kashima and his colleagues (2004) found that RelSC was associated with contextualized self-description for Japanese participants but not among members of Western societies (Australia, the United Kingdom, and Germany) and was negatively related to context-sensitive self-descriptions among Korean participants. This inconsistency may be due in part to methods that make it more likely that Western participants will feel a press to describe themselves consistently across situations (e.g., a one-time questionnaire).

Context-Dependent Cognition

Researchers have extended research on self-construal and context-dependent cognition beyond self-description. In early work, people with high InterSC tended to report greater attention to the context described in social scenarios and were more likely to attribute outcomes in the scenarios to contextual effects than were others (Singelis, 1994). In an experimental study with German students, InterSC-primed participants were more sensitive to context effects on questions in a questionnaire than were IndSC-primed participants (Haberstroh, Oyserman, Schwarz, Kühnen, & Ji, 2002).

Kühnen, Hannover, and Schubert (2001) found that priming the IndSC (using sentence-completion and other tasks) resulted in context-independent processing and that priming the InterSC resulted in context-dependent processing. For example, when the IndSC was primed, German and American participants were quicker to find geometric figures embedded within more complex geometric designs. In contrast, InterSC-primed participants performed better than IndSC-primed participants on a task that was especially sensitive to context-dependent thinking. In another study, InterSC-primed North American participants were more sensitive to contextual information presented in a causal reasoning induction task than were IndSC-primed participants (Kim, Grimm, & Markman, 2007).

Hannover, Pöhlmann, Springer, and Roeder (2005) have examined additional cognitive consequences of priming self-construals. In one series of studies, they used a modified Stroop task to examine the association between self-construal and attentional focus.

They found more contextual interference effects for participants high in InterSC than for participants high in IndSC. In addition, in a paradigm that involved switching frequently between two different cognitive tasks, participants high in InterSC were less facile in their switches than were the participants high in IndSC. This suggests that IndSC allows the person to quickly and easily focus on a specific task and to inhibit attention to previous or irrelevant tasks.

Relational Self-Construal and Information Processing

Cross, Morris, and Gore (2002) have argued that the RelSC should influence information processing without conscious control, and they examined the role of RelSC in a variety of implicit cognitive processes that centered on relationship-oriented material. They found that North American participants with chronically high RelSC responded more positively to relationship-oriented terms in an Implicit Association Test (IAT) task (Greenwald, McGhee, & Schwartz, 1998) and had denser associative networks for relationship-oriented terms than did those low in RelSC. Cross and her colleagues also found that participants high in RelSC remembered more relationship-related information about a target person and organized information about others in terms of their relationships. In short, persons with chronically high RelSC are "tuned" to pay attention to and to organize their worlds in terms of relationships.

Memory

A focus on the IndSC or InterSC also influences what one remembers. In one study, both European American and Asian or Asian American participants were primed with IndSC or InterSC and asked to recall their earliest memories (Wang & Ross, 2005). The IndSC-primed participants tended to describe more individual-focused memories, whereas the InterSC-primed participants tended to describe more group-focused memories and memories that focused on social interaction. In a follow-up study in which European American and Asian American participants read a child's picture book about a bear going to market, InterSC-primed participants again were more likely than IndSC-primed participants to remember details about social interactions in the story. In other research, InterSC-primed participants had better memory for incidental contextual information when asked to remember the location of items in an array than did IndSC-primed participants (Kühnen & Oyserman, 2002).

Contrast versus Assimilation

Self-construal also influences information-processing styles. For example, priming the IndSC results in contrast or differentiation effects (distinguishing oneself from others), and priming the InterSC results in assimilation or integration effects (connecting oneself to others; Stapel & Koomen, 2001). Furthermore, chronic differences in the activation of these self-construals influence perceived similarity with others (Cross et al., 2002). North American participants rated the descriptiveness of multiple traits, values, and abilities for themselves and a same-sex friend. Similarity scores were calculated by computing intraclass correlations for each person's pair of ratings in each domain (traits, values, and abilities). In regression analyses that controlled for self-esteem, RelSC scores significantly predicted each type of similarity.

Perspective Taking

If others are connected to the self and viewed as self-defining, then a person will tend to take the other's perspective in social interaction and decision making. Cross and colleagues (2000) found that students with high RelSC were more likely to consider the needs and wishes of friends and family members when making decisions than were students with low RelSC. Likewise, Gore and Cross (2006) found that North Americans with high RelSC were more likely to include other people in their rationale for pursuing important goals. People whose InterSC is chronically activated (or primed) tend to give more weight to others' views or opinions about their goals and behaviors than do people with high IndSC (e.g., Ybarra & Trafimow, 1998). In priming studies, Haberstroh and colleagues (2002) showed that InterSC-primed Western participants were

more likely than IndSC-primed participants to take a target person's prior knowledge into account.

Self-Construal Influences Affect

Despite interest in cultural differences in emotion, little research has actually measured self-construals to investigate how they relate to emotion. The few studies that have tend to find that IndSC is associated with lower levels of depression (e.g., Lam, 2005; Okazaki, 1997; Sato & McCann, 1998), unhappiness (Kim, Kasser, & Lee, 2003), general anxiety (e.g., Hardin, Varghese, Tran, & Carlson, 2006; Kim et al., 2003), and social anxiety (Hardin et al., 2006; Okazaki, 1997), whereas InterSC is often associated with higher levels of these negative affects (Hardin et al., 2006; Okazaki, 1997; Sato & McCann, 1998).

Such results raise the question of *why* these relations exist. The relation of self-construal to social anxiety is intuitive; it is not surprising that individuals high in InterSC, for whom interpersonal relationships are central, would express more concern about appropriate behavior in social contexts. Interestingly, IndSC is often found to be a better predictor of social anxiety than InterSC. "In other words, those who were more concerned with asserting one's own judgment and emphasizing autonomy from others were less likely to be socially avoidant, distressed in social situations, and fearful of social evaluations" (Okazaki, 1997, p. 58). But what of the relation of self-construal to other types of negative affect, such as unhappiness and depression? These relations are likely artifactual, explained by the high correlations between social anxiety and other types of negative affect. Okazaki (1997) demonstrated that once social anxiety is controlled, neither IndSC nor InterSC is related to depression.

Such failure to control for social anxiety may account for other findings that, on the surface, appear to contradict predictions of self-construal theory. For example, given that InterSC is consistent with collectivist values, we might expect interdependence to be associated with positive outcomes in collectivist cultures. Some evidence does support this hypothesis: InterSC was associated with greater life satisfaction in Hong

Kong but was unrelated to life satisfaction in the United States (Kwan, Bond, & Singelis, 1997). Surprisingly, then, greater relative InterSC predicted greater unhappiness and less happiness in South Koreans but was unrelated to unhappiness in the United States (Kim et al., 2003). If the measures of happiness and unhappiness used in this study are correlated with social anxiety, the finding that interdependence predicts unhappiness in South Korea may be an artifact of interdependence predicting social anxiety. These results, however, must be interpreted with caution, as they are based on unidimensional self-construal scores.

Other researchers have explored mediators of the relation between self-construal and affect. Given the importance of interpersonal relationships for interdependent people and the importance of internal, private self-evaluations for independent people, Kwan and colleagues (1997) argued—and demonstrated—that relationship harmony fully mediates the relation between InterSC and life satisfaction, whereas global self-esteem fully mediates the relation between IndSC and life satisfaction in samples from Hong Kong and the United States.

Using the same measures of global self-esteem and self-construal in a sample of Vietnamese American adolescents, Lam (2005) also found that self-esteem fully mediates the relation between IndSC and depression. Contrary to the results of Kwan and colleagues (1997), however, self-esteem also fully mediated the relation between InterSC and depression. As in other samples, IndSC in Lam's sample was associated with greater self-esteem (Kwan et al., 1997) and less depression (Okazaki, 1997; Sato & McCann, 1998); contrary to past research, however, InterSC was also associated with greater self-esteem and less depression. This is likely due to the more bicultural nature of Lam's adolescent sample, which, in contrast to other studies that have used college students (Kwan et al., 1997; Okazaki, 1997; Sato & McCann, 1998), consisted of adolescents living in ethnically enculturated families. Thus Lam argued that higher interdependence reflected an important cultural consistency with the participants' home environments, which in turn was associated with greater self-esteem and less depression.

Finally, Lam (2005) argued that family cohesion should be more important to the self-esteem of interdependent adolescents, whereas peer support should be more important to the self-esteem of independent adolescents. Indeed, family cohesion fully mediated the relation between InterSC and global self-esteem, whereas peer support partially mediated the relation between IndSC and self-esteem.

Relational Self-Construal and Affect

Although RelSC is not associated with general psychological well-being among predominantly European American college students, it is associated with greater *relational* well-being (Cross et al., 2003). RelSC is related to general well-being in other samples. Berkel and Constantine (2005) argued that a need for affiliation may be stronger and more beneficial to women of color in predominantly white environments and hypothesized that RelSC would predict life satisfaction among these women of color. Indeed, in their sample of African American and Asian American women recruited from a predominantly white university, greater RelSC predicted greater life satisfaction, even after controlling for relationship harmony and family conflict.

Self-Construal Influences Motivation and Self-Regulation

Markus and Kitayama's (1991) conceptualization has several implications for the manifestation of motivations. First, for the InterSC, being a part of social groups and maintaining harmonious relationships with important others are of great importance, in contrast to the autonomy-related needs of the IndSC. To date, however, only a few studies have used measures or manipulations of self-construal to examine motivational processes. One such study found that cultural orientation of individualism–collectivism and self-construal were both related to sensitivity to a partner's concerns for saving face in conflict situations (Oetzel & Ting-Toomey, 2003). Moreover, InterSC was positively related to avoiding confrontation in a conflict and engaging in integrative behavior. IndSC, on the other hand, was related to dominating behavior in such a situation. These results imply that people with high InterSC are motivated to avoid potentially harmful behavior in order to maintain harmony.

Second, agency for these two self-systems results from different motivational sources. For the IndSC, personal goals, desires, and abilities become the fuel for action, whereas for the InterSC, goals, desires, and needs of relational others coordinated with those of the self are the sources of agency (Markus & Kitayama, 2004). These motivational differences were illustrated in a study by Iyengar and Lepper (1999), which found that European American children performed best when given the opportunity to select tasks for themselves, whereas Asian American children performed best when tasks were presumably selected by their mothers. The children from collectivistic and individualistic backgrounds were equally agentic, but the sources of the motivation that grounds agency were different for the two groups.

Unfortunately, Iyengar and Lepper (1999) did not assess the self-construals of their participants. Gore and Cross (2006), however, examined the relations between RelSC and two reasons for pursuing goals: relational and personal reasons. For example, a person could pursue a goal for a personally autonomous reason (e.g., "because it is important to me") or for a relationally autonomous reason (e.g., "because it is important to someone who is close to me"). A similar distinction was made for controlled reasons for goals. People with higher RelSC indicated more relational autonomous reasons for their goals compared with those with lower RelSC, and both personal and relational autonomous reasons for goals affected perceived progress and effort. Moreover, a second longitudinal study showed that relational autonomous reasons were influential in goal pursuits over time. The results of these studies indicate that autonomous reasons can be both personal and relational, which fits with the concept of interdependent agency proposed by Markus and Kitayama (2004).

A third important implication of self-construals concerns self-related motives. Motives that are directly related to the self (i.e., self-motives) are expected to be experienced very differently depending on one's self-construal. One such self-motive, self-enhancement, has attracted a significant amount of research and has prompted a lively debate.

Self-Enhancement

In social-psychological theorizing, the needs to view oneself with positive regard and to protect oneself from negative information have long been considered to be basic tendencies of the self. As Heine, Lehman, Markus, and Kitayama (1999) argued, however, enhancing one's positive internal attributes and seeing oneself with positive regard bring one closer to the cultural ideal of an independent self in individualistic societies. In cultural contexts conducive to the development of interdependent selves, group harmony is encouraged, and the self's needs are expected to be sacrificed if they conflict with group needs. Being a good group member requires self-improvement, which depends largely on self-monitoring and a self-critical attitude. In such a cultural environment, self-enhancement would be detrimental to basic social needs such as maintaining harmonious relationships.

Most research on self-enhancement has relied only on group comparisons, using the individualism–collectivism of the given culture as a proxy for self-construal. This line of research has proven valuable in providing evidence for the claim of cultural variation in self-enhancement with a range of self-enhancing behaviors (e.g., Heine, Kitayama, & Lehman, 2001). Others, however, have argued that self-enhancement is a universal motivation (e.g., Sedikides, Gaertner, & Toguchi, 2003). Unfortunately, very few of the studies testing this hypothesis have employed measures or manipulations of self-construal, leaving unclear whether differences in self-construal account for observed differences in self-enhancement.

One exception to this oversight is provided in research by Kurman (2001), who examined the better-than-average effect among Israeli Druze (an Arabic minority), Israeli Jews, and Singaporean Chinese. Kurman found that when trait adjectives used in better-than-average studies were differentiated according to their value for collectivistic and individualistic settings (e.g., *intelligent* for the IndSC, *agreeable* for the InterSC), self-enhancement occurred on attributes consistent with the individual's cultural background. Analyses at the individual level revealed that IndSC, but not InterSC, was related to self-enhancement on agentic traits. Self-enhancement on communal traits was related to InterSC, but not to IndSC. A cautionary note is in order, however: Correlating self-construal scores of individual participants with their standing on the better-than-average measure does not provide us with the appropriate information concerning the presence of a self-serving bias (see Heine & Hamamura, 2007, for a discussion of this problem).

Implicit comparisons with others also influence self-esteem, but the impact of these comparisons may depend on self-construal. Gardner, Gabriel, and Hochschild (2002) examined Tesser's (1980) self-evaluation maintenance (SEM) model, which predicts that self-esteem is threatened when a close other outperforms oneself in a personally important domain. These effects are reversed when the target of comparison is not close or when the performance is not personally important. Gardner and colleagues' results revealed that the expected SEM effects occurred only for participants in an IndSC prime condition, not for those in the InterSC prime condition. This implies that for people with an InterSC, comparing oneself with a close other is not a source of threat but instead is an opportunity to bask in the reflected glory of the relational other (see also Cheng & Lam, 2007).

Self-Regulation

Self-regulation is an essential element in any goal-directed behavior, and, as such, it is extremely relevant to the dynamic relation between motivation and self-construal. According to Higgins (1996, 1997), there are two basic self-regulatory foci: a promotion focus, which is characterized by an approach motivation toward desired end states, and a prevention focus, which is characterized by an avoidance motivation away from undesired end states. For people with an InterSC, failing to live up to one's obligations or to the expectations of significant others is a constant concern, which can create a prevention focus. People with an IndSC, in contrast, are socialized to pursue personal aspirations, which can create a promotion focus. Indeed, when presented with scenarios that provided the same information with either a promotion or prevention framing, participants with an InterSC evaluated loss-framed information as more important than gain-framed information, and participants with an IndSC evaluated gain-framed information as more important than loss-framed information (Lee, Aaker, & Gardner, 2000).

Challenged by a stressful situation, people can cope with it by either changing the environment to fit their personal needs (primary control) or by altering their own feelings and cognitions to adjust to the objective environment (secondary control; Weisz, Rothbaum, & Blackburn, 1984). In their description of primary and secondary control, Weisz and his colleagues (1984) pointed to Japan as an example of a society that promotes adjustment to the environment rather than control over it. Building on their work, researchers have hypothesized that people who construe themselves in relation to others would prefer secondary control over primary control and that the reverse would be true of people who construe themselves as independent of others. In one study, Asian participants scored higher than Americans on a self-report measure of secondary control, whereas American participants scored higher than Asians on primary control (Lam & Zane, 2004). IndSC was positively related to primary control, while the InterSC was related to secondary control, and self-construal accounted for cultural differences in preferences for types of control.

These results point to the willingness of people with high InterSC to change themselves to adjust to the situation. This willingness to adjust may cause one to develop stronger self-control over time. According to Baumeister and his colleagues, self-regulatory strength is analogous to the strength of a muscle in that recent use leads to temporary exhaustion, or "ego depletion" (Baumeister & Vohs, 2003). Although it is exhaustible, the strength of this "muscle" can be improved by chronic use. For this reason, one would expect people with high InterSC to experience less ego depletion after a self-regulatory task. The results of a study by Seeley and Gardner (2003) supported this hypothesis: Regulatory depletion was greater for participants with high IndSC than for those with high InterSC, and it was more pronounced for Americans than for Asians. These findings suggest that for individuals with high InterSC, self-regulation may be construed as primarily serving social goals.

Self-Construal Shapes Interpersonal Behavior

How does variation in self-construal shape interaction with other people? People with high InterSC should seek to maintain connectedness and harmony in relationships, whereas those with high IndSC should seek to maintain individuality and separateness from others (Markus & Kitayama, 1991). Pursuit of these goals may be relatively automatic or nonconscious when the associated self-construal is chronically or temporarily activated. For example, people who have chronically high InterSC (or who are primed with InterSC) tend to sit closer to another person in a lab situation than do those with a primed or chronically high IndSC (Holland, Roeder, van Baaren, Brandt, & Hannover, 2004). Similarly, priming the InterSC results in a greater likelihood of an individual's imitating the behavior of another person, compared with priming the IndSC or with a control condition (van Baaren, Maddux, Chartrand, de Bouter, & van Knippenberg, 2003). The association between self-construal and mimicry is bidirectional: People who are imitated by others also come to describe themselves more interdependently than do people who are not mimicked (Ashton-James, van Baaren, Chartran, Decety, & Karremans, 2007).

These laboratory studies of proximity and mimicry provide compelling confirmation that InterSC promotes positive relational behavior, because there is no prior relationship between the partners. When there is an ongoing relationship, however, individuals with high RelSC should tend to engage in behaviors that promote closeness and harmony. Cross and her colleagues (Cross & Morris, 2003; Gore, Cross, & Morris, 2006) have investigated how North Americans with varying levels of RelSC (as measured by the RISC scale; Cross et al., 2000) interact with strangers who were assigned to be their roommates. They found that measures of the RelSC were positively associated with participants' self-reports of open self-disclosure and with their partners' reports of feeling supported and encouraged by the participant (Gore et al., 2006). In a prospective study that examined these processes over a 1-month period, Gore and colleagues (2006, Study 2) found that both highly re-

lational individuals and their roommates reported enhanced relationship quality after 1 month. Furthermore, the participants with high RelSC were better able than others to predict their roommates' responses to statements assessing their values and beliefs (Cross & Morris, 2003). In short, the participants with high RelSC interacted with their roommates in ways that created a supportive environment for the relationship to develop.

To date, researchers have paid little attention to the role of variation in self-construal in romantic relationships. In one of the few studies, Sinclair and Fehr (2005) examined the association between self-construal and responses to dissatisfaction in romantic relationships. Whether measured or primed, IndSC was positively associated with the preference for using the active, constructive strategy of *voice* when one was dissatisfied with the relationship. InterSC was positively associated with the passive, constructive strategy of *loyalty*, in which the person waits for things to improve. These findings are consistent with research that suggests that IndSC is associated with a promotion focus and that InterSC is associated with a prevention focus (Lee et al., 2000) and with other studies showing that individuals with high InterSCs avoid dominating forms of conflict resolution (see the next subsection).

Self-Construal and Communication Processes

The focus on harmonious relationships among those with high InterSC should result in a preference for indirect communication, sensitivity to the context in social interaction, attention to others' thoughts and feelings, and nonconfrontational conflict resolution styles (Singelis & Brown, 1995). In contrast, for individuals with high IndSC, the goal of communication is to express the person's unique goals, wishes, thoughts, and feelings. As a result, the IndSC should be associated with direct communication styles, little attention to contextual aspects of social interaction, attention to one's own thoughts and feelings, and willingness to engage in confrontational dispute resolution styles.

Researchers have made several inroads into investigating these theoretical consequences of self-construal for communication. For example, InterSC is positively related to concern for a conversation partners' feelings and possible negative evaluation of the self (Gudykunst et al., 1996; Kim, Sharkey & Singelis, 1994), as well as to communication apprehension, a desire to avoid arguments (Kim, Aune, Hunter, Kim, & Kim, 2001), and the use of cooperative strategies in group discussions (Oetzel, 1998). IndSC is positively related to a concern for clarity or directness in communication (Gudykunst et al., 1996; Kim et al., 1994), open and expressive communication (Gudykunst et al., 1996), and the use of assertive or dominating strategies in group discussions (Oetzel, 1998). Unfortunately, most studies of self-construal and communication employ cross-sectional designs and use only self-report data. New advances may be made by using experimental paradigms in which self-construal is manipulated and behavioral measures of direct or indirect, confrontive or nonconfrontive communication strategies are used (see Seeley Howard, Gardner, & Thompson, 2007, for an example of such a study).

Self-Construals and Organizational Justice

Finally, a few researchers have begun to consider the role of self-construal in organizational justice. For example, Brockner, De Cremer, van den Bos, and Chen (2005) argued that because procedural fairness communicates that individuals are respected and valued, it therefore reflects the importance of relational values. Thus people who tend to define themselves in terms of their relationships may be especially sensitive to procedural fairness in organizations. Brockner and his colleagues found that perceptions of procedural fairness (e.g., the degree to which one has a voice in decisions or the fairness of interpersonal treatment) were more strongly related to a variety of outcomes (e.g., cooperation, positive affect, and desire to interact with the other party) for people who had high InterSC than for those who scored low on this dimension. Others have found that the degree to which the three dimensions of self-construal (independent, relational, and collective) moderate the association between procedural justice and work-related outcomes differs depending on the specific forms of procedural justice under investigation (Johnson, Selenta, & Lord, 2006).

Conclusions

Many theoretical, measurement, and empirical questions remain in research on self-construals. Theoretically, researchers need to agree on a common definition of RelSC and InterSC. Initially, the term *interdependent* applied to both relational and group-oriented self-construals. Some researchers have begun to disentangle the two (e.g., Brewer & Chen, 2007), but not everyone recognizes this distinction. In addition, research would be advanced with further developments of manipulations that are targeted specifically at relational versus collective InterSCs. As we mentioned, it is quite likely that the manipulations initially developed to prime InterSC actually activate relational selves (rather than group-oriented collective selves). Finally, advances in measurement that focus on specific dimensions of IndSC, RelSC, and InterSC (such as autonomy, behavioral consistency, or primacy of self) will allow researchers to distinguish the specific processes, values, and beliefs that underlie different forms of being independent or interdependent.

The distinction that Markus and Kitayama (1991) made between the IndSC and the InterSC, and the later addition of the RelSC, have generated considerable research and fruitful theories. Although not all that research could be reviewed here, we have attempted to provide an overview of those efforts and a snapshot of the current status of these constructs. This snapshot is somewhat fuzzy now, but the details of the picture will become sharper, clearer, and much more intriguing as researchers continue to puzzle over how self-construal shapes behavior.

References

Aaker, J. L. (2000). Accessibility or diagnosticity?: Disentangling the influence of culture on persuasion processes and attitudes. *Journal of Consumer Research, 26,* 340-357.

Ashton-James, C., van Baaren, R. B., Chartrand, T. L., Decety, J., & Karremans, J. (2007). Mimicry and me: The impact of mimicry on self-construal. *Social Cognition, 25,* 518-535.

Baumeister, R. F., & Vohs, K. D. (2003). Self-regulation and the executive function of the self. In M. R. Leary & J. P. Tangney (Eds.), *Handbook of self and identity* (pp. 197–217). New York: Guilford Press.

Berkel, L. A., & Constantine, M. G. (2005). Relational

variables and life satisfaction in African American and Asian American college women. *Journal of College Counseling, 8,* 5–13.

Bresnahan, M. J., Levine, T. R., Shearman, S. M., Lee, S. Y., Park, C., & Kiyomiya, T. (2005). A multimethod multitrait validity assessment of self-construal in Japan, Korea, and the United States. *Human Communication Research, 31,* 33–59.

Brewer, M. B., & Chen, Y. (2007). Where (who) are collectives in collectivism?: Toward conceptual clarification of individualism and collectivism. *Psychological Review, 114,* 133–151.

Brewer, M. B., & Gardner, W. (1996). Who is this "we"?: Levels of collective identity and self representations. *Journal of Personality and Social Psychology, 71,* 83–93.

Brockner, J., De Cremer, D., van den Bos, K., & Chen, Y. R. (2005). The influence of interdependent self-construal on procedural fairness effects. *Organizational Behavior and Human Decision Processes, 96,* 155–167.

Cheng, R. W., & Lam, S. (2007). Self-construal and social comparison effects. *British Journal of Educational Psychology, 77,* 197–211.

Cross, S. E., Bacon, P. L., & Morris, M. L. (2000). The relational–interdependent self-construal and relationships. *Journal of Personality and Social Psychology, 78,* 791–808.

Cross, S. E., Gore, J. S., & Morris, M. L. (2003). The relational–interdependent self-construal, self-concept consistency, and well-being. *Journal of Personality and Social Psychology, 85,* 933–944.

Cross, S. E., & Madson, L. (1997). Models of the self: Self-construals and gender. *Psychological Bulletin, 122,* 5–37.

Cross, S. E., & Morris, M. L. (2003). Getting to know you: The relational self-construal, relational cognition, and well-being. *Personality and Social Psychology Bulletin, 29,* 512–523.

Cross, S. E., Morris, M. L., & Gore, J. S. (2002). Thinking about oneself and others: The relational–interdependent self-construal and social cognition. *Journal of Personality and Social Psychology, 82,* 399–418.

Gabriel, S., & Gardner, W. L. (1999). Are there "his" and "hers" types of interdependence?: The implications of gender differences in collective versus relational interdependence for affect, behavior, and cognition. *Journal of Personality and Social Psychology, 77,* 642–655.

Gardner, W. L., Gabriel, S., & Hochschild, L. (2002). When you and I are "we," you are not threatening: The role of self-expansion in social comparison. *Journal of Personality and Social Psychology, 82,* 239–251.

Gardner, W. L., Gabriel, S., & Lee, A. Y. (1999). "I" value freedom, but "we" value relationships: Self-construal priming mirrors cultural differences in judgment. *Psychological Science, 10,* 321–326.

Gore, J. S., & Cross, S. E. (2006). Pursuing goals for us: Relationally autonomous reasons in long-term goal pursuit. *Journal of Personality and Social Psychology, 90,* 848–861.

Gore, J. S., Cross, S. E., & Morris, M. L. (2006). Let's be friends: Relational self-construal and the development of intimacy. *Personal Relationships, 13,* 83–102.

Grace, S. L., & Cramer, K. L. (2003). The elusive nature of self-measurement: The self-construal scale versus the twenty statements test. *Journal of Social Psychology, 143,* 649–668.

Greenwald, A. G., McGhee, D. E., & Schwartz, J. L. K. (1998). Measuring individual differences in implicit cognition: The Implicit Association Test. *Journal of Personality and Social Psychology, 74,* 1464–1480.

Gudykunst, W. B., Matsumoto, Y., Ting-Toomey, S., Nishida, T., Kim, K., & Heyman, H. (1996). The influence of cultural individualism–collectivism, self-construals, and individual values on communication styles across cultures. *Human Communication Research, 22,* 510–543.

Haberstroh, S., Oyserman, D., Schwarz, N., Kühnen, U., & Ji, L. (2002). Is the interdependent self more sensitive to question context than the independent self?: Self-construal and the observation of conversational norms. *Journal of Experimental Social Psychology, 38,* 323–329.

Hannover, B., Pöhlmann, C., Springer, A., & Roeder, U. (2005). Implications of independent versus interdependent self-knowledge for motivated social cognition: The semantic procedural interface model of the self. *Self and Identity, 4,* 159–175.

Harb, C., & Smith, P. B. (2008). Self-construals across cultures: Beyond independence–interdependence. *Journal of Cross-Cultural Psychology, 39,* 178–197.

Hardin, E. E. (2006). Convergent evidence for the multidimensionality of self-construal. *Journal of Cross-Cultural Psychology, 37,* 516–521.

Hardin, E. E., Leong, F. T. L., & Bhagwat, A. A. (2004). Factor structure of the Self-Construal Scale revisited: Implications for the multidimensionality of self-construal. *Journal of Cross-Cultural Psychology, 35,* 327–345.

Hardin, E. E., Varghese, F. V., Tran, U. V., & Carlson, A. Z. (2006). Anxiety and career exploration: Gender differences in the role of self-construal. *Journal of Vocational Behavior, 69,* 346–358.

Heine, S. J., & Hamamura, T. (2007). In search of East Asian self-enhancement. *Personality and Social Psychology Review, 11,* 4–27.

Heine, S. J., Kitayama, S., & Lehman, D. R. (2001). Cultural differences in self-evaluation: Japanese readily accept negative self-relevant information. *Journal of Cross-Cultural Psychology, 32,* 434–443.

Heine, S. J., Lehman, D. R., Markus, H. R., & Kitayama, S. (1999). Is there a universal need for positive self-regard? *Psychological Review, 106,* 766–794.

Heine, S. J., Lehman, D. R., Peng, K., & Greenholtz, J. (2002). What's wrong with cross-cultural comparisons of subjective Likert scales?: The reference-group effect. *Journal of Personality and Social Psychology, 82,* 903–918.

Higgins, E. T. (1996). The "self-digest": Self-knowledge serving self-regulatory functions. *Journal of Personality and Social Psychology, 71,* 1062–1083.

Higgins, E. T. (1997). Beyond pleasure and pain. *American Psychologist, 52,* 1280–1300.

Holland, R. W., Roeder, U., van Baaren, R. B., Brandt, A. C., & Hannover, B. (2004). Don't stand so close to me: The effects of self-construal on interpersonal closeness. *Psychological Science, 15,* 237–242.

Hong, Y., Morris, M. W., Chiu, C., & Benet-Martínez, V. (2000). Multicultural minds: A dynamic constructivist approach to culture and cognition. *American Psychologist, 55*, 709–720.

Iyengar, S. S., & Lepper, M. R. (1999). Rethinking the value of choice: A cultural perspective on intrinsic motivation. *Journal of Personality and Social Psychology, 76*, 349–366.

Johnson, R. E., Selenta, C., & Lord, R. G. (2006). When organizational justice and the self-concept meet: Consequences for the organization and its members. *Organizational Behavior and Human Decision Processes, 99*, 175–201.

Kanagawa, C., Cross, S. E., & Markus, H. R. (2001). "Who am I?": The cultural psychology of the conceptual self. *Personality and Social Psychology Bulletin, 27*, 90–103.

Kashima, Y., Kashima, E., Farsides, T., Kim, U., Strack, F., Werth, L., et al. (2004). Culture and context-sensitive self: The amount and meaning of context sensitivity of phenomenal self differ across cultures. *Self and Identity, 3*, 125–141.

Kim, K., Grimm, L. R., & Markman, A. B. (2007). Self-construal and the processing of covariation information in causal reasoning. *Memory and Cognition, 35*, 1337–1343.

Kim, M., Aune, K. S., Hunter, J. E., Kim, H., & Kim, J. (2001). The effect of culture and self-construals on predispositions toward verbal communication. *Human Communication Research, 27*, 382–408.

Kim, M., Sharkey, W. F., & Singelis, T. M. (1994). The relationships between individuals' self-construals and perceived importance of interactive constraints. *International Journal of Intercultural Relations, 18*, 117–140.

Kim, Y., Kasser, T., & Lee, H. (2003). Self-concept, aspirations, and well-being in South Korea and the United States. *Journal of Social Psychology, 143*, 277–290.

Kuhn, M. H., & McPartland, T. (1954). An empirical investigation of self-attitudes. *American Sociological Review, 19*, 58–76.

Kurman, J. (2001). Self-enhancement: Is it restricted to individualistic cultures? *Personality and Social Psychology Bulletin, 27*, 1705–1716.

Kühnen, U., & Hannover, B. (2000). Assimilation and contrast in social comparisons as a consequence of self-construal activation. *European Journal of Social Psychology, 30*, 799–811.

Kühnen, U., Hannover, B., & Schubert, B. (2001). The semantic–procedural interface model of the self: The role of self-knowledge for context-dependent versus context-independent modes of thinking. *Journal of Personality and Social Psychology, 80*, 397–409.

Kühnen, U., & Oyserman, D. (2002). Thinking about the self influences thinking in general: Cognitive consequences of salient self-concept. *Journal of Experimental Social Psychology, 38*, 492–499.

Kwan, V. S. Y., Bond, M. H., & Singelis, T. M. (1997). Pancultural explanations for life satisfaction: Adding relationship harmony to self-esteem. *Journal of Personality and Social Psychology, 73*, 1038–1051.

Lam, A. G., & Zane, N. W. S. (2004). Ethnic differences in coping with interpersonal stressors: A test of self-construals as cultural mediators. *Journal of Cross-Cultural Psychology, 35*, 446–459.

Lam, B. T. (2005). Self-construal and depression among Vietnamese American adolescents. *International Journal of Intercultural Relations, 29*, 239–250.

Lee, A. Y., Aaker, J. L., & Gardner, W. L. (2000). The pleasures and pains of distinct self-construals: The role of interdependence in regulatory focus. *Journal of Personality and Social Psychology, 78*, 1122–1134.

Levine, T. R., Bresnahan, M. J., Park, H. S., Lapinski, M. K., Wittenbaum, G. M., Shearman, S. M., et al. (2003). Self-construal scales lack validity. *Human Communication Research, 29*, 210–252.

Markus, H. R., & Kitayama, S. (1991). Culture and the self: Implications for cognition, emotion, and motivation. *Psychological Review, 98*, 224–253.

Markus, H. R., & Kitayama, S. (2004). Models of agency: Sociocultural diversity in the construction of action. In V. Murphy-Berman & J. J. Berman (Eds.), *Nebraska Symposium on Motivation: Vol. 49. Cross-cultural differences in perspectives on the self* (pp. 1–57). Lincoln: University of Nebraska Press.

Matsumoto, D. (1999). Culture and self: An empirical assessment of Markus and Kitayama's theory of independent and interdependent self-construal. *Asian Journal of Social Psychology, 2*, 289–310.

Oetzel, J. G. (1998). Explaining individual communication processes in homogeneous and heterogeneous groups through individualism–collectivism and self-construal. *Human Communication Research, 25*, 202–224.

Oetzel, J. G., & Ting-Toomey, S. (2003). Face concerns in interpersonal conflict: A cross-cultural empirical test of face negation theory. *Communication Research, 30*, 599–624.

Okazaki, S. (1997). Sources of ethnic differences between Asian American and white American college students on measures of depression and social anxiety. *Journal of Abnormal Psychology, 106*, 52–60.

Oyserman, D., Coon, H. M., & Kemmelmeier, M. (2002). Rethinking individualism and collectivism: Evaluation of theoretical assumptions and meta-analyses. *Psychological Bulletin, 128*, 3–72.

Sato, T., & McCann, D. (1998). Individual differences in relatedness and individuality: An exploration of two constructs. *Personality and Individual Differences, 24*, 847–859.

Sedikides, C., & Brewer, M. B. (Eds.). (2001). *Individual self, relational self, collective self.* New York: Psychology Press.

Sedikides, C., Gaertner, L., & Toguchi, Y. (2003). Pancultural self-enhancement. *Journal of Personality and Social Psychology, 84*(1), 60–79.

Seeley, E. A., & Gardner, W. L. (2003). The "selfless" and self-regulation: The role of chronic other-orientation in averting self-regulatory depletion. *Self and Identity, 2*, 103–117.

Seeley Howard, E., Gardner, W. L., & Thompson, L. (2007). The role of the self-concept and the social context in determining the behavior of power holders: Self-construal in intergroup versus dyadic dispute resolution negotiations. *Journal of Personality and Social Psychology, 93*, 614–631.

Sinclair, L., & Fehr, B. (2005). Voice vs. loyalty: Self-construals and responses to dissatisfaction in romantic relationships. *Journal of Experimental Social Psychology, 41*, 298–304.

Singelis, T. M. (1994). The measurement of independent and interdependent self-construals. *Personality and Social Psychology Bulletin, 20*, 580–591.

Singelis, T. M., & Brown, W. J. (1995). Culture, self, and collectivist communication: Linking culture to individual behavior. *Human Communication Research, 21*, 354–389.

Singelis, T. M., Triandis, H. C., Bhawuk, D., & Gelfand, M. J. (1995). Horizontal and vertical dimensions of individualism and collectivism: A theoretical and measurement refinement. *Cross-Cultural Research: The Journal of Comparative Social Science, 29*, 240–275.

Somech, A. (2000). The independent and the interdependent selves: Different meanings in different cultures. *International Journal of Intercultural Relations, 24*, 161–172.

Stapel, D. A., & Koomen, W. (2001). I, we, and the effects of others on me: How self-construal level moderates social comparison effects. *Journal of Personality and Social Psychology, 80*, 766–781.

Suh, E. M. (2002). Culture, identity consistency, and subjective well-being. *Journal of Personality and Social Psychology, 83*, 1378–1391.

Tesser, A. (1980). Self-esteem maintenance in family dynamics. *Journal of Personality and Social Psychology, 39*, 77–91.

Trafimow, D., Triandis, H. C., & Goto, S. G. (1991). Some tests of the distinction between the private self and the collective self. *Journal of Personality and Social Psychology, 60*, 649–655.

van Baaren, R. B., Maddux, W. W., Chartrand, T. L., de Bouter, C., & van Knippenberg, A. (2003). It takes two to mimic: Behavioral consequences of self-construals. *Journal of Personality and Social Psychology, 84*, 1093–1102.

Wang, Q., & Ross, M. (2005). What we remember and what we tell: The effects of culture and self-priming on memory representations and narratives. *Memory, 13*, 594–606.

Weisz, J. R., Rothbaum, F. M., & Blackburn, T. C. (1984). Standing out and standing in: The psychology of control in America and Japan. *American Psychologist, 39*, 955–969.

Ybarra, O., & Trafimow, D. (1998). How priming the private self or collective self affects the relative weights of attitudes and subjective norms. *Personality and Social Psychology Bulletin, 24*, 362–370.

CHAPTER 36

■ ● ▲ ◆ ■ ● ▲ ◆

Self-Esteem

JENNIFER K. BOSSON
WILLIAM B. SWANN, JR.

Self-esteem refers to people's evaluations of themselves. It is, at once, one of psychology's most important and controversial constructs. It has inspired a vast literature, including scores of books and thousands of articles. At the same time, it has attracted a small but vocal cadre of critics who argue that it is essentially useless and adds little, if anything, to our ability to predict important social outcomes. We suggest here that the checkered reputation of self-esteem owes, in part, to disagreements regarding what it is and how its consequences ought to be assessed. In this chapter, we offer a compromise by proposing a broad definition of self-esteem and discussing its nature, origins, and consequences. To set the stage for this discussion, we begin with a brief history of the construct.

A Brief History of Self-Esteem

Like the proverbial blind men who formed very different impressions of an elephant based on the part of the elephant's body that they touched, different authors have focused on different aspects of self-esteem and, accordingly, come away with dramatically different views of it. William James (1890/1950), for example, noted that people can stake their self-worth on strikingly dis-tinct qualities, with the result that anyone can achieve high self-esteem so long as they emphasize their strengths and devalue their weaknesses. In contrast, Cooley (1902) focused on the interpersonal processes that generate and sustain people's beliefs about themselves and concluded that we rely on the reactions of others, particularly significant others, in forming impressions of ourselves.

Within mainstream American psychology, interest in self-esteem waned during the first half of the 20th century. This dip in interest occurred, in large measure, because of the dominance of behaviorism and its hostility toward mentalistic constructs such as self-esteem. Progress was made during this era, however, in conceptualizing narcissism, which is a disorder of self-esteem. Freud (1914/1957) introduced the idea of narcissism, or excessive self-love, to the psychoanalytical literature. He believed that whereas self-love was a normal feature of the developing child, it could grow into a pathological condition if it became excessive. Over the years theorists have offered many variations on Freud's original arguments, but there seems to be some agreement that narcissism emerges when troubled interpersonal relationships undermine individuals' certainty in their own self-worth. Such doubts cause narcissists to overreact when they encounter challenges to the self (e.g., American Psychiatric Association, 2000; Morf & Rhodewalt, 2001; Paulhus, Robins, Trzesniewski, & Tracy, 2004; Raskin, Novacek, & Hogan, 1991; Westen, 1990).

By the late 1950s, behaviorism was beginning to lose its grip on psychology in America. As a result, more and more theorists began focusing on issues related to the self, although most avoided using the language of self-esteem. In his theory of social comparison, for example, Festinger (1954) posited that people learn about their abilities and opinions by comparing themselves with others. Although Festinger did not state that social comparison could serve as a basis for self-esteem, such a conclusion is surely compatible with his formulation. Similarly, although Bem (1972) refrained from discussing self-esteem in his self-perception theory, his notion that people derive self-knowledge from observing their own behavior and the conditions under which it occurs can be understood as a means through which people develop self-esteem.

Not long after the introduction of Bem's (1972) theory, there was an explosion of interest in the self within social psychology. There were several reasons for this emerging interest, but one factor seems to have been the success of efforts to draw parallels between self-knowledge and other cognitive structures (e.g., Kuiper & Rogers, 1979; Markus, 1977). By drawing on well-researched cognitive phenomena—such as mental schemas, encoding, and priming effects—research on the self and self-esteem earned new credibility.

Independent of these developments in academia, a self-esteem movement emerged within the lay community in the late 1960s (Branden, 1994; see also Twenge & Campbell, 2001). The movement peaked in the 1980s with the formation of the California Task Force to Promote Self-Esteem and Personal and Social Responsibility (1990). On the basis of no empirical evidence (in fact, evidence pointed to the contrary), the movement characterized self-esteem as a panacea that would cure a wide range of social ills, from teenage pregnancy and welfare dependency to juvenile delinquency and low educational attainment. As a result, thousands of Americans came to believe not only that raising self-esteem could cure all of society's

problems but also that it could be accomplished by merely reciting a few affirmations such as "I am lovable and capable."

Members of the academic community challenged the extravagant claims of the self-esteem movement, noting that they lacked a solid basis in reality (e.g., Dawes, 1994; Swann, 1996). Some authors recently took the argument a step further, not only echoing the criticisms of the self-esteem movement but also questioning the viability of the self-esteem construct itself. Most significantly, after reviewing a subset of the self-esteem literature, Baumeister, Campbell, Krueger, and Vohs (2003) asserted that measures of self-esteem fail to offer strong predictions of socially important behaviors, as promised by the California Task Force. Some have taken this gloomy assessment to mean that self-esteem is not a viable construct and that its effects should no longer be studied (Scheff & Fearon, 2004).

Others, however, took issue with Baumeister and colleagues' (2003) conclusions regarding the viability of the self-esteem construct (e.g., Marsh & Craven, 2006; Swann, Chang-Schneider, & McClarty, 2007, 2008). For example, Swann, Chang-Schneider, and McClarty (2007) countered Baumeister and colleagues' claims by proposing that, in evaluating the capacity of a global construct (self-esteem) to predict a host of specific behaviors, Baumeister and colleagues had failed to heed a widely recognized doctrine of psychometrics (see Ajzen & Fishbein, 2005). We elaborate on this issue and related ones in the course of discussing the nature of self-esteem.

The Nature of Self-Esteem

A key aspect of understanding self-esteem is recognizing its relationship to self-concepts and other cognitive structures. Some authors contend that self-esteem is the "affective" component of self-representation (i.e., what people *feel* about themselves) and that self-concepts are "cognitive" components of self-representation (i.e., what people *believe* about themselves). Although the affective–cognitive distinction is useful in some contexts, we do not believe that it is the most useful means of distinguishing self-esteem from self-concepts, as empirical support for this distinction is lacking (Marsh, 1986; Marsh & Hattie, 1996; Shavelson, Hubner, & Stanton, 1976). It is not difficult to see why. After all, many of the self-concepts that social–personality psychologists study are strongly affectively charged. People often care a great deal, for example, about their beliefs that they are intelligent, athletic, or dominant. Likewise, *social* self-concepts (self-concepts that align people to groups, such as Christian, American, or teacher) are sometimes held so passionately that their bearers make huge sacrifices for them, even to the point of giving up their lives. Not only do self-concepts often have an affective component, but self-esteem also has a belief component; it is, after all, a belief about one's worth. Using the affective–cognitive distinction to distinguish self-esteem from self-concepts thus rests on shaky conceptual as well as empirical grounds.

In this chapter we define self-esteem as a global view of the self and self-concepts as relatively specific views of the self along various dimensions (e.g., honest, clumsy, mathematically inclined). Rather than making categorical distinctions between self-esteem and self-concepts, we suggest that they represent different levels of specificity within the superordinate category of *self-views* (see also Swann, Chang-Schneider, & McClarty, 2007).

This conceptualization of self-esteem has clear implications for how its consequences should be assessed. Specifically, if self-esteem and self-concepts are simply more or less specific members of the same overarching category, it makes little sense to consider the predictive validity of one without simultaneously considering the predictive utility of the other. This point is related to a key insight from the past three decades of research on attitudes (e.g., Ajzen & Fishbein, 2005) and traits (e.g., Epstein, 1979; Fleeson, 2004), dubbed the *specificity-matching principle*. To compensate for the fact that outcomes in naturally occurring settings are often caused by multiple factors other than the predictor variable of interest, the specificity-matching principle holds that the specificity of predictors and criteria should be matched. When a predictor variable is relatively specific, the impact of rival influences on the predictor–criterion relationship can be minimized by selecting an equally specific criterion variable (e.g., attitudes toward action films predict how many action films people watch in a given year, but not the total number of movies they watch). Conversely, when a predictor variable is relatively general, the impact of rival influences can be averaged out by combining numerous behaviors into the criterion variable (e.g., attitudes toward movies in general predict how many movies of all types that people watch in a given year, but not necessarily how many action films they watch). In short, specific predictors should be used to predict specific outcomes, and general predictors should be used to predict general outcomes.

Applied to research on self-esteem, the specificity-matching principle suggests that researchers who use global self-esteem as a predictor should focus on global outcome measures, such as several outcomes bundled together (see also Rosenberg, Schooler, Schoenbach, & Rosenberg, 1995). From the perspective of the specificity-matching principle, then, Baumeister and colleagues' (2003) review of the self-esteem literature most likely underestimated the potential importance of self-esteem because it focused on the capacity of global self-esteem to predict specific outcomes (e.g., Does self-esteem predict grades in a math class?).

The intricate interplay between self-concepts and self-esteem also figures importantly in understanding the relationship between constructs that have recently been integrated into the psychological literature. Whereas the terms *self-esteem* and *self-concept* have traditionally been used to refer to characteristics of single individuals, theorists have recently popularized "groupier" variations on these constructs, such as collective self-esteem and group identity. As we discuss next, the key difference between these distinct but related self-views lies in how global (vs. specific) and group-like (vs. personal) their referents are.

The Dimensions of Self-Esteem and Self-Concepts

We suggest that the referents of self-esteem and self-concepts can be organized along the two orthogonal dimensions of *globality* and *groupiness*. As seen in Figure 36.1, self-concepts or identities (we use these terms interchangeably) refer to personal qualities

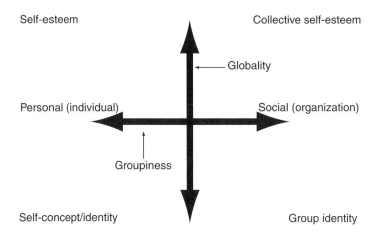

FIGURE 36.1. Self-views organized along the dimensions of globality and groupiness.

that are relatively specific; hence they reside in the lower left-hand quadrant of the figure. Pelham and Swann's (1989) Self-Attributes Questionnaire, which asks respondents to rank themselves relative to others along several dimensions (e.g., social skills, physical attractiveness, artistic ability), measures this type of self-view. Similarly, Marsh and Shavelson's (1985) Self-Description Questionnaire assesses people's self-concepts along relatively specific dimensions, such as academic, social, emotional, and physical. Self-esteem also refers to a personal quality, but it is global in nature; hence it is located in the upper left-hand quadrant of the figure. To measure self-esteem, investigators have people respond to statements such as "I feel that I am a person of worth, at least on an equal basis with others" (Rosenberg, 1965).

To the right are self-views that are social rather than personal in nature. Because group identity refers to relatively specific qualities of groups (e.g., "Germans are industrious," "Students care about their grades"), it appears in the lower right-hand quadrant of Figure 36.1. Although we are not aware of any scales designed explicitly to measure group identity, measures of self-stereotyping (e.g., Biernat, Vescio, & Green, 1996) and infrahumanization (e.g., Cortes, Demoulin, Rodriguez, Rodriguez, & Leyens, 2005) can be used to assess people's beliefs about the qualities that link them to their ingroups. Finally, collective self-esteem refers to glob-

al feelings of worth that derive from one's memberships in social groups. As such, it occupies the upper right-hand quadrant of Figure 36.1. An example of a scale that measures this type of self-view is Luhtanen and Crocker's (1992) Collective Self-Esteem Scale, which asks respondents to indicate their agreement with statements such as "I am a worthy member of the social groups I belong to" and "I'm glad to be a member of the social groups I belong to."

Certainty and Stability of Self–Esteem and Self–Concepts

In addition to varying along the dimensions of globality and groupiness, self-esteem and self-concepts differ in other meaningful ways. For instance, people differ in the extent to which their self-views are held with certainty and are stable across time.

Generally speaking, the more converging evidence people have to support a given belief, the more certain of that belief they will be. Applying this principle to self-views, the more consistent evidence that people have to support a particular view of themselves, the more certain that self-view will be (e.g., Pelham, 1991). The certainty with which people hold self-views, in turn, has important implications. For example, increases in the certainty and confidence of people's self-knowledge predict increases in global self-esteem (Baumgardner, 1990; Campbell, 1990).

The earliest consideration of the implications of self-certainty was offered in the literature on narcissism. In particular, theorists contended that people who were uncertain of their self-worth would be easily threatened. Furthermore, they proposed that people low in certainty would respond to threats by engaging in compensatory activity, sometimes resulting in high levels of defensiveness and vigorous attacks on the source of the threat. This early theorizing on narcissism led to several distinct lines of contemporary research. Aside from current discussions of narcissism in clinical populations (e.g., Westen, 1990), the most direct descendant of early treatments of narcissism is the Narcissistic Personality Inventory (NPI; Raskin & Hall, 1981), a scale designed to measure narcissistic tendencies within normal, non-pathological populations (see also Ames, Rose, & Anderson, 2006). As expected, scores on the NPI predict a host of defensive behaviors, including derogating others who outperform oneself, derogating the source of negative feedback, self-handicapping, and distorting memory for past events (see Morf & Rhodewalt, 2001).

Although it is true that narcissism and self-esteem are correlated, the relationship between these constructs is modest ($\approx .30$; Campbell, 1999). Moreover, both narcissism and self-esteem are multifaceted constructs, and research suggests that the facets of each correlate differently with one another. For instance, narcissism correlates strongly and positively with self-esteem scales that capture dominance and agency (Brown & Zeigler-Hill, 2004), but not at all with measures of communal self-concepts (Campbell, Bosson, Goheen, Lakey, & Kernis, 2007). Similarly, self-esteem correlates with the socially benign components of narcissism, such as vanity and authority, but it is largely independent of the socially noxious aspects of narcissism such as entitlement and exploitativeness (Trzesniewski et al., 2006). It should, therefore, come as no surprise that, just as narcissism predicts maladaptive tendencies toward defensiveness and aggression, self-esteem predicts a wide array of prosocial behaviors (Bushman & Baumeister, 1998; Donnellan, Trzesniewski, Robins, Moffitt, & Caspi, 2005; Paulhus et al., 2004; Webster, 2007).

Deficits in the certainty of self-knowledge may also manifest themselves in unstable self-assessments across time. Kernis (2005), for example, finds that people with unstable high self-esteem—that is, high baseline levels of global self-esteem but relatively large changes in moment to moment feelings of self-worth—exhibit some of the characteristics of narcissists. For example, both narcissists and individuals with unstable high self-esteem are hypervigilant for social feedback and highly reactive to events that have evaluative significance for the self. A major difference between these two types of individuals, however, lies in the extent to which their high self-esteem is overinflated (unrealistically positive). Kernis (2001) notes that whereas narcissists' self-esteem is inflated, the self-esteem of people with unstable high self-esteem is poorly anchored but not unrealistic. Moreover, unlike people with unstable high self-esteem, narcissists tend to manipulate and exploit relationship partners to meet their own ends. Confirming the idea that narcissism and unstable high self-esteem are independent constructs, the results of a meta-analysis showed no correlation between them (Bosson et al., 2008; but see Rhodewalt, Madrian, & Cheney, 1998). Thus, although narcissism and unstable high self-esteem are both fragile forms of self-esteem (Kernis, 2003) that may have their roots in uncertain self-knowledge, they should be considered distinct.

Components of Global Self-Esteem

Since the publication of the first self-esteem instrument 58 years ago (Raimy, 1948), researchers have developed a wide range of self-esteem measures. Of these, the vast majority are self-report scales (for a review, see Blascovich & Tomaka, 1991). Exceptions to this general rule include a pictorial self-esteem measure that was developed for use with children (Harter & Pike, 1971) and instruments that attempt to circumvent respondents' ability to "fake" high self-esteem. Examples of the latter category of instruments include experience-sampling measures of self-esteem (Savin-Williams & Jaquish, 1981) and measures based on observer judgments (Waters, Noyes, Vaughn, & Ricks, 1985) or peer ratings (Demo,

1985). More recently, the quest for a measure of uncontaminated, "true" self-esteem led researchers to develop implicit tests of self-esteem (e.g., Greenwald, McGhee, & Schwartz, 1998).

Still, as noted, most self-esteem research relies on respondents' self-reports. This practice makes sense given that self-esteem is, by definition, the esteem that one has for oneself. Asking people directly about their feelings toward themselves is therefore a reasonable strategy for assessing such feelings. Among researchers who utilize self-report measures, however, there are widely divergent ideas about the number of distinct components or aspects that presumably underlie global self-esteem. We group these diverging perspectives here into single-component, two-component, and multiple-component approaches.

The Single-Component Approach

Probably the most common approach to measuring self-esteem is based on the assumption that it consists of a single, general dimension that can be measured with a modest number of items (e.g., Coopersmith, 1967). This assumption is evident in the most commonly used measure of self-esteem, Rosenberg's (1965) Self-Esteem Scale. Taking the unifactorial assumption even further, some researchers recently developed a one-item self-esteem scale that consists of the single statement "I have high self-esteem" (Robins, Hendin, & Trzesniewski, 2001).

The Two-Component Approach

In recent years, it became increasingly popular to divide global self-esteem into two components. One approach—which harks back to Osgood's (1952) early work on the evaluative and potency components of social judgments, as well as Bakan's (1966) distinction between communal and agentic aspects of personality—distinguishes between people's assessments of their lovability (*self-liking*) and competence (*self-competence*). Several scales capture these components (e.g., Diggory, 1966; Franks & Marolla, 1976; Gecas, 1971), but the one that does so most explicitly is Tafarodi and Swann's (2001) Self-Liking and Self-Competence Scale. Tafar-

odi, Swann, and their colleagues note that although self-liking and self-competence are correlated, the correlation is moderate, and, more important, each component predicts unique outcomes (e.g., Bosson & Swann, 1999; Tafarodi & Milne, 2002).

Another two-component approach distinguishes between *trait self-esteem*, which refers to people's baseline level of global self-esteem that remains fairly stable across time, and *state self-esteem*, which fluctuates on a moment-to-moment basis in response to self-relevant experiences. Heatherton and Polivy (1991) developed the State Self-Esteem Scale (SSES) to capture people's immediate feelings about themselves within several domains (performance, social, and appearance). However, this scale's substantial correlation with trait measures of self-esteem ($r \approx .75$) raises questions about whether it truly captures a distinct component of self-esteem. Others (e.g., Kernis, 2005) measure state self-esteem by administering trait self-esteem scales multiple times throughout the day, with the instruction to "respond according to how you feel about yourself *right now*." Indeed, many standard trait self-esteem scales can be modified to assess state self-esteem by rewording their instructions or by adding the phrase "at this moment ... " to individual items.

Another popular two-component approach is based on the distinction between implicit and explicit attitudes. Although different authors make different assumptions about the precise nature of explicit and implicit attitudes, one common view holds that *explicit self-esteem* is controllable, deliberate, and easy to verbalize, whereas *implicit self-esteem* is uncontrollable, automatic, and difficult to verbalize (Epstein & Morling, 1995). Several unobtrusive methods are used to capture implicit self-esteem, including measures of people's preferences for their own initials relative to other letters (e.g., the Name Letter Task; Koole, Dijksterhuis, & van Knippenberg, 2001) and reaction-time tasks that assess the speed with which people associate positive versus negative stimuli with the self (e.g., the Implicit Association Test; Greenwald et al., 1998). The consistently low or nonexistent correlations between explicitly and implicitly assessed self-esteem lend credence to the notion that they are distinct while simultaneously raising questions about whether implicit and explicit scales truly tap the same underlying construct. Currently, theorists disagree on this point (see Buhrmester, Blanton, & Swann, 2008; Olson, Fazio, & Hermann, 2007) and may continue to do so until further research sheds more light on this issue.

The Multiple-Component Approach

Shavelson and colleagues (1976) were among the first to articulate a multidimensional and hierarchically structured self, with *global* self-esteem at the top of the hierarchy and *domain-specific* self-esteem—self-views nested within relatively specific dimensions, such as academic, physical, and social—falling beneath it. As originally theorized by Shavelson and colleagues, the different types of domain-specific self-esteem should correlate with each other, but some empirical work fails to support this hypothesis. For example, Marsh and Hattie (1996) found that specific self-concepts are only weakly associated with each other, although self-concepts as a whole combine to form a superordinate global self-esteem factor.

In a slight variation on this theme, some theorists treat domain-specific self-esteem as people's feelings of worth within separate domains (e.g., "I feel good about my physical appearance") rather than simply their beliefs about themselves within those domains (e.g., "I am physically attractive"). Heatherton and Polivy's (1991) SSES, for example, measures this type of domain-specific self-esteem in performance, social, and appearance domains. Similarly, Hoyle's (1991) Domain-Specific Self-Esteem Inventory measures people's feelings about their worth within social, ability, physical, and public domains.

The multiple-component approach poses a possible solution to the ongoing debate over the usefulness of self-esteem in predicting important outcomes (e.g., Baumeister et al., 2003; Swann, Chang-Schneider, & McClarty, 2007). As noted, matching the specificity of predictor and criterion variables maximizes the strength of predictor–criterion relationships. Thus academic self-concepts are more predictive of academic achievement than is global self-esteem (Marsh & Craven, 2006), and global self-esteem predicts aggregated outcomes better than specific self-concepts do (e.g., Trzesniewski et al., 2006). These patterns are consistent with the multiple-component approach, which theorizes both global and specific dimensions of the self-concept.

Perspectives on the Origins and Functions of Self-Esteem and Self-Concepts

Having considered many of the fundamental questions regarding the nature of self-esteem and self-concepts, we now turn to related issues, such as where these self-views come from and how they relate to various aspects of people's lives. In what follows, we first summarize influential perspectives on how people acquire a stable sense of self-esteem and then consider why self-esteem may be important for human functioning.

Nature

As with many individual-difference variables, people's self-esteem levels reflect both biological (genetic) and sociocultural (environmental) factors. Concerning the biology of global self-esteem, results of twin studies suggest that self-esteem is heritable (McGuire et al., 1999), with a heritability estimate of about .30 (Kendler, Gardner, & Prescott, 1998). This suggests that genes explain approximately 30% of the population variance in global self-esteem levels. Heredity also appears to explain a substantial amount of the variance in changes in self-esteem across time (Neiss, Sedikides, & Stevenson, 2002). Given the strong negative correlations between self-esteem and neuroticism or negative affectivity (Judge, Erez, Bono, & Thoresen, 2002), and particularly depression (Watson, Suls, & Haig, 2002), some speculate that genes influence neuroticism, which in turn influences self-esteem (Neiss et al., 2002). More specifically, recent evidence points to a potentially important role played by the short alleles of the serotonin transporter gene (Swann, Beavers, & McGeary, 2007). At present, however, behavioral-genetic studies of self-esteem are relatively scarce as compared with studies that focus on the sociocultural origins of self-esteem.

Nurture

If genes explain approximately 30% of the population variance in self-esteem, then this leaves roughly 70% of the variance to be explained by other factors, including environmental influences and gene × environment interactions. Much of the research on environmental influences on self-esteem explores how specific relationship partners—such as parents, siblings, peers, and teachers—as well as the broader culture shape individuals' self-esteem.

According to attachment theory (Bowlby, 1969), infants begin to formulate schemas (working models) about their worth, based on the treatment they receive from caregivers, before they even have self-awareness. During infancy and early childhood, working models reflect the consistency and responsiveness of caregivers' treatment. Specifically, consistent and responsive caregiving should instill in children the rudimentary foundations of high self-esteem and favorable self-concepts by teaching them that they are worthy of love and capable of efficacious action (Bowlby, 1973; Mikulincer, 1995; Verschueren, Marcoen, & Schoefs, 1996).

During middle childhood (around the age of 8), relatively sophisticated cognitive processes further refine children's self-esteem and self-concepts (Harter, 1990). For instance, children at this age begin developing specific self-concepts by comparing their traits and abilities with those of their peers (Festinger, 1954). They also begin looking to others for feedback about the extent to which they are valued (Cooley, 1902; Mead, 1934), and they internalize their perceptions of others' approval (or disapproval) as feelings of self-esteem. Thus, across childhood, high self-esteem is associated with positive self-concepts in valued domains and perceptions of approval from significant relationship partners (Harter, 1999). Importantly, the type of approval that children receive from others can influence their developing self-views. Whereas approval that is contingent on the child accomplishing specific goals or meeting specific standards can foster self-esteem that is unstable and fragile, approval

that values the child's inherent worth should foster authentic feelings of true self-esteem (Deci & Ryan, 1995).

Continuing through adolescence and into adulthood, individuals continue to develop specific self-concepts through comparisons with others (Festinger, 1954), as well as observations of their own behavior (Bem, 1972). The positivity versus negativity of specific self-concepts, in turn, may influence self-esteem via the importance that individuals place on them. For example, individuals who place importance on success in a given domain and who have positive self-concepts in this domain will enjoy higher global self-esteem than those who have negative self-concepts in valued domains (Higgins, 1987; James, 1890/1950; Pelham, 1991). Moreover, given the multidimensionality of the self, successes in a given domain may predict increases in the positivity of specific self-concepts *without* also influencing global feelings of self-esteem (Marsh & Craven, 2006).

On a broader level, self-concepts and self-esteem reflect the culture in which people are socialized. One consistent finding is that, on average, people who are raised in individualistic cultures report substantially higher self-esteem and more favorable self-concepts than do people raised in collectivistic cultures (Heine & Hamamura, 2007). Indeed, in analyses that treat culture as the unit of analysis, there is a strong positive correlation between a culture's individualism and the average self-esteem of its members (Oyserman, Coon, & Kemmelmeier, 2002). Furthermore, as the length of exposure to an individualistic culture increases, so does the self-esteem of visitors from a collectivistic culture (Heine & Lehman, 1997).

These cross-cultural findings raise an interesting—and currently unresolved—question about the "true" self-esteem of people from individualistic versus collectivistic cultures. Some theorists suggest, for example, that the tendency toward high self-esteem and positive self-concepts is universal and that people from collectivistic cultures merely appear (relatively) low in self-esteem because of the value they place on modest self-presentation and "fitting in" rather than "standing out" (Sedikides, Gaertner, & Toguchi, 2003). In support of this view, Sedikides and his colleagues report that people from collectivistic cultures display highly favorable views of themselves on communal self-concepts that are valued within their culture, such as loyalty (Sedikides, Gaertner, & Vevea, 2005). Likewise, Tafarodi and Swann (1996) found that Chinese participants scored higher than American participants on the self-liking dimension of global self-esteem, whereas they scored lower than Americans on the self-competence dimension. In contrast, other theorists call the tendency toward high self-esteem and positive self-concepts "strikingly elusive" among people from collectivistic East Asian cultures (Heine & Hamamura, 2007, p. 22) and argue that such individuals instead display a tendency toward self-criticism (Heine, Lehman, Markus, & Kitayama, 1999). Although this debate is still going strong, one promising resolution involves the development of a method for separating the self-presentational component of self-esteem from "true" self-esteem. For example, Kwan and Mandisodza (2007) identified three components of self-esteem: benevolence, merit, and bias. The bias component is conceptually similar to self-enhancement bias, whereas the benevolence and merit components seem to reflect "true" self-esteem. This approach may provide a starting point from which to pursue questions about the nature of self-esteem across cultures.

Functional Perspectives

Rather than focusing on the origins of individuals' self-esteem, several perspectives take a broader look by focusing on the origins of self-esteem itself. These perspectives ask: Why do humans have self-esteem in the first place, and what function(s) are served by self-esteem? One such perspective proposes that self-esteem and self-concepts reflect the operation of psychological mechanisms that evolved because they helped humans negotiate the social world (Kirkpatrick & Ellis, 2001). According to this perspective, self-esteem and self-concepts provide people with information about, for example, their dominance status (Barkow, 1989), social inclusion versus exclusion (Leary & Baumeister, 2000), prestige (Henrich & Gil-White, 2001), and mate value

(Kenrick, Groth, Trost, & Sadalla, 1993). When goals relevant to success in these social domains are not met, negative self-assessments and feelings of low self-esteem motivate the individual to either renew efforts toward goal achievement or redirect energies elsewhere.

Another functional perspective suggests that self-esteem feelings protect people from the existential anxiety that accompanies awareness of their own mortality (Hart, Shaver, & Goldenberg, 2005; Pyszczynski, Greenberg, Solomon, Arndt, & Schimel, 2004). According to this view, high self-esteem and positive self-concepts signal that one meets or exceeds the value standards associated with one's role(s) within a larger system of meaning. Conversely, low self-esteem and negative self-concepts signal a breakdown in the psychological "armor" that protects people from their deep-rooted fear of death and its accompanying unknowns. Thus drops in self-esteem and negative self-assessments motivate behaviors geared toward restoring one's value in the eyes of others and shoring up support for human-made systems of meaning.

Whereas the aforementioned perspectives suggest that self-esteem and self-concepts confer survival benefits, such arguments seem to come perilously close to mistaking an abstraction (i.e., self-esteem) for a thing (i.e., a psychological entity that shapes rather than merely reflects reality). From this vantage point, the survival benefits associated with self-esteem may merely reflect those qualities that give rise to self-esteem rather than self-esteem itself (cf. Baumeister et al., 2003). Furthermore, excessive focus on self-esteem may be problematic in and of itself. Crocker and Park (2004), for example, suggest that preoccupation with one's achievements in self-esteem-relevant domains can divert attention from other important needs, such as the needs for relatedness, competence, autonomy, and self-regulation. Note, however, that this view is not necessarily incompatible with the functional views described previously. Although self-esteem may have evolved to serve the informational and/or protective functions noted earlier, valuing self-esteem *for its own sake* may indeed yield the maladaptive outcomes noted by Crocker and Park. Moreover, although self-esteem is an abstraction, it can have motivational properties. For example, people who enjoy high self-esteem are likely to persist on tasks in the wake of failure (McFarlin, Baumeister, & Blascovich, 1984), and those who suffer from negative self-views are prone to tolerate various forms of poor treatment (Swann, De La Ronde, & Hixon, 1994; Wiesenfeld, Swann, Brockner, & Bartel, 2007).

Correlates of Self-Esteem and Self-Concepts

Research on the correlates of self-esteem and self-concepts is abundant. Given the expansiveness of the literature, we can do little more than summarize broadly some of the key findings. We organize these findings temporally, beginning with the metacognitive features of self-knowledge and then proceeding through goal setting, environment and partner selection, self-presentation, and cognitive and affective reactions and ending with real-world outcomes. Note that in keeping with our conviction that self-esteem and self-concepts are members of the larger self-view category, we include investigations of both in our review.

Before proceeding, we must acknowledge the inherent difficulty of establishing causality when discussing individual-difference variables such as self-esteem and self-concepts. Although it is certainly possible that self-esteem causes some of the variables with which it is associated, it is also possible that self-esteem is caused by some of these variables. Other possibilities include the "third variable problem"—that is, the notion that a third, unmeasured variable causes changes in both self-esteem and the variables with which it correlates—and the prospect of dynamic interrelations in which self-esteem causes some outcome, which then influences self-esteem, and so on. Because of these difficulties, we avoid causal language when describing the correlates of self-esteem and self-concepts.

Metacognitive Features of Self-Knowledge

Metacognitive features include qualities such as the content and structure of, and links among, different pieces of self-knowledge. For example, global self-esteem shows ro-

bust correlations with the valence of people's specific self-concepts, such that higher self-esteem is associated with more positive evaluations of the self along specific dimensions (Brown, Dutton, & Cook, 2001; Pelham & Swann, 1989), as well as smaller discrepancies between actual and ideal beliefs about the self (Higgins, 1987). Higher self-esteem is also associated with smaller overall proportions of negative, relative to positive, self-concepts (Hoyle, 2006; Showers, 1992), and the negative self-concepts of people with high self-esteem tend to be relatively less complex and differentiated (Morgan & Janoff-Bulman, 1994; Woolfolk, Novalany, Gara, Allen, & Polino, 1995). These structural features buffer people who have primarily favorable beliefs about themselves from the painful effects of negative self-relevant information (such as negative feedback, memories of undesirable past behavior, etc.). Unfortunately, these same features do little to protect those who have many negative self-views from painful reminders of their deficits (Showers, 1992).

Decisions and Goals

When it comes to decision making, research paints a portrait of people with low self-esteem as being less decisive (Rosenberg & Owens, 2001) and more likely to procrastinate (Ferrari, 1994) than those high in self-esteem. Persons lower in self-esteem are also more easily persuaded than those high in self-esteem (Gibson, 1981), particularly in response to forceful or heavy-handed communications, which tend to yield reactance effects among those high in self-esteem (Brockner & Elkind, 1985). In a similar vein, people low as compared with high in self-esteem are also more risk averse when making decisions, most likely because they have relatively low expectations of success (Wray & Stone, 2005) and are motivated to avoid feelings of regret should a risky decision yield negative consequences (Josephs, Larrick, Steele, & Nisbett, 1992).

In addition to making riskier decisions, people high in self-esteem also tend to set higher goals for themselves and to persist more doggedly through setbacks than those low in self-esteem. Indeed, some research suggests that persons high in self-esteem pursue goals with an eye to achieving excellence, whereas those low in self-esteem seek merely to attain adequacy (Baumeister & Tice, 1985). Moreover, higher self-esteem is associated with superior self-regulation during goal pursuit. For example, people with high self-esteem persist more than those with low self-esteem after a single failure, but they persist less than persons low in self-esteem after repeated failures (Di Paula & Campbell, 2002). People with high self-esteem also persist more than those low in self-esteem if they believe that persistence is linked with success at a particular task, but not if they believe that persistence is irrelevant to success (McFarlin, 1985). These findings suggest that persons high in self-esteem are particularly adept at modifying their goal-pursuit strategies to reflect the likelihood of goal attainment.

Creating a Niche

Once people make decisions and set goals, they must select the environments and relationships within which to pursue those goals. According to self-verification theory, the need for psychological coherence—or a sense that the world fits with past experiences—is a primary motive behind the selection of settings and interaction partners (Swann, Rentfrow, & Guinn, 2003). That is, people actively seek and embed themselves within social environments that sustain their stable self-views. Evidence of this tendency appears in people's choices of relationship partners, careers, home and work environments, group memberships, and even home and office décor (Gosling, Ko, Mannarelli, & Morris, 2002; Sadalla, Vershure, & Burroughs, 1987).

To illustrate, people low in self-esteem tend to withdraw and isolate themselves from others, whereas those high in self-esteem more readily seek others' company (Rosenberg & Owens, 2001). Once they enter social settings, people's stable self-views predict their preferences for specific interaction partners. Whereas people with favorable self-concepts tend to seek out relationship partners who view them favorably, those with negative self-concepts prefer the companionship of those who view them unfavorably (Swann et al., 1994; Swann & Pelham, 2002). Similarly, people high in self-esteem seek work environments that offer them more positive feedback (in the form of financial compensation), whereas those low in self-esteem seek work environments that offer fewer such financial rewards (Schroeder, Josephs, & Swann, 2006). Such tendencies should ensure that people surround themselves with relationship partners, feedback sources, and environments that bolster, rather than challenge, their self-esteem and self-concepts. Moreover, to the extent that a given relationship or environment *discon*firms people's self-concepts or self-esteem, they are likely to leave in search of a better fitting niche (Schroeder et al., 2006; Swann & Pelham, 2002).

Self-Presentation

Within their chosen relationships and environments, people's self-esteem and self-concepts relate predictably to the manner in which they present themselves. For example, whereas persons high in self-esteem seek to impress others—and thereby enhance themselves—by presenting themselves in a highly favorable manner, those low in self-esteem present themselves in a more modest, self-protective fashion (Baumeister, Tice, & Hutton, 1989). Ironically, one of the ways in which people high in self-esteem present a favorable image is by self-handicapping, or creating obstacles to their own success so as to create plausible external attributions for poor performance (Jones & Berglas, 1978). To illustrate this phenomenon, Tice and Baumeister (1990) measured the amount of time that people high versus low in self-esteem spent practicing for an upcoming test, under public versus private conditions. Only when they thought that others would know how much time they practiced did people high in self-esteem self-handicap by engaging in less preparation than people low in self-esteem. Thus the desire to present the self favorably may, at times, lead persons with high self-esteem to behave in ways that undermine their own performances.

Social Cognition

Social interactions provide the raw material for a host of social-cognitive processes that differ as a function of self-esteem and self-concepts. In this section, we consider the links between self-views and social-cognitive processes such as information seeking, attention, recall, interpretation, and mental simulation.

Information Seeking

Within their interactions, people tend to seek self-relevant information that is consistent with their chronic, firmly held self-views (e.g., Swann, 1983, 1990). Despite early findings suggesting that global self-esteem did not predict people's reactions to positive or negative feedback (Swann, Pelham, & Krull, 1989), later studies revealed strong links between specific self-concepts and information-seeking tendencies regarding those self-concepts. Thus, when researchers uphold the specificity-matching principle, they find that people generally seek positive information about their favorable self-views and negative information about their unfavorable self-views (e.g., Bosson & Swann, 1999).

Attention

Just as people seek information that is consistent with their self-views, they pay more attention to evaluatively consistent than inconsistent information. In general, people low as compared with high in self-esteem attend more to negative information and events (Leitenberg, Yost, & Carroll-Wilson, 1986). When it comes to self-relevant information, people with negative self-concepts pay more attention to unfavorable than favorable evaluations of themselves, whereas the reverse is true among those with positive self-concepts (Swann & Read, 1981). In the wake of failure feedback, persons with low self-esteem focus attention on their weaknesses, whereas those high in self-esteem increase attention to their strengths (Dodgson & Wood, 1998). Finally, people high in self-esteem are more likely than those low in self-esteem to focus on the ways in which their own outcomes compare favorably to the outcomes obtained by the friends, acquaintances, and strangers that they encounter in daily life (Wheeler & Miyake, 1992).

Recall

Perhaps reflecting these differences in attention, people display better memory for feedback and experiences that are congruent relative to incongruent with the valence of their self-esteem, and they recall incongruent feedback and experiences as more congruent than they really were (Christensen, Wood, & Barrett, 2003; Story, 1998). Similar effects have been found at the level of self-concepts, with people displaying better memory for feedback that is congruent than incongruent with the positivity or negativity of their self-perceived likeability (Swann & Read, 1981). Interestingly, these congruency effects in memory for self-relevant information appear to be moderated by self-esteem level, such that people high in self-esteem exhibit a stronger congruency bias (i.e., tendency to recall past behavior in a manner congruent with self-concepts) than those low in self-esteem (Campbell, 1990).

Self-esteem differences in recall also emerge during threatening experiences. For example, people high in self-esteem are more likely than those low in self-esteem to remember *other people's* negative behaviors following their own failure experiences (Crocker, 1993), and persons high in self-esteem spontaneously recall more positive autobiographical memories than do persons low in self-esteem when in an experimentally-induced negative mood (Setliff & Marmurek, 2002). Such recall biases presumably facilitate and hamper mood repair efforts among people with high and low self-esteem, respectively.

Interpretation

The manner in which people interpret their own and other people's behaviors and outcomes is linked predictably with their self-esteem and self-concepts. For instance, people interpret feedback that is congruent with their self-concepts as accurate, whereas they dismiss incongruent feedback as inaccurate (Markus, 1977; Shrauger & Lund, 1975; Swann, Griffin, Predmore, & Gaines, 1987). Moreover, a large body of research on attribution processes shows that people high in self-esteem take credit for their successes and blame their failures on external factors (for reviews, see Blaine & Crocker, 1993; Campbell & Sedikides, 1999). In contrast, people low in self-esteem are less inclined to take credit for their successes and more inclined to assume responsibility for their failures (e.g., Fitch, 1970).

Self-esteem also relates to the manner in which people interpret ambiguous social stimuli. To illustrate, people who are high as compared with low in self-esteem are more likely to interpret ambiguous phrases ("Is this how you want it?") as conveying positive feelings toward them (Bosson, Swann, & Pennebaker, 2000; Tafarodi, 1998). Furthermore, people with low self-esteem may not even interpret their own success experiences as successes unless a credible outsider tells them explicitly that they have done well (Josephs, Bosson, & Jacobs, 2003).

Mental Simulation

Paralleling these self-esteem differences in interpretation are differences in people's mental simulations, or thoughts regarding alternative possible outcomes for themselves. Whereas people low in self-esteem tend to think more about how future outcomes "could be better," those high in self-esteem think more about how future outcomes "could be worse" (Sanna & Meier, 2000). Similar self-esteem differences emerge when people generate alternative outcomes for past events, with people low in self-esteem simulating more "could have been better" scenarios and those high in self-esteem simulating more "could have been worse" scenarios (Sanna, Turley-Ames, & Meier, 1999).

Affect

Given the aforementioned differences in self-knowledge, choice of partners and environments, and cognitive responses to their worlds, it should come as no surprise that people's self-esteem and self-concepts are closely tied to their chronic and moment-to-moment affective states. As noted, global self-esteem is strongly negatively correlated with neuroticism (Judge et al., 2002) and negative affectivity (Suls, 2006), both of which reflect people's stable tendencies to experience unpleasant emotions. Thus people who are higher in self-esteem tend to experience fewer negative emotions such as depression, anxiety, and hostility. Indeed, the negative association between self-esteem and depression is so strong ($r \approx .80$; Watson et al., 2002) that some suggest conceptualizing self-esteem and depression as end points of a bipolar continuum (Suls, 2006). Like-

wise, people higher in self-esteem tend to score higher in extraversion and positive affectivity (Watson et al., 2002), which reflect chronic tendencies toward positive emotions such as enthusiasm and joy. Not surprisingly, research reveals strong and consistent positive links between self-esteem and reports of subjective happiness (e.g., Diener & Diener, 1995), leading Baumeister and colleagues (2003) to conclude—in the midst of their otherwise disparaging review—that "high self-esteem may pay off handsomely for the individual in terms of subjective happiness" (p. 26). Related to this self-esteem–happiness link is a strong positive correlation between self-esteem and optimism, or the tendency to anticipate positive future outcomes for the self (Lyubomirsky, Tkach, & DiMatteo, 2005).

Considerably less research explores the links between self-esteem and self-conscious emotions, but the existing work points to strong negative correlations between self-esteem and shame proneness (Leith & Baumeister, 1998), moderate negative correlations between self-esteem and hubristic (all-encompassing) pride, and strong positive correlations between self-esteem and authentic (achievement-oriented) pride (Tracy & Robins, 2007). Thus people high in self-esteem neither react to their own failures and transgressions with painful feelings of disgrace nor react to their successes with overblown feelings of arrogance. Instead, they appear to feel good or bad about their actions in a given context, rather than feeling good or bad about themselves as a whole.

Life Outcomes

In this section, we consider some of the ways in which the self-esteem and self-concept differences summarized here predict real-world outcomes in terms of people's relationship functioning, academic and athletic performances, criminal activity, health behaviors, and finances.

As noted earlier, some theorists propose that self-esteem evolved to alert people to survival-relevant fluctuations in their relationship status (Leary & Baumeister, 2000). According to this sociometer hypothesis, painful drops in self-esteem inform people about possible threats to their social inclusion (Leary, Tambor, Terdal, & Downs,

1995). Consistent with this idea, people low in self-esteem exhibit an attentional bias toward information that conveys interpersonal rejection, whereas those high in self-esteem pay particular attention to information that conveys acceptance (Dandeneau & Baldwin, 2004). Unfortunately for those low in self-esteem, their heightened sensitivity to rejection cues can have harmful implications for their close relationships. To illustrate, the heightened rejection sensitivity of those low in self-esteem undermines their confidence in romantic partners' love for them, which then leads them to withdraw psychologically from partners (Murray, Holmes, MacDonald, & Ellsworth, 1998). Moreover, people low in self-esteem may react to relationship conflict in ways that anger and frustrate their partners, ultimately eliciting the very rejection they fear most (Downey, Freitas, Michaelis, & Khouri, 1998). In contrast, the expectations of acceptance of persons high in self-esteem allow them to use their romantic relationships as sources of self-affirmation in the face of failure, thus furthering their confidence in their partners' positive regard and increasing their commitment to those partners (Murray et al., 1998).

People's specific self-concepts also figure importantly in relationship functioning. Self-concepts predict the types of appraisals that people seek and prefer from their partners, as well as their feelings of commitment to and intimacy with partners who offer them congruent appraisals. In relationships ranging from college roommates to long-term married partners, people with positive self-concepts prefer partners who view them favorably, whereas those with negative self-concepts prefer partners who view them negatively (Swann & Pelham, 2002; Swann et al., 1994). Indeed, people experience higher levels of marital distress to the extent that their spouses' views of them disconfirm their stable self-concepts (Schafer, Wickrama, & Keith, 1996). As such, securing relationship partners who confirm their self-views may be important for people's psychological well-being (e.g., Swann et al., 2003).

In the academic domain, there are strong links between people's relatively specific academic self-concepts and outcomes such as academic achievement, college grade point average, and persistence at academic pursuits (e.g., Marsh & Craven, 2006; Robbins,

Lauver, Le, Langley, & Carlstrom, 2004; Valentine, DuBois, & Cooper, 2004). In the domain of athletics, physical self-concepts predict future exercise behavior, gymnastic self-concepts predict future gymnastic performance, and swimming self-concepts predict performance during elite swimming competitions (for a review, see Marsh & Craven, 2006). It is worth noting that these effects emerge even when controlling for past performance in the domain of interest, indicating that self-concepts explain unique variance in people's behavioral outcomes. Conversely—and consistent with the specificity-matching principle—global self-esteem predicts bundled outcomes, or summary indices that combine multiple behavioral observations. Some work, for example, shows that people lower in self-esteem during adolescence are more likely to develop physical and mental health difficulties, to use tobacco, to commit crimes, to drop out of school, and to suffer money and work problems in adulthood (Trzesniewski et al., 2006). Thus many important life outcomes can be predicted by people's specific self-concepts and global self-esteem.

Future Directions

We began this chapter by acknowledging the deep doubts that several influential critics expressed recently regarding the self-esteem construct (e.g., Baumeister et al., 2003; Crocker & Park, 2004). Although we agree that simpleminded characterizations of self-esteem as a panacea for all of society's ills are wrongheaded, we believe that some critics have gone too far in arguing for the abandonment of the self-esteem construct. In support of this viewpoint, we summarized a vast literature that suggests that self-esteem and self-concepts are predictive of people's behaviors, thoughts, feelings, and life outcomes. We now outline three suggestions for improving the study of self-esteem.

First, when addressing matters related to predictive validity, self-esteem should be reunited with other members of the self-view family. This will mean moving away from the knee-jerk use of Rosenberg's (1965) global self-esteem scale and toward assessing the key components of self-esteem (self-liking vs. self-competence, implicit vs. explicit self-esteem), as well as the specific self-concepts that are most relevant to researchers' outcome variables. In addition, researchers may benefit from assessing the metacognitive features of self-esteem and self-concepts, such as their certainty, importance, clarity, extremity, accessibility, organizational structure, and temporal stability, to name a few. Such shifts not only make sound conceptual sense, but they are also consistent with the way that related psychological constructs, such as attitudes and traits, have been conceptualized and studied. Furthermore, once other members of the self-view family are thrown into the mix, specificity matching becomes possible, and following this psychometric principle will lead to assessments that are simultaneously more meaningful and more optimistic. Note, however, that we do not recommend that researchers blur the distinction between global self-esteem and specific self-concepts. To the contrary, we are simply pointing out the importance of recognizing that self-esteem and self-concepts are members of the same self-view category and that following the specificity-matching principle will undoubtedly improve researchers' ability to predict the outcomes of self-esteem.

Second, as in research on attitudes, theoretical models of the factors that constrain the links between self-views and behavior should be developed. Attitude researchers have approached this challenge in two distinct ways. First, in their reasoned-action model, Ajzen and Fishbein (2005) identified the many normative, contextual, and personal variables that moderate the links between attitudes and behaviors, thus allowing for heightened precision when predicting behavioral outcomes from attitudes. Second, in his motivation and opportunity as determinants (MODE) model, Fazio (1990) offered a process model of the chain of events that determines when attitudes will become translated into behaviors. Fazio and his colleagues (e.g., Olson et al., 2007) have made progress in applying the MODE model to the study of self-esteem, but additional work is needed. For example, their initial work focuses primarily on the conditions under which people's global self-esteem (an attitude) translates into self-reports of self-esteem (a behavior). It is important to know as well the conditions under which both global self-esteem and specific self-concepts

translate into behaviors and outcomes outside of the laboratory.

Finally, in light of the debilitating predictive outcomes of low self-esteem and negative self-concepts, it is critical to learn more about how they can be changed. We recognize, of course, the irony of ending this chapter with the question of how to change self-views, as changing self-views was the original (and almost comically misguided) goal of the much-maligned California task force. While acknowledging this irony, we also defend our position by pointing out that self-esteem change, when based on empirically substantiated strategies, can theoretically produce large improvements in people's well-being and overall functioning. In this regard, we are encouraged by recent evidence that self-esteem can be improved via elaborate programs (e.g., DuBois & Flay, 2004; Haney & Durlak, 1998). Of course, self-esteem programs are not for everyone—after all, most people in the general population have high self-esteem and thus do not require self-esteem interventions. Furthermore, successful self-esteem improvement programs have all been multifaceted, and it is not clear which of their many components are effective in generating change, or how they do so. Rather than boosting self-esteem directly, it is possible that these programs have their effects by increasing people's social skills and interpersonal problem-solving abilities, for example, which then leads to increases in social acceptance, which in turn improves self-esteem (e.g., Leary, 1999). Rigorous empirical work is needed to pinpoint the strategies that most effectively increase self-esteem, to uncover the underlying mechanism(s) that drive this change, and to explore whether increasing the positivity of self-esteem and self-concepts can, in fact, engender some of the beneficial outcomes that inspired the original efforts of the task force.

References

Ajzen, I., & Fishbein, M. (2005). The influence of attitudes on behavior. In D. Albarracín, B. T. Johnson, & M. P. Zanna (Eds.), *The handbook of attitudes* (pp. 173–221). Mahwah, NJ: Erlbaum.

American Psychiatric Association. (2000). *Diagnostic and statistical manual of mental disorders* (4th ed., text rev.). Washington, DC: Author.

Ames, D. R., Rose, P., & Anderson, C. P. (2006). The NPI-16 as a short measure of narcissism. *Journal of Research in Personality, 40,* 440–450.

Bakan, D. (1966). *The duality of human existence: An essay on psychology and religion.* Oxford, UK: Rand McNally.

Barkow, J. H. (1989). *Darwin, sex, and status: Biosocial approaches to mind and culture.* Toronto, Ontario, Canada: University of Toronto Press.

Baumeister, R. F., Campbell, J. D., Krueger, J. I., & Vohs, K. D. (2003). Does high self-esteem cause better performance, interpersonal success, happiness, or healthier lifestyles? *Psychological Science in the Public Interest, 4,* 1–44.

Baumeister, R. F., & Tice, D. M. (1985). Self-esteem and responses to success and failure: Subsequent performance and intrinsic motivation. *Journal of Personality, 53,* 450–467.

Baumeister, R. F., Tice, D. M., & Hutton, D. G. (1989). Self-presentational motivations and personality differences in self-esteem. *Journal of Personality, 57,* 547–579.

Baumgardner, A. H. (1990). To know oneself is to like oneself: Self-certainty and self-affect. *Journal of Personality and Social Psychology, 58,* 1062–1072.

Bem, D. J. (1972). Self-perception theory. In L. Berkowitz (Ed.), *Advances in experimental social psychology* (Vol. 6, pp. 1–62). New York: Academic Press.

Biernat, M., Vescio, T. K., & Green, M. L. (1996). Selective self-stereotyping. *Journal of Personality and Social Psychology, 71,* 1194–1209.

Blaine, B., & Crocker, J. (1993). Self-esteem and self-serving biases in reactions to positive and negative events. In R. F. Baumeister (Ed.), *Self-esteem: The puzzle of low self-regard* (pp. 55–85). New York: Plenum Press.

Blascovich, J., & Tomaka, J. (1991). Measures of self-esteem. In J. Robinson, P. Shaver, & L. Wrightsman (Eds.), *Measures of personality and social psychological attitudes* (pp. 115–160). San Diego, CA: Academic Press.

Bosson, J. K., Lakey, C. E., Campbell, W. K., Zeigler-Hill, V., Jordan, C. H., & Kernis, M. H. (2008, April). Untangling the links between narcissism and self-esteem: A theoretical and empirical review. *Social and Personality Psychology Compass,* p. 2.

Bosson, J. K., & Swann, W. B., Jr. (1999). Self-liking, self-competence, and the quest for self-verification. *Personality and Social Psychology Bulletin, 25,* 1230–1241.

Bosson, J. K., Swann, W. B., Jr., & Pennebaker, J. W. (2000). Stalking the perfect measure of implicit self-esteem: The blind men and the elephant revisited? *Journal of Personality and Social Psychology, 79,* 631–643.

Bowlby, J. (1969). *Attachment and loss: Vol. 1. Attachment.* New York: Basic Books.

Bowlby, J. (1973). *Attachment and loss: Vol. 2. Separation, anxiety, and anger.* London: Penguin Books.

Branden, N. (1994). *The six pillars of self-esteem.* New York: Bantam Books.

Brockner, J., & Elkind, M. (1985). Self-esteem and reactance: Further evidence of attitudinal and motivational consequences. *Journal of Experimental Social Psychology, 21,* 346–361.

Brown, J. D., Dutton, K. A., & Cook, K. E. (2001). From the top down: Self-esteem and self-evaluation. *Cognition and Emotion, 15,* 615–631.

Brown, R. P., & Zeigler-Hill, V. (2004). Narcissism and the non-equivalence of self-esteem measures: A matter of dominance? *Journal of Research in Personality, 38,* 585–592.

Buhrmester, M., Blanton, H., & Swann, W. B., Jr. (2008). *Measuring implicit self-esteem: Not there yet.* Unpublished manuscript, University of Texas at Austin.

Bushman, B. J., & Baumeister, R. F. (1998). Threatened egotism, narcissism, self-esteem, and direct and displaced aggression: Does self-love or self-hate lead to violence? *Journal of Personality and Social Psychology, 75,* 219–229.

California Task Force to Promote Self-Esteem and Personal and Social Responsibility. (1990). *Toward a state of self-esteem.* Sacramento: California State Department of Education.

Campbell, J. D. (1990). Self-esteem and clarity of the self-concept. *Journal of Personality and Social Psychology, 59,* 538–549.

Campbell, W. K. (1999). *Narcissism in everyday life.* Unpublished manuscript, Case Western Reserve University.

Campbell, W. K., Bosson, J. K., Goheen, T. W., Lakey, C. E., & Kernis, M. H. (2007). Do narcissists dislike themselves "deep down inside"? *Psychological Science, 18,* 227–229.

Campbell, W. K., & Sedikides, C. (1999). Self-threat magnifies the self-serving bias: A meta-analytic integration. *Review of General Psychology, 3,* 23–43.

Christensen, T. C., Wood, J. V., & Barrett, L. F. (2003). Remembering everyday experience through the prism of self-esteem. *Personality and Social Psychology Bulletin, 29,* 51–62.

Cooley, C. H. (1902). *Human nature and the social order.* New York: Scribner's.

Coopersmith, S. (1967). *The antecedents of self-esteem.* San Francisco: Freeman.

Cortes, B. P., Demoulin, S., Rodriguez, R. T., Rodriguez, A. P., & Leyens, J.-P. (2005). Infrahumanization or familiarity?: Attribution of uniquely human emotions to the self, the ingroup, and the outgroup. *Personality and Social Psychology Bulletin, 31,* 243–253.

Crocker, J. (1993). Memory for information about others: Effects of self-esteem and performance feedback. *Journal of Research in Personality, 27,* 35–48.

Crocker, J., & Park, L. E. (2004). The costly pursuit of self-esteem. *Psychological Bulletin, 130,* 392–414.

Dandeneau, S. D., & Baldwin, M. W. (2004). The inhibition of socially rejecting information among people with high versus low self-esteem: The role of attentional bias and the effects of bias reduction training. *Journal of Social and Clinical Psychology, 23,* 584–602.

Dawes, R. M. (1994). *House of cards: Psychology and psychotherapy built on myth.* New York: Free Press.

Deci, E. L., & Ryan, R. M. (1995). Human autonomy: The basis for true self-esteem. In M. H. Kernis (Ed.), *Efficacy, agency, and self-esteem* (pp. 31–49). New York: Plenum Press.

Demo, D. H. (1985). The measurement of self-esteem:

Refining our methods. *Journal of Personality and Social Psychology, 48,* 1490–1502.

Di Paula, A., & Campbell, J. D. (2002). Self-esteem and persistence in the face of failure. *Journal of Personality and Social Psychology, 83,* 711–724.

Diener, E., & Diener, M. (1995). Cross-cultural correlates of life satisfaction and self-esteem. *Journal of Personality and Social Psychology, 68,* 653–663.

Diggory, J. C. (1966). *Self-evaluation: Concepts and studies.* New York: Wiley.

Dodgson, P. G., & Wood, J. V. (1998). Self-esteem and the cognitive accessibility of strengths and weaknesses after failure. *Journal of Personality and Social Psychology, 75,* 178–197.

Donnellan, B., Trzesniewski, K., Robins, R., Moffitt, T., & Caspi, A. (2005). Low self-esteem is related to aggression, antisocial behavior, and delinquency. *Psychological Science, 16,* 328–335.

Downey, G., Freitas, A. L., Michaelis, B., & Khouri, H. (1998). The self-fulfilling prophecy in close relationships: Rejection sensitivity and rejection by romantic partners. *Journal of Personality and Social Psychology, 75,* 545–560.

DuBois, D. L., & Flay, B. R. (2004). The healthy pursuit of self-esteem: Comment on and alternative to the Crocker and Park (2004) formulation. *Psychological Bulletin, 130,* 415–420.

Epstein, S. (1979). Stability of behavior: On predicting most of the people much of the time. *Journal of Personality and Social Psychology, 37,* 1097–1126.

Epstein, S., & Morling, B. (1995). Is the self motivated to do more than enhance and/or verify itself? In M. H. Kernis (Ed.), *Efficacy, agency, and self-esteem* (pp. 9–29). New York: Plenum Press.

Fazio, R. H. (1990). Multiple processes by which attitudes guide behavior: The MODE model as an integrative framework. *Advances in Experimental Social Psychology, 23,* 75–109.

Ferrari, J. R. (1994). Dysfunctional procrastination and its relationship with self-esteem, interpersonal dependency, and self-defeating behaviors. *Personality and Individual Differences, 17,* 673–679.

Festinger, L. (1954). A theory of social comparison processes. *Human Relations, 7,* 117–140.

Fitch, G. (1970). Effects of self-esteem, perceived performance, and choice on causal attributions. *Journal of Personality and Social Psychology, 16,* 311–315.

Fleeson, W. (2004). Moving personality beyond the person–situation debate: The challenge and opportunity of within-person variability. *Current Directions in Psychological Science, 13,* 83–87.

Franks, D. D., & Marolla, J. (1976). Efficacious action and social approval as interacting dimensions of self-esteem: A tentative formulation through construct validation. *Sociometry, 39,* 324–341.

Freud, S. (1914/1957). On narcissism: An introduction. In J. Strachey (Ed. & Trans.), *The standard edition of the complete psychological works of Sigmund Freud* (Vol. 14, pp. 67–104). London: Hogarth Press. (Original work published 1914)

Gecas, V. (1971). Parental behavior and dimensions of adolescent self-evaluation. *Sociometry, 34,* 466–482.

Gibson, J. L. (1981). Personality and elite political behavior: The influence of self-esteem on judicial decision making. *Journal of Politics, 43,* 104–125.

Gosling, S. D., Ko, S. J., Mannarelli, T., & Morris, M. E. (2002). A room with a cue: Personality judgments based on offices and bedrooms. *Journal of Personality and Social Psychology, 82,* 379–398.

Greenwald, A. G., McGhee, D. E., & Schwartz, J. L. K. (1998). Measuring individual differences in implicit cognition: The Implicit Association Test. *Journal of Personality and Social Psychology, 74,* 1464–1480.

Haney, P., & Durlak, J. A. (1998). Changing self-esteem in children and adolescents: A meta-analytic review. *Journal of Clinical Child Psychology, 27,* 423–433.

Hart, J., Shaver, P. R., & Goldenberg, J. R. (2005). Attachment, self-esteem, worldviews, and terror management: Evidence for a tripartite security system theory. *Journal of Personality and Social Psychology, 88,* 999–1013.

Harter, S. (1990). Causes, correlates, and the functional role of global self-worth: A life-span perspective. In J. Kolligian & R. Sternberg (Eds.), *Perceptions of competence and incompetence across the life-span* (pp. 67–98). New Haven, CT: Yale University Press.

Harter, S. (1999). *The construction of the self: A developmental perspective.* New York: Guilford Press.

Harter, S., & Pike, R. (1971). The pictorial scale of Perceived Competence and Social Acceptance for Young Children. *Child Development, 55,* 1969–1982.

Heatherton, T. F., & Polivy, J. (1991). Development and validation of a scale for measuring state self-esteem. *Journal of Personality and Social Psychology, 60,* 895–910.

Heine, S. J., & Hamamura, D. R. (2007). In search of East Asian self-enhancement. *Personality and Social Psychology Review, 11,* 1–24.

Heine, S. J., & Lehman, D. R. (1997). The cultural construction of self-enhancement: An examination of group-serving biases. *Journal of Personality and Social Psychology, 72,* 1268–1283.

Heine, S. J., Lehman, D. R., Markus, H. R., & Kitayama, S. (1999). Is there a universal need for positive self-regard? *Psychological Review, 106,* 766–794.

Henrich, J., & Gil-White, F. J. (2001). The evolution of prestige: Freely conferred deference as a mechanism for enhancing the benefits of cultural transmission. *Evolution and Human Behavior, 22,* 165–196.

Higgins, E. T. (1987). Self-discrepancy: A theory relating self and affect. *Psychological Review, 94,* 319–340.

Hoyle, R. H. (1991). Evaluating measurement models in clinical research: Covariance structure analysis of latent variable models of self-conception. *Journal of Consulting and Clinical Psychology, 59,* 67–76.

Hoyle, R. H. (2006). Self-knowledge and self-esteem. In M. H. Kernis (Ed.), *Self-esteem issues and answers: A sourcebook of current perspectives* (pp. 208–215). New York: Psychology Press.

James, W. (1950). *The principles of psychology.* New York: Dover. (Original work published 1890)

Jones, E. E., & Berglas, S. (1978). Control of attributions about the self through self-handicapping strategies: The appeal of alcohol and the role of underachievement. *Personality and Social Psychology Bulletin, 4,* 200–206.

Josephs, R. A., Bosson, J. K., & Jacobs, C. G. (2003). Self-esteem maintenance processes: Why low self-esteem may be resistant to change. *Personality and Social Psychology Bulletin, 29,* 920–933.

Josephs, R. A., Larrick, R. P., Steele, C. M., & Nisbett, R. E. (1992). Protecting the self from the negative consequences of risky decisions. *Journal of Personality and Social Psychology, 62,* 26–37.

Judge, T. A., Erez, A., Bono, J. E., & Thoresen, C. J. (2002). Are measures of self-esteem, neuroticism, locus of control, and generalized self-efficacy indicators of a common core construct? *Journal of Personality and Social Psychology, 83,* 693–710.

Kendler, K. S., Gardner, C. O., & Prescott, C. A. (1998). A population-based twin study of self-esteem and gender. *Psychological Medicine, 28,* 1403–1409.

Kenrick, D. T., Groth, G. E., Trost, M. R., & Sadalla, E. K. (1993). Integrating evolutionary and social exchange perspectives on relationships: Effects of gender, self-appraisal, and involvement level on mate selection criteria. *Journal of Personality and Social Psychology, 64,* 951–969.

Kernis, M. H. (2001). Following the trail from narcissism to fragile self-esteem. *Psychological Inquiry, 12,* 223–226.

Kernis, M. H. (2003). Toward a conceptualization of optimal self-esteem. *Psychological Inquiry, 14,* 1–26.

Kernis, M. H. (2005). Measuring self-esteem in context: The importance of stability of self-esteem in psychological functioning. *Journal of Personality, 73,* 1–37.

Kirkpatrick, L. A., & Ellis, B. J. (2001). An evolutionary–psychological perspective on self-esteem: Multiple domains and multiple functions. In G. J. O. Fletcher & M. S. Clark (Eds.), *Blackwell handbook of social psychology: Vol. 2. Interpersonal processes* (pp. 411–436). Oxford, UK: Blackwell.

Koole, S. L., Dijksterhuis, A., & van Knippenberg, A. (2001). What's in a name: Implicit self-esteem and the automatic self. *Journal of Personality and Social Psychology, 80,* 669–685.

Kuiper, N. A., & Rogers, T. B. (1979). Encoding of personal information: Self–other differences. *Journal of Personality and Social Psychology, 37,* 499–514.

Kwan, V. S. Y., & Mandisodza, A. N. (2007). Self-esteem: On the relation between conceptualization and measurement. In C. Sedikides & S. Spencer (Eds.), *Frontiers in social psychology: The self* (pp. 259–282). Philadelphia: Psychology Press.

Leary, M. R. (1999). The social and psychological importance of self-esteem. In R. M. Kowalski & M. R. Leary (Eds.), *The social psychology of emotional and behavioral problems: Interfaces of social and clinical psychology* (pp. 197–221). Washington, DC: American Psychological Association.

Leary, M. R., & Baumeister, R. F. (2000). The nature and function of self-esteem: Sociometer theory. In M. Zanna (Ed.), *Advances in experimental social psychology* (Vol. 32, pp. 1–62). San Diego, CA: Academic Press.

Leary, M. R., Tambor, E. S., Terdal, S. K., & Downs, D. L. (1995). Self-esteem as an interpersonal monitor: The sociometer hypothesis. *Journal of Personality and Social Psychology, 68,* 518–530.

Leitenberg, H., Yost, L. W., & Carroll-Wilson, M. (1986). Negative cognitive errors in children: Questionnaire development, normative data, and comparisons between children with and without self-reported symptoms of depression, low self-esteem, and evaluation anxiety. *Journal of Consulting and Clinical Psychology, 54,* 528–536.

Leith, K. P., & Baumeister, R. F. (1998). Empathy, shame, guilt, and narratives of interpersonal conflicts: Guilt-prone people are better at perspective taking. *Journal of Personality, 66,* 1–37.

Luhtanen, R., & Crocker, J. (1992). A collective self-esteem scale: Self-evaluation of one's social identity. *Personality and Social Psychology Bulletin, 18,* 302–318.

Lyubomirsky, S., Tkach, C., & DiMatteo, M. R. (2005). What are the differences between happiness and self-esteem? *Social Indicators Research, 78,* 363–404.

Markus, H. (1977). Self-schemas and processing information about the self. *Journal of Personality and Social Psychology, 35,* 63–78.

Marsh, H. W. (1986). Global self-esteem: Its relation to specific facets of self-concept and their importance. *Journal of Personality and Social Psychology, 51,* 1224–1236.

Marsh, H. W., & Craven, R. G. (2006). Reciprocal effects of self-concept and performance from a multidimensional perspective: Beyond seductive pleasure and unidimensional perspectives. *Perspectives on Psychological Science, 1,* 133–163.

Marsh, H. W., & Hattie, J. (1996). Theoretical perspectives on the structure of self-concept. In B. Bracken (Ed.), *Handbook of self-concept* (pp. 38–90). New York: Wiley.

Marsh, H. W., & Shavelson, R. (1985). Self-concept: Its multifaceted, hierarchical structure. *Educational Psychologist, 20,* 107–125.

McFarlin, D. B. (1985). Persistence in the face of failure: The impact of self-esteem and contingency information. *Personality and Social Psychology Bulletin, 11,* 153–163.

McFarlin, D. B., Baumeister, R. F., & Blascovich, J. (1984). On knowing when to quit: Task failure, self-esteem, advice, and nonproductive persistence. *Journal of Personality, 52,* 138–155.

McGuire, S., Manke, B., Saudino, K. J., Reiss, D., Hetherington, E. M., & Plomin, R. (1999). Perceived competence and self-worth during adolescence: A longitudinal behavioral genetic study. *Child Development, 70,* 1283–1296.

Mead, G. H. (1934). *Mind, self and society.* Chicago: University of Chicago Press.

Mikulincer, M. (1995). Attachment style and the mental representation of the self. *Journal of Personality and Social Psychology, 69,* 1203–1215.

Morf, C. C., & Rhodewalt, F. (2001). Unraveling the paradoxes of narcissism: A dynamic self-regulatory processing model. *Psychological Inquiry, 12,* 177–196.

Morgan, H. J., & Janoff-Bulman, R. (1994). Positive and negative self-complexity: Patterns of adjustment following traumatic versus non-traumatic life experiences. *Journal of Social and Clinical Psychology, 13,* 63–85.

Murray, S. L., Holmes, J. G., MacDonald, G., & Ellsworth, P. (1998). Through the looking glass darkly?: When self-doubts turn into relationship insecurities. *Journal of Personality and Social Psychology,* 75, 1459–1480.

Neiss, M. B., Sedikides, C., & Stevenson, J. (2002). Self-esteem: A behavioural genetic perspective. *European Journal of Personality,* 16, 351–367.

Olson, M. A., Fazio, R. H., & Hermann, A. D., Sr. (2007). Reporting tendencies underlie discrepancies between implicit and explicit measures of self-esteem. *Psychological Science,* 18, 267–291.

Osgood, C. E. (1952). The nature and measurement of meaning. *Psychological Bulletin,* 49, 197–237.

Oyserman, D., Coon, H. M., & Kemmelmeier, M. (2002). Rethinking individualism and collectivism: Evaluation of theoretical assumptions and meta-analyses. *Psychological Bulletin,* 128, 3–72.

Paulhus, D. L., Robins, R. W., Trzesniewski, K. H., & Tracy, J. L. (2004). Two replicable suppressor situations in personality research. *Multivariate Behavioral Research,* 39, 303–329.

Pelham, B. W. (1991). On confidence and consequence: The certainty and importance of self-knowledge. *Journal of Personality and Social Psychology,* 60, 518–530.

Pelham, B. W., & Swann, W. B., Jr. (1989). From self-conceptions to self-worth: The sources and structure of self-esteem. *Journal of Personality and Social Psychology,* 57, 672–680.

Pyszczynski, T., Greenberg, J., Solomon, S., Arndt, J., & Schimel, J. (2004). Why do people need self-esteem?: A theoretical and empirical review. *Psychological Bulletin,* 130, 435–468.

Raimy, V. C. (1948). Self reference in counseling interviews. *Journal of Consulting Psychology,* 12, 153–163.

Raskin, R. N., & Hall, C. S. (1981). The Narcissistic Personality Inventory: Alternative form reliability and further evidence of construct validity. *Journal of Personality and Social Psychology,* 45, 159–162.

Raskin, R. N., Novacek, J., & Hogan, R. (1991). Narcissism, self-esteem, and defensive self-enhancement. *Journal of Personality,* 59, 19–38.

Rhodewalt, F., Madrian, J. C., & Cheney, S. (1998). Narcissism, self-knowledge organization, and emotional reactivity: The effect of daily experiences on self-esteem and affect. *Personality and Social Psychology Bulletin,* 24, 75–87.

Robbins, S. B., Lauver, K., Le, H., Langley, R., & Carlstrom, A. (2004). Do psychosocial and study skill factors predict college outcomes?: A meta-analysis. *Psychological Bulletin,* 130, 261–288.

Robins, R. W., Hendin, H. M., & Trzesniewski, K. H. (2001). Measuring global self-esteem: Construct validation of a single-item measure and the Rosenberg Self-Esteem Scale. *Personality and Social Psychology Bulletin,* 27, 151–161.

Rosenberg, M. (1965). *Society and the adolescent self-image.* Princeton, NJ: Princeton University Press.

Rosenberg, M., & Owens, T. J. (2001). Low self-esteem people: A collective portrait. In T. J. Owens, S. Stryker, & N. Goodman (Eds.), *Extending self-esteem theory and research: Sociological and psychological currents* (pp. 400–436). New York: Cambridge University Press.

Rosenberg, M. R., Schooler, C., Schoenbach, C., & Rosenberg, F. (1995). Global self-esteem and specific self-esteem: Different concepts, different outcomes. *American Sociological Review,* 60, 141–156.

Sadalla, E. K., Vershure, B., & Burroughs, J. (1987). Identity symbolism in housing. *Environment and Behavior,* 19, 569–587.

Sanna, L. J., & Meier, S. (2000). Looking for clouds in a silver lining: Self-esteem, mental simulations, and temporal confidence changes. *Journal of Research in Personality,* 34, 236–251.

Sanna, L. J., Turley-Ames, K. J., & Meier, S. (2000). Mood, self-esteem, and simulated alternatives: Thought-provoking affective influences on counterfactual direction. *Journal of Personality and Social Psychology,* 76, 543–558.

Savin-Williams, R. C., & Jaquish, G. A. (1981). The assessment of adolescent self-esteem: A comparison of methods. *Journal of Personality,* 49, 324–336.

Schafer, R. B., Wickrama, K. A. S., & Keith, P. M. (1996). Self-concept disconfirmation, psychological distress, and marital happiness. *Journal of Marriage and the Family,* 58, 167–177.

Scheff, T. J., & Fearon, D. S. (2004). Cognition and emotion?: The dead end in self-esteem research. *Journal for the Theory of Social Behaviour,* 34, 73–91.

Schroeder, D. G., Josephs, R. A., & Swann, W. B., Jr. (2006). *Foregoing lucrative employment to preserve low self-esteem.* Unpublished manuscript.

Sedikides, C., Gaertner, L., & Toguchi, Y. (2003). Pancultural self-enhancement. *Journal of Personality and Social Psychology,* 84, 60–79.

Sedikides, C., Gaertner, L., & Vevea, J. (2005). Pancultural self-enhancement reloaded: A meta-analytic reply to Heine (2005). *Journal of Personality and Social Psychology,* 89, 539–551.

Setliff, A. E., & Marmurek, H. H. C. (2002). The mood regulatory function of autobiographical recall is moderated by self-esteem. *Personality and Individual Differences,* 32, 761–771.

Shavelson, R. J., Hubner, J. J., & Stanton, G. C. (1976). Validation of construct interpretations. *Review of Educational Research,* 46, 407–441.

Showers, C. J. (1992). Compartmentalization of positive and negative self-knowledge: Keeping bad apples out of the bunch. *Journal of Personality and Social Psychology,* 62, 1036–1049.

Shrauger, J. S., & Lund, A. K. (1975). Self-evaluation and reactions to evaluations from others. *Journal of Personality,* 43, 94–108.

Story, A. L. (1998). Self-esteem and memory for favorable and unfavorable personality feedback. *Personality and Social Psychology Bulletin,* 24, 51–64.

Suls, J. (2006). On the divergent and convergent validity of self-esteem. In M. H. Kernis (Ed.), *Self-esteem issues and answers: A sourcebook of current perspectives* (pp. 36–43). New York: Psychology Press.

Swann, W. B., Jr. (1983). Self-verification: Bringing social reality into harmony with the self. In J. Suls & A. G. Greenwald (Eds.), *Psychological perspectives on the self* (Vol. 2, pp. 33–66). Hillsdale, NJ: Erlbaum.

Swann, W. B., Jr. (1990). To be adored or to be known?: The interplay of self-enhancement and self-verification. In E. T. Higgins & R. M. Sorrentino (Eds.), *Handbook of motivation and cognition: Vol. 2. Foundations of social behavior* (pp. 408–448). New York: Guilford Press.

Swann, W. B., Jr. (1996). *Self-traps: The elusive quest for higher self-esteem.* New York: Freeman.

Swann, W. B., Jr., Beavers, C., & McGeary, J. (2007). *Genetic influences on self-esteem.* Unpublished manuscript, University of Texas.

Swann, W. B., Jr., Chang-Schneider, C., & McClarty, K. (2007). Do our self-views matter?: Self-concept and self-esteem in everyday life. *American Psychologist, 62,* 84–94.

Swann, W. B., Jr., Chang-Schneider, C., & McClarty, K. (2008). Yes, cavalier attitudes can have pernicious consequences: A reply to Krueger, Vohs, & Baumeister. *American Psychologist, 63,* 65–66.

Swann, W. B., Jr., De La Ronde, C., & Hixon, J. G. (1994). Authenticity and positivity strivings in marriage and courtship. *Journal of Personality and Social Psychology, 66,* 857–869.

Swann, W. B., Jr., Griffin, J. J., Predmore, S. C., & Gaines, B. (1987). The cognitive–affective crossfire: When self-consistency confronts self-enhancement. *Journal of Personality and Social Psychology, 52,* 881–889.

Swann, W. B., Jr., & Pelham, B. W. (2002). Who wants out when the going gets good?: Psychological investment and preference for self-verifying college roommates. *Self and Identity, 1,* 219–233.

Swann, W. B., Jr., Pelham, B. W., & Krull, D. S. (1989). Agreeable fancy or disagreeable truth?: Reconciling self-enhancement and self-verification. *Journal of Personality and Social Psychology, 57,* 782–791.

Swann, W. B., Jr., & Read, S. J. (1981). Self-verification processes: How we sustain our self-conceptions. *Journal of Experimental Social Psychology, 17,* 351–372.

Swann, W.B., Jr., Rentfrow, P. J., & Guinn, J. (2003). Self-verification: The search for coherence. In M. R. Leary & J. P. Tangney (Eds.), *Handbook of self and identity* (pp. 367–383). New York: Guilford Press.

Tafarodi, R. W. (1998). Paradoxical self-esteem and selectivity in the processing of social information. *Journal of Personality and Social Psychology, 74,* 1181–1196.

Tafarodi, R. W., & Milne, A. B. (2002). Decomposing global self-esteem. *Journal of Personality, 70,* 443–483.

Tafarodi, R. W., & Swann, W. B., Jr. (1996). Individualism–collectivism and global self-esteem: Evidence for a cultural trade off. *Journal of Cross-Cultural Psychology, 27,* 651–672.

Tafarodi, R. W., & Swann, W. B., Jr. (2001). Two-dimensional self-esteem: Theory and measurement. *Personality and Individual Differences, 31,* 653–673.

Tice, D. M., & Baumeister, R. F. (1990). Self-esteem, self-handicapping, and self-presentation: The strategy of inadequate practice. *Journal of Personality, 58,* 443–464.

Tracy, J. L., & Robins, R. W. (2007). The psychological structure of pride: A tale of two facets. *Journal of Personality and Social Psychology, 92,* 506–525.

Trzesniewski, K., Donnellan, B., Moffitt, T., Robins, R., Poulton, R., & Caspi, A. (2006). Low self-esteem during adolescence predicts poor health, criminal behavior, and limited economic prospects during adulthood. *Developmental Psychology, 42,* 381–390.

Twenge, J. M., & Campbell, W. K. (2001). Age and birth cohort differences in self-esteem: A cross-temporal meta-analysis. *Personality and Social Psychology Review, 5,* 321–344.

Valentine, J. C., DuBois, D. L., & Cooper, H. (2004). The relation between self-beliefs and academic achievement: A meta-analytic review. *Educational Psychologist, 39,* 111–133.

Verschueren, K., Marcoen, A., & Schoefs, V. (1996). The internal working model of the self, attachment, and competence in five-year-olds. *Child Development, 67,* 2493–2511.

Waters, E., Noyes, D. M., Vaughn, B. E., & Ricks, M. (1985). Q-sort definitions of social competence and self-esteem: Discriminant validity of related constructs in theory and data. *Developmental Psychology, 21,* 508–522.

Watson, D., Suls, J., & Haig, J. (2002). Global self-esteem in relation to structural models of personality and affectivity. *Journal of Personality and Social Psychology, 83,* 185–197.

Webster, G. D. (2007). Is the relationship between self-esteem and physical aggression necessarily U-shaped? *Journal of Research in Personality, 41,* 977–982.

Westen, D. (1990). The relations among narcissism, egocentrism, self-concept, and self-esteem: Experimental, clinical, and theoretical considerations. *Psychoanalysis and Contemporary Thought, 13,* 183–239.

Wheeler, L., & Miyake, K. (1992). Social comparison in everyday life. *Journal of Personality and Social Psychology, 62,* 760–773.

Wiesenfeld, B. M., Swann, W. B., Jr., Brockner, J., & Bartel, C. (2007). Is more fairness always preferred?: Self-esteem moderates reactions to procedural justice. *Academy of Management Journal, 50,* 1235–1253.

Woolfolk, R. L., Novalany, J., Gara, M. A., Allen, L. A., & Polino, M. (1995). Self-complexity, self-evaluation, and depression: An examination of form and content within the self-schema. *Journal of Personality and Social Psychology, 68,* 1108–1120.

Wray, L. D., & Stone, E. R. (2005). The role of self-esteem and anxiety in decision making for self versus others in relationships. *Journal of Behavioral Decision Making, 18,* 125–144.

CHAPTER 37

■ ● ▲ ◆ ■ ● ▲ ◆

Narcissism

FREDERICK RHODEWALT
BENJAMIN PETERSON

In his review of theory and research on narcissism, Pulver (1970) concluded that narcissism ranks among psychoanalysis's most important contributions—but also among its most confusing. Although clinical psychology continues to be the wellspring of theory and data on pathological narcissism, interest in narcissism has spread to other areas in the social and behavioral sciences. Emmons (1987) described two trends in the study of narcissism. First, he noted that narcissism is sometimes discussed as a social or cultural tendency (see Lasch, 1979). Emmons suggested that to the extent that a society is "self-seeking," the less it is willing to pursue common societal goals and the more it is willing to abide egocentric biases such as racism, sexism, fundamentalism, and nationalism, as well as conflict stemming from these biases. The second trend Emmons noted is research in social psychology on "self-serving" biases and processes, such as those exemplified in Greenwald's (1980) classic essay, "The Totalitarian Ego." In this view, we are all a little narcissistic, taking credit for successes and shunning responsibility for failures.

A third trend in theory and research on narcissism has developed largely in the 20 years since Emmons's (1987) work. Growing out of the work in psychoanalysis, clinical psychology, and social psychology, this newest trend involves the study of the narcissistic personality type, or individual differences in narcissistic style at the subclinical level. This direction in the study of narcissism is indebted to two related advances. First, psychiatry and psychology agreed on a clinical description of narcissistic personality disorder (DSM-III; American Psychiatric Association, 1980), which, in turn, allowed measurement instruments to be developed and validation work to be undertaken. This advance then spawned the interest of contemporary social and personality psychologists in the expression of narcissism in nonclinical populations, allowing the placement of narcissism within current social-cognitive, self-regulatory frameworks. In this chapter we focus on issues and assumptions involving the conceptualization and assessment of narcissism in *nonclinical* populations, outline some current theoretical and measurement issues, and propose some important future directions for research on narcissism.

Clinical Theory and Background

Havelock Ellis (1898) is credited with transporting the concept "narcissus-like" from Greek mythology to his writings on sexual behavior. He used the term to refer to autoeroticism, a condition in which a person regards his or her body as a sexual object. Psychoanalysts Freud (1914/1953), Kernberg (1975), and Kohut (1971), however, made the most substantial contributions in terms of placing the construct of narcissism within the lexicon of psychiatry and clinical psychology. Their positions are elaborate and complex and differ from one another in significant ways. A full description of the Freud, Kernberg, and Kohut writings on narcissism is beyond the scope of this chapter, and the reader is referred to an edited volume by Morrison (1986), which contains many of the original sources and several excellent overviews.

Here we extract what we view as their essential ideas, those that have formed the foundation for contemporary work on the narcissistic personality type. Collectively, Freud's, Kernberg's, and Kohut's central theoretical positions described the narcissist as an individual who, as a result of a history of unsatisfactory social relationships, possesses a grandiose and defensive self-concept that contains a conflicted psychological dependence on other people. Rhodewalt and Morf (2005) characterized psychoanalytic views on narcissism as agreeing that adult narcissism results from a childhood history of problematic interpersonal relationships. As a consequence, narcissistic adults appear to possess a grandiose self-concept and invulnerability on the outside but emptiness and isolation on the inside. This combination leads to a highly conflicted overdependence on others to maintain self-esteem.

Perhaps the theorist who best bridges classic psychoanalytic and contemporary views on narcissism is Annie Reich (1960). Her discussion of narcissism as pathological self-esteem regulation anticipates recent work on social-cognitive self-regulatory models of narcissism (Morf & Rhodewalt, 2001; Rhodewalt & Morf, 2005). In accord with the psychoanalytic views of the time, Reich described narcissism as an overinvestment of libido in the self at the expense of investment in others (objects). Reich took a contemporary view of self-esteem, stating that it is the harmony or discrepancy between one's self-representations and one's wishful concept of the self—in other words, a discrepancy between actual and ideal selves (cf. Higgins, 1987). Given that narcissists' ideal self-images are grandiose and unrealistic, they must go to extraordinary lengths to create an actual self that is close to these self-standards in order to experience high self-regard. Reich described behaviors such as compensatory self-inflation, aggression, and overdependence on social approval as part of the narcissist's repertoire of self-esteem regulation behaviors. In brief, narcissists embrace grandiose self-images to compensate for deficits in their early interpersonal experiences and spend their lives managing the problem of grandiose but fragile self-esteem resulting from the pursuit of such self-ideals.

Definition and Operationalization

Despite the richness of clinical theory and description, they did not generate systematic research on narcissism because there was little consensus among theorists on the defining features of narcissism. Consequently, there was no consistently accepted manner of assessing the presence (or degree) of narcissism that would allow the empirical study of the thoughts and behaviors of such individuals. Thus the field was left with a body of work that was highly theoretical and based mainly on clinical description.

This situation changed with the publication of the third edition of the *Diagnostic and Statistical Manual of Mental Disorders* (DSM-III, American Psychiatric Association, 1980), which organized clinical description into a working "definition" of narcissism with criteria that could be used for assessment and research. In this edition of the DSM-III, narcissism was included as an Axis II personality disorder. The specific criteria that were ultimately adopted reflected the major influence of the theoretical models of Kernberg (1975) and Kohut (1971).

As is the tradition for all DSM disorders, an individual is considered to be a "narcissist" (classified as having narcissistic personality disorder [NPD]) if he or she meets a certain level of the criteria set forth. In other words, there is a certain cutoff point between individuals who are narcissistic and others who fall just shy, with a qualitative difference assumed between the two groups (see Foster & Campbell, 2007, for further discussion of the taxonic vs. dimensional description of narcissism). The initial criteria included in the DSM-III for narcissism were as follows:

(1) Grandiose sense of self-importance and uniqueness, e.g., exaggeration of achievements and talents, focus on the special nature of one's problems.
(2) Preoccupation with fantasies of unlimited success, power, brilliance, beauty, or ideal love.
(3) Exhibitionism: the person requires constant attention and admiration.
(4) Cool indifference or marked feelings of rage, inferiority, shame, humiliation, or emptiness in response to criticism, indifference of others, or defeat.
(5) At least two of the following characteristic of disturbances in interpersonal relationships:
  a. Entitlement: expectation of special favors without assuming reciprocal responsibilities, e.g., surprise and anger that people will not do what is wanted;
  b. Interpersonal exploitativeness: taking advantage of others to indulge own desires or for self-aggrandizement; disregard for the personal integrity and rights of others;
  c. Relationships that characteristically alternate between the extremes of overidealization and devaluation;
  d. Lack of empathy: inability to recognize how others feel, e.g., unable to appreciate the distress of someone who is seriously ill. (American Psychiatric Association, 1980)

This definition clearly emphasizes the narcissist's characteristic grandiosity in relation to his or her self-image, and this emphasis has continued through subsequent revisions to the criteria (DSM-III-R [American Psychiatric Association, 1987], DSM-IV [American Psychiatric Association, 1994], DSM-IV-TR [American Psychiatric Association, 2000]). It is this grandiosity aspect of narcissism that most effectively distinguishes it from other "Cluster B" personality disorders (such as histrionic, antisocial, and borderline personalities) when DSM criteria are evaluated for their ability to categorize disorders properly (Gunderson, Ronningstam, & Smith, 1991). Such distinctions are important for psychiatric diagnosis, though this process may exclude important features of the construct that are potentially important to other researchers.

The establishment of criteria for NPD was important in many ways, most significantly in facilitating the development of self-report scales that were based on these criteria—which, in turn, stimulated research on the construct. Some scales were based on existing large-scale personality inventories such as the Minnesota Multiphasic Personality Inventory (MMPI) (e.g., Ashby, Lee, & Duke, 1979; Morey, Waugh, & Blashfield, 1985; Wink & Gough, 1990), and other new scales were subsequently created (e.g., the Margolis–Thomas Measure of Narcissism—Mullins & Kopelman, 1988; the Millon Clinical Multiaxial Inventory narcissism subscale—Millon & Davis, 1997), but the one that has received by far the most empirical attention is the Narcissistic Personality Inventory (NPI; Raskin & Hall, 1979, 1981). Using the DSM-III criteria directly as a guide, Raskin and Hall (1979) originally developed a 54-item scale that used a forced-choice format, such that the respondent had to choose the one of two statements that was most self-descriptive. Unlike some of the other scales that were developed, the stated purpose of the NPI was to assess narcissism in the subclinical general population (as a personality "trait"). Thus narcissism was seen as falling on a general continuum of personality such that only extreme levels may be considered to characterize NPD in the clinical sense. Even though certain elevated "subthreshold" narcissism scores may not be considered as constituting NPD in a clinical sense, high levels of subclinical narcissism should promote similar outcomes and problems as does NPD.

A great deal of research has been conducted on the construct validity, reliability, internal consistency, and factor structure of the NPI. From the original 54-item version, two commonly used versions have been put forth, each paring off several of the original items and proposing varying factor structures (Emmons, 1987; Raskin & Terry, 1988). Emmons's (1984, 1987) 37-item version comprises four underlying factors: Leadership/Authority, Self-Absorption/Self-Admiration, Superiority/Arrogance, and Exploitativeness/Entitlement. Using this version, Emmons and others have argued that exploitativeness and entitlement may represent the most maladaptive aspects of NPI-based narcissism. Raskin and Terry (1988) also revised and improved on the original NPI with a 40-item version that could be divided into seven subscales: Authority, Self-Sufficiency, Superiority, Exhibitionism, Exploitativeness, Vanity, and Entitlement. Even though the description of the underlying structure varies between the two versions, the proposed elements that make up the overall narcissism score are very similar (and also relatively consistent with the DSM criteria on which the scale is based). Additionally, there is essentially no difference in the item pool of the two versions, with all of the items in the 37-item version found in the 40-item set.

Both of these versions are commonly used in research, and in most cases, researchers simply use the full-scale narcissism score and disregard the subscale scores. Although the subscales are different across the two versions, a common outcome that hampers their use is low internal consistency (del Rosario & White, 2005; Emmons, 1987; Raskin & Terry, 1988). Additionally, there have been problems in attempting to replicate the factor structure of both versions. For example, Kubarych (2004) proposed that the NPI could be represented across three factors, which he named Power, Exhibitionism, and Special Person.

Even so, the NPI continues to be the measure of choice. Although the NPI has not undergone any large-scale revisions to its item content or response format, it has been translated into several languages (e.g., Kansi, 2003) and adapted for use with children (Ang & Yusof, 2006) and juvenile offenders (Calhoun, Glaser, Stefurak, & Bradshaw, 2000). Additionally, a shorter, 16-item version was recently developed to cut down on administration time (Ames, Rose, & Anderson, 2006), although further testing is necessary to see whether this shorter scale effectively captures the essence of the full version. Questions about the psychometrics and appropriate breadth of the NPI (e.g., Pimentel, Ansell, Pincus, & Cain, 2006), as well as debates over subforms of narcissism and the development of instruments that isolate certain underlying characteristics of narcissism (e.g., Campbell, Bonacci, Shelton, Exline, & Bushman, 2004) might challenge the supremacy of the NPI as the measure of choice. For now, a substantial amount of research attests to the construct validity of the NPI as a measure of the narcissistic personality type.

Contemporary Models

The NPI has been used to produce a wealth of correlational and experimental data (see Rhodewalt & Sorrow, 2003, for a review). As mentioned, such data provide compelling evidence for the NPI's construct validity. More important, social and personality psychologists have begun to mine these findings to construct theories of narcissism that highlight the coherence of the broad range of its defining characteristics. These theories expand on earlier psychoanalytic perspectives by incorporating contemporary social-cognitive and motivational constructs in an attempt to characterize the psychological *processes* that underlie narcissism.

The most expansive attempt in this area is Morf and Rhodewalt's dynamic self-regulatory model of narcissism (Morf & Rhodewalt, 2001; Rhodewalt, 2001; Rhodewalt & Morf, 2005). This model captures the convergence among clinical theorists that narcissism is energized by concerns about self-esteem maintenance and enhancement. Moreover, the model recognizes that narcissists' self-esteem concerns are played out (and satisfied or frustrated) through social interaction. As a consequence of this interpersonal regulation of the self, the narcissistic self-concept is highly contextually variable. As situations change with respect to self-enhancement affordances, narcissists redirect their attention and behavior to new opportunities. One situation may offer the opportunity to garner admiration for a particular competency, and the next may offer the opportunity to enhance in a different domain. The focal goal for the narcissist is polymorphous self-enhancement, regardless of the relevance of the attribute to his or her self-definition.

Narcissism in the Morf–Rhodewalt model reflects a set of self-regulatory processes that comprise both interpersonal gambits for admiration and intrapersonal strategies for self-protection and enhancement. The key idea is that it is the *self* (self-concept and attached self-worth) that is regulated, maintained, and defended in the interpersonal context. Narcissists are seen to possess transient, overblown, and fragile self-images that can be sustained only through social validation. Narcissists are active rather than passive in their efforts at self-protection and enhancement, employing interpersonal strategies designed to manipulate impressions that others hold of them, as well as the feedback they receive from others. They also are active with regard to the intrapersonal strategies they employ, distorting and biasing their interpretations of outcomes and selectively recalling past events in self-enhancing ways.

The dynamic aspect of the model is captured in its recursive quality. Narcissistic self-esteem regulation is shaped and molded by ongoing and changing self-concerns and social contexts. In turn, narcissistic individuals behave in accord with their current concerns about self-definition, and these behaviors influence the social context. The social context provides affordances for addressing issues involving self-concept and self-worth by highlighting, intensifying, or redirecting attention to specific aspects of the self. Rhodewalt and Morf (2005) argued that the narcissistic self is context bound and that transitions from one social context to another lend to the fragility and vulnerability of such individuals' self-views.

The model has been helpful in organizing research findings and generating new hypotheses. The research is too extensive to review here (see Rhodewalt & Sorrow, 2003), so we highlight some key examples of the intra- and interpersonal self-regulation in which narcissists engage. Perhaps the clearest example of narcissistic intrapersonal self-regulation is their pronounced tendency to make self-aggrandizing attributions for positive outcomes even when those outcomes are response noncontingent (Rhodewalt & Morf, 1995, 1998). In line with Jones and Berglas's (1978) reasoning about the genesis of self-handicapping, this self-aggrandizing attributional style in all likelihood contributes to narcissists' positive but fragile self-conceptions, as well as to their emotional and interpersonal reactions to threats to the self. Rhodewalt and colleagues (Rhodewalt & Morf, 1998; Rhodewalt, Tragakis, & Finnerty, 2006) contend that narcissists claim identities that, although highly positive, are uncertain and easily threatened. This unspoken uncertainty about the self lies behind the narcissist's apparently insatiable drive for admiration and regard from others. Interpersonal strategies include aggrandizing self-presentations (Morf, 1994), derogation of those who threaten them (Kernis &

Sun, 1994), and self-handicapping (Rhodewalt et al., 2006).

Morf and Rhodewalt (2001) also included the narcissist's social relationships and contexts as an element in the model. Narcissists have an impact on their social worlds through their actions, interpretations, and choices of interaction partners, so their social environments are objectively different from those of less narcissistic individuals. Relationships and social contexts are attractive to narcissists to the extent that they provide self-enhancement opportunities, and it appears that they manage these with at least some short-term success. Paulhus (1998) reported that narcissists are successful in garnering admiration and positive regard early in their relationships but that, over time, these same interpersonal tactics result in rejection and hostility. The reason is that interaction partners come to see the narcissists as acting in ways that are self-promoting and aggrandizing while also putting others down (Buss & Chiodo, 1991).

The final element in the model is the narcissistic self-concept. Akhtar and Thomson (1982) summarized the clinical literature as indicating that narcissists' public grandiosity overlays an underlying fragility and feelings of worthlessness. A challenge that has clear implications for the assessment of narcissism is to understand the coexistence of grandiosity and vulnerability within the narcissistic self-concept.

Following the publication of the Morf–Rhodewalt model, others have offered extensions or alternatives to the dynamic self-regulatory processing framework. Baumeister and Vohs (2001) offered the analogy of addiction to describe narcissists' pursuit of self-esteem. They suggested that narcissists *crave* feelings of superiority and approval, build up a tolerance to such feedback (thus requiring more and more), and exhibit withdrawal (distress) when they fail to receive what they crave. This perspective is descriptive but not yet subjected to empirical test. In our view, it is a way of restating the self-regulation model and may not be substantially different in the final analysis.

More recently, Campbell and Foster (2007) proposed the extended-agency model. They noted that narcissists have positive self-images that are based on admiration and success rather than on social acceptance and approval (Raskin, Novacek, & Hogan, 1991). Additionally, narcissists are not invested in warm communal relationships, and their self-regulatory strategies center on attempts to make themselves look powerful and competent. Campbell and Foster argued that, collectively, these characteristics are accounted for by the narcissist's high agency and low communion. An interesting contribution is their notion that narcissism waxes and wanes as a function of whether self-esteem needs are currently satisfied. That is, narcissism is more state-like than trait-like. One corollary of their model is that narcissism is not driven by the pursuit of an overarching goal such as self-enhancement or self-esteem regulation. Rather, narcissists' goals are context dependent. This is a provocative idea that contrasts with the Rhodewalt–Morf assumption that protecting, maintaining, and enhancing the self are chronically accessible goals that may be fulfilled polymorphously in any social context that affords the opportunity to experience positive self-esteem. Distinguishing between these two models would provide an important advance in the understanding of self-esteem regulation. This discussion may also shed light on gender differences in the incidence of narcissism observed in clinical populations. The higher incidence of NPD among men may reflect compatibility between narcissism and the agentic features of the male gender role. Narcissism in women may be masked by the fact that narcissism is not compatible with the expression of communion, the hallmark of the female gender role.

Several theorists have taken the approach that narcissism is best accounted for through its association with certain dispositions. Paulhus (2001) proposed that the combination of extraversion and low agreeableness (high antagonism) is equivalent to narcissism. Evidence suggests that narcissism occupies the high extraversion/low agreeableness location in "Big Five" space (Wiggins & Pincus, 1989). Ruiz, Smith, and Rhodewalt (2001) projected measures of hostility and narcissism onto the interpersonal circumplex (IASR-B5; Trapnell & Wiggins, 1990) and found that both hostility and narcissism were associated with low affiliation (low agreeableness) but that only narcissism was associated with high dominance (extraversion). When the NPI subscales were projected onto the circumplex, however, Leadership/Authority and Self-Absorption/Self-Admiration were associated with dominance but not low affiliation, Superiority/Arrogance was associated with both dominance and low affiliation, and Exploitativeness/Entitlement was associated with dominance, low affiliation, and high neuroticism. Ruiz and colleagues suggested caution in the interpretation of composite scores that may contain distinct personality characteristics. That caution notwithstanding, in our view, reducing narcissism to a combination of extraversion (or dominance) and low agreeableness (or low affiliation) does not account for the specific patterns of motivation and self-regulatory behaviors indicated in the literature. That is, narcissists may be high in extraversion and low in agreeableness, but this description does not account for their being so sensitive to threats to the self and relentless in seeking admiration.

In a meta-analysis of studies that included measures of narcissism and measures of impulsivity, Vazire and Funder (2006) reported a mean effect size of $r = .34$ across 10 independent samples and concluded that impulsivity is a defining characteristic of narcissism. Impulsivity, they contend, accounts for much of narcissists' self-enhancing as well as self-defeating behavior. Vazire and Funder suggested that impulsivity should be included in self-regulatory models of narcissism, and we agree, with two important caveats. First, the correlations between NPI-defined narcissism and impulsivity, extraversion, and low agreeableness are significant but modest, and many people who possess these dispositions would not be considered narcissists. Second, we suspect that the linkages between narcissism and these dispositions reflect their common associations with temperament; all have significant heritability quotients. Thus a child who is temperamentally disposed toward extraversion, impulsivity, and/or low agreeableness is more likely to become narcissistic given a set of parent–child interactions than is an introverted, agreeable, well-controlled child placed in the same socialization context.

In sum, a number of contemporary models of narcissism draw on either social-cognitive processing constructs (Morf & Rhodewalt, 2001) or dispositional models (Paulhus, 2001; Vazire & Funder, 2006) to account for the psychological features that underlie the construct. This work largely relies on narcissism as assessed by the NPI, which, in turn, is based on clinical definitions of narcissism (DSM-IV-TR; American Psychiatric Association, 2000). The research is extensive and supports the view that narcissism is fundamentally a pattern of interpersonal self-esteem regulation. However, pieces of the puzzle require further explanation and elaboration. One central question is whether these models characterize all narcissists or whether there are different forms of the characteristic.

Building on NPI Description and Self-Regulatory Models: Some Integrative Issues

Personality and social psychology researchers have successfully taken the construct of narcissism as described in the psychoanalytic literature and translated it into the narcissistic personality type, an individual difference in dynamic, defensive self-regulation found in nonclinical populations. This burgeoning literature relies almost exclusively on the NPI as its measure of narcissism. Although the overall characterization of narcissism as pathological self-esteem regulation is both compelling and consistent with clinical research and theory, puzzling inconsistencies and paradoxes raise difficult questions and calls for further refinement of narcissism theory and measurement. For example, researchers are debating the true nature of narcissism: Should it be considered a unitary or multidimensional construct? Does it contain both adaptive and maladaptive aspects? How might potentially discrepant "inner" and "outer" self-beliefs be assessed and incorporated into theory? What needs to be assessed to capture the possible multifaceted nature of narcissism? In this section, we address the current state of some of these debates and provide some analysis and integration in the hope of organizing and stimulating future research.

Is There More Than One Type of Narcissism?

The DSM definition of narcissism (developed for NPD) focuses on grandiosity as its essen-

tial feature. The NPI was developed using this definition, and, as noted, the NPI has been used in the vast majority of research on narcissism within personality and social psychology. Thus this research is based on an interpersonal type of narcissism that Akhtar and Thomson (1982) labeled *overt* narcissism. Overt narcissists openly seek admiration and use their interpersonal relationships for self-aggrandizement.

Although this conceptualization has produced a large and coherent research base, it may tell only half the narcissism story, because there may be a second "type" of narcissist, one that was also described by Kernberg (1975) and Kohut (1971). This narcissist has been variously termed *covert* (Akhtar & Thomson, 1982; Kernberg, 1975; Wink, 1991), *vulnerable* (Dickinson & Pincus, 2003; Wink, 1991), *hypersensitive* (Hendin & Cheek, 1997), and *hypervigilant* (Gabbard, 1998), as the individual tends to be reserved and withdrawn interpersonally while harboring some elements of characteristic narcissistic expectations for self and others (e.g., entitlement). In other words, the grandiose type of narcissist does not hide his or her narcissistic expectations from others (he or she is "overt"), whereas the vulnerable type of narcissist may present in a different, more modest manner (he or she keeps his or her grandiosity needs more "covert"). Because of this difference, some clinical theorists and practitioners believe that the narcissist captured by the DSM criteria and the NPI (and thus most social-personality research that uses the NPI) is incongruent with what they see in therapy (see Cain, Pincus, & Ansell, 2008, for a review).

There is support for the position that narcissism occurs in several types. For example, Wink (1991) examined several MMPI narcissism scales, including some that focus on grandiose aspects and others that focus on more sensitive aspects. In a factor analysis of the six scales, Wink found that the two sets loaded on separate factors, which he called Grandiosity-Exhibitionism and Vulnerability-Sensitivity. Importantly, the two factors had very distinct patterns of correlates. Whereas the grandiose pattern resembled much of what has been discussed up to this point (i.e., dominance, assertiveness, aggressiveness), the vulnerable pattern was one of "defensive, hypersensitive, anxious, and socially reticent individuals whose personal relations, however, were marked by self-indulgence, conceit, and arrogance, and an insistence on having their own way" (Wink, 1991, p. 596). More recent research by Dickinson and Pincus (2003) found similar patterns using the NPI and its subscales. At the clinical level, Fossati and colleagues (2005) found evidence for two clusters of symptoms reflecting overt and covert expressions in a structural examination of DSM-IV NPD criteria. Thus there appears to be support for more than one type of narcissism and for the idea that the overwhelming focus on grandiose aspects does not capture the full nature of the construct.

The picture of the covert, vulnerable, and hypersensitive narcissist is one of a "seething" individual who expects a great deal from him- or herself and the world but who has not experienced a great deal of confirmation of those expectations. As a result, this person becomes anxious and depressed and withdraws from social interaction, out of fear of further narcissistic injury in the form of lack of admiration and rejection from others. Even though this picture is in stark contrast to that of its more overt and grandiose counterpart, the two types do share some commonalities. Most prominently, assessments of covert narcissism tend to correlate to a greater extent with overt (e.g., NPI) elements involving entitlement and exploitativeness (Emmons, 1987). Dickinson and Pincus (2003), citing consistencies with clinical theory (e.g., Akhtar & Thomson, 1982) and empirical research (e.g., Emmons, 1987), proposed that entitlement may be the "core element" of narcissism that contributes to difficulties in regulating self-esteem. Thus overt/grandiose and covert/vulnerable narcissism may be different manifestations of this underlying core. Future research should look for ways of recognizing these two "types," as well as attempting to integrate their core elements.

Researchers are often urged to report relations between NPI subscales and dependent variables, as well as the relations between the NPI total score and these outcomes. The logic is that such analyses will allow researchers to identify the "toxic" component of narcissism and perhaps reveal different forms of narcissism, but we are not certain that this practice addresses the subtype

question. First, the NPI is based on the DSM definition of narcissism, which recognizes that pathological narcissism is a syndrome of characteristics. Would a person who has a sense of leadership and authority in the absence of entitlement, exploitativeness, superiority, arrogance, self-absorption, and self-admiration be categorized as a narcissist? (We think not.) Second, in research using the NPI, the subscales are always correlated. Thus a person categorized as a narcissist is, in all likelihood, scoring somewhat highly on all subscales. It is important to develop assessment instruments that allow researchers to distinguish between overt and covert narcissism, but we do not believe that decomposing the NPI will prove to be the most useful means of doing so.

Are "Normal" Narcissists More Psychologically Healthy?

Research has generally found that narcissists report that they possess many positive psychological resources, such as self-esteem, happiness, optimism, and life satisfaction, as well as a lack of negative psychological outcomes, such as depression, loneliness, anxiety, and neuroticism. Although we do not find these results surprising, the more interesting question may be, What do they truly tell us about narcissism and its adaptive versus maladaptive features?

Sedikides, Rudich, Gregg, Kumashiro, and Rusbult (2004) suggested that such findings tell us that self-esteem is the key to the overall psychological "health" of narcissists. Similarly, Rose and Campbell (2004) pointed to the appetitive goals that narcissists pursue, combined with their subjective appraisals that they are successfully negotiating their interpersonal environments in pursuit of such goals. We agree that narcissists display a positive bias in self-related accounts but question whether this indicates positive mental health. First, the pattern of hyperresponsiveness to threats to the self belies a secure, confident, and mentally healthy individual. Furthermore, narcissists' self-views are quite positive, but evidence shows that their self-evaluations are *inflated* compared with objective reality (Gabriel, Critelli, & Ee, 1994; John & Robins, 1994; Rhodewalt & Eddings, 2002; Rhodewalt & Morf, 1998). Finally, many of the empirical findings relating narcissism to maladaptive outcomes (aggression, hostility, and defensive self-aggrandizement) statistically control for self-esteem (e.g., Bushman & Baumeister, 1998; Morf & Rhodewalt, 1993; Rhodewalt & Morf, 1998). The evidence thus suggests that although narcissists' self-descriptions *appear* to reflect a mentally healthy person, the coexistence of vulnerability calls into question the proposition that "normal narcissism" involves high self-esteem and mental health. Again, this debate suggests that more refined assessment methods are needed to capture the juxtaposition of grandiosity and vulnerability that defines narcissism.

On the other side, whereas overt and grandiose narcissists tell us that they are doing well, covert and vulnerable narcissists display poor psychological health, reporting low self-esteem and high rates of depressive and anxious symptomology, among other indicators (e.g., Dickinson & Pincus, 2003; Rose, 2002; Watson, Sawrie, Greene, & Arredondo, 2002; Wink, 1991). Why do overt narcissists seem to be so "healthy" psychologically whereas covert narcissists appear considerably less so?

In an attempt to reconcile this question, Watson and his colleagues proposed a "continuum hypothesis" that places narcissism at varying levels of adjustment along a continuum related to self-esteem (e.g., Watson, Little, Sawrie, & Biderman, 1992; Watson et al., 2002). This continuum ranges from purely maladaptive narcissism at the "unhealthy" pole followed by an overlap between maladaptive and adaptive narcissism to more adaptive narcissism alone followed by an overlap between more adaptive narcissism and healthy self-esteem and finally to a fully healthy self-esteem at the "healthy" pole (Watson et al., 2002, p. 86). Watson and colleagues (2002) found that the maladaptive part of the continuum (greater covert narcissism) is strongly related to depression, whereas healthy self-esteem is negatively related to depression (with the overt narcissists on the more "adaptive" part in between). Furthermore, these researchers suggest that one's position along this continuum should not be considered stable; rather, situational changes and changes in life circumstances can lead to movement up or down the continuum of narcissism. This is consistent with the view of narcissism as a self-esteem regulation system, one that is sensitive to contextual demands and threats.

So narcissists, especially those who may be characterized as overt and grandiose, display high self-esteem and apparent psychological adjustment, but is this a tenuous state they find themselves in? Even if such individuals are "better off" than those low in narcissism on certain occasions, are they potentially setting themselves up for a hard fall? Are the patterns of maladjustment that we see in covert and vulnerable narcissists not far removed from the happier existence of the overt and grandiose narcissist? The grandiose and inflated self-views that promote perceptions of psychological adjustment may also leave the individual more open to difficulties that threaten self-esteem and well-being. As noted previously, (overt) narcissists are self-aggrandizing in their attributions for positive outcomes, even outcomes that they in fact did not produce. Although this tendency to self-aggrandize appears to reflect positive mental health, it backfires when the narcissist cannot sustain success (e.g., Rhodewalt & Morf, 1998). These findings suggest that the propensity to describe oneself positively contributes to the emotional instability that is one of the hallmarks of covert narcissism.

Are All Narcissists Defending against Underlying Vulnerabilities?

An additional question concerns whether grandiosity and vulnerability are actually found in the same individuals. In other words, are overt and covert narcissists qualitatively different from one another at the level of subjective experience and defensiveness? The work of Watson and his colleagues (e.g., 2002) with the continuum hypothesis is a step in the direction of integrating the two "types" as opposite ends of the same spectrum, but this idea needs to go further to discuss the common basis of the two. Whereas covert narcissists have vulnerabilities that are displayed through a combination of a sense of entitlement and explicitly stated feelings of worthlessness, the vulnerabilities of overt narcissists include entitlement and hypersensitivity to threat. Still, these vulnerabilities may be another common theme that binds the two forms together, with overt and grandiose narcissists simply more effective at defending against these concerns.

The recent conceptualization and development of techniques for assessing implicit cognition and automatic evaluations (e.g., Greenwald & Banaji, 1995) have been extended to the construct of self-esteem. Thus researchers can explore discrepancies between explicit and implicit self-esteem as a way to track narcissistic vulnerability. Consistent with this hypothesis, Jordan, Spencer, Zanna, Hoshino-Browne, and Correll (2003) showed that the combination of high explicit (self-reported) and low implicit self-esteem significantly predicted higher scores on the NPI (see also Ziegler-Hill, 2006). Other research has shown that high explicit–low implicit individuals are extremely defensive and self-serving, as well as reactive to threats to self-esteem, similar to narcissists (e.g., Brown, Bosson, Ziegler-Hill, & Swann, 2003; Jordan et al., 2003; Kernis et al., 2005; McGregor & Marigold, 2003). But narcissism is not necessarily so easily explained by the combination of high explicit and low implicit self-esteem.

Campbell, Bosson, Goheen, Lakey, and Kernis (2007) pointed out that narcissism has not been found to be *negatively* associated with implicit self-esteem; rather, its level is simply not *as* high as would be expected by narcissists' explicit reports of self-esteem. Also, this latter work demonstrates that the implicit self-esteem of narcissists tends to be higher when participants are provided with agentic as opposed to communal words to evaluate in the Implicit Association Test (IAT). Thus research on the implicit self-views of narcissists has provided inconsistent support for the idea that narcissistic grandiosity is a defense against an underlying vulnerability and sense of worthlessness, as indexed by implicit self-esteem. Of course, the weak and inconsistent findings may reflect a combining of covert and overt narcissism, and it may be that only covert narcissists display the explicit–implicit self-esteem discrepancy.

Another way to assess the possible underlying vulnerability of narcissists is through an examination of their grandiose self-views over time. In other words, the relative stability or instability of high self-esteem across time, within different situations, and in response to challenges and threats may point

to how secure and confidently held these grandiose opinions are (e.g., Kernis, 2003). In a series of daily diary studies, Rhodewalt and his colleagues (Rhodewalt, Madrian, & Cheney, 1998) had participants high and low in NPI provide daily descriptions of events and state self-esteem across a number of days. Narcissists not only displayed greater day-to-day fluctuations in their self-esteem than less narcissistic individuals, but their self-esteem was also more strongly related to the quality of their social interactions than it was for less narcissistic individuals. In particular, narcissists' daily self-esteem was more highly correlated with the extent to which the day's social interactions were perceived as positive or negative, the extent to which the interactions made them feel like themselves, and, surprisingly, the extent to which they felt accepted by the audience. Evidence of greater self-esteem instability among narcissists suggests that their grandiosity masks feelings of vulnerability that are brought to the surface in challenging social contexts.

Other research shows that narcissistic self-esteem is highly contingent on the individual's ability to self-enhance through other people (Morf & Rhodewalt, 2001). Thus the positive self-views of narcissists in many ways depend on confirmation by others in their social environment. On top of this, narcissistic self-esteem is based to a high degree on competition (Crocker, Luhtanen, Cooper, & Bouvrette, 2003) such that outperforming others and the ability to make favorable social comparisons is essential to maintaining grandiose self-views. Such contingencies may contribute to the vulnerability of all narcissists, as it would take an extremely high level of self-regulatory resources and skill to continually affect the social environment in desired ways that maintain self-esteem.

Such ideas about the vulnerability of the narcissistic self, even the grandiose type, find support in self-regulatory models such as that set forth by Morf and Rhodewalt (2001). It is also indicative of more general models of the "fragile" self (e.g., Kernis, 2003; Rhodewalt & Peterson, 2008). The model recently described by Rhodewalt and Peterson (2008) may help to reconcile the potential vulnerabilities of both covert and overt narcissists, as well as discrepancies in the psychological adjustment of the two types. In this model, self-esteem is seen as both an outcome of and input to effective self-regulation toward important goals. Importantly, both the content and structure of self-beliefs can influence regulatory effectiveness and thus have implications for both the level and stability of one's self-esteem. A "fragile" self is one that is organized such that it is difficult to sustain and effectively regulate toward important goals, leaving the individual vulnerable to threat, low and/ or unstable self-esteem, and, potentially, depression. Applied to narcissism, the core features of the construct (e.g., entitlement and beliefs in superiority, whether overtly expressed or not) will promote interpersonal self-regulation toward the confirmation of such content. What may come to distinguish the overt narcissist (relatively unstable high self-esteem) from the covert narcissist (relatively unstable low self-esteem) is each one's history of self-regulatory effectiveness in the pursuit of similar underlying goals. Whereas overt/grandiose narcissists enjoy a relatively high (though somewhat imperfect) level of success at confirming their grandiose self-beliefs, covert/vulnerable narcissists may have encountered frustration in their attempts to affect their environment in desired ways, leaving them with low self-esteem and hypersensitive to further failure in these pursuits. In this account, self-esteem regulation is the key to differences between overt and covert narcissists.

How Should Narcissism Be Assessed Most Effectively?

Given such questions in theory and research, there are obvious limitations to the current methods of assessing narcissism. The NPI, the most commonly used instrument in research, appears to assess a narcissism that is mostly descriptive of the grandiose pole. Additionally, it has not been updated in more than 20 years, and its reliability and internal consistency have been questioned (e.g., del Rosario & White, 2005; Kubarych, 2004). Until recently, researchers were forced to look to the MMPI to find an assessment instrument that captured the vulnerable pole of narcissism (with the exception of entitlement and exploitativeness subscales in the NPI). A new Vulnerable Narcissism Scale (VNS; Pimental et al., 2006) was recently created,

though the initial version (56 items and eight subscales) is burdensome for researchers and awaits further validation. At this point, the VNS appears to display a small positive correlation with the NPI (Peterson & Rhodewalt, 2007; Pimental et al., 2006), combined with a moderately negative correlation with self-esteem. Thus, although there is some overlap, the NPI and VNS appear to capture different points on a potential continuum of self-esteem and regulatory effectiveness. However, for the sake of integrated assessment of an overall narcissism construct, research would benefit from an instrument that included overt, covert, and shared elements in one scale that is less cumbersome to administer than both the NPI and VNS together. An integrated narcissism scale would allow researchers to test some of the potential relationships described here, such as whether more covert/vulnerable elements emerge over time as self-regulatory effectiveness and self-esteem decrease and whether more overt/grandiose elements emerge with more effective self-regulation and higher self-esteem.

Additionally, elements that have been identified as potential "core" descriptors of an integrated construct would be expected to remain more stable over time. In line with thinking about core aspects of narcissism, Campbell and colleagues (2004) have created a short Psychological Entitlement Scale (PES), the validity of which was established over nine studies. These researchers explicitly defined entitlement as "a stable and pervasive sense that one deserves more and is entitled to more than others" (p. 31). They found that high scorers on this 9-item scale not only reported that they deserved more pay in a hypothetical employment setting but also displayed interpersonal behaviors similar to those found in studies of narcissists, including competition, selfishness in relationships, and aggression. From this and other research (e.g., Dickinson & Pincus, 2003; Emmons, 1987), it appears that entitlement would be an important part of any fully integrated scale of narcissism.

Thus researchers now have several options when choosing an assessment instrument for narcissism and its associated features. The choice at this point depends on the questions being asked, as there is not yet an integrated tool that captures all parts of the picture being painted by theory and research. It remains to be seen whether this is a viable endeavor or whether scales assessing only the core features of narcissism (i.e., entitlement) are appropriate considering the wide spectrum of associated features that define narcissism, from the vulnerable to the grandiose ends.

Conclusion

On its journey from the clinic to the laboratory, the construct of narcissism has taken an interesting and, we would argue, quite fruitful path. Personality and social psychologists have expanded the construct, originally a psychoanalytically defined personality disorder, to describe a subclinical personality type. This effort has been facilitated by consensus among clinicians concerning narcissism's defining characteristics, as well as face-valid assessment devices based on this consensual definition. Contemporary researchers have proposed and validated process models of narcissism that focus on interpersonal self-esteem regulation. In this regard, narcissism is clearly an interpersonally embedded individual difference. As progress toward understanding the process of narcissistic self-esteem regulation advances, however, some of the controversies that divided the psychoanalytic community have reemerged. In particular, the various psychoanalytic perspectives disagreed about how to best conceptualize the coexistence of narcissistic grandiosity and vulnerability. In this chapter we have discussed state-of-the-art theory and research on the narcissistic personality type with attention to measurement issues and offered recommendations for conceptualizing and assessing overt and covert narcissism within contemporary frameworks.

References

Akhtar, S., & Thomson, J. A. (1982). Overview: Narcissistic personality disorder. *American Journal of Psychiatry, 139*, 12–20.

American Psychiatric Association. (1980). *Diagnostic and statistical manual of mental disorders* (3rd ed.). Washington, DC.

American Psychiatric Association. (1987). *Diagnostic and statistical manual of mental disorders* (3rd ed., revised). Washington, DC: Author.

American Psychiatric Association. (1994). *Diagnostic and statistical manual of mental disorders* (4th ed.). Washington, DC: Author.

American Psychiatric Association. (2000). *Diagnostic and statistical manual of mental disorders* (4th ed., text rev.). Washington, DC: Author.

Ames, D. R., Rose, P., & Anderson, C. P. (2006). The NPI-16 as a short measure of narcissism. *Journal of Research in Personality, 40*, 440–450.

Ang, R. P., & Yusof, N. (2006). Development and initial validation of the Narcissistic Personality Questionnaire for Children: A preliminary investigation using school-based Asian samples. *Educational Psychology, 26*, 1–18.

Ashby, H. U., Lee, R. R., & Duke, E. H. (1979, August). *A narcissistic personality disorder MMPI scale.* Paper presented at the annual convention of the American Psychological Association, New York.

Baumeister, R. F., & Vohs, K. D. (2001). Narcissism as an addiction to esteem. *Psychological Inquiry, 12*, 206–210.

Brown, R. P., Bosson, J. K., Zeigler-Hill, V., & Swann, W. B. (2003). Self-enhancement tendencies among people with high explicit self-esteem: The moderating role of implicit self-esteem. *Self and Identity, 2*, 169–187.

Bushman, B., & Baumeister, R. F. (1998). Threatened egotism, narcissism, self-esteem, and direct and displaced aggression: Does self-love or self-hate lead to violence? *Journal of Personality and Social Psychology, 75*, 219–229.

Buss, D. M., & Chiodo, L. M. (1991). Narcissistic acts in everyday life. *Journal of Personality, 19*, 179–215.

Cain, N. M., Pincus, A. L., & Ansell, E. B. (2008). Narcissism at the crossroads: Phenotypic description of pathological narcissism across clinical theory, social/personality psychology, and clinical diagnosis. *Clinical Psychology Review, 28*, 638–656.

Calhoun, G. B., Glaser, B. A., Stefurak, T., & Bradshaw, C. P. (2000). Preliminary validation of the Narcissistic Personality Inventory—Juvenile Offender. *International Journal of Offender Therapy and Comparative Criminology, 44*, 564–580.

Campbell, W. K., Bonacci, A. M., Shelton, J., Exline, J. J., & Bushman, B. J. (2004). Psychological entitlement: Interpersonal consequences and validation of a self-report measure. *Journal of Personality Assessment, 83*, 29–45.

Campbell, W. K., Bosson, J. K., Goheen, T. W., Lakey, C. E., & Kernis, M. H. (2007). Do narcissists dislike themselves "deep down inside"? *Psychological Science, 18*, 227–229.

Campbell, W. K., & Foster, J. D. (2007). The narcissistic self: Background, an extended-agency model, and ongoing controversies. In C. Sedikides & S. J. Spencer (Eds.), *The self* (pp. 115–138). New York: Psychology Press.

Crocker, J., Luhtanen, R. K., Cooper, M. L., & Bouvrette, A. (2003). Contingencies of self-worth in college students: Theory and measurement. *Journal of Personality and Social Psychology, 85*, 894–908.

del Rosario, P. M., & White, R. M. (2005). The Narcissistic Personality Inventory: Test–retest stability and internal consistency. *Personality and Individual Differences, 39*, 1075–1081.

Dickinson, K. A., & Pincus, A. L. (2003). Interpersonal analysis of grandiose and vulnerable narcissism. *Journal of Personality Disorders, 17,* 188–207.

Ellis, H. (1878). Autoeroticism: A psychological study. *Alienist and Neurologist, 19,* 260–299.

Emmons, R. A. (1984). Factor analysis and construct validity of the Narcissistic Personality Inventory. *Journal of Personality and Social Psychology, 48,* 291–300.

Emmons, R. A. (1987). Narcissism: Theory and measurement. *Journal of Personality and Social Psychology, 52,* 11–17.

Fossati, A., Beauchaine, T. P., Grazioli, F., Carretta, L., Cortinovis, F., & Maffei, C. (2005). A latent structure analysis of *Diagnostic and Statistical Manual of Mental Disorders, Fourth Edition,* narcissistic personality disorder criteria. *Comprehensive Psychiatry, 46,* 361–367.

Foster, J. D., & Campbell, W. K. (2007). Are there such things as "narcissists" in social psychology?: A taxometric analysis of the Narcissistic Personality Inventory. *Personality and Individual Differences, 43,* 1321–1332.

Freud, S. (1953). On narcissism: An introduction. In J. Strachey (Ed. & Trans.), *The standard edition of the complete psychological works of Sigmund Freud* (Vol. 14, pp. 69–102). London: Hogarth Press. (Original work published 1914)

Gabbard, G. O. (1998). Transference and countertransference in the treatment of narcissistic patients. In E. Ronningstam (Ed.), *Disorders of narcissism: Diagnostic, clinical, and empirical implications* (pp. 125–145). Washington, DC: American Psychiatric Press.

Gabriel, M. T., Critelli, J. W., & Ee, J. S. (1994). Narcissistic illusions in self-evaluations of intelligence and attractiveness. *Journal of Personality, 62,* 143–155.

Greenwald, A. G. (1980). The totalitarian ego: Fabrication and revision of personal history. *American Psychologist, 35,* 603–618.

Greenwald, A. G., & Banaji, M. R. (1995). Implicit social cognition: Attitudes, self-esteem, and stereotypes. *Psychological Review, 102,* 4–27.

Gunderson, J. G., Ronningstam, E., & Smith, L. E. (1991). Narcissistic personality disorder: A review of data on DSM-III-R descriptions. *Journal of Personality Disorders, 5,* 167–177.

Hendin, H. M., & Cheek, J. M. (1997). Assessing hypersensitive narcissism: A reexamination of Murray's narcism scale. *Journal of Research in Personality, 31,* 588–599.

Higgins, E. T. (1987). Self-discrepancy: A theory relating self and affect. *Psychological Review, 80,* 307–336.

John, O. P., & Robins, R. (1994). Accuracy and bias in self-perception: Individual differences in self-enhancement and the role of narcissism. *Journal of Personality and Social Psychology, 66,* 206–219.

Jones, E. E., & Berglas, S. (1978). Control of attributions about the self through self-handicapping strategies: The appeal of alcohol and the role of underachievement. *Personality and Social Psychology Bulletin, 4,* 200–206.

Jordan, C. H., Spencer, S. J., Zanna, M. P., Hoshino-Browne, E., & Correll, J. (2003). Secure and defensive high self-esteem. *Journal of Personality and Social Psychology, 85,* 969–978.

Kansi, J. (2003). The Narcissistic Personality Inventory: Applicability in a Swedish population sample. *Scandinavian Journal of Psychology, 44,* 441–448.

Kernberg, O. F. (1975). *Borderline conditions and pathological narcissism.* New York: Aronson.

Kernis, M. H. (2003). Toward a conceptualization of optimal self-esteem. *Psychological Inquiry, 14,* 1–26.

Kernis, M. H., Abend, T. A., Goldman, B. M., Shrira, I., Paradise, A. N., & Hampton, C. (2005). Self-serving responses arising from discrepancies between explicit and implicit self-esteem. *Self and Identity, 4,* 311–330.

Kernis, M. H., & Sun, C.-R. (1994). Narcissism and reactions to interpersonal feedback. *Journal of Research in Personality, 28,* 4–13.

Kohut, H. (1971). *The analysis of the self.* New York: International Universities Press.

Kubarych, T. S. (2004). The Narcissistic Personality Inventory: Factor structure in a nonclinical sample. *Personality and Individual Differences, 36,* 857–872.

Lasch, C. (1979). *The culture of narcissism: American life in an age of diminishing expectations.* New York: Norton.

McGregor, I., & Marigold, D. C. (2003). Defensive zeal and the uncertain self: What makes you so sure? *Journal of Personality and Social Psychology, 85,* 838–852.

Millon, T., & Davis, R. D. (1997). The MCMI-III: Present and future directions. *Journal of Personality Assessment, 68,* 69–85.

Morey, L. C., Waugh, M. H., & Blashfield, R. K. (1985). MMPI scales for DSM-III personality disorders: Their derivation and correlates. *Journal of Personality Assessment, 52,* 610–625.

Morf, C. C. (1994). *Interpersonal consequences of narcissists' continual efforts to maintain and bolster self-esteem.* Unpublished doctoral dissertation, University of Utah.

Morf, C. C., & Rhodewalt, F. (1993). Narcissism and self-evaluation maintenance: Explorations in object relations. *Personality and Social Psychology Bulletin, 19,* 668–676.

Morf, C. C., & Rhodewalt, F. (2001). Unraveling the paradoxes of narcissism: A dynamic self-regulatory processing model. *Psychological Inquiry, 12,* 177–196.

Morrison, A. P. (1986) Introduction. In A. P. Morrison (Ed.), *Essential papers on narcissism* (p. 11). New York: New York University Press.

Mullins, L. S., & Kopelman, R. E. (1988). Toward an assessment of the construct validity of four measures of narcissism. *Journal of Personality Assessment, 52,* 610–625.

Paulhus, D. L. (1998). Interpersonal and intrapsychic adaptiveness of trait self-enhancement: A mixed blessing? *Journal of Personality and Social Psychology, 74,* 1197–1208.

Paulhus, D. L. (2001). Normal narcissism: Two minimalist views. *Psychological Inquiry, 12,* 228–230.

Peterson, B., & Rhodewalt, F. (2007). [The ostracized narcissist: Differential reactions to being ignored]. Unpublished raw data, University of Utah.

Pimentel, C. A., Ansell, E. B., Pincus, A. L., & Cain, N. M. (2006). *Initial validation and derivation of the Vulnerable Narcissism Scale*. Unpublished manuscript, Pennsylvania State University.

Pulver, S. (1970). Narcissism: The term and concept. *Journal of the American Psycho-Analytic Association, 18,* 319–341.

Raskin, R., & Hall, C. S. (1979). A narcissistic personality inventory. *Psychological Reports, 40,* 590.

Raskin, R., & Hall, C. S. (1981). The Narcissistic Personality Inventory: Alternate form reliability and further evidence of construct validity. *Journal of Personality Assessment, 45,* 159–162.

Raskin, R., Novacek, J., & Hogan, R. (1991). Narcissism, self-esteem, and defensive self-enhancement. *Journal of Personality, 59,* 20–38.

Raskin, R., & Terry, H. (1988). A principal-components analysis of the Narcissistic Personality Inventory and further evidence for its construct validity. *Journal of Personality and Social Psychology, 54,* 890–902.

Reich, A. (1960). Pathologic forms of self-esteem regulation. *Psychoanalytic Study of the Child, 18,* 218–238.

Rhodewalt, F. (2001). The social mind of the narcissist: Cognitive and motivational aspects of interpersonal self-construction. In J. P. Forgas, K. Williams, & L. Wheeler (Eds.), *The social mind: Cognitive and motivational aspects of interpersonal behavior* (pp. 177–198). New York: Cambridge University Press.

Rhodewalt, F., & Eddings, S. (2002). Narcissus reflects: Memory distortion in response to ego relevant feedback in high and low narcissistic men. *Journal of Research in Personality, 36,* 97–116.

Rhodewalt, F., Madrian, J. C., & Cheney, S. (1998). Narcissism, self-knowledge organization, and emotional reactivity: The effect of daily experiences on self-esteem and affect. *Personality and Social Psychology Bulletin, 24,* 75–87.

Rhodewalt, F., & Morf, C. C. (1995). Self and interpersonal correlates of the Narcissistic Personality Inventory: A review and new findings. *Journal of Research in Personality, 29,* 1–23.

Rhodewalt, F., & Morf, C. C. (1998). On self-aggrandizement and anger: A temporal analysis of narcissism and affective reactions to success and failure. *Journal of Personality and Social Psychology, 74,* 672–685.

Rhodewalt, F., & Morf, C. C. (2005). Reflections in troubled waters: Narcissism and the vicissitudes of an interpersonally contextualized self. In A. Tesser, J. V. Wood, & D. A. Staper (Eds.), *On building, defending, and regulating the self* (pp. 127–152). New York: Psychology Press.

Rhodewalt, F., & Peterson, B. (2008). The self and social behavior: The fragile self and interpersonal self-regulation. In F. Rhodewalt (Ed.), *Personality and social behavior* (pp. 49–78). New York: Taylor & Francis.

Rhodewalt, F., & Sorrow, D. L. (2003). Interpersonal self-regulation: Lessons from the study of narcissism. In M. R. Leary & J. P. Tangney (Eds.) *Handbook of self and identity* (pp. 519–535). New York: Guilford Press.

Rhodewalt, F., Tragakis, M., & Finnerty, J. (2006). Narcissism and self-handicapping: Linking self-aggrandizement to behavior. *Journal of Research in Personality, 40,* 573–597.

Rose, P. (2002). The happy and unhappy faces of narcissism. *Personality and Individual Differences, 33,* 379–391.

Rose, P., & Campbell, W. K. (2004). Greatness feels good: A telic model of narcissism and subjective well-being. In S. P. Shohov (Ed.), *Advances in psychology research* (Vol. 31, pp. 3–27). Hauppauge, NY: Nova Science.

Ruiz, J. M., Smith, T. W., & Rhodewalt, F. (2001). Distinguishing narcissism and hostility: Similarities and differences in interpersonal circumplex and five-factor correlates. *Journal of Personality Assessment, 76,* 537–555.

Sedikides, C., Rudich, E. A., Gregg, A. P., Kumashiro, M., & Rusbult, C. (2004). Are normal narcissists psychologically healthy?: Self-esteem matters. *Journal of Personality and Social Psychology, 87,* 400–416.

Trapnell, P. D., & Wiggins, J. S. (1990). Extension of the interpersonal adjective scales to include the Big Five dimensions of personality. *Journal of Personality and Social Psychology, 59,* 781–790.

Vazire, S., & Funder, D. (2006). Impulsivity and the self-defeating behavior of narcissists. *Personality and Social Psychology Review, 10,* 154–165.

Watson, P. J., Little, T., Sawrie, S. M., & Biderman, M. D. (1992). Measures of the narcissistic personality: Complexity of relationships with self-esteem and empathy. *Journal of Personality Disorders, 6,* 434–449.

Watson, P. J., Sawrie, S. M., Greene, R. L., & Arredondo, R. (2002). Narcissism and depression: MMPI-2 evidence for the continuum hypothesis in clinical samples. *Journal of Personality Assessment, 79,* 85–109.

Wiggins, J. S., & Pincus, A. L. (1989). Conceptions of personality disorders and dimensions of personality. *Journal of Clinical and Consulting Psychology, 1,* 305–316.

Wink, P. (1991). Two faces of narcissism. *Journal of Personality and Social Psychology, 61,* 590–597.

Wink, P., & Gough, H. G. (1990). New narcissism scales for the California Psychological Inventory and MMPI. *Journal of Personality Assessment, 54,* 446–462.

Ziegler-Hill, V. (2006). Discrepancies between implicit and explicit self-esteem: Implications for narcissism and self-esteem instability. *Journal of Personality, 74,* 119–143.

CHAPTER 38

■ ◆ ▲ ◆ ■ ◆ ▲ ◆

Self-Compassion

KRISTIN NEFF

In the West, compassion is mainly conceptualized in terms of compassion for others. As defined by Webster's online dictionary, compassion is "the humane quality of
understanding the suffering of others and
wanting to do something about it." In Eastern traditions such as Buddhism, however,
it is considered equally important to offer
compassion to oneself (Brach, 2003; Salzberg, 1997). Recent psychological research
suggests that individuals vary on the personality trait of self-compassion, and numerous studies suggest that self-compassion is
strongly linked to psychological well-being.

What Is Self-Compassion?

Neff (2003a, 2003b) proposed that self-
compassion involves three main components: self-kindness versus self-judgment, a
sense of common humanity versus isolation,
and mindfulness versus overidentification.
These components combine and mutually
interact to create a self-compassionate frame
of mind. Compassion can be extended toward the self when suffering occurs through
no fault of one's own—when the external
circumstances of life are simply painful or
difficult to bear. Self-compassion is equally
relevant, however, when suffering stems
from one's own foolish actions, failures, or

personal inadequacies. Whereas most people
say that they are less kind and harsher toward themselves than they are with other
people (Neff, 2003a), self-compassionate individuals report being equally kind to themselves and others.

Self-kindness refers to the tendency to be
caring and understanding with oneself rather than being harshly critical or judgmental.
When noticing some disliked aspect of one's
personality, for example, the flaw is treated
gently, and the emotional tone of language
used toward oneself is soft and supportive.
Rather than attacking and berating oneself for being inadequate, the self is offered
warmth and unconditional acceptance (even
though the particular personality feature
may be identified as problematic and in need
of change). Similarly, when life circumstances are difficult and painful, instead of merely
"soldiering on" with an outward focus that
tries to control or solve the problem, self-
compassionate people turn inward to offer
themselves soothing and comfort. Self-
compassion involves being moved by one's
own distress, so that the desire to heal and
ameliorate suffering is experienced.

The sense of common humanity central to
self-compassion involves recognizing that all
humans are imperfect, that all people fail,
make mistakes, and engage in unhealthy behaviors. Self-compassion connects one's own

flawed condition to the shared human condition, so that one's own characteristics and experiences are considered from a broad, inclusive perspective. In the same way, life difficulties and struggles are framed in light of the shared human experience, so that one feels connected to others when experiencing pain. Often, however, people feel isolated and cut off from others when considering their personal flaws, as if the failing were an aberration not shared by the rest of humankind. Similarly, people often fall into the trap of believing that they are the only ones struggling when they experience difficult life circumstances, and they feel a sense of isolation and separation from other people who are presumably leading "normal," happy lives.

Mindfulness, the third component of self-compassion, involves being aware of present-moment experience in a clear and balanced manner so that one neither ignores nor ruminates on disliked aspects of oneself or one's life (Brown & Ryan, 2003). First, it is necessary to recognize that one is suffering in order to be able to extend compassion toward the self. While it might seem that personal suffering is blindingly obvious, people do not always pause to acknowledge their own pain when they are busy judging themselves or coping with life's challenges. Mindfulness involves a sort of stepping out of oneself, taking a metaperspective on one's own experience so that it can be considered with greater objectivity and perspective. Thus mindfulness enables a way of relating to oneself that involves one aspect of the self giving compassion to another aspect of the self. Mindfulness also prevents being swept up in and carried away by the story line of one's own pain, a process that Neff (2003b) has termed *overidentification*. When caught up in this manner, one tends to ruminate and obsessively fixate on negative self-relevant thoughts and emotions, so that the mental space needed to be self-compassionate is unavailable.

Other Conceptualizations of Self-Compassion

It should be noted that other ways of defining self-compassion exist in the literature. Gilbert (1989, 2005) views self-compassion through the lens of evolutionary psychol-ogy and especially attachment theory. Gilbert argues that self-compassion taps into an evolved mammalian physiological system guiding attachment and caregiving behavior. When accessed via external signals (other people's behavior) or internal signals (self-directed thoughts and emotions) of kindness and caring, individuals experience feelings of connectedness and soothing. In contrast, self-criticism taps into the threat-focused physiological systems of social ranking, which involve aggressive dominance and fearful submission (Gilbert, 1989, 2005). From this perspective, self-compassion involves an interdependent set of motives and competencies that relate to prototypic caring: concern for individuals' well-being, sensitivity to individuals' distress and needs, sympathy, distress tolerance, empathy, and nonjudgment. These are called the compassion circle and are directed toward others or toward oneself.

Research on Self-Compassion

Much of the research on self-compassion has been conducted using the Self-Compassion Scale (SCS; Neff, 2003a), though researchers are also starting to use mood inductions or therapeutic interventions as a means of examining the impact of self-compassion on functioning (e.g., Gilbert & Proctor, 2006; Leary, Tate, Adams, Allen, & Hancock, 2007). The SCS is a 26-item self-report scale that is composed of six subscales: self-kindness, self-judgment, common humanity, perceived isolation, mindfulness, and overidentification. The subscales are highly intercorrelated, however, and confirmatory factor analyses have indicated that these intercorrelations can be explained by a single overarching factor termed "Self-Compassion" (Neff, 2003a). Most research to date has focused on overall self-compassion scores rather than examining the various subcomponents of self-compassion separately. The SCS evidences strong internal reliability (consistently above .90), as well as test–retest reliability (.93 over a 3-week interval) (Neff, 2003a). Convergent validity for the scale is strong, with self-reported SCS scores substantially overlapping with observer reports (either by romantic partners or therapists) (Neff, 2006; Neff, Kirkpatrick, & Rude, 2007). The scale also shows discriminant validity: Practicing Buddhists report higher SCS scores than non-Buddhists (Neff, 2003a), for instance.

Self-Compassion and Psychological Resilience

One of the most robust and consistent findings in the research literature is that greater self-compassion (as reported on the SCS) is linked to lower anxiety and depression, with zero-order correlations typically falling in the range of –.50 to –.60 for depression and –.60 to –.70 for anxiety (Neff, 2003a; Neff, Hseih, & Dejitthirat, 2005; Neff, Kirkpatrick, & Rude, 2007; Neff, Pisitsungkagarn, & Hseih, 2008). Of course, a key feature of self-compassion is that individuals do not harshly judge and criticize themselves when they notice something about themselves they do not like, and self-criticism is known to be an important predictor of anxiety and depression (Blatt, 1995). However, self-compassion is still a robust negative predictor of anxiety and depression even after controlling for self-criticism (Neff, 2003a), suggesting that self-compassion provides unique buffering effects. Similarly, self-compassion is a negative predictor of anxiety even when controlling for negative affect (Neff, Kirkpatrick, & Rude, 2007). Thus self-compassion is not merely a matter of looking on the bright side of experiences and avoiding negative feelings. Self-compassionate individuals recognize when they are suffering, but when doing so they provide themselves feelings of warmth, kindness, and interconnectedness with the rest of humanity. As Gilbert and Irons (2005) suggested, self-compassion may help activate the self-soothing system (related physiologically to the parental caregiving system), and therefore help reduce feelings of fear and isolation.

In support of this proposition, Neff, Kirkpatrick, and Rude (2007) conducted a study involving a mock interview task in which participants were asked to write their answers to a difficult interview question: "Please describe your greatest weakness." Individuals with higher levels of self-compassion experienced less anxiety after the task. They also tended to use less isolating language when writing about their weaknesses, using fewer first-person singular pronouns such as I, using more first-person plural pronouns such

as we, and making more social references to friends, family, and other humans.

Similarly, Leary and colleagues (2007) investigated the way that self-compassionate people deal with negative life events using experience-sampling techniques, asking participants to report about problems they experienced over a 20-day period. Individuals with higher levels of self-compassion had more perspective on their problems and were less likely to feel isolated by them. For example, they were more likely to feel that their struggles were not any worse than what lots of other people go through and were less likely to think that their lives were more "screwed up" than those of others. They also experienced less anxiety and self-consciousness when thinking about their problems.

The emotional resilience provided by self-compassion is further evidenced by findings that self-compassionate individuals tend to engage in less rumination and thought suppression than those scoring low on the trait (Neff, 2003a; Neff, Kirkpatrick, & Rude, 2007). Self-compassion entails taking a balanced approach to one's emotional experience—so that one neither runs away from or away with one's feelings. Thus it appears that self-compassionate individuals can face up to personal weaknesses and life challenges with fewer emotional overreactions. Similarly, self-compassion is related to emotional intelligence. Individuals with higher levels of self-compassion report greater emotional coping skills, clarity of feelings, and ability to repair negative emotional states (Neff, 2003a).

Self-Compassion and Psychological Strengths

In addition to providing protection against negative mental states, self-compassion also appears to bolster positive emotional mindsets. For instance, self-compassion has been linked to greater feelings of social connectedness and life satisfaction, important elements of a meaningful life (Neff, 2003a; Neff, Kirkpatrick, & Rude, 2007; Neff et al., 2008). It has also been associated with feelings of autonomy, competence, and relatedness (Neff, 2003a), indicating that self-compassion helps meet basic psychological needs that Deci and Ryan (1995) identified as fundamental to well-being. Self-compassionate people have been shown to possess many of the psychological strengths associated with the positive psychology movement (Seligman & Csikzentmihalyi, 2000) such as greater happiness, optimism, wisdom, curiosity and exploration, personal initiative, and positive affect (Neff, Rude, & Kirkpatrick, 2007). Although self-compassion is associated with positive affect, however, it is not merely a form of "positive thinking." Rather, self-compassion refers to the ability to hold difficult negative emotions in nonjudgmental awareness without having to suppress or deny negative aspects of one's experience. For instance, self-compassionate individuals do *not* use fewer negative emotion words when describing personal weaknesses; they are just less anxious when considering their weaknesses (Neff, Kirkpatrick, & Rude, 2007).

Self-Compassion, Motivation, and Health

People often express concerns about the possible downsides of self-compassion; they worry that if they are too self-compassionate, they will lack motivation or become passive and self-indulgent (Neff, 2003b). This does not appear to be the case, however. Self-compassion involves the desire for the health and well-being of the self and is associated with greater personal initiative to make needed changes in one's life (Neff, Rude, & Kirkpatrick, 2007). Although self-compassion is negatively related to neurotic perfectionism (Neff, 2003a), in which individuals are driven by the need to escape feelings of inferiority, it has no association with the level of performance standards adopted for oneself. In other words, self-compassionate individuals are motivated to achieve, but this goal is not driven by the desire to bolster one's self-image. Rather, it is driven by the compassionate desire to maximize one's potential and well-being.

Because self-compassionate individuals do not berate themselves when they fail, they are more able to learn, grow, and take on new challenges. This can be seen in the general orientation of self-compassionate individuals toward learning in academic settings. Educational psychologists often make a distinction between learning goals that are mastery based or performance based (Dweck, 1986).

Students with mastery goals are intrinsically motivated by curiosity, and they desire to develop skills and master new material. They tend to make effort attributions for success and failure and view the making of mistakes as a part of the learning process. Students with performance goals, on the other hand, are motivated to defend or enhance their sense of self-worth. They tend to make ability attributions for success and failure and to evaluate their ability through social comparisons with others. Mastery goals appear to be more academically adaptive than performance goals, being linked to greater effort and persistence at tasks, willingness to seek needed help, and less anxiety and fear of failure (Elliot & Church, 1997).

In a study of self-compassion and learning goals, Neff and colleagues (2005) found that self-compassion is positively associated with mastery goals and negatively associated with performance goals. This relationship was mediated by the lower fear of failure of self-compassionate individuals and also by their greater perceived competence (which is likely related to lessened self-criticism). Thus self-compassionate individuals are motivated to learn and grow, but for intrinsic reasons—not because they want to garner social approval. The research also examined the reactions of students who had recently failed a midterm exam, and found that self-compassionate individuals were better able to cope with and accept their failure as a learning experience. Rather than being complacent and merely accepting the status quo, it appears that self-compassion enables people to grow from their failures because they do not interpret failure as an indictment of their self-worth.

Because people with self-compassion care about themselves, they *want* to engage in healthy behaviors. They do not need to motivate themselves by fear of self-punishment or the judgments of others; their motivation stems from the intrinsic desire for well-being. Support for this proposition comes from a study that examined women's goals for exercising (Magnus, 2007). Results indicated that women with higher levels of self-compassion had greater intrinsic rather than extrinsic motivation to exercise, and their goals for exercising were less related to ego concerns. Women with higher levels of self-compassion also reported feeling more comfortable with their bodies and had less anxiety regarding social evaluations of their physiques.

Self-compassion may help people learn to deal with the intense pressures to be thin and attractive in Western society, while still promoting healthy eating patterns. One study investigated whether inducing a state of self-compassion attenuates certain disordered eating behaviors. Highly restrictive eaters (i.e., dieters) often display a paradoxical tendency—if they break their diets and eat high-calorie foods, they tend to eat even more afterward (a process known as the disinhibition effect). Heatherton and Polivy (1990) proposed that this pattern of overeating is an attempt to reduce the negative affect associated with the lapse of a desired goal. Adams and Leary (2007) asked college women to eat an unhealthy food (a doughnut) as part of an experiment and either induced them to think self-compassionately about eating the donut or else gave them no intervention. Participants were later given the opportunity to eat as much candy as they wanted while unobserved. Results showed that the self-compassion induction reduced negative affect and attenuated the amount of candy eaten after the doughnut among highly restrictive eaters (who displayed similar patterns to nondieters). In contrast, highly restrictive eaters in the control condition ate more candy afterward. Again, having compassion for mistakes and failures allows such lapses to be taken less personally (in other words, they do not define the self as "bad" or "unworthy"). Thus self-compassionate individuals are able to emotionally recover from transgressions more quickly and to continue to work toward their goals of growth and change.

Self-Compassion and Interpersonal Functioning

Just as there is a fair amount of evidence that self-compassion psychologically benefits oneself, there are also some indications that self-compassion also benefits others within interpersonal relationships. In a study of heterosexual couples (Neff, 2006), self-compassionate individuals were described by their partners as being more emotionally connected, accepting, and autonomy supporting while being less detached, control-

ling, and verbally or physically aggressive. Self-compassion was also associated with more relationship satisfaction (as reported by participants and their partners) and greater attachment security. Because self-compassionate people give themselves caring, understanding, and support, they appear to have more emotional resources available to give to their romantic partners. Also, the ability to admit mistakes without ego defensiveness means that self-compassionate people may have less need to project their faults onto partners via angry accusations (Feldman & Gowen, 1998).

An interesting question concerns whether self-compassionate people are more compassionate toward others in general. On the one hand, cultivating an openhearted stance toward oneself that recognizes human interconnectedness should theoretically facilitate being kind, forgiving, and empathetic toward others. On the other hand, given that people who lack self-compassion say they are much kinder to others than they are to themselves (Neff, 2003a), it may be that the tendency to be kind and giving toward others is relatively independent from the tendency to be compassionate toward oneself. Although there is very little research on this topic, preliminary findings suggest that the link between self-compassion and other-focused concern is mixed. Neff (2008) found that individuals with higher levels of self-compassion reported a significantly greater tendency to forgive others than those low in self-compassion. They also reported being more likely to take others' perspectives and to feel less personal distress when considering other people's misfortunes. However, self-compassion had only a very weak association with the tendency to experience compassionate love toward others (Sprecher & Fehr, 2005). Also, self-compassion was not significantly linked to empathy for others or to altruism. These results suggest that there may be some aspects of other-focused concern that are facilitated by self-compassion—such as the ability to detach oneself from one's own point of view and take another's perspective or to recognize that all humans make mistakes and are worthy of forgiveness. However, self-compassion does not appear to predict general emotional responsiveness toward others in terms of kindness, compassionate love, or empathy. Clearly, more research will be needed to examine these issues, and it will be important to examine the impact of self-compassion on behavior in experimental settings rather than relying solely on self-reports.

Self-Compassion in Therapeutic Settings

An exciting area of research concerns the application of self-compassion in clinical contexts. Neff, Kirkpatrick, and Rude (2007) conducted a study that tracked changes in self-compassion experienced by therapy clients over a 1-month interval. Therapists used a Gestalt two-chair technique designed to help clients lessen self-criticism and have greater compassion for themselves (Greenberg, 1983; Safran, 1998). Results indicated that increased self-compassion levels over the month-long period (which were assessed under the guise of an unrelated study) were linked to fewer experiences of self-criticism, depression, rumination, thought suppression, and anxiety.

Gilbert and Procter (2006) have developed a group-based therapy intervention called "compassionate mind training" (CMT). The model is designed to help people develop skills of self-compassion, especially when their more habitual form of self-relating involves self-attacking. In a pilot study of CMT among patients in a day treatment program for people suffering from intense shame and self-criticism, individuals were led through weekly 2-hour CMT sessions for 12 weeks. Participants were instructed about the qualities involved in self-compassion (e.g., developing empathy for one's own distress), explored their fears of being too self-compassionate (e.g., "it makes me feel vulnerable"), and were helped to understand their own self-critical tendencies without judgment. Participants were also invited to create an ideal image of caring and compassion, a figure embodying qualities of wisdom, strength, warmth, and nonjudgmental acceptance. The training resulted in significant pre–post changes in depression, self-attacking, feelings of inferiority, submissive behavior, and shame. Moreover, almost all of the participants felt ready to be discharged from their hospital day program at the end of the study. This demonstration of the healing qualities of self-compassion in a real-life setting provides strong support for the link between self-compassion and psychological well-being.

Self-Compassion versus Self-Esteem

Interest in self-compassion has been spurred by the observation that self-compassion is associated with many of the benefits of high self-esteem, while having fewer of the downsides associated with self-esteem pursuit. For instance, Leary and colleagues (2007) examined self-compassionate individuals' reactions to a mildly awkward and embarrassing task—being videotaped while looking into a camera and making up a children's story that began "Once upon a time there was a little bear." Self-compassionate people rated their tapes more favorably and felt better while watching their tapes than those who were low in self-compassion, indicating that, like self-esteem, self-compassion is a source of positive emotions toward the self. However, self-compassionate individuals also rated how they appeared on the tape (e.g., awkward, competent, attractive, nervous) in a similar way to objective observers. This suggests that self-compassionate individuals did not display the type of self-enhancement bias often associated with high self-esteem (Robins & Beer, 2001).

Research indicates that people sometimes engage in dysfunctional behaviors in order to maintain a sense of high self-worth (for reviews, see Blaine & Crocker, 1993; Crocker & Park, 2004). People who are highly invested in having high self-esteem often display narcissistic tendencies (Morf & Rhodewalt, 2001), a maladaptive pattern that causes interpersonal problems (Campbell & Baumeister, 2001). Those wanting to maintain high self-esteem sometimes trivialize personal failings or blame them on external causes, hindering their ability to grow and change (Sedikides, 1993). Other ways to protect high self-esteem involve becoming angry toward those who threaten one's ego (Baumeister, Smart, & Boden, 1996), or engaging in downward social comparisons (Fein & Spencer, 1997). The motivation to protect feelings of self-worth can also lead to a type of closed-mindedness known as "need for cognitive closure" (Jost, Glaser, Kruglanski, & Sulloway, 2003; Taris, 2000), in which alternative viewpoints are not tolerated.

Because global self-esteem rests in part on evaluations of self-worth in various life domains, high self-esteem is often contingent on particular outcomes (Crocker, Luhtanen, Cooper, & Bouvrette, 2003). This means that self-esteem can fluctuate according to particular circumstances. Even though trait levels of global self-esteem tend to remain relatively constant over time, state feelings of self-worth may be highly unstable and change quite frequently (Kernis, Paradise, Whitaker, Wheatman, & Goldman, 2000). In fact, individuals with high levels of competence may be most vulnerable to experiencing drops in state self-esteem (Crocker & Park, 2004), because they have more opportunities to fall short of their personal standards (e.g., the A student who receives a B+ on an exam). As the Hollywood saying goes, you're only as good as your latest success (at least when viewing the world through the lens of self-esteem).

Research indicates that self-compassion is moderately associated with trait levels of global self-esteem, with correlations around .55–.60 using the Rosenberg (1965) measure (Leary et al., 2007; Neff, 2003a; Neff et al., 2008). This is unsurprising given that both constructs represent a positive emotional stance toward the self. Similarly, self-esteem and self-compassion are both associated with emotional well-being, such as lower levels of anxiety and depression, as well as higher levels of happiness, optimism, and life satisfaction. Unlike self-esteem, however, the healthy states of mind associated with self-compassion do not stem from positive evaluations of the self, meeting set standards, or favorable comparisons with others. Rather, they stem from recognizing the need to be kind to oneself in instances of suffering and framing one's experience in light of the shared human experience—fragile and imperfect as it is. Thus self-compassion appears to provide emotional resilience over and above that attributable to self-esteem.

For example, when controlling for self-esteem, self-compassion is still a robust predictor of happiness, optimism, and positive affect (Neff & Vonk, 2009), and it also negatively predicts depression and anxiety (Neff, 2003a). The two constructs differ in important ways, moreover. Whereas high self-esteem depends on successful performances and positive self-evaluations, self-compassion is relevant precisely when self-esteem tends to falter—when one fails or feels inadequate. Thus self-compassion provides a way of dealing with negative life experiences that self-esteem cannot provide. In the Neff, Kirkpatrick, and Rude (2007) mock interview study asking people to describe their greatest weaknesses, for instance, self-compassion provided a significant buffer against anxiety, whereas trait self-esteem did not.

Leary and colleagues (2007) found that when considering hypothetical scenarios involving failure or embarrassment (e.g., being responsible for losing an athletic competition for one's team), participants with greater self-compassion reported less negative affect (e.g., sadness or humiliation) and more emotional equanimity (e.g., remaining calm and unflustered). In contrast, global levels of trait self-esteem predicted no variance in emotional reactions after controlling for self-compassion levels. In another study, participants were asked to give a brief introduction of themselves on video (describing interests, future plans, etc.) and were then given positive or negative feedback about the introduction that was ostensibly made by an observer. Participants' reactions to the feedback were then assessed, including their attributions for the observer's feedback. Individuals with low self-compassion gave defensive attributions. They were more likely to attribute the observer's feedback to their own personalities when the feedback was positive rather than negative. Individuals high in self-compassion, however, were equally likely to attribute the feedback to their personalities regardless of whether the feedback was positive or negative. An opposite pattern was found for self-esteem. Individuals with low self-esteem were equally likely to attribute the feedback to their personalities when feedback was positive or negative, but participants with high self-esteem were more likely to attribute the feedback to their own personalities when feedback was positive rather than negative. This suggests that self-compassion enables people to admit and accept negative as well as positive aspects of their personalities. In contrast, high self-esteem appears to involve a desire to bolster and protect a positive self-identity.

Leary and colleagues (2007) also compared self-compassion and self-esteem using mood inductions. Participants were instructed to recall a previous failure, rejection, or loss that made them feel bad about themselves and were then asked a series of questions that assessed their feelings about the event. In the self-compassion condition, participants responded in writing to prompts designed to lead them to think about the negative event in ways that tapped into the three components of self-compassion: self-kindness, common humanity, and mindful acceptance. In the self-esteem condition, participants responded to prompts that were designed to protect or bolster their self-esteem: reminding them of their positive characteristics and leading them to interpret the negative event in a way that did not reflect badly on themselves. Two types of control condition were also included: a standard control and a writing control in which participants were instructed to "really let go" and explore their deepest emotions as they wrote about the event. The latter condition was included because merely writing about negative events in a self-disclosing manner has been shown to reduce negative emotions (Pennebaker, Colder, & Sharp, 1990). Participants who received the self-compassion induction reported less negative affect when thinking about the past events than those in the self-esteem or control conditions (ratings of how bad the event was did not differ across conditions). Similarly, those in the self-compassion condition took more personal responsibility for the event than those in the control conditions (and also the self-esteem condition, but this may have been an artifact of how self-esteem was induced.) Results from this study buttress the claim that self-compassion allows for the processing and acceptance of negative self-relevant emotions in a way that leads to greater emotional equanimity, whereas self-esteem does not. It also suggests that self-compassion does not lead to complacency, as it allows people to take personal responsibility for their actions without the need to shield the truth from themselves in order to maintain positive self-affect.

A survey conducted with a large Web-based community sample in Denmark (Neff & Vonk, 2009) demonstrated that self-compassion is a stronger predictor of stable, noncontingent self-worth than global self-esteem. Self-compassion predicted more stability in state feelings of self-worth over an 8-month period (assessed 12 different times) than global self-esteem, which was *not* associated with self-worth stability after accounting for self-compassion levels. Self-compassion was also negatively associated with general self-worth contingency, as well as contingency on physical attractiveness or successful performances (global self-esteem was not). These findings indicate that the sense of self-worth associated with self-compassion is less likely to fluctuate according to external circumstances, perhaps because self-compassion does not depend on personal success and positive self-judgments for its self-soothing qualities. (To date, research has not examined fluctuations in state self-compassion itself, and this is an issue that should be examined in the future.)

Results from the Neff and Vonk (2009) study also indicated that self-compassion was a stronger negative predictor of social comparison, public self-consciousness, self-rumination, anger, and need for cognitive closure than global self-esteem. The one exception to this pattern was narcissism: Self-esteem had a significant positive association with narcissism, whereas self-compassion had no association with narcissism when controlling for self-esteem. These findings suggest that self-compassion involves less intense self-evaluation and ego defensiveness than self-esteem. One might say that with self-compassion, the ego moves from the foreground into the background. In contrast to individuals with high self-esteem, self-compassionate individuals are less focused on evaluating themselves, feeling superior to others, worrying about whether or not others are evaluating them, or angrily reacting against those who disagree with them.

Gilbert and Irons (2005) suggested that self-compassion enhances well-being because it helps people feel a greater sense of interpersonal connection. They propose that self-compassion deactivates the threat system (associated with feelings of insecure attachment, defensiveness, and the limbic system) and activates the self-soothing system (associated with feelings of secure attachment, safeness, and the oxytocin–opiate system). In contrast, self-esteem is thought to be an evaluation of superiority–inferiority that helps to establish social-rank stability and is related to alerting, energizing impulses and dopamine activation (Gilbert & Irons, 2005). Self-compassion, therefore, enhances feelings of interconnectedness, whereas self-esteem positions the self in competition with others and amplifies feelings of distinctiveness and separation.

Self-compassion may be a more useful way to conceptualize a healthy way of relating to oneself than the more ubiquitous construct of self-esteem, as it provides a more stable foundation of positive self-regard that is less ego reactive and contingent on external sources. In fact, self-compassion may be a key source of the "optimal" or "true" self-esteem extolled by some theorists. Deci and Ryan (1995) have proposed that some people possess "true self-esteem," a self-determined and autonomous way of evaluating oneself that is not dependent on particular outcomes or social approval. Similarly, Kernis (2003) has proposed the concept of "optimal self-esteem," which is founded on stable and noncontingent self-evaluations. Self-compassion provides greater self-worth stability and noncontingency than trait self-esteem because its source is internal rather than external and because it avoids processes of self-judgment and evaluation altogether. For this reason, self-compassion does not require feeling "above average" or superior to others, and it provides emotional stability when facing up to personal inadequacies.

The Origins of Self-Compassion

Although there is evidence that self-compassion is associated with psychological well-being and that individuals can be taught to be more self-compassionate, less is known about why people have greater or lesser levels of self-compassion in the first place. Some variation may be due to broader personality traits. In an examination of self-compassion and major personality traits as measured by the NEO-FFI (Neff, Rude, & Kirkpatrick, 2007), it was found that self-compassion had the strongest association with neuroticism ($r = -.65$), with greater self-compassion

linked to significantly lower levels of neuroticism. This is perhaps unsurprising, given that the feelings of self-judgment, isolation, and ruminative emotional processing inherent in the *lack* of self-compassion are similar to those described by the neuroticism construct. Self-compassion was also positively associated with agreeableness, extraversion, and conscientiousness (correlations ranged from .32–.42), but no association was found with openness to experience. The socially oriented nature of people high in agreeableness and extraversion may help them to be kind to themselves and to take a broader human perspective on their negative experiences. Similarly, being conscientious may help individuals to pay greater attention to their own needs and to respond to difficult situations in a responsible and nonreactive manner. Importantly, however, self-compassion still predicted positive psychological functioning after controlling for the "Big Five," suggesting that self-compassion is not reducible to these personality traits. It should also be remembered that the directionality of the link between these personality traits and self-compassion probably goes both ways, and it is possible that developing greater self-compassion leads to a healthier personality (e.g., lessened neuroticism).

Early family experiences are also likely to play a key role in the development of self-compassion or lack thereof. Gilbert (2005) suggested that self-compassion stems largely from the attachment system, so that individuals who are raised in safe, secure environments and who experience supportive and validating relationships with caregivers are more able to relate to themselves in a caring and compassionate manner. In contrast, individuals who are raised in insecure, stressful, or threatening environments and who experience constant criticism and aggression from caregivers tend to be self-critical rather than self-compassionate (Gilbert & Proctor, 2006). This occurs because individuals with insecure attachment relationships have an insufficiently developed self-soothing system and few internalized models of compassion to draw on. Also, children may develop defense mechanisms of self-attacking because it is too risky to blame powerful others for their punitive or neglectful behavior. Recent data collected with a sample of adolescents and young adults gives some tentative support to these propositions. Neff and McGe-hee (2008) found that maternal criticism and stressful family relationships were negatively related to self-compassion among youths. Those who felt accepted and validated by their parents, on the other hand, reported having greater self-compassion. Secure attachment was positively associated with self-compassion, whereas preoccupied or fearful attachment was negatively linked to self-compassion, supporting the notion that attachment schemas play a role in the ability to be self-compassionate. Another way that familial environments might affect the development of self-compassion is the extent to which parents model self-compassionate versus self-critical reactions to their own failures or life difficulties, although this proposition has yet to be empirically examined.

Cross–Cultural Variations in Self–Compassion

There has been a small amount of research exploring whether self-compassion differs across cultures. Neff and colleagues (2008) examined self-compassion, independent and interdependent self-construal, and psychological well-being in Thailand, Taiwan, and the United States. Mean self-compassion levels were highest in Thailand and lowest in Taiwan, with the United States falling in between (all cultures differed significantly from one another, although within-culture variations in self-compassion were as great as between-culture variations). These cross-cultural differences may be explained by the fact that Thais are strongly influenced by Buddhism and that the value of compassion is emphasized in parenting practices and everyday interactions in Thailand. In contrast, the Taiwanese are more influenced by Confucianism, and shame and self-criticism is more strongly emphasized as a means of parental and social control in Taiwan. Americans may have reported middling levels of self-compassion because U.S. culture displays more mixed messages with regard to self-compassion (e.g., a strong emphasis on positive self-affect but also an isolating, competitive ethos).

Interestingly, cross-cultural differences remained even when controlling for self-construal, suggesting that self-construal dif-ferences did not explain group differences in self-compassion. Self-construal theory has been used to argue that Asians are more self-critical than Westerners (Heine, Lehman, Markus, & Kitayama, 1999), which implies that they should also be less self-compassionate. Because people with interdependent self-construals are more invested in conforming the self's behavior to the requirements of social relationships, the theory goes, they tend to constantly criticize themselves in order to keep themselves in line. This did not appear to hold true for Thais, however, who had almost identical levels of interdependent self-construal as did Taiwanese yet were much more self-compassionate. Moreover, the link between self-construal and self-compassion itself varied across cultures. Self-compassion was associated with interdependent self-construal in Thailand but with independent self-construal in Taiwan and the United States. This suggests that the meanings of independence and interdependence may vary across cultures. Interdependence involves being deeply embedded in a particular social system. If that system promotes the value of self-compassion, as it does in Thailand, then being more interdependent within that system may promote self-compassion and decrease self-judgment. If the culture does not actively promote self-compassion, however, which appears to be the case in Taiwan and the United States, being independent of the prevailing cultural ethos may facilitate the type of self-understanding and self-care required to be compassionate toward oneself. In all three cultures, however, greater self-compassion significantly predicted less depression and greater life satisfaction, suggesting that there may be universal benefits to self-compassion despite cultural differences in its prevalence.

Summary and Conclusions

Self-compassion is a relatively new construct in personality and social psychology, but the data gathered so far suggest that the ability to be self-compassionate is linked to greater emotional resilience and psychological well-being. Self-compassionate people are less depressed and anxious, have better emotional coping skills, are less afraid of failure, are more intrinsically motivated to learn and grow, are happier, are more curious and wise, and feel more connected to others. Importantly, these mental health benefits are not obtained through a process of judging or evaluating the self—by stuffing oneself into a box labeled "good" versus "bad." This type of self-evaluation often requires comparing oneself to others, with cognitive distortion being used to overevaluate one's own competencies and underevaluate those of others (Taylor & Brown, 1988). The need to feel special and above average can lead to increased feelings of isolation and separation from fellow humans and is counterproductive to feelings of interconnectedness. With self-compassion, however, the boundaries between self and other are softened. All human beings are worthy of compassion, oneself included. Thus self-compassion is a useful alternative to self-esteem when conceptualizing healthy forms of self-relating. It provides similar mental health benefits to high self-esteem without being linked to patterns of narcissism, social comparison, ego defensiveness, or self-worth contingency and instability that have been associated with self-esteem pursuit (Crocker & Park, 2004).

Even if the quest for high self-esteem were not so potentially problematic, it has proved difficult to raise people's levels of self-esteem in any case (Baumeister, Campbell, Krueger, & Vohs, 2003). The reason is partly that people with low self-esteem identify with their perceived lack of competence and often prefer to verify and maintain their identities rather than engaging in the positive self-illusions that are common among those high in self-esteem (Swann, 1996). It may be more possible to raise people's levels of self-compassion, given that it requires them to merely acknowledge and accept their human limitations with kindness, rather than changing their self-evaluations from negative to positive. Research demonstrates that self-compassion can be enhanced in the short and long term (Gilbert & Proctor, 2006; Leary et al., 2007; Neff, Kirkpatrick, & Rude, 2007), suggesting that programs designed to increase self-compassion have some chance of success. In fact, there is increasing interest in mindfulness-based interventions for their ability to reduce stress and improve mental health (Baer, 2003). Mindfulness-based stress reduction (MBSR; Kabat-Zinn, 1982) is the best known of these interventions and is aimed at the management of chronic pain and the treatment of stress disorders (Grossman, Niemann, Schmidt, & Walach, 2004). Although MBSR training primarily focuses on teaching mindfulness skills, it also teaches meditation practices aimed at developing compassion for self and others and has been shown to increase self-compassion among participants (Shapiro, Astin, Bishop, & Cordova, 2005; Shapiro, Brown, & Biegel, 2007). Future research should be aimed at determining whether self-compassion can be successfully taught to children and adolescents in the schools, as it might provide youths with greater emotional resilience when facing the problems and difficulties of living a human life.

References

Adams, C. E., & Leary, M. R. (2007). Promoting self-compassionate attitudes toward eating among restrictive and guilty eaters. *Journal of Social and Clinical Psychology, 26,* 1120–1144.

Baer, R. A. (2003). Mindfulness training as a clinical intervention: A conceptual and empirical review. *Clinical Psychology: Science and Practice, 10,* 125–143.

Baumeister, R. F., Campbell, J. D., Krueger, J. I., & Vohs, K. D. (2003). Does high self-esteem cause better performance, interpersonal success, happiness, or healthier lifestyles? *Psychological Science in the Public Interest, 4,* 1–44.

Baumeister, R. F., Smart, L., & Boden, J. M. (1996). Relation of threatened egotism to violence and aggression: The dark side of high self-esteem. *Psychological Review, 103,* 5–33.

Blaine, B., & Crocker, J. (1993). Self-esteem and self-serving biases in reactions to positive and negative events: An integrative review. In R. F. Baumeister (Ed.), *Self-esteem: The puzzle of low self-regard* (pp. 55–85). Hillsdale, NJ: Erlbaum.

Blatt, S. J. (1995). Representational structures in psychopathology. In D. Cicchetti & S. Toth (Eds.), *Rochester symposium on developmental psychopathology: Emotion, cognition, and representation* (Vol. 6, pp. 1–34). Rochester, NY: University of Rochester Press.

Brach, T. (2003). *Radical acceptance: Embracing your life with the heart of a Buddha.* New York: Bantam Books.

Brown, K. W., & Ryan, R. M. (2003). The benefits of being present: Mindfulness and its role in psychological well-being. *Journal of Personality and Social Psychology, 84,* 822–848.

Campbell, W. K., & Baumeister, R. F. (2001). Is loving the self necessary for loving another?: An examination of identity and intimacy. In M. Clark & G. Fletcher (Eds.), *Blackwell handbook of social psychology: Vol. 2. Interpersonal processes* (pp. 437–456). London: Blackwell.

Crocker, J., Luhtanen, R. K., Cooper, M. L., & Bou- vrette, S. (2003). Contingencies of self-worth in col- lege students: Theory and measurement. *Journal of Personality and Social Psychology, 85*, 894–908.

Crocker, J., & Park, L. E. (2004). The costly pursuit of self-esteem. *Psychological Bulletin, 130*, 392– 414.

Deci, E. L., & Ryan, R. M. (1995). Human autonomy: The basis for true self-esteem. In M. H. Kernis (Ed.), *Efficacy, agency, and self-esteem* (pp. 31–49). New York: Plenum Press.

Dweck, C. S. (1986). Motivational processes affecting learning. *American Psychologist, 41*, 1040–1048.

Elliot, A. J., & Church, M. A. (1997). A hierarchical model of approach and avoidance achievement mo- tivation. *Journal of Personality and Social Psychol- ogy, 72*, 218–232.

Fein, S., & Spencer, S. J. (1997). Prejudice as self-image maintenance: Affirming the self through derogating others. *Journal of Personality and Social Psychol- ogy, 73*, 31–44.

Feldman, S. S., & Gowen, L. K. (1998). Conflict ne- gotiation tactics in romantic relationships in high school students. *Journal of Youth and Adolescence, 27*, 691–717.

Gilbert, P. (1989). *Human nature and suffering*. Hove, UK: Erlbaum.

Gilbert, P. (2005). Compassion and cruelty: A biop- sychosocial approach. In P. Gilbert (Ed.), *Compas- sion: Conceptualisations, research and use in psy- chotherapy* (pp. 9–74). London: Routledge.

Gilbert, P., & Irons, C. (2005). Therapies for shame and self-attacking, using cognitive, behavioural, emo- tional imagery and compassionate mind training. In P. Gilbert (Ed.), *Compassion: Conceptualisations, research and use in psychotherapy* (pp. 263–325). London: Routledge.

Gilbert, P., & Proctor, S. (2006). Compassionate mind training for people with high shame and self-criticism: Overview and pilot study of a group therapy approach. *Clinical Psychology and Psycho- therapy, 13*, 353–379.

Greenberg, L. S. (1983). Toward a task analysis of con- flict resolution in gestalt therapy. *Psychotherapy: Theory, Research and Practice, 20*(2), 190–201.

Grossman, P., Niemann, L., Schmidt, S., & Walach, H. (2004). Mindfulness-based stress reduction and health benefits: A meta-analysis. *Journal of Psycho- somatic Research, 57*, 35–43.

Heatherton, T. F., & Polivy, J. (1990). Chronic diet- ing and eating disorders: A spiral model. In J. H. Crowther, D. L. Tennenbaum, S. E. Hobfoll, & M. A. P. Stephens (Eds.), *The etiology of bulimia ner- vosa: The individual and familial context* (pp. 133– 155). Washington, DC: Hemisphere.

Heine, S. J., Lehman, D. R., Markus, H. R., & Kitaya- ma, S. (1999). Is there a universal need for positive self-regard? *Psychological Review, 106*, 766–795.

Jost, J. T., Glaser, J., Kruglanski, A. W., & Sulloway, F. J. (2003). Political conservatism as motivated social cognition. *Psychological Bulletin, 129*, 339–375.

Kabat-Zinn, J. (1982). An outpatient program in be- havioral medicine for chronic pain patients based on the practice of mindfulness meditation: Theoret- ical considerations and preliminary results. *General Hospital Psychiatry, 4*, 33–47.

Kernis, M. H. (2003). Optimal self-esteem and authen-

ticity: Separating fantasy from reality, *Psychologi- cal Inquiry, 14*, 83–89.

Kernis, M. H., Paradise, A. W., Whitaker, D. J., Wheatman, S. R., & Goldman, B. N. (2000). Mas- ter of one's psychological domain?: Not likely if one's self-esteem is unstable. *Personality and Social Psychology Bulletin, 26*, 1297–1305.

Leary, M. R., Tate, E. B., Adams, C. E., Allen, A. B., & Hancock, J. (2007). Self-compassion and reactions to unpleasant self-relevant events: The implications of treating oneself kindly. *Journal of Personality and Social Psychology, 92*, 887–904.

Magnus, C. M. (2007). *Does self-compassion matter beyond self-esteem for women's self-determined motives to exercise and exercise outcomes?* Unpub- lished master's thesis, University of Saskatchewan, Saskatoon, Canada.

Morf, C. C., & Rhodewalt, F. (2001). Unraveling the paradoxes of narcissism: A dynamic self-regulatory processing model. *Psychological Inquiry, 12*, 177– 196.

Neff, K. D. (2003a). Development and validation of a scale to measure self-compassion. *Self and Identity, 2*, 223–250.

Neff, K. D. (2003b). Self-compassion: An alternative conceptualization of a healthy attitude toward one- self. *Self and Identity, 2*, 85–102.

Neff, K. D. (2006, August). *The role of self-compassion in healthy relationship interactions*. Paper presented at the annual meeting of the American Psychologi- cal Association, New Orleans, LA.

Neff, K. D. (2008, February). *Self-compassion and other-focused responding*. Paper presented at the annual convention of the Society for Personality and Social Psychology, Albuquerque, NM.

Neff, K. D., Hseih, Y., & Dejitthirat, K. (2005). Self- compassion, achievement goals, and coping with academic failure. *Self and Identity, 4*, 263–287.

Neff, K. D., Kirkpatrick, K., & Rude, S. S. (2007). Self-compassion and its link to adaptive psychologi- cal functioning. *Journal of Research in Personality, 41*, 139–154.

Neff, K. D., & McGehee, P. (2008, June). *Self- compassion among adolescents and young adults*. Paper presented at the annual meeting of the Jean Piaget Society, Quebec City, Canada.

Neff, K. D., Pisitsungkagarn, K., & Hseih, Y. (2008). Self-compassion and self-construal in the United States, Thailand, and Taiwan. *Journal of Cross- Cultural Psychology, 39*, 267–285.

Neff, K. D., Rude, S. S., & Kirkpatrick, K. (2007). An examination of self-compassion in relation to posi- tive psychological functioning and personality traits. *Journal of Research in Personality, 41*, 908–916.

Neff, K. D., & Vonk, R. (2009). Self-compassion ver- sus global self-esteem: Two different ways of relat- ing to oneself. *Journal of Personality, 77*, 23–50.

Pennebaker, J. W., Colder, M., & Sharp, L. K. (1990). Accelerating the coping process. *Journal of Person- ality and Social Psychology, 58*, 528–537.

Robins, R. W., & Beer, J. S. (2001). Positive illusions about the self: Short-term benefits and long-term costs. *Journal of Personality and Social Psychology, 80*, 340–352.

Rosenberg, M. (1965). *Society and the adolescent self- image*. Princeton, NJ: Princeton University Press.

Safran, J. D. (1998). *Widening the scope of cognitive*

therapy: The therapeutic relationship, emotion, and the process of change. Northvale, NJ: Aronson.

Salzberg, S. (1997). *Lovingkindness: The revolutionary art of happiness.* Boston: Shambala.

Sedikides, C. (1993). Assessment, enhancement, and verification determinants of the self-evaluation process. *Journal of Personality and Social Psychology, 65,* 317–338.

Seligman, M. E., & Csikzentmihalyi, M. (2000). Positive psychology: An introduction. *American Psychologist, 55,* 5–14.

Shapiro, S. L., Astin, J. A., Bishop, S. R., & Cordova, M. (2005). Mindfulness-based stress reduction for health care professionals: Results from a randomized trial. *International Journal of Stress Management, 12,* 164–176.

Shapiro, S. L., Brown, K. W., & Biegel, G. M. (2007). Teaching self-care to caregivers: Effects of mindfulness-based stress reduction on the mental health of therapists in training. *Training and Education in Professional Psychology, 1,* 105–115.

Sprecher, S., & Fehr, B. (2005). Compassionate love for close others and humanity. *Journal of Social and Personal Relationships, 22,* 629–651.

Swann, W. B. (1996). *Self-traps: The elusive quest for higher self-esteem.* New York: Freeman.

Taris, T. W. (2000). Dispositional need for cognitive closure and self-enhancing beliefs. *Journal of Social Psychology, 140,* 35–50.

Taylor, S. E., & Brown, J. D. (1988). Illusion and well-being: A social psychological perspective on mental health. *Psychological Bulletin, 103,* 193–210.

CHAPTER 39

■ ● ▲ ◆ ■ ● ▲ ◆

Self-Monitoring

PAUL T. FUGLESTAD
MARK SNYDER

In its most basic conceptualization, the psychological construct of self-monitoring refers to the regulation of expressive and self-presentational behaviors in social situations. Self-monitoring theory proposes that individuals systematically vary in the extent to which they are willing and able to monitor and control their expressive behaviors and public appearances. Individuals known as high self-monitors are particularly aware of and responsive to social cues. The images that they present are variable and tailored to situational context. In contrast, low self-monitors value consistent behavior that reflects what they perceive to be their true selves. Low self-monitors are typically less reactive to their social circumstances and possess smaller repertoires of self-presentational skills. Self-monitoring is related to a diverse set of behavioral domains such as expressive control, attitude–behavior consistency, responsiveness to different types of persuasion and advertising, organizational behavior, and interpersonal relationships (Gangestad & Snyder, 2000; Snyder, 1987). In this chapter, we begin with a brief overview of the self-monitoring construct, including a discussion of its measure and the development of self-monitoring orientations. Next, we review major areas of empirical inquiry, focusing on applications to social worlds and interpersonal contexts. Finally, drawing on recent theorizing and research emphasiz-

ing the role of affect and status concerns, we discuss the evolution of the self-monitoring construct and the motivational underpinnings of self-monitoring orientations.

The Construct of Self-Monitoring

Theorizing about self-monitoring begins with the proposition that, in most contexts, one can utilize two kinds of information to construct a pattern of action and self-presentation: (1) external cues such as situational and interpersonal features and (2) internal cues such as affective states, dispositions, and attitudes. The prototypical high self-monitor is thought to draw extensively on features of the situation to construct desired self-presentations, whereas the prototypical low self-monitor draws on salient inner dispositions and attitudes to guide behavior.

The construct of self-monitoring was introduced to psychological discourse at the time of the "person–situation" debate, which (succinctly put) was a debate between proponents of trait explanations of behavior and proponents of situational explanations of behavior. Self-monitoring was a way to specify, in the domain of expressive behavior, individuals for whom situations would have greater influence (high self-monitors) and those for whom dispositions would have greater influence (low self-monitors).

Research generated by self-monitoring theorizing was initially focused on basic processes, such as consistency across channels of expression (e.g., facial expression, tone of voice), cross-situational variability of behavior, control of emotional expression, attitude–behavior consistency, and attention to social comparison information. From its initial focus, self-monitoring research evolved to explore the links between self-monitoring and interpersonal relationships, advertising, persuasion, organizational behavior, and consumer behavior. These later lines of research focus on the divergent self-conceptions and motivations of low and high self-monitors, as well as the processes of image cultivation. Individual differences in monitoring of public appearances and self-presentation go well beyond influencing expressive behavior and the links between inner dispositions and behavior to shape many facets of people's lives.

The Measurement of Self–Monitoring

The most frequently used measures of self-monitoring are the 25-item, true-false Self-Monitoring Scale and the 18-item modification of it (Snyder, 1974; Snyder & Gangestad, 1986). The items of the Self-Monitoring Scale sample from interrelated facets of self-monitoring processes: (1) concern with social appropriateness, (2) attention to cues to appropriate self-presentation, (3) ability to tailor one's self-presentations, (4) the use of this ability in specific situations, and (5) the extent to which one's self-presentation and expressive behavior is cross-situationally variable. The Self-Monitoring Scale is a reliable and valid measure (see Snyder, 1974, and Snyder & Gangestad, 1986, for details of scale construction and validity).

Some have argued that the Self-Monitoring Scale does not measure a unitary construct but rather distinct dimensions (Briggs & Cheek, 1988; Lennox & Wolfe, 1984). Indeed, the 25-item measure generally yields three factors (e.g., Briggs & Cheek, 1986; Gangestad & Snyder, 1985; Lennox & Wolfe, 1984; Snyder & Gangestad, 1986), labeled Acting (e.g., "I would probably make a good actor"), Extraversion (e.g., "In a group of people I am rarely the center of attention"), and Other-Directedness (e.g., "I guess I put

on a show to impress or entertain people"). A key question has been whether findings in the literature are driven by different factors rather than by the unitary construct of self-monitoring. However, Gangestad and Snyder (1985) showed that the structure of the self-monitoring items corresponds to a common latent variable that correlates with all three subscales (Acting, Extraversion, and Other-Directedness) and reflects two classes of individuals (high and low self-monitors). Additionally, the full scale has performed better than the subscales in a number of data sets (Snyder & Gangestad, 1986). However, based on these analyses, Snyder and Gangestad (1986) proposed a revised 18-item Self-Monitoring Scale that better reflects the general latent self-monitoring factor.

Another challenge to the self-monitoring construct suggests that the general self-monitoring factor tapped by the revised Self-Monitoring Scale should be interpreted in terms of extraversion and social surgency (e.g., Briggs & Cheek, 1988). However, the Self-Monitoring Scale is only modestly or not at all correlated with measures of extraversion, need for approval, Machiavellianism, public self-consciousness, private self-consciousness, and locus of control (Jones & Baumeister, 1976; Lippa, 1976; Snyder, 1974, 1979; Snyder & Monson, 1975).

To further address issues of measurement and validity, Gangestad and Snyder (2000) quantitatively examined the self-monitoring literature to see whether the phenomena associated with self-monitoring cluster together in a coherent way to suggest that self-monitoring is a unitary construct and not a set of dimensions each related to a class of criterion variables. To do so, they placed the Self-Monitoring Scale and self-monitoring criterion variables in a two-factor self-monitoring space (Public Performing and Other-Directedness factors) as defined by factor analyses of the 18-item Self-Monitoring Scale (Briggs & Cheek, 1988; Snyder & Gangestad, 1986). The first step was to locate the Self-Monitoring Scale and its subscales in this space. After establishing the location of the general self-monitoring axis, the other-directedness axis, and the extraversion axis (the acting axis was nearly identical to the general self-monitoring axis), criterion variables from the literature were placed in the two-factor space. In this way, the researchers could ascertain whether particular phenomena (e.g., attitude–behavior consistency) were associated with particular dimensions (e.g., Other-Directedness) or whether diverse phenomena would cluster together and load most highly on the general self-monitoring axis. Of the nine groups of criteria, seven clustered around the self-monitoring axis. The axis defined by the average of these seven categories was displaced only 3° from the self-monitoring axis. Furthermore, 78% of the criterion variables correlated most highly with the self-monitoring axis, 13% with the extraversion axis, and 9% with the other-directedness axis. Clearly, the results suggest that self-monitoring represents a unified construct related to a wide range of self-presentational behaviors.

The Origins of Self-Monitoring

How do differences in self-monitoring emerge? Are high and low self-monitors born or made? Is self-monitoring a product of culture? Such questions address self-monitoring's origins.

Self-Monitoring in Childhood

Gangestad and Snyder (1985) suggest that self-monitoring differences in adulthood may partially emerge because of differences in childhood communication patterns and/or receiving differential treatment from adults in childhood. They propose that initially small differences between individuals become amplified over time, producing larger differences (i.e., divergent causality; Meehl, 1978). These differences have a substantial genetic component (Dworkin, 1977; Gangestad, 1984), and the development of early self-monitoring orientations may be sensitive to some specific environmental parameter, such as attention received from caretakers. It could be that children who receive little attention from their caretakers develop a strategy designed to gain the attention and regard of others—a high self-monitoring strategy. Predispositions may influence the effects of environmental factors on self-monitoring. For example, for some individuals, a lack of parental attention may need to be somewhat extreme to influence the adoption of a high self-monitoring strategy.

Nelson (1981) has noted two distinct patterns in language acquisition by children ages 2–3. Some children, labeled *referential*, first learn to use language as a referential system for the communication of happenings in the world. Other children, labeled *expressive*, learn early on that linguistic expressions are dependent on social context and that language can be used to obtain attention from others. It is possible that these early differences in language acquisition patterns reflect the same underlying trait that manifests itself in adult self-monitoring orientations.

Graziano, Leone, Musser, and Lautenschlager (1987) developed the Junior Self-Monitoring Scale to differentiate self-monitoring propensities in children (see also Eder, 1987, for a self-monitoring scale to be used with children as young as age 3). Like the original Self-Monitoring Scale, items were designed to tap five related domains of self-presentation and expressive behavior. In one study they found that high self-monitoring children were more likely to examine social comparison information than were low self-monitoring children while completing an opinion survey and anticipating a discussion with other students.

Musser and Browne (1991) examined the stability of self-monitoring scores for first-, third-, and fifth-graders over 15 months, as well as relations of self-monitoring to other personality variables, competence, and peer acceptance. They found that self-monitoring scores were stable over time for each age group. Similar to the findings for adults, self-monitoring was modestly related to extraversion, but not to other aspects of personality. For boys, especially older boys, self-monitoring was positively related to number of friends, peer popularity, and self-esteem; self-monitoring was not reliably related to these measures for girls. The positive association of self-monitoring with popularity and self-esteem for boys may reflect the gender appropriateness of high self-monitoring behavior. Boys tend to associate in large groups, but girls tend to have more intimate, two-person friendships over longer periods of time (Rubin, 1980). If children's self-monitoring friendship patterns are similar to those of adults in that high self-monitors tend to engage in particular activities with particular people and low self-monitors tend to engage in most activities with the same well-liked people (Snyder, Gangestad, & Simpson, 1983), then high self-monitoring would be more gender appropriate for boys than for girls. This could be one possible explanation for the consistent trend for men to score slightly higher than women on the Self-Monitoring Scale (Day, Schleicher, Unckless, & Hiller, 2002; Snyder, 1987).

The Influence of Culture

Does self-monitoring vary by culture? Is it influenced by individualism and collectivism? One could argue that collectivistic cultures pull for high self-monitoring because of a focus on social context and status in these cultures. Similarly, one could characterize individualistic cultures as pulling for low self-monitoring because of a focus on self and the expression of one's unique beliefs, attitudes, and dispositions.

However, such an analysis does not necessarily fit with self-monitoring theory. Because low self-monitors try to be themselves, they draw on self-conceptions of their characteristic behaviors that are relevant across situations (Snyder, 1979). Although behavior may be more dictated by social context in a collectivistic culture, one may still draw on enduring conceptions of self to develop plans of action in a particular context. In a collectivistic culture, enduring self-conceptions are heavily influenced by connections to other people, and these conceptions in relation to others will play an important role in shaping one's behavior (Markus & Kitayama, 1991). Instead of focusing on enduring self-conceptions, high self-monitors draw on their knowledge of prototypic persons and behaviors for a given situation and attempt to be that person (Snyder, 1979). As noted by Gangestad and Snyder (2000), the self-presentations of high self-monitors do not reflect a passive conformity to others but an active and strategic means of image projection and status cultivation.

It follows from this line of reasoning that individualistic cultures should exhibit greater high-self-monitoring tendencies. In fact, cross-cultural research on self-monitoring has revealed that people from more individualistic cultures (e.g., United States, Australia) have greater self-monitoring scores than people from more collectivistic cultures (e.g., Japan, Taiwan) (Gudykunst et al., 1989; Gudykunst, Yang, & Nishida, 1987). Although it appears that strategic self-presentation as captured by the Self-Monitoring Scale is somewhat more prevalent in individualistic cultures, future studies are needed to examine developmental and behavioral differences in self-monitoring across cultures.

Psychophysiology of Self-Monitoring

Hofmann (2006) examined psychophysiological correlates of self-monitoring during an impromptu speech task on a controversial topic. Not only did high self-monitors report less distress than low self-monitors, but they also had lower skin conductance levels and lower frontal and parietal activation as measured by electroencephalogram. This ability to remain calm in the face of stressful social interactions allows high self-monitors to control expressive behaviors and project desired images. These findings are consistent with research by Bono and Vey (2007) on emotional regulation. Across two role-playing tasks, high self-monitors had better emotional performances than low self-monitors, and this effect was partially mediated by high self-monitors' experiences of less stress. Physiological investigations, as well as brain imaging studies, are fertile areas for research that can contribute to a full understanding of self-monitoring processes (e.g., Do high and low self-monitors exhibit differential brain activation when making social judgments?) and the development of self-monitoring (e.g., Do physiological differences emerge in early childhood?).

Major Areas of Inquiry

Basic Processes

Expressive Control and Self-Presentation

High self-monitors exhibit greater expressive control than do low self-monitors and are better able to recognize emotional displays in others (e.g., Bono & Vey, 2007; Lippa, 1976; Mill, 1984; Snyder, 1974). For example, Snyder (1974) found that high self-monitors were better able than low self-monitors to communicate various types of emotions in both facial and vocal channels. Similarly, Lippa (1976) found that high self-monitors can more effectively assume the mannerisms of a typical extravert and introvert.

High self-monitors, relative to low self-monitors, project a general self-presentation that is more friendly and outgoing and less worried and anxious (Lippa, 1976). Onto this general background, high self-monitors project specific images that are tailored to situational features and, therefore, display more behavioral variability across situations than do low self-monitors (Lippa & Donaldson, 1990; Snyder, 1979). In studies of social interaction, high self-monitors, more so than low self-monitors, choose clearly defined situations, use scripts for typical situations, formulate effective plans of action before social interaction, use other people's behavior as guides to their own behavior, and actively facilitate smooth and pleasing conversations (e.g., Douglas, 1983; Ickes & Barnes, 1977; Jordan & Roloff, 1997; Snyder & Gangestad, 1982). In an examination of impression-management tactics, Bolino and Turnley (2003) found that high self-monitors were likely to be classified as positive impression managers (i.e., using ingratiation, self-promotion, and exemplification, but not supplication and intimidation), whereas low self-monitors were likely to be classified as aggressive (i.e., using all tactics to some extent) or passive impression managers (eschewing self-presentational tactics).

Social-Cognitive Processes

High and low self-monitors also diverge in social-cognitive and attributional processes. For example, in a study in which participants were allowed to observe a potential dating partner, high self-monitors were more likely than low self-monitors to remember information about their partners and to infer their partners' dispositions; that is, they were able to construct clear images of their partners (Berscheid, Graziano, Monson, & Dermer, 1976). Furthermore, high self-monitors pay particular attention to social comparison information, are more responsive to expectations, and are more likely to look to others for guidance in unfamiliar social situations (e.g., Harris & Rosenthal, 1986; Rarick, Soldow, & Geizer, 1976; Snyder, 1974). In a study of evaluations of people in dyadic interactions, high self-monitors based judgments not only on a person's actual behavior but also on the motivational context of the interaction (certain participants were instructed to either gain affection or win respect; Jones & Baumeister, 1976). On the other hand, low self-monitors generally accepted people's behavior at face value, irrespective of the motivational context.

Self-Conceptions

Self-monitoring orientations relate to basic understandings of what constitutes a "self." High self-monitors regard themselves as adaptive individuals who pragmatically tailor their expressive behavior to features of interpersonal contexts. They tend to attribute their own behavior to situational influences and to define their identities in terms of situational features (Sampson, 1978; Snyder, 1976). On the other hand, low self-monitors think of themselves as principled individuals who value consistency between who they are and what they do. They tend to attribute their own behavior to dispositional influences and to define their identities in terms of enduring dispositions (Sampson, 1978; Snyder, 1976).

When deciding how to express and present oneself in a social situation, the prototypical high self-monitor is thought to ask, "Who does this situation want me to be and how can I be that person?" In this way, the behavior of high self-monitors is shaped by knowledge of the prototypical person called for by a given situation. For example, when faced with a party, a high self-monitor may conjure up the image of an "ideal extravert" and engage in expressive behavior that is outgoing, witty, and friendly. In contrast, when deciding how to express and present oneself in a social situation, the prototypical low self-monitor is thought to ask, "Who am I and how can I be me in this situation?" In this way, the behavior of a prototypical low self-monitor is shaped by knowledge of his or her self-conceptions and typical ways of behaving in a given situation. In support of these conceptions of self-monitoring processes, Snyder and Cantor (1980) found that low self-monitors have richer and better articulated self-images in a wide variety of social situations, whereas high self-monitors have richer and better articulated images of prototypic persons in the same situations. For both high and low self-monitors, self-monitoring processes involve linking thoughts and self-conceptions to actions in social situations. However, what guides these processes (e.g., a desire to be oneself) and what information figures more prominently (e.g., inner feelings and attitudes) varies by self-monitoring (Snyder, 1979).

Attitudinal Processes and the Dispositional and Situational Determinants of Behavior

Issues of attitude–behavior consistency and situational variability in self-presentations are central to self-monitoring theory and research (Snyder, 1974, 1987). In support of self-monitoring theory, low self-monitors are more aware of and sensitive to internal states and display more attitude–behavior consistency (e.g., Snyder & Cantor, 1980; Snyder & Swann, 1976; Zanna, Olson, & Fazio, 1980). Conversely, high self-monitors do not necessarily display consistency between attitudes and behaviors and are more comfortable with discrepancies between what they do and what they believe (e.g., Snyder, 1974; Snyder & Monson, 1975). For example, in a study of attitudes toward affirmative action and verdicts in a mock court case involving alleged sexual discrimination, the privately held attitudes of low self-monitors were predictive of their verdicts in the case; the attitudes of high self-monitors were not related to their verdicts (Snyder & Swann, 1976). To demonstrate the "situational" nature of high self-monitors, Snyder and Monson (1975) assigned students to engage in group discussions of student issues in either a "public" condition with norms favoring autonomy or a "private" condition with norms favoring conformity and group harmony. High self-monitors adjusted their self-presentations to match the situational norms of each condition (i.e., autonomy in the public condition and conformity in the private conditions); the behavior of low self-monitors was unaffected by condition.

In a related line of research, DeMarree, Wheeler, and Petty (2005) examined the moderating role of self-monitoring in the effects of primes on self-judgments and behavior. Consistent with an "active-self" account of the effects of priming (i.e., an activated prime such as *elderly* becomes linked to or part of a person's self-concept, and/or the prime activates prime-consistent self-

content), low self-monitors displayed more prime-consistent self-judgments and behaviors, presumably because low self-monitors are more likely to modify their self-concepts in response to self-relevant information (to be more aware of and responsive to internal states) and to use dispositions and internal states to guide behavior.

Because low self-monitors tend to act on their attitudes and are more sensitive to their internal states, one might expect them to be more affected by performing counterattitudinal behaviors. Indeed, Snyder and Tanke (1976) found that low self-monitors displayed attitudes more in line with views expressed in a counterattitudinal essay than did high self-monitors; inconsistencies between internal attitudes and freely chosen behaviors resulted in more attitude change (and presumably dissonance) for low self-monitors, but not for high self-monitors. In examining the contextual nature of dissonance, DeBono and Edmonds (1989) had high and low self-monitors write freely chosen counterattitudinal essays in a peer-relevant context (i.e., the essay was at odds with the attitudes of the majority of their peers). In contrast to prior results on dissonance and self-monitoring, high self-monitors showed more dissonance reduction by expressing postessay attitudes in line with their essays. Although interpreted in terms of dissonance, this result is consistent with the Snyder and Monson (1975) study described earlier (high self-monitors behaved autonomously when norms favored autonomy), which suggests a more self-presentational account of the attitudes expressed by high self-monitors. In both studies, high self-monitors appear to be projecting images in line with situational norms.

Extending research on self-monitoring and cognitive consistency, Spangenberg and Sprott (2006) examined the self-prophecy effect. When people make predictions about whether or not they will perform a normative behavior, the likelihood that they will perform the behavior is increased. This effect is thought to be driven by dissonance aroused by discrepancies between values and actions. Therefore, low self-monitors should be particularly susceptible to self-prophecy effects because their values are closely linked to their behavior. Indeed, low self-monitors are more likely than high self-monitors to commit to normative behaviors (e.g., donating time to the American Cancer Society) following self-prediction of these behaviors.

Building on the ideas of low self-monitors as more attuned to internal states and dispositions and high self-monitors as more attuned to the social environment, Gonnerman, Parker, Lavine, and Huff (2000) predicted that self-discrepancies based on personal beliefs about oneself (i.e., the discrepancy between one's actual self-views and views of what one ought to be like) would influence the emotional well-being of low self-monitors, whereas self-discrepancies based on perceptions of what another person believes one ought to be like should influence the emotional well-being of high self-monitors. Their results confirmed these predictions. For low self-monitors, greater self-discrepancies from one's own standpoint, but not from that of others, predicted greater depression and anxiety. The opposite pattern was found for high self-monitors; greater self-discrepancies from the standpoint of others (e.g., parents, romantic partners), but not from one's own standpoint, predicted greater depression and anxiety.

Extension to Important Life Domains

A fundamental distinction between low and high self-monitors is a differential focus on the internal world of dispositions, attitudes, and affect versus the external world of appearances, images, and roles. High self-monitors display behaviors consistent with the roles and situations in which they find themselves, whereas low self-monitors display behaviors consistent with their attitudes and values regardless of roles and situations. Applying these concepts to social worlds, high self-monitors focus on the external qualities of people (e.g., physical appearance) so they can create social worlds that allow them to play clear, desirable roles with complementary casts of characters. In contrast, low self-monitors focus on the internal qualities of people (e.g., shared values) so they can create social worlds that allow them to be themselves. These fundamental differences have broad implications for the nature and structure of social worlds (friendships, romantic relationships), as well as consumer and organizational behavior.

Interpersonal Orientations and Social Worlds

High and low self-monitors have very different conceptions of what friendships are and how they function. High self-monitors base their friendships on shared activities, engage in utilitarian interactions, have relatively superficial, short-term exchanges, limit friendships to specific contexts, and restrict the amount of nurturance. In contrast, low self-monitors base their friendships on shared values, have deeper, long-term exchanges, generalize friendships across contexts, and are unrestricted in nurturance. These characterizations are borne out by a study in which participants wrote essays about their friendships (Snyder & Smith, 1984). High self-monitors described friendship in terms of activities done with friends; conversely, low self-monitors described friendship in terms of affect, general compatibility, and nurturance.

In examining the overall nature of the social worlds of high and low self-monitors, Snyder and colleagues (1983) found high self-monitors to have segmented worlds in which they engage in specific activities with specific people. Given the choice of doing an activity with a friend who is good at the activity or with a more liked friend who is bad at the activity, high self-monitors choose the friend who is better at the activity. In contrast, low self-monitors have relatively homogenous social worlds, choosing to engage in multiple activities with a few people. When choosing between a friend who is good at an activity or a more liked friend who is bad at the activity, low self-monitors choose the more liked friend. These findings suggest that high self-monitors want partners who will allow them to project images that are consistent with given roles and allow them to express desired aspects of self. On the other hand, low self-monitors are not concerned with the role congruence of potential partners but rather with similarity and global liking.

Romantic Relationships

From relationship initiation to dissolution, low and high self-monitors differ in terms of what they seek in mates (e.g., Jones, 1993; Snyder, Berscheid, & Glick, 1985), in the growth of trust, commitment, and satisfaction (e.g., Norris & Zweigenhaft, 1999; Snyder & Simpson, 1984), in sexual behavior in short-term relationships (e.g., Snyder, Simpson, & Gangestad, 1986), in relationship longevity (e.g., Leone & Hall, 2003; Snyder & Simpson, 1984), and in reactions to relationship dissolution (e.g., Snyder & Simpson, 1984), among other relationship processes.

In a study by Snyder and colleagues (1985), men examined the profiles (which contained information about personality and attitudes, as well as photos) of potential dating partners. High self-monitors spent more time examining the photos, whereas low self-monitors spent more time examining the personal information. In a study that forced a choice between a possible date with a good personality and an unattractive appearance and a date with a bad personality and an attractive appearance, high self-monitors chose the attractive date and low self-monitors chose the date with the good personality (Snyder & Simpson, 1984). In an examination of dating motivations, low self-monitors reported greater desire for similar values, honesty, loyalty, and kindness in a potential dating partner, whereas high self-monitors expressed greater desire for attractiveness, sex appeal, and social status (Jones, 1993).

The patterns of low and high self-monitors in romantic relationships reflect two distinct orientations toward close relationships—the restricted sociosexual orientation of low self-monitors and the unrestricted sociosexual orientation of high self-monitors (Snyder et al., 1986). In romantic relationships, low self-monitors strive to cultivate intimate, long-term relationships with partners chosen on the basis of dispositional compatibility. In contrast, high self-monitors are more willing to "play the field" of potential dating partners. High self-monitors view love as a social game and believe there may be more than one person whom they can love (Neto, 1993; Snyder, 1987). In contrast, low self-monitors are more likely to view love as a psychologically close and emotionally intense endeavor or as a quest to find a similar other who will be a compatible life partner; they are also more likely to believe that there is only one person who is ideally suited to them (Neto, 1993; Snyder, 1987).

Because trust is often a function of predictability and faith (Holmes & Rempel, 1989), low self-monitors should be more likely to develop trust in their romantic relationships, because they prefer partners with traits that foster these attributes (e.g., kindness, honesty, loyalty; Jones, 1993). High self-monitors, on the other hand, desire attributes such as social status and physical attractiveness to a greater extent (Jones, 1993; Snyder et al., 1985). Indeed, Norris and Zweigenhaft (1999) found that low-self-monitoring couples had greater trust than did high-self-monitoring couples and were more likely to see their relationships developing into marriage.

In marriage, there is no assortative mating with respect to self-monitoring (Leone & Hawkins, 2006; Snyder, 1987). However, similar to dating relationships, self-monitoring orientations influence marital satisfaction and functioning (Leone & Hall, 2003; Leone & Hawkins, 2006). Low self-monitors, relative to high self-monitors, report greater consensus in matters such as finances and religion, greater partner engagement in positive relationship activities such as calm problem solving, greater displays of affection to their partners, greater investment of resources, more commitment, more psychological intimacy, and greater marital satisfaction. Moreover, currently married high self-monitors are more likely than currently married low self-monitors to have been divorced.

Consumer Behavior

Self-monitoring processes have also been linked to consumer decision making and behavior (e.g., DeBono, 2006; DeBono & Snyder, 1989). Advertisements for consumer products tend to emphasize one of two broad themes—images associated with the product or utilitarian features of the product itself (Fox, 1984). Because high self-monitors are concerned with image projection and the social appropriateness of their behavior, they should be responsive to advertisements that emphasize desired images. Conversely, because low self-monitors value consistency between believing and doing, they should be responsive to advertisements that emphasize a product's actual qualities. In studies of self-monitoring and advertising, high self-monitors generally find image-based advertisements more appealing, whereas low self-monitors generally respond more favorably to quality-based appeals (e.g., Snyder & DeBono, 1985). However, as discussed by DeBono (2006), the results of these and subsequent studies paint a more complex picture. For example, Snyder and DeBono (1985) found that the image-versus-quality results were stronger for some products (e.g., Canadian Club whiskey) than others (e.g., Irish Mocha Mint coffee). Other research has found little or no support for the association between self-monitoring and advertising appeals (e.g., Bearden, Shuptrine, & Teel, 1989).

In attempting to account for these discrepant findings, DeBono (2006) suggests that information processing plays a role in the persuasiveness of advertising appeals. The elaboration likelihood model of persuasion (Petty & Cacioppo, 1986) posits that the persuasiveness of a given message will depend on the strength of the arguments as well as the ability and motivation of the recipient to process the message. One factor that can influence motivation to process is whether or not the content of a message matches the functional basis of individuals' attitudes (Lavine & Snyder, 2000; Petty & Wegener, 1998). When there is a match, individuals are more motivated to process messages, and argument quality will play a more crucial role in persuasion than when there is not a match. In support of these ideas, Petty and Wegener (1998) found that when participants were exposed to ads that functionally matched (i.e., high self-monitors exposed to image-based ads; low self-monitors exposed to quality-based ads), the strength of the arguments played a crucial role in determining the effectiveness of the ads. Specifically, high self-monitors reacted favorably to image-based ads with strong arguments and unfavorably to image-based ads with weak arguments, and low self-monitors reacted favorably to quality-based ads with strong arguments and unfavorably to quality-based ads with weak arguments.

Beyond responses to advertising, self-monitoring is also related to product evaluation strategies and the influence of brand and self-concept matching on product judgments. For example, DeBono and Rubin (1995) found that high self-monitors based their quality judgments of cheese solely on the country of origin (an image-based strat-

egy), whereas low self-monitors based their judgments solely on the actual taste of the cheese (a performance- based strategy). Similarly, high self-monitors are influenced by packaging attractiveness, whereas low self-monitors are not (DeBono, Leavitt, & Backus, 2003; DeBono & Snyder, 1989).

Aaker (1999) has demonstrated that low self-monitors are more likely than high self-monitors to prefer products with brand images (e.g., exciting, rugged) that match their own self-images. In contrast, high self-monitors are more likely to prefer products with brand images that match hypothetical social situations (e.g., preferring rugged brands for an informal barbecue after river rafting). It appears that low self-monitors prefer products that consistently reflect who they are, whereas high self-monitors prefer to match specific products to specific situations. Using a theatrical metaphor, high self-monitors prefer to have the right props for the role.

Other research suggests that high self-monitors, relative to low self-monitors, prefer products that match their own self-images when the products are used in public (e.g., Chevy Camaros, Reebok shoes) as opposed to private settings (e.g., *Reader's Digest*, Budweiser beer) (Graeff, 1996). The discrepancy between this finding and studies by Aaker (1999) may be explained by the fact that products such as the car one drives are relatively invariant to the situation, and high self-monitors should prefer such items to the extent that they convey desired images. On the other hand, for items that can be consumed or used in a wide variety of contexts (e.g., beverages), high self-monitors may base usage decisions on relevant situational cues.

Employment Decisions and Organizational Behavior

Self-monitoring figures prominently in work-related behaviors and decisions. Just as high self-monitors focus on the appearances of prospective romantic partners, they also use appearance in making employment decisions (e.g., Jawahar & Mattsson, 2005; Snyder, Berscheid, & Matwychuk, 1988). In one study, participants made hiring decisions for either a sales clerk or camp counselor (Snyder et al., 1988). The information on potential candidates varied in terms of personality and appearance (in each case, more or less appropriate to the job). High self-monitors were more likely to base their decisions on *looking the part*, whereas low self-monitors were more likely to base decisions on *being the part*. A recent experiment examined the hiring decisions of human resource professionals. Consistent with Snyder and colleagues (1988), high self-monitoring human resource professionals, relative to their low self-monitoring counterparts, were more willing to hire attractive candidates and applicants whose sex matched the sex typing of the job (e.g., hiring women as social workers; Jawahar & Mattsson, 2005). In addition, when making decisions about jobs to pursue, high self-monitors are more willing to apply for clearly defined positions (allowing them to play a good part), whereas low self-monitors are more willing to apply for jobs that match their personalities (Snyder & Gangestad, 1982).

Self-monitoring has also been implicated in organizational behavior (e.g., Day & Kilduff, 2003; Day et al., 2002). In a meta-analysis, Day and colleagues (2002) examined the relation of self-monitoring to work-related criteria such as job attitudes, job performance, and leadership. High self-monitors reported greater job involvement/identification, greater role ambiguity/conflict, and less commitment to the job than low self-monitors. Job satisfaction did not vary by self-monitoring. High self-monitors had consistently better job performance ratings than low self-monitors, especially on subjective measures of performance, and were seen as more leader-like by themselves and others. These findings suggest that high self-monitors are better able to manage impressions and cultivate desired images in the minds of coworkers and supervisors.

In a review of self-monitoring and work behavior, Day and Schleicher (2006) examined the literature through the motivational perspective of socioanalytic theory (Hogan, 1991), which proposes three broad motivational patterns in life and work—"getting along" with others, "getting ahead" in terms of status, and "making sense" of the world. As organizational settings afford the opportunity for a myriad of self-presentational behaviors and the development of a wide variety of interpersonal relationships, self-monitoring should play a crucial role in behaviors related to these motivational patterns.

In terms of "getting along" in dyadic interactions and getting-acquainted situations, high self-monitors generally display a friendly self-presentation, are responsive to the expectations of others, and work to be flexible and adaptive (Snyder, 1979, 1987). Thus they are likely to appear likeable and supportive to coworkers and bosses. In support of these contentions, high self-monitors, relative to low self-monitors, are seen as more helpful by coworkers and tend to occupy central positions in social networks at work (Flynn, Reagans, Amanatullah, & Ames, 2006; Mehra, Kilduff, & Brass, 2001). The penchant of low self-monitors to behave in disposition-consistent ways and to eschew impression-management tactics may make them appear rigid, especially to high-self-monitoring bosses who value projecting positive images. A low self-monitor may develop close, nurturing relationships with people who share similar values and interests but may come across as relatively unlikeable to people who do not have similar values, attitudes, and strategies of self-presentation.

In regard to "getting ahead," high self-monitors are more adept than low self-monitors at achieving status in organizational settings, as evidenced by better performance and leadership ratings (Day et al., 2002). In addition, high self-monitors exhibit less organizational commitment and are more willing to pursue other positions, which can be beneficial for moving up the corporate ladder. The proclivity of high self-monitors to "get along" may contribute to perceptions of performance, leadership, and status (Flynn et al., 2006). The tendency for low self-monitors to develop deep bonds with others may actually inhibit their desire to pursue opportunities at other organizations (Day & Kilduff, 2003). Interestingly, Day and Schleicher (2006) point out that the high-self-monitoring tendencies (e.g., cultivating favorable images, responding to expectations) that lead to the top may not be the traits that are most needed at the top. They argue that issues such as setting the strategic direction of a company and negotiating ethical issues may be responsibilities that are best suited to the low self-monitor.

Research by Flynn and Ames (2006) has shown that high-self-monitoring women outperform low-self-monitoring women in settings that are stereotypically masculine. Because many performance contexts in organizations are gender stereotyped in that men are expected to outperform women (Eagly & Karau, 2002), they hypothesized that high-self-monitoring women should be better able to counteract the negative expectations of others by cultivating social images that convey competence. High self-monitoring should be less advantageous for men in these situations because gender-typed behaviors are the norm and because others may be inclined to perceive them in expectation-congruent ways. Additionally, to be viewed as competent, women must act in agentic ways (e.g., being assertive, controlling, confident), but this behavior violates gender norms and may result in backlash from others (Eagly & Karau, 2002). Because women are faced with self-presentational dilemmas in the workplace, the ability to manage conflicting expectations is vital for successful performance. In Flynn and Ames's first study, small groups of MBA students completed a semester-long project. At the end of the semester, high self-monitoring women were seen as more influential and more valuable to the group than low self-monitoring women; self-monitoring did not predict group evaluations for men. Moreover, in a mixed-sex negotiation task, high self-monitoring women outperformed low self-monitoring women. As a whole, these results suggest that the self-presentational flexibility and skills of the high self-monitor are quite beneficial for women working in masculine-typed settings.

Day and Schleicher (2006) also speculate on Hogan's (1991) third broad motivational aspect of "making sense." The relatively more variable behavior of high self-monitors could be seen as unpredictability by others. As such, a high self-monitor who is in a top-level position could be seen as an inconsistent leader, which could undermine workers' trust and commitment. Additionally, if high self-monitors are ethically pragmatic, they may have difficulty in consistently dealing with ambiguous ethical dilemmas. Low self-monitors, drawing on principles and values, may more effectively deal with ethi-cal issues in organizations, provided they have the *right* principles and values. From the perspective of the individual, high self-monitors may be in a better position than low self-monitors to obtain information and opportunities within organizations because they tend to occupy central positions in their social networks at work (Mehra et al., 2001). Having access to information could contribute to "making sense" of the workplace, which could lead to "getting along" and "getting ahead."

The Evolution of Self-Monitoring Theory and Research

Originally, self-monitoring theorizing proposed that high self-monitors have a concern for the social appropriateness of their expressive behavior and that low self-monitors do not have such a concern for social appropriateness but are instead driven from internal states and dispositions. Although concern for social appropriateness has been at the heart of self-monitoring theorizing, self-monitoring should not be confused with need for social approval (Crowne & Marlowe, 1964), as evidenced by small correlations between the Self-Monitoring Scale and the Marlowe–Crowne Social Desirability Scale (in the –.2 range) and differential prediction of criterion behaviors such as emotional expression and attention to social comparison information (e.g., Snyder, 1974). Hence the concern for social appropriateness of the high self-monitor is distinct from defensive posturing to avoid disapproval. Early self-monitoring theorizing did not precisely and explicitly address the motivations behind self-monitoring propensities. However, as theory and research on the self-monitoring construct have progressed over the past 30 years, so, too, have conceptions of self-monitoring processes and ideas regarding the motivational underpinnings of both low- and high-self-monitoring orientations.

In considering the evolution of self-monitoring, we first present Gangestad and Snyder's (2000) reappraisal of the self-monitoring construct. We then discuss several lines of empirical work that directly relate to Gangestad and Snyder's analysis of self-monitoring with regard to status-related concerns and motivations. Last, we consider a recent theoretical view emphasizing the motivational role of affect in self-monitoring processes.

Self-Monitoring Reappraisal

Beyond addressing the construct validity of self-monitoring, Gangestad and Snyder's (2000) quantitative review further refined the construct by showing what phenomena are unrelated and what phenomena are most closely related to self-monitoring. In regard to specifying what self-monitoring is not, two areas of inquiry were not related to self-monitoring. First, self–peer ratings of traits did not vary by self-monitoring; that is, agreement between self-ratings of one's traits and peer ratings of traits were similar for low and high self-monitors. This suggests that self-monitoring cannot resolve the person–situation debate as it specifically pertains to trait consistency. However, as evidenced by the empirical review and prior research, self-monitoring does relate to attitude–behavior consistency and behavioral variability. The idea that high self-monitors would show consistency in traits is not antithetical to self-monitoring theory. As argued by Snyder (1979) and supported by research (Lippa, 1976, 1978; Snyder & Monson, 1975), high self-monitors show cross-situational consistency in background self-presentation, appearing friendly and nonanxious, and cross-situational variability in foreground self-presentation based on the specifics of a given interaction or situation.

Another set of criterion behaviors that are unrelated to self-monitoring are impression-management behaviors involving close attention and responsivity to others. People who engage in this type of impression management are socially anxious, concerned about negative social evaluation, and seek to appease others. It appears as though vigilantly attending to others and being highly responsive to others' behavior are tendencies associated with a defensive self-presentational style, which is not related to self-monitoring. Those with defensive self-presentational styles may adapt to others, but, unlike a high self-monitor, they engage in restrained and appeasing social behavior that may be relatively consistent across situations.

As discussed, seven of nine criterion categories were related to self-monitoring and can help to clarify the construct of self-monitoring. Of those, four categories were most strongly related to self-monitoring: behavioral variability, sensitivity to expectations and other cues, interpersonal orientations, and responses to physical appearance. Together, these criteria suggest that the specific impression management engaged in by high self-monitors involves actively constructing public appearances that lead to favorable outcomes and social cachet (e.g., knowing what image to project based on situational cues, choosing friends based on playing a role). Additionally, other categories of phenomena related to self-monitoring include expressive control and nonverbal decoding skills, both of which are skills useful to image cultivation, and attitude–behavior consistency, which involves the correspondence between public images and private beliefs. As a whole, these criteria relate to image management and cultivation, concerns that have been central to self-monitoring theory.

Gangestad and Snyder (2000) further suggested that high self-monitors engage in *assimilative* (vs. accommodative; Ickes, Reidhead, & Patterson, 1986) and *acquisitive* (vs. self-protective; Wolfe, Lennox, & Cutler, 1986) forms of self-presentation to enhance status (i.e., one's social and occupational standing) and effectively operate within perceived hierarchical social structures (i.e., perceptions of relative influence and/or power in relationships or groups). Research on the interpersonal orientations of high and low self-monitors supports this view—high self-monitors, relative to low self-monitors, generally have less committed and stable social relationships, choose friends based on activity expertise, and desire high-status romantic partners (e.g., Jones, 1993; Snyder et al., 1983, 1986; Snyder & Simpson, 1984). High self-monitors may be more invested in negotiating status within unequal-status social structures, whereas low self-monitors may be more invested in establishing equal-status bonds in which they are free to be themselves and in which trust can develop. Furthermore, low self-monitors, instead of being unconcerned with public images, may actively try to cultivate images of genuineness and sincerity.

Empirical Investigations of Status Concerns

Perceptions of Status and Status Cultivation in Exchange Relationships

In a direct examination of self-monitoring and status concerns, Flynn and colleagues (2006) found that high self-monitors reported greater desire than did low self-monitors for social status and were more accurate in perceiving status in dyadic exchange relationships. In addition, high self-monitors were perceived by former coworkers to have had higher social status and to have displayed greater generosity than low self-monitors. A mediational analysis suggested that high self-monitors were able to achieve status, at least in part, by helping others in workplace networks. In a study of exchange relations of MBA students, each student indicated to whom he or she would go for help or advice and who would be most likely to come to him or her for help and advice. Additionally, students provided ratings of who would go to whom for help among a subset of their peers. High self-monitors were particularly accurate in their perceptions of exchange relationships (i.e., they knew who would go to whom for help), less likely seek out help, and more likely to be sought out for help. Additionally, high self-monitors were likely to occupy positions of higher status (i.e., being sought for help from someone, but not seeking help from that person). By more accurately perceiving exchange relationships and developing a positive reputation and social standing, high self-monitors may be in a better position than low self-monitors to obtain resources and influence others in the workplace.

Status and Nonconscious Mimicry

Although the interaction behavior of high self-monitors is often quite deliberate and effortful (see Ickes, Holloway, Stinson, & Hoodenpyle, 2006, for a discussion), other research suggests that high self-monitors also engage in nonconscious behaviors that facilitate social interactions and self-presentational goals (Cheng & Chartrand, 2003). People tend to nonconsciously engage in behavioral mimicry (Chartrand & Bargh, 1999). For example, if one person in a dyadic interaction engages in face touching or foot shaking, the other person will tend to engage in these same behaviors. Importantly, priming an affiliation goal (either consciously or nonconsciously) leads peoples to engage in more mimicry (Lakin & Chartrand, 2003). Because high self-monitors tend to be more responsive to situational cues and desire to make favorable impressions and cultivate status, they should be more likely to engage in nonconscious mimicry when situations call for affiliation.

Cheng and Chartrand (2003) examined mimicry in dyadic interactions in which participants' interaction partners were ostensibly either high school students, fellow psychology students, or graduate students. Because a psychology student is someone with whom participants could have future contact, affiliation should be relevant. In this study, high self-monitors engaged in more mimicry than low self-monitors, but only when they thought they were interacting with a psychology student. However, high self-monitors did not pay particular attention to the psychology student, were not consciously aware of foot shaking, and did not explicitly report a greater desire to affiliate. A second study examined mimicry in the context of leader–worker interactions. High self-monitors engaged in more mimicry when interacting with a more powerful versus less powerful other; low self-monitors did not vary by condition. This finding provides further evidence for the contention that high self-monitors are attuned to and motivated by social status (Gangestad & Snyder, 2000). By engaging in conscious processes such as help giving and nonconscious processes such as behavioral mimicry, high self-monitors are better able to facilitate smooth social interactions and cultivate desired images.

Attractiveness and Self-Evaluation

Physical appearance is an important and salient feature of high self-monitors' social worlds (e.g., Snyder et al., 1985, 1988). Low self-monitors, however, seem relatively unconcerned with physical appearance in the ways they view and structure their social worlds. Accordingly, why are high self-monitors so attentive to and influenced by the physical appearance of others? Fuglestad and Snyder (2005) suggest that physical appearance is an important instrument in the facilitation of social status and should be an important aspect of self to high self-monitors but of lesser importance to low self-monitors.

A meta-analysis by Langlois and colleagues (2000) demonstrated that physically attractive people are treated more favorably (have less negative and more positive interactions) and achieve more occupational and interpersonal rewards (e.g., greater income, more popularity) than unattractive people. Given that physical attractiveness has these implications for how one is treated by others, it follows that attractiveness would affect how one feels about oneself. However, overall correlations between attractiveness and self-evaluations are small (Langlois et al., 2000). Because high self-monitors place greater importance on physical appearance, the relation between attractiveness and self-evaluations should be stronger for them than for low self-monitors. Indeed, self-monitoring does moderate the relation between attractiveness and self-evaluations (Fuglestad & Snyder, 2005). Attractiveness and self-evaluations are positively related for high self-monitors but unrelated for low self-monitors. Thus attractiveness appears to be a more important and salient aspect of self for high self-monitors than for low self-monitors.

Balance of Power in Romantic Relationships

Oyamot, Fuglestad, and Snyder (in press) examined balance of power and relationship quality in romantic relationships. They hypothesized that low self-monitors, out of a concern for cultivating intimate and trusting relationships, would perceive their relationships as relatively egalitarian (i.e., the partners have equal influence) and that, for them, balance of power would be a crucial element in determining relationship quality (i.e., closeness, satisfaction, investment). In contrast, they hypothesized that high self-monitors would perceive greater power asymmetries in their relationships (i.e., one person having more influence) and might actually prefer hierarchical ones. Therefore, although equal balance of power is generally associated with greater relationship quality

(e.g., Gray-Little & Burks, 1983), an attenuation of this association was expected for high self-monitors. In line with these hypotheses, low self-monitors perceived greater power equality than did high self-monitors; they also reported greater relationship quality in symmetrical relationships and less relationship quality in asymmetrical relationships. For high self-monitors, the negative effects of power asymmetries were attenuated. Thus power and influence asymmetries may be more of a happenstance for high self-monitors or even an integral feature of their relationships. And high self-monitors' tolerance for asymmetries could lead to long-term relationships less satisfying than those of low self-monitors. Low and high self-monitors in shorter relationships did not differ in their perceptions of asymmetries in the relationship. However, in longer relationships, high self-monitors perceived more asymmetries (results consistent with the finding that high self-monitors are less satisfied in their marriages than are low self-monitors; Leone & Hall, 2003).

The Role of Affect in Self-Monitoring Processes

In a review of self-monitoring processes in dyadic interactions, Ickes and colleagues (2006) presented a perspective on the motivations behind self-monitoring; they propose that high self-monitors are motivated to express and evoke positive affect in social situations and to regulate their affect through impression management. The idea of monitoring the affective tone of an interaction is not antithetical to cultivating image and status; rather, it specifies a mechanism to facilitate positive interactions and make favorable impressions. Indeed, research on job performance suggests that high self-monitors are good at "getting along" and "getting ahead" and that getting along facilitates getting ahead (e.g., Day & Schleicher, 2006; Flynn et al., 2006).

In a study on the role of self-monitoring in unstructured interactions, Ickes and Barnes (1977) found that high self-monitors, relative to low self-monitors, were more motivated to make the interaction go well and reported being more self-conscious if the conversation did not go well. Furthermore, high self-monitors also consciously develop self-presentational plans and use clear scripts to enact appropriate self-presentation (Douglas, 1983; Jordan & Roloff, 1997). Ickes and colleagues (2006) suggest that these findings are not simply due to a desire to facilitate a positive interaction but to the desire to cultivate and maintain positive self-affect during interaction. However, the primary motivation of high self-monitors may be to cultivate images and status, and the monitoring of self-affect may serve as a guide to how well that goal is being achieved.

In support of the centrality-of-affect view, high self-monitors tend to express and evoke more positive affect and less negative affect in dyadic interactions than low self-monitors (Levine & Feldman, 1997; Lippa, 1978). Interestingly, in the studies by Levine and Feldman (1997), not only did high self-monitors express less negative affect and cultivate images of happiness, but they were also more successful in creating impressions of competence and likeability. As such, the expression and evocation of positive affect may be a tool for the cultivation of desired images.

Applying sociometer theory (Leary, Tambor, Terdal, & Downs, 1995) to self-monitoring, Ickes and colleagues (2006) suggested that high self-monitors possess "sociometers" finely tuned to the effects of their self-presentations on others. Depending on the perceived effects of their expressive behavior (acceptance and validation vs. dismissal and rejection), high self-monitors will experience positive or negative affect. On the other hand, low self-monitors' "sociometers" may be relatively insensitive to the effects of their expressive behaviors on others. As noted by Ickes and colleagues, an alternative account could be that low self-monitors have sensitive "sociometers" in regard to self-presentation but that, instead of responding to feedback regarding social appropriateness, they respond to feedback regarding self-verification. In this view, the low self-monitor is not oblivious to or unconcerned about impression management, but he or she seeks to gain validation of his or her own self-image and attempts to cultivate an image of genuineness.

Another interpretation of the self-monitoring and interaction literature is that low self-monitors have relatively insensitive sociometers in *brief* encounters with strangers but

have highly attuned sociometers in *long-term* relationships. That is, the observed pattern of results in interaction studies could mean that low self-monitors are not concerned with superficial encounters and relationships, whereas high self-monitors are concerned with cultivating desired images in these brief encounters. Indeed, high self-monitors do seem to benefit in the workplace from engaging in such encounters with coworkers (Day & Schleicher, 2006).

Hoyle and Sowards (1993) have also discussed the role of affect in self-monitoring. In their view, high self-monitors should experience positive affect to the extent that their behavior matches perceived standards of social appropriateness and negative affect to the extent that their behavior does not correspond to these standards. On the other hand, low self-monitors should experience positive affect to the extent that their behavior matches their self-concepts and negative affect to the extent that it violates their self-concepts. Alternatively, Gangestad and Snyder's (2000) reappraisal of self-monitoring suggests that high self-monitors should experience positive affect to the extent that they are able to cultivate desired images (especially status-related images), not merely to the extent that their behavior is socially appropriate.

As pointed out by Ickes and colleagues (2006), more research is needed to address these competing accounts of motivation and affect in self-monitoring processes. Thus a sociometer account would suggest that the affective experiences of high self-monitors should be more variable during social interactions than those of low self-monitors. On the other hand, if the perspective of Hoyle and Sowards (1993) is correct, low and high self-monitors should be equally variable, but the affect of high self-monitors should vary with the appropriateness of their behavior (or their success in cultivating images and status), and the affect of low self-monitors should vary with the self-concept consistency of their behavior. Additionally, the relative status of interaction partners should be crucially important to high self-monitors' affective responses (e.g., being more responsive to higher status partners), whereas the relative closeness of interaction partners should be critical to low self-monitors' affective responses (e.g., being more responsive with a friend than a stranger).

Conclusion

The influence of self-monitoring extends well beyond regulating expressive behaviors in social interaction to affect people's basic self-conceptions, interactions with the marketplace, workplace behavior, and friendships and romantic relationships. High self-monitors, out of a concern for social appropriateness and image cultivation, focus on exterior features of self and others to create social worlds that allow them to play many roles with complementary casts of characters. Low self-monitors, out of a concern for consistency between what they do and who they are, focus on interior qualities of self and others to create social worlds that allow them to be themselves with close, similar others. Although much is known about self-monitoring, researchers are investigating new areas of inquiry, such as the motivational underpinnings of self-monitoring orientations, the role of affect in self-monitoring processes, the nonconscious aspects of self-monitoring, the physiological correlates of self-monitoring, and the influence of status and power dynamics in self-monitoring processes. As these areas of research develop and expand in new directions, so too (we anticipate) will the construct of self-monitoring.

References

Aaker, J. L. (1999). The malleable self: The role of self-expression in persuasion. *Journal of Marketing Research, 36,* 45–57.

Bearden, W. O., Shuptrine, F. K., & Teel, J. E. (1989). Self-monitoring and reactions to image appeals and claims about product quality. *Advances in Consumer Research, 16,* 703–710.

Berscheid, E., Graziano, W., Monson, T. C., & Dermer, M. (1976). Outcome dependency: Attention, attribution, and attraction. *Journal of Personality and Social Psychology, 34,* 978–989.

Bolino, M. C., & Turnley, W. H. (2003). More than one way to make an impression: Exploring profiles of impression management. *Journal of Management, 29,* 141–160.

Bono, J. E., & Vey, M. A. (2007). Personality and emotional performance: Extraversion, neuroticism, and self-monitoring. *Journal of Occupational Health Psychology, 12,* 177–192.

Briggs, S. R., & Cheek, J. M. (1986). The role of factor analysis in the development and evaluation of personality scales. *Journal of Personality, 54,* 106–148.

Briggs, S. R., & Cheek, J. M. (1988). On the nature of self-monitoring: Problems with assessment, problems with validity. *Journal of Personality and Social Psychology, 54,* 663–678.

Chartrand, T. L., & Bargh, J. A. (1999). The chameleon effect: The perception–behavior link and social interaction. *Journal of Personality and Social Psychology, 76,* 893–910.

Cheng, C. M., & Chartrand, T. L. (2003). Self-monitoring without awareness: Using mimicry as a nonconscious affiliation strategy. *Journal of Personality and Social Psychology, 85,* 1170–1179.

Crowne, D. P., & Marlowe, D. (1964). *The approval motive.* New York: Wiley.

Day, D. V., & Kilduff, M. (2003). Self-monitoring personality and work relationships: Individual differences in social networks. In M. R. Barrick & A. M. Ryan (Eds.), *Personality and work: Reconsidering the role of personality in organizations* (pp. 205–228). San Francisco: Jossey-Bass.

Day, D. V., & Schleicher, D. J. (2006). Self-monitoring at work: A motive-based perspective. *Journal of Personality, 74,* 685–713.

Day, D. V., Schleicher, D. J., Unckless, A. L., & Hiller, N. J. (2002). Self-monitoring personality at work: A meta-analytic investigation of construct validity. *Journal of Applied Psychology, 87,* 390–401.

DeBono, K. G. (2006). Self-monitoring and consumer psychology. *Journal of Personality, 74,* 715–737.

DeBono, K. G., & Edmonds, A. E. (1989). Cognitive dissonance and self-monitoring: A matter of context? *Motivation and Emotion, 13,* 259–270.

DeBono, K. G., Leavitt, A., & Backus, J. (2003). Product packaging and product evaluation: An individual difference approach. *Journal of Applied Social Psychology, 33,* 513–521.

DeBono, K. G., & Rubin, K. (1995). Country of origin and perceptions of product quality: An individual difference perspective. *Basic and Applied Social Psychology, 17,* 239–247.

DeBono, K. G., & Snyder, M. (1989). Understanding consumer decision-making processes: The role of form and function in product evaluation. *Journal of Applied Social Psychology, 19,* 416–424.

DeMarree, K. G., Wheeler, S. C., & Petty, R. E. (2005). Priming a new identity: Self-monitoring moderates the effects of nonself primes on self-judgments and behavior. *Journal of Personality and Social Psychology, 89,* 657–671.

Douglas, W. (1983). Scripts and self-monitoring: When does being a high self-monitor really make a difference? *Human Communication Research, 10,* 81–86.

Dworkin, R. H. (1977, August). *Genetic influences on cross-situational consistency.* Paper presented at the Second International Congress on Twin Studies, Washington, DC.

Eagly, A., & Karau, S. (2002). Role congruity theory of prejudice toward female leaders. *Psychological Review, 109,* 573–598.

Eder, R. (1987, April). *Individual differences in children's sensitivity to social cues: The emergence of self-monitoring.* Paper presented at the annual meeting of the Society for Research in Child Development, Baltimore.

Flynn, F. J., & Ames, D. R. (2006). What's good for the goose may not be as good for the gander: The benefits of self-monitoring for men and women in task groups and dyadic conflicts. *Journal of Applied Psychology, 91,* 272–281.

Flynn, F. J., Reagans, R. E., Amanatullah, E. T., & Ames, D. R. (2006). Helping one's way to the top: Self-monitors achieve status by helping others and knowing who helps whom. *Journal of Personality and Social Psychology, 91,* 1123–1137.

Fox, S. (1984). *The mirror makers.* New York: Morrow.

Fuglestad, P. T., & Snyder, M. (2005, January). *Looking good and feeling good: The relationship of self-monitoring to attractiveness and self-evaluations.* Poster session presented at the annual meeting of the Society for Personality and Social Psychology, New Orleans, LA.

Gangestad, S., & Snyder, M. (1985). "To carve nature at its joints": On the existence of discrete classes in personality. *Psychological Review, 92,* 317–349.

Gangestad, S. W. (1984). *On the etiology of individual differences in self-monitoring and expressive self-control: Testing the case of strong genetic influence.* Unpublished doctoral dissertation, University of Minnesota.

Gangestad, S. W., & Snyder, M. (2000). Self-monitoring: Appraisal and reappraisal. *Psychological Bulletin, 126,* 530–555.

Gonnerman, M. E., Jr., Parker, C. P., Lavine, H., & Huff, J. (2000). The relationship between self-discrepancies and affective states: The moderating roles of self-monitoring and standpoints on the self. *Personality and Social Psychology Bulletin, 26,* 810–819.

Graeff, T. R. (1996). Image congruence effects on product evaluations: The role of self-monitoring and public/private consumption. *Psychology and Marketing, 13,* 481–499.

Gray-Little, B., & Burks, N. (1983). Power and satisfaction in marriage: A review and critique. *Psychological Bulletin, 93,* 513–538.

Graziano, W., Leone, C., Musser, L., & Lautenschlager, G. (1987). Self-monitoring in children: A differential approach to social development. *Developmental Psychology, 23,* 571–576.

Gudykunst, W. B., Gao, G., Nishida, T., Bond, M. H., Kwok, L., & Wang, G. (1989) A cross-cultural comparison of self-monitoring. *Communication Research Reports, 6,* 7–12.

Gudykunst, W. B., Yang, S., & Nishida, T. (1987). Cultural differences in self-consciousness and self-monitoring. *Communication Research, 14,* 7–36.

Harris, M. J., & Rosenthal, R. (1986). Counselor and client personality as determinants of counselor expectancy effects. *Journal of Personality and Social Psychology, 50,* 362–369.

Hofmann, S. G. (2006). The emotional consequences of social pragmatism: The psychophysiological correlates of self-monitoring. *Biological Psychology, 73,* 169–174.

Hogan, R. T. (1991). Personality and personality measurement. In M. D. Dunnette & L. M. Hough (Eds.), *Handbook of industrial and organizational psychology* (2nd ed., Vol. 2, pp. 873–919). Palo Alto, CA: Consulting Psychologists.

Holmes, J. G., & Rempel, J. K. (1989). Trust in close relationships. In C. Hendrick (Ed.), *Close relationships* (Vol. 10, pp. 187–220). London: Sage.

Hoyle, R. H., & Sowards, B. A. (1993). Self-monitoring and the regulation of social experience: A control-process model. *Journal of Social and Clinical Psychology, 12,* 280–306.

Ickes, W., & Barnes, R. D. (1977). The role of sex and self-monitoring in unstructured dyadic interactions. *Journal of Personality and Social Psychology, 35,* 315–330.

Ickes, W., Holloway, R., Stinson, L. L., & Hoodenpyle, T. G. (2006). Self-monitoring in social interaction: The centrality of self-affect. *Journal of Personality, 74,* 659–684.

Ickes, W., Reidhead, S., & Patterson, M. (1986). Machiavellianism and self-monitoring: Different as "me" and "you." *Social Cognition, 4,* 58–74.

Jawahar, I. M., & Mattsson, J. (2005). Sexism and beautyism effects in selection as a function of self-monitoring level of decision maker. *Journal of Applied Psychology, 90,* 563–573.

Jones, E. E., & Baumeister, R. (1976). The self-monitor looks at the ingratiator. *Journal of Personality, 44,* 654–674.

Jones, M. (1993). Influence of self-monitoring and dating motivations. *Journal of Research in Personality, 27,* 197–206.

Jordan, J. M., & Roloff, M. E. (1997). Planning skills and negotiator goal accomplishment. *Communication Research, 24,* 31–63.

Lakin, J. L., & Chartrand, T. L. (2003). Using nonconscious behavioral mimicry to create affiliation and rapport. *Psychological Science, 14,* 334–339.

Langlois, J. H., Kalakanis, L., Rubenstein, A. J., Larson, A., Hallam, M., & Smoot, M. (2000). Maxims or myths of beauty?: A meta-analytic and theoretical review. *Psychological Bulletin, 126,* 390–423.

Lavine, H., & Snyder, M. (2000). Cognitive processes and the functional matching effect in persuasion: Studies of personality and political behavior. In G. M. Maio & J. M. Olson (Eds.), *Why we evaluate: Functions of attitudes* (pp. 97–132). Mahwah, NJ: Erlbaum.

Leary, M. R., Tambor, E. S., Terdal, S. K., & Downs, D. L. (1995). Self-esteem as an interpersonal monitor: The sociometer hypothesis. *Journal of Personality and Social Psychology, 68,* 518–530.

Lennox, R., & Wolfe, R. (1984). Revision of the Self-Monitoring Scale. *Journal of Personality and Social Psychology, 46,* 1349–1364.

Leone, C., & Hall, I. (2003). Self-monitoring, marital dissatisfaction, and relationship dissolution: Individual differences in orientations to marriage and divorce. *Self and Identity, 2,* 189–202.

Leone, C., & Hawkins, L. B. (2006). Self-monitoring and close relationships. *Journal of Personality, 74,* 739–788.

Levine, S. P., & Feldman, R. S. (1997). Self-presentational goals, self-monitoring, and nonverbal behavior. *Basic and Applied Social Psychology, 19,* 505–518.

Lippa, R. (1976). Expressive control and the leakage of dispositional introversion–extraversion during role-played teaching. *Journal of Personality, 44,* 541–559.

Lippa, R. (1978). Expressive control, expressive consistency, and the correspondence between expressive behavior and personality. *Journal of Personality, 46,* 438–461.

Lippa, R., & Donaldson, S. I. (1990). Self-monitoring and idiographic measures of behavioral variability across interpersonal relationships. *Journal of Personality, 58,* 465–479.

Markus, H. R., & Kitayama, S. (1991). Culture and the self: Implications for cognition, emotion, and motivation. *Psychological Review, 98,* 224–253.

Meehl, P. E. (1978). Theoretical risks and tabular asterisks: Sir Karl, Sir Ronald, and the slow progress of soft psychology. *Journal of Consulting and Clinical Psychology, 46,* 806–834.

Mehra, A., Kilduff, M., & Brass, D. J. (2001). The social networks of high and low self-monitors: Implications for workplace performance. *Administrative Science Quarterly, 46,* 121–146.

Mill, J. (1984). High and low self-monitoring individuals: Their decoding skills and empathic expression. *Journal of Personality, 52,* 372–388.

Musser, L. M., & Browne, B. (1991). Self-monitoring in middle childhood: Personality and social correlates. *Developmental Psychology, 27,* 994–999.

Nelson, K. (1981). Individual differences in language development: Implications for development and language. *Developmental Psychology, 17,* 170–187.

Neto, F. (1993). Love styles and self-representations. *Personality and Individual Differences, 14,* 795–803.

Norris, S. L., & Zweigenhaft, R. L. (1999). Self-monitoring, trust, and commitment in romantic relationships. *Journal of Social Psychology, 139,* 215–220.

Oyamot, C. M., Jr., Fuglestad, P. T., & Snyder, M. (in press). Self-monitoring and perceptions of balance of power in romantic relationships: Who influences whom, and with what effect? *Journal of Social and Personal Relationships.*

Petty, R. E., & Cacioppo, J. T. (1986). The elaboration likelihood model of persuasion. In L. Berkowitz (Ed.), *Advances in experimental social psychology* (Vol. 19, pp. 123–205). New York: Academic Press.

Petty, R. E., & Wegener, D. T. (1998). Matching versus mismatching attitude functions: Implications for scrutiny of persuasive messages. *Personality and Social Psychology Bulletin, 24,* 227–240.

Rarick, D. L., Soldow, G. F., & Geizer, R. S. (1976). Self-monitoring as a mediator of conformity. *Central States Speech Journal, 27,* 267–271.

Rubin, Z. (1980). *Children's friendships.* Cambridge, MA: Harvard University Press.

Sampson, E. E. (1978). Personality and the location of identity. *Journal of Personality, 46,* 552–568.

Snyder, M. (1974). Self-monitoring of expressive behavior. *Journal of Personality and Social Psychology, 30,* 526–537.

Snyder, M. (1976). Social perception and social causation. In J. H. Harvey, W. J. Ickes, & R. F. Kidd (Eds.), *New directions in attribution research* (Vol. 1). Hillsdale, NJ: Erlbaum.

Snyder, M. (1979). Self-monitoring processes. In L. Berkowitz (Ed.), *Advances in experimental social psychology* (Vol. 12, pp. 85–128). New York: Academic Press.

Snyder, M. (1987). *Public appearances/private realities: The psychology of self-monitoring.* New York: Freeman.

Snyder, M., Berscheid, E., & Glick, P. (1985). Focusing on the exterior and the interior: Two investigations of the initiation of personal relationships. *Journal of Personality and Social Psychology, 48,* 1427–1439.

Snyder, M., Berscheid, E., & Matwychuk, A. (1988). Orientations toward personnel selection: Differential reliance on appearance and personality. *Journal of Personality and Social Psychology, 54,* 972–979.

Snyder, M., & Cantor, N. (1980). Thinking about ourselves and others: Self-monitoring and social knowledge. *Journal of Personality and Social Psychology, 39,* 222–234.

Snyder, M., & DeBono, K. G. (1985). Appeals to image and claims about quality: Understanding the psychology of advertising. *Journal of Personality and Social Psychology, 49,* 586–597.

Snyder, M., & Gangestad, S. (1982). Choosing social situations: Two investigations of self-monitoring processes. *Journal of Personality and Social Psychology, 43,* 123–135.

Snyder, M., & Gangestad, S. (1986). On the nature of self-monitoring: Matters of assessment, matters of validity. *Journal of Personality and Social Psychology, 51,* 125–139.

Snyder, M., Gangestad, S., & Simpson, J. A. (1983). Choosing friends as activity partners: The role of self-monitoring. *Journal of Personality and Social Psychology, 45,* 1061–1072.

Snyder, M., & Monson, T. C. (1975). Persons, situations, and the control of social behavior. *Journal of Personality and Social Psychology, 32,* 637–644.

Snyder, M., & Simpson, J. A. (1984). Self-monitoring and dating relationships. *Journal of Personality and Social Psychology, 47,* 1281–1291.

Snyder, M., Simpson, J. A., & Gangestad, S. (1986). Personality and sexual relations. *Journal of Personality and Social Psychology, 51,* 181–190.

Snyder, M., & Smith, D. (1984, May). *Self-monitoring and conceptions of friendship.* Paper presented at the annual meeting of the Midwestern Psychological Association, Chicago.

Snyder, M., & Swann, W. B. (1976). When actions reflect attitudes: The politics of impression management. *Journal of Personality and Social Psychology, 34,* 1034–1042.

Snyder, M., & Tanke, E. D. (1976). Behavior and attitude: Some people are more consistent than others. *Journal of Personality, 44,* 501–517.

Spangenberg, E. R., & Sprott, D. E. (2006). Self-monitoring and susceptibility to the influence of self-prophecy. *Journal of Consumer Research, 32,* 550–556.

Wolfe, R., Lennox, R., & Cutler, B. L. (1986). Getting along and getting ahead: Empirical support for a theory of protective and acquisitive self-presentation. *Journal of Personality and Social Psychology, 44,* 1069–1074.

Zanna, M. P., Olson, J. M., & Fazio, R. H. (1980). Attitude–behavior consistency: An individual difference perspective. *Journal of Personality and Social Psychology, 38,* 432–440.

Author Index

Subject Index

Page numbers followed by *f* indicate figure, *n* indicate note, and *t* indicate table